PERIODONTICS

MEDICINE, SURGERY, *and* IMPLANTS

PERIODONTICS
MEDICINE, SURGERY, *and* IMPLANTS

Louis F. Rose, DDS, MD
Clinical Professor of Periodontics, School of Dental Medicine, University of
Pennsylvania; Professor of Surgery, Drexel University College of Medicine,
Philadelphia, Pennsylvania; Clinical Professor of Periodontics, School of Dental
Medicine, New York University, New York, New York; Faculty, Harvard University
School of Dental Medicine, Boston, Massachusetts

Brian L. Mealey, DDS, MS
Chairman and Graduate Program Director, Department of Periodontics, Wilford Hall
Medical Center, Lackland Air Force Base, Texas; Clinical Assistant Professor,
Department of Periodontics, University of Texas Health Science Center, San Antonio,
Texas; Adjunct Associate Professor, Baylor College of Dentistry, Texas A&M
University System, Dallas, Texas

Robert J. Genco, DDS, PhD
Distinguished Professor and Chair, School of Dental Medicine, Department of Oral
Biology, State University of New York, Buffalo, New York

D. Walter Cohen, DDS
Dean Emeritus and Professor Emeritus of Periodontics, School of Dental Medicine,
University of Pennsylvania, Philadelphia, Pennsylvania

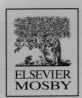

ELSEVIER
MOSBY

ELSEVIER
MOSBY

11830 Westline Industrial Drive
St. Louis, Missouri 63146

Notice

Dentistry is an ever-changing field. Standard safety precautions must be followed, but as new research and clinical experience broaden our knowledge, changes in treatment and drug therapy may become necessary or appropriate. Readers are advised to check the most current product information provided by the manufacturer of each drug to be administered to verify the recommended dose, the method and duration of administration, and contraindications. It is the responsibility of the licensed prescriber, relying on experience and knowledge of the patient, to determine dosages and the best treatment for each individual patient. Neither the publisher nor the author assumes any liability for any injury and/or damage to persons or property arising from this publication.

Library of Congress Cataloging-in-Publication Data
Periodontics: medicine, surgery, and implants/[edited by] Louis F. Rose . . . [et al.].
  p.   ; cm.
    Includes bibliographical references and index.
    ISBN 0-8016-7978-8
  1. Periodontics. 2. Periodontal disease. 3. Periodontium—Surgery. 4. Dental implants.
    I. Rose, Louis F.
    [DNLM: 1. Periodontal Diseases—diagnosis. 2. Periodontal Diseases—surgery.
    WU 240 P4477 2004]
RK361.P466 2004
617.6′32—dc22

    2003065160

Executive Editor: Penny Rudolph
Senior Developmental Editor: Jaime Pendill
Associate Developmental Editor: Julie Nebel
Publishing Services Manager: Melissa Lastarria
Associate Project Manager: Bonnie Spinola
Senior Designer: Julia Dummitt

Printed in China

Last digit is the print number: 9 8 7 6 5 4 3 2 1

Section Editors

Gary C. Armitage, DDS, MS
R. Earl Robinson Distinguished Professor, UCSF School of Dentistry; Division of Periodontology, San Francisco, California

John Kois, DMD
Private Practice, Seattle and Tacoma, Washington; Director of Creating Excellence Center for Dental Learning; Affiliate Professor, University of Washington, Graduate Restorative Department

Louis F. Rose, DDS, MD
Clinical Professor of Periodontics, School of Dental Medicine, University of Pennsylvania; Professor of Surgery, Drexel University College of Medicine, Philadelphia, Pennsylvania; Clinical Professor of Periodontics, School of Dental Medicine, New York University, New York, New York; Faculty, Harvard University School of Dental Medicine, Boston, Massachusetts

Brian L. Mealey, DDS, MS
Chairman and Graduate Program Director, Department of Graduate Periodontics, Wilford Hall Medical Center, Lackland Air Force Base, Texas; Clinical Assistant Professor, Department of Periodontics, University of Texas Health Science Center, San Antonio, Texas; Adjunct Associate Professor, Baylor College of Dentistry, Texas A&M University System, Dallas, Texas

Leonard S. Tibbetts, DDS, MSD
Private Practice and Affiliate Associate Professor of Periodontics, University of Washington School of Dentistry, Seattle, Washington; Private Practice, Arlington, Texas

Contributors

Leonard Abrams, DDS
Clinical Professor, Department of Periodontics, School of
Dental Medicine, University of Pennsylvania, Philadelphia,
Pennsylvania

Alfredo Aguirre, DDS, MS
Director, Advanced Oral and Maxillofacial Pathology; Professor,
Department of Oral Diagnostic Sciences, School of Dental
Medicine, State University of New York, Buffalo, New York

William F. Ammons, Jr., DDS, MSD
Professor Emeritus, Department of Periodontics, School of
Dentistry, University of Washington, Seattle, Washington

Gary C. Armitage, DDS, MS
R. Earl Robinson Distinguished Professor, USCF School of
Dentistry, Division of Periodontology, San Francisco, California

Sebastian G. Ciancio, DDS, PhD
Distinguished Professor and Chair, Department of
Periodontics and Endodontics, School of Dental Medicine,
State University of New York, Buffalo, New York

D. Walter Cohen, DDS
Dean Emeritus and Professor Emeritus of Periodontics,
School of Dental Medicine, University of Pennsylvania,
Philadelphia, Pennsylvania; Chancellor Emeritus,
Drexel University College of Medicine, Philadelphia,
Pennsylvania.

Connie L. Drisko, DDS
Dean, School of Dentistry, Medical College of Georgia,
Augusta, Georgia

Becky DeSpain Eden, BSDH, MEd
Associate Professor, Public Health Sciences, Baylor College of
Dentistry, Texas A&M University System Health Science
Center, Dallas, Texas

Cyril I. Evian, DMD
Private Practice, King of Prussia, Pennsylvania; Acting Chair,
Department of Periodontics, University of Pennsylvania School
of Dental Medicine, Philadelphia, Pennsylvania

Mark E. Glover, DDS, MSD
Private Practice, Dallas, Texas

Henry Greenwell, DMD, MSD
Professor, Chairman, and Director, Graduate Periodontics,
Department of Periodontics, Endodontics, and
Dental Hygiene, School of Dentistry, University of Louisville,
Louisville, Kentucky

Sara G. Grossi, DDS, MS
Senior Research Scientist, Department of Oral Biology,
School of Dental Medicine, State University of New York,
Buffalo, New York

Margaret Hill, DMD
Associate Professor, Department of Periodontics, Endodontics,
and Dental Hygiene, School of Dentistry, University of
Louisville, Louisville, Kentucky

Richard T. Kao, DDS, PhD
Associate Adjunct Professor, Department of Periodontology,
School of Dentistry, University of the Pacific, San Francisco,
California

David G. Kerns, DMD, MS
Associate Professor and Director of Postdoctoral Periodontics,
Department of Periodontics, Baylor College of Dentistry,
Texas A&M University System Health Science Center, Dallas,
Texas

Denis F. Kinane, BDS, PhD
Associate Dean for Research and Enterprise, School of
Dentistry, University of Louisville, Louisville, Kentucky

John Kois, DMD
Private Practice, Seattle and Tacoma, Washington;
Director of Creating Excellence Center for Dental Learning,
Affiliate Professor, University of Washington,
Graduate Restorative Department

Vincent G. Kokich, DDS, MSD
Professor, Department of Orthodontics, School of Dentistry,
University of Washington, Seattle, Washington

Vincent O. Kokich, DMD, MSD
Affiliate Assistant Professor, Department of Orthodontics,
School of Dentistry, University of Washington, Seattle,
Washington

Peter M. Loomer, DDS, PhD, MRCD (C)
Assistant Professor of Clinical Periodontology, Division of
Periodontology, School of Dentistry, University of California
at San Francisco, San Francisco, California

Howard T. McDonnell, DDS, MS
Director of Periodontal Research, United States Air Force
Periodontics Residency, Department of Periodontics,
Wilford Hall Medical Center, Lackland Air Force Base,
Texas; Clinical Assistant Professor, Department of
Periodontics, University of Texas Health Science Center,
San Antonio, Texas

Brian L. Mealey, DDS, MS
Chairman and Graduate Program Director, Department of Periodontics, Wilford Hall Medical Center, Lackland Air Force Base, Texas; Clinical Assistant Professor, Department of Periodontics, University of Texas Health Science Center, San Antonio, Texas; Adjunct Associate Professor, Baylor College of Dentistry, Texas A&M University System, Dallas, Texas

Bryan S. Michalowicz, DDS
Associate Professor, Department of Preventive Sciences, School of Dentistry, University of Minnesota, Minneapolis, Minnesota

Dale A. Miles, DDS, MS
Associate Dean for Clinical Affairs and Faculty Development, Arizona School of Dentistry and Oral Health, Mesa, Arizona

Michael P. Mills, DMD, MS
Clinical Associate Professor, Department of Periodontics, University of Texas Health Science Center, San Antonio, Texas

Laura Minsk, DMD
Assistant Professor, Department of Periodontics, School of Dental Medicine, University of Pennsylvania, Philadelphia, Pennsylvania

Regan L. Moore, DDS, MSD
Associate Professor, Department of Periodontics, Endodontics, and Dental Hygiene, School of Dentistry, University of Louisville, Louisville, Kentucky

Jacqueline M. Plemons, DDS, MS
Associate Professor, Department of Periodontics, Baylor College of Dentistry, Texas A&M University Health Science Center, Dallas, Texas

Stephen R. Potashnick, DMD
Private Practice, Chicago, Illinois

John W. Rapley, DDS, MS
Director, Graduate Periodontics and Chairman, Department of Periodontics, University of Missouri-Kansas City School of Dentistry, Kansas City, Missouri

Terry D. Rees, DDS
Professor and Former Chair, Department of Periodontics, Baylor College of Dentistry, Texas A&M University System Health Science Center, Dallas, Texas

Jill Rethman, RDH
Clinical Instructor, Department of Dental Hygiene, School of Dental Medicine, University of Pittsburgh, Pittsburgh, Pennsylvania

Paul Rhodes, DDS, MSD
Private Practice, Walnut Creek, California

Mauricio Ronderos, DDS, MS, MPH
Assistant Professor, Department of Periodontics, School of Dentistry, University of the Pacific, San Francisco, California

Louis F. Rose, DDS, MD
Clinical Professor of Periodontics, School of Dental Medicine, University of Pennsylvania; Professor of Surgery, Drexel University College of Medicine, Philadelphia, Pennsylvania; Clinical Professor of Periodontics, School of Dental Medicine, New York University, New York, New York; Faculty, Harvard University School of Dental Medicine, Boston, Massachusetts

Edwin S. Rosenberg, BDS, H.DipDent, DMD
Clinical Professor of Periodontics and Director, Postdoctoral Periodontics, Periodontal Prosthesis and Implant Dentistry, University of Pennsylvania, Philadelphia, Pennsylvania

Louis E. Rossman, DMD
Diplomate, American Board of Endodontics; Clinical Associate Professor, Department of Endodontics, School of Dental Medicine, University of Pennsylvania; Chairman Emeritus IB Bender Division of Endodontics, Albert Einstein Medical Center, Philadelphia, Pennsylvania

Randal W. Rowland, MS, DMD, MS
Director, Postgraduate Periodontology, and Professor, Clinical Periodontology, School of Dentistry, University of California at San Francisco, San Francisco, California

Mark I. Ryder, DMD
Professor and Chair, Division of Periodontology, School of Dentistry, University of California at San Francisco, San Francisco, California

Robert E. Schifferle, DDS, MMSc, PhD
Associate Professor, Departments of Periodontics, Endodontics, and Oral Biology, School of Dental Medicine, State University of New York at Buffalo, Buffalo, New York

Dennis A. Shanelac, DDS
Director, Microsurgery Training Institute, Santa Barbara, California

Neil L. Starr, DDS
Adjunct Clinical Assistant Professor, Department of Periodontics, School of Dental Medicine, University of Pennsylvania, Philadelphia, Pennsylvania; Private Practice in Prosthodontics, Washington, DC

Jose Luis Tapia, DDS, MS
Professor, Department of Oral Pathology, Facultad de Odontologia, Universidad Nacional Autonoma de Mexico

Mark V. Thomas, DMD
Assistant Professor and Division Chief, Department of Periodontics, College of Dentistry, University of Kentucky, Lexington, Kentucky

Leonard S. Tibbetts, DDS, MSD
Private Practice and Affiliate Associate Professor of Periodontics, University of Washington School of Dentistry, Seattle, Washington; Private Practice, Arlington, Texas

Arnold S. Weisgold, DDS, FACD
Clinical Professor and Director of Postdoctoral Periodontal Prosthesis, Department of Periodontics, School of Dental Medicine, University of Pennsylvania, Philadelphia, Pennsylvania

M. Robert Wirthlin, DDS
Clinical Professor Emeritus, Division of Periodontology, Department of Stomatology, School of Dentistry, University of California at San Francisco, San Francisco, California; Captain (DC) US Navy, retired

*To my wife and best friend, Claire, who has always supported
and encouraged my desire to pursue every endeavor I dreamed possible.
To my wonderful children, Michael, David, and Hedy,
for their ever-present love and devotion.
To my beautiful granddaughters Cameron Sara and Halle Kate,
who have brought so much love and joy into my life,*

and

*to the memory of my mother and father and mother-in-law,
who taught me the importance of family.*

*Also, a special debt of gratitude to D. Walter Cohen, my mentor,
friend, and partner in practice who has shaped my education
and continues to do so.
His thirst for life-long learning and commitment to innovation
and educational contributions are second to none.*

L F R

To my wife, Carla,

and

*to my wonderful children, Colleen and Patrick,
in appreciation for their constant love and support.
I also dedicate the text to my steadfast mentors,
Dr. William W. Hallmon and Dr. Michael P. Mills, whose encouragement
has brought me far and whose powerful intellects have humbled me
and shown me how much farther I have to go.*

B L M

*To the memory of one of the great leaders in our field,
Henry M. Goldman,*

and

in honor of Dorothy A. Goldman.

D W C

*In honor of my wife, Sandra, and my parents;
to my children, Deborah, Robert, and Julie;*

and

to my grandchildren and students.

R J G

Dental medicine, especially periodontics, has changed dramatically during the past 80 years. Much of this progress has been the result of research findings carried out in laboratories, dental practices, and clinical research settings around the world. Investigations in periodontics have been supported by the National Institute for Dental and Craniofacial Research, industry, foundations, and academic institutions. The first Department of Periodontics was established at New York University in 1924, and most dental curricula did not include this subject until after World War II. In 1940, at the age of 39, Dr. Henry M. Goldman published the first edition of *Periodontia*. That volume might be considered the great-great ancestor of this text since D. Walter Cohen joined Dr. Goldman in the fourth edition of *Periodontia* in 1957, followed by *Periodontal Therapy* in 1959, which included Saul Schluger and Lewis Fox as co-authors. In 1990, the book *Contemporary Periodontics* by Genco, Goldman, and Cohen continued this lineage. These volumes formed the foundations upon which this current textbook, *Periodontics: Medicine, Surgery, and Implants*, is laid. But this book is not simply a look to the past. Quite the opposite, it embraces a vision of the future for the practice of periodontics in dentistry. This vision asks not only "Where are we *today* in the field of periodontics?" but also "Where are we going *in the next 10 or 20 years?*" Guided by a firm understanding of the pathobiology of periodontal diseases and other oral infections, this book details new knowledge in the field of periodontal medicine, periodontal surgery and nonsurgical care, oral plastic and reconstructive surgical techniques, and dental implant therapy.

Dentistry is no longer a profession whose driving force is the "saving of teeth." Rather, dental diagnosis and treatment is directed toward controlling infection and establishing an oral environment that is conducive to the overall health and well-being of the patient. This is particularly true of the field of periodontology. The new evidence that has been made available to the profession has been the inspiration for this volume, which is designed for all oral health professionals who have the opportunity to treat patients. A group of distinguished contributors has made the text one that can be used by dental students, postdoctoral students, generalists, dental hygienists, and specialists. The goal of the book is to bring this knowledge into the dental practice and into the day-to-day activities of all oral health care providers. The book is about possibilities: possibilities to reinforce what one may already have learned in the field of periodontology, to examine one's current level of understanding in light of today's expanded knowledge base, and to look to the future with confidence that periodontics will play a major role in one's dental practice and will help address many of the problems cited in the recent Surgeon General's report on the nation's oral health.

In this textbook, chapters have been grouped into five sections for ease of reference:

Part I, *Basic Concepts in Periodontal Pathobiology*, introduces the reader to the anatomy and physiology of the periodontium, the most current diagnoses and classification of periodontal diseases, epidemiology and risk factors, the microbiology of periodontal lesions, immuno-inflammatory responses in periodontal diseases, dental plaque and calculus, microbial biofilms, and other factors that contribute to the onset and progression of periodontal diseases.

Part II, *Periodontal Evaluation, Treatment Planning, and Nonsurgical Therapy*, discusses clinical and radiographic diagnostic techniques, management of acute periodontal conditions, oral physiotherapy, nonsurgical therapy and instrumentation, periodontal and dental implant maintenance care, and use of locally acting and systemic chemotherapeutic agents. This section contains a first-of-its-kind chapter on digital record keeping in the dental practice and serves as a guide to the future "paperless" dental office.

Part III, *Surgical Therapy*, addresses the surgical aspects of therapy and includes principles and practice of periodontal surgery, periodontal plastic and reconstructive surgery, principles of periodontal microsurgery, resective surgical techniques, and management of molar furcation problems. Included in this section is a detailed chapter on conscious sedation and anxiety control. The section ends with an extensive chapter on dental implant therapy.

Part IV, *Multidisciplinary Care*, includes several chapters on multidisciplinary dental therapy, including the topics of diagnosis and treatment planning of the compromised dentition, periodontal-restorative and periodontal-prosthetic associations, occlusion, and considerations in the relationships between periodontics, orthodontics, and endodontics.

Part V, *Periodontal Medicine*, addresses systemic considerations and contains the latest information on systemic factors impacting the periodontium, the effects of periodontal infection on a number of systemic conditions, medications impacting the periodontium, tumors and other pathology involving the periodontium, the effects of smoking and other habits on the periodontium and on

periodontal therapy, and proper execution of the medical/dental history. The final chapter contains a detailed and exhaustive review of clinical dental/periodontal management of the medically compromised patient.

Louis F. Rose
Brian L. Mealey
Robert J. Genco
D. Walter Cohen

Acknowledgments

This book came into existence only because of the dedicated efforts of its many contributors. Each clinician and scientist who played a part in its writing and editing has given of his or her time and knowledge, exactly as one might expect of these fine educators. Their efforts are extremely valuable in making this text much more readable for the numerous audiences that will have this opportunity. We acknowledge the special efforts of our Section Editors, Drs. John Kois, Leonard Tibbetts, and Gary Armitage, who provided outstanding review and editorial input.

Two individuals, Dr. Leonard Tibbetts and Dr. Gary Armitage, require exceptional recognition. As Section Editors of major parts of this book, the work would have simply been impossible without their commitment and dedication to seeing the project to its fruition. They served not only as Section Editors but also as counselors and guides to each of us. They made themselves available at all times of day and night to give feedback, provide ideas, and spur the project along. Their many years as clinicians, researchers, and teachers toiling in the field of periodontology were invaluable, and their broad experience forms the ties that bind this book together. We can do little more than say, "thank you," but these men know how deeply we appreciate all of their help.

We are also indebted to Elsevier, and especially to Penny Rudolph, Executive Editor; Julie Nebel, Associate Developmental Editor; and Jaime Pendill, Senior Developmental Editor. They were our constant sounding boards, sifting through countless ideas and separating wheat from chaff. Their attention to detail contributed immensely to the quality of the book.

ABOUT THE COVER

The theme of the cover reflects the mission of our specialty—advancing oral health and well-being through expertise in Periodontal Medicine, Plastic and Reconstructive Surgery, and Implants. The cover drawing was originally conceived and designed by Dr. Leonard Tibbetts. The editors greatly appreciate his artistic gifts.

Contents

PERIODONTICS

MEDICINE, SURGERY, *and* IMPLANTS

Basic
Concepts in
Periodontal
Pathobiology

Gary C. Armitage

1 Anatomy, Development, and Physiology of the Periodontium

Mark I. Ryder

THE NORMAL PERIODONTIUM

DEVELOPMENT OF THE PERIODONTAL ATTACHMENT

CEMENTUM AND ALVEOLAR BONE: FORMATION, STRUCTURE, AND PHYSIOLOGY

PERIODONTAL LIGAMENT AND GINGIVAL CONNECTIVE TISSUE: FORMATION, STRUCTURE, AND PHYSIOLOGY

GINGIVAL EPITHELIUM: FORMATION, STRUCTURE, AND PHYSIOLOGY

IMPLICATIONS FOR PERIODONTAL REGENERATION

This chapter presents an overview and in depth examination of the structure, development, and physiology of the periodontal tissues. In other texts, these topics are traditionally divided over several chapters devoted to such areas as the gingiva, periodontal support, macroanatomy of the periodontium, microanatomy of the periodontium, and development. Integrating these topics into a single chapter was done in the hope that the reader will gain a comprehensive understanding of the relations between these topics. Such an integration is important for our understanding as to how normal tissues change during the pathologic processes of periodontal diseases. In addition, by integrating the story of the development of the periodontium into the macroanatomy and the microanatomy of the periodontium, the reader may understand the often confusing and complex terminologies used for periodontal tissues. This integration of the discussion of periodontal development into periodontal anatomy can also help the reader understand how investigators are developing new regeneration strategies based on these developmental principles. Thus in this chapter, the microanatomy, macroanatomy, physiology, and development of the periodontium will be presented in such a way that the reader can carry this knowledge forward to the subsequent chapters in this textbook. Therefore, these anatomic, developmental, and physiologic topics will be presented in the following sequence:

- A description of the normal clinical, radiographic, and gross microscopic appearance of the periodontal tissues that support, protect, and nourish the tooth.
- An overview of the development of the periodontal attachment.
- A more detailed discussion of the development, structure, and physiology of each of the principal periodontal tissues: the cementum and alveolar bone, the periodontal ligament and gingival connective tissues, and the gingival epithelium and epithelial attachment.

THE NORMAL PERIODONTIUM

The periodontium consists of those tissues that surround and anchor the tooth in the maxillary and mandibular alveolar process. These tissues include the gingiva and gingival attachment to the tooth, cementum, periodontal ligament, and alveolar bone. When viewed clinically, the only portion of periodontium that is visible to the unaided eye is the oral aspect of the gingival epithelium (Fig. 1-1). When healthy, this area of gingiva is normally coral pink with variations in melanin pigmentation among different racial groups.[1,2] The firm, pink, coronally located gingiva is distinguished from the more pliable and more red oral mucosa on the buccal aspect of the maxillary teeth and on the buccal and lingual aspect of the mandibular teeth by a distinct mucogingival line or mucogingival junction.

On the palatal aspect, the firm pink gingiva is continuous with the firm pink palatal mucosa. In areas of the dentition where there is contact between adjacent teeth, the gingiva has a typical scalloped profile coming to a triangular point in the interproximal embrasure. In areas where there is no contact between teeth, this gingival profile is flatter in appearance. In cross section, the margin of the gingiva comes to a tapered point or knife edge. On the surface of the oral gingival epithelium there is a characteristic dimpled pattern or stippled pattern formed from invaginations of the oral gingival epithelium into the underlying connective tissue. A shallow gingival groove is seen on approximately 50% of the gingival surface, which runs a few millimeters below the gingival margin profile at approximately the level of the base of the gingival sulcus.

The remaining periodontal structures can best be appreciated in low-power buccal-lingual sections or diagrams of the tooth and surrounding bone (see Fig. 1-1).[3,4] In this type of section, one can discern a thin covering of mineralized tissue over the root dentin, termed the *cementum*. Fibers of the periodontal ligament insert into the cementum on the tooth side and into the alveolar bone on the opposite side. The periodontal ligament thus provides the principal anchoring mechanism of the tooth to the alveolar bone. The width of the space occupied by the periodontal ligament often can be visualized on standard dental radiographs (Fig. 1-2). This width ranges from 0.1 to 0.25 mm and is generally narrowest at the midpoint of the root. The periodontal ligament space also has a blood supply to provide nutrients to the surface and the alveolar bone; cells for repair and remodeling the cementum, ligament, and surface of the alveolar bone; and a sensory nerve network to provide tactile information on the position of the tooth. Thus the periodontal ligament and associated structures have supportive, nutritive, regenerative, and sensory functions.

In a buccal-lingual cross section, the gingival epithelium forms a crevice around the tooth.[5] This epithelium can be distinguished into three regions covering the underlying gingival connective tissue (Fig. 1-3). In all cases, the basal lamina of the basal epithelial layer attaches to the underlying connective tissue through anchoring fibrils. The three regions include:

- A thicker keratinized (orthokeratinized) or parakeratinized oral gingival epithelium (see Fig. 1-3, A).
- A thinner and flatter parakeratinized or nonkeratinized lining of the crevice itself, termed the *crevicular epithelium* (see Fig. 1-3, B).
- An area apical to the unattached crevicular epithelium, termed the *junctional epithelium*, which forms an epithelial attachment to the tooth surface itself (see Fig. 1-3, C).

This epithelial attachment is therefore the most coronal portion of the periodontal attachment apparatus. When

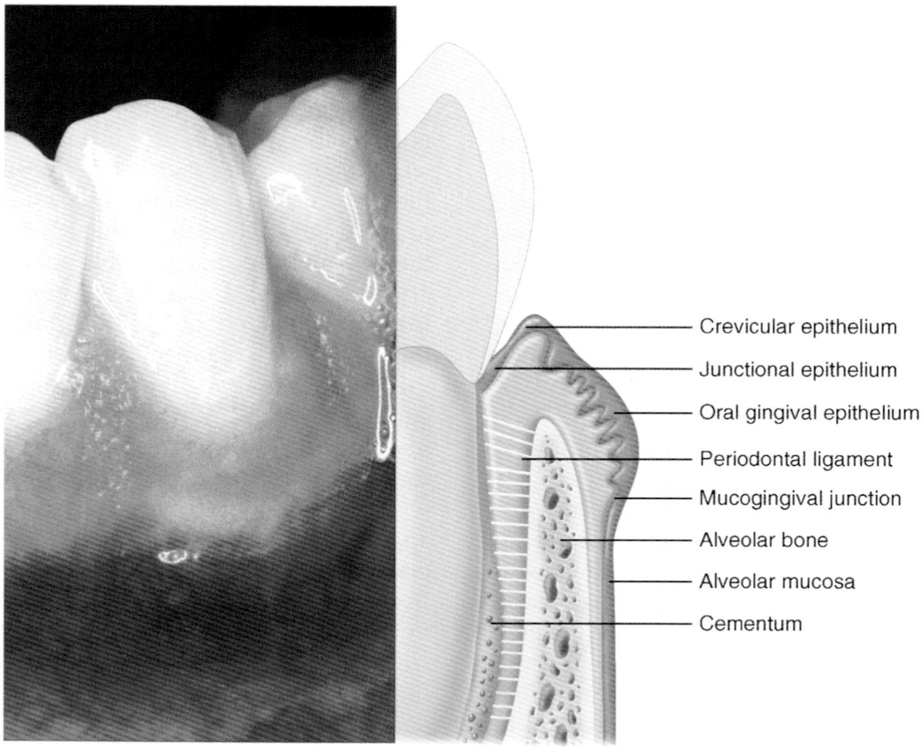

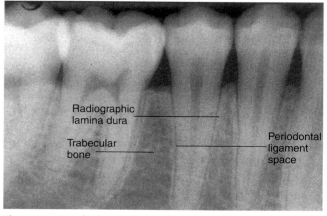

Crevicular epithelium

Junctional epithelium

Oral gingival epithelium

Periodontal ligament

Mucogingival junction

Alveolar bone

Alveolar mucosa

Cementum

Figure 1-1. Clinical view and diagrammatic representation of the major elements of the periodontium. A diagram of what a buccal-lingual cross section of the clinical view might look like is presented to the right of the clinical photograph. The buccal-lingual scale is exaggerated to illustrate some of the much thinner regions of the periodontium. (*Redrawn from Rateitschak KH, Rateitschak EM, Wolf HF, Hassell TM: Color atlas of dental medicine/periodontology, ed 2, New York, 1994, Thieme Medical Publishers.*)

healthy, the level of the epithelium attachment to the tooth is usually at or slightly coronal to the level of the border between the apical extent of the enamel and coronal extent of the cementum. This area on the tooth is called the *cementoenamel junction*. The connective tissue

Radiographic lamina dura

Trabecular bone

Periodontal ligament space

Figure 1-2. Standard periapical radiograph of the tooth and alveolar bone support. The more radiodense lamina dura and radiolucent periodontal ligament space can be seen.

underlying the gingival epithelium can be divided into a less collagen-dense papillary layer directly beneath the gingival epithelium and a deeper more collagen-dense reticular layer.

The blood supply for the periodontium comes from the inferior and superior alveolar arteries, respectively.[3,5] Branches of these arteries extend coronally into the ligament from the apices of the teeth and from branches that extend coronally into the central trabecular areas of the alveolar bone, or over the oral side of the periosteum, and then penetrate perpendicularly through the alveolar bone and into the periodontal ligament (Fig. 1-4). When the surface of the bony socket is viewed face on, numerous small holes can be seen that correspond to the penetration of these small blood vessels and nerves into the periodontal ligament. This perforated appearance of the alveolar bone is similar to the appearance of the cribriform plate of the ethmoid bone above the nasal cavity.

Some branches of the blood supply run directly into the periodontal ligament and into the alveolar bone. Other branches run along the surface of the bone. These various arterial branches continue into the gingival tissue and terminate in numerous capillary loops in the superficial area of the gingival connective tissue adjacent to the gingival

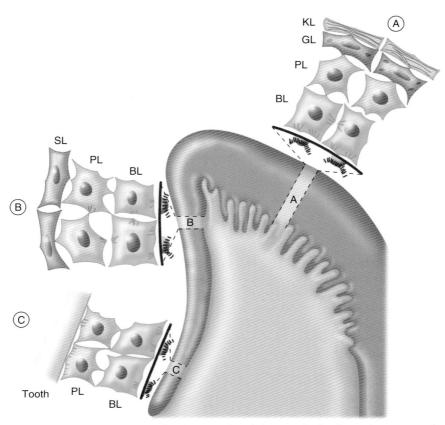

Figure 1-3. The three major types of epithelial organization within the gingival epithelium. *a,* The four layers characteristic of orthokeratinized gingiva are seen. These include the cuboidal cells of the basal layer (BL), a prickle cell layer or spinous layer (PL), a granular layer (GL) with flattened cells containing keratohyaline granules, and a keratinized layer (KL) with flattened cells packed with keratin filaments. When dark nuclei are present in the KL, the epithelium is termed *parakeratinized.* When no nuclei can be seen in the KL, the epithelium is "orthokeratinized." *b,* Nonkeratinized epithelium. Although a BL and PL are still present, the cells in the more superficial layers (SL) are not as flat as the parakeratinized or orthokeratinized epithelium, contain fewer keratin filaments, and still have nuclei. *c,* Junctional epithelium. Only two layers are seen: a BL and a PL. The cells of the most SL of the PL attach to the tooth in part through hemidesmosomes. Note that in all types of epithelium (*a, b,* and *c*), the basal layer is anchored to the underlying connective tissue through hemidesmosomes, which interdigitate with anchoring collagen fibrils extending from the connective tissue.

epithelium (the papillary region of the gingival connective tissue) (see Fig. 1-4). Within the gingival tissue, there are numerous anastomoses among these three blood supplies. This extensive collateral circulation enables the clinician to perform a variety of surgical procedures on the gingiva without significantly compromising its blood supply.

The nerve supply to the periodontium is derived from branches of the trigeminal nerve and thus is sensory in function. Nerve branches terminate in the periodontal ligament, surface of the alveolar bone, and within the gingival connective tissue in four different morphologies of nerve endings that receive stimuli for pain (nociceptors) and position and pressure (mechanoreceptors or proprioreceptors).

Because the alveolar bone that lines the tooth socket has numerous small perforations and is mixed in with calcified fiber bundles of the periodontal ligament, it is termed *woven bone.* The buccal and lingual plates on the buccal or lingual external surface of the alveolar process is composed of compact bone (see Fig. 1-1). Between the buccal or lingual plates and the alveolar bone socket, the bone is more trabecular in appearance. These three bone regions are usually clearly visible on standard dental radiographs (see Fig. 1-2). The height of this alveolar bone or alveolar crest is usually 1.0 to 1.5 mm apical to the radiographic cementoenamel junction. In conventional radiographs of teeth and the supporting alveolar bone, the alveolar bone that lines the bony socket and extends over the alveolar crest often appears as a radiodense line, termed the *lamina dura.* The appearance of this radiodense lamina dura may be because of an increased density of bone in this area, or superimposition of the bony curvatures of the bony socket, or both. In periodontal diseases accompanied by loss of alveolar bone, this radiographic lamina dura is often not seen.

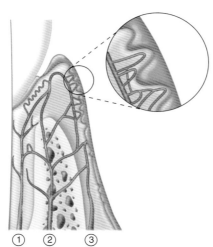

Figure 1-4. Blood supply of the periodontal tissues. From the apical aspect of the periodontal tissues, arterial branches course through the periodontal ligament (*1*), through the alveolar bone (*2*), and along the surface of the periosteum (*3*). The terminal branches of each of the three arterial sources form numerous anastomoses and capillary loops. These arterial loops are especially prominent within the connective tissue that interdigitates with the oral gingival epithelium (*inset* enlargement).

DEVELOPMENT OF THE PERIODONTAL ATTACHMENT

The story of the development of the periodontal attachment and supporting tissues begins at the earliest stages of tooth development at 4 to 5 weeks gestation.[5-7] At this stage, the oral cavity consists of a simple cavity known as the *primitive stomatodeum*. This primitive stomatodeum is lined by a single layer of ectoderm with an underlying ectomesenchyme. At 4 to 5 weeks, a horseshoe-shaped thickening of this ectoderm can be seen along the developing mandibular and maxillary arches. This thickening is formed through the focal division of the ectoderm and is called the *primary epithelial band*. At the site of each developing primary tooth, this primary epithelial band will extend as a dental lamina into the underlying ectomesenchyme and will form a knoblike projection or *tooth bud* at its terminal end (Fig. 1-5, A). Deeper within this ectomesenchyme, rudimentary woven bone will begin to form around each of these developing tooth buds. This first woven bone will be the structural framework for the developing alveolar bone support. The epithelium of the tooth bud will begin to differentiate into

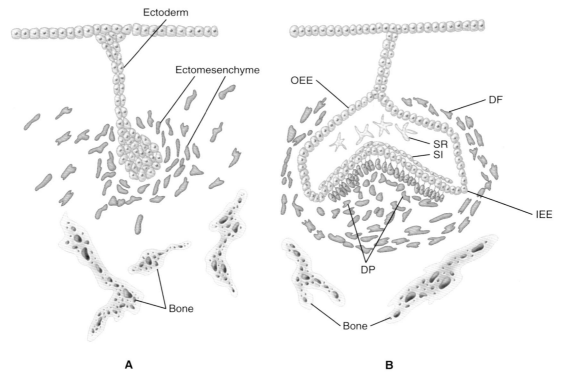

A   **B**

Figure 1-5. Two early stages of the development of the tooth and periodontium. **A,** At approximately 4 to 5 weeks into development there is downgrowth of the ectoderm of the primitive oral stomatodeum into the underlying ectomesenchyme. At the terminal end of this downgrowth, the cells form a knoblike structure or bud. Cells in the surrounding ectomesenchyme begin to concentrate around this bud. **B,** Several weeks later, this ectodermal bud has developed into a caplike structure with four distinct layers: an outer enamel epithelium (OEE), an inner enamel epithelium (IEE), a stellate reticulum (SR), and a stratum intermedium (SI). Directly beneath the inner enamel epithelium, cells of the underlying ectomesenchyme have condensed into a dental papilla (DP). Surrounding these two structures is a third condensation, the dental follicle (DF), which will give rise to most of the cementum, periodontal ligament, and alveolar bone.

a *dental organ* with four distinct layers (see Fig. 1-5, B): an inner enamel epithelium that will first differentiate into a columnar secretory ameloblast layer, an overlying layer of one to two cells of stratum intermedium, a wide area of stellate reticulum, and an outer enamel epithelium.

Directly beneath this dental organ, the underlying ectomesenchyme will condense into a *dental papilla*, which will give rise to the crown and root dentin and most of the cellular elements of the pulp (see Fig. 1-5, B). At this time, a second spherical condensation of ectomesenchyme will form to surround the developing dental organ and dental papilla (see Fig. 1-5, B). This surrounding spherical condensation is called the *dental follicle*. Cells of the dental follicle will eventually differentiate into cementoblasts to lay down cementum, periodontal ligament fibroblasts to lay down the fibers of the periodontal ligament, and osteoblasts to lay down the alveolar bone adjacent to the periodontal ligament. The central question of development of the periodontal attachment is how the root dentin, cementum, periodontal ligament, and alveolar bone integrate to form this critical anchor for the tooth in the supporting bone. To understand this process, the development of the root dentin and cementum will be presented first.

At the apical extent of the developing crown, the inner and outer epithelium come together in close apposition. The **loop** formed by the inner and outer enamel epithelium is termed the *cervical loop* and will play a pivotal role in directing the formation of both the root dentin and the periodontal attachment (Figs. 1-6 and 1-7). As the dental organ begins to assume a more bell shape and then lays down the first enamel and dentin matrix at the incisal tip

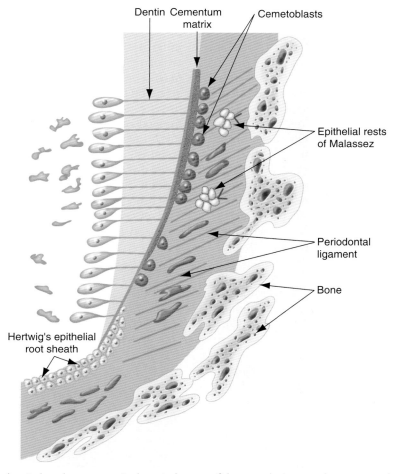

Figure 1-6. Developing root and periodontal structures. At the apical extent of the root, the inner and outer enamel epithelium have fused to form the Hertwig's epithelial root sheath (HES). More coronally, this root sheath breaks down to form islands of epithelial cells in the developing periodontal ligament space, the epithelial rests of Malassez (ERM). The breakdown of the root sheath and subsequent exposure of the dentin (D) to the dental follicle allows cells in the dental follicle nearest the developing root surface to differentiate into cementoblasts (CB) and lay down the first cementum matrix (CM). Further away from the tooth follicle, cells differentiate into fibroblasts and lay down the first bundles of collagen in the periodontal ligament (PDL).

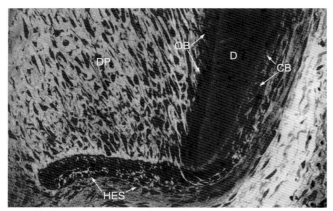

Figure 1-7. Low-power micrograph of the apical extent of a developing human root. At the apical extent of the developing root dentin is Hertwig's epithelial root sheath (HES). On the more coronal aspect of the root dentin (D), this sheath has been replaced by cementoblasts (CB) derived from the dental follicle. Odontoblasts (OB) derived from the dental papilla (DP) produce dentin matrix, whereas cementoblasts (CB) from the dental follicle produce cementum. (*Courtesy Dr. Max Listgarten, Foster City, Calif.*)

area, cells in the cervical loop begin to divide and extend apically as a cylindrical sheath called *Hertwig's epithelial root sheath* (see Figs. 1-6 and 1-7). This root sheath migrates apically around the dental papilla. Cells in the dental papilla in direct contact with the sheath differentiate into odontoblasts and lay down the first dentin matrix of the surface of the root. At about the same time, the root sheath secretes an amorphous hyaline-like layer that contains among other things, embryonic enamel proteins. This protein is similar to the protein laid down more coronally by the inner enamel epithelium. After this initial secretion of dentin matrix by cells of the dental papilla and the amorphous enamel-like matrix of the root sheath, this root sheath breaks down to form small islands of epithelial cells in the developing periodontal ligament space called the *epithelial rests of Malassez* (see Fig. 1-6).

When this root sheath breaks down, it leaves the developing root in direct contact with the cells of the surrounding dental follicle.[8-11] Cells nearest the developing root dentin will differentiate into a layer of cementoblasts that will lay down a fibrillar cementum matrix. This layer of cementoblasts will move away from the tooth leaving a layer of calcifying cementum that slowly grows in thickness. Meanwhile, cells in the dental follicle nearest the developing alveolar process will differentiate into a layer of osteoblasts and will lay down bone matrix over the developing alveolar bone process. Between the developing root and alveolar bone, cells of the dental follicle will differentiate into fibroblasts and will lay down the first short lengths of periodontal ligament fibers (see Fig. 1-6). Periodontal ligament fibroblasts will continuously

remodel lengths of ligament fibers into longer and thicker bundles. As the cementum and alveolar bone both thicken by apposition of their respective matrices and narrow the periodontal ligament space, periodontal ligament fibers will become trapped and will calcify within these thickening matrices (Fig. 1-8). These trapped calcified bundles of collagen fibers are termed *Sharpey's fibers*. It is primarily through the entrapment of these ligament fibers by the bone and cementum matrices that a periodontal connection is made between the root of the tooth and the supporting alveolar bone.

At first the orientation of these early bundles of collagen fibers is nearly parallel to the longitudinal root surface, with fibers oriented in a steep oblique angle coronally from the alveolar bone to apically into the root cementum. Fibroblasts within this steep oblique orientation are attached, through the adhesion protein *fibronectin*, to the segments of collagen bundles through a specialized attachment called the *fibronexus*. These periodontal ligament fibroblasts have the ability to contract, and thereby bring these collagen fibers closer together. Because the alveolar bone is fixed in the developing mandible and maxilla relative to the unanchored developing root, this action on the segments of periodontal ligament fibers has the effect of pulling the developing tooth upward toward the oral cavity. This phenomenon has been shown to be the primary force for tooth eruption and is called *active eruption*.

As discussed in the overview section, the most coronal portion of the periodontal attachment is the epithelial attachment extending apically from the base of the gingival crevice. The development of this unique attachment begins at the completion of enamel formation.[7] At this

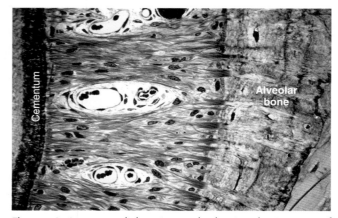

Figure 1-8. Low-power light micrograph showing the insertion of periodontal ligament fiber bundles into root cementum on the left and alveolar bone on the right in a monkey. The ligament fibers insert in thicker and more widely spaced bundles on the alveolar bone side, whereas fiber bundles are smaller but more numerous on the cementum side. (*Courtesy Dr. Max Listgarten, Foster City, Calif.*)

stage, the columnar layer of inner enamel epithelium differentiates into a flat layer of reduced enamel epithelium (Fig. 1-9). This layer of reduced enamel epithelium attaches to the entire enamel surface of the crown through "spot weld"-like attachments along the epithelial cell membrane called *hemidesmosomes*. These hemidesmosomes appear as thickenings in the cell membrane that are anchored to the underlying cell structure through intermediate filaments. Above this layer of reduced enamel epithelium, the more superficial stratum intermedium and stellate reticulum break down. This results in the outer enamel epithelium coming in direct contact with the reduced inner enamel epithelium. This attachment of the inner enamel epithelium to the enamel surface is called the *primary epithelial attachment.*

As the tooth erupts toward the oral cavity, this bilayer of reduced enamel epithelium derived from the dental organ makes contact with epithelium originating from the lining of the oral cavity. This epithelium from the oral cavity extends into the connective tissue by cell division (Fig. 1-10). The epithelial cells of the primary epithelial attachment

begin to break down (see Fig. 1-9) and are replaced by these epithelial cells from the oral cavity (see Fig. 1-10). These oral epithelial cells migrate from the cusp tips in an apical direction down the enamel crown to the cemento-enamel junction. The result is a multilayered covering of the crown with oral epithelial cells that are attached to the tooth through hemidesmosomes (Fig. 1-11). This attachment of oral epithelium to the tooth surface is called the *secondary epithelial attachment.*

As the tooth erupts into the oral cavity, this multilayered secondary epithelial attachment will split between its layers, leaving a layer or several layers adjacent to the tooth surface, which will abrade off the tooth surface. The layer of cells on the opposite side of the split will recede away in an apical direction along with the underlying connective tissue. This splitting and recession of the epithelial cell layers more distant from the tooth results in more clinical exposure of the crown. Because this process does not involve an actual displacement of the tooth as in active eruption, it is called *passive eruption.* In the normal passive eruption process, this epithelial splitting process will continue in a coronal direction until the split approaches the normal clinical attachment level at the cementoenamel junction. The epithelium on the opposite side of the split will continue to recede until it is slightly coronal to the cementoenamel junction. This splitting

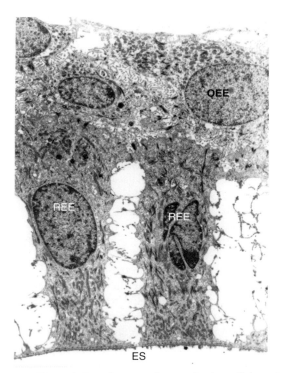

Figure 1-9. Transmission electron microscopic view of the primary epithelial attachment. In this section of demineralized tissue, two reduced enamel epithelial (REE) cells that derive from the inner enamel epithelium attach to the demineralized enamel, which appears as an enamel space (ES). Directly above these reduced enamel epithelial cells, cells of the original outer enamel epithelium (OEE) are juxtaposed directly adjacent to these REE cells. (*Courtesy Dr. Max Listgarten, Foster City, Calif.*)

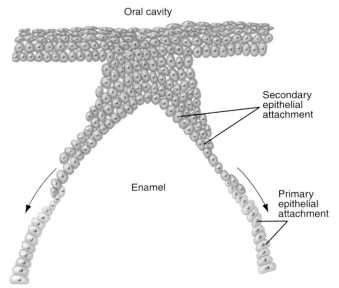

Figure 1-10. Diagrammatic representation of the formation of the primary and secondary epithelial attachment. At the more apical aspect of the tooth crown, the epithelial attachment is formed by cells of the inner enamel epithelium (the primary epithelial attachment). As the enamel crown approaches the oral cavity, epithelial cells from the oral cavity grow downward, replace these inner enamel epithelial cells from the cusp tips to the cemento-enamel junction, and form the secondary epithelial attachment.

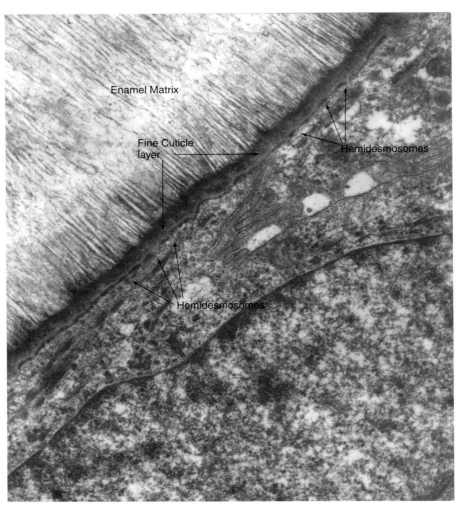

Enamel Matrix

Fine Cuticle
layer

Hemidesmosomes

Hemidesmosomes

Figure 1-11. High-power transmission electron microscopic view of the junctional epithelium at the region of the epithelial attachment to a section of enamel. In this demineralized section, the enamel matrix can still be seen covered by a fine cuticle layer. On the epithelial cell side, numerous hemidesmosomal attachment complexes can be seen. They appear as small, dark "spot welds." When numerous hemidesmosomes lie side-by-side, they may appear as a more continuous dark line (see hemidesmosomes, *bottom left*). (*Courtesy Dr. Max Listgarten, Foster City, Calif.*)

and recession thus results in the formation of the gingival crevice.

CEMENTUM AND ALVEOLAR BONE: FORMATION, STRUCTURE, AND PHYSIOLOGY

The deposition of cementum on the root surface that gradually thickens toward the periodontal ligament space is somewhat similar to the deposition of alveolar bone that thickens the alveolar bone support from the opposite side of the ligament space. As a result, the cementum does have some structural and biochemical similarities (as well as some critical differences) with alveolar bone.[9-11] As with the development of the alveolar bone proper, an organic matrix of cementum composed primarily of type

I and type III collagen is secreted by a layer of formative cells (the cementoblasts) over the thin hyaline-like layer secreted by Hertwig's epithelial root sheath covering the root dentin. This fine fibrillar matrix calcifies to form a relatively uniform and well organized layer of cementum free of cellular elements called *primary acellular cementum*.[10] This first thin layer of mineralized cementum contains only the fibrillar matrix from the cementoblasts themselves. These fibers are therefore called *intrinsic fibers* of cementum.

As the cementum continues to thicken by apposition of cementum by the cementoblast layers, this thickening cementum will encounter and incorporate bundles of the forming periodontal ligament. These ligament bundles incorporated into the cementum surface will calcify along with the surrounding intrinsic fibers to form a significant portion of the more superficial layers of the cementum. These insertions of calcified ligament fibers are termed *extrinsic fibers* of the cementum.[11] A similar entrapment and calcification process occurs on the forming alveolar bone side. The general term for these calcified insertions of bundles of ligament fibers into the cementum and bone are *Sharpey's fibers*. On the cementum side, these *Sharpey's fibers* are much thinner in diameter and insert at closer intervals when compared with the alveolar bone side (see Fig. 1-8). These differences in the pattern of insertion have clinical importance in the distribution of forces that are generated within the periodontal ligament during occlusion, tooth movement, and traumatic forces. Specifically, these forces are more evenly distributed along the cementum surface and are more concentrated along the more widely spaced insertions on the alveolar bone side. As a result, in response to mechanical forces, there is generally a remodeling of the periodontal housing on the alveolar bone side and not on the cementum side. This prevents the possibility of significant cementum and root resorption. In addition, the root cementum is protected from this relatively extensive remodeling because it is avascular, and therefore not as exposed to osteoclast-like precursor cells in the circulation. Although small areas of microscopic cementum resorption and repair have been frequently observed in histologic sections, more extensive resorption of cementum is usually not seen unless there is a force on the tooth of a high enough magnitude, or duration, or both, that cannot be accommodated by the remodeling of the alveolar bone.

As the tooth completes active eruption into the oral cavity and meets its opposing tooth in the other arch, the formation of cementum becomes somewhat less regular and organized. This type of cementum formation that occurs over the more organized primary cementum is called *secondary cementum*. It occurs mainly along the apical one third of the root. During the formation of secondary cementum, cells in the layer of secreting cementoblasts will often become entrapped within the cementum matrix (Fig. 1-12). These entrapped cementoblasts become cementocytes similar in appearance to the entrapped osteoblasts that become osteocytes on the alveolar bone side (Fig. 1-13). These areas of cementum that contain cementocytes are called *cellular cementum*. Layers of cellular cementum are generally seen in the apical one third of the root surface. In secondary cementum, these layers of cellular cementum often alternate with layers of acellular cementum.

By understanding how cementum forms, it can be understood how areas of cementum can be termed *acellular* or *cellular cementum*, *primary* or *secondary cementum*, and can contain intrinsic fibers, extrinsic fibers, or a mixture of these fibers. There is one final terminology of

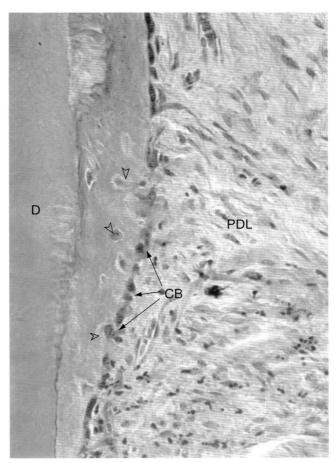

Figure 1-12. Low-power light micrograph of an area of cementum between root dentin (D) and periodontal ligament (PDL). Numerous cementoblasts can be seen lining the cementum surface (CB). In some areas (*arrowheads*), the cementoblasts appear partially trapped in the cementum. (*Courtesy Dr. Gary Armitage, San Francisco, Calif.*)

cementum that needs to be introduced to complete this discussion: the formation of a thin layer of cementum at the junction of the enamel and the root surface.[12] This form of cementum lacks a fibrillar organization and is therefore called *afibrillar cementum*. It is usually formed after root eruption when the connective tissue comes in direct contact with the enamel and dentin at the cementoenamel junction without an intervening layer of cementoblasts. In approximately 30% of teeth, the coronal extent of the cementum ends in a "butt" joint adjacent to the enamel, whereas in 60% to 65% of teeth, the cementum may overlap the enamel, and in 5% to 10% of teeth, the cementum will end short of the enamel thereby exposing the root surface dentin. This latter situation may have clinical importance in that patients with this type of gap may experience root sensitivity during instrumentation or exposure to extreme temperatures.

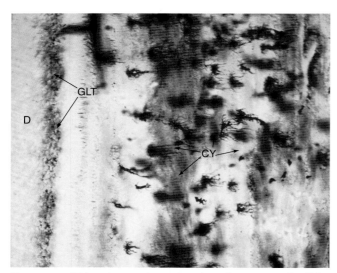

Figure 1-13. Light micrograph section through an area of cellular cementum in a monkey. The dentin (D) and granular layer of tomes (GLT) are on the *left* and the periodontal ligament space on the *right*. Numerous cementocytes (CY) are seen within this layer of cellular cementum. Note the orientation of the cementocyte cell processes toward the periodontal ligament side. (*Courtesy Dr. Max Listgarten, Foster City, Calif.*)

From the time the tooth has erupted to the occlusal plane, cementum will continue to be deposited throughout life.[13] This thickening of cementum with age is usually greatest around the apical one third of the tooth. This apical thickening may partially maintain the overall length of the tooth during the natural attrition of the crown and may therefore retard the collapse of the vertical bite dimension with aging. Abnormal thickening of the cementum is often observed in certain metabolic bone diseases such as Paget's disease.[14]

On the other side of the future periodontal ligament, the alveolar bone is forming.[15] The alveolar bone is similar in chemical composition to fibrillar cementum, particularly cellular fibrillar cementum. As discussed in the overall development section, the alveolar bone begins to first form by an intramembranous ossification within the ectomesenchyme surrounding the developing tooth. This first bone formed is less organized woven bone that will be replaced with a more organized lamellar bone. Within this forming lamellar bone, individual osteons with blood and nerve supplies can be observed. As cells in the dental follicle between this first alveolar bone and developing root differentiate into cementoblasts on the root dentin side and fibroblasts in the future periodontal ligament space, the cells in the dental follicle near the alveolar bone side differentiate into osteoblasts. This layer of osteoblasts will lay down bone matrix to form the outer wall of the alveolar bone support.

During the life of the periodontium, the alveolar bone continuously remodels its shape in response to mechanical forces on the tooth and inflammation. As a result, on the surface of the alveolar bone the following can be observed:

1. *Bone synthesis* with areas of bone covered with cuboidal-shaped osteoblasts secreting bone matrix,
2. *Bone resorption* with areas of bone covered by multinucleated bone resorbing osteoclasts (Fig. 1-14), and
3. Areas of no synthetic or resorptive activity with bone covered by flattened cells.

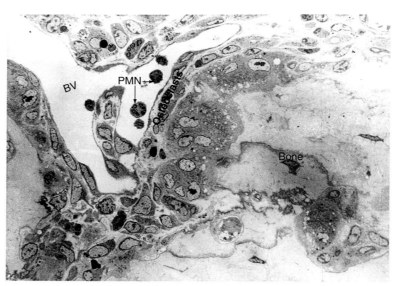

Figure 1-14. Low-power trypan blue stained section from an advanced periodontal lesion in the rice rat. Several multinucleated osteoclasts are seen on the bone surface. Polymorphonuclear leukocytes (PMN) can be seen in the adjacent blood vessel (BV) and in the connective tissue.

PERIODONTAL LIGAMENT AND GINGIVAL CONNECTIVE TISSUE: FORMATION, STRUCTURE, AND PHYSIOLOGY

In this section, the periodontal ligament and gingival connective tissue structures will be considered together because there is some overlap in their respective structure and function. When the early development of the periodontal ligament was discussed previously, the ligament *per se* was in the form of short lengths of collagen bundles oriented in a near parallel direction to the tooth surface. As discussed in the previous section on the development of cementum, the bundles closest to the developing and expanding cementum on one side and alveolar bone on the other side are incorporated into the matrix of these forming hard tissues. The fibroblasts that form the collagen in these ligament bundles will continue to extend and remodel these ligament fiber bundles, through secretion of new collagen and resorption of older collagen, until they form a continuous network of fibers between the cementum and bone. As the tooth erupts into the oral cavity by the process of active eruption, the erupting root connected to the ligament fibers will move the orientation of the fibers to a generally more perpendicular orientation to the root surface (Fig. 1-15).[5] At the coronal extent of the ligament near the alveolar crest, the ligament will be oriented more obliquely from an apical

insertion at the alveolar crest to a coronal insertion at the root near the cementoenamel junction (see Fig. 1-15). More apically these fibers will orient in a more horizontal and perpendicular direction to the root surface, whereas near the root apex and within the furcations of molars, these fibers will orient more vertically and perpendicularly to the root surface. Thus periodontal ligament fiber groups can be classified based on their orientation (see Fig. 1-15). However, these distinct fiber orientations are not always observed on routine histologic sections.

The collagen fiber bundles themselves are made up primarily of type I collagen (80%) with a smaller percentage of type III collagen (20%).[7] As with collagen fiber structures in other connective tissues of the body, each fiber bundle is composed of smaller diameter collagen fibrils (Fig. 1-16). Each collagen fibril is in turn composed of individual bundles of collagen molecules that are secreted by the fibroblasts as procollagen α helices. These procollagen molecules are assembled and modified extracellularly into bundles that are staggered in a regular linear manner to give the characteristic cross-banding pattern seen in the collagen fibril.

In addition, the periodontal ligament also contains immature forms of other connective tissue fibers, such as an immature form of elastin fiber known as *elaunin*, and *oxytalan fibers*. Elaunin fibers and oxytalan fibers form a more reticular-like network that is generally oriented

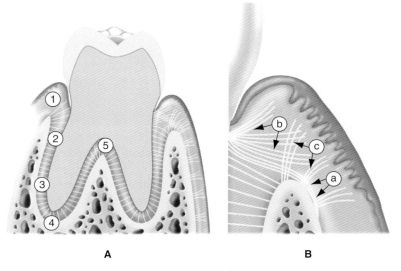

A   B

Figure 1-15. The major periodontal ligament and gingival fiber groups. **A,** In this low-power diagram, periodontal ligament fibers can be divided into several groupings depending on their orientation. These include: (1) an alveolar crest group, (2) a horizontal fiber group, (3) an oblique fiber group, (4) an apical group, and (5) a radicular group. **B,** In this magnified view of the alveolar crest, the gingival fibers can also be classified based on their orientation, origin, and insertion. These groups include: (a) fibers that run from the root surface and over the oral periosteum, (b) fibers that run from the root surface and into the gingiva, and (c) fibers that run from the alveolar bone and into the gingiva. Not shown are fibers that run in a circumferential or semicircumferential direction around the tooth within the gingiva, as well as the transseptal fiber group that runs from the root surface of one tooth over the alveolar crest and into the root surface of the adjacent tooth.

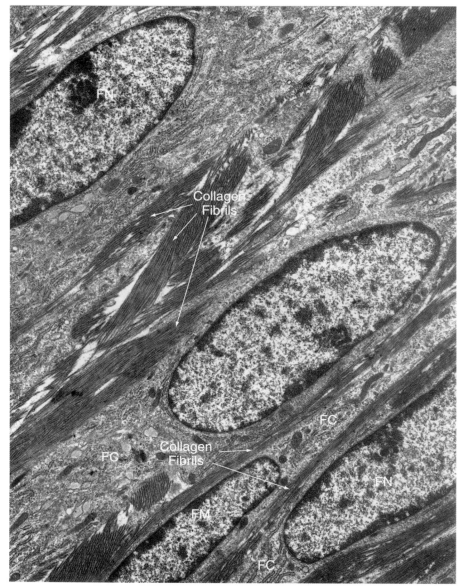

Figure 1-16. High-power transmission electron microscopic view of a periodontal ligament in the rice rat. Bundles of collagen fibrils that make up collagen fibers are seen running parallel to elongated fibroblasts. FC, fibroblast cytoplasm; FN, fibroblast nucleus.

perpendicular to the collagen fiber bundles. Although the role of these elaunin and oxytalan fibers still remains unknown, they may play a role in the spatial organization of the principal collagen fibers and blood vessel elements in the periodontal ligament. At intervals along the periodontal ligament near the root surface, remnants of Hertwig's epithelial root sheath, the *epithelial rests of Malassez*, can be observed (see Fig. 1-6). Although several theories regarding the future fate of these cells in periodontal development and periodontal disease have been proposed, the significance of these epithelial remnants has yet to be determined.[7]

Between the fiber elements of the ligament, there is a ground substance consisting of glycosaminoglycans,

laminin, and fibronectin. The ground substance itself has the potential to retain aqueous fluid and is composed of 70% water. As an aqueous "cushion," the ground substance may help the ligament absorb mechanical forces placed on the tooth and periodontal support.

As discussed in the overview of the periodontium, the gingival connective tissue coronal to the periodontal ligament area is called the *reticular area* of the gingival connective tissue. This area shares many of the same structural features as the periodontal ligament. It is an area composed of a dense network of collagen fibers (primarily of type I) surrounded by a similar composition of ground substance seen in the periodontal ligament. As with the periodontal ligament, these bundles of collagen fibers have distinct orientations that can be classified as gingival fiber groups (see Fig. 1-15). These groups include fibers that run from the alveolar crest into the gingiva; fibers that run from the tooth surface and over the buccal or lingual periosteum; fibers that run in a circular or semicircular pattern around the tooth; and fibers that run interproximally from the root surface of one tooth, over the alveolar crest, and into the root surface of the adjacent tooth (the transseptal fibers).[1,5] These organized gingival fiber groups enable the gingiva to form a rigid cuff around the tooth that can add stability, especially when a significant portion of the periodontal ligament and alveolar support is lost. This may explain in part the increased mobility in periodontally involved teeth immediately after surgical procedures because these procedures often significantly disrupt or remove these gingival fiber groups. In addition, after tooth movement, these fiber groups may exert forces on the tooth to move it toward its original position. Therefore, after tooth movement procedures, a "fiberotomy" to cut the gingival fiber attachments to the tooth is sometimes performed.[16]

The portion of the gingival connective tissue above the dense reticular layer and underlying the gingival epithelium itself is called the *papillary layer* of the gingival connective tissue. In this layer, the distribution of collagen is sparser and less organized than in the reticular layer. Between the epithelial cells and the connective tissue lies the basal lamina (basement membrane), which is critical to the attachment between the two tissues.[7] At the electron microscopic level, the basal lamina consists of a dark band called the *lamina densa* and a more translucent band known as the *lamina lucida*. The portion of the papillary layer adjacent to the basal lamina has small anchoring fibrils of type IV collagen that anchor the lamina densa of the basal lamina of the gingival epithelium (also composed of type IV collagen) to the gingival connective tissue. In addition to the collagen types I, III, and IV, ground substance, blood vessels, neural and lymphatic elements, and small numbers of inflammatory cells such as neutrophils, monocytes, lymphocytes, mast cells, and macrophages are routinely observed. During the inflammatory process of periodontal diseases, the number of these cells increases within this papillary layer. The clinical importance of this inflammatory cell infiltrate is discussed in later chapters.

GINGIVAL EPITHELIUM: FORMATION, STRUCTURE, AND PHYSIOLOGY

As described in the section on development of the periodontium, the erupting enamel crown of the tooth is covered with several layers of epithelium that are first derived from the inner enamel epithelium (the primary epithelial attachment) and are then replaced from the incisal tips to the cementoenamel junction with epithelial cells from the oral cavity (the secondary epithelial attachment) (see Fig. 1-1o). During the process of passive eruption, a natural gingival crevice is formed around the circumference of the tooth. Within this gingival crevice, three distinct zones of epithelium can be seen on routine buccal-lingual sections of the tooth and surrounding periodontal tissues (see Fig. 1-3). These include a thick orthokeratinized or parakeratinized oral gingival epithelium that faces the oral cavity, an unattached thinner and parakeratinized or nonkeratinized crevicular epithelium, and an area of junctional epithelium where the gingiva actually attaches to the tooth through hemidesmosomes and adhesion proteins such as laminins (Fig. 1-17, see also Figs. 1-3 and 1-11). Each of these three zones of gingival epithelium is distinct in the organization, stratification, and characteristics of the keratinocytes that make up each strata.

The oral gingival epithelium resembles the epidermis in structure and has multiple layers (see Fig. 1-3).[5-7] The basal layer has one or two layers of cuboidal-shaped cells that divide and migrate toward the superficial layers of epithelium. Outside of the basal layers is the prickle layer consisting of more spinous-shaped cells with large intercellular spaces (also known as the *spinous layer,* or *stratum spinosum*). Cells of both the basal and prickle cell layers attach to each other in part through desmosomes. These desmosome "spot-weld" junctions appear on transmission electron micrographs as thickenings of the inner membranes of both apposing cells. In the intercellular space between these membrane thickenings, a central dark line is often discernible, which may be an area of protein links between the two cell membranes. As with hemidesmosomes, these membrane thickenings are anchored to the underlying cell structures through intermediate filaments. Above the prickle layer there is a layer of flattened granular cells with flattened and condensed nuclei, increased accumulation of intracellular keratin within keratin filaments and keratohyaline granules, and intracellular and extracellular membrane-coated granules (also known as the *stratum granulosum*). Above the granular layer there is a keratinized layer of flattened cells packed with keratin (also known as the *stratum corneum*). In some instances, the cells of the keratinized layer have no discernible nuclei (orthokeratinized), whereas in others, dense nuclei are visible (parakeratinized). The superficial cells of this keratinized layer will continuously slough off into the oral cavity to be replaced by cells migrating from the deeper layers.

Within the oral gingival epithelium, there are several other cells not derived from keratinocytes. These include melanocytes that transfer melanin pigment granules to the surrounding basal layer of keratinocytes, Langerhans cells that are part of the reticuloendothelium system and

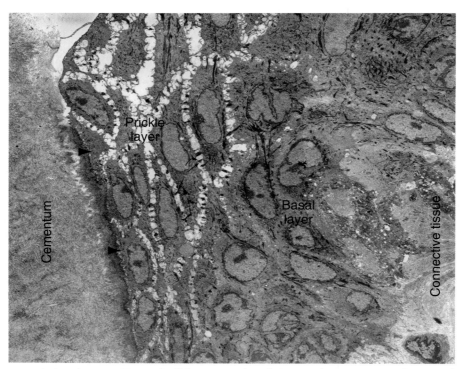

Figure 1-17. Low-power transmission electron micrograph of the junctional epithelium in the rice rat. As in humans, this junctional epithelium consist of solely two layers: a basal layer and a prickle (spinous) layer. In this view, the most superficial layer of the prickle layer is seen to attach to the root cementum (*arrowheads*), which has been decalcified in the preparation of this section. In humans, this attachment level can be on enamel alone, the junction of enamel and root cementum or root dentin, or on the root cementum or dentin alone. The basal layer has numerous desmosomes between the individual cells, making intercellular spaces very narrow and almost indistinguishable. Conversely, the cells of the prickle layer have fewer desmosomal attachments (*small arrows*) and wider, more visible intercellular spaces.

are responsible for processing and presenting foreign antigens to the immune system, and Merkel cells that may be responsible for perception of sensation in the gingiva.

The crevicular epithelium is generally nonkeratinized, although some parakeratinized cells may be seen in the most coronal region. As with the oral gingival epithelium, the crevicular epithelium has a basal layer and a prickle layer; however, a distinct granular layer and keratinized layer are not present (see Fig. 1-3). Rather the most superficial layers of the crevicular epithelium have some keratin filaments and an intact flattened nucleus. Several investigators have proposed the idea that in the complete absence of bacterial plaque and inflammation, the crevicular epithelium may become more orthokeratinized with a distinct stratum basale and granulosum layer. Conversely, in the presence of significant inflammation, this layer of crevicular epithelium can become quite thin to the extent that breaks may form in the epithelium to allow substances in the gingival crevice to penetrate into the underlying connective tissue.

The junctional epithelium consists of only two layers: a basal layer and a prickle layer. The prickle layer of the junctional epithelium is oriented parallel to the tooth surface (see Figs. 1-3 and 1-17). The prickle layer attaches to the tooth surface through hemidesmosomes (see Fig. 1-11) and through adhesion proteins such as laminin. Within this prickle layer, inflammatory cells from the granulocyte or mononuclear blood cell lines can be observed migrating from the underlying connective tissue and into the gingival crevice. In the natural course of inflammatory changes in the periodontium there is a marked increase in the numbers of these inflammatory cells within the junctional epithelium. The presence of inflammatory cells in the prickle layer of the junctional epithelium disrupts desmosomal attachments between keratinocytes and creates even larger intercellular spaces. Because the coronal aspect of this layer is exposed to the gingival crevice with the typically larger intercellular spaces exposed to the crevicular environment, this area may be a critical entry for bacteria and bacterial products into the deeper connective tissues.

IMPLICATIONS FOR PERIODONTAL REGENERATION

By presenting the microstructure of the periodontium through the story of the development of the periodontium, it is hoped that the reader not only has gained an appreciation of the origins of the different terminologies for the various periodontal tissues, but can also gain an understanding for the rationale for several approaches in periodontal therapy. In the concluding section of this chapter, several examples of periodontal regeneration treatment approaches are discussed that draw on this understanding of periodontal development.

To begin, there are several types of periodontal surgical procedures during which the epithelial attachment of the gingiva is severed and the gingiva is reflected away from the tooth to give the operator a better view of the underlying tissues. At the end of the procedure, the gingiva is repositioned on the tooth with sutures. In the postsurgical healing process, the gingiva reforms its epithelial attachment on the tooth surface. This reformation of the epithelial attachment after flap surgery involves processes similar to the formation of the gingival crevice and epithelial attachment during development. Specifically, these processes involve the formation of an attachment of the epithelium to the tooth surface, apical proliferation of the epithelium along the root surface, and splitting of the epithelium within its strata to form a crevice. In postsurgical healing, this process often leads to the formation of a "long epithelial attachment" along the root surface. This long epithelial attachment is less desirable in some procedures because it may lead to epithelial splitting and formation of a deeper crevice. In addition, this long attachment may prevent mesenchymal cells from the periodontal ligament from reaching the root surface.[17] As with the embryonic development of cementum, ligament, and alveolar bone from the mesenchymal cells of the dental follicle, these mesenchymal cells from the ligament have the potential to differentiate into cementoblasts, fibroblasts, and osteoblasts if they can reach the root surface.[18]

One approach to prevent this formation of a long epithelial attachment is to place some form of barrier between the reapposed gingival epithelial flap and the underlying bone and connective tissue.[17] This "guided tissue regeneration approach" with a membrane barrier will prevent the downgrowth of the epithelial attachment and allow cells from the periodontal ligament, remaining cementum, and bone to migrate into the wound to form new cementum, ligament, and bone.

From this example of guided tissue regeneration, it can be seen that in the proper environment or with the proper stimulus, cells derived from the dental follicle have the potential to migrate to areas of lost periodon-tium and to lay down new tissue.[19] One of these stimuli for new periodontal tissue formation may be cementum itself. Some investigators have stressed the importance of retaining as much healthy cementum as possible during surgical and nonsurgical debridement procedures to create an environment in which new cementum can form and induce new periodontal ligament attachment. In addition, several investigators have reported gains in periodontal support by coating the root surface with an enamel matrix derivative to stimulate the formation of new cementum.[20] The rationale for this approach can be understood from periodontal development. Specifically, the very first hyaline-like layer deposited on the root dentin from the inner enamel epithelium of the *Hertwig's epithelial root sheath* contains enamel matrix proteins. This enamel matrix derivative coating, applied to the roots during periodontal surgery, may induce the surrounding cells to reenact the developmental process of periodontal attachment formation.

In the future, it is possible that clinicians will use other forms of tissue engineering to regenerate lost portions of the periodontium based on these concepts of periodontal development. For example, several investigators are developing tissue engineering approaches whereby cells from a patient's periodontal ligament are harvested and cultured in the laboratory to form monolayers of less differentiated cells with characteristics of dental follicle stem cells, and then are reimplanted into areas of periodontal loss. These types of therapeutic approaches based on the development, anatomy, and microanatomy of the periodontium have considerable potential.

REFERENCES

1. Ainamo J, Loe H: Anatomical characteristics of gingiva. A clinical and microscopic study of the free and attached gingival, *J Periodontol* 37:5-13, 1966.
2. Itoiz ME, Carranza FA: The gingiva. In Newman MG, Takei HM, Carranza FA, editors: *Carranza's clinical periodontology*, ed 9, Philadelphia, 2002, WB Saunders (pp 16-35).
3. Carranza FA, Bernard GW: The tooth-supporting structures. In Newman MG, Takei HM, Carranza FA, editors: *Carranza's clinical periodontology*, ed 9, Philadelphia, 2002, WB Saunders (pp 36-57).
4. Rateitschak KH, Rateitschak EM, Wolf HF, Hassell TM: *Color atlas of dental medicine/periodontology*, ed 2, New York, 1994, Thieme Medical Publishers.
5. Cho MI, Garant PR: Development and general structure of the periodontium, *Periodontol 2000* 24:9-27, 2000.
6. Berkovitz BKB, Holland GR, Moxham BJ: *Color atlas and textbook of oral anatomy histology and embryology*, ed 2, St. Louis, 1992, Mosby Year-Book.
7. Ten Cate AR: *Oral histology, development, structure and function*, ed 5, St. Louis, 1998, Mosby.

8. Listgarten MA: A light and electron microscopic study of coronal cementogenesis, *Arch Oral Biol* 13:93-114, 1968.

9. Diekwisch TG: The developmental biology of cementum, *Int J Dev Biol* 45:695-706, 2001.

10. Bosshardt DD, Schroeder HE: Establishment of acellular extrinsic fiber cementum on human teeth. A light- and electron-microscopic study, *Cell Tissue Res* 263:325-336, 1991.

11. Saygin NE, Giannobile WV, Somerman MJ: Molecular and cell biology of cementum, *Periodontol 2000* 24:73-98, 2000.

12. Schroeder HE, Scherle WF: Cemento-enamel junction revisited, *J Periodont Res* 23:53-59, 1988.

13. Van der Velden U: Effect of age on the periodontium, *J Clin Periodontol* 11:281-294, 1984.

14. Soni NN: A microradiographic and polarized light study of cementum in Paget's disease, *J Oral Med* 24:27-30, 1969.

15. Sodek J, McKee MD: Molecular and cellular biology of alveolar bone, *Periodontol 2000* 24:99-126, 2000.

16. Kaplan RG: Supracrestal fiberotomy, *J Am Dent Assoc* 95:1127-1132, 1977.

17. Karring T, Nyman S, Gottlow J, Laurell L: Development of the biological concept of guided tissue regeneration—animal and human studies, *Periodontol 2000* 1:26-35, 1993.

18. Lekic PC, Rajshankar D, Chen H et al: Transplantation of labeled periodontal ligament cells promotes regeneration of alveolar bone, *Anat Rec* 262:193-202, 2001.

19. Bartold PM, McCulloch CA, Narayanan AS, Pitaru S: Tissue engineering: a new paradigm for periodontal regeneration based on molecular and cell biology, *Periodontol 2000* 24:253-269, 2000.

20. Hakki SS, Berry JE, Somerman MJ: The effect of enamel matrix protein derivative on follicle cells in vitro, *J Periodontol* 72:679-687, 2001.

2 Diagnosis and Classification of Periodontal Diseases

Gary C. Armitage

COMPONENTS OF A PERIODONTAL DIAGNOSIS

One of the first steps in the management of a patient with periodontal disease is to take thorough medical and dental histories and to perform a complete oral/periodontal examination. On the basis of the information collected, a diagnosis (Greek: *dia* "through," *gnosis* "knowledge") can be made. Plaque-induced periodontal diseases can be divided into two general diagnostic categories—*gingivitis* or *periodontitis*—based on the presence or absence of attachment loss. Gingivitis is the presence of gingival inflammation without loss of connective tissue attachment.[1] Periodontitis is the presence of gingival inflammation at sites where there has been apical migration of the junctional epithelium onto the root surface with the concomitant loss of connective tissue and alveolar bone.[1] In making a periodontal diagnosis, a clinician must answer three simple questions:

1. What disease (if any) is present?
2. Where is the disease (e.g., localized vs. generalized)? In answering this question, an assessment of the extent of the disease is made.
3. How severe is the disease (e.g., slight, moderate, severe)?

Although these questions are simple, they are sometimes difficult to answer. To decide on a diagnosis one must use previous clinical experiences and apply current concepts of the etiology and pathogenesis of periodontal diseases. A diagnosis is in reality the clinician's educated guess as to what disease or condition the patient has (see Chapter 11). All experienced clinicians have, at one time or another, been wrong in their initial assignment of a diagnosis. Therefore, it is good practice to develop what is known as a *differential diagnosis*, which lists the possible diagnoses from most likely to least likely. Even in cases in which there is considerable certainty about the initial diagnostic impression, it is always a good idea to acknowledge that other possibilities exist.

The separation of plaque-induced periodontal diseases into two categories (i.e., gingivitis and periodontitis) is not as simple as it might seem at first. For example, if sites with periodontitis have been successfully treated they can be assigned a post-treatment diagnosis of "periodontal health on a reduced periodontium." A reduced periodontium is one in which there has been loss of attachment that is usually induced by periodontitis. Much of this periodontal damage is permanent, even in successfully treated cases of periodontitis. If such sites develop gingival inflammation at a later date, do those sites now have recurrent periodontitis or gingivitis superimposed on a reduced but stable periodontium? Unfortunately, there is no answer to this question. However, it has been clearly established that only a small percentage of sites with gingivitis actually progress to periodontitis.[2] Therefore, it can

be assumed that gingivitis can occur on a reduced periodontium in which additional attachment loss is not occurring. Because it is not possible to determine if attachment loss is occurring from the findings of a single examination, most clinicians err on the side of caution and assign the diagnosis of "periodontitis" to inflamed sites that have experienced loss of attachment and bone in the past. This is particularly the case if there are periodontal pockets at the inflamed sites.

The *extent* of a periodontal disease is a general description of its location or distribution throughout the mouth. There is no fixed rule regarding when a periodontal disease is designated as localized or generalized. However, it has been recommended that distribution of the disease be designated as: localized if less than 30% of the sites are involved, and generalized if more than 30% of the sites are affected.[3] There is a practical rationale behind this recommendation because if the disease is characterized as "localized," then in correspondence to colleagues (such as a referring dentist) it is necessary to itemize all of the sites where the disease is present. This can simply be done in cases of localized aggressive periodontitis (LAP) for which the disease is frequently localized to the permanent first molars and incisors; it is not excessively time-consuming to list the affected teeth. However, in cases of generalized aggressive periodontitis (GAP) in which most teeth in all sextants might be affected, it becomes impractical to list them all in a letter to a colleague. This is especially true because a copy of the periodontal chart showing the precise location of affected sites is usually attached to any correspondence with colleagues. It should be emphasized that the 30% cutoff point between localized and generalized categories is arbitrary, because in cases of LAP, if all permanent first molars and incisors are affected, then approximately 43% (12 of 28 teeth excluding third molars) would be involved. Clearly, strict adherence to the "30% rule" would lead one to the ambiguous conclusion that LAP is a generalized disease.

The *severity* of a periodontal disease is usually characterized as slight, moderate, or severe. Sometimes the terms *initial* or *mild* are used instead of *slight*, and *advanced* is used interchangeably with *severe*. It does not make a difference what terms are used to designate the severity of involvement as long as they are understood by clinicians who may be treating the patient and have access to your records. In cases of periodontitis, it has been recommended that severity be characterized on the basis of the amount of clinical attachment loss (CAL) as follows: slight = 1 or 2 mm of CAL, moderate = 3 to 4 mm of CAL, and severe = 5 mm or more of CAL.[3] CAL is measured with a periodontal probe and is the distance from the cementoenamel junction to the base of the probeable crevice. The rationale behind this recommendation is that 5 mm of CAL means that more than 40%

of the periodontal attachment at that site has been lost (assuming an average root length of 12 mm). In cases of gingivitis the terms slight, moderate, and severe are sometimes used to indicate the intensity of the clinical inflammation (mild vs. intense). Again what is important is minimal or no ambiguity in the terms used so that other clinicians will understand what is written.

When entering the periodontal diagnosis in a patient's chart or in written correspondence, one usually writes the extent followed by severity and then the name of the disease (Box 2-1). There are, of course, many other possible periodontal diagnoses (Box 2-2). In most instances it is useful for purposes of clarity to specify the disease name, its extent, and its severity.

VALUE OF ESTABLISHING A DIAGNOSIS

Deciding on a diagnosis has several practical purposes: (1) it sets the stage or context for treatment planning, (2) it helps in estimating outcomes (prognosis), (3) it facilitates

Box 2-1	Examples of Typical Diagnoses for Plaque-Induced Periodontal Diseases	
Extent	**Severity**	**Disease**
Localized	Slight	Gingivitis
Localized	Moderate	Gingivitis
Localized	Severe	Gingivitis
Generalized	Slight	Gingivitis
Generalized	Moderate	Gingivitis
Generalized	Severe	Gingivitis
Localized	Slight	Aggressive periodontitis
Localized	Moderate	Aggressive periodontitis
Localized	Severe	Aggressive periodontitis
Generalized	Slight	Aggressive periodontitis
Generalized	Moderate	Aggressive periodontitis
Generalized	Severe	Aggressive periodontitis
Localized	Slight	Chronic periodontitis
Localized	Moderate	Chronic periodontitis
Localized	Severe	Chronic periodontitis
Generalized	Slight	Chronic periodontitis
Generalized	Moderate	Chronic periodontitis
Generalized	Severe	Chronic periodontitis

communication with colleagues and patients, and (4) it reassures investigators in a research setting that they are studying the same disease rather than multiple diseases under one umbrella. In addition, some third-party (insurance) plans link the level of reimbursement to the diagnosis.

The label that one puts on a disease conjures up the entire reservoir of a clinician's knowledge and past experience with that particular form of disease. Numerous important questions begin to be answered when careful thought is given to making a diagnosis. In different cases in which the same diagnosis was assigned, did the disease respond to treatment as expected? What was done last time that worked? What didn't work? How much time did treatment take? Was there a problem with patient compliance? For example, if one assigns a diagnosis of generalized moderate chronic periodontitis, most clinicians would expect that the disease will respond well to oral hygiene instructions and thorough scaling and root planing, followed by a program of periodic periodontal maintenance care. In addition, a good long-term prognosis for the affected teeth would be anticipated. Conversely, in many cases of generalized severe chronic periodontitis a more complicated and costly course of therapy might be anticipated. There is an increased likelihood that periodontal surgery might be needed. A less favorable prognosis for some of the severely affected teeth might be predicted. These scenarios are, of course, oversimplified because many factors impact treatment outcomes. Nevertheless, a wide spectrum of anticipated events in the management of periodontal disease all start with a carefully developed and well thought-out diagnosis. (A detailed discussion of formulating a diagnosis and prognosis appears in Chapter 11.)

CLASSIFICATION SYSTEMS

In the last 130 years, many classification systems for periodontal diseases have been used.[4] Over time, classification systems have been changed to reflect new knowledge about the nature of periodontal infections. In 1989, a classification system was developed that included five types of periodontitis: **(i) adult periodontitis, (ii) early onset periodontitis, (iii) periodontitis associated with systemic disease, (iv) necrotizing ulcerative periodontitis, and (v) refractory periodontitis.**[5] Even though this system had some serious flaws, it was widely accepted and is still occasionally used by some authors. The main problems with this classification were: (1) considerable overlap in disease categories, (2) absence of a gingival disease component, (3) inappropriate emphasis on age of onset of disease and rates of progression, and (4) inadequate or unclear classification criteria.[3] The currently accepted classification system (see Box 2-2), developed in 1999, attempts to correct some of the deficiencies of the 1989 classification. It is based on an infection/host response paradigm

| Box 2-2 | Classification of Periodontal Diseases and Conditions (1999 International Workshop for a Classification of Periodontal Diseases and Conditions) |

I. Gingival Diseases

A. Dental Plaque-Induced Gingival Diseases*

1. Gingivitis associated with dental plaque only
   a. without other local contributing factors
   b. with local contributing factors (see section VIII, part A)
2. Gingival diseases modified by systemic factors
   a. associated with the endocrine system
      1) puberty-associated gingivitis
      2) menstrual cycle–associated gingivitis
      3) pregnancy-associated
         a) gingivitis
         b) pyogenic granuloma
      4) diabetes mellitus–associated gingivitis
   b. associated with blood dyscrasias
      1) leukemia-associated gingivitis
      2) other
3. Gingival diseases modified by medications
   a. drug-influenced gingival diseases
      1) drug-influenced gingival enlargements
      2) drug-influenced gingivitis
         a) oral contraceptive–associated gingivitis
         b) other
4. Gingival diseases modified by malnutrition
   a. ascorbic acid–deficiency gingivitis
   b. other

B. Nonplaque-Induced Gingival Lesions

1. Gingival diseases of specific bacterial origin
   a. *Neisseria gonorrhea*–associated lesions
   b. *Treponema pallidum*–associated lesions
   c. *Streptococcal* species–associated lesions
   d. other
2. Gingival diseases of viral origin
   a. herpes virus infections
      1) primary herpetic gingivostomatitis
      2) recurrent oral herpes
      3) varicella zoster infections
   b. other
3. Gingival diseases of fungal origin
   a. *Candida* species infections
      1) generalized gingival candidiasis
   b. linear gingival erythema
   c. histoplasmosis
   d. other
4. Gingival lesions of genetic origin
   a. hereditary gingival fibromatosis
   b. other
5. Gingival manifestations of systemic conditions
   a. mucocutaneous disorders
      1) lichen planus
      2) pemphigoid
      3) pemphigus vulgaris
      4) erythema multiforme

Box 2-2   **Classification of Periodontal Diseases and Conditions (1999 International Workshop for a Classification of Periodontal Diseases and Conditions)—cont'd**

       5) lupus erythematosus
       6) drug induced
       7) other
     b. allergic reactions
       1) dental restorative materials
         a) mercury
         b) nickel
         c) acrylic
         d) other
       2) reactions attributable to
         a) toothpastes/dentifrices
         b) mouthrinses/mouthwashes
         c) chewing gum additives
         d) foods and additives
       3) other
   6. Traumatic lesions (factitious, iatrogenic, accidental)
     a. chemical injury
     b. physical injury
     c. thermal injury
   7. Foreign body reactions
   8. Not otherwise specified

II. Chronic Periodontitis†

  A. Localized
  B. Generalized

III. Aggressive Periodontitis†

  A. Localized
  B. Generalized

IV. Periodontitis as a Manifestation of Systemic Diseases

  A. Associated with hematologic disorders
    1. Acquired neutropenia
    2. Leukemias
    3. Other
  B. Associated with genetic disorders
    1. Familial and cyclic neutropenia
    2. Down syndrome
    3. Leukocyte adhesion deficiency syndromes
    4. Papillon-Lefèvre syndrome
    5. Chediak-Higashi syndrome
    6. Histiocytosis syndromes
    7. Glycogen storage disease
    8. Infantile genetic agranulocytosis
    9. Cohen syndrome
    10. Ehlers-Danlos syndrome (types IV and VIII AD)
    11. Hypophosphatasia
    12. Other
  C. Not otherwise specified (NOS)

V. Necrotizing Periodontal Diseases

  A. Necrotizing ulcerative gingivitis (NUG)
  B. Necrotizing ulcerative periodontitis (NUP)

Continued

Box 2-2   **Classification of Periodontal Diseases and Conditions (1999 International Workshop for a Classification of Periodontal Diseases and Conditions)—cont'd**

VI. Abscesses of the Periodontium

A. Gingival abscess
B. Periodontal abscess
C. Pericoronal abscess

VII. Periodontitis Associated With Endodontic Lesions

A. Combined periodontal-endodontic lesions

VIII. Developmental or Acquired Deformities and Conditions

A. Localized tooth-related factors that modify or predispose to plaque-induced gingival diseases/periodontitis
   1. tooth anatomic factors
   2. dental restorations/appliances
   3. root fractures
   4. cervical root resorption and cemental tears

B. Mucogingival deformities and conditions around teeth

   1. gingival/soft tissue recession
      a. facial or lingual surfaces
      b. interproximal (papillary)
   2. lack of keratinized gingiva
   3. decreased vestibular depth
   4. aberrant frenum/muscle position
   5. gingival excess
      a. pseudopocket
      b. inconsistent gingival margin
      c. excessive gingival display
      d. gingival enlargement (see section I, parts A.3 and B.4)
   6. abnormal color

C. Mucogingival deformities and conditions on edentulous ridges

   1. vertical and/or horizontal ridge deficiency
   2. lack of gingiva/keratinized tissue
   3. gingival/soft tissue enlargement
   4. aberrant frenum/muscle position
   5. decreased vestibular depth
   6. abnormal color

D. Occlusal trauma

   1. primary occlusal trauma
   2. secondary occlusal trauma

Can occur on a periodontium with no attachment loss or on a periodontium with attachment loss that is not progressing.
†*Can be further classified on the basis of extent and severity. As a general guide, extent can be characterized as localized (<30% of sites involved) or generalized (≥30% of sites involved). Severity can be characterized on the basis of the amount of clinical attachment loss (CAL) as follows: slight = 1 to 2 mm of CAL, moderate = 3 to 4 mm of CAL, and severe ≥5 mm of CAL.*
Modified from Armitage GC: Development of a classification system for periodontal diseases and conditions, Ann Periodontol 4:1-6, 1999.

that follows the concept that plaque-induced periodontal diseases are infections, and much of the destruction observed in these infections occurs as a result of host inflammatory and immunologic responses to dental plaque bacteria.[4] By far, the most common periodontal diseases listed in the current classification system are plaque-induced gingivitis and chronic periodontitis.

GINGIVAL DISEASES

Dental Plaque-Induced Gingival Diseases

Gingival diseases include several subcategories in which dental plaque plays an important etiologic role. The simplest and most common of these subcategories is plaque-induced gingivitis with no other local or systemic complicating factors. In the three other subcategories in this group—that is, plaque-induced gingival diseases modified by systemic factors, medications, or malnutrition—dental plaque still plays a central etiologic role, but the harmful effects of plaque bacteria are enhanced or modified by perturbations in host–parasite interactions.[6] Examples of this are regularly encountered in clinical practice and include pregnancy-associated gingivitis in which endogenous hormone fluctuations promote the growth of certain members of the plaque flora[7] and medication-influenced gingival enlargement.[8,9] In the presence of plaque-induced gingival inflammation certain medications can promote the development of gingival enlargement. Meticulous plaque control can often reduce,[10,11] but not completely prevent,[12] the severity of this side effect. Drugs with this side effect include certain anticonvulsants (e.g., phenytoin),[13,14] immunosuppressive agents (e.g., cyclosporin),[15] and a variety of calcium channel blockers (e.g., nefedipine, verapamil, diltiazem).[13]

Patients with diabetes mellitus under poor metabolic control tend to develop more intense plaque-induced gingival inflammation than individuals without diabetes.[6,16] The reasons for this are not entirely clear, but alterations in antibacterial host defenses such as decreased neutrophil adherence, chemotaxis, and phagocytosis have been reported.[17-19] Such patients are occasionally seen in general dental practices and the pronounced inflammatory response of the gingiva is sometimes assigned the diagnosis of "diabetes mellitus–associated gingivitis."[6] Severe malnutrition is unusual in well developed countries, and therefore the effects of nutritional deficiencies as modifiers of plaque-induced gingival inflammation are rarely encountered. The effects of slight dietary deficiencies on the periodontium have not been well studied, but it is unlikely that they have any significant impact on the course of periodontal infections. However, during early phases of experimental ascorbic acid deficiency, modest increases in gingival inflammation and bleeding on probing have been reported.[6,20]

Nonplaque-Induced Gingival Diseases

In nonplaque-induced gingival diseases dental plaque does not have an etiologic role. These diseases can present difficulties in making the correct diagnosis because the observed gingival inflammation might be caused by specific bacterial, viral, or fungal infections.[21] Specific bacteria that can infect gingival tissues and cause a form of gingivitis include medically important exogenous pathogens such as *Neisseria gonorrhea, Treponema pallidum*, as well as other nonoral species.[22] In addition, some types of gingivitis can be caused by a number of viruses with the most important being herpes simplex virus types 1 and 2[21,23,24] and the varicella zoster virus.[21,25] Papillomaviruses can also infect gingival tissues, but the growths (i.e., squamous papillomas)

do not have any of the clinical characteristics of gingivitis.[26] Although rare in otherwise healthy individuals, gingival lesions can also be caused by fungal infections such as candidosis[21] and histoplasmosis.[27] In addition, there are some gingival lesions with a genetic etiology that are not infections at all, such as hereditary gingival fibromatosis.[28]

A wide variety of gingival lesions, some resembling plaque-induced gingivitis, can occur as manifestations of systemic conditions such as mucocutaneous disorders and allergic reactions.[21] Among these mucocutaneous disorders are lichen planus,[29,30] pemphigoid,[31,32] pemphigus vulgaris,[33,34] erythema multiforme,[35] lupus erythematosus,[36] and psoriasis.[37] The diagnosis of these disorders is based on their clinical features and histopathologic characteristics of biopsy specimens. Hypersensitivity (allergic) reactions to dental restorative materials, oral care products (e.g., mouthrinses), and foods are occasionally encountered.[21] Allergic reactions to restorative materials can present a considerable diagnostic quandary because the allergen–gingiva contact frequently results in an inflammatory response that clinically looks exactly like plaque-induced gingivitis. In such cases, the gingival inflammation does not resolve when plaque control procedures are instituted. Sometimes the only way to determine if the patient is allergic to the restorative material is to remove the restoration and replace it with a different material.

CHRONIC PERIODONTITIS

Chronic periodontitis is a common plaque-induced periodontal infection that is a major cause of tooth loss throughout the world. This form of periodontitis was once called *adult periodontitis* because it was thought to be primarily found in adults.[5] However, epidemiologic data suggest that the disease can also be found in children and adolescents.[38] Chronic periodontitis has been historically considered as a slowly progressive disease and there are data to support this view.[39-41] However, there are also data indicating that some patients may experience short periods of rapid progression.[42,43] Some of the more important clinical features of the disease are listed in Box 2-3.[44]

Although chronic periodontitis can be distributed in localized and generalized patterns throughout the mouth, the two forms appear to be identical with regard to their etiology and pathogenesis. There is a general consensus that chronic periodontitis is initiated and sustained by dental plaque biofilms, but host responses to plaque bacteria are responsible for most of the tissue destruction. The extent and severity of the disease can be increased by several host-modifying factors including poorly controlled diabetes mellitus,[45] cigarette smoking,[46] and emotional stress.[46] The progression of the disease can only be confirmed by repeated examinations that show additional

Box 2-3 | **Main Clinical Features and Characteristics of Chronic Periodontitis**

Most prevalent in adults, but can occur in children and adolescents
Amount of destruction is consistent with the presence of local factors
Subgingival calculus is a frequent finding
Associated with a variable microbial pattern
Slow to moderate rate of progression, but may have periods of rapid progression
Can be associated with local predisposing factors (e.g., tooth-related or iatrogenic factors)
May be modified by or associated with systemic diseases (e.g., diabetes mellitus)
Can be modified by factors other than systemic disease such as cigarette smoking and emotional stress

From Lindhe J, Ranney R, Lamster I, et al: Consensus report: chronic periodontitis, Ann Periodontol 4:38, 1999.

connective attachment loss and resorption of alveolar bone. It is generally assumed that the risk for progression is increased if the disease is untreated.[44] Treatment for chronic periodontitis is directed against disruption, removal, and control of subgingival plaque biofilms. Reduction in probing depths is a desirable outcome of treatment because periodontal pockets are the primary habitat of bacteria that cause the disease.[1] However, pocket reduction is not an absolute requirement for successful treatment of the disease.

AGGRESSIVE PERIODONTITIS

Aggressive periodontitis is much less common than chronic periodontitis and affects a narrower range of young patients. It is generally acknowledged that it occurs in localized and generalized forms, and the two forms differ in many respects with regard to their etiology and pathogenesis.[47] LAP and GAP were once called *localized* and *generalized juvenile periodontitis*, respectively.[5] However, these terms were replaced with the LAP and GAP terminology because they do not depend on questionable age-based classification criteria.[3] There is a consensus that both forms of aggressive periodontitis share the following common features:

- Except for the presence of periodontitis, patients are otherwise clinically healthy
- Rapid attachment loss and bone destruction
- Familial aggregation[47]

Some of the more important secondary features of both forms of aggressive periodontitis are:

- Amounts of microbial deposits are inconsistent with the severity of periodontal tissue destruction
- Increased proportions of *Actinobacillus actinomycetemcomitans* and, in some populations, *Porphyromonas gingivalis* may be increased
- Phagocyte abnormalities
- Hyperresponsive macrophage phenotype, including increased levels of prostaglandin E_2 and interleukin-1β
- Progression of attachment loss and bone loss may be self-arresting[47]

All of these characteristics do not need to be present to make a diagnosis that is usually based on clinical, radiographic, and historical information.[47]

As in the case of chronic periodontitis, both forms of aggressive periodontitis are plaque-induced infections, and host responses to plaque bacteria are responsible for most of the tissue destruction. The plaque biofilms are, however, often clinically thinner than with chronic periodontitis. This is particularly true in cases of LAP. Host-modifying factors that increase the extent and severity of chronic periodontitis can also adversely affect the clinical course of both forms of aggressive periodontitis.[45-47] Treatment for aggressive periodontitis is directed toward controlling subgingival biofilms. In many cases, successful treatment requires mechanical disruption of the biofilms supplemented with systemic antibiotics.[48]

On the basis of several specific clinical and host-response differences between LAP and GAP, it is clear that LAP is not merely a localized form of GAP. Features that are said to be specific for each of these forms of aggressive periodontitis are shown in Box 2-4. Importantly, LAP generally has a circumpubertal onset or is first detected and diagnosed during puberty, whereas GAP is usually detected and diagnosed in patients younger than 30 years; however, some patients with GAP may be older than 30 years. It has been suggested that patients with LAP usually mount a robust serum antibody response to periodontal pathogens, whereas patients with GAP exhibit a poor antibody response to the infecting agents.[47] (A detailed discussion of host responses in periodontal diseases can be found in Chapter 5.)

PERIODONTITIS AS A MANIFESTATION OF SYSTEMIC DISEASES

There are two general categories of systemic diseases that have periodontitis as a frequent manifestation: (1) certain hematologic disorders (e.g., acquired neutropenia, leukemia) and (2) some genetic diseases (e.g., familial/cyclic neutropenia, Down syndrome, leukocyte adhesion deficiency syndromes, Papillon-Lefèvre syndrome).[49] In

Box 2-4	Specific Features of Localized and Generalized Aggressive Periodontitis

Localized Aggressive Periodontitis

Circumpubertal onset
Robust serum antibody to infecting agents
Localized first molar/incisor presentation with interproximal attachment loss on at least two permanent teeth, one of which is a first molar, and involving no more than two teeth other than first molars and incisors

Generalized Aggressive Periodontitis

Usually affecting individuals younger than 30 years, but patients may be older
Poor serum antibody response to infecting agents
Pronounced episodic nature of the destruction of attachment and alveolar bone
Generalized interproximal attachment loss affecting at least three permanent teeth other than first molars and incisors

From Lang N, Bartold PM, Cullinan M, et al: Consensus report: aggressive periodontitis, Ann Periodontol 4:53, 1999.

most of these systemic diseases there is either a significant impairment in the ability of neutrophils to fight infections or a severe reduction in the number of functional neutrophils. Dental plaque biofilms are etiologically important in this group of periodontal infections. However, the severely decreased host resistance associated with the systemic disease is a major determinant in the development of the observed periodontitis, and therefore the periodontal condition is usually referred to as a manifestation of the systemic disease. In such cases, the systemic disease is such a dominant modifier of the periodontal infection that the infection is considered a secondary feature of the systemic disease.

There are no established criteria governing when a host-modifying factor, such as a systemic disease, is so important in the development of periodontitis that it should be a principal part of the disease classification.[4] Indeed, sometimes it is difficult to make this decision. For example, although the presence of poorly controlled diabetes mellitus can modify or alter the clinical course and expression of periodontitis, most authorities believe that there are insufficient data to conclude that "diabetic periodontitis" is a valid term.[3] The current view is that diabetes under poor metabolic control is simply an important modifier of all forms of periodontitis. In other words, chronic periodontitis in a patient with poorly controlled diabetes might be more severe than in an individual without diabetes, but both patients still have chronic periodontitis.

There are some rare genetic disorders (e.g., hypophosphatasia,[50] Ehlers-Danlos syndrome[51]) of connective tissue and bone metabolism in which periodontitis-like bone loss occurs around the teeth. In these disorders plaque is of minimal etiologic importance in the observed bone loss. Finally, plaque does not play an important etiologic role in the periodontal bone loss frequently found in Langerhans cell disease (idiopathic histiocytosis) in which there is an uncontrolled proliferation of Langerhans cells.[52] The clinical appearance of periodontal lesions of Langerhans cell disease often mimics plaque-induced periodontitis and can present the clinician with a difficult diagnostic challenge.[53]

NECROTIZING PERIODONTAL DISEASES

Necrotizing periodontal infections include necrotizing ulcerative gingivitis (NUG)[54] and necrotizing ulcerative periodontitis (NUP),[55] which share many of the same clinical characteristics. In both conditions there is a rapid onset of pain associated with the development of necrotic and ulcerative lesions of the marginal gingiva, particularly involving interproximal sites. In addition, they both appear to share certain predisposing factors that lead to diminished systemic resistance to bacterial infection of periodontal tissues.[56] There is some uncertainty about the relation between NUG and NUP. It is possible that they are fundamentally different diseases. Alternatively, they could be two stages of a single disease process. Until this issue is resolved they have been grouped under the single disease category of "necrotizing periodontal diseases."[3]

Necrotizing Ulcerative Gingivitis

NUG is an acute periodontal infection that has been described since ancient times.[54] Over the years many terms have been used for this clinically distinct periodontal infection (e.g., "trench mouth," Vincent's infection, Gilmer's disease, Vincent-Plaut disease, Vincent's ulceromembranous gingivostomatitis, fusospirochetal stomatitis). The diagnosis of NUG is made on the basis of findings from the clinical examination and history. The two most significant criteria used for the diagnosis of NUG are: (1) the presence of interproximal necrosis and ulceration, and (2) a history of rapid onset of gingival soreness and pain. The interproximal necrosis and ulceration take the form of eroded crater-like depressions of one or more interproximal gingival papillae, sometimes referred to as having a "punched-out" appearance.[57]

Marked halitosis is present in most patients with NUG. Numerous other signs and symptoms have been associated with the disease, but they are not present in every case. Some patients have a pseudomembrane covering the ulcerated areas of the gingiva. It is a heterogeneous film composed of fibrin, bacteria, sloughed epithelial cells, and other debris. It can be easily wiped off or removed by the frictional forces of eating and is, therefore, frequently absent. Also occasionally associated with NUG are lymphadenopathy, increased salivation, fever, malaise, and anorexia.[57] The diagnosis is usually easy to make from the clinical presentation of the disease. However, cicatricial pemphigoid involving the gingiva may sometimes clinically resemble NUG.[58]

Factors that have been implicated as predisposing factors for NUG in adult patients from North America and Europe include: (1) emotional stress, (2) heavy cigarette smoking, (3) lack of sleep, (4) poor dietary habits, and (5) immunosuppression.[54,57] In children from underdeveloped countries, NUG appears to be associated with malnutrition or the debilitating and immunosuppressive effects of viral or parasitic infections.[57,59] The common feature of all of the predisposing factors for NUG is that they decrease host resistance to periodontal infections. Indeed, in severely immunosuppressed children, NUG is believed to be the first stage of noma or cancrum oris, a severe necrotic infection that causes massive destruction of the tissues of the oral cavity and face.[60-62]

Necrotizing Ulcerative Periodontitis

The principal clinical difference between NUG and NUP is that the latter disease always involves considerable loss of periodontal attachment and alveolar bone.[55] In most cases of NUG loss of clinical attachment is not generally found; however, some attachment loss can probably occur in untreated NUG or with recurrent attacks of the disease.[63]

The term *necrotizing ulcerative periodontitis* did not appear in classification systems for periodontal diseases until the late 1980s at the peak of the AIDS epidemic.[5] It was added to classification systems primarily because of the increasing appearance of a rapidly destructive and intensely painful form of periodontitis in HIV-infected patients. In some patients with NUP there is exposure and sequestration of alveolar bone. In addition to HIV infection, severe immunosuppression from other sources such cancer chemotherapy[1] and advanced protein-energy malnutrition[64] can lead to the development of NUP. It could be argued that NUP should be classified as a periodontal manifestation of those specific systemic diseases that decrease host resistance and allow NUP to develop. However, only a relatively small subset of HIV-infected patients or those with protein-energy malnutrition actually experience NUP development. Until more is known about how severe immunosuppression leads to NUP, this periodontal disease is grouped with NUG because they share so many clinical characteristics.

ABSCESSES OF THE PERIODONTIUM

An abscess is a circumscribed collection of pus (i.e., purulent exudate). Bacteria in subgingival dental plaque biofilms attract enormous quantities of neutrophils from the highly vascularized and inflamed soft tissue side of a periodontal pocket. Most of the time the neutrophil-laden inflammatory exudate slowly oozes unnoticed into the oral cavity through the pocket orifice. However, when this drainage is blocked or impeded, the exudate collects in the soft tissue wall of the pocket and forms a periodontal abscess. A tooth with a periodontal abscess may exhibit one or more of the following: gingival swelling, a draining fistula, pain on percussion, and increased mobility. Occasionally, the abscess is asymptomatic. Some of the common situations that predispose to abscess formation are: (1) deep periodontal pockets,[65-67] (2) incomplete removal of subgingival calculus during scaling and root planing,[65-68] (3) occlusion of the pocket orifice by foreign bodies,[66,69,70] and (4) administration of antibiotics to patients with periodontitis in the absence of mechanical therapy.[71]

Abscesses of the periodontium are classified primarily on the basis of their location. *Gingival abscesses* are those localized to the marginal gingiva and interdental papilla. *Periodontal abscesses* are those localized within the tissues adjacent to the periodontal pocket that may lead to nearby portions of the periodontal ligament and alveolar bone. Of the three types of abscesses of the periodontium, periodontal abscesses are the ones most frequently encountered in clinical practice. *Pericoronal abscesses* develop within tissue surrounding the crown of a partially erupted tooth.[72]

Uncomplicated periodontal abscesses are usually, but not always, easy to diagnose. In some instances, painful gingival swellings with signs and symptoms identical to those of a periodontal abscess may be of endodontic origin.[73] In rare cases, malignancies[74,75] and periodontal lesions of Langerhans cell disease[76] have been mistaken for periodontal abscesses.

PERIODONTITIS ASSOCIATED WITH ENDODONTIC LESIONS

Infections of periapical tissues caused by pulpal death (i.e., endodontic lesions) can often locally join with separate infections emanating from periodontal pockets. This coalescence of endodontic and periodontal infections has been termed *combined periodontal-endodontic lesions.*[73,77] In some cases, an existing periapical (endodontic) infection spreads into a periodontal pocket, whereas in other situations, infection from the periodontal pocket spreads to the apex of the tooth and joins a periapical lesion. (A detailed discussion of the relation between periodontal and endodontic lesions appears in Chapter 30.)

DEVELOPMENTAL OR ACQUIRED DEFORMITIES AND CONDITIONS

There are many developmental or acquired deformities and conditions of periodontal tissues that technically are not diseases. They are included in most classifications of periodontal diseases because they may be important modifiers of susceptibility to periodontal infections or can dramatically influence treatment outcomes.[3] Some are included because dentists are routinely called on to treat many of these conditions.

Localized Tooth-Related Factors That Modify or Predispose to Plaque-Induced Periodontal Diseases

Tooth-related factors that can be associated with an increased risk for development of plaque-induced periodontal diseases include cervical enamel projections, enamel pearls, furcation anatomy, tooth position, root proximity, and anomalous grooves in roots. In addition, defects in dental restorations such as poor contours and marginal discrepancies can increase the risk of periodontal infections.[78] (A detailed discussion of this topic appears in Chapter 7.)

Mucogingival Deformities and Conditions Around Teeth

Mucogingival deformities refer to a group of congenital, developmental, or acquired defects in the normal relation between keratinized gingival tissues and nonkeratinized alveolar mucosa.[79] (A detailed description of these deformities and their treatment appears in Chapter 21.)

Mucogingival Deformities and Conditions on Edentulous Ridges

Mucogingival problems associated with edentulous ridges are similar to those associated with teeth. (A detailed discussion of this topic appears in Chapter 21.)

Occlusal Trauma

Damage to periodontal tissues can occur during a variety of conditions involving occlusal loads and forces that exceed the capacity of the periodontium to withstand them.[80] (A detailed discussion of this topic appears in Chapter 29.)

FUTURE REVISIONS TO PERIODONTAL DISEASE CLASSIFICATIONS

All classification systems should be considered as works in progress. There has never been a perfect and permanent disease classification in *any* medical or dental disci-

pline, and there probably never will be. Classification systems are merely tools to study the etiology, pathogenesis, and treatment of diseases in an orderly fashion. In addition, such systems provide clinicians a way to organize their approach to the health care needs of patients.[3] The classification system presented in this chapter was developed in 1999 and has been widely accepted by the international community. However, it is certain that as more is learned about the nature of periodontal diseases evidence-based revisions will be necessary.

REFERENCES

1. Armitage GC: Clinical evaluation of periodontal diseases, *Periodontol 2000* 7:39-53, 1995.
2. Armitage GC: Periodontal diseases: diagnosis, *Ann Periodontol* 1:37-215, 1996.
3. Armitage GC: Development of a classification system for periodontal diseases and conditions, *Ann Periodontol* 4:1-6, 1999.
4. Armitage GC: Classifying periodontal diseases—A longstanding dilemma, *Periodontol 2000* 30:9-23, 2002.
5. American Academy of Periodontology: Consensus report. Discussion section I, *Proceedings of the World Workshop in Clinical Periodontics*. Chicago, 1989, American Academy of Periodontology, pp I-23-I-32.
6. Mariotti A: Dental plaque-induced gingival diseases, *Ann Periodontol* 4:7-17, 1999.
7. Amar S, Chung KM: Influence of hormonal variation on the periodontium in women, *Periodontol 2000* 6:79-87, 1994.
8. Seymour RA, Thomason JM, Ellis JS: The pathogenesis of drug-induced gingival overgrowth, *J Clin Periodontol* 23:165-175, 1996.
9. Seymour RA, Ellis JS, Thomason JM: Risk factors for drug-induced gingival overgrowth, *J Clin Periodontol* 27:217-223, 2000.
10. Pihlstrom BL, Carlson JF, Smith QT, et al: Prevention of phenytoin associated gingival enlargement—A 15-month longitudinal study, *J Periodontol* 51:311-317, 1980.
11. Somacarrera ML, Hernández G, Acero J, et al: Factors related to the incidence and severity of cyclosporin-induced gingival overgrowth in transplant patients. A longitudinal study, *J Periodontol* 65:671-675, 1994.
12. Dahllöf G, Modéer T: The effect of a plaque control program on the development of phenytoin-induced gingival overgrowth. A 2-year longitudinal study, *J Clin Periodontol* 13:845-849, 1986.
13. Marshall RI, Bartold PM: Medication induced gingival overgrowth, *Oral Dis* 4:130-151, 1998.
14. Thomason J, Seymour RA, Rawlins MD: Incidence and severity of phenytoin-induced gingival overgrowth in epileptic patients in general medical practice, *Community Dent Oral Epidemiol* 20:288-291, 1992.

15. Spratt H, Boomer S, Irwin CR, et al: Cyclosporin associated gingival overgrowth in renal transplant patients, *Oral Dis* 5:27-31, 1999.

16. Ervasti T, Knuuttila M, Pohjamo L, et al: Relation between control of diabetes and gingival bleeding, *J Periodontol* 56:154-157, 1985.

17. Marhoffer W, Stein M, Maeser E, et al: Impairment of polymorphonuclear leukocyte function and metabolic control of diabetes, *Diabetes Care* 15:256-260, 1992.

18. Gallacher SJ, Thomson G, Fraser WD, et al: Neutrophil bactericidal function in diabetes mellitus: Evidence for association with blood glucose control, *Diabet Med* 12:916-920, 1995.

19. Delamaire M, Maugendre D, Moreno M, et al: Impaired leucocyte function in diabetic patients, *Diabet Med* 14:29-34, 1997.

20. Leggott PJ, Robertson PB, Rothman DL, et al: The effect of controlled ascorbic acid depletion and supplementation on periodontal health, *J Periodontol* 57:480-485, 1986.

21. Holmstrup P: Non-plaque-induced gingival lesions, *Ann Periodontol* 4:20-29, 1999.

22. Siegel MA: Syphilis and gonorrhea, *Dent Clin N Am* 40:369-383, 1996.

23. Miller CS, Redding SW: Diagnosis and management of orofacial herpes simplex virus infections, *Dent Clin N Am* 36:879-895, 1992.

24. Scully C, Epstein JB, Porter SR, et al: Viruses and chronic diseases of the oral mucosa, *Oral Surg Oral Med Oral Pathol* 72:537-544, 1991.

25. Straus SE, Ostrove JM, Inchauspé G, et al: Varicella-zoster infections. Biology, natural history, treatment, and prevention, *Ann Intern Med* 108:221-237, 1988.

26. Jimenez C, Correnti M, Salma N, et al: Detection of human papillomavirus DNA in benign oral squamous epithelial lesions in Venezuela, *J Oral Pathol Med* 30:385-388, 2001.

27. Loh FC, Yeo JF, Tan WC, et al: Histoplasmosis presenting as hyperplastic gingival lesion, *J Oral Pathol Med* 18:533-536, 1989.

28. Hart TC, Zhang Y, Gorry MC, et al: A mutation in the *SOS1* gene causes hereditary gingival fibromatosis type 1, *Am J Hum Genet* 70:943-954, 2002.

29. Gorsky M, Raviv M, Moskona D, et al: Clinical characteristics and treatment of patients with oral lichen planus in Israel, *Oral Surg Oral Med Oral Pathol Oral Radiol Endod* 82:644-649, 1996.

30. Thorn JJ, Holmstrup P, Rindum J, et al: Course of various clinical forms of oral lichen planus. A prospective follow-up of 611 patients, *J Oral Pathol* 17:213-218, 1988.

31. Damoulis PD, Gagari E: Combined treatment of periodontal disease and benign mucous membrane pemphigoid. Case report with 8 years of maintenance, *J Periodontol* 71:1620-1629, 2000.

32. Kurihara M, Nishimura F, Hashimoto T, et al: Immunopathological diagnosis of cicatricial pemphigoid with desquamative gingivitis, *J Periodontol* 72:243-249, 2001.

33. Barnett ML: Pemphigus vulgaris presenting as a gingival lesion. A case report, *J Periodontol* 59:611-614, 1988.

34. Mignogna MD, Lo Muzio L, Bucci E: Clinical features of gingival pemphigus vulgaris, *J Clin Periodontol* 28:489-493, 2001.

35. Farthing PM, Maragou P, Coates M, et al: Characteristics of the oral lesions in patients with cutaneous recurrent erythema multiforme, *J Oral Pathol Med* 24:9-13, 1995.

36. Schiødt M: Oral manifestations of lupus erythematosus, *Int J Oral Surg* 13:101-147, 1984.

37. Yamada J, Amar S, Pertungaro P: Psoriasis-associated periodontitis: A case report, *J Periodontol* 63:854-857, 1992.

38. Papapanou PN: Periodontal diseases: Epidemiology, *Ann Periodontol* 1:1-36, 1996.

39. Brown LJ, Löe H: Prevalence, extent, severity and progression of periodontal disease, *Periodontol 2000* 2:57-71, 1993.

40. Papapanou PN, Wennström JL, Gröndahl K: A 10-year retrospective study of periodontal disease progression, *J Clin Periodontol* 16:403-411, 1989.

41. Löe H, Anerud A, Boysen H, et al: Natural history of periodontal disease in man. Rapid, moderate and no loss of attachment in Sri Lankan laborers 14 to 46 years of age, *J Clin Periodontol* 13:431-440, 1986.

42. Socransky SS, Haffajee AD, Goodson JM, et al: New concepts of destructive periodontal disease, *J Clin Periodontol* 11:21-32, 1984.

43. Jeffcoat MK, Reddy MS: Progression of probing attachment loss in adult periodontitis, *J Periodontol* 62:185-189, 1991.

44. Lindhe J, Ranney R, Lamster I, et al: Consensus report: chronic periodontitis, *Ann Periodontol* 4:38, 1999.

45. Taylor GW: Bidirectional interrelationships between diabetes and periodontal diseases: an epidemiological perspective, *Ann Periodontol* 6:99-112, 2001.

46. Salvi GE, Lawrence HP, Offenbacher S, et al: Influence of risk factors on the pathogenesis of periodontitis, *Periodontol 2000* 14:173-201, 1997.

47. Lang N, Bartold PM, Cullinan M, et al: Consensus report: aggressive periodontitis, *Ann Periodontol* 4:53, 1999.

48. Slots J, Ting M: Systemic antibiotics in the treatment of periodontal disease, *Periodontol 2000* 28:106-176, 2002.

49. Kinane DF: Periodontitis modified by systemic factors, *Ann Periodontol* 4:54-63, 1999.

50. Chapple ILC: Hypophosphatasia: dental aspects and mode of inheritance, *J Clin Periodontol* 20:615-622, 1993.

51. Hartsfield JK Jr, Kousseff BG: Phenotypic overlap of Ehlers-Danlos syndrome types IV and VIII, *Am J Med Genet* 37:465-470, 1990.

52. Ardekian L, Peled M, Rosen D, et al: Clinical and radiographic features of eosinophilic granuloma in the jaws. Review of 41 lesions treated by surgery and low-dose radiotherapy, *Oral Surg Oral Med Oral Pathol Oral Radiol Endod* 87:238-242, 1999.

53. Nicopoulou-Karayianni K, Mombelli A, Lang NP: Diagnostic problems of periodontitis-like lesions caused by eosinophilic granuloma, *J Clin Periodontol* 16:505-509, 1989.

54. Rowland RW: Necrotizing ulcerative gingivitis, *Ann Periodontol* 4:65-73, 1999.

55. Novak MJ: Necrotizing ulcerative periodontitis, *Ann Periodontol* 4:74-77, 1999.

56. Lang N, Soskolne WA, Greenstein G, et al: Consensus report: Necrotizing periodontal diseases, *Ann Periodontol* 4:78, 1999.

57. Armitage GC: Acute periodontal lesions. In: *Biologic basis of periodontal maintenance therapy*, Berkeley, Calif, 1980, Praxis Publishing.

58. Musa NJ, Kumar V, Humphreys L, et al: Oral pemphigoid masquerading as necrotizing ulcerative gingivitis in a child, *J Periodontol* 73:657-663, 2002.

59. Osuji OO: Necrotizing ulcerative gingivitis and cancrum oris (noma) in Ibadan, Nigeria, *J Periodontol* 61:769-772, 1990.

60. Enwonwu CO: Epidemiological and biochemical studies of necrotizing ulcerative gingivitis and noma (cancrum oris) in Nigerian children, *Arch Oral Biol* 17:1357-1371, 1972.

61. Enwonwu CO, Falkler WA Jr, Idigbe EO, et al: Noma (cancrum oris): questions and answers, *Oral Diseases* 5:144-149, 1999.

62. Falkler WA Jr, Enwonwu CO, Idigbe EO: Microbiological understandings and mysteries of noma (cancrum oris), *Oral Dis* 5:150-155, 1999.

63. MacCarthy D, Claffey N: Acute necrotizing ulcerative gingivitis is associated with attachment loss, *J Clin Periodontol* 18:776-779, 1991.

64. Enwonwu CO: Cellular and molecular effects of malnutrition and their relevance to periodontal diseases, *J Clin Periodontol* 21:643-657, 1994.

65. Kahldahl WB, Kalkwarf KL, Patil KD, et al: Long-term evaluation of periodontal therapy: I. Response to 4 treatment modalities, *J Periodontol* 67:93-102, 1996.

66. Meng HX: Periodontal abscess, *Ann Periodontol* 4:79-82, 1999.

67. Herrera D, Roldán S, González I, et al: The periodontal abscess (I). Clinical and microbiological findings, *J Clin Periodontol* 27:387-394, 2000.

68. Dello Russo NM: The post-prophylaxis periodontal abscess: etiology and treatment, *Int J Periodontics Restorative Dent* 5(1):28-37, 1985.

69. Abrams H, Kopczyk RA: Gingival sequela from a retained piece of dental floss, *J Am Dent Assoc* 106:57-58, 1983.

70. O'Leary TJ, Standish SM, Bloomer RS: Severe periodontal destruction following impression procedures, *J Periodontol* 44:43-48, 1973.

71. Helovuo H, Hakkaraainen K, Paunio K: Changes in the prevalence of subgingival enteric rods, staphylococci and yeasts after treatment with penicillin and erythromycin, *Oral Microbiol Immunol* 8:75-79, 1993.

72. Lang N, Soskolne WA, Greenstein G, et al: Consensus report: Abscesses of the periodontium, *Ann Periodontol* 4:83, 1999.

73. Meng HX: Periodontic-endodontic lesions, *Ann Periodontol* 4:84-89, 1999.

74. Kirkham DB, Hoge HW, Sadeghi EM: Gingival squamous cell carcinoma appearing as a benign lesion: report of a case, *J Am Dent Assoc* 111:767-769, 1985.

75. Selden HS, Manhoff DT, Hatges NA, et al: Metastatic carcinoma to the mandible that mimicked pulpal/periodontal disease, *J Endod* 24:267-270, 1998.

76. Girdler NM: Eosinophilic granuloma presenting as a chronic lateral periodontal abscess: a lesson in diagnosis? *Br Dent J* 170:250, 1991.

77. Lang N, Soskolne WA, Greenstein G, et al: Consensus report: periodontic-endodontic lesions, *Ann Periodontol* 4:90, 1999.

78. Blieden TM: Tooth-related issues, *Ann Periodontol* 4:91-96, 1999.

79. Pini Prato GP: Mucogingival deformities, *Ann Periodontol* 4:98-100, 1999.

80. Hallmon WW: Occlusal trauma: effect and impact on the periodontium, *Ann Periodontol* 4:102-107, 1999.

3

Epidemiology of Periodontal Diseases and Risk Factors

Mauricio Ronderos and Bryan S. Michalowicz

Epidemiology is the science and practice concerned with the distribution and determinants of states of health and disease in populations, and the application of this knowledge to control health problems.[1] As the basic method of public health, the goals of epidemiology are to understand the natural course of a disease and the factors that influence its distribution. On the basis of this knowledge, the epidemiologist looks for effective ways to reduce the occurrence or sequelae of disease in the population.

In contrast to the clinical practice of dentistry or medicine, epidemiologists focus on groups of people rather than on individuals. Epidemiology is an interdisciplinary field that uses methods from biostatistics, social and behavioral sciences, immunology, genetics, microbiology, clinical dentistry, and medicine. There are two basic types of epidemiologic research: observational and experimental. During the past decades the methods of epidemiologic research have evolved significantly, giving rise to subspecialties within the field, including behavioral epidemiology, molecular epidemiology, and genetic epidemiology. Box 3-1 contains terms and definitions that are frequently used in epidemiologic research and will be used throughout this chapter.

OBSERVATIONAL STUDIES

In observational studies, the researcher acts as a spectator who documents the natural course of events and draws conclusions. One of the most important limitations of all observational studies is that the effect of confounders can never be completely ruled out as a possible explanation for any observations. A confounder is an extraneous factor that distorts the effect of the exposure or characteristic of interest. For example, in the United States, chronic periodontitis is more prevalent, extensive, and severe among **ethnic** minorities.[4] Such differences are not likely to be caused by genetic differences that exist among races; they are most likely because of **racial discrepancies in access to preventive dental care, education, and other behavioral factors**. Therefore, it could be said that access to dental care and to education are confounders of the association between prevalence of chronic periodontitis and race.

Observational studies are frequently subclassified as descriptive or analytic. However, most observational studies in periodontics have both components. Purely *descriptive studies* are used to provide basic knowledge about the characteristics, frequency, and distribution of a health-related condition. These studies characterize the occurrence of the disease with respect to personal (e.g., age, sex, race/ethnicity), geographic (i.e., geographic distribution), and time characteristics. Such knowledge regarding the general characteristics of those at increased risk for disease in a given population is essential for the formulation of a

hypothesis regarding the etiology of the disease and for the implementation of rational and cost-effective health care programs. Descriptive studies are also valuable in establishing a baseline assessment for future evaluation of preventive and therapeutic interventions. Cross-sectional studies, case reports, and case series are the most common study designs used for purely descriptive purposes. In contrast, *analytic studies* are used to test a specific hypothesis regarding etiologic or nonetiologic factors that may be associated with the presence of the disease or factors that may predict the future occurrence of the disease. The most common study designs used for hypothesis testing are the case-control studies, cohort studies, and ecologic studies. Cross-sectional studies are also frequently used for testing a specific hypothesis.

Cross-Sectional Studies

In cross-sectional studies, the researcher examines a group of subjects with an unknown history of exposure or disease and assesses their health status, as well as the presence of factors that may be associated with disease. The subjects are evaluated only at a single point in time. Cross-sectional studies are traditionally classified as being purely descriptive. However, data gathered from most cross-sectional studies in periodontics are used for descriptive and analytical (i.e., hypothesis testing) purposes. For example, the U.S. National Health and Nutrition Examination Surveys (NHANES) are a series of cross-sectional studies designed to obtain information on the health and nutritional status of the population of the United States. This series of surveys included periodontal examinations that were primarily collected to describe the periodontal status of the entire U.S. population, as well as the periodontal condition of people in different age groups, geographic locations, races/ethnicities, and sex categories. However, data gathered in the surveys have also been used by investigators to analyze the possible association between periodontitis and various dietary, behavioral, and environmental factors, as well as to assess associations between periodontitis and systemic diseases (e.g., diabetes mellitus, osteoporosis, cardiovascular diseases). To look for such associations the researcher compares the frequency or level of the exposure of interest (e.g., smoking, calcium intake, etc.) between patients with disease and healthy subjects. The basic unit of observation and analysis is the individual. Cross-sectional studies are valuable at studying chronic diseases that affect a large proportion of the population (e.g., chronic periodontitis), but they are not efficient to study rare conditions or conditions that may only last for short periods (e.g., periodontitis associated with Papillon-Lefèvre syndrome). Repeated cross-sectional studies are often conducted to examine changes in the prevalence of a disease or risk factors that can vary over time. Such information may be valuable to demonstrate trends of the disease over time or to evaluate the effects of preventive or therapeutic programs. The main limitation of cross-sectional studies is that they do not follow the population over time. It is, therefore, difficult to assess whether a given factor preceded the onset of a disease. Because this study design assesses the presence of the disease and the risk factors at the same time, in most cases it is not appropriate to make inferences of cause-and-effect relations on the basis of cross-sectional studies.

Case-Control Studies

In case-control studies, the investigator starts with a group of individuals who have the disease (cases) and a group of subjects without disease (control subjects). Both groups are assessed for the history of exposure or the presence of putative risk factors. The frequency, or levels, or both, of the exposure among the cases and control subjects are compared statistically to assess if there are associations between the exposure of interest and the presence of the disease.

Box 3-1 | Basic Terminology Used in Epidemiology of Periodontal Diseases

- *Incidence:*
  - Number of new cases that occur in a population over a given period of time.[1]
- *Prevalence:*
  - Number or percentage of affected persons in a population. For example, the prevalence of periodontal disease in populations may be characterized by assessing the percentage of persons with at least one site with clinical attachment loss ≥ 2 mm, ≥ 4 mm, or ≥ 7 mm.
- *Extent:*
  - Number or proportion of teeth or examined sites that are affected with a given condition.
- *Severity:*
  - How advanced or serious a given condition is. For example, periodontal disease may be classified as being slight, moderate or severe, depending on the amount of attachment loss present.
- *Exposure:*
  - A factor that may possibly lead to disease or may be protective against a disease (e.g., cigarette smoking, a specific microorganism, calcium intake, or dental care). Depending on the nature of the factor being measured, subjects may be classified according to the level of exposure or as having been exposed or nonexposed to the factor of interest.
- *Risk factor:*
  - A characteristic that is associated with a disease. The association may or may not be causal, although the use of this term often implies causality.[1] In the periodontal literature, this term is usually reserved for environmental, behavioral or biologic exposures or characteristics that have been related to the disease through longitudinal/cohort studies. If present, the factor directly increases the probability of disease occurrence, and if absent, reduces the probability.[2,3]
- *Risk indicator:*
  - A probable or putative risk factor that has been associated with the disease through cross-sectional studies. Risk indicators identified in cross-sectional studies are not always confirmed as risk factors in longitudinal studies.[2,3]
- *Risk predictor/marker:*
  - A factor that is associated with increased probability of future disease, but where causality is usually not implied.[2]
- *Odds ratio:*
  - *Odds* represent the ratio of the probability of occurrence of an event to that of nonoccurrence and *odds ratio* (OR) is the ratio of two odds.[1] Consider the following situation:

	Exposed	Nonexposed
Disease	a	b
Healthy	c	d

The odds ratio is equal to the odds of being exposed among the subjects with disease divided by the odds of being exposed among the healthy subjects.

$$OR = (a/b)/(c/d) = ad/cd$$

Odds ratios are frequently used as measures of association between exposures and disease in cross-sectional studies, case-control studies that deal with dichotomous outcomes (i.e., where the subjects are classified as either having the disease or not having the disease). An odds ratio equal to 1.0 indicates lack of an association. An odds ratio greater than 1.0 indicates that subjects were more likely to have been exposed than the healthy subjects and an odds ratio less than 1.0 indicates that the level of exposure was greater for the healthy group.

| Box 3-1 | Basic Terminology Used in Epidemiology of Periodontal Diseases—cont'd |

Risk ratio:

Risk is the probability that a disease or event will occur and risk ratio (RR) is the ratio of two risks.[1] Consider the following situation:

	Developed disease	Did not develop disease
Exposed	a	b
Nonexposed	c	d

The risk ratio is equal to the risk for development of disease among the exposed (i.e., a/a + b) divided by the risk for development of disease among the nonexposed subjects (i.e., c/c + d).

$$RR = (a/a + b)/(c/c + d)$$

Risk ratios are frequently used as measures of association between exposures and disease in cohort studies that deal with dichotomous outcomes (i.e., where the subjects are classified as either having the disease or not having the disease). A risk ratio equal to 1.0 indicates that the exposure is unrelated to the occurrence of disease. A risk ratio more than 1.0 indicates that exposed subjects are at greater risk for development of the disease (i.e., the exposure is detrimental). A risk ratio less than 1.0 indicates that exposed subjects are at lower risk for development of the disease (i.e., the exposure is protective).

This study design is the most efficient way to study conditions that are not highly prevalent. Case-control studies do not follow the subjects over time; therefore, it is difficult to assess if the exposure preceded the onset of disease. A major difficulty in conducting a case-control study is selecting a control group of individuals without disease that is representative of the general population from which the cases were recruited. Case-control studies have been used extensively to study chronic and aggressive periodontitis.

Cohort Studies

In the classic cohort study design, the researcher will gather a group of individuals without disease and will classify them according to the presence or levels of exposures of interest (e.g., specific bacteria, smoking, oral hygiene, diabetes, and others). The subjects are then followed over time. If the incidence of the disease is greater among the subjects who were exposed to a given factor, this factor may be considered to predict the development of the disease. Cohort studies can establish if exposure to some environment or behavior preceded the onset of disease.

Performing cohort studies for the study of periodontitis is difficult and expensive. To recruit a group of individuals without disease who are representative of the overall population, it would be necessary to enroll a very large group of young individuals. Because periodontitis is generally a slowly progressing, late-onset disease, cohorts would need to be followed for several years. Variations in the exposure of interest over the follow-up period would further complicate interpretation of the results. Many longitudinal studies have been conducted to study periodontitis, but no

study has assessed exclusively disease-free individuals at baseline. A limitation of periodontal studies that follow mixed populations of subjects with disease and healthy individuals is that they cannot ascertain if the exposure of interest preceded the onset of the disease. However, these longitudinal studies have provided valuable information regarding predictors of disease progression.

Ecologic Studies

In ecologic studies, the unit of analysis is a group of persons rather than an individual. This study design has not been frequently used in the study of periodontal diseases. There are two basic types of ecologic studies: ecologic comparisons and ecologic trends. In ecologic comparison studies, the researcher gathers information regarding the overall prevalence or incidence of the disease in various populations and categorizes these populations according to their level of exposure or characteristic of interest. Subsequently, the researcher assesses associations between the exposure or characteristic of interest and the disease rates among the different groups or populations. In ecologic trend studies, the researcher studies possible relations between changes in exposure and changes of disease level over time in a given population.

EXPERIMENTAL STUDIES

In observational studies, the researcher is a spectator of the natural course of disease. In contrast, in experimental studies, the researcher has control over the exposure of interest and assigns subjects to exposed or nonexposed groups, or to different treatment and no treatment groups. The researcher may also control the characteristics of the exposure and factors that may influence the subject's response to such an exposure. Experimental studies may be used to assess the role of potential determinants of a disease or the effectiveness of therapeutic or preventive interventions. In experimental designs, the study group(s) receive an intervention and the outcome is compared with concurrent observations conducted in a control group that may be receiving another intervention or no intervention. Therefore, experimental studies produce stronger evidence of the effects of an exposure than observational studies. The two most common types of experimental designs are clinical and community trials.

Clinical trials are primarily used to assess the safety and efficacy of new drugs, therapies, and procedures used for the treatment of a disease. In periodontics, most clinical trials fall into three main categories: (1) randomized parallel-arm design, (2) crossover design, and (3) the split-mouth design. Studies in which subjects are randomly assigned to either an experimental or a control group and subsequently followed over time are generally described as parallel-arm studies. In parallel-arm studies, each subject will be part of one treatment group and there may be two or more study groups. The response to the intervention of each group will be compared with the response of the other groups. Crossover designs are only used to test the effects of interventions that are fully reversible and do not have a lasting effect (e.g., antiplaque agents). Crossover studies have three phases: experimental phase I, washout period, and experimental phase II. During the experimental phase I, each subject is assigned to either an experimental or a control group and the response to the intervention is documented. Thereafter, interventions are discontinued for a time to ensure that the effects of the interventions of phase I have completely disappeared (i.e., washout period). Subsequently, the subjects who received the experimental treatment during phase I will be part of the control group during phase II. In this way, the responses of each subject during phase I of the study will be compared with his/her response during phase II. In split-mouth designs, each subject will receive two or more types of therapy to treat lesions of similar characteristics that are located in different parts of the mouth. A classic application of split-mouth designs is in studies conducted to compare the effects of surgical versus nonsurgical therapy in the treatment of chronic periodontitis.[5] For example, subjects with generalized moderate to severe chronic periodontitis received scaling and root planing followed by surgical therapy in one half of the mouth and scaling and root planing alone on the contralateral side. The cases were followed for several years to compare the long-term response of the quadrants treated with surgery to those treated with root planing alone.[5]

Community trials examine the impact of an intervention on the overall health status of a group or community. This study design is most commonly used to evaluate the effects of educational campaigns, behavior change, or policy change on the health status of a population as a whole. A typical example of a community trial is a study of residents of the South Pacific islands of Tonga.[6] The effects of different preventive strategies on the overall periodontal condition of three village communities were determined. One village received free toothbrushes and toothpaste, health education, and periodic dental scaling at no cost; another village received the same except that dental scaling was not provided; and a third village did not receive any services. A sample of each community was examined at baseline and 3 years later. It was concluded that unsupervised self-care promoted at the community level, when supplemented with periodic scaling, significantly improves the periodontal health of the overall community.[6] The main limitation of community trials is that it is impossible to control for the possible influence of differences among populations over the outcome of the study.

MEASURES OF ASSOCIATION

Measures of association are used to assess the presence of a relation between an exposure and the occurrence of the disease and to describe the direction and magnitude of such an association. Odds ratios and risk ratios are measures of association that are frequently used in the periodontal literature to describe relations between exposures and the presence or absence of disease (see Box 3-1). Other measures used to evaluate the performance of tests at determining the presence or absence of pathology or at predicting future disease occurrence are presented in Box 3-2. Notably, close associations or statistically significant correlations between putative etiologic factors and disease occurrence, as established on the basis of epidemiologic surveys, may be suggestive but are not proof of cause and effect.

Assessment of Periodontal Diseases

Periodontal tissue destruction is generally a gradual process, unevenly distributed within the mouth, and often presents great variability of severity from site to site. Therefore, when characterizing periodontal disease in a population, it is not feasible to independently analyze the prevalence, severity, and extent of the periodontal condition. A major limitation in estimating the prevalence of periodontal disease in a population is the difficulty in establishing a valid threshold to distinguish health from disease. There is no consensus about the number of sites or teeth that should meet a given threshold for an individual to be considered as having disease. The lack of

Box 3-2	Terminology Frequently Used in Evaluation of Screening Tests

- *Reliability:*   The degree to which the results of a measurement can be replicated. Also referred to as *reproducibility* or *repeatability*.
- *Validity:*   A measure of the degree to which a test measures what it purports to measure. Specificity and sensitivity are measurements of the validity of a test.
- *Sensitivity:*   The proportion of truly diseased persons in a screened population who are identified as diseased by the screening test. Sensitivity is the true positive rate, a measure of the probability of correctly diagnosing or predicting disease, or the probability that any given case will be identified by a test.
- *Specificity:*   The proportion of truly nondiseased persons who are so identified by the screening test. Specificity is the true negative rate, a measure of the probability of correctly identifying a nondiseased person with a screening test.
- *Positive predictive value:*   Probability that a person with a positive test is truly diseased.
- *Negative predictive value:*   Probability that a person with a negative test is truly nondiseased.

Summary

	True status	
Test results	Diseased	Nondiseased
Positive	a	b
Negative	c	d

a: true positives
b: false positives
c: false negatives
d: true negatives

Sensitivity = a/a + c
Specificity = d/b + d
Positive predictive value = a/a + b
Negative predictive value = d/c + d

Adapted from Last JM, Abramson JH—International Epidemiological Association: A dictionary of epidemiology, ed 3, New York (1995): Oxford University Press.

uniform criteria to define disease has resulted in great variability in the literature. Differences among studies can also be attributed to examiner variability, the use of different partial-mouth recording systems, differences in the parameters scored and indexes used, variation in the instruments used, or differences in examination conditions.

Until the 1940s, the epidemiology of periodontal diseases was mainly based on subjective and nonnumeric descriptions of populations. Thereafter, numerous indexes and examination protocols were developed. The main purpose of such recording systems was to express the gingival and/or periodontal condition in numerical values. Each of these index systems and examination protocols had properties, assumptions, and limitations that influenced the study results. The selection of the most appropriate approach is determined by the research question and the study design. The following discussion of specific measures for assessing periodontal diseases includes the most widely used indexes. Many of these indexes and disease definitions that were developed for epidemiologic purposes are not necessarily adequate or practical for the clinical practice of periodontics.

Assessment of Gingival Inflammation

There are several methods for categorizing and quantifying gingival inflammation. Most of these methods categorize the extent and severity of gingival inflammation based on the assessment of gingival color, contour, and bleeding. Some authors have also proposed the use of more sensitive techniques including measurements of laser-Doppler readings,[7] subgingival temperature,[8] or gingival crevicular fluid flow.[9,10] However, these methods are impractical for large-scale epidemiologic surveys.

Perhaps the first index described to assess the extent of gingival inflammation was the PMA (papilla, margin, and attached gingiva) index.[11] This simple method was based on a count of the number of facial interdental papillae, marginal gingival sites, and attached gingival units that were inflamed. The sum of the affected units was used as the PMA score for a given person. The PMA was also the first system that used the examination of a subset of index teeth as representative of the periodontal condition of the entire dentition, a concept that became important in the epidemiology of periodontal disease.

The most widely used systems to characterize gingival inflammation in observational and experimental epidemiology are the Gingival Index (GI) of Löe and Silness[12] and the bleeding on probing index. The GI is sensitive enough to detect small differences in gingival inflammation, and for this reason it is the most widely used method in clinical trials for antigingivitis agents. The gingival areas surrounding each selected tooth are scored according to the criteria described in Box 3-3. The scores are frequently averaged to determine a mean GI score for each individual. Various protocols for assessing gingival inflammation based on gingival bleeding have been described. Most use a periodontal probe to induce bleeding, whereas others use wooden wedges or floss. Some indexes score the amount of bleeding observed after mechanical stimulation. However, most investigators today simply assess the presence or absence of bleeding at each site and compute the percentage of sites that bleed on probing. This is a practical method to characterize gingival inflammation in large-scale population studies. Variation in probing force, type of probe used, and angulations of the probe can influence the results of a study.[13] The time between probing and the assessment of bleeding may also influence the results. For example, it has been reported that 14% of sites examined among attendants of a large health maintenance organization in the Minneapolis-St. Paul area bled immediately after probing. However, when sites that exhibited more delayed bleeding were also considered, the percentage increased to 55%.[14]

Bleeding on mechanical stimulation is highly correlated with gingival inflammation.[10,15] Although some categorical indexes, like the GI,[12] use redness and swelling as the initial signs for gingival inflammation, others suggest that bleeding precedes redness and swelling. Histologic[15] and clinical findings[16,17] indicate that bleeding on probing (i.e., to the base of the sulcus) is an earlier and more sensitive sign of inflammation than redness and swelling. However, sites with obvious edema and erythema may not bleed on gentle probing. Furthermore, bleeding may appear to be an early or later sign of inflammation depending on the nature of the mechanical stimulus used to elicit bleeding. In some studies bleeding is assessed after gently running the probe in a mesiodistal direction one millimeter subgingivally, whereas in other studies the probe is inserted to the depth of the gingival sulcus. It is possible that more severe inflammation is necessary to elicit bleeding when the probe is not inserted to the depth of the pocket.

Assessment of Periodontitis

The Periodontal Index (PI), described by Russell in 1956,[18] was the first widely used index system in periodontal epidemiology. The World Health Organization (WHO) adopted this method as the standard, and the index was used in several studies worldwide. The PI combined assessments of gingival inflammation, periodontal pockets, and tooth mobility into a single score (Box 3-4). A score was assigned to each tooth in the mouth, and the average score for the patient was calculated. The population mean and the percentage of persons with scores greater than a given threshold were usually reported. However, the PI has important limitations. It does not distinguish between gingivitis and periodontitis, and the assessment of periodontal pockets is made visually **without the aid of a periodontal probe**, which yields very subjective and unreliable results.

In 1959, Ramfjord introduced the Periodontal Disease Index (PDI).[19] Like Russell's PI, the PDI includes both gingivitis and periodontitis in a single index system that summarizes the presence and severity of periodontal disease in a population. Although never widely used, the PDI introduced important concepts to periodontal epidemiology. It used a subset of teeth as representative of the overall periodontal condition. This tooth subset (i.e., 3, 9, 12, 19, 25, 28), often referred to as the "Ramfjord teeth," is still frequently used in epidemiologic research and clinical trials. In addition, it incorporated the concept of clinical attachment level (CAL) to estimate periodontal destruction. The clinical attachment level of a site is assessed by using a periodontal probe to measure the distance in millimeters from the cementoenamel junction (CEJ) to the base of the probeable gingival sulcus. Recession or formation of periodontal pockets may accompany clinical attachment loss. Therefore, it is important to describe the

---

Box 3-3	Criteria for the Gingival Index

Score	Criteria
0	*Normal gingiva*
1	*Mild inflammation:* slight change in color, slight edema, no bleeding on probing
2	*Moderate inflammation:* redness, edema and glazing, bleeding on probing
3	*Severe inflammation:* marked redness and edema, ulcerations; tendency toward spontaneous bleeding

From Löe H, Silness J: Periodontal disease in pregnancy. 1. Prevalance and severity, Acta Odontol Scand 21:533, 1963.

Box 3-4	**Criteria for the Periodontal Index**

Score	Criteria
0	*Normal gingiva:* There is neither overt inflammation in the investing tissues nor loss of function because of destruction of supporting tissues.
1	*Mild gingivitis:* There is an overt area of inflammation in the free gingiva, but this area does not circumscribe the tooth.
2	*Gingivitis:* Inflammation completely circumscribes the tooth, but there is no apparent break in the epithelial attachment.
6	*Gingivitis with pocket formation:* The epithelial attachment has been broken and there is a pocket (not merely a deepened gingival crevice caused by swelling in the free gingiva). There is no interference with normal masticatory function.
8	*Advanced destruction with loss of masticatory function:* The tooth may be loose, may have drifted, may sound dull on percussion with a metallic instrument, or may be depressible in its socket.

From Russell AL: *A system of classification and scoring for prevalence surveys of periodontal disease,* J Dent Res, 35:350, 1956.

presence of periodontal pockets and gingival recession. Currently, clinical attachment level remains the "gold standard" for scoring periodontitis.

In contemporary epidemiology, the description of the periodontal condition of populations is generally based on full- or partial-mouth assessments of probing depths (PDs), CALs, and gingival recession. Because of the lack of a consensus definition for disease and the use of different research methodologies, it is difficult to compare results from the literature on epidemiology of periodontal diseases. In the description of periodontal disease in a population, three features should be described: prevalence, extent, and severity of periodontal destruction. The prevalence of slight, moderate, and severe periodontitis could be characterized, for example, by the percentage of persons with at least one site with CAL **2 to less than 3 mm**, 3 to 4 mm, or 5 mm or more, respectively. Different cutoffs and thresholds may be used to estimate the prevalence of periodontal pockets or recession and to assess the proportion of affected teeth or sites (i.e., extent). The mean clinical attachment loss (average across all examined sites) is also frequently used to characterize the periodontal condition. This measurement, often regarded as a measurement of severity, is a combined estimate of disease prevalence, extent, and severity.

Attachment level measurements and bone loss reflect the effects of prior damage caused by periodontal disease but do not necessarily indicate ongoing progression of disease. Currently, there are no reliable methods to distinguish between progressing and nonprogressing sites. The finding of additional attachment loss or radiographic bone loss between two examination periods confirms that the disease has progressed but does not reliably predict future destructive events. Considerable work is in progress to develop assays that identify ongoing periodontal destruction. Levels of inflammatory mediators, host-derived enzymes, tissue-breakdown products, and other biochemical markers in gingival crevicular fluid are possible sources for future tests to accurately detect progressive periodontitis.[20]

Determination of PD and CAL remain the standard assessments for epidemiologic studies of periodontal disease. However, periodontal probing does not precisely measure the level of the connective tissue attachment.[21] Because of the large variability in repeated probing measurements, 2 to 3 mm changes in PD and CAL are necessary to determine with confidence that change has actually occurred. The rate of false-positive findings increases if smaller thresholds are used to define disease progression.[22] In longitudinal studies (i.e., cohort designs and clinical trials), periodontal disease progression is generally characterized by assessment of increases in clinical attachment levels of at least 2 mm.

Computer-assisted subtraction radiography is a very precise method to measure small changes in alveolar bone level.[23] It is able to detect bone level differences as small as 0.5 mm between two radiographs. In this method, the computer superimposes initial and follow-up radiographs that have been obtained in a standardized way. Subsequently, a computer program detects and quantifies differences in bone levels and bone density between the two digitized radiographs. Subtraction radiography is a useful tool for clinical trials. The evaluation of bone loss in radiographs and the quantitative assessment of progressive bone loss through computer-assisted subtraction radiography are currently not practical for population-based studies. These approaches are technique-sensitive, expensive, and time-consuming. Furthermore, radiographic bone levels are closely related to clinical attachment levels,[20] which can be more easily obtained with a periodontal probe. The assessment of the periodontal condition in epidemiologic studies may dramatically change in the future as more precise and practical imaging techniques and computer software for analysis of such images evolve.

Assessment of Periodontal Treatment Needs

To allocate resources, estimate manpower needs, and design effective public health programs, public health practitioners need to assess the treatment needs of the population. Investigators have attempted to develop specific measures to assess a population's periodontal treatment needs. In 1978, the WHO recommended the Community Periodontal Index of Treatment Needs (CPITN) for use in epidemiologic surveys.[24] Since then, the CPITN has been used extensively to assess the treatment needs of populations around the world. This system combines assessments of gingival health, calculus, and the presence of periodontal pockets (Box 3-5).

Although it is simple and practical, the validity of the CPITN for determining treatment needs has been challenged.[25] In theory, the CPITN is a reversible index (i.e., after adequate treatment the CPITN score of a person should be 0). However, this is not true in practice and the index is unable to distinguish between pretreatment and posttreatment conditions.[26] Furthermore, it overestimates certain treatment needs in the population. For example, the CPITN assumes that a sextant with a pocket 6 mm or deeper will require periodontal surgery. However, as a public health strategy, surgical therapy is not always cost-effective, and in most cases scaling and root planing alone are effective.[5]

Assessment of Plaque

Various plaque index systems have been described. Many estimate the quantity of plaque in terms of tooth area covered with plaque, whereas other systems simply score the presence or absence of plaque. Some indexes require the use of plaque disclosing solutions. Although the use of disclosing solutions may improve the accuracy of the plaque assessment, this is not practical for population-based studies and its use is mainly reserved for clinical trials that require accurate documentation of small changes in oral cleanliness.

The Turesky modification of the Quigley and Hein plaque index[27,28] is perhaps the index system most frequently used in clinical trials that evaluate antiplaque measures such as toothbrushing, flossing, and mouthrinses (Box 3-6). The most frequently used plaque indexes in observational epidemiologic studies are the Plaque Index (Box 3-7)[29,30] or less elaborate systems that only score plaque as being present or absent at each examined surface. The most significant problem with most plaque indexes is that their criteria are somewhat subjective; they require well trained and experienced examiners to obtain reliable data.[31]

Full-Mouth Versus Partial-Mouth Examinations

A full-mouth examination, including individual recordings of six sites (i.e., mesiofacial, facial, distofacial, mesiolingual, lingual, and distolingual) on each of the teeth present in the mouth, is the ideal method to characterize periodontal conditions. However, in epidemiologic investigations, conducting full-mouth examinations is frequently not feasible because of limited resources and time. A variety of tooth subsets have been proposed for partial-mouth examinations, but the most frequently used are the tooth subsets originally proposed for the CPITN index, the Ramfjord teeth, and the half-mouth examination protocol (Box 3-8).[19,24] The Ramfjord teeth and half-mouth subsets are used to estimate the average extent and severity of the disease of the entire dentition. The CPITN tooth subsets, however, are primarily designed to assess periodontal treatment needs and score the most severely involved sites in the mouth. These partial-mouth evaluation protocols are meant to be used as research tools and are not appropriate for the clinical practice of periodontics.

Box 3-5	Community Periodontal Index of Treatment Needs (CPITN)

Score	Criteria
0	Normal gingiva
1	Bleeding after probing. No calculus and the periodontal pockets are less than 4 mm.
2	Calculus felt during probing but pockets are less than 4 mm.
3	Pocket 4 or 5 mm.
4	Pocket ≥ 6 mm.

The following index teeth are examined and a single score is given for each tooth:

Persons ≤ 20 years-old				Persons 20 years or older				
3	8	14		2	3	8	14	15
30	24	19		31	30	24	19	18

Among young people the second molars are not examined to avoid classifying the deepened crevices associated with eruption as periodontal pockets. For the same reason, the World Health Organization does not recommend the recording of pockets for children younger than 15 (i.e., only bleeding and calculus should be considered).

Box 3-6   Quigley & Hein, Turesky Modification

Score	Criteria
0	No plaque in gingival area.
1	Noncontinuous flecks of plaque at the cervical margin of the tooth.
2	Thin continuous band of plaque at the cervical margin of the tooth (up to 1 mm).
3	A continuous band of plaque wider than 1 mm but covering less than one third of the crown.
4	Plaque covering at least one third but less than two thirds of the crown of the tooth.
5	Plaque covering more than two thirds of the crown of the tooth.

Note: A disclosing solution should be used prior to the assessment.
From Quigley G, Hein J: Comparative cleansing efficiency of manual and power brushing, J Am Dent Assoc 65:26, 1962; and Turesky S, Gilmore ND, Glickman I: Reduced plaque formation by the chloromethyl analogue of vitamin C, J Periodontol 41:41, 1970.

The use of partial-mouth recording systems may underestimate or overestimate the prevalence, severity, or extent of disease. Examination of the Ramfjord teeth and half-mouth examinations produce accurate estimates of extent and severity of periodontitis and gingivitis.[32-35] Meanwhile, because of the predominance of molar teeth, the CPITN subset grossly overestimates the **severity** and the **extent** of PD, gingivitis, and plaque.[32]

All partial-mouth examination protocols grossly underestimate the **prevalence** of periodontal disease.[33,35] The degree of underestimation is dependent on the cut-off established to discriminate between health and disease, and on the extent and distribution of disease within the sample population. The more extensive the disease, the lower the relative bias and vice versa. As a result, disease is more likely to be underestimated in younger age groups and in periodontally healthier populations.[33,35] If the disease is extensive in a sample population, a partial-mouth examination is likely to find diseased sites. By contrast, when the disease is less extensive, it is less likely that diseased sites will be detected through a partial-mouth examination.

Similarly, the relative bias of a partial-mouth index is inversely related to the severity and extent of the disease among the sample population. As the definition of "disease" becomes more stringent, the proportional difference between prevalence estimates obtained from full and partial-mouth examinations increase.[33] This is because more severe conditions generally involve fewer sites in the mouth and, therefore, partial-mouth examinations are less likely to detect affected sites. In general, examination of the CPITN-2 subset of teeth generally renders a better estimate of the true prevalence of the disease than examination of the Ramfjord teeth or half-mouth examinations.[35] The Ramfjord teeth and half-mouth examinations underestimate the prevalence of the disease to a similar degree.[35]

Buccal tooth sites are more often directly visible than lingual sites and are therefore more reliably measured.[36] Examination protocols used in epidemiologic surveys are often limited to scoring buccal sites. Although these measures are more reliable, this scheme also underestimates the prevalence of periodontal disease.[33,34] Furthermore, lingual sites are generally more susceptible to periodontal disease than buccal sites.[35] Therefore, a

Box 3-7   Criteria for the Plaque Index (PlI)

Score	Criteria
0	No plaque in gingival area.
1	No plaque visible by the unaided eye, but plaque is made visible on the point of the probe after it has been moved across surface at entrance of gingival crevice.
2	Gingival area is covered with a thin to moderately thick layer of plaque; deposit is visible to the naked eye.
3	Heavy accumulation of soft matter, the thickness of which fills out niche produced by gingival margin and tooth surface: interdental area is stuffed with soft debris.

Note: There is no need for the use of disclosing solution before the assessment.
(From Silness P, Löe H: Periodontal disease in pregnancy, Acta Odontol Scand 22:123, 1964; and Löe H: The gingival index, the plaque index and the retention index systems, J Periodontol 38:610, 1967.)

Box 3-8   Most Frequently Used Partial Mouth Examination Protocols

Subset	Examined Teeth					Comments
Half-mouth	All teeth in one upper and one lower, randomly selected, quadrants.					Examination of these subsets produces accurate estimates of **extent** and **severity** of periodontal disease and gingivitis (e.g., extent: % sites with CAL > 2 mm, % sites bleeding after probing, etc.; Severity: mean attachment levels, mean probing depths, mean gingival index scores, etc.). However, examination of these tooth subsets results in gross underestimation of the true **prevalence** of periodontal conditions.
Ramfjord teeth	3	9	12			
	28	25	19			
CPITN-2	2 3	8	14 15			Mainly used with the CPITN index for studies of adult populations. Overestimates the severity and the extent of probing depth, gingivitis and plaque. Underestimates the prevalence of periodontal diseases to a lesser degree than the Ramfjord teeth or half-mouth examinations.
	31 30	24	19 18			

method that only includes facial sites tends to make the population look healthier than it is.[33-35] Regardless of the subset used, it is recommended to measure as many sites per tooth as possible.

EPIDEMIOLOGY OF GINGIVITIS

Gingivitis is defined as gingival inflammation in the absence of clinical attachment loss or in the presence of reduced but stable attachment levels.[37] Attachment level stability can only be demonstrated through longitudinal monitoring, which is generally not feasible in epidemiologic surveys. In most epidemiologic studies, no distinction is made between gingival inflammation with or without attachment loss (i.e., gingivitis as a clinical sign rather than gingivitis as a diagnosis). This discrepancy in the clinical and epidemiologic uses of the term *gingivitis* should be considered when evaluating the epidemiologic literature.

Most people have clinical signs of gingival inflammation in one or more sites of their mouth. However, the extent and severity of inflammation vary greatly from person to person and from one population to another. Such variability is mainly the reflection of personal differences in oral hygiene. Virtually all epidemiologic studies conducted in treated and untreated populations have shown that the prevalence, extent, and severity of gingivitis are strongly associated with the levels of plaque. Clear evidence of a cause-and-effect relation between undisturbed bacterial plaque and gingivitis came from a classic "experimental gingivitis" study of Löe and coworkers in 1965.[38] In this study, young healthy individuals with normal gingiva were asked to refrain from all oral hygiene practices during a 3-week period. All subjects showed rapid accumulation of plaque and distinct changes in the composition of the bacterial flora that were followed by gingival

inflammation. The time necessary to develop visible signs of gingivitis varied from 10 to 21 days of plaque accumulation. When good oral hygiene was reinstituted, the original microflora was reestablished and the inflamed gingiva returned to health. Such findings have been confirmed in different populations.[39,40] Intraorally, the distribution of gingivitis reflects the areas of the mouth where patients are less effective at controlling plaque accumulation. Gingivitis most frequently affects the interdental areas of posterior teeth.[41,42]

According to the 1988-1994 U.S. National Health and Nutrition Examination Survey (NHANES III), 50% of the adult population in the United States has gingival inflammation (i.e., at least one site with bleeding on probing (**BOP**).[43] This percentage represents a gross underestimation of the true prevalence of gingival inflammation, because this study was based on half-mouth examinations of the mesiofacial and facial sites. Gingival bleeding occurred in 13.5% of the teeth of all the adult subjects examined and in 26.8% of teeth in people with gingival inflammation.[43]

In the United States, as in most industrialized populations, males tend to have more plaque and gingivitis than females.[43] Gingivitis is also more prevalent, extensive, and severe in groups with low socioeconomic status, groups with limited access to dental care, groups with less education, adolescents (especially males), and mentally handicapped individuals. In the United States, gingival inflammation is more prevalent among African Americans, Mexican Americans, and other underserved minorities than in white individuals.[43] Aside from undisturbed plaque, various local and host-related factors influence the occurrence of gingivitis by influencing plaque accumulation or the inflammatory response of the host. Factors that favor gingival inflammation by increasing plaque accumulation and retention include calculus, ill-fitting restorations, crowding, and tooth malalignment. Aging, smoking, diabetes mellitus, HIV infection, and hormonal changes may influence gingival inflammation by altering the host response to bacterial plaque.

Age

Gingivitis is a highly prevalent condition that can begin in early childhood. The reported prevalence of gingivitis varies greatly among studies. Between 35% to 85% of 3- to 6-year-old children have been reported to have gingivitis.[42,44-46] Such a large range in the reported prevalence of gingivitis mainly results from differences in study methodology and in the parameters used to define the disease. The prevalence, extent, and severity of gingivitis gradually increase during childhood, peaking in severity during puberty.[42,46-48] After puberty, the extent and severity of gingival inflammation decrease. Throughout adulthood, the extent and severity of gingivitis appear to remain stable or slightly increase with increasing age.[43,47-53]

The apparent increase in gingivitis that occurs during puberty has been reported for boys and girls. Such increase may be influenced by the effect of increasing levels of sex hormones on tissue physiology and the colonization of periodontal bacteria.[12,54-56] The gradual decrease in the extent and severity that occurs during the late teenage years is most likely associated with an improvement of oral hygiene. Of 161 independent studies included in the WHO Oral Health Data Bank, 115 (71.4%) found that more than 80% of the subjects had sites that bleed after probing or had pockets 4 mm or greater.[57] Other studies have reported that 90% to 100% of teenagers have detectable levels of gingival inflammation.[48,58-60]

Age appears to modify the initial clinical response of the gingiva to bacterial plaque. In the absence of oral hygiene, younger subjects tend to develop gingivitis slightly faster than older persons.[61] However, age does not appear to significantly affect how quickly gingivitis resolves after oral hygiene is reinstituted.[40,61]

Tobacco Use

A clear delay in inflammatory response to plaque accumulation has been documented for smokers.[62,63] The intensity of the vascular reaction to plaque-induced gingivitis in smokers is suppressed compared with the response of nonsmokers.[64]

Diabetes Mellitus

Given the same amount of plaque and calculus, patients with diabetes tend to present more gingival inflammation than groups without diabetes.[65] Furthermore, among people with diabetes, those with complications such as retinopathy and nephropathy also tend to have more gingival inflammation.[66]

Pregnancy

Gingival inflammation and PDs gradually increase during pregnancy, with resolution after parturition.[12,67,68] Such an increase in gingivitis is unrelated to the amount of plaque present and is not accompanied by increased rates of bone loss or attachment loss.[12,68] Increases in gingival inflammation have also been reported for women during periods of ovulation and during puberty (i.e., puberty-associated gingivitis and menstrual cycle-associated gingivitis).[37] An even more exaggerated inflammatory response to local irritants that occurs during pregnancy is the pregnancy-associated pyogenic granuloma. This lesion, also referred to as pregnancy tumor, may occur in as many as 0.5% to 5% of pregnant women.[37] It may start to develop during the first trimester and frequently reduces in size or completely disappears after parturition.

Worldwide Distribution

Gingivitis associated with extensive plaque and calculus deposits is most prevalent, extensive, and severe in developing countries and populations with limited access to health education and dental care (Fig. 3-1).[50,51,53,69-75] Data from national surveys in the United States suggest that improvements in overall oral hygiene and access to preventive dental care have resulted in a tendency toward a decline in gingival inflammation.[76]

EPIDEMIOLOGY OF AGGRESSIVE PERIODONTITIS

Aggressive periodontitis, which occurs in otherwise healthy patients, is characterized by rapid clinical attachment loss and bone destruction.[77,78] The true incidence or even prevalence of aggressive periodontitis is difficult to determine from published reports for many of the same reasons that will be discussed in the context of chronic periodontitis. These include the following:

- Most surveys were cross sectional in nature, making it impossible to determine the *rate* of disease progression. Rates of disease progression can only be determined through prospective or careful retrospective evaluations of individuals. Furthermore, the extent to which the rate of disease in aggressive periodontitis must exceed that seen in chronic lesions has not been specified.
- Different tools (e.g., probes, radiographs) have been used to assess participants.
- A variety of diagnostic criteria have been used to define this disease.
- In many surveys, especially the largest ones, cases were identified using partial-mouth examination protocols. Although data from such evaluations can be used to estimate the *severity* of disease (i.e., mean clinical attachment loss) or treatment needs in a population, they can grossly underestimate the *prevalence* of disease.[72]

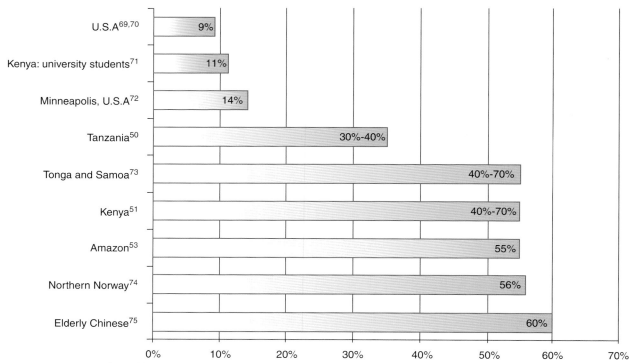

Figure 3-1. Mean percent of sites bleeding on probing per person in adult populations.

These substantive differences among studies also limit the ability to make rigorous comparisons across studies. Furthermore, surveys that relied solely on radiographic findings likely underestimated the prevalence of the disease because early lesions may not be visible on radiographs. The reliability of pocket probing also limits accurate reporting of individuals with incipient disease. Between 2 and 3 mm of clinical attachment level must be recorded before a site is considered, with statistical confidence, to be diseased or progressing. Reliability of the assessment method is a particularly critical issue in longitudinal surveys designed to identify risk factors or prognostic factors, because few tooth sites or individuals experience more than 2 mm of attachment loss over 1 to 2 years.[79]

Because the diagnosis of aggressive periodontitis is based principally on the rate of progression rather than the pattern or severity of disease, it may be inadequate to establish a diagnosis based on data collected at a single time point. For example, in a six-year follow-up of a national survey of aggressive periodontitis, initial disease classifications were not predictive of the rate of progression over the next 6 years.[80] More specifically, one third to one half of adolescents originally diagnosed with localized or generalized disease showed minimal or no disease progression during the follow-up period. The authors concluded that localized and generalized aggressive periodontitis consist of both rapidly and slowly progressing forms within each classification.

Finally, there have been no studies that followed clinically healthy subjects to determine the incidence of aggressive periodontitis. It has been estimated that the incidence rate of radiographic bone loss in young adults (but not necessarily aggressive periodontitis) is 6% over 8 years.[81] Unfortunately, only a small fraction of subjects originally examined in this study were available for follow-up assessments. Rather surprisingly, only 3 of 26 subjects with bone loss at baseline had persistent lesions 8 years later. Such findings are either because of error in the assessment method or the transiency of some lesions. Either cause makes it difficult to accurately estimate from radiographs the incidence of bone loss in adolescents.

Worldwide Distribution

Worldwide, aggressive periodontitis appears to be more prevalent in black individuals, including those of African, African-American, or Afro-Caribbean heritage, than in white individuals (Table 3-1). Scandinavians and whites individuals of northern European descent are infrequently affected. There is insufficient evidence, however, to determine if these differences are attributable to disparities in socioeconomic factors or access to dental care.

Age

Aggressive periodontitis can occur at any age. Most surveys, however, focus on disease forms previously referred

TABLE 3-1	Estimated Prevalence of Aggressive Periodontitis in Selected Populations	
POPULATION	**PREVALENCE**	**REFERENCES**
• U.S. African Americans	• 2.1-2.6%	• 82, 83
• U.S. whites	• 0.09-0.17%	• 82, 83
• Swiss	• 0.1%	• 84
• Dutch	• 0.1-0.2%	• 85
• Norwegian	• 0-0.2%	• 86, 87
• Finnish	• 0.1%	• 88
• Danish	• 0.1%	• 89
• Chileans	• 0.32%	• 90
• Brazilians	• 0.32-3.7%	• 91, 92
• Saudis	• 0.42%	• 93
• Japanese	• 0.47%	• 94
• Italians	• 0.51%	• 95
• Nigerians	• 0.75-0.8%	• 96
• Afro-Caribbean	• 0.80%	• 97
• Ugandans (blacks)	• 6.5%	• 98

to as juvenile or early-onset periodontitis, which by definition occur only in adolescents and young adults. Among adolescents, the frequency of affected individuals usually increases from puberty to about 25 years of age.[88] Unfortunately, there are no good estimates of the prevalence in adults, which makes it impossible to determine the age-dependent risk for the disease in individuals older than about 25 years.

Aggressive disease in adolescents usually starts as a localized condition, affecting primarily the first molars and incisors. The disease can remain localized, or spread over time to affect teeth other than incisors and first molars.[99] In younger adolescents, therefore, the localized form is usually found more frequently than the generalized form.[83] A follow-up study of aggressive disease in adolescents and young adults highlights this point.[99] Over a 6-year period, the disease became more severe and extensive. Existing lesions became more advanced and more of the teeth unaffected at baseline exhibited periodontal attachment loss at follow-up, thus changing the disease characteristics and the basis for the clinical classification. About 35% of the subjects with localized aggressive disease at baseline experienced disease progression around teeth other than first molars and incisors and were hence reclassified at the follow-up visit as having generalized disease. About one fourth of subjects who initially had some attachment loss—but whose pattern did not meet the criteria for localized or generalized disease—developed localized or generalized periodontitis in the ensuing period. These findings indicate that the localized and generalized forms of aggressive periodontitis may be variants of the same condition and not distinct

entities, and that cases need to be followed over time before definitive diagnoses are established.

Sex

Although few studies have identified enough cases to make robust comparisons between male and female cases, it appears there is no sex predilection for aggressive periodontitis. Although some investigators found the disease to be more common in female than male cases,[92,100] others claim the opposite.[83,98] In a large survey of U.S. adolescents, male adolescents were found to be more likely than female adolescents to have generalized but not localized disease.[83]

Most early surveys of aggressive periodontitis, which report a preponderance of affected female cases, sampled subjects from dental clinic populations. When this selection bias is eliminated, however, the number of affected male and female individuals in the population is found to be similar.[101]

Race/Ethnicity

Does the prevalence of aggressive periodontitis differ by race or ethnicity? The answer seems simple; one could simply compare the frequency of disease among ethnic or racial groups. Most surveys, however, either sample from a single racial or ethnic group or do not sample adequate numbers of subjects from separate groups. As discussed previously, because of substantive methodologic differences, comparisons across studies must be made cautiously.

Only two surveys, both conducted in the United States, have been large enough to permit a robust comparison among racial groups. Between 5,000 and 11,000 youths or young adults were included in these surveys. Although one used clinical probing and the other radiographs to screen subjects, both reported that black individuals were more likely than white individuals to have aggressive periodontitis.[82,83] The prevalence of aggressive periodontitis in these studies ranged from 2.1% to 2.9% in black and 0.09% to 0.17% in white individuals (see Table 3-1). Similar conclusions can be gleaned from the literature, where black individuals, including those of African, African-American or Afro-Caribbean heritage, and Hispanics appear to be at greater risk than white individuals. Whereas the prevalence in white youths is generally 0.2% or less,[83,102] the disease has been reported to affect up to 6.5% of African[98] and 3.7 % of South American youths.

Socioeconomic Status

In the general population, the extent and severity of periodontitis is inversely related to educational level attained and income. Children from low socioeconomic strata (SES) also appear to be at greater risk for attachment loss, but not necessarily aggressive periodontitis. That is, the pattern of disease in these children is more consistent with an early presentation of chronic periodontitis rather than aggressive periodontitis.[95] This increased risk likely reflects income-related differences in access to dental care, and socioeconomic factors could be considered, at best, risk indicators and not risk factors for disease. That is, lack of education or income or low SES status *per se* does not cause disease.

A few studies have examined whether SES is a risk indicator for aggressive periodontitis, and the findings have been mixed. Although the disease is reportedly more common in impoverished than nonimpoverished South American populations,[90,103] it has recently been reported that no association exists between risk for disease and SES in schoolchildren in Uganda.[98] Before drawing specific conclusions from such surveys, however, one should carefully consider both the sampling strategy used and the number of cases identified. For example, although aggressive periodontitis was reported to be greater in schoolchildren in Chile from lower rather than upper income strata, only eight cases were identified in the entire survey.[90]

Disease Trends

Although there are a number of reports detailing changes in prevalence rates of gingivitis, attachment loss, and bone loss in children and adults over time, none has addressed aggressive periodontitis specifically. Currently, it is unknown if the prevalence of this disease has increased, decreased, or remained unchanged over the years. One study of 16-year-old cohorts found that the prevalence rate of marginal bone loss was unchanged from 1975 to 1988,[104] but this study was not limited to aggressive periodontitis.

Diabetes Mellitus

Although people with diabetes, especially those with long-standing poor metabolic control, may be at increased risk for periodontitis in general,[105] diabetes mellitus has not been established as a risk factor for aggressive periodontitis. Adolescents with type 1 (insulin-dependent) diabetes generally have more gingival inflammation than healthy control subjects; a finding that may be more closely related to metabolic control than the presence of diabetes *per se*.[106,107] Currently, there are no data from large-scale epidemiologic surveys to determine if patients with diabetes (either type 1 or type 2) are more or less likely to have aggressive periodontitis.

Tobacco Use

There is strong evidence that smoking is a risk factor for chronic periodontitis. The role of smoking in aggressive periodontitis, however, is less clear. One reason is that many individuals with aggressive disease may be too young to smoke or to have significant pack-year smoking histories.

Nonetheless, there is some evidence that smoking can alter the severity and extent of generalized aggressive disease.[108] When compared with nonsmokers, the disease tends to be more extensive and severe in the maxilla of smokers with generalized aggressive disease.[109,110] Smokers with aggressive periodontitis also tend to harbor more periodontal pathogens than nonsmokers with disease.[110] Overall, smoking also tends to suppress serum immunoglobulin levels, including those specific against periodontal pathogens. The impact of smoking on IgG levels is particularly pronounced in black smokers with generalized aggressive disease.[111] Smoking does not appear to influence the severity of disease in subjects with localized aggressive periodontitis.[108] In summary, it is unclear if smoking is a risk factor for aggressive periodontitis. Among persons with the disease, however, smokers tend to have more severe and widespread disease, especially in the maxilla.

Oral Hygiene

Currently, no associations between aggressive periodontitis and oral hygiene have been established, and it is unknown whether good oral hygiene by itself can reduce the incidence of aggressive periodontitis. Clinicians have recognized that aggressive periodontitis can occur in otherwise healthy young individuals who display good oral hygiene. However, most surveys have not reported measures of plaque or calculus. It is entirely possible that many cases reported in the literature were associated with heavy plaque and calculus, and were thus more likely to represent chronic rather than aggressive disease.

Genetic Epidemiology of Aggressive Periodontitis

The evidence that genetic factors affect risk for aggressive periodontitis can be summarized as follows:

- The prevalence rate of disease is greater in first-degree relatives (parents, siblings, and offspring) of affected individuals than in the general population.
- The disease is a consistent feature in several genetic or inherited disorders.
- Segregation analyses implicate the role of a major gene.
- Several genetic polymorphisms have been associated with the disease.
- At least one form of disease, which cosegregates with dentinogenesis imperfecta, has been linked to a specific region on a chromosome.

Aggressive periodontitis clearly tends to run in families.[112] Familial clustering alone, however, does not prove that genes or inheritance affects the risk for disease. Clustering can occur if the disease has an heritable or genetic component or if important environmental or behavioral risk factors are shared within families. Significantly, the transmission of pathogenic microorganisms within families may explain part of the observed familial aggregation for this disease. Currently, genetic studies have examined the role of genes or microbes, but not both. More sophisticated models that address both inherited factors and family-correlated environmental risk factors must be applied to begin to understand how genes and the environment act and interact to affect risk for these diseases.

Segregation analyses are used to determine whether the occurrence of disease in families is consistent with the action of autosomal or sex-linked genes, and whether the putative disease alleles are dominant or recessive. Results from such analyses of aggressive periodontitis have implicated the role of a major gene effect.[112-114] Statistical models that assume the disease is caused by environmental factors alone, or by the additive action of many genes, do not adequately explain the distribution of the disease within families. The specific mode of inheritance, however, is less clear. Autosomal dominant, autosomal recessive, and X-linked dominant modes of inheritance have been proposed for this disease.[112-117] In the largest U.S. study to date, autosomal dominant inheritance was favored in both African-American and white populations.[112] The estimated frequency of the disease allele was significantly greater in African Americans, which reflects the greater prevalence of disease in this group. The disparate results from segregation analyses may be because of inadequate statistical power, the use of inadequate statistical models for this complex multifactorial disease, or true genetic heterogeneity. *Genetic heterogeneity* means that there are multiple underlying genetic causes that lead to the same clinical presentation of disease. Given that clinical criteria and not biologic markers define the periodontal diseases, it is likely that aggressive periodontitis, as currently defined, is indeed a group of genetically heterogeneous conditions.

Linkage analyses are used to localize disease-causing alleles to specific locations on a chromosome. In linkage studies, individuals are characterized both phenotypically (i.e., by disease status) and genotypically (through typing of polymorphic genetic markers). There have been few linkage studies of aggressive periodontitis. In one such study of a multigenerational, triracial family, linkage between the putative aggressive periodontitis allele and a region on the long arm of chromosome 4 was established.[116] The family members in this report, however, also had dentinogenesis imperfecta, which is not associated with aggressive periodontitis in the general population. Linkage to this chromosomal region could not be verified in another sample population.[118] Despite its implied existence from segregation analyses, no major disease allele has been identified for aggressive periodontitis in outbred populations.

Aggressive periodontitis is a consistent feature in a number of inherited or genetic disorders (Box 3-9). The rapid periodontal destruction associated with these disorders demonstrates that genetic mutations can substantially affect risk for aggressive periodontitis. Typically, however, affected individuals have a number of systemic or organ problems in addition to aggressive periodontitis. Fortunately, these disorders are not common and the particular mutations that cause these conditions are too rare to be of value in predicting risk in the general population. Researchers instead have studied more common genetic variations, or polymorphisms. Whereas the term *gene mutation* usually connotes a sequence alteration that produces a deleterious phenotype, common polymorphisms often do not profoundly affect phenotype. Rather, they code for the variations that can be considered to define the range of "normal" within a population.

Given the vast extent of variation in the human genome—there are an estimated three million single nucleotide polymorphisms in the human genome—random searches for associations with aggressive periodontitis are unlikely to be productive. Rather, investigators have focused on polymorphisms that reside in or near candidate genes—that is, those that play some role in pathogenesis of disease. For periodontitis, candidate genes are typically those that control the expression of tissue-degrading enzymes or inflammatory mediators (e.g., cytokines) or that code for receptors or proteins activated by bacterial antigens. These candidate gene polymorphisms may be located in the coding, promoter, or regulatory regions of genes, and alter either the amino acid sequence of the protein product or the efficiency of gene transcription. The case-control study design has been exploited in the search for associations between such candidate markers and aggressive periodontitis. However, these analyses are less powerful and unreliable than the genetic linkage studies.

Polymorphisms in genetic regions that encode interleukin-1 (IL-1),[119] the vitamin D receptor,[120] the N-formyl-methionyl-leucyl-phenylalanine (FMLP) receptor,[121] and the Fcγ receptor[122] have been associated with either localized or generalized aggressive periodontitis (Table 3-2). Results from these and other studies, however, have been both inconsistent and often contradictory. Currently, the risk for aggressive periodontitis attributed to any single genetic polymorphism has not been reliably determined. For example, an IL-1B allele—specifically, the more common allele 1 at a polymorphic site 3,954 base pairs "downstream" from the start of the *IL-1B* gene—has been reported to be in linkage disequilibrium with generalized aggressive periodontitis.[119] This finding suggests that at least one disease allele is at or very close to this polymorphism. This "high-risk" IL-1B allele, however, was not found to be associated with generalized disease in a northern European population[127] and may be too common in African Americans to be of any predictive value.[128]

Box 3-9   Aggressive Periodontitis Associated with Genetic Disorders

Disorder	Protein Affected by Gene Mutation
Leukocyte adhesion deficiencies:	
Type I	CD18 (β2 integrin chain of the LFA molecule)
Type II	CD15 (neutrophil ligand for E and P selectins)
Acatalasia	Catalase enzyme
Chediak-Higashi syndrome	Unknown, the mutation in the lysosomal trafficking regulator gene results in abnormal transport of vesicles to neutrophil lysosomes
Ehler-Danlos syndrome [types IV and VIII]	Type III collagen
Papillion-Lefèvre syndrome	Cathepsin C (dipeptidyl aminopeptidase I)
Hypophosphatasia	Tissue nonspecific alkaline phosphatase
Prepubertal periodontitis (nonsyndromic)	Cathepsin C

TABLE 3-2   Associations (Linkage Disequilibrium) between Aggressive Periodontitis (Localized and/or Generalized) and Genetic Polymorphisms

GENES	FINDING CONFIRMED BY MORE THAN ONE POPULATION OR STUDY?	REFERENCES
IL-1A, IL-1B	No	119
HLA-DRB1 and DQB1	No	123
Vitamin D receptor	Partially*	120, 124
N-formyl peptide receptor	No	121
Fc γ receptor	No	122
IL-1 receptor antagonist	No	125
IL-4	No	126

*Both studies reported greater carriage rates for the minor (t) allele in cases than control subjects, although Hennig and colleagues[120] found the association in localized, but not generalized, aggressive disease. HLA, human leukocyte antigen; IL, interleukin.

The human leukocyte antigens (HLAs) have long been considered candidate markers for aggressive periodontitis. Again, however, there have been few consistent findings among the many studies of these antigens. This inconsistency may be because of false-positive findings, differences in the racial or ethnic makeup of the study groups, differences in the clinical criteria used to define cases, or true heterogeneity. Only two antigens, HLA-A9 and HLA-B15, repeatedly have been found to occur more frequently in cases than control subjects.[129] In contrast, the HLA-A2 antigen appears less frequently in cases than in control subjects, which suggests this antigen may somehow be protective against disease.[130,131] The DR4 (a Class II) antigen has also been reported to be more prevalent in Israeli and Turkish patients than control subjects,[132,133] although others have not found this association in other populations.[134]

It is important to remember that aggressive periodontitis is a complex, multifactorial disease. It seems rather simplistic to believe that one disease-allele will be found to confer more than a mild increase in risk for disease in the general population. It is likely that several or many disease alleles act and interact to affect risk for disease. Furthermore, alleles that confer some increased risk in one population may not do so in another. The search for disease alleles for aggressive periodontitis remains a daunting task. It is imperative that, before any genetic marker or allele is considered a risk factor for aggressive periodontitis, its association (or linkage) is confirmed in multiple studies, preferably of different populations. The importance of recognizing and controlling important environmental risk factors for aggressive periodontitis must not be overlooked.

EPIDEMIOLOGY OF CHRONIC PERIODONTITIS

Most epidemiologic studies conducted between 1950 and 1970 used Russell's PI to characterize the periodontal conditions of populations. Periodontitis was found to be strongly associated with poor oral hygiene, calculus, low SES, and lack of access to dental care and education.[135-139]

These studies also reported that U.S. adults had very low disease scores,[135,137] Latin-American countries had intermediate scores, and most Middle Eastern and Asian populations had very high scores.[137] Interestingly, the periodontal conditions of "primitive Eskimos" from rural Alaska were similar to U.S. adults and significantly better than that of urban Eskimos.[137] In general, however, groups with limited access to dental care and those from developing nations were found to have more disease than populations from industrialized countries.[135,137] These differences were attributed primarily to differences in plaque control among the groups.[137] However, these results and conclusions should be viewed with caution. As previously discussed, differences in disease levels, especially when scored using Russell's PI, may be driven by differences in plaque levels leading to gingivitis rather than true differences in attachment levels or bone loss.

The model of the pathogenesis of periodontitis in the 1950s to 1970s was predicated on the following beliefs:
- All individuals were equally susceptible to periodontitis.
- Long-standing gingivitis invariably progresses to periodontitis with subsequent tooth loss. Gingivitis and periodontitis were regarded as different stages of the same disease.
- Susceptibility to periodontal disease increases with increasing age.
- Risk for periodontal disease was determined by environmental factors alone. Poor oral hygiene and age were believed to account for 90% of the differences among individuals.[137]

These concepts have been challenged by more recent research indicating the following: (1) all individuals are *not* equally susceptible to periodontitis; (2) only a small percentage of sites with untreated gingivitis will develop periodontitis; (3) even though periodontitis is more prevalent, extensive, and severe among older persons, the susceptibility to future periodontal breakdown seems to be independent of age; and (4) periodontal disease is a complex disease and only a portion of the variability of disease in the population can be attributed to environmental exposures (e.g., Gram-negative bacteria, oral hygiene, dental care, smoking, and others), whereas the remaining variation is attributed to differences in host susceptibility.

All individuals are not equally susceptible to development of periodontal disease. In a longitudinal study of Sri Lankan tea laborers with no access to dental care and poor oral hygiene, it was observed that subgroups of individuals could be defined based on their rates of disease progression.[140] In this environmentally homogeneous population, some persons had disease development at rapid rates, whereas others experienced little progression. A total of 11% of the subjects had slow progression, 81% were categorized as having "moderate" progression, and the remaining 8% experienced "rapid" progression (Fig. 3-2). In both

the rapidly and moderately progressing disease groups, the disease process was not self-limiting; it progressed until multiple teeth or the entire dentition was lost (Fig. 3-3).[140]

When these individuals from Sri Lanka were compared with a group of Norwegian scholars and students with optimal personal and professional dental care,[140-142] the rate of clinical attachment loss was found to be two to four times greater in the Sri Lankan sample. Even persons with "moderate" progression by age 41 to 45 years had a mean clinical attachment loss of 5.4 mm. In contrast, the mean clinical attachment loss in U.S. adults in this age group ranges from 1.1 to 1.6 mm.[70]

These classic reports on the natural history of periodontitis elucidated two important features of this disease: (1) severe disease tends to cluster in a small fraction of the population; and (2) there may be pronounced differences in disease susceptibility within a population that are independent of the environment. Both principles have been subsequently documented in treated and untreated populations.* However, the findings in these Sri Lankan individuals may not be representative of all untreated populations. Although extensive and early onset disease has also been reported in persons in Nigeria[145] and Polynesia[73] with limited access to dental care, other studies suggest that people in developing countries do not necessarily have severe periodontal destruction, despite having extensive plaque, calculus, and gingivitis. An analysis of 154 independent surveys conducted in 79 countries revealed little differences between developing and industrialized countries in the prevalence of periodontal pockets 6 mm or deeper among 35- to 44-year-old persons.[146] Furthermore, studies of Tanzanians, Kenyans and Guinea-Bissauans, and Amazonians revealed that the extent and severity of disease in these populations was only slightly worse than that found in industrialized countries or regions.[50-53,147] Figure 3-4 compares the mean clinical attachment loss for various untreated and treated populations; similar relations are observed when the extent of clinical attachment loss of these populations is compared.

It is apparent from the study of skull specimens that humans have experienced alveolar bone loss since at least the Neolithic period (5800-3000 BC).[148] Studies of ancient populations indicate that, despite the presence of massive calculus deposits, only a small fraction of individuals had severe periodontal destruction.[149,150] An evaluation of 1,149 ancient skulls from around the world revealed that only 10% to 26% of the teeth studied displayed severe bone loss; 65% of the teeth in people 46 years age or older had only slight bone loss.[149] Prehistoric remains from

---

*See References 35, 50, 51, 53, 75, 143, and 144.

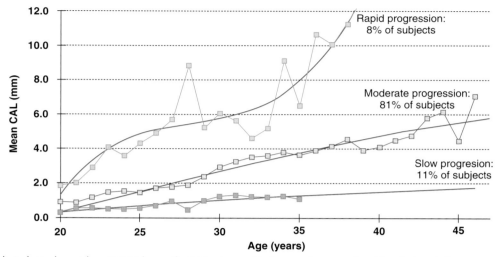

Figure 3-2. Mean clinical attachment loss (CAL)* by age for Sri Lankans with slow, moderate, and rapid periodontal disease progression (n = 480). Solid lines represent trends in mean CAL generated by second- and third-degree polynomial functions. (*From Löe H, Anerud A, Boysen H: Natural history of periodontal disease in man. Rapid, moderate and no loss of attachment in Sri Lankan laborers 14 to 46 years of age,* J Clin Periodontol 13:431, 1986.)

Eskimos[150] and archeological material from Scottish medieval populations (900-1600 AD) and more recent English populations (1645-1852 AD) also reveal that relatively few individuals had severe periodontal destruction.[151,152] Such archeological material also suggests that the prevalence or severity of periodontal diseases has not changed significantly throughout human history.

In summary, when compared with groups with ready access to dental care, individuals with limited access to dental care and those from underdeveloped or undevel-

oped regions have, on average, more plaque, calculus, and gingival inflammation. Although they also tend to have more severe periodontal disease (i.e., clinical attachment loss, bone loss, and pockets), these differences are less pronounced. The majority of individuals in these untreated populations have extensive plaque, calculus, and long-standing gingivitis, yet do not develop severe periodontitis. Therefore, destructive periodontal disease should not be considered as an invariable consequence of long-standing gingival inflammation.[153] Periodontitis is,

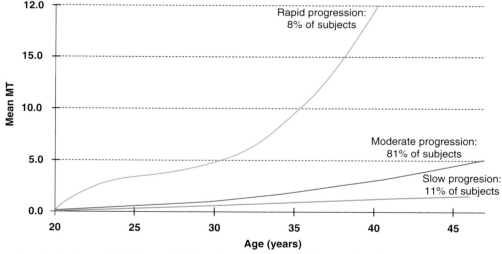

Figure 3-3. Mean number of missing teeth (MT) by age for Sri Lankans with slow, moderate, and rapid periodontal disease progression (n = 480). Lines represent trends in mean CAL generated by linear (for slow progression group), second- (for moderate progression group), and third-degree (for rapid progression group) polynomial functions. (*From Löe H, Anerud A, Boysen H: Natural history of periodontal disease in man. Rapid, moderate and no loss of attachment in Sri Lankan laborers 14 to 46 years of age,* J Clin Periodontol 13:431, 1986.)

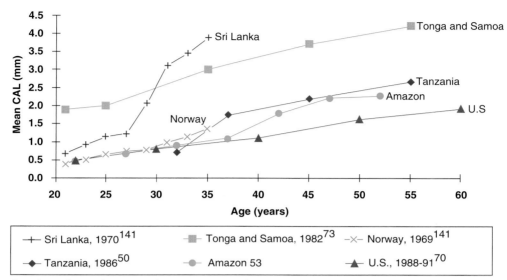

Figure 3-4. Mean clinical attachment loss (CAL) by age in six population samples. (*Adapted from Ronderos M, Pihlstrom BL, Hodges JS: Periodontal disease among indigenous people in the Amazon rain forest, J Clin Periodontol 28:995, 2001.*)

however, almost invariably preceded by gingivitis, and gingival inflammation (i.e., BOP) has some predictive value for determining future attachment loss among patients receiving supportive periodontal therapy.[154]

Although it has been suggested that the extent and severity of periodontitis has gradually declined in the United States and Norway,[76,155] the evidence to support this claim is not strong. Furthermore, despite improvements in oral hygiene and access to dental care, the absolute number and the percentage of U.S. adults with periodontitis may be on the increase because of increases in life expectancies, decreases in caries rates, and increase in the percentage of dentate seniors.[156]

According to the most recent U.S. national survey, 35% of adults older than 30 years have periodontitis, with 22% having a mild form and 13% having moderate to severe forms (Fig. 3-5).[4] As previously discussed, however, the estimated prevalence of diseases depends on the threshold used to define affected teeth and individuals and on the examination methods used in the study. Because only a portion of the dentition was examined in this national survey, these figures are an underestimation of the true prevalence of disease.

The following sections describe the population distribution of periodontal disease and various risk factors and risk indicators for the disease (Table 3-3).

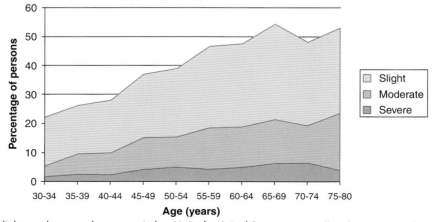

Figure 3-5. Prevalence of slight, moderate, and severe periodontitis in the United States. (*From Albandar JM, Brunelle JA, Kingman A: Destructive periodontal disease in adults 30 years of age and older in the United States, 1988-1994, J Periodontol 70:13, 1999.*)

TABLE 3-3	Factors Associated with Chronic Periodontitis	
VARIABLE	TYPE OF ASSOCIATION	COMMENTS
Age	Positive association *Risk indicator*	As age increases, the prevalence, extent and severity of chronic periodontitis also increase. However, the rate of progression or the likelihood of disease progression is not related to the age of an individual. Age is a poor predictor of future disease.
Sex	Males tend to have more periodontal disease than females. *Risk indicator*	This association has been observed in the United States and other populations from industrialized nations. However, this association is not consistently found in populations with limited access to dental care. This association is most likely related to behavioral differences between males and females.
Socioeconomic status (SES), education, and access to dental care	Negative association *Risk indicator*	Groups of lower SES, less education, and limited access to dental care have more periodontal tissue destruction.
Race-ethnicity	In the United States the prevalence, extent, and severity of periodontal tissue destruction is greatest among African Americans, intermediate among Mexican Americans and lowest among white individuals. *Risk indicator*	Such differences may be because of discrepancies in access to dental care and education.
Tobacco use	Positive association *Risk factor*	Strongest modifiable risk factor and predictor of future disease and periodontal treatment outcomes.
Diabetes	Positive association *Risk factor*	Patients with diabetes, especially those with poor glycemic control and type 1 (insulin-dependent) diabetes, tend to have more periodontal tissue destruction.
HIV-infection	Positive association *Risk factor*	HIV-positive patients, especially those who are not receiving medical treatment, those with CD4+ counts <200 cells/μl and those who are severely immunocompromised, are at increased risk for periodontitis.
Osteoporosis	Positive association *Possible risk factor*	Among females with high calculus scores, those with osteoporosis and osteopenia have more attachment loss than control subjects with normal bone density.
Psychological stress	Positive association *Possible risk factor*	Weak association.

Age

Clinical attachment loss and alveolar bone loss become more prevalent, extensive, and severe with advancing age.[4] Figures 3-6 to 3-9 summarize the prevalence and extent of clinical attachment loss and periodontal pockets for U.S. adults.[4] Although early loss can occur before the age of 20 years,[141] by 30 to 39 years of age at least two thirds of U.S. adults have 1 or more sites with clinical attachment loss of 2 mm or more (see Fig. 3-6).[4] By contrast, the prevalence, extent, and severity of pathologic pocketing increase only slightly with increasing age (see Figs. 3-8 and 3-9).[53,70] On average, therefore, clinical attachment loss appears to be more commonly associated with gingival recession than with pocket deepening.

Although age is strongly associated with periodontal disease, aging *per se* is not likely to be a predisposing factor for periodontal disease. Because attachment loss and bone loss are not fully reversible with treatment, they may reflect the cumulative effects of past tissue destruction more so than current disease activity. The association between age and disease is strong because age, more than any other variable, directly reflects how long an individual has been exposed to etiologic factors. In fact, even in untreated populations, young and older adults lose periodontal support at similar rates.[157-160]

Aging also does not appear to affect the outcome of periodontal therapy. Despite this, however, age should always be considered when assessing a patient's susceptibility to periodontitis. For example, a 35-year-old patient

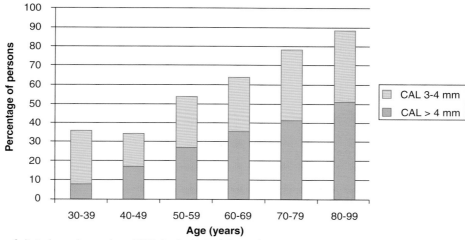

Figure 3-6. Prevalence of clinical attachment loss (CAL) in the United States by age. (*From Albandar JM, Brunelle JA, Kingman A: Destructive periodontal disease in adults 30 years of age and older in the United States, 1988-1994,* J Periodontol *70:13, 1999.*)

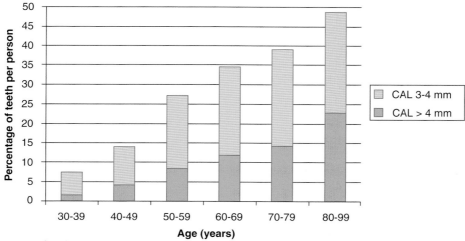

Figure 3-7. Extent: Percentage of teeth with clinical attachment loss (CAL) in the United States by age. (*From Albandar JM, Brunelle JA, Kingman A: Destructive periodontal disease in adults 30 years of age and older in the United States, 1988-1994,* J Periodontol *70:13, 1999.*)

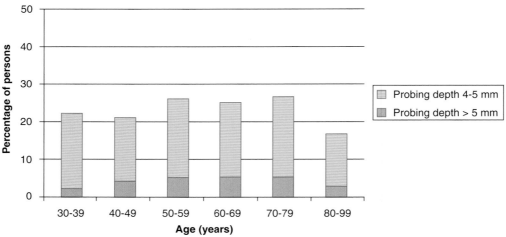

Figure 3-8. Prevalence of periodontal pockets in the United States by age. (*From Albandar JM, Brunelle JA, Kingman A: Destructive periodontal disease in adults 30 years of age and older in the United States, 1988-1994,* J Periodontol 70:13, 1999.)

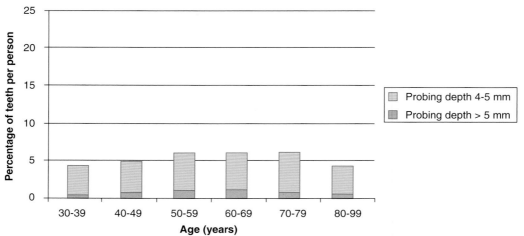

Figure 3-9. Extent: Percentage of teeth with periodontal pockets in the United States by age. (*From Albandar JM, Brunelle JA, Kingman A: Destructive periodontal disease in adults 30 years of age and older in the United States, 1988-1994,* J Periodontol 70:13, 1999.)

with generalized moderate periodontitis is more susceptible to disease than a 55-year-old patient with the same severity and extent of disease. Furthermore, more cases of aggressive forms of periodontitis are generally seen in younger age groups.

Sex

In the United States and in most industrialized populations, male individuals of every age group have more attachment loss, deeper pockets, and more bleeding on probing than females.[4] However, such differences have not been observed in all untreated populations and developing nations.[33,161] This suggests that sex differences arise from behavioral differences, culturally related or otherwise, and not because of true differences in predisposition to the disease. For example, it has been reported

that in the United States male individuals have poorer oral hygiene and more calculus than females.[162,163]

Socioeconomic Status, Dental Care, and Race

Personal income, educational level, and occupation all contribute to designation of SES. In most societies, access to health care is intimately related to SES. Periodontitis is more severe and widespread in groups from low SES strata, in those with less education, and in those who visit the dentist infrequently.[69,144,164-166] Socioeconomic differences may also be the root of racial differences in the prevalence of periodontal diseases that have been consistently reported in the United States. The prevalence, extent, and severity of periodontitis in the United States are greatest in black, intermediate in Mexican American, and least in white individuals.[4]

Interestingly, attachment loss in white individuals tends to be most severe on the facial aspect of teeth and is frequently associated with gingival recession. In black individuals, however, the most severe loss is found on proximal tooth surfaces and is associated with periodontal pockets.[4] All of these racial/ethnic differences are most likely the result of socioeconomic differences, education, and disparity in access to health care rather than true differences in disease susceptibility (e.g., genetic differences). Racial minorities also tend to have more plaque, calculus, and gingivitis. When the periodontal conditions of white, black, and Mexican American individuals are compared after standardizing for income, frequency of dental visits, and calculus, most of the differences in disease severity disappear (Fig. 3-10).[163]

Oral Hygiene, Calculus, and Gingival Inflammation

Bacterial plaque is both necessary and sufficient to cause *gingivitis*. However, undisturbed bacterial plaque alone is not sufficient to cause *periodontitis*. Plaque plays a central role in the initiation of gingival inflammation[38] and calculus formation,[167] and poor plaque control has been shown to have a deleterious effect on the success of periodontal treatment.[168] Furthermore, periodontal disease is preventable in most individuals through a combination of frequent professional care and improved oral hygiene.[169] However, the independent effect of oral hygiene in preventing periodontitis has not been established. A few reports indicate that persons with greater plaque scores are more likely to experience progressive periodontal disease.[159,170] Most longitudinal[22,160,171] and cross-sectional studies of treated[144,166,172-175] and untreated[50-53,73,75,176] populations, however, indicate that supragingival plaque scores correlate poorly with periodontal destruction. Furthermore, a recent study failed to detect an association between oral hygiene practices reported by subjects and the presence of periodontitis.[177] Although supragingival

plaque plays a central role in the occurrence and prevention of gingivitis, it has not been clearly established as a strong risk factor for periodontitis.[2]

In treated and untreated populations, persons with high calculus scores tend to have the most clinical attachment loss and bone loss.[53,144,176] In fact, calculus may be more strongly associated with attachment loss and bone loss than supragingival plaque.[53,178] Similarly, gingival inflammation appears to be a good clinical predictor of future loss of attachment.[159] It is not surprising that calculus and gingival inflammation are better predictors of periodontal disease than plaque scores. Calculus and gingival indexes are generally the result of the presence of undisturbed mature plaque and the lack of preventive periodontal therapy.[38,167] In most cases, calculus and gingival inflammation are surrogate indicators of the quality of the plaque control performed by a subject during the weeks before the examination. Meanwhile, plaque scores represent a point estimate of the oral hygiene at the examination. The lack of association between plaque scores and clinical attachment loss may be because plaque-scoring systems are poor "predictors." However, this does not necessarily mean that bacterial plaque itself is not an important determinant.

Tobacco Use

Cigarette smoking is the strongest modifiable risk factor for the occurrence of periodontal disease. People who smoke are two to six times more likely to have periodontitis than those who do not smoke.[144,160,179-181] This relation is independent of potential confounders including oral hygiene. In other words, even in subjects with good oral hygiene, smokers have significantly more bone loss than nonsmokers.[182] Smoking is related to periodontal disease in a dose-related manner. As the number of years exposed to tobacco and the number of cigarettes smoked per day increase, so does the risk for development of severe periodontitis.[144] Cigar and pipe smoking also seem to have a harmful effect

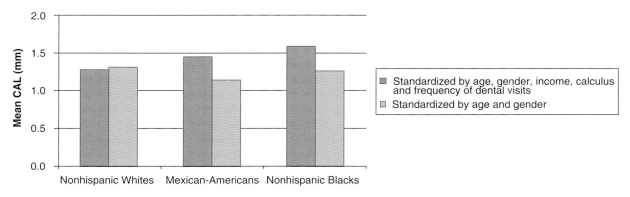

Figure 3-10. Effect of poverty-income ratio, frequency of dental visits, and calculus scores on the racial differences in mean clinical attachment levels (CAL) in the United States. (*From the U.S. Department of Health and Human Services (DHHS), Centers for Disease Control and Prevention. National Center for Health Statistics. Third National Health and Nutrition Examination Survey, 1988-1994, NHANES III Data File (CD ROM). Public Use Data File Documentation No. 76200. Hyattsville, Md, 1996, Centers for Disease Control and Prevention.*)

on the periodontium.[183,184] Furthermore, smokeless tobacco (e.g., chewing tobacco, snuff) has been associated with gingival recession and attachment loss at tooth sites that come into direct contact with the tobacco.[185] Tobacco use has also been proven to adversely affect the outcomes of periodontal treatment and increase the chances of disease recurrences among treated populations.[186]

The deleterious effects of tobacco on periodontal health are most likely because of an induced impairment in the host immune response.[187,188] Although constituents of tobacco smoke may directly or indirectly influence bacterial colonization in the oral cavity, this pathway to increased disease risk is debatable. Some studies have reported that the periodontal microbiota is different in smokers and nonsmokers,[189,190] whereas studies have shown that the rate of recovery of periodontal pathogens from relatively shallow pockets is greater in smokers.[191] However, not all studies have found the microbiota to be different in smokers and nonsmokers.[14,192]

Diabetes Mellitus

Individuals with diabetes, especially those with poor metabolic control, have more extensive and severe periodontal destruction than otherwise healthy persons[144,193,194] (see Chapter 31). The most prevalent forms of diabetes are type 1 (formerly insulin-dependent) and type 2 (formerly noninsulin-dependent) diabetes mellitus. The onset of type 1 diabetes generally occurs before 30 years of age, whereas the more common type 2 diabetes peaks in incidence during the fifth decade of life. Patients with either type are at increased risk for periodontitis. However, the deleterious effect of diabetes on the periodontium appears to be cumulative, because patients with long-term diabetes tend to have greater attachment or bone loss than those who have had diabetes for shorter periods.[195]

The metabolic control of diabetes is also strongly related to the incidence and severity of periodontal disease.[196,197] Patients with diabetes who have retinopathy, nephropathy, and other complications (all signs of less than ideal glycemic control) have significantly more periodontal destruction than patients with well controlled diabetes.[66] In contrast, patients with well controlled diabetes have similar levels of periodontitis to individuals without diabetes.[198]

Perhaps the most comprehensive epidemiologic studies of type 2 diabetes and periodontitis have been conducted among the Pima Indians in Arizona. The incidence of diabetes in this population is extremely high, and the risk for losing clinical attachment and alveolar bone loss among the individuals with diabetes is approximately three times greater than among healthy persons from the community.[199,200]

More recent evidence suggests that there may be a reciprocal relation between diabetes and periodontitis;

each may influence the development and natural history of the other. As described earlier, diabetes appears to increase the risk for periodontitis. It has been hypothesized, however, that periodontal inflammation itself may increase insulin resistance, which leads to increases in blood glucose. This fledgling hypothesis is supported by recent studies that show small, but in some cases significant, improvements in glucose control after periodontal treatment in patients with diabetes.[201-203]

HIV Infection

Some reports published during the early stages of the AIDS epidemic in the United States suggest that HIV-positive patients, especially those with AIDS and low counts of T lymphocytes ($CD4^+ < 200$ cells/μl), were at increased risk for severe chronic periodontitis (see Chapter 31). Most recent epidemiologic studies, however, suggest that HIV infection alone does not increase the risk for periodontal disease.[204-207] Still other studies have reported a slightly greater prevalence of bone loss and attachment loss in HIV-infected patients accompanied by gingival recession and shallow pocket depths.[208-210] The disparate findings among these studies may be attributable to the gradual yet significant improvements in the medical management of HIV-positive patients or to variations in sampling strategies among these studies (i.e., selection bias). Most early reports focus on severely immunocompromised patients who went to treatment centers for the management of oral symptoms. Recent studies, however, have obtained more representative samples of the general HIV-positive population.

Necrotizing periodontal diseases and other intraoral lesions have been described in HIV-positive and AIDS patients. However, the development of more effective therapies for the management of HIV infection has been accompanied by a precipitous decline in the incidence of oral manifestations of the disease such as candidiasis, hairy leukoplakia, and necrotizing periodontal diseases.[211,212]

Osteoporosis

It has long been hypothesized that individuals with osteoporosis (i.e., low skeletal bone density) are also at increased risk for periodontitis (see Chapter 31). These conditions share some common pathways in their pathogeneses. For example, systemic up-regulation and increased production of IL-1α and IL-1β, tumor necrosis factor-α, and IL-6 induce osteoclastic activity and increase bone turnover rates that lead to loss of bone mass and osteoporosis.[213,214] Increased concentrations of these cytokines in the periodontal tissues also lead to alveolar bone loss and periodontal disease.[215] It is possible that patients who are at risk for osteoporosis because of a systemically up-regulated cytokine response may also be more susceptible to periodontitis in the presence of local irritants.

Although this theory is appealing, the relation between osteoporosis and periodontal disease is not well understood. Although most observational studies conclude that patients with low skeletal bone mineral density have slightly more periodontal disease than healthy control subjects,[216-218] other studies have found no association between the two conditions.[219,220] Finally, it has been reported that female individuals with low bone density and gross amounts of calculus were at an increased risk for attachment loss.[221] No such association was observed among women with low or intermediate levels of calculus. Currently, no definitive statements can be made concerning the relation between osteoporosis and periodontitis.

Nutrition

Persons with severe nutritional deficiencies are at an increased risk for development of acute periodontal lesions (see Chapter 31). For example, severe vitamin C deficiency (i.e., scurvy) leads to gingival lesions characterized by severe inflammation and spontaneous bleeding. Necrotizing lesions involving the periodontium and deeper tissues (i.e., cancrum oris or noma) have been reported in severely malnourished children. However, most epidemiologic studies have failed to find significant relations between nutritional status and chronic periodontal disease in more general populations.[132,138,222-225] In these studies, the periodontal conditions of malnourished individuals or those with specific vitamin deficiencies were not different from well nourished individuals. A recent cross-sectional study indicated that adults in the United States who reported low dietary intake of calcium and vitamin C tended to have more clinical attachment loss than those with high intakes.[226] The lack of evidence regarding the relations between nutritional factors and chronic periodontitis may result from a shortage of properly designed epidemiologic studies rather than the actual unimportance of nutrition in the development and progression of periodontitis.[227] Most of the studies currently available have evaluated dietary intake from 24-hour recall questionnaires or from nutrient levels in single serum samples. Although these methods are useful to assess the overall dietary and nutritional status of a population, they do not accurately represent the long-term dietary patterns of an individual.

Other Factors

Hormone Replacement Therapy

Women who use hormone replacement therapy have slightly less gingival inflammation[228] and clinical attachment loss[221,228] than age-matched women who do not (see Chapter 31). In postmenopausal women, estrogen supplementation appears to prevent loss of skeletal and alveolar bone.[229,230] Estrogen may exert its protective effect against bone loss and infectious diseases by acting as a metabolic mediator of cytokine expression.[231] Systemic levels of inflammatory mediators (i.e., IL-1, IL-6, and tumor necrosis factor-α), which increase after menopause, are lower in women who receive estrogen and progesterone supplementation.[231-233] This association, however, may be caused by confounders and not the result of a cause-and-effect relationship. Women who choose to receive hormone replacement therapy may be more health conscientious and, therefore, may be more likely to receive preventive periodontal therapy and to have better oral health behaviors.

Psychological Factors

Recent epidemiologic studies suggest that periodontal disease is more prevalent and severe among persons who report being psychologically stressed or depressed.[234-236] It has further been suggested that a person's ability to cope with stress is more important for determining risk for periodontitis than the level of stress *per se*.[237,238] (See Chapter 31.) It is hypothesized that stress leads to immune or behavioral changes, or both, that make a person more susceptible to infections. Emotional stress or depression may also lead to changes in oral health-related behaviors, including oral hygiene.

Genetic Epidemiology of Chronic Periodontitis

Measures of periodontitis and gingivitis are correlated within families.[239,240] The nature of this clustering effect has been investigated using a number of study designs. Studies using family correlations (e.g., sibling, parent-offspring) to estimate genetic and environmental variances suggest that similarities within families are mainly because of cultural inheritance and the common family environment, but not shared genes.[239,241] Meanwhile, twin studies have supported the theory that genetic factors significantly influence the risk for chronic periodontitis.[242-244] More specifically, these studies have found that a significant portion of the variance in PD and clinical attachment loss measures is attributable to genetic variance. Although such estimates should be interpreted with caution because they are not precise, it has been estimated that approximately 50% of the variance in disease can be attributable to genetic variance (i.e., heritability is about 50%).

Oral bacteria can be transmitted within families. This finding could explain, in part, why some forms of periodontitis are familial. Although the introduction of bacteria into the oral cavity is an environmental event, long-term colonization may be determined by both host genetic and environmental factors. In groups of adolescent twins, genetically related individuals were found to be more similar microbiologically than pairs of unrelated individuals.[245] In adults, however, neither host genes nor the early family environment appear to significantly influence the presence of periodontal bacteria in plaque.[246] These findings support the theory that, although host genes may influence early bacterial colonization of the oral cavity, the effect does not persist into adulthood.

As with aggressive periodontitis, the case-control study design has been used to search for specific genetic risk factors for chronic periodontitis. Various candidate genes including tumor necrosis factor-α polymorphisms, HLA antigens, FcγR genotypes and others, have been evaluated for their association with chronic periodontitis, but the overall results have been equivocal.[247-256] Table 3-4 summarizes the studies that have found associations between candidate markers and periodontitis. However, most of these findings have not been corroborated by other investigators or in multiple or racially mixed populations.

In 1997, Kornman and colleagues[251] first reported that a "composite" IL-1 genotype, consisting of at least one copy of the less frequent allele 2 at both IL-1α (-889) and IL-1β (+3954) loci, was associated with severe periodontitis in a small group of nonsmoking Northern European adults. Those with the composite genotype were 6.8 times more likely to have severe disease, as opposed to mild or no disease. There was no association in smokers, which suggests that some environmental risk factors appear to overwhelm any genetically determined susceptibility or resistance to disease. Furthermore, neither of the two alleles, independently, was associated with disease. These findings have not been consistently supported by subsequent research. Although some studies support an association between the IL-1 composite genotype and periodontitis,[252] others have reported no association[257] or inconsistencies in the specific alleles found to be associated with periodontitis. For example, Gore and colleagues[258] found the less common IL-1B allele, but not the composite genotype, to be more prevalent in patients with severe chronic periodontitis.

There is some evidence that the IL-1 composite genotype may be useful as a prognostic factor—that is, it may be useful, along with smoking history and the presence of *P. gingivalis*, for predicting those at greatest risk for disease occurrence, progression, or tooth loss.[259,260] Two Fcγ receptor polymorphisms have also been associated with recurrent chronic disease in adults in Japan.[248] All of these studies, however, involved a relatively small number of subjects, and the use of this or any other genotype has not been examined in large or diverse populations. In fact, no association was found between these same FcγR polymorphisms and refractory disease in a U.S. study.[249] Currently, information about genotypes must be considered cautiously when assessing risk for chronic periodontitis. Certainly, environmental factors, such as smoking and specific bacteria, must be given equal if not greater weight in determining an individual's overall risk for disease.

It remains to be seen if these or any genetic markers will be useful for predicting risk for chronic periodontitis in the general population. Chronic periodontitis is a complex and multifactorial disease in which the host's genetic makeup can modify the course of disease rather than cause it outright. Disease will not ensue in the absence of pathogenic microorganisms, and like hypertension and coronary artery disease, it is possible to mitigate the influence of high- or low-risk genotypes through exposure to favorable or deleterious environments.

PATTERNS OF DISEASE AND TOOTH LOSS

In some persons or sites, attachment loss is accompanied by pocket formation, whereas in others it tends to be associated with gingival recession. On average, clinical attachment level appears to be more commonly associated with gingival recession than with pocket deepening. This general pattern of periodontal destruction has been reported in the United States and in groups with limited

TABLE 3-4   Associations between Genetic Polymorphisms and Chronic Periodontitis

GENES	VERIFIED BY OTHER INVESTIGATORS OR IN OTHER POPULATIONS?	REFERENCES
IL-1α and IL-1β	Yes*	251, 252
N-acetyl transferase	No	253, 254
RAGE	No	255
Tumor necrosis factor (TNF)-α	No	250
Fcγ receptor (IIIa and IIIb)	No	248
TNF-α, ACE, and ET-1	No	256

*Verified in some but not all studies. ACE, angiotensin-converting enzyme; ET-1, endothelin-1, IL, interleukin; RAGE, receptor for advanced glycation endproducts; TNF, tumor necrosis factor.

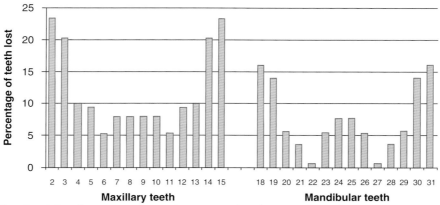

Figure 3-11. Percentage of total teeth lost during maintenance phase in periodontal practices by tooth type. Percentages represent unweighted averages of the percentage of teeth lost reported by Hirschfeld and Wasserman (1978),[265] McFall (1982),[266] and Goldman and colleagues (1986).[267]

or no access to dental care.* In a longitudinal study of elderly subjects, only 58% of sites that lost attachment demonstrated an increase in PD. The remaining 42% of progressing sites in this study experienced concurrent gingival recession with no increase in pocketing.[261] It has also been reported that facial sites tend to have attachment loss accompanied by recession, whereas proximal sites are more prone to develop periodontal pockets.

It is generally thought that recession in industrialized societies results from traumatic oral hygiene or periodontal treatment.[36,262] However, these reasons do not explain the recession-associated loss of attachment that has been reported in various untreated populations who do not practice regular oral hygiene. In such populations, recession tends to be more pronounced in individuals with extensive calculus. The association between calculus and gingival recession, which has been reported in a number of diverse populations,[53,142,263,264] could be because of the following reasons: (1) calculus acts as a plaque-retentive factor; (2) recessed sites facilitate the formation of calculus; and/or (3) it is simply easier to detect calculus when the gingiva is recessed.

Severe periodontitis is most frequently found in the posterior teeth, and the distribution appears to be symmetric in both jaws.[49] Such distribution is clearly reflected in the patterns of tooth loss observed among patients with moderate to severe periodontal disease. Figure 3-11 summarizes the percentage of teeth lost among patients with moderate to severe periodontal disease who were treated and managed through long-term maintenance care. Such percentages have been stratified by tooth type, excluding third molars. In general, upper teeth are more frequently lost than lower teeth. The teeth most frequently lost were the upper second molars, followed by the upper first

molars, lower second and first molars, upper premolars, and upper and lower incisors. The lower canines were by far the teeth least frequently lost.

In industrialized countries and many developing nations, the rates of tooth loss and edentulism have declined drastically since the 1960s. Such decline is most likely related to reducing caries rates and improvements in dental care. Between 20% and 50% of the permanent teeth extracted in industrialized nations are extracted for periodontal reasons.[268] Various studies have indicated that periodontitis is the leading cause of tooth loss in the United States among adults 40 years and older.[269] As part of a U.S. survey in 1981, examiners were asked to indicate which teeth currently in the mouth should be extracted and whether the extraction was required because of caries, periodontal disease, or other reasons.[270] Only 1% of adults 19 to 44 years old had a tooth that required extraction because of periodontal problems; this percentage increased to 10% for adults 45 years or older. They also assessed the reasons for the extraction of teeth that were missing at the time of examination. Caries accounted for approximately 70% of the extractions, slightly less than 20% of the teeth were reported to be lost because of periodontal disease, and prosthetic, orthodontic, and other causes had led to the loss of approximately 11%. The mean number of teeth lost because of periodontal reasons increased from 0.2 teeth per person for the 19- to 44-year-old group to 1.9 teeth per person for the 45- to 64-year-old group, reaching a high of 4.7 teeth per person in older age groups. However, even among the elderly, only 29% of missing teeth were because of periodontal disease. Obviously, the percentage of tooth loss associated with periodontal disease is highly dependent on the caries rates of the population. If caries rates continue to decrease faster than the rates of periodontal diseases, the percentage of teeth lost for periodontal reasons will increase even if the absolute number of teeth lost declines.

---

*See References 4, 43, 50, 51, 53, and 75.

PERIODONTITIS AS A RISK FACTOR FOR OTHER DISEASES

During the last decade several epidemiologic studies have been conducted to assess the potential effect of periodontal diseases as risk factors for other systemic diseases. It has been hypothesized that persons with periodontitis are at increased risk for development of cardiovascular diseases (e.g., myocardial infarction and stroke) and respiratory diseases. In addition, pregnant women with periodontal disease may be at increased risk for having preterm delivery or giving birth to neonates that are small according to their gestational age. Furthermore, among patients with diabetes, periodontal disease may lead to increased glucose levels. (See Chapter 32 for a complete discussion regarding the possible effects of periodontal health on the general health of a patient.)

CAUSALITY OF PERIODONTAL DISEASES

In epidemiologic studies of infectious diseases, people often search for a single deterministic factor that causes the disease. Pure determinism specifies that a single agent, behavior, or exposure is considered to be an etiologic factor if it is both necessary (i.e., the disease will not appear without it) and sufficient (i.e., the factor alone can be causative) to produce disease. Some infectious diseases (e.g., varicella zoster virus as a cause of chickenpox) and Mendelian disorders (e.g., trisomy 21 as a cause of Down syndrome) fit this model of causation. Such a model may also be applicable to the study of plaque-related gingivitis. Undisturbed bacterial plaque is both a necessary and sufficient cause of gingivitis. Nevertheless, gingivitis is caused by a nonspecific infection and no single microorganism can be deemed as the single etiologic agent. A purely deterministic model, however, is too simplistic to explain the occurrence of chronic or aggressive periodontitis. No single factor—behavioral, microbial, or genetic—is both necessary *and* sufficient to cause periodontitis.

In the past, periodontitis was thought to be caused strictly by environmental factors (e.g., poor oral hygiene). However, only a fraction of the differences among individuals in a population can be explained by differences in exposure to these environments. There is mounting evidence indicating that genetic factors play a role in the etiology of aggressive and chronic periodontitis. Diseases with etiologies that include various genetic and environmental factors are referred to as *multifactorial*. Chronic and aggressive periodontitis are clearly multifactorial in nature. The "sufficient cause" model is a useful approach for understanding diseases of multifactorial etiology.[271] A *sufficient cause* represents a set group of minimal conditions or events that invariably lead to disease occurrence. A sufficient cause for chronic or aggressive periodontitis is most likely the combination of various genetic and environmental factors. Furthermore, these diseases appear to have etiologic heterogeneity, which means that more than one sufficient cause can be involved in the occurrence of the disease. For example, chronic periodontitis is more likely to occur in individuals who smoke. However, not all smokers will have periodontitis, and therefore only a portion of smokers possess other components of a sufficient cause for periodontitis. Moreover, severe periodontitis occurs in nonsmokers; therefore, sufficient causes that do not include smoking exist. This example is applicable to all other risk factors, including microbial risk factors, for periodontitis. The interaction between the different components of a given sufficient cause may also have an important effect on disease occurrence (e.g., two risk factors may have a synergistic effect).

In establishing whether a factor should be considered as part of the causality of the disease the following should be evaluated: (1) the strength of the association between the factor in question and the occurrence of the disease, (2) the presence of dose-response effects, (3) temporal consistency (i.e., the exposure should consistently precede the occurrence of disease), (4) consistency of findings, (5) biologic plausibility, (6) specificity of the association, and (7) the overall coherence of the evidence. Various environmental factors that may play a role in chronic periodontal disease causation have been identified. Risk factors for chronic periodontitis include smoking, poorly controlled diabetes, and lack of preventive periodontal care (i.e., oral hygiene and professional care). In addition, a significant portion of the variation in the population can be attributable to genetic variation. The roles that specific genes play in the etiology of these diseases, however, are largely unknown. In rare cases, single gene mutations lead to aggressive periodontitis as one of the characteristics of an overall syndrome (e.g., Papillon-Lefèvre syndrome, Leukocyte Adhesion Deficiency syndrome, Chédiak-Higashi syndrome). However, it is not likely that a single gene causes the most common presentations of chronic or aggressive periodontitis. Most likely few or many disease alleles interact with environmental factors to affect individual risk for chronic or aggressive periodontitis. Future epidemiologic research assessing the interaction of host susceptibility factors (e.g., genetic risk factors) and environmental factors are necessary.

REFERENCES

1. Last JM, Abramson JH, International Epidemiological Association: *A Dictionary of Epidemiology*, ed 3, New York, 1995, Oxford University Press.
2. American Academy of Periodontology: Epidemiology of periodontal diseases (position paper), *J Periodontol* 67:935, 1996.

3. World Workshop in Periodontics: Consensus report on periodontal diseases: epidemiology and diagnosis, *Ann Periodontol* 1:216, 1996.

4. Albandar JM, Brunelle JA, Kingman A: Destructive periodontal disease in adults 30 years of age and older in the United States, 1988-1994, *J Periodontol* 70:13, 1999.

5. Pihlstrom BL, McHugh RB, Oliphant TH: Comparison of surgical and nonsurgical treatment of periodontal disease. A review of current studies and additional results after 6 1/2 years, *J Clin Periodontol* 10:524, 1983.

6. Cutress TW, Powell RN, Kilisimasi S, et al: A 3-year community-based periodontal disease prevention program for adults in a developing nation, *Int Dent J* 41:323, 1991.

7. Hinrichs JE, Jarzembinski C, Hardie N, Aeppli D: Intrasulcular laser Doppler readings before and after root planing, *J Clin Periodontol* 22:817, 1995.

8. Holthuis AF, Gelskey SC, Chebib FS: The relationship between gingival tissue temperatures and various indicators of gingival inflammation, *J Periodontol* 52:187, 1981.

9. Hancock EB, Cray RJ, O'Leary TJ: The relationship between gingival crevicular fluid and gingival inflammation: a clinical and histologic study, *J Periodontol* 50:13, 1979.

10. Oliver RC, Holm-Pedersen P, Löe H: The correlation between clinical scoring, exudate measurements and microscopic evaluation of inflammation in the gingiva, *J Periodontol* 40:201, 1969.

11. Schour I, Massler M: Gingival disease in postwar Italy (1945). 1. Prevalence of gingivitis in various age groups, *J Am Dent Assoc* 35:475, 1947.

12. Löe H, Silness J: Periodontal disease in pregnancy. 1. Prevalence and severity, *Acta Odontol Scand* 21:533, 1963.

13. Hassell TM, Germann MA, Saxer UP: Periodontal probing: investigator discrepancies and correlations between probing force and recorded depth, *Helv Odontol Acta* 17:38, 1973.

14. Stoltenberg JL, Osborn JB, Pihlstrom BL, et al: Association between cigarette smoking, bacterial pathogens, and periodontal status, *J Periodontol* 64:1225, 1993.

15. Greenstein G, Caton J, Polson AM: Histologic characteristics associated with bleeding after probing and visual signs of inflammation, *J Periodontol* 52:420, 1981.

16. Hirsch RS, Clarke NG, Townsend GC: The effect of locally released oxygen on the development of plaque and gingivitis in man, *J Clin Periodontol* 8:21, 1981.

17. Mühlemann HR, Son S: Gingival sulcus bleeding: a leading symptom in initial gingivitis, *Helv Odontol Acta* 15:107, 1971.

18. Russell AL: A system of classification and scoring for prevalence surveys of periodontal disease, *J Dent Res* 35:350, 1956.

19. Ramfjord SP: Indices for prevalence and incidence of periodontal disease, *J Periodontol* 30:51, 1959.

20. Armitage GC: Periodontal diseases: diagnosis, *Ann Periodontol* 1:37, 1996.

21. Armitage GC, Svanberg GK, Löe H: Microscopic evaluation of clinical measurements of connective tissue attachment levels, *J Clin Periodontol* 4:173, 1977.

22. Haffajee AD, Socransky SS, Goodson JM: Clinical parameters as predictors of destructive periodontal disease activity, *J Clin Periodontol* 10:257, 1983.

23. Jeffcoat MK, Reddy MS: Advances in measurements of periodontal bone and attachment loss, *Monogr Oral Sci* 17:56, 2000.

24. Ainamo J, Barmes D, Beagrie G, et al: Developement of the World Health Organization (WHO) Community Periodontal Index of Treatment Needs (CPITN), *Int Dent J* 32:281, 1982.

25. Oliver RC, Brown J, Löe H: Periodontal treatment needs, *Periodontology 2000*, 2:150, 1993.

26. Butterworth M, Sheiham A: Changes in the Community Periodontal Index of Treatment Needs (CPITN) after periodontal treatment in a general practice, *Br Dent J* 171: 363, 1991.

27. Quigley G, Hein J: Comparative cleansing efficiency of manual and power brushing, *J Am Dent Assoc* 65:26, 1962.

28. Turesky S, Gilmore ND, Glickman I: Reduced plaque formation by the chloromethyl analogue of vitamin C, *J Periodontol* 41:41, 1970.

29. Silness P, Löe H: Periodontal disease in pregnancy, *Acta Odontol Scand* 22:123, 1964.

30. Löe H: The gingival index, the plaque index and the retention index systems, *J Periodontol* 38:610, 1967.

31. Mandel ID: Indices for measurement of soft accumulations in clinical studies of oral hygiene and periodontal disease, *J Periodont Res* 9:7, 1974.

32. Silness J, Røynstrand T: Partial mouth recording of plaque, gingivitis and probing depth in adolescents, *J Clin Periodontol* 15:189, 1988.

33. Kingman A, Morrison E, Löe H, Smith J: Systematic errors in estimating the prevalence and severity of periodontal disease, *J Periodontol* 59:707, 1988.

34. Gettinger G, Patters MR, Testa MA, et al: The use of six selected teeth in population measures of periodontal status, *J Periodontol* 54:155, 1983.

35. Diamanti-Kipioti A, Papapanou PN, Mooraitaki-Tsami A: Comparative estimation of periodontal conditions by means of different index systems, *J Clin Periodontol* 20:656, 1993.

36. Kingman A, Löe H, Anerud A: Errors in measuring parameters associated with periodontal health and disease, *J Periodontol* 62:477, 1991.

37. Mariotti A: Dental plaque-induced gingival diseases, *Ann Periodontol*, 4:7-19, 1999.

38. Löe H, Theilade E, Jensen SB: Experimental gingivitis in man, *J Periodontol* 36:177, 1965.

39. Theilade E, Wright WH, Jensen SB, et al: Experimental gingivitis in man. II. A longitudinal clinical and bacteriological investigation, *J Periodont Res* 1:1, 1966.

40. Holm-Pedersen P, Agerbaek P, Theilade E: Experimental gingivitis in young and elderly individuals, *J Clin Periodontol* 2:14, 1975.

41. Lang NP, Cumming BR, Löe HA: Oral hygiene and gingival health in Danish dental students and faculty, *Community Dent Oral Epidemiol* 5:237, 1977.

42. Hugoson A, Koch G, Hallonsten AL, et al: Dental health 1973 and 1978 in individuals aged 3-20 years in the community of Jönköping, Sweden. A cross-sectional study, *Swed Dent J* 4:217, 1980.

43. Albandar JM, Kingman A: Gingival recession, gingival bleeding, and dental calculus in adults 30 years of age and older in the United States, 1988-1994, *J Periodontol* 70:30, 1999.

44. Spencer AJ, Beighton D, Higgins TJ: Periodontal disease in five and six year old children, *J Periodontol* 54:19, 1983.

45. Gibson A, Gelbier S, Bhatia S: Dental health and treatment needs of 5-year-old children in the health area of Lambeth, Southwark and Lewisham, England, *Community Dent Oral Epidemiol* 9:5, 1981.

46. Hugoson A, Koch G, Bergendal T, et al: Oral health of individuals aged 3-80 years in Jönköping, Sweden, in 1973 and 1983, *Swed Dent J* 10:175, 1986.

47. Sutcliffe P: A longitudinal study of gingivitis and puberty, *J Periodont Res* 7:52, 1972.

48. Curilovic Z, Mazor Z, Berchtold H: Gingivitis in Zurich schoolchildren. A reexamination after 20 years, *SSO Schweiz Monatsschr Zahnheilkd* 87:801, 1977.

49. Löe H, Anerud A, Boysen H: The natural history of periodontal disease in man. Study design and baseline data, *J Periodont Res* 13:550, 1978.

50. Baelum V, Fejerskov O, Karring T: Oral hygiene, gingivitis and periodontal breakdown in adult Tanzanians, *J Periodont Res* 21:221, 1986.

51. Baelum V, Fejerskov O, Manji F: Periodontal diseases in adult Kenyans, *J Clin Periodontol* 15:445, 1988.

52. Lembariti BS, Frencken JE, Pilot T: Prevalence and severity of periodontal conditions among adults in urban and rural Morogoro, Tanzania, *Community Dent Oral Epidemiol* 16:240, 1988.

53. Ronderos M, Pihlstrom BL, Hodges JS: Periodontal disease among indigenous people in the Amazon rain forest, *J Clin Periodontol* 28:995, 2001.

54. Gusberti FA, Mombelli A, Lang NP et al: Changes in subgingival microbiota during puberty. A 4-year longitudinal study, *J Clin Periodontol* 17:685, 1990.

55. Mombelli A, Lang NP, Burgain WB, et al: Microbial changes associated with the development of puberty gingivitis, *J Periodont Res* 25:3, 1990.

56. Nakagawa S, Fujii H, Machida Y, et al: A longitudinal study from prepuberty to puberty gingivitis. Correlation between the occurrence of puberty Prevotella Intermedia and sex hormones, *J Clin Periodontol* 21:658, 1994.

57. World Health Organization (WHO), Division of Noncommunicable Diseases, Oral Health WHO Collaborating Center, School of Dentistry, Niigata University, Japan. WHO Oral Health Country/Area Profile Program. Observed periodontal conditions measured by CPITN at age 15-19 years. Available online at: http://www.dent.niigata-u.ac.jp/ prevent/ perio/m1519a.html. [Accessed July 1, 2002].

58. Bjorby A, Löe H: Gingival and oral hygiene conditions in school children in Gothenburg, Sweden, *Sverig Tandlak Tidn* 61:561, 1969.

59. Ramfjord SP: Survey of the periodontal status of boys 11 to 17 years old in Bombay, India, *J Periodontol* 32:237, 1961.

60. Rosenzweig KA: Gingivitis in children of Israel, *J Periodontol* 31:404, 1960.

61. van der Valden U, Abbas F, Hart AAM: Experimental gingivitis in relationship to susceptibility to periodontal disease, *J Clin Periodontol* 12:61, 1985.

62. Bergstrom J, Preber H: The influence of cigarette smoking on the development of experimental gingivitis, *J Periodont Res* 21:668, 1986.

63. Bergstrom J: Oral hygiene compliance and gingivitis expression in cigarette smokers, *Scand J Dent Res* 98:497, 1990.

64. Bergstrom J, Persson L, Preber H: Influence of cigarette smoking on vascular reaction during experimental gingivitis, *Scand J Dent Res* 96:34, 1988.

65. Sznajder N, Carraro JJ, Rugna S, et al: Periodontal findings in diabetic and nondiabetic patients, *J Periodontol* 49:445, 1978.

66. Rylander H, Ramberg P, Blohme G: Prevalence of periodontal disease in young diabetics, *J Clin Periodontol* 14:38, 1986.

67. Cohen DW, Friedman L, Shapiro J, et al: A longitudinal investigation of the periodontal changes during pregnancy, *J Periodontol* 40:563, 1969.

68. Hugoson A: Gingival inflammation and female sex hormones. A clinical investigation of pregnant women and experimental studies in dogs, *J Periodont Res Suppl* 5:1, 1970.

69. U.S. Public Health Service, National Institute of Dental Research: Oral Health of United States Adults; National Findings, NIH Publ No 87-2868, Bethesda, MD, NIDR, 1987.

70. Brown LJ, Brunelle JA, Kingman A: Periodontal status in the United States, 1988-91: prevalence, extent and demographic variation, *J Dent Res* 75:672, 1996.

71. Chindia ML, Vandererhaug J, Ng'ang'a PM: Oral health habits and periodontal health among a group of university students in Kenya, *East Afr Med J* 69:337, 1992.

72. Stoltenberg JL, Osborn JB, Pihlstrom BL, et al: Prevalence of periodontal disease in a health maintenance organization and comparisons to the national survey of oral health, *J Periodontol* 64:853, 1993.

73. Cutress TW, Powell RN, Ball ME: Differing profiles of periodontal disease in two similar South Pacific island populations, *Community Dent Oral Epidemiol* 10:193, 1982.

74. Norheim PW: Oral health status in a population in Northern Norway, *Acta Odontol Scand* 37:293, 1979.

75. Baelum V, Wen-Min L, Fejerskov O: Tooth mortality and periodontal conditions in 60-80-year-old Chinese, *Scand J Dent Res* 96:99, 1988.

76. Capilouto ML, Douglass CW: Trends in the prevalence and severity of periodontal diseases in the US: a public health problem, *J Public Health Dent* 48:245, 1988.

77. Armitage GC: Development of a classification system for periodontal diseases and conditions, *Ann Periodontol* 4:1, 1999.

78. American Academy of Periodontology: Parameter on aggressive periodontitis. American Academy of Periodontology, *J Periodontol* 71:867, 2000.

79. Lindhe J, Haffajee AD, Socransky SS: Progression of periodontal disease in adult subjects in the absence of periodontal therapy, *J Clin Periodontol* 10:433, 1983.

80. Albandar JM, Brown LJ, Genco RJ, Löe H: Clinical classification of periodontitis in adolescents and young adults, *J Periodontol* 68:545, 1997.

81. Aass AM, Rossow I, Preus HR, Gjermo P: Incidence of early periodontitis in a group of young individuals during 8 years: associations with selected potential predictors, *J Periodontol* 65:814, 1994.

82. Melvin WL, Sandifer JB, Gray JL: The prevalence and sex ratio of juvenile periodontitis in a young racially mixed population, *J Periodontol* 62:330, 1991.

83. Löe H, Brown LJ: Early onset periodontitis in the United States of America, *J Periodontol* 62:608, 1991.

84. Kronauer E, Borsa G, Lang NP: Prevalence of incipient juvenile periodontitis at age 16 years in Switzerland, *J Clin Periodontol* 13:103, 1986.

85. Van der Velden U, Abbas F, Van Steenbergen TJ, et al: Prevalence of periodontal breakdown in adolescents and presence of Actinobacillus actinomycetemcomitans in subjects with attachment loss, *J Periodontol* 60:604, 1989.

86. Hansen BF, Gjermo P, Bergwitz-Larsen KR: Periodontal bone loss in 15-year-old Norwegians, *J Clin Periodontol* 11:125, 1984.

87. Aass AM, Albandar J, Aasenden R, et al: Variation in prevalence of radiographic alveolar bone loss in subgroups of 14-year-old schoolchildren in Oslo, *J Clin Periodontol* 15:130, 1988.

88. Saxen L: Prevalence of juvenile periodontitis in Finland, *J Clin Periodontol* 7:177, 1980.

89. Hoover JN, Ellegaard B, Attstrom R: Radiographic and clinical examination of periodontal status of first molars in 15-16-year-old Danish schoolchildren, *Scand J Dent Res* 89:260, 1981.

90. Lopez NJ, Rios V, Pareja MA, Fernandez O: Prevalence of juvenile periodontitis in Chile, *J Clin Periodontol* 18:529, 1991.

91. Tinoco EM, Beldi MI, Loureiro CA, et al: Localized juvenile periodontitis and Actinobacillus actinomycetemcomitans in a Brazilian population, *Eur J Oral Sci* 105:9, 1997.

92. Albandar JM, Baghdady VS, Ghose LJ: Periodontal disease progression in teenagers with no preventive dental care provisions, *J Clin Periodontol* 18:300, 1991.

93. Nassar MM, Afifi O, Deprez RD: The prevalence of localized juvenile periodontitis in Saudi subjects, *J Periodontol* 65:698, 1994.

94. Kowashi Y: Prevalence of juvenile periodontitis among students at Nagasaki University, *Adv Dent Res* 2:395, 1988.

95. Paolantonio M, di Bonaventura G, di Placido G, et al: Prevalence of Actinobacillus actinomycetemcomitans and clinical conditions in children and adolescents from rural and urban areas of central Italy, *J Clin Periodontol* 27:549, 2000.

96. Harley AF, Floyd PD: Prevalence of juvenile periodontitis in schoolchildren in Lagos, Nigeria, *Community Dent Oral Epidemiol* 16:299, 1988.

97. Saxby MS: Juvenile periodontitis: an epidemiological study in the west Midlands of the United Kingdom, *J Clin Periodontol* 14:594, 1987.

98. Albandar JM, Muranga MB, Rams TE: Prevalence of aggressive periodontitis in school attendees in Uganda, *J Clin Periodontol* 29:823, 2002.

99. Brown LJ, Albandar JM, Brunelle JA, Löe H: Early-onset periodontitis: progression of attachment loss during 6 years, *J Periodontol* 67:968, 1996.

100. Albandar JM: Juvenile periodontitis—pattern of progression and relationship to clinical periodontal parameters, *Community Dent Oral Epidemiol* 21:185, 1993.

101. Hart TC, Marazita ML, Schenkein HA, et al: No female preponderance in juvenile periodontitis after correction for ascertainment bias, *J Periodontol* 62:745, 1991.

102. Horning GM, Hatch CL, Lutskus J: The prevalence of periodontitis in a military treatment population, *J Am Dent Assoc* 121:616, 1990.

103. Albandar JM, Buischi YA, Barbosa MF: Destructive forms of periodontal disease in adolescents. A 3-year longitudinal study, *J Periodontol* 62:370, 1991.

104. Kallestal C, Matsson L: Marginal bone loss in 16-year-old Swedish adolescents in 1975 and 1988, *J Clin Periodontol* 18:740, 1991.

105. Oliver RC, Brown LJ, Löe H: Periodontal diseases in the United States population, *J Periodontol* 69:269, 1998.

106. Bernick SM, Cohen DW, Baker L, Laster L: Dental disease in children with diabetes mellitus, *J Periodontol* 46:241, 1975.

107. de Pommereau V, Dargent-Pare C, Robert JJ, Brion M: Periodontal status in insulin-dependent diabetic adolescents, *J Clin Periodontol* 19:628, 1992.

108. Schenkein HA, Gunsolley JC, Koertge TE, et al: Smoking and its effects on early-onset periodontitis, *J Am Dent Assoc* 126:1107, 1995.

109. Mullally BH, Breen B, Linden GJ: Smoking and patterns of bone loss in early-onset periodontitis, *J Periodontol* 70:394, 1999.

110. Kamma JJ, Nakou M, Baehni PC: Clinical and microbiological characteristics of smokers with early onset periodontitis, *J Periodont Res* 34:25, 1999.

111. Gunsolley JC, Pandey JP, Quinn SM, et al: The effect of race, smoking and immunoglobulin allotypes on IgG subclass concentrations, *J Periodont Res* 32:381, 1997.

112. Marazita ML, Burmeister JA, Gunsolley JC, et al: Evidence for autosomal dominant inheritance and race-specific heterogeneity in early-onset periodontitis, *J Periodontol* 65:623, 1994.

113. Long JC, Nance WE, Waring P, et al: Early onset periodontitis: a comparison and evaluation of two proposed modes of inheritance, *Genet Epidemiol* 4:13, 1987.

114. Beaty TH, Boughman JA, Yang P, et al: Genetic analysis of juvenile periodontitis in families ascertained through an affected proband, *Am J Hum Genet* 40:443, 1987.

115. Melnick M, Shields ED, Bixler D: Periodontosis: a phenotypic and genetic analysis, *Oral Surg Oral Med Oral Pathol* 42:32, 1976.

116. Boughman JA, Halloran SL, Roulston D, et al: An autosomal-dominant form of juvenile periodontitis: its localization to chromosome 4 and linkage to dentinogenesis imperfecta and Gc, *J Craniofac Genet Dev Biol* 6:341, 1986.

117. Saxen L, Nevanlinna HR: Autosomal recessive inheritance of juvenile periodontitis: test of a hypothesis, *Clin Genet* 25:332, 1984.

118. Hart TC, Marazita ML, McCanna KM, et al: Reevaluation of the chromosome 4q candidate region for early onset periodontitis, *Hum Genet* 91:416, 1993.

119. Diehl SR, Wang Y, Brooks CN, et al: Linkage disequilibrium of interleukin-1 genetic polymorphisms with early-onset periodontitis, *J Periodontol* 70:418, 1999.

120. Hennig BJ, Parkhill JM, Chapple IL, et al: Association of a vitamin D receptor gene polymorphism with localized early-onset periodontal diseases, *J Periodontol* 70:1032, 1999.

121. Gwinn MR, Sharma A, De Nardin E: Single nucleotide polymorphisms of the N-formyl peptide receptor in localized juvenile periodontitis, *J Periodontol* 70:1194, 1999.

122. Kobayashi T, Sugita N, van der Pol WL, et al: The Fc gamma receptor genotype as a risk factor for generalized early-onset periodontitis in Japanese patients, *J Periodontol* 71:1425, 2000.

123. Ohyama H, Takashiba S, Oyaizu K, et al: HLA Class II genotypes associated with early-onset periodontitis: DQB1 molecule primarily confers susceptibility to the disease, *J Periodontol* 67:888, 1996.

124. Yoshihara A, Sugita N, Yamamoto K, et al: Analysis of vitamin D and Fcgamma receptor polymorphisms in Japanese patients with generalized early-onset periodontitis, *J Dent Res* 80:2051, 2001.

125. Tai H, Endo M, Shimada Y, et al: Association of interleukin-1 receptor antagonist gene polymorphisms with early onset periodontitis in Japanese, *J Clin Periodontol* 29:882, 2002.

126. Michel J, Gonzales JR, Wunderlich D, et al: Interleukin-4 polymorphisms in early onset periodontitis, *J Clin Periodontol* 28:483, 2001.

127. Hodge PJ, Riggio MP, Kinane DF: Failure to detect an association with IL1 genotypes in European Caucasians with generalised early onset periodontitis, *J Clin Periodontol* 28:430, 2001.

128. Walker SJ, Van Dyke TE, Rich S, et al: Genetic polymorphisms of the IL-1alpha and IL-1beta genes in African-American LJP patients and an African-American control population, *J Periodontol* 71:723, 2000.

129. Sofaer JA: Genetic approaches in the study of periodontal diseases, *J Clin Periodontol* 17:401, 1990.

130. Terasaki PI, Kaslick RS, West TL, Chasens AI: Low HL-A2 frequency and periodontitis, *Tissue Antigens* 5:286, 1975.

131. Kaslick RS, West TL, Chasens AI: Association between ABO blood groups, HL-A antigens and periodontal diseases in young adults: a follow-up study, *J Periodontol* 51:339, 1980.

132. Katz J, Goultschin J, Benoliel R, Brautbar C: Human leukocyte antigen (HLA) DR4. Positive association with rapidly progressing periodontitis, *J Periodontol* 58:607, 1987.

133. Firatli E, Kantarci A, Cebeci I, et al: Association between HLA antigens and early onset periodontitis, *J Clin Periodontol* 23:563, 1996.

134. Klouda PT, Porter SR, Scully C, et al: Association between HLA-A9 and rapidly progressive periodontitis, *Tissue Antigens* 28:146, 1986.

135. Waerhaug J: Prevalence of periodontal disease in Ceylon. Association with age, sex, oral hygiene, socio-economic factors, vitamin deficiencies, malnutrition, betel and tobacco consumption and ethnic group. Final Report, *Acta Odontol Scand* 25:205, 1967.

136. Bukley LA, Crowley MJ: A longitudinal study of untreated periodontal disease, *J Clin Periodontol* 11:523, 1984.

137. Russell AL: Epidemiology of periodontal disease, *Int Dent J* 17:282, 1967.

138. Barros L, Witkop CJ: Oral and genetic study of Chileans, 1960-V. Factors that influence the severity of periodontal disease, *Arch Oral Biol* 8:765, 1963.

139. Burt BA, Ismail AI, Eklund SA: Periodontal disease, tooth loss, and oral hygiene among older Americans, *Community Dent Oral Epidemiol* 13:93, 1985.

140. Löe H, Anerud A, Boysen H: Natural history of periodontal disease in man. Rapid, moderate and no loss of

attachment in Sri Lankan laborers 14 to 46 years of age, *J Clin Periodontol* 13:431, 1986.

141. Löe H, Anerud A, Boysen H, et al: The natural history of periodontal disease in man: the rate of periodontal destruction before 40 years of age, *J Periodontol* 49:607, 1978.

142. Löe H, Anerud A, Boysen H: The natural history of periodontal disease in man: prevalence, severity and extent of gingival recession, *J Periodontol* 63:489, 1992.

143. Hugoson A, Laurell L, Lundgren D: Frequency distribution of individuals aged 20-70 years according to severity of periodontal disease experience in 1973 and 1983. *J Clin Periodontol* 19:227, 1992.

144. Grossi SG, Zambon JJ, Ho AW, et al: Assessment of risk for periodontal disease I. Risk indicators for attachment loss, *J Periodontol* 65:260, 1994.

145. MacGregor IDM, Sheiham A: Patterns of periodontal pocketing in Western Nigerian populations, *J Periodontol* 45:402, 1974.

146. Miyazaki H: A global overview of periodontal epidemiology. In Pack ARC, Newman HN, editors: *Periodontal needs of developing nations*, Middlesex, NJ, 1996, International Academy of Periodontology, Science Reviews Limited.

147. Matthesen M, Baelum V, Aasrlev I: Dental health of children and adults in Guinea-Bissau, West Africa in 1986, *Community Dent Health* 7:123, 1990.

148. Mitsis FJ, Taramidis G: Alveolar bone loss on neolithic man remains on 38 skulls of Khirokitia's (Cyprus) inhabitants, *J Clin Periodontol* 22:788, 1995.

149. Clarke NG, Carey SE, Srikandi W: Periodontal disease in ancient populations, *Am J Phys Antropol* 71:173, 1986.

150. Costa RL: Periodontal disease in the prehistoric Ipiutak and Tigara skeletal remains from Point Hope, Alaska, *Am J Phys Antropol* 59:97, 1982.

151. Kerr NW: Prevalence and natural history of periodontal disease in Scotland-the medieval period (900-1600 AD), *J Periodont Res* 26:346, 1991.

152. Kerr NW: Prevalence and natural history of periodontal disease in a London, Spitalfields, population (1645-1852 AD), *Arch Oral Biol* 39:581, 1994.

153. Listgarten MA, Schifter CC, Laster L: 3-year longitudinal study of the periodontal status of an adult population with gingivitis, *J Clin Periodontol* 12:225, 1985.

154. Lang NP, Joss A, Orsanic T, et al: Bleeding on probing. A predictor for the progression of periodontal disease, *J Clin Periodontol* 13:590, 1986.

155. Hansen BF, Bjertness E, Gjermo P: Changes in periodontal disease indicators in 35-year-old Oslo citizens from 1973 to 1984, *J Clin Periodontol* 17:249, 1990.

156. Douglass CW, Fox CH: Cross-sectional studies in periodontal disease: current status and implications for dental practice, *Adv Dent Res* 7:25, 1993.

157. Brown LJ, Oliver RC, Löe H: Evaluating periodontal status of U.S. employed adults, *J Am Dent Assoc* 121:226, 1990.

158. Papapanou PN, Wenstrom JL, Grondhal K: A 10-year retrospective study of periodontal disease progression, *J Clin Periodontol* 16:403, 1989.

159. Haffajee AD, Socransky SS, Lindhe J: Clinical risk indicators for periodontal attachment loss, *J Clin Periodontol* 18:117, 1991.

160. Ismail AI, Morrison EC, Burt BA: Natural history of periodontal disease in adults: findings from the Tecumseh Periodontal Disease Study, 1959-87, *J Dent Res* 69:430, 1990.

161. Waerhaug J: Epidemiology of periodontal disease. In Ramfjord SP, Keer DA, Ash MM, editors: *Workshop in periodontics*, Ann Arbor, 1966, University of Michigan Press.

162. U.S. Public Health Service, National Center for Health Statistics, Oral Hygiene in Adults, United States 1960-1962, PHS Publ. No. 1000, Series 11 No. 16. Washington, DC, 1966, U.S. Government Printing Office.

163. U.S. Department of Health and Human Services (DHHS), Centers for Disease Control and Prevention: National Center for Health Statistics. Third National Health and Nutrition Examination Survey, 1988-1994, NHANES III Data File (CD ROM). Public Use Data File Documentation No. 76200, Hyattsville, Md, 1996, Centers for Disease Control and Prevention.

164. Beck JD, Koch GG, Rozier RG, et al: Prevalence and risk indicators for periodontal attachment loss in a population of older community-dwelling blacks and whites, *J Periodontol* 61:521, 1990.

165. Locker D, Leake JL: Risk indicators and risk markers for periodontal disease experience in older adults living independently in Ontario, Canada, *J Dent Res* 72:9, 1993.

166. Grossi SG, Genco RJ, Machtei EE, et al: Assessment of risk for periodontal disease. II. Risk indicators for alveolar bone loss, *J Periodontol* 66:23, 1995.

167. Waerhaug J: Effect of toothbrushing on subgingival plaque formation, *J Periodontol* 52:30, 1981.

168. Nyman S, Lindhe J, Rosling B: Periodontal surgery in plaque-infected dentitions, *J Clin Periodontol* 4:240, 1977.

169. Axelsson P, Lindhe J, Nystrom B: On the prevention of caries and periodontal disease. Results of a 15-year longitudinal study, *J Clin Periodontol* 18:182, 1991.

170. Papapanou PN, Wenstrom JL: A 10-year retrospective study of periodontal disease progression. Clinical characteristics of subjects with pronounced and minimal disease development. *J Clin Periodontol* 17:78, 1990.

171. Claffey N, Nylund K, Kiger R, et al: Diagnostic predictibility of scores of plaque, bleeding, suppuration and probing depth for probing attachment loss. $3^{1}/_{2}$ years of observation following initial periodontal therapy, *J Clin Periodontol* 17:108, 1990.

172. Haffajee AD, Socransky SS, Dzink JL, et al: Clinical, microbiological and immunological features of subjects

with destructive periodontal diseases, *J Clin Periodontol* 15:240, 1988.

173. Lindhe J, Okamoto H, Yoneyama T, et al: Longitudinal changes in periodontal disease in untreated subjects, *J Clin Periodontol* 16:662, 1989.

174. Machtei EE, Christersson LA, Zambon JJ, et al: Alternative methods for screening periodontal disease in adults, *J Clin Periodontol* 20:81, 1993.

175. Ramfjord SP, Morrison EC, Burgett FG, et al: Oral hygiene and maintenance of periodontal support, *J Periodontol* 53:26, 1982.

176. Neely AL, Holford TR, Löe H, et al: The natural history of periodontal disease in man. Risk factors for progression of attachment loss in individuals receiving no oral health care, *J Periodontol* 72:1006, 2001.

177. Merchant A, Pitiphat W, Douglass CW, et al: Oral hygiene practices and periodontitis in health care professionals, *J Periodontol* 73:531, 2002.

178. Wouters FR, Salonen LW, Fithiof L, et al: Significance of some variables on interproximal bone height based on cross-sectional epidemiologic data, *J Clin Periodontol* 20:199, 1993.

179. Bergstrom J: Cigarette smoking as risk factor in chronic periodontal disease, *Community Dent Oral Epidemiol* 17:245, 1989.

180. Haber J, Wattles J, Crowley M, et al: Evidence for cigarette smoking as a major risk factor for periodontitis, *J Periodontol* 64:16, 1993.

181. Papapanou PN: Periodontal diseases: epidemiology, *Ann Periodontol* 1:1, 1996.

182. Bergstrom J, Eliasson S: Cigarette smoking and alveolar bone height in subjects with high standard of oral hygiene, *J Clin Periodontol* 14:466, 1987.

183. Krall EA, Garvey AJ, Garcia RI: Alveolar bone loss and tooth loss in male cigar and pipe smokers, *J Am Dent Assoc* 130:57, 1999.

184. Albandar JM, Streckfus CF, Adesanya MR, Winn DM: Cigar, pipe, and cigarette smoking as risk factors for periodontal disease and tooth loss. *J Periodontol* 71:1874, 2000.

185. Robertson PB, Walsh M, Greene J, et al: Periodontal effects associated to the use of smoking tobacco, *J Periodontol* 61:438, 1990.

186. American Academy of Periodontology: Position paper: Tobacco use and the periodontal patient, *J Periodontol* 70:1419, 1999.

187. Mooney J, Hodge PJ, Kinane DF: Humoral immune response in early-onset periodontitis: influence of smoking, *J Periodont Res* 36:227, 2001.

188. Persson L, Bergstrom J, Ito H, et al: Tobacco smoking and neutrophil activity in patients with periodontal disease, *J Periodontol* 72:90, 2001.

189. van Winkelhoff AJ, Bosch-Tijhof CJ, Winkel EG, et al: Smoking affects the subgingival microflora in periodontitis, *J Periodontol* 72:666, 2001.

190. Haffajee AD, Socransky SS: Relationship of cigarette smoking to the subgingival microbiota, *J Clin Periodontol* 28:377, 2001.

191. Haffajee AD, Socransky SS: Relationship of cigarette smoking to attachment level profiles, *J Clin Periodontol* 28:283, 2001.

192. Preber H, Bergstrom J, Linder LE: Occurrence of periopathogens in smoker and non-smoker patients, *J Clin Periodontol* 19:667, 1992.

193. Shlossman M, Knowler WC, Pettitt DJ, et al: Type 2 diabetes mellitus and periodontal disease, *J Am Dent Assoc* 121:532, 1990.

194. Cianciola LJ, Park BH, Bruck E, et al: Prevalence of periodontal disease in insulin-dependent diabetes mellitus (juvenile diabetes), *J Am Dent Assoc* 104:653, 1982.

195. Glavind L, Lund B, Löe H: The relationship between periodontal state and diabetes duration, insulin dosage and retinal changes, *J Periodontol* 39:341, 1968.

196. Tsai C, Hayes C, Taylor GW: Glycemic control of type 2 diabetes and severe periodontal disease in the US adult population, *Community Dent Oral Epidemiol* 30:182, 2002.

197. Oliver RC, Tervonen T: Diabetes—a risk factor for periodontitis in adults, *J Periodontol* 65:530, 1994.

198. Tervonen T, Oliver RC: Long term control of diabetes mellitus and periodontitis, *J Clin Periodontol* 20:431, 1993.

199. Emrich LJ, Shlossman M, Genco RJ: Periodontal disease in non-insulin dependent diabetes mellitus, *J Periodontol* 62:123, 1991.

200. Nelson RG, Shlossman M, Budding LM, et al: Periodontal disease and non-insulin dependent diabetes mellitus in Pima Indians, *Diabetes Care* 13:836, 1990.

201. Aldridge JP, Lester V, Watts TL, et al: Single-blind studies of the effects of improved periodontal health on metabolic control in type 1 diabetes mellitus, *J Clin Periodontol* 22:271, 1995.

202. Stewart JE, Wager KA, Friedlander AH, et al: The effect of periodontal treatment on glycemic control in patients with type 2 diabetes mellitus, *J Clin Periodontol* 28:306, 2001.

203. Grossi SG: Treatment of periodontal disease and control of diabetes: an assessment of the evidence and need for future research, *Ann Periodontol* 6:138, 2001.

204. Friedman RB, Gunsolley J, Gentry A, et al: Periodontal status of HIV-seropositive and AIDS patients, *J Periodontol* 62:623, 1991.

205. Klein RS, Quart AM, Small CB: Periodontal disease in heterosexuals with acquired immunodeficiency syndrome, *J Periodontol* 62:535, 1991.

206. Swango PA, Kleinman DV, Konzelman JL: HIV and periodontal health. A study of military personnel with HIV, *J Am Dent Assoc* 122:49, 1991.

207. Smith GL, Cross DL, Wray D: Comparison of periodontal disease in HIV seropositive subjects and controls (I). Clinical features, *J Clin Periodontol* 22:558, 1995.

208. Barr C, Lopez MR, Rua-Dobles A: Periodontal changes by HIV serostatus in a cohort of homosexual and bisexual men, *J Clin Periodontol* 19:794, 1992.

209. Yeung SC, Stewart GJ, Cooper DA, et al: Progression of periodontal disease in HIV seropositive patients, *J Periodontol* 64:651, 1993.

210. McKaig RG, Patton LL, Thomas JC, et al: Factors associated with periodontitis in an HIV-infected southeast USA study, *Oral Dis* 6:158, 2000.

211. Dios PD, Ocampo A, Miralles C, et al: Changing prevalence of human immunodeficiency virus-associated oral lesions, *Oral Surg Oral Med Oral Pathol Oral Radiol Endod* 90:403, 2000.

212. Ceballos-Salobreña A, Gaitán-Cepeda LA, Ceballos-Garcia L, et al: Oral lesions in HIV/AIDS patients undergoing highly active antiretroviral treatment including protease inhibitors: a new face of oral AIDS, *AIDS Patient Care STDS* 14:627, 2000.

213. Girasole G, Jilka RL, Passeri G, et al: 17-estradiol inhibits interleukin-6 production by bone marrow-derived stromal cells and osteoblasts in vitro: A potential mechanism for the antiosteoporotic effect of estrogens, *J Clin Invest* 89:883, 1992.

214. Jilka RL, Hangoc G, Girasole G, et al: Increased osteoclast development after estrogen loss: mediation by interleukin-6, *Science* 257:88, 1992.

215. American Academy of Periodontology: The pathogenesis of periodontal diseases, *J Periodontol* 70:457, 1999.

216. Inagaki K, Kurosu Y, Kamiya T, et al: Low metacarpal bone density, tooth loss, and periodontal disease in Japanese women, *J Dent Res* 80:1818, 2001.

217. Wactawski-Wende J, Grossi SG, Trevisan M, et al: The role of osteopenia in oral bone loss and periodontal disease, *J Periodontol* 67:1076, 1996.

218. Tezal M, Wactawski-Wende J, Grossi SG, et al: The relationship between bone mineral density and periodontitis in postmenopausal women, *J Periodontol* 71:1492, 2000.

219. Elders PJ, Habets LL, Netelenbos JC, et al: The relation between periodontitis and systemic bone mass in women between 46 and 55 years of age, *J Clin Periodontol* 19:492, 1992.

220. Weyant RJ, Pearlstein ME, Churak AP, et al: The association between osteopenia and periodontal attachment loss in older women, *J Periodontol* 70:982, 1991.

221. Ronderos M, Jacobs DR, Himes JH, et al: Associations of periodontal disease with femoral bone mineral density and estrogen replacement therapy: cross-sectional evaluation of US adults from NHANES III, *J Clin Periodontol* 27:778, 2000.

222. Russell AL, Consolazio CF, White CL: Periodontal disease and nutrition in Eskimo scouts of the Alaska national guard, *J Dent Res* 40:604, 1961.

223. Wertheimer FW, Brewster RH, White CL: Periodontal disease and nutrition in Thailand, *J Periodontol* 38:100, 1967.

224. Ramfjord SP, Emslie RD, Greene JC, et al: Epidemiological studies of periodontal diseases, *Am J Public Health* 58:1713, 1968.

225. Russell AL: Periodontal disease in well and malnourished populations, *Arch Environ Health* 5:153, 1962.

226. Nishida M, Grossi SG, Dunford RG, et al: Calcium and the risk for periodontal disease, *J Periodontol* 71:1057, 2000.

227. Mangan DF: Nutrition and oral infectious diseases: connections and future research, *Compend Contin Educ Dent* 23:416, 2002.

228. Reinhardt RA, Payne JB, Maze CA: Influence of estrogen and osteopenia/osteoporosis on clinical periodontitis in postmenopausal women, *J Periodontol* 70:823, 1999.

229. Payne JB, Zachs NR, Reinhardt RA, et al: The association between estrogen status and alveolar bone density changes in postmenopausal women with a history of periodontitis, *J Periodontol* 68:24, 1997.

230. Jacobs R, Ghyselen J, Koninckx P, et al: Long-term bone mass evaluation of mandible and lumbar spine in a group of women receiving hormone replacement therapy, *Eur J Oral Sci* 104:10, 1996.

231. Pacifici R, Brown C, Rifas L: TNF-α and GM-CSF secretion from human blood monocytes: effects of menopause and estrogen replacement, *J Bone Miner Res* 5:145, 1990.

232. Pacifici R, Rifas L, McCraken R, et al: Ovarian steroid treatment blocks a postmenopausal increase in blood monocyte interleukin 1 release, *Proc Natl Acad Sci USA* 86:2398, 1989.

233. Bismar H, Diel I, Ziegler R: Increased cytokine secretion by human marrow cells after menopause or discontinuation of estrogen replacement, *J Clin Endocrinol Metab* 80:3351, 1995.

234. Genco RJ, Ho AW, Grossi SG: et al: Relationship of stress, distress and inadequate coping behaviors to periodontal disease, *J Periodontol* 70:711, 1999.

235. Anttila SS, Knuuttila ML, Sakki TK: Relationship of depressive symptoms to edentulousness, dental health, and dental health behavior, *Acta Odontol Scand* 59:406, 2001.

236. Aleksejuniene J, Holst D, Eriksen HM: Psychosocial stress, lifestyle and periodontal health, *J Clin Periodontol* 29:326, 2002.

237. Genco RJ, Ho AW, Kopman J, et al: Models to evaluate the role of stress in periodontal disease, *Ann Periodontol* 3:288, 1998.

238. Wimmer G, Janda M, Wieselmann-Penkner K, et al: Coping with stress: its influence on periodontal disease, *J Periodontol* 73:1343, 2002.

239. Beaty TH, Colyer CR, Chang YC, et al: Familial aggregation of periodontal indices, *J Dent Res* 72:544, 1993.

240. van der Velden U, Abbas F, Armand S, et al: The effect of sibling relationship on the periodontal condition, *J Clin Periodontol* 20:683, 1993.

241. Chung CS, Kau MC, Chung SS, Rao DC: A genetic and epidemiologic study of periodontal disease in Hawaii. II. Genetic and environmental influence, *Am J Hum Genet* 29:76, 1977.

242. Corey LA, Nance WE, Hofstede P, Schenkein HA: Self-reported periodontal disease in a Virginia twin population, *J Periodontol* 64:1205, 1993.

243. Michalowicz BS, Aeppli D, Virag JG, et al: Periodontal findings in adult twins, *J Periodontol* 62:293, 1991.

244. Michalowicz BS, Diehl SR, Gunsolley JC, et al: Evidence of a substantial genetic basis for risk of adult periodontitis, *J Periodontol* 71:1699, 2000.

245. Moore WE, Burmeister JA, Brooks CN, et al: Investigation of the influences of puberty, genetics, and environment on the composition of subgingival periodontal floras, *Infect Immun* 61:2891, 1993.

246. Michalowicz BS, Wolff LF, Klump D, et al: Periodontal bacteria in adult twins, *J Periodontol* 70:263, 1999.

247. Goteiner D, Goldman MJ: Human lymphocyte antigen haplotype and resistance to periodontitis, *J Periodontol* 55:155, 1984.

248. Kobayashi T, Yamamoto K, Sugita N, et al: The Fc gamma receptor genotype as a severity factor for chronic periodontitis in Japanese patients, *J Periodontol* 72:1324, 2001.

249. Colombo AP, Eftimiadi C, Haffajee AD, et al: Serum IgG2 level, Gm(23) allotype and FcgammaRIIa and FcgammaRIIIb receptors in refractory periodontal disease, *J Clin Periodontol* 25:465, 1998.

250. Galbraith GM, Hendley TM, Sanders JJ, et al: Polymorphic cytokine genotypes as markers of disease severity in adult periodontitis, *J Clin Periodontol* 26:705, 1999.

251. Kornman KS, Pankow J, Offenbacher S, et al: Interleukin-1 genotypes and the association between periodontitis and cardiovascular disease, *J Periodont Res* 34:353, 1999.

252. McDevitt MJ, Wang HY, Knobelman C, et al: Interleukin-1 genetic association with periodontitis in clinical practice, *J Periodontol* 71:156, 2000.

253. Kocher T, Sawaf H, Fanghanel J, et al: Association between bone loss in periodontal disease and polymorphism of N-acetyltransferase (NAT2), *J Clin Periodontol* 29:21, 2002.

254. Meisel P, Timm R, Sawaf H, et al: Polymorphism of the N-acetyltransferase (NAT2), smoking and the potential risk of periodontal disease, *Arch Toxicol* 74:343, 2000.

255. Holla LI, Kankova K, Fassmann A, et al: Distribution of the receptor for advanced glycation end products gene polymorphisms in patients with chronic periodontitis: a preliminary study, *J Periodontol* 72:1742, 2001.

256. Holla LI, Fassmann A, Vasku A, et al: Interactions of lymphotoxin alpha (TNF-beta), angiotensin-converting enzyme (ACE), and endothelin-1 (ET-1) gene polymorphisms in adult periodontitis, *J Periodontol* 72:85, 2001.

257. Mark LL, Haffajee AD, Socransky SS, et al: Effect of the interleukin-1 genotype on monocyte IL-1b expression in subjects with adult periodontitis, *J Periodont Res* 35:172, 2000.

258. Gore EA, Sanders JJ, Pandey JP, et al: Interleukin-1beta [13953] allele 2: association with disease status in adult periodontitis, *J Clin Periodontol* 25:781, 1998.

259. McGuire MK, Nunn ME: Prognosis versus actual outcome. IV. The effectiveness of clinical parameters and IL-1 genotype in accurately predicting prognoses and tooth survival, *J Periodontol* 70:49, 1999.

260. Cullinan MP, Westerman B, Hamlet SM, et al: A longitudinal study of interleukin-1 gene polymorphisms and periodontal disease in a general adult population, *J Clin Periodontol* 28:1137, 2001.

261. Brown LF, Beck JD, Rozier RG: Incidence of attachment loss in community-dwelling older adults, *J Periodontol* 65:316, 1994.

262. Khocht A, Simon G, Person P: Gingival recession in relation to history of hard toothbrush use, *J Periodontol* 64:900, 1993.

263. van Palstein Helderman WH, Lembariti BS, van der Weijden GA: Gingival recession and its association with calculus in subjects deprived of prophylactic dental care, *J Clin Periodontol* 25:106, 1998.

264. Rustogi KN, Triratana T, Kietprajuk C, et al: The association between supragingival [correction of subgingival] calculus deposits and the extent of gingival recession in a sample of Thai children and teenagers, *J Clin Dent* 3(Suppl B):6, 1991.

265. Hirschfeld L, Wasserman B: A long-term survey of tooth loss in 600 treated periodontal patients, *J Periodontol* 49:225, 1978.

266. McFall WT: Tooth loss in 100 treated patients with periodontal disease, *J Periodontol* 53:539, 1982.

267. Goldman MJ, Ross IF, Goteiner D: Effect of periodontal therapy on patients maintained for 15 years or longer. A retrospective study, *J Periodontol* 57:347, 1986.

268. Ong G: Periodontal disease and tooth loss, *Int Dent J* 48 (3 Suppl 1):233, 1998.

269. Oliver RC, Brown LJ: Periodontal diseases and tooth loss, *Periodontol 2000* 2:117, 1993.

270. Brown LJ Oliver RC, Löe H: Periodontal disease in the U.S. in 1981: prevalence, severity, extent and role in tooth mortality, *J Periodontol* 60:363, 1989.

271. Khoury MJ, Beaty TH, Cohen BH: *Fundamentals of genetic epidemiology*, ed 1, New York, 1993, Oxford University Press.

4

Microbiology of Periodontal Diseases

Peter M. Loomer and Gary C. Armitage

MICROBIAL ECOSYSTEMS OF THE ORAL CAVITY
Dorsum of the Tongue
Epithelial Surfaces (Excluding Dorsum of Tongue)
Supragingival Tooth Surfaces
Subgingival Tooth Surfaces and the Epithelium Lining
  the Gingival Crevice
Saliva

**EVIDENCE FOR A BACTERIAL ETIOLOGY
OF PERIODONTAL DISEASES**
Clinical Observations
Periodontal Disease in Germfree Animals
Periodontal Disease in Monoinfected Gnotobiotic Animals
Experimental Periodontal Diseases
Therapeutic Effect of Plaque Control on Human
  Periodontitis

Epidemiologic Studies on the Relation Between
  Oral Hygiene and Periodontitis
Pathogenic Potential of Plaque Bacteria
"Proof" That Bacteria Cause Periodontal Diseases
Nonspecific and Specific Plaque Hypotheses

PERIODONTAL MICROFLORA IN HEALTH AND DISEASE
Polymicrobial Nature of Periodontal Infections
Periodontal Health
Gingivitis
Chronic Periodontitis
Localized Aggressive Periodontitis
Generalized Aggressive Periodontitis
Refractory Chronic Periodontitis
Necrotizing Ulcerative Gingivitis/Periodontitis
Periodontal Abscesses

MICROBIAL ECOSYSTEMS OF THE ORAL CAVITY

The oral cavity contains multiple ecologic milieus that provide unique environments for the diverse communities of microorganisms that reside in it. Although the mouth contains hundreds of microecosystems, for purposes of discussion it can be divided into four to five major ecosystems on the basis of anatomic, environmental, and microbiologic factors.

Dorsum of the Tongue

The dorsal surface of the tongue is covered with both shallow and deep fissures associated with such anatomic features as the foramen cecum, lingual follicles, and four types of papillae (i.e., filiform, fungiform, vallate, foliate). On a site-by-site basis the normal flora of the tongue has not been well characterized. However, gram-positive bacteria account for approximately 70% of the lingual flora.[1] Prominent among these are *Streptococcus sanguis* and *Streptococcus salivarius*. Low levels of cariogenic bacteria (*S. mutans*)[1] and gram-negative putative (suspected) periodontal pathogens (e.g., *Porphyromonas gingivalis*, *Prevotella intermedia*, *Campylobacter rectus*) have been found as part of the resident lingual flora in some healthy individuals.[2]

Epithelial Surfaces (Excluding Dorsum of Tongue)

Epithelial surfaces include the buccal epithelium, ventral surface of the tongue, alveolar mucosa, gingival surfaces exposed to saliva, and the palate (hard and soft). Colonization of epithelial cells depends on subtle differences in cell surface receptors for bacteria and other microorganisms. Epithelial receptors for oral microorganisms are very specific and differences exist between keratinized and nonkeratinized surfaces. In general, the normal flora of epithelial surfaces is dominated by streptococci, but not in the same proportions as those found on the tongue.

Supragingival Tooth Surfaces

The bacterial flora that colonizes supragingival tooth surfaces is of considerable interest because this is the environment in which dental caries develops. Supragingival tooth surfaces are constantly bathed in saliva. In vivo, tooth surfaces are rapidly coated with specific salivary proteins that form a coating called the *acquired pellicle*. The composition of the pellicle depends on a variety of factors including the genetic make-up of the host and free surface energies of the surface.[3,4] Subtle differences can be found in the pellicles that form on enamel, cementum, dentin, and restorative materials. These differences have a significant impact on the types of microorganisms that colonize the teeth. The composition and properties of acquired pellicles are discussed in greater detail in **Chapter 6**.

Subgingival Tooth Surfaces and the Epithelium Lining the Gingival Crevice

The ecosystem of subgingival tooth surfaces and the epithelium lining the gingival crevice is also of considerable interest because it is the environment in which periodontal diseases develop. During most conditions, subgingival surfaces are not bathed in saliva. Instead, these surfaces are exposed to serum proteins found in gingival crevicular fluid, which is an inflammatory exudate. Gingival crevicular fluid is a rich source of antibodies (e.g., IgG, IgM, IgA) and other antibacterial proteins. In addition, it contains cellular elements such as neutrophils that can significantly affect microbial colonization at subgingival sites. Microorganisms that colonize subgingival sites frequently have the ability to bypass or counteract these and other host defenses.

Saliva

The ecosystem of saliva is a turbulent environment with no fixed surface for microorganisms to reside. Indeed, some authors do not consider it a separate ecosystem because it contains shed components of the other four ecosystems. Nevertheless, important interactions of bacteria with each other and the host occur in saliva; these interactions have an impact on the overall ecology of the mouth.

EVIDENCE FOR A BACTERIAL ETIOLOGY OF PERIODONTAL DISEASES

In the last century numerous lines of evidence have emerged supporting the concept that, in susceptible hosts, bacteria cause periodontal diseases. Strong arguments favoring this concept can be made, including the following seven lines of evidence: (1) clinical observations, (2) germfree animal studies, (3) observations in monoinfected gnotobiotic animals, (4) data from studies of experimental periodontal diseases in animals and humans, (5) results of periodontal therapy in humans, (6) epidemiologic data, and (7) pathogenic potential of dental plaque bacteria.

Clinical Observations

Testimonials from the empiric observations of clinicians are the weakest form of evidence. Nevertheless, careful observations by astute clinicians have led to significant advances in our understanding of disease. In the past 250 years numerous individuals expressed the clinical opinion that periodontal diseases are caused by uncleanliness of the mouth.[5,6] After 1876, when Koch[7] showed that bacteria could cause disease, many clinicians used the terms *uncleanliness* and *bacteria* interchangeably.[8-10] Most scientific evidence, however, supporting the clinical impression that bacteria cause periodontal diseases is of recent vintage, emerging only within the past four to five decades.

Periodontal Disease in Germfree Animals

Since the initial studies of Orland and colleagues in 1954,[11] it has been known that dental caries cannot develop in germfree animals. The development of periodontal disease in animals maintained in a germfree environment is not as clear-cut. In the absence of microorganisms, several strains of mice and rats have alveolar bone loss with apical migration of the junctional epithelium.[12-14] It is generally believed, however, that this loss of attachment is attributable to mechanical irritation from hair and food impaction.[15-18] Slight gingival inflammation without attachment loss has also been reported in germfree beagle dogs.[19,20] Such inflammation is believed to be an immune-mediated response caused by exposure of the animals to foreign proteins and endotoxins in their sterilized diets.[19] Conventional beagles with a naturally acquired oral flora, however, develop severe gingival inflammation and extensive attachment loss.[21-23] Without question, these investigations show that, during some circumstances, a limited amount of periodontal destruction can occur in the absence of microorganisms. But because this tissue destruction only bears a superficial resemblance to that observed in conventional animals and humans with periodontitis, such studies do not disprove the hypothesis that bacteria are necessary for the development of periodontal disease.

Periodontal Disease in Monoinfected Gnotobiotic Animals

Gnotobiotic animals are those in which the microbial flora is known (Greek: *gnotos*, "know" + *bios*, "life"). A germfree animal is gnotobiotic because it is known that no microbial flora is present. Germfree animals are rarely screened for the presence of viruses and rickettsiae; therefore, strictly speaking, they may not be germfree. However, in general, use of the term *germfree* indicates animals free of bacteria, yeasts, fungi, and protozoa. Some, but not all bacteria, when introduced into environments of germfree animals, can colonize them. In such cases, the colonized animals are also termed *gnotobiotic* because their flora is known. Monoinfected animals are those colonized by a single microbial species or strain. Monoinfected animals have been widely used as a model for studying the pathogenic potential of certain microorganisms.[24] Several strains of bacteria can produce caries, or periodontal disease, or both when implanted in gnotobiotic animals. In some cases, the clinical characteristics produced by monoinfection of experimental animals closely resemble those found in the human disease from which the microorganism was obtained. For example, *Actinomyces viscosus*, a species associated with gingival inflammation and root caries in humans, produces these pathologic conditions in monoinfected rats.[25]

Experiments with monoinfected animals generally support the concept that microorganisms can cause periodontal disease. The gnotobiotic animal is, however, a somewhat artificial situation.[24] In many instances, bacteria that are suspected periodontopathogens in humans will not cause disease in gnotobiotic animals because of an inability to successfully colonize oral tissues of the animals. Conversely, disease production in monoinfected animals may have no direct relation to pathologic events occurring in human periodontal tissues. Unlike humans, monoinfected animals have no endogenous or normal oral flora to interfere with, or enhance, the pathogenic properties of the infecting microorganisms, and their immune system has not been conditioned for microbial assaults. Furthermore, bone loss in monoinfected animals is frequently localized to areas of hair impaction, a situation not found in humans.

Experimental Periodontal Diseases

One of the strongest lines of evidence supporting an etiologic role for bacteria in human periodontal disease comes from an elegantly simple *experimental gingivitis* model introduced by Löe in 1965. The original studies of experimental gingivitis were performed on Danish dental students.[26-30] The model has three stages:

- *Preparatory period:* Through an intensive plaque control program, plaque-free mouths and healthy gingivae are produced in healthy volunteers.
- *Period of no plaque control:* The disease-free volunteers cease all efforts toward oral cleanliness. As plaque accumulates, the onset and severity of disease is monitored. Gingivitis produced during these conditions is termed *experimental gingivitis*.
- *Period of plaque control:* Efforts are made to once again remove plaque. The influence of plaque removal on the experimental gingivitis is monitored.

This model has been used to study the sequential changes in the microbial flora of developing plaque and the relation of these changes to the time required for the onset of gingivitis. It was clearly shown that gingivitis could be experimentally produced in humans by deliberately allowing plaque to accumulate, and reversal of experimental gingivitis could be accomplished by plaque control procedures. The major findings of these studies were:

- The *time* necessary for the development of clinically detectable marginal gingivitis varied from 10 to 21 days.[26,27]
- With the reinstitution of oral hygiene procedures experimental gingival inflammation resolved in about 1 week.[26,27]
- As dental plaque from the gingival margin matured, its composition changed from a predominantly gram-positive flora (90% to 100%) to one rich in gram-negative forms (40% to 50%) (Table 4-1).[27]

TABLE 4-1   Summary of Bacteriological Data from the Original Experimental Gingivitis Studies

HEALTHY GINGIVA (DAY 0)	EXPERIMENTAL GINGIVITIS (DAYS 10-21)
G+ cocci and rods: 90% to 100%	G+ cocci and rods: 45-60% G− cocci and rods: 22% (range 11-31%) G+ filaments: 10% (range 5-16%) Fusobacteria (G−): 10% (range 4-15%) Vibrios (G−): 6% (range 1-12%) Spirochetes: 1% (range 0-2%)

Data from References 26 and 27.
Totals are about 40% to 50% G− bacteria.

- The appearance of the gram-negative flora *preceded* the onset of clinically detectable gingivitis by about 3 to 10 days.[27]
- Despite the use of antibiotics to selectively suppress portions of the plaque flora, gingival inflammation still developed, albeit at a slower rate.[28,29]

The bacteriological data from the original experimental gingivitis studies were based on microscopic examination of smears and impression preparations of supragingival plaque near the gingival margin.[26] The impression technique involved pressing a thin plastic film against the gingival margin region. Plaque adhering to the film was Gram-stained and examined microscopically. These methods provide only a rough approximation of the composition of the flora. Therefore, the studies were repeated using bacteriological culturing techniques to better analyze the microbial composition of developing supragingival plaque associated with experimental gingivitis.[31,32] The principal findings (Table 4-2) from this series of studies were:

- The flora was predominantly gram-positive at all time periods (0, 1, 2, and 3 weeks)
- *A. viscosus* (G+ filament) was significantly associated with the development of marginal gingivitis
- *Actinomyces* species dominated in the 2- and 3-week-old plaques (i.e., 40% to 50% of the colony-forming units).

Results of these cultural studies[31,32] differ somewhat from those based on examination of crude smears of plaque.[26,27] The cultural studies showed no increase in the gram-negative flora of developing supragingival plaque, a result that has been confirmed by other authors.[33,34] However, the overall clinical findings of most experimental gingivitis studies are the same.

Unlike experimental gingivitis studies, for ethical reasons *experimental periodontitis* studies have not been performed in humans. However, data are available from studies in animals. In a series of studies, young beagle dogs were brought to a state of gingival health through a rigorous plaque control regimen.[22,23] Dogs in one group had their teeth brushed twice daily for 4 years. Another group was allowed to form plaque during the same time period. Both groups were periodically examined clinically, radiographically, and histologically. At the end of 4 years animals receiving daily plaque control had no gingival inflammation or attachment loss. All of the animals that had been allowed to form plaque had extensive gingival inflammation and most of them (i.e., 8 of 10) also had attachment loss at the end of the 4-year observation period.[23] These important studies unequivocally show that, in beagles, experimental gingivitis can progress to periodontitis. They further show that the entire series of pathologic events associated with periodontitis can be prevented by rigorous plaque control. It is likely that similar results would be obtained in humans. Importantly, the finding that 2 of the 10 animals in this series of studies had severe gingivitis, but did not develop attachment loss, allowed researchers to begin to understand that gingivitis does not *always* lead to periodontitis.

Therapeutic Effect of Plaque Control on Human Periodontitis

If bacteria are important in the etiology of periodontitis, then periodic plaque removal in humans should control and/or prevent the disease. Indeed, longitudinal studies of periodontal therapy indicate that this is the case. In the last 35 years several important clinical studies have shown that *plaque control* and *maintenance* are the most important steps in the treatment of periodontitis.[35-37] Plaque control is the daily mechanical removal of plaque by the patient. Maintenance involves the periodic removal of supragingival and subgingival plaque and calculus by a dentist or dental hygienist. Plaque control and maintenance can be viewed as *mechanical* forms of antimicrobial therapy.[38] That they are effective in the clinical management of periodontitis supports the concept that periodontal diseases are of microbial origin.

Further evidence that bacteria cause periodontal diseases comes from numerous studies demonstrating the value of antimicrobial chemicals when used as adjuncts to mechanical periodontal therapy.[39] Antimicrobial agents

TABLE 4-2 Summary of Bacteriological Data from Cultural Studies on Experimental Gingivitis	
HEALTHY GINGIVA (DAY 0)	MARGINAL GINGIVITIS (DAYS 14-21)
G+ streptococci: 62% *Veillonella* (G− cocci): 15-20%	G+ streptococci: 26-32% *Veillonella* (G− cocci): 15-20% Other G− forms: 5% *Actinomyces* sp. (G+ filaments): 40-50%

Data from References 31 and 32.
Percentages represent colony-forming units.

that have been shown to add to the beneficial effects of mechanical periodontal treatment include: antiseptic mouthrinses,[40] systemically administered antibiotics,[41] and subgingivally applied antiseptics and antibiotics.[42] For a variety of reasons, none of the antimicrobial agents used in periodontal treatment is sufficient when used alone to adequately treat periodontal diseases.

Epidemiologic Studies on the Relation Between Oral Hygiene and Periodontitis

Numerous epidemiologic studies have examined the relation between gingivitis or periodontitis and such variables as: oral hygiene, age, race, sex, socioeconomic factors, education, occupation, tobacco consumption, nutrition, and vitamin deficiencies.[43-55] In general, there is a strong relation between poor oral hygiene and gingivitis. The relation between poor oral hygiene and the risk for development of periodontitis is not as strong. Indeed, many studies indicate that there is a poor correlation between severe periodontitis and the amount of plaque and calculus.[48-54] The probable reason for this observation is that periodontitis is a multifactorial disease that requires the presence of plaque bacteria, a genetically susceptible host, and one or more risk factors such as aging or smoking. In other words, because some people have substantial amounts of plaque but no major periodontal destruction, the statistical relation between plaque and periodontitis is weakened. Nevertheless, it is rare to find individuals with periodontitis who also have excellent oral hygiene and very little plaque.

Overall, epidemiologic studies provide considerable support for the hypothesis that bacteria are a cause of gingivitis and periodontitis. People with very clean teeth do not usually have these diseases. Epidemiologic studies also clearly show that, in addition to plaque, there are other equally important risk factors for the development of periodontitis. (A detailed discussion of risk factors for periodontal diseases appears in **Chapter 3**.)

Pathogenic Potential of Plaque Bacteria

The final line of evidence supporting a role for microorganisms in the pathogenesis of periodontitis deals with their potential to directly or indirectly cause tissue damage.[56-60] Although this potential is immense, it is difficult to pinpoint the exact mechanisms by which plaque bacteria damage periodontal tissues because so many injurious agents emanate from plaque.

Whereas frank invasion of gingival tissues does not occur in most cases of periodontitis, their *products* readily enter the gingiva. Entry of these products is facilitated by increased permeability of sulcular and pocket epithelia. In addition, in cases of periodontitis, microulcerations in the epithelial lining of the pocket wall are common. These ulcerations allow microbial products to come into direct contact with gingival connective tissue.

There are numerous ways in which bacterial products from dental plaque might theoretically be involved in the development and progression of periodontitis, including the following:

- *Direct destruction of periodontal tissues* (e.g., by enzymes of microbial origin)
- *Activation of endogenous or host-oriented lytic systems* (e.g., activation of endogenous enzymes, generation of chemotactic factors)
- *Local alterations in tissue integrity* (e.g., increased permeability of sulcular epithelium)
- *Enhancement or perpetuation of the inflammatory response* (e.g., generation of chemotactic factors, alterations in vascular permeability, formation of antigen-antibody complexes, sensitization of lymphocytes)
- *Inhibition of host-repair processes* (e.g., interference with collagen synthesis)
- *Local suppression of host defenses* (e.g., blockage of the antimicrobial responses of neutrophils, production of enzymes that lyse antibacterial antibodies).

"Proof" That Bacteria Cause Periodontal Diseases

Koch's postulates

In 1876, Robert Koch presented formal criteria for proving that a specific microorganism can cause a given disease.[7] These criteria were: (1) the organism must be found in lesions of the disease, (2) it must be isolated and grown in pure culture on artificial media, (3) inoculation of this culture into experimental animals must produce lesions similar to those observed in cases of the disease in humans, and (4) the organism must be recovered from the lesions in the experimental animals. In the "Golden Age of Medical Microbiology" (1876-1940) these criteria were valuable in identifying human pathogens. However, in some diseases, Koch's postulates cannot be satisfied because some pathogens cannot be grown on artificial media and some microorganisms are only pathogenic for humans (i.e., are species-specific).

Alternative criteria

In 1979, alternative criteria were suggested for establishing an etiologic role of a microorganism in periodontal diseases.[61] These criteria include:

1. *Association with Disease:* The putative pathogen must be at significantly greater levels at diseased sites than at healthy sites. This is a slight modification of Koch's first postulate. (Weighting Factor = 0.3.)

2. *Elimination of the Organism:* If a putative pathogen is eliminated from or suppressed in a periodontal lesion by therapy, progression of the lesion should be arrested. (Weighting Factor = 0.3.)

3. *Host Response:* Compared with host responses against nonpathogens, the response to pathogens should be increased or decreased. For example, a heightened immune response to an organism in cases of active periodontal disease suggests a possible etiologic role for that organism. (Weighting Factor = 0.2.)

4. *Animal Pathogenicity:* If the putative pathogen can colonize the mouths of either germfree or conventional animals, it should cause a disease similar to that observed in humans from which it was originally isolated (e.g., gingival inflammation, bone loss, and others). (Weighting Factor = 0.1.)

5. *Mechanisms of Pathogenicity:* The putative pathogen should possess characteristics that could allow it to contribute to the pathogenesis of the disease. (Weighting Factor = 0.1.)

Application of these alternative criteria can be useful in objectively evaluating if certain components of the periodontal flora play a causative role in the disease. If a given microorganism performs well during these criteria, then it is highly suggestive that the organism is etiologically important.

Nonspecific and Specific Plaque Hypotheses

Two major hypotheses have been proposed to explain the role of bacterial plaque in the initiation and progression of periodontal diseases: the nonspecific plaque hypothesis and the specific plaque hypothesis. The *nonspecific plaque hypothesis* proposes that with plaque accumulation on tooth surfaces and in the gingival crevice, it is not specific bacteria but the entire microbial community, through the production of virulence factors, that collectively induce inflammation and the subsequent destruction

of periodontal tissue.[62] Despite the increase in proportions of gram-negative anaerobic bacteria at periodontally diseased sites, these same microorganisms are also present at healthy sites; thus it is not any specific microorganism that is responsible for inducing disease, but a general nonspecific increase in the amount of plaque.

Alternatively, the *specific plaque hypothesis* states that despite the detection of several hundred different species of microorganisms in periodontal pockets, less than 20 are routinely found in increased proportions at periodontally diseased sites. According to this hypothesis, only certain bacteria whose levels increase during the development and progression of periodontal disease are causative.[63,64]

Although there is support for both hypotheses, probably neither completely explains the role bacteria play in all diseased sites at all times. For example, it is conceivable that the levels of one or two specific bacteria may be increased at one site, whereas at another site no increases in any specific bacterium is detected. The combined effect of slight or nondetectable increases or shifts in the proportions of many different bacteria may be enough to initiate disease. Furthermore, the host's immune defenses and the local pocket environmental niche may modify the composition of the microbial community. Thus the multifactorial nature of periodontal disease probably contributes to the validity of both hypotheses depending on the individual circumstances.

Irrespective of which theory applies, our understanding of the microbiology of periodontal disease is limited by our inability to completely characterize the composition of the subgingival flora. It has been estimated that only 50% of the subgingival flora has been identified; the remainder cannot even be cultivated.[65] The use of newer molecular techniques, such as examination of well conserved 16S ribosomal RNA gene sequences in the oral flora, has led to the recognition of previously undetected microorganisms in subgingival plaque.[66-74] The role that these uncultivable microorganisms may play in the pathogenesis of periodontal diseases remains unknown, largely because of our technologic inability to grow them. Clearly, as 16S rRNA gene technology is more widely applied to the characterization of the oral flora in health and disease, our current view of the nature of the disease-producing microflora will change.

PERIODONTAL MICROFLORA IN HEALTH AND DISEASE

Although some periodontal infections can be caused by bacteria that are not ordinarily residents of the oral cavity (i.e., *exogenous* bacteria),[75,76] most forms of gingivitis and periodontitis are caused by members of the normal flora (i.e., *endogenous* bacteria).[77] Indeed, most of the putative periodontal pathogens are frequently found, albeit in low numbers, in the oral flora of patients without periodontitis.[78-85]

Microorganisms associated with periodontal diseases have been identified through cross-sectional and longitudinal studies in which specific bacteria are detected in subgingival plaque samples taken from diseased and nondiseased sites. The presence or absence of bacteria or their components has been determined using a variety of methodologies, including culture, nucleic acid (DNA, RNA) probes, direct and indirect immunofluorescence, 16S rRNA gene sequences, and polymerase chain reaction. These methods have different thresholds in their ability to detect specific bacteria.[86] Although the same species that are believed to cause periodontal diseases are also often found at healthy sites, it is differences in the quantities and proportions of the bacteria that often determine whether the microorganism is considered a pathogen. Interestingly, it has been reported that fewer putative pathogens are found in healthy sites of people with no periodontal disease than in healthy sites of individuals with chronic periodontitis.[85]

Some of the characteristics that determine whether a bacterial species is pathogenic are presence at diseased sites, increased levels in these sites, and possession of an array of virulence factors (Table 4-3). These virulence factors give the bacteria an advantage over the host by helping the bacteria adhere to host tissue, avoiding the host's immune defense systems, penetrating into host tissue, or by producing compounds that are capable of damaging host tissue or inducing host-mediated inflammation. The structure and organization of the plaque biofilm itself also imparts virulence to the community of pathogenic microorganisms by enabling bacteria to act synergistically to provide nutrients to each other, safely remove waste products, and provide physical and chemical barriers to avoid the host immune defenses or antimicrobial agents (see **Chapter 6**).

The results of microbiologic studies are greatly influenced by the methods used to collect and process plaque samples. The two most common methods for obtaining subgingival plaque samples for laboratory analysis are using curettes or endodontic paper points. There are often major differences in the microbial profiles of plaque samples collected by the two methods. One main reason for the disparate results from plaque samples collected by curettes versus paper points is that the two methods sample different portions of the biofilm. Paper points primarily harvest bacteria from loosely adherent portions of the biofilm, whereas curettes collect bacteria from most tooth-associated portions. It is important to remember that bacteria are not evenly distributed throughout plaque biofilms and the sampling strategy used will affect the outcome of microbiologic analysis of the clinical specimen. In addition, the specific laboratory procedures used to process the plaque samples and the laboratories themselves can also lead to widely varying results.[87,88]

Polymicrobial Nature of Periodontal Infections

An important characteristic of all periodontal infections is that they are associated with, and probably caused by, multiple pathogens. In other words they are mixed infections. There are no forms of dental plaque-induced

TABLE 4-3 Virulence Factors of Bacteria Associated With Periodontal Infections	
VIRULENCE FACTOR	**MECHANISM OF ACTION**
Fimbriae, pili, fibrillae	Bacterial attachment, prevention of bacterial phagocytosis
Capsule, exopolysaccharide, glycocalyx	Bacterial attachment, prevention of bacterial phagocytosis, protection from complement and immune system
Peptidoglycan, muramyl peptides	Immunodilation, induction of inflammatory mediators
Endotoxin	Activation of inflammatory response, activation of cytokine production, induction of bone resorption
Proteolytic enzymes: collagenase, gelatinase, hyaluronidase, fibrolysin, immunoglobulin proteases. H_2S and volatile sulfur compounds.	Breakdown of host connective tissue; host tissue invasion
Inorganic acids: butyric acid, propionic acid	Host cell toxicity
Superoxide dismutase	Breakdown of oxygen products, protecting anaerobes

periodontal diseases that are caused by a single pathogen. Although certain microbial combinations and patterns are frequently associated with a given form of periodontal disease, considerable variation in the recoverable subgingival flora is usually encountered.

An additional complicating factor in the microbiology of periodontal infections is the extensive genetic and clonal diversity of each putative periodontal pathogen.[59,89-96] For example, in one study of 33 clinical isolates of *P. gingivalis*, 29 had different DNA fingerprints as assessed with restriction endonuclease analysis.[89] Observations such as this suggest that it would be a mistake to assume that two patients harboring *P. gingivalis* are necessarily infected by identical microorganisms. Polymerase chain reaction analyses make it possible to detect clonal variations in putative periodontal pathogens and it is clear that enormous variations exist.[89-96] It has preliminarily been shown that certain clonal types of putative periodontal pathogens are more important in the etiology of chronic periodontitis than other clonal types.[95]

Periodontal Health

At periodontally healthy sites the microbial load is low with only 10^2 to 10^3 bacteria typically being isolated from plaque samples in a healthy gingival sulcus.[59] Although extensive variation exists across studies, there is general agreement that the cultivable bacteria at healthy sites are mostly gram-positive and belong to the *Streptococcus* and *Actinomyces* genera (Box 4-1).[97-99] In health, approximately 75% to 80% of the recoverable microflora is gram-positive with most of the remainder belonging to gram-negative species of the *Veillonella* and *Fusobacterium* genera. It is not surprising that these bacteria are associated with healthy sites because they are prominent early colonizers of tooth surfaces and gingival crevices. It should be pointed out that an average of approximately 40% to 50% of the subgingival flora at healthy sites of people with periodontitis[100] and periodontitis-free individuals older than age 55[98] have been reported to be composed of gram-negative bacteria. It should also be emphasized that bacteria associated with periodontal diseases are often found in the subgingival microflora at healthy sites, although they are normally present in small proportions. Finally, the microflora in health is mostly of a nonmotile nature.[101]

Gingivitis

As discussed earlier, studies of changes in the cultivable microflora during the development of experimental gingivitis in humans indicate that gram-positive bacteria dominated at all time periods.[31-34] In general, this finding is also true in cases of naturally occurring gingivitis in which the disease may have been present for months or even years.[102] Studies of naturally occurring gingivitis indicate that, compared with periodontally healthy sites,

---

Box 4-1   Prominent Subgingival Bacteria Found in Biofilms at Sites Exhibiting Periodontal Health and Naturally Occurring Gingivitis

Periodontal Health

Gram-positive:

Streptococcus sanguis	*Actinomyces naeslundii*
Streptococcus gordonii	*Actinomyces israelii*
Streptococcus oralis	*Actinomyces viscosus*
Streptococcus mitis	

Gram-negative:

Veillonella parvula
Fusobacterium nucleatum

Naturally Occurring Gingivitis

Gram-positive:

Streptococcus sanguis	*Actinomyces naeslundii*
Streptococcus oralis	*Actinomyces israelii*
Streptococcus mitis	*Actinomyces odontolyticus*
Streptococcus intermedius	*Eubacterium brachy*
Peptostreptococcus micros	*Eubacterium timidum*

Gram-negative:

Veillonella parvula	*Capnocytophaga ochracea*
Fusobacterium nucleatum	*Capnocytophaga gingivalis*
*Campylobacter rectus**	*Capnocytophaga sputigena*
Bacteroides gracilis	*Selenomonas noxia**
Prevotella nigrescens	*Eikenella corrodens*
Prevotella loeschii	

Other (Gram stain not useful in separating bacterial types):

*Treponema denticola** (and many other spirochetes)

*Motile bacteria

---

the microbial load at diseased sites is greater, with approximately 10^4 to 10^6 bacteria being typically isolated from subgingival plaque samples.[59] In addition to the increased microbial load at sites with gingivitis, there is a general shift toward increasing proportions of gram-negative bacteria (Box 4-1). Compared with healthy sites, noticeable increases also occur in the numbers of motile bacteria, including cultivable and uncultivable treponemes (spirochetes).[102,103] It is not possible to name a specific subset of bacteria that cause gingivitis because a very diverse group of microorganisms appear to be capable of producing gingival irritation. Nevertheless, there are significant differences in the subgingival flora of healthy and gingivitis sites, and the bacteria believed to be responsible for periodontitis are already present at sites with gingivitis.[102]

Chronic Periodontitis

The microflora of sites displaying the clinical features of chronic periodontitis exhibit a spectrum of bacterial species similar to that found in naturally occurring

---

Box 4-2 | **Prominent Subgingival Bacteria Found in Biofilms at Sites with Chronic Periodontitis and Bacteria in These Biofilms That Have Been Etiologically Linked to Chronic Periodontitis**

Chronic Periodontitis (prominent members of subgingival biofilms)

Gram-positive:

Streptococcus sanguis
Streptococcus oralis
Streptococcus intermedius
Peptostreptococcus micros
Lactobacillus uli
Lactobacillus rimae

Actinomyces naeslundii
Actinomyces odontolyticus
Eubacterium nodatum
Eubacterium timidum

Gram-negative:

Fusobacterium nucleatum
Bacteroides gracilis

Campylobacter concisus
Selenomonas sputigena

Other (Gram stain not useful in separating bacterial types):

Treponema denticola (and many other spirochetes)

Chronic Periodontitis (biofilm bacteria of probable etiologic importance)

Gram-positive:

Streptococcus intermedius
Peptostreptococcus micros

Eubacterium nodatum
Lactobacillus uli

Gram-negative:

Porphyromonas gingivalis
*Campylobacter rectus**
Fusobacterium nucleatum[†]
*Selenomonas noxia**
*Selenomonas flueggii**

Tannerella forsythensis [Bacteroides forsythus]
Prevotella intermedia
Actinobacillus actinomycetemcomitans
Eikenella corrodens

Other (Gram-stain not useful in separating bacterial types):

*Treponema denticola** (and many other spirochetes)

*Motile bacteria.
[†]Subspecies of probable etiologic importance are F. nucleatum *subsp.* nucleatum, F. nucleatum *subsp.* vincentii, *and* F. nucleatum *subsp.* polymorphum.

---

gingivitis. However, the proportions of the individual bacteria usually vary between the two diseases.[102,103] Because it is believed that gingivitis precedes all cases of chronic periodontitis, the microflora of the latter represents a further maturation of subgingival plaque biofilms. In general, sites with chronic periodontitis will be populated with greater proportions of gram-negative organisms and motile bacteria (e.g., *Treponema denticola* and other spirochetes) (Box 4-2). Although gram-positive bacteria represent a substantial proportion of subgingival biofilms in cases of chronic periodontitis, certain gram-negative bacteria with pronounced virulence properties have been strongly implicated as etiologic agents (e.g., *P. gingivalis* and *Tannerella forsythensis* [formerly *Bacteroides forsythus*]).[104] An important feature of the microbiology of periodontal infections is that the putative pathogens rarely constitute a major component of the entire dental plaque biofilm.

Indeed, usually the suspected pathogen is less than 5% of the recoverable isolates from the entire plaque biomass.[103] Coaggregating bacteria such as *Actinomyces naeslundii, S. sanguis,* and *Fusobacterium nucleatum* are among the most numerous bacteria isolated from dental plaque irrespective of disease status.[103]

Coaggregation of bacteria or the cell-to-cell adherence of microorganisms is a basic characteristic or feature of dental plaque biofilms. Importantly, coaggregation of bacteria in plaque biofilms is not a random occurrence.[105,106] It has been determined that there are at least six specific microbial groups or complexes within subgingival plaque. For purposes of discussion they have been given color designations to reflect developmental stages of biofilm formation and the association of certain bacterial complexes with periodontal infections. Four groups referred to as the blue, yellow, green, and purple complexes are composed of early colonizers of the subgingival niche (Table 4-4). Late colonizers associated with climax microbial communities of mature subgingival biofilms are called the orange and red complexes (Table 4-4). The presence of these complexes emphasizes that bacteria do not colonize or proliferate in subgingival sites as isolated species. The colonization of gingival crevices by microbial complexes gives the bacteria within them an ecological advantage over an isolated bacterial species in the process of colonization. It is of interest that some bacteria in four of the six complexes contain putative periodontal pathogens (Table 4-4).

TABLE 4-4   Microbial Complexes of Late and Early Colonizers in Subgingival Biofilms Reflecting the Nonrandom Associations of Bacteria

COLONIZERS	GRAM STAIN/MOTILITY
Early Colonizers	
Blue Complex:	
Various *Actinomyces* species	G+, nonmotile
Purple Complex:	
Veillonella parvula	G−, nonmotile
Actinomyces odontolyticus	G+, nonmotile
Green Complex:	
Eikenella corrodens	G−, nonmotile
Capnocytophaga gingivalis	G−, nonmotile
Capnocytophaga sputigena	G−, nonmotile
Capnocytophaga ochracea	G−, nonmotile
Capnocytophaga concisus	G−, nonmotile
Actinobacillus actinomycetemcomitans (serotype a)*	G−, nonmotile
Yellow Complex:	
Streptococcus mitis	G+, nonmotile
Streptococcus oralis	G+, nonmotile
Streptococcus sanguis	G+, nonmotile
Streptococcus gordonii	G+, nonmotile
*Streptococcus intermedius**	G+, nonmotile
Late Colonizers	
Orange Complex:	
Campylobacter gracilis	G−, motile
*Campylobacter rectus**	G−, motile
Campylobacter showae	G−, motile
*Eubacterium nodatum**	G+, nonmotile
Fusobacterium nucleatum, subsp. *nucleatum**	G−, nonmotile
Fusobacterium nucleatum, subsp. *polymorphum**	G−, nonmotile
*Prevotella intermedia**	G−, nonmotile
*Peptostreptococcus micros**	G+, nonmotile
*Prevotella nigrescens**	G−, nonmotile
Streptococcus constellatus	G+, nonmotile
Red Complex:	
*Porphyromonas gingivalis**	G−, nonmotile
*Tannerella forsythensis (Bacteroides forsythus)**	G−, nonmotile
*Treponema denticola**	NA, motile

Data from Reference 106.
Putative periodontal pathogens.
G+, Gram-positive; G−, Gram-negative; NA, not applicable.

Localized Aggressive Periodontitis

Localized aggressive periodontitis (LAP) is the diagnostic term used for periodontal diseases that are characterized by severe attachment loss over a short period of time, occurring mostly around permanent incisors and first molars in young individuals (see Chapter 2). Taken as a whole, the microflora of subgingival biofilms from patients with LAP is similar to that of patients with chronic periodontitis.[103,107-109] On a percentage basis, the most numerous isolates are several species from the genera *Eubacterium, A. naeslundii, F. nucleatum, C. rectus,* and *Veillonella parvula.*[103,107] In some populations, a strong case can be made for *Actinobacillus actinomycetemcomitans* playing a causative role in LAP, especially in cases in which patients harbor highly leukotoxic strains of the organism.[77,104,109-113] However, some populations of patients with LAP do not harbor *A. actinomycetemcomitans,*[114] and in still others *P. gingivalis* may be etiologically more important.[104,107,111,115] It should be remembered, however, that all dental plaque-induced periodontal diseases are mixed infections and none of them is caused by a single pathogen.

Generalized Aggressive Periodontitis

Generalized aggressive periodontitis is an unusually severe form of periodontal disease that affects young individuals. It differs clinically from LAP in several ways, but one of the main differences is that periodontitis develops in many more teeth than in cases of LAP (see Chapter 2). The subgingival flora in patients with generalized aggressive periodontitis resembles that in other forms of periodontitis in that the predominant bacteria in subgingival plaque are *Eubacterium* species, *F. nucleatum, A. naeslundii,* and *Lactobacillus uli.*[103,116] However, this only holds true in situations in which a large portion of the subgingival biofilm is collected with a curet.[103,116] If the plaque is sampled with sterile paper points, as is commonly done, the microflora appears to be dominated by a different spectrum of bacteria.[117] For example, when collected with paper points the predominant subgingival bacteria in patients with generalized aggressive periodontitis are *P. gingivalis, T. forsythensis* [*B. forsythus*], *A. actinomycetemcomitans,* and *Campylobacter* species.[117]

Refractory Chronic Periodontitis

Treatment of chronic periodontitis by conventional methods is usually effective. However, in a small subset of patients therapy fails to stop progression of disease despite excellent patient compliance. Patients who have unexpectedly not responded to therapy are referred to as having *refractory* periodontitis.[118] In fact, patients who are given this diagnosis represent a very heterogeneous group clinically and microbiologically. The microflora taken from progressing sites in some of these patients is unusually diverse and may contain enteric rods, staphy-

lococci, and *Candida.*[119-123] In other patients, persistently high levels are found of one or more of the following bacteria: *P. gingivalis, T. forsythensis* [*B. forsythus*], *S. intermedius, P. intermedia, Peptostreptococcus micros,* and *Eikenella corrodens.*[124-128] Persistence of *Streptococcus constellatus* has also been reported.[129] From a microbiological point of view it is clear that refractory chronic periodontitis is not a single entity.

Chronic periodontitis patients with refractory disease are candidates for microbial testing to identify subgingival bacteria that might be responsible for the continuing infection. In such cases, one to two paper points are inserted into representative therapy-resistant pockets for approximately 20 seconds, withdrawn, and immediately placed in reduced transport fluid, and then sent to a licensed clinical laboratory for analysis. Cultivable putative pathogens are identified and their sensitivity to various antibiotics determined. Clinicians can use the laboratory report as a guide for possible adjunctive antimicrobial therapy in treating the patient's refractory periodontitis. Cultural analysis and antibiotic sensitivity testing are not done in most cases of chronic periodontitis because the disease usually responds to conventional mechanical therapy.[130]

Necrotizing Ulcerative Gingivitis/Periodontitis

Necrotizing ulcerative gingivitis/periodontitis is clinically characterized by painful and highly destructive ulcerative lesions in which the protective epithelial barrier has been destroyed (see Chapter 2). This breach enhances access of the resident microflora to the underlying connective tissues. Invasion up to 250 μm into the exposed connective tissue by spirochetes has been demonstrated in cases of necrotizing ulcerative gingivitis.[131,132] The majority of the spirochetes (treponemes) associated with necrotizing ulcerative gingivitis are uncultivable, but it is clear that they constitute a very large and diverse group.[68,70,133,134] A cultural study of subgingival plaque from necrotizing ulcerative gingivitis lesions revealed that on average more than 50% of the bacteria were gram-negative, with the most frequently encountered groups being *P. intermedia, Fusobacterium,* and *Selenomonas* species.[135] In another study, approximately 78% of the cultivated species were gram-negative, most of which could not be identified. More than 50% of the isolated species were strict anaerobes with *P. gingivalis* and *F. nucleatum* accounting for 7.8% and 3.4%, respectively.[136]

The microbiology of necrotizing ulcerative periodontitis (NUP) has not been studied in medically healthy individuals because of difficulties in assembling a large enough population. However, the microbial profiles of NUP-like lesions from immunosuppressed HIV-infected patients have been preliminarily examined. In one group of HIV-positive patients with NUP, analysis of subgingival plaque samples using 16S rRNA gene techniques revealed 108 distinct species of bacteria, 65 of which were uncultivable, and 26 were novel to NUP. In addition, in the cases of NUP-like lesions studied, the classical periodontal pathogens such as *T. forsythensis* and *P. gingivalis* were not detected.[72]

Periodontal Abscesses

The microflora associated with periodontal abscesses has not been extensively studied. However, as might be expected, because periodontal abscesses develop in the soft tissue walls of periodontal pockets, the bacteria isolated from abscesses are similar to those associated with chronic and aggressive forms of periodontitis. An average of approximately 70% of the cultivable flora in exudates from periodontal abscesses are gram-negative and about 50% are anaerobic rods.[137] Analysis of microbial samples collected by placing paper points into pockets with periodontal abscesses revealed a high prevalence of the following putative pathogens: *F. nucleatum* (70.8%), *P. micros* (70.6%), *P. intermedia* (62.5%), *P. gingivalis* (50.0%), and *T. forsythensis* (47.1%). At positive sites, proportions of these bacteria as a percentage of the total flora were 13.6% *P. gingivalis*, 9.3% *P. micros*, 8.5% *P. intermedia*, 3.6% *T. forsythensis*, and 2.6% *F. nucleatum*.[138] Similar results have been found by others.[139-141] Enteric bacteria, coagulase-negative staphylococci, and *Candida albicans* have also been detected in patients with development of periodontal abscesses after taking antibiotics for medical reasons.[120] This latter observation suggests that the microflora associated with periodontal abscesses can be highly variable.

REFERENCES

1. Socransky SS, Manganiello SD: The oral microbiota of man from birth to senility, *J Periodontol* 42:485-494, 1971.
2. Dahlén G, Manji F, Baelum V, Fejerskov O: Putative periodontopathogens in "diseased" and "non-diseased" persons exhibiting poor oral hygiene, *J Clin Periodontol* 19:35-42, 1992.
3. De Jong HP, De Boer P, Busscher HJ, et al: Surface free energy changes of human enamel during pellicle formation: an *in vivo* study, *Caries Res* 18:408-415, 1984.
4. Quirynen M, Marechal M, Busscher HJ, et al: The influence of surface free-energy on planimetric plaque growth in man, *J Dent Res* 68:796-799, 1989.
5. Bryan AW: Progress in the recognition of etiologic factors of periodontal diseases, *J Periodontol* 10:25-30, 1939.
6. Fauchard P: *The surgeon dentist*, ed 2, New York, 1746, Pound Ridge (Translated by L Lindsay L).
7. Koch R: Die aetiologie der Milzbrand-Krankheit, Begrundet auf die Entwick lungsgeschichte des bacillus Anthracis. *Beitrage zur Biologie Pflanzen* 2:277-310, 1876.

8. Harlan AW: Treatment of pyorrhea alveolaris, *Dental Cosmos* 25:517-521, 1883.
9. Miller WD: *Original investigations concerning pyorrhea alveolaris. The micro-organisms of the human mouth*, Philadelphia, 1890, The SS White Dental Mfg. Co., p. 328-334.
10. Talbot ES: Pyorrhea alveolaris, *Dental Cosmos* 28:689-692, 1886.
11. Orland FJ, Blayney JR, Harrison RW, et al: Use of the germfree animal technic in the study of experimental dental caries. I. Basic observations on rats reared free of all microorganisms, *J Dent Res* 33:147-174, 1954.
12. Baer PN, Newton WL: The occurrence of periodontal disease in germ-free mice, *J Dent Res* 38:1238, 1959.
13. Baer PN, Newton WL: Studies on periodontal disease in the mouse. III. The germ-free mouse and it conventional control, *Oral Surg Oral Med Oral Pathol* 13:1134-1144, 1960.
14. Baer PN, Newton WL, White CL: Studies on periodontal disease in the mouse. VI. The older germ-free mouse and its conventional control, *J Periodontol* 35:388-396, 1964.
15. Baer PN, Fitzgerald RJ: Periodontal disease in the 18-month-old germ-free rat, *J Dent Res* 45:406, 1966.
16. Eckersberg T: Periodontal disease in germ-free white rats, *J Periodont Res* 2:241, 1967 (abstract).
17. Fitzgerald RJ, Jordan HV, Stanley HR: Experimental caries and gingival pathologic changes in the gnotobiotic rat, *J Dent Res* 39:923-935, 1960.
18. Rovin S, Costich ER, Gordon HA: The influence of bacteria and irritation in the initiation of periodontal disease in germfree and conventional rats, *J Periodont Res* 1:193-203, 1966.
19. Listgarten MA, Heneghan JB: Chronic inflammation in the gingival tissues of germfree dogs, *Arch Oral Biol* 16:1207-1213, 1971.
20. Listgarten MA, Heneghan JB: Observations on the periodontium and acquired pellicle of adult germfree dogs, *J Periodontol* 44:85-91, 1973.
21. Saxe SR, Greene JC, Bohannan HM, et al: Oral debris, calculus, and periodontal disease in the beagle dog, *Periodontics* 5:217-225, 1968.
22. Lindhe J, Hamp S-E, Löe H: Experimental periodontitis in the beagle dog, *J Periodont Res* 8:1-10, 1973.
23. Lindhe J, Hamp S-E, Löe H: Plaque induced periodontal disease in beagle dogs. A 4-year clinical, roentgenographical and histometrical study, *J Periodont Res* 10:243-255, 1975.
24. Socransky SS: Microbiology of periodontal disease—present status and future considerations, *J Periodontol* 48:497-504, 1977.
25. Jordan HV, Keyes PH, Bellack S: Periodontal lesions in hamsters and gnotobiotic rats infected with *Actinomyces* of human origin, *J Periodont Res* 7:21-28, 1972.
26. Löe H, Theilade E, Jensen SB: Experimental gingivitis in man, *J Periodontol* 36:177-187, 1965.

27. Theilade E, Wright WH, Jensen SB, Löe H: Experimental gingivitis in man. II. A longitudinal clinical and bacteriological investigation, *J Periodont Res* 1:1-13, 1966.

28. Löe H, Theilade E, Jensen SB, Schiött CR: Experimental gingivitis in man. III. The influence of antibiotics on gingival plaque development, *J Periodont Res* 2:282-289, 1967.

29. Jensen SB, Löe H, Schiött CR, Theilade E: Experimental gingivitis in man. IV. Vancomycin induced changes in bacterial plaque composition as related to the development of gingival inflammation, *J Periodont Res* 3:284-292, 1968.

30. Zachrisson BU: A histological study of experimental gingivitis in man, *J Periodont Res* 3:293-302, 1968.

31. Syed SA, Loesche WJ: Bacteriology of human experimental gingivitis: Effect of plaque age, *Infect Immun* 21:821-829, 1978.

32. Loesche WJ, Syed WJ: Bacteriology of human experimental gingivitis: Effect of plaque and gingivitis score, *Infect Immun* 21:830-839, 1978.

33. Moore WEC, Holdeman LV, Smibert RM, et al: Bacteriology of experimental gingivitis in young adult humans, *Infect Immun* 38:651-667, 1982.

34. Moore WEC, Holdeman LV, Smibert RM, et al: Bacteriology of experimental gingivitis in children, *Infect Immun* 46:1-6, 1984.

35. Hancock EB: Prevention, *Ann Periodontol* 1:223-249, 1996.

36. Cobb CM: Non-surgical pocket therapy: mechanical, *Ann Periodontol* 1:443-490, 1996.

37. Palcanis KG: Surgical pocket therapy, *Ann Periodontol* 1:589-617, 1996.

38. Petersilka GJ, Ehmke B, Flemmig TF: Antimicrobial effects of mechanical debridement, *Periodontol 2000* 28:56-71, 2002.

39. Drisko CH: Non-surgical pocket therapy: Pharmacotherapeutics, *Ann Periodontol* 1:491-566, 1996.

40. Quirynen M, Teughels W, De Soete M, et al: Topical antiseptics and antibiotics in the initial therapy of chronic adult periodontitis: microbiological aspects, *Periodontol 2000* 28:72-90, 2002.

41. Slots J, Ting M: Systemic antibiotics in the treatment of periodontal disease, *Periodontol 2000* 28:106-176, 2002.

42. Greenstein G, Polson A: The role of local drug delivery in the management of periodontal diseases: a comprehensive review, *J Periodontol* 69:507-520, 1998.

43. Russell AL: International nutrition surveys: a summary of preliminary findings, *J Dent Res* 42:233-244, 1963.

44. Waerhaug J: Prevalence of periodontal disease in Ceylon. Association with age, sex, oral hygiene, socioeconomic factors, vitamin deficiencies, malnutrition, betel and tobacco consumption and ethnic group, *Acta Odontol Scand* 25:205-231, 1967.

45. Ismail AI, Morrison EC, Burt BA, et al: Natural history of periodontal disease in adults: findings from the Tecumseh Periodontal Disease Study, 1959-1987, *J Dent Res* 69:430-435, 1990.

46. Haffajee AD, Socransky SS, Lindhe J, et al: Clinical risk indicators for periodontal attachment loss, *J Clin Periodontol* 18:117-125, 1991.

47. Burt BA: Epidemiology of periodontal diseases, *J Periodontol* 67:935-945, 1996.

48. Löe H, Anerud A, Boysen H, et al: Natural history of periodontal disease in man. Rapid, moderate and no loss of attachment in Sri Lankan laborers 14 to 46 years of age, *J Clin Periodontol* 13:431-440, 1986.

49. Baelum V, Fejerskov O, Karring T: Oral hygiene, gingivitis and periodontal breakdown in adult Tanzanians, *J Periodont Res* 21:221-232, 1986.

50. Baelum V, Fejerskov O, Manji F: Periodontal disease in adult Kenyans, *J Clin Periodontol* 15:445-452, 1988.

51. Baelum V, Wen-Min L, Fejerskov O, et al: Tooth mortality and periodontal conditions in 60-80-year-old Chinese, *Scand J Dent Res* 96:99-107, 1988.

52. Ismail AI, Burt BA, Brunelle JA: Prevalence of total tooth loss, dental caries, and periodontal disease in Mexican-American adults: results from the Southwestern HHANES, *J Dent Res* 66:1183-1188, 1987.

53. Grossi SG, Zambon JJ, Ho AW, et al: Assessment of risk for periodontal disease. I. Risk indicators for attachment loss, *J Periodontol* 65:260-267, 1994.

54. Grossi SG, Genco RJ, Machtei EE, et al: Assessment of risk for periodontal disease. II. Risk indicators for alveolar bone loss, *J Periodontol* 66:23-29, 1995.

55. Albandar JM: Global risk factors and risk indicators for periodontal diseases, *Periodontol 2000* 28:177-206, 2002.

56. Socransky SS, Haffajee AD: Microbial mechanisms in the pathogenesis of destructive periodontal diseases: a critical assessment, *J Periodont Res* 26:195-212, 1991.

57. Socransky SS, Haffajee AD: Evidence of bacterial etiology: a historical perspective, *Periodontol 2000* 5:7-25, 1994.

58. Offenbacher S: Periodontal diseases: pathogenesis, *Ann Periodontol* 1:821-878, 1996.

59. Darveau RP, Tanner A, Page RC: The microbial challenge in periodontitis, *Periodontol 2000* 14:12-22, 1997.

60. Kornman KS, Page RC, Tonetti MS: The host response to the microbial challenge in periodontitis: assembling the players, *Periodontol 2000* 14:33-53, 1997.

61. Socransky SS: Criteria for the infectious agents in dental caries and periodontal disease, *J Clin Periodontol* 6(7):16-21, 1979.

62. Theilade E: The non-specific theory in microbial etiology of inflammatory periodontal diseases, *J Clin Periodontol* 13:905-911, 1986.

63. Loesche WJ: Chemotherapy of dental plaque infections, *Oral Sci Rev* 9:65-107, 1976.

64. Loesche WJ: DNA probe and enzyme analysis in periodontal diagnostics, *J Periodontol* 63:1102-1109, 1992.

65. Wilson MJ, Weightman AJ, Wade WG: Applications of molecular ecology in the characterisation of uncultured

microorganisms associated with human disease, *Rev Med Microbiol* 8:91-101, 1997.

66. Choi BK, Paster BJ, Dewhirst FE, et al: Diversity of cultivable and uncultivable oral spirochetes from a patient with severe destructive periodontitis, *Infect Immun* 62:1889-1895, 1994.

67. Spratt DA, Weightman AJ, Wade WG: Diversity of oral asaccharolytic *Eubacterium* species in periodontitis—identification of novel phylotypes representing uncultivated taxa, *Oral Microbiol Immunol* 14:56-59, 1999.

68. Dewhirst FE, Tamer MA, Ericson RE, et al: The diversity of periodontal spirochetes by 16S rRNA analysis, *Oral Microbiol Immunol* 15:196-202, 2000.

69. Sakamoto M, Umeda M, Ishikawa I, et al: Comparison of the oral bacterial flora in saliva from a healthy subject and two periodontitis patients by sequence analysis of 16S rDNA libraries, *Microbiol Immunol* 44:643-652, 2000.

70. Paster BJ, Boches SK, Galvin JL, et al: Bacterial diversity in human subgingival plaque, *J Bacteriol* 183:3770-3783, 2001.

71. Paster BJ, Falkler WA Jr, Enwonwu CO, et al: Predominant bacterial species and novel phylotypes in advanced noma lesions, *J Clin Microbiol* 40:2187-2191, 2002.

72. Paster B, Russell MK, Alpagot T, et al: Bacterial diversity in necrotizing ulcerative periodontitis in HIV-positive subjects, *Ann Periodontol* 7:8-16, 2002.

73. Kulik EM, Sandmeier H, Hinni K, et al: Identification of archaeal rDNA from subgingival dental plaque by PCR amplification and sequence analysis, *FEMS Microbiol Letters* 196:129-133, 2001.

74. Brinig MM, Lepp PW, Ouverney CC, et al: Prevalence of bacteria of division TM7 in human subgingival plaque and their association with disease, *Appl Environ Microbiol* 69:1687-1694, 2003.

75. Armitage GC, Newbrun E, Hoover CI, et al: Periodontal disease associated with *Shigella flexneri* in rhesus monkeys. Clinical, microbiologic and histopathologic findings, *J Periodont Res* 17:131-144, 1982.

76. Holmstrup P: Non-plaque-induced gingival lesions, *Ann Periodontol* 4:20-29, 1999.

77. Haffajee AD, Socranskyy SS: Microbial etiological agents of destructive periodontal diseases, *Periodontol 2000* 5:78-111, 1994.

78. Simonson LG, Goodman CH, Bial JJ, et al: Quantitative relationship of *Treponema denticola* to severity of periodontal disease, *Infect Immun* 56:726-728, 1988.

79. Dahlèn G, Manji F, Baelum V, et al: Black-pigmented *Bacteroides* species and *Actinobacillus actinomycetemcomitans* in subgingival plaque of adult Kenyans, *J Clin Periodontol* 16:305-310, 1989.

80. McNabb H, Mombelli A, Gmür R, et al: Periodontal pathogens in shallow pockets of immigrants from developing countries, *Oral Microbiol Immunol* 7:267-272, 1992.

81. Wilson M, Lopatin D, Osborne G, et al: Prevalence of *Treponema denticola* and *Porphyromonas gingivalis* in plaque from periodontally-healthy and periodontally-diseased sites, *J Med Microbiol* 38:406-410, 1993.

82. Gmür R, Guggenheim B: Interdental supragingival plaque—a natural habitat of *Actinobacillus actinomycetemcomitans*, *Bacteroides forsythus*, *Campylobacter rectus*, and *Prevotella nigrescens*, *J Dent Res* 73: 1421-1428, 1994.

83. Zimmer W, Wilson M, Marsh PD, et al: *Porphyromonas gingivalis*, *Prevotella intermedia* and *Actinobacillus actinomycetemcomitans* in the plaque of children without periodontitis, *Microbiol Ecol Health Dis* 4:329-336, 1991.

84. Di Murro C, Paolantonio M, Pedrazzoli V, et al: Occurrence of *Porphyromonas gingivalis*, *Bacteroides forsythus*, and *Treponema denticola* in periodontally healthy and diseased subjects determined by an ELISA technique, *J Periodontol* 68:18-23, 1997.

85. Choi B-K, Park S-H, Yoo Y-J, et al: Detection of major putative periodontopathogens in Korean advanced adult periodontitis patients using a nucleic acid-based approach, *J Periodontol* 71:1387-1394, 2000.

86. Armitage GC: Periodontal diseases: diagnosis, *Ann Periodontol* 1:37-215, 1996.

87. Mellado JR, Freedman AL, Salkin LM, et al: The clinical relevance of microbiologic testing: a comparative analysis of microbiologic samples secured from the same sites and cultured in two independent laboratories, *Int J Periodont Rest Dent* 21:233-239, 2001.

88. Suchett-Kaye G, Morrier JJ, Barsotti O: Clinical usefulness of microbiological diagnostic tools in the management of periodontal disease, *Res Microbiol* 152:631-639, 2001.

89. Loos BG, Mayrand D, Genco RJ, et al: Genetic heterogeneity of *Porphyromonas (Bacteroides) gingivalis* by genomic DNA fingerprinting, *J Dent Res* 69:1488-1493, 1990.

90. Loos BG, Dyer DW, Whittman TS, et al: Genetic structure of populations of *Porphyromonas gingivalis* associated with periodontitis and other oral infections, *Infect Immun* 61:204-212, 1993.

91. Chen C, Slots J: Clonal analysis of *Porphyromonas gingivalis* by the arbitrarily primed polymerase chain reaction, *Oral Microbiol Immunol* 9:99-103, 1994.

92. Griffen AL, Leys EJ, Fuerst PA: Strain identification of *Actinobacillus actinomycetemcomitans* using the polymerase chain reaction, *Oral Microbiol Immunol* 7: 240-243, 1992.

93. Preus HR, Haraszthy VI, Zambon JJ, et al: Differentiation of strains of *Actinobacillus actinomycetemcomitans* by arbitrarily primed polymerase chain reaction, *J Clin Microbiol* 31:2773-2776, 1994.

94. DiRienzo JM, Slots J, Sixou M, et al: Specific genetic variants of *Actinobacillus actinomycetemcomitans* correlate with disease and health in a regional population of families with localized juvenile periodontitis, *Infect Immun* 62:3058-3065, 1994.

95. Zhang YJ, Yasui S, Yoshimura F, et al: Multiple restriction length polymorphism genotypes of *Porphyromonas*

gingivalis in single periodontal pockets, *Oral Microbiol Immunol* 10:125-128, 1995.

96. Pearce MA, Devine Dam Dixon RA, et al: Genetic heterogeneity in *Prevotella intermedia, Prevotella nigrescens, Prevotella corporis* and related species isolated from oral and nonoral sites, *Oral Microbiol Immunol* 15:89-95, 2000.

97. Slots J: Microflora in the healthy gingival sulcus in man, *Scand J Dent Res* 85:247-254, 1977.

98. Newman MG, Grinenco V, Weiner M, et al: Predominant microbiota associated with health in the aged, *J Periodontol* 49:553-559, 1978.

99. Tanner A, Kent R, Maiden MFJ, et al: Clinical, microbiological and immunological profile of healthy, gingivitis and putative active periodontal subjects, *J Periodont Res* 31:195-204, 1996.

100. Slots J: The predominant cultivable organisms in juvenile periodontitis, *Scand J Dent Res* 84:1-10, 1976.

101. Listgarten MA, Helldèn L: Relative distribution of bacteria at clinically healthy and periodontally diseased sites in humans, *J Clin Periodontol* 5:115-132, 1978.

102. Moore LVH, Moore WEC, Cato EP, et al: Bacteriology of gingivitis, *J Dent Res* 66:989-995, 1987.

103. Moore WEC, Moore LVH: The bacteria of periodontal diseases, *Periodontol 2000* 5:66-77, 1994.

104. Genco R, Kornman K, Williams R, et al: Consensus report: periodontal diseases: pathogenesis and microbial factors, *Ann Periodontol* 1:926-932, 1996.

105. Socransky SS, Haffajee AD, Cugini MA, et al: Microbial complexes in subgingival plaque, *J Clin Periodontol* 25:134-144, 1998.

106. Socransky SS, Haffajee AD: Dental biofilms: difficult therapeutic targets, *Periodontol 2000* 28:12-55, 2002.

107. Moore WEC, Holdeman LV, Cato EP, et al: Comparative bacteriology of juvenile periodontitis, *Infect Immun* 48:507-519, 1985.

108. Nonnenmacher C, Mutters R, de Jacoby LF: Microbiological characteristics of subgingival microbiota in adult periodontitis, localized juvenile periodontitis and rapidly progressive periodontitis subjects, *Clin Microbiol Infect* 7:213-217, 2001.

109. Yano-Higuchi K, Takamatsu N, He T, et al: Prevalence of *Bacteroides forsythus, Porphyromonas gingivalis* and *Actinobacillus actinomycetemcomitans* in subgingival microflora of Japanese patients with adult and rapidly progressive periodontitis, *J Clin Periodontol* 27:597-602, 2000.

110. Zambon JJ, Haraszthy VI, Hariharan G, et al: The microbiology of early-onset periodontitis: association of highly toxic *Actinobacillus actinomycetemcomitans* strains with localized juvenile periodontitis, *J Periodontol* 67:282-290, 1996.

111. López NJ, Mellado JC, Leighton GX: Occurrence of *Actinobacillus actinomycetemcomitans, Porphyromonas gingivalis* and *Prevotella intermedia* in juvenile periodontitis, *J Clin Periodontol* 23:101-105, 1996.

112. Slots J, Ting M: *Actinobacillus actinomycetemcomitans* and *Porphyromonas gingivalis* in human periodontal disease: occurrence and treatment, *Periodontol 2000* 20: 82-121, 1999.

113. Mullally BH, Dace B, Shelburne CE, et al: Prevalence of periodontal pathogens in localized and generalized forms of early-onset periodontitis, *J Periodont Res* 35:232-241, 2000.

114. Han N, Xiao X, Zhang L, et al: Bacteriological study of juvenile periodontitis in China, *J Periodont Res* 26:409-414, 1991.

115. Albandar JM, Brown LJ, Löe H: Putative periodontal pathogens in subgingival plaque of young adults with and without early-onset periodontitis, *J Periodontol* 68:973-981, 1997.

116. Moore WEC, Holdeman LV, Smibert RM, et al: Bacteriology of severe periodontitis in young adult humans, *Infect Immun* 37:1137-1148, 1982.

117. Kamma JJ, Nakou M, Manti FA: Predominant microflora of severe, moderate and minimal periodontal lesions in young adults with rapidly progressing periodontitis, *J Periodont Res* 30:66-72, 1995.

118. American Academy of Periodontology: Consensus report. Discussion section I. Nevins M, Becker W, Kornman K, editors: *Proceedings of the World Workshop in Clinical Periodontics.* Chicago: 1989, American Academy of Periodontology, pp. I-23-I-32.

119. Dahlén G, Wikström M: Occurrence of enteric rods, staphylococci and *Candida* in subgingival samples, *Oral Microbiol Immunol* 10:42-46, 1995.

120. Helovuo H, Hakkarainen K, Paunio K: Changes in the prevalence of subgingival enteric rods, staphylococci and yeasts after treatment with penicillin and erythromycin, *Oral Microbiol Immunol* 8:75-79, 1993.

121. Listgarten MA, Lai C-H, Young V: Microbial composition and pattern of antibiotic resistance in subgingival microbial samples from patients with refractory periodontitis, *J Periodontol* 64:155-161, 1993.

122. Rams TE, Babalola OO, Slots J: Subgingival occurrence of enteric rods, yeasts and staphylococci after systemic doxycycline therapy, *Oral Microbiol Immunol* 5:166-168, 1990.

123. Rams TE, Feik D, Young V, et al: Enterococci in human periodontitis, *Oral Microbiol Immunol* 7:249-252, 1992.

124. Haffajee AD, Socransky SS, Dzink JL, et al: Clinical, microbiological and immunological features of subjects with refractory periodontal diseases, *J Clin Periodontol* 15:390-398, 1988.

125. Edwardsson S, Bing M, Axtelius B, et al: The microbiota of periodontal pockets with different depths in therapy-resistant periodontitis, *J Clin Periodontol* 26:143-152, 1999.

126. Choi J-I, Nakagawa T, Yamada S, et al: Clinical, microbiological and immunological studies on recurrent periodontal disease, *J Clin Periodontol* 17:426-434, 1990.

127. Lee H-J, Kang I-K, Chung C-P, et al: The subgingival microflora and gingival crevicular fluid cytokines in refractory periodontitis, *J Clin Periodontol* 22:885-890, 1995.

128. Magnusson I, Marks RG, Clark WB, et al: Clinical, microbiological and immunological characteristics of subjects with "refractory" periodontal disease, *J Clin Periodontol* 18:291-299, 1991.

129. Colombo AP, Haffajee AD, Dewhirst FE, et al: Clinical and microbiological features of refractory periodontitis subjects, *J Clin Periodontol* 25:169-180, 1998.

130. Rosenberg ES, Torosian JP, Hammond BF, et al: Routine anaerobic bacterial culture and systemic antibiotic usage in the treatment of adult periodontitis: a 6-year longitudinal study, *Int J Periodont Rest Dent* 13:213-243, 1993.

131. Listgarten MA: Electron microscopic observations on the bacterial flora of acute necrotizing ulcerative gingivitis, *J Periodontol* 36:328-339, 1965.

132. Heylings RT: Electron microscopy of acute ulcerative gingivitis (Vincent's type). Demonstration of the fusospirochetal complex of bacteria within pre-necrotic gingival epithelium, *Br Dent J* 122:51-56, 1967.

133. Riviere GR, Wagoner MA, Baker-Zander SA, et al: Identification of spirochetes related to *Treponema pallidum* in necrotizing ulcerative gingivitis and chronic periodontitis, *N Engl J Med* 325:539-543, 1991.

134. Riviere GR, Weisz KS, Simonson LG, et al: Pathogen-related spirochetes identified within gingival tissue from patients with acute necrotizing ulcerative gingivitis, *Infect Immun* 59:2653-2657, 1991.

135. Loesche WJ, Syed SA, Laughon BE, et al: The bacteriology of acute necrotizing ulcerative gingivitis, *J Periodontol* 53:223-230, 1982.

136. Falkler WA Jr, Martin SA, Vincent JW, et al: A clinical, demographic and microbiologic study of ANUG patients in an urban dental school, *J Clin Periodontol* 14:307-314, 1987.

137. Newman MG, Sims TN: The predominant cultivable microbiota of the periodontal abscess, *J Periodontol* 50:350-354, 1979.

138. Herrera D, Roldán S, González I, et al: The periodontal abscess (I). Clinical and microbiological findings, *J Clin Periodontol* 27:387-394.

139. Umeda M, Tominaga Y, He T, et al: Microbial flora in the acute phase of periodontitis and the effect of local administration of minocycline, *J Periodontol* 67:422-427, 1996.

140. Van Winkelhoff AJ, Carlee AW, de Graaff J: *Bacteroides endodontalis* and other black-pigmented *Bacteroides* species in odontogenic abscesses, *Infect Immun* 49:494-497, 1985.

141. Topoll HH, Lange DE, Müller RF: Multiple periodontal abscesses after systemic antibiotic therapy, *J Clin Periodontol* 17:268-272, 1990.

5

Immunoinflammatory Response in Periodontal Diseases

Randal W. Rowland

HISTORICAL PERSPECTIVE

During the past two decades, extraordinary advances have been made in understanding the etiologic mechanisms and pathogenesis of infectious diseases. As a result, the role of the immunoinflammatory response in periodontal diseases has become clearer. The tissue destruction found in periodontal disease results, for the most part, from the actions of the immune system and related effector mechanisms.[1-7] Microorganisms, especially bacteria in dental plaque, cause periodontal diseases. Although these microorganisms produce enzymes and other factors that can directly cause degradation of periodontal tissues, the progression and severity of tissue destruction are mostly caused by host immune responses to infecting bacteria. This concept was not always thought to be the case. The development of this tenet has been a dramatic, albeit slow, evolution in the understanding of the pathogenesis of periodontal diseases.

Historically, the understanding of the pathogenesis of periodontal diseases began with histologic evaluations of periodontal clinical presentations. The transition from health (Fig. 5-1) to gingivitis was described as the development of an inflammatory state exhibiting polymorphonuclear leukocytes (PMNs) in close approximation to the dental plaque and sulcular epithelium with lymphocytes in the lamina propria. A limited destruction of the collagen fiber network was also noted. Histologic evaluation of specimens from experimental gingivitis and chronic periodontitis provided considerable insight into the immunopathogenic processes involved in periodontal diseases.[8,9] Gingivitis lesions were classified as initial, early, or established lesions based on their histology. The initial lesion was found to exhibit signs of acute

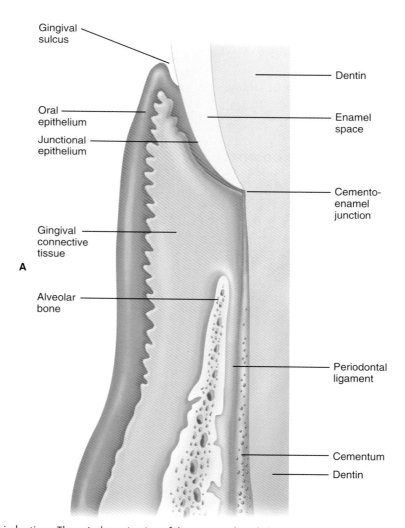

Figure 5-1. A, The healthy periodontium. The apical termination of the junctional epithelium (JE) is at the cementoenamel junction (CEJ). There are very few, if any, inflammatory cells in the gingival connective tissue underlying the JE.

Continued

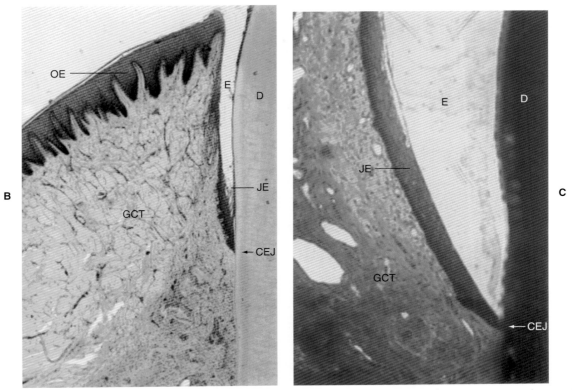

Figure 5-1. cont'd B, Healthy dentogingival junction of a monkey (*Macaca mulatta*). Original magnification approximately × 16. **C,** Healthy dentogingival junction of a beagle dog. Note the absence of inflammatory cells adjacent to the JE. Original magnification approximately × 25. D, dentin; E, enamel; GCT, gingival connective tissue; OE, oral epithelium. (*A, Redrawn from Armitage GC: Biologic basis of periodontal maintenance therapy, Berkeley, 1980, Praxis Publishing; B and C, courtesy of Dr. G.C. Armitage*).

inflammation with vascular changes such as vessel dilation, increased intercellular spacing, and high numbers of PMNs. The early lesion contained increased numbers of lymphocytes, especially thymus-derived lymphocytes known as T lymphocytes or T cells. The established lesion contained increased numbers of lymphocytic cells derived from the bone marrow known as B lymphocytes or B cells and plasma cells that differentiate to produce immunoglobulins, also known as antibodies (Fig. 5-2). An increasing degradation of collagen was noted from the initial to the early to the established lesion. As the disease progressed to periodontitis, it exhibited destruction of the periodontal fiber network and supporting bone with an apical migration of the junctional epithelium and a marked inflammatory infiltrate (Fig. 5-3). This infiltrate included numerous immune cells, lymphocytes, macrophages, and PMNs, with plasma cells predominating.[10,11]

Subsequent to these early studies, two developments emerged that complicated this model of periodontal pathogenesis. First was a paradigm shift from the assumption that all humans were equally susceptible to periodontitis to the awareness of individual differences in susceptibility (see Chapters 3 and 4).[12] Second, and perhaps more important to our understanding of periodontitis, a shift occurred in infectious disease pathology in general. It began to emerge that immune mechanisms rather than infecting agents played a dominant role in the tissue destruction associated with infectious diseases. In part, this was driven by observations that the histologic presentations of some autoimmune diseases were similar to the histologic presentation of some infectious diseases. It was not long before it was noted that the histologic appearance of periodontal diseases also resembled some of these diseases with immunologic mechanisms of tissue destruction.[13,14] Since these early observations, numerous studies have evaluated the involvement of immune phenomena in the pathogenesis of periodontal diseases.

Many of the initial studies investigated the possibilities of tissue damage resulting from autoimmune or hypersensitivity types of immune reactions.[1,15,16] Such immunologic phenomena are commonly known as allergic reactions. There are four basic types of hypersensitivity—three are classified as immediate types and one as a delayed type of hypersensitivity. The immediate hypersensitivities are antibody-dependent, whereas the

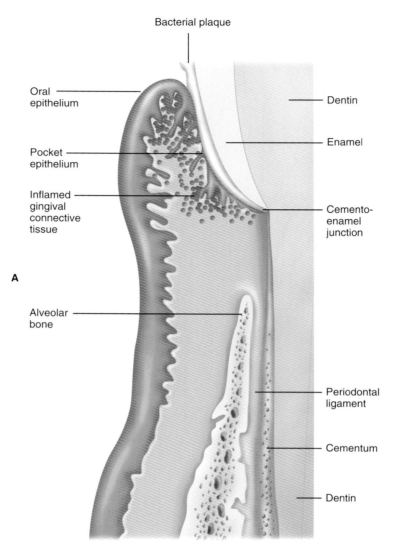

Figure 5-2. A, Schematic drawing of gingivitis. The apical termination of the junctional epithelium (JE) is at the cementoenamel junction (CEJ). The gingival sulcus has deepened and much of the JE has been transformed into pocket epithelium (PE). The gingival connective tissue (IGCT) near the PE is heavily infiltrated with inflammatory cells (i.e., T lymphocytes, some plasma cells and neutrophils). Proliferation of the PE into the inflamed CT is a prominent feature. No apical migration of the JE or resorption of alveolar bone (AB) has occurred.

Continued

delayed is a cell-mediated–dependent immune response. The initial studies of hypersensitivity reactions and their historical relation to the pathogenesis of periodontal diseases have been reviewed.[1] These studies were before the advent of current molecular biology with techniques such as polymerase chain reaction or molecular identifiers such as cell surface markers. With our current understanding of immune responses it is unlikely that hypersensitivity type reactions play an important role in the immunopathogenesis of periodontal diseases. However, these studies, along with histologic evaluations, provided the initial foundation for our current body of knowledge. Given this historical perspective, let's now look at our current understanding of the functions of immune cells and components of the host response and their involvement in the immunopathogenesis of periodontal diseases.

FUNCTIONS OF INNATE IMMUNITY AND PERIODONTAL DISEASES

Soluble Factors, Polymorphonuclear Leukocytes, Monocytes/Macrophages, Modifying Factors

Innate immunity provides the body's natural resistance to infection. Innate immunity as its name implies is intrinsic and therefore immediate, reacting on recognition of

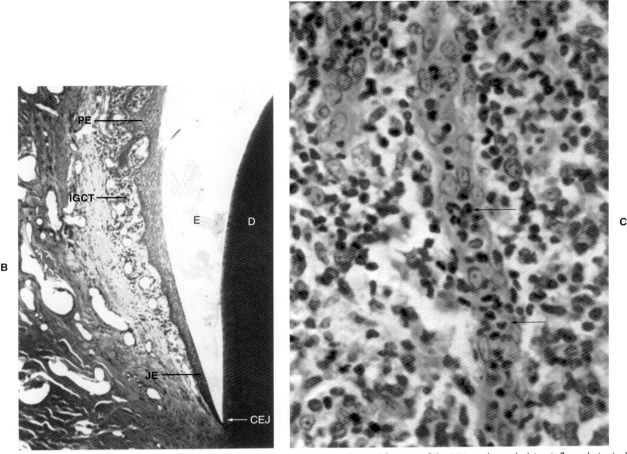

Figure 5-2. cont'd B, Dentogingival junction of a beagle dog with gingivitis. Note the proliferation of the PE into the underlying inflamed gingival connective tissue (IGCT). Original magnification approximately ✕ 16. **C,** Inflammatory infiltrate from a human gingival biopsy specimen taken from a site with gingivitis. Note the numerous neutrophils in the blood vessel (*arrows*). The inflammatory cells in the surrounding area are primarily T lymphocytes with a lesser number of plasma cells. Most of the gingival connective tissue has been destroyed and replaced by the inflammatory infiltrate. Original magnification approximately ✕ 40. D, dentin; E, enamel; OE, oral epithelium; PDL, periodontal ligament. (**A,** *Redrawn from Armitage GC: Biologic basis of periodontal maintenance therapy, Berkeley, 1980, Praxis Publishing;* **C,** *courtesy of Dr. G.C. Armitage*).

foreign or nonself elements. Various factors and cells make up the innate immune system. Soluble factors, such as those found circulating in plasma, function in the innate immune system.[17] They include complement, acute-phase proteins, and interferons. These soluble factors have a wide range of activity. Basically, complement and acute-phase proteins function intrinsically against bacteria and fungi, whereas interferons defend against viral infections.[18] Concentrations of these soluble factors may increase up to 100-fold during infections. This increase is associated with inflammation, which is characterized by increased blood flow caused by vessel dilation and increased vascular permeability, which allows transport of factors and cells between the endothelial cells lining blood vessels.[17-19]

Complement is an aggregate system composed of serum proteins that function primarily to control inflam-

mation. Inflammation is controlled by complement through the activation of immune cells, clearance of microorganisms, and an enhanced development of immunity. The proteins of complement interact with each other in a sequential fashion during a process known as complement activation. Activation occurs through two basic processes. There is a specific activation in response to antibodies, which is known as the classical pathway. There is also a nonspecific activation known as the alternative pathway, which occurs in response to microbial infection. Complement activation results in production of various peptides that have antibacterial and immunomodulating properties. Three antibacterial actions of complement have been well elucidated. First, some of the complement system proteins have the intrinsic ability to lyse bacterial cell membranes resulting in bacterial death. These components form what has been

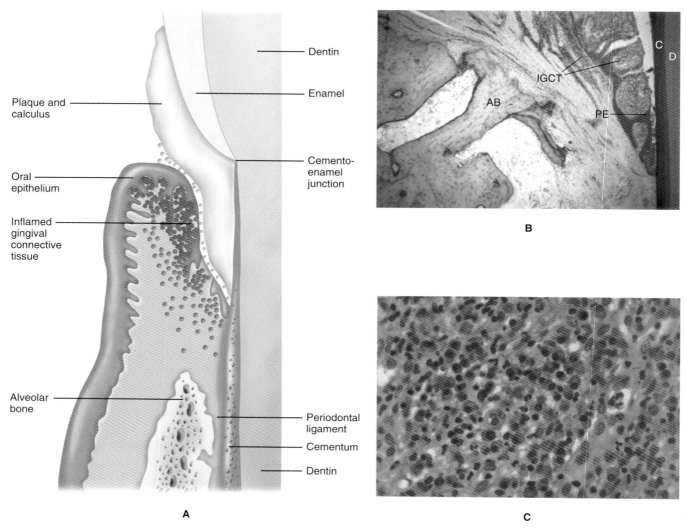

Figure 5-3. A, Periodontitis. Major features include apical migration of the junctional epithelium (JE) onto the root surface, bone loss, and recession of the gingival margin. The inflamed gingival connective tissue (IGCT) adjacent to the pocket epithelium (PE) is heavily infiltrated with inflammatory cells of which plasma cells are a prominent component. **B,** Human autopsy specimen of the dentogingival junction showing the histopathologic features of an infrabony lesion caused by chronic periodontitis. The JE has been converted to an ulcerated PE that is located on the root surface apical to the crest of the alveolar bone (AB). The connective tissue (IGCT) underlying the PE has been replaced with a heavy inflammatory infiltrate. Original magnification approximately × 16. **C,** Inflammatory infiltrate in chronic periodontitis from a human gingival autopsy specimen. The inflammatory infiltrate is richly populated with plasma cells; some lymphocytes are also present. Most of the surrounding connective tissue has been destroyed and replaced by the inflammatory infiltrate. Original magnification approximately × 40. C, Cementum; D, dentin. (**A,** *Redrawn from Armitage GC: Biologic basis of periodontal maintenance therapy, Berkeley, 1980, Praxis Publishing;* **B** and **C,** *courtesy of Dr. G.C. Armitage*).

known as membrane attack complexes that bind to cell membranes resulting in lysis. Second, some complement system proteins act as chemoattractants for phagocytic cells resulting in the migration of phagocytic cells to the site of injury or infection. These components also result in dilation of blood vessels and increase vascular permeability. Together these properties result in the localization of immune cells to the area of infection. Third, comple-

ment opsonizes, or coats bacteria, thus enhancing the phagocytosis and removal of bacteria by phagocytic cells.[18,19]

Given the actions of complement it is not surprising that many have sought to define the role of complement in periodontal diseases. Early studies of patients exhibiting periodontal diseases found activation of the complement system by periodontal bacteria and bacterial degradation of complement components.[20-26] More recent studies have focused on the potential role of complement components in specific periodontal diseases, sometimes investigating specific putative pathogenic bacteria.[27-31] The complement system appears to be down-regulated in patients with periodontal diseases. The decrease in complement function results from both bacterial and host actions and may increase the susceptibility of the host to periodontal disease.

Acute-phase proteins include: α_2-macroglobulin (α_2-M), α_1-antitrypsin (α_1-AT), iron-binding proteins transferrin (TF) and lactoferrin (LF), serum amyloid A (SAA), ceruloplasmin, α_1-acid-glycoprotein (AAG), α_1-antichymotrypsin (ACT), and C-reactive protein (CRP).[17,18] The highly investigated CRP typifies acute-phase proteins. It is named for its ability to bind the C protein of *Streptococcus pneumoniae*. CRP opsonizes bacteria, which facilitates the binding of complement and makes the bacteria more easily phagocytized. It has been long known that acute-phase proteins are often increased with periodontal diseases. Early studies indicated that the increase of CRP may be associated with either periodontal disease activity or untreated periodontal disease.[32-36]

Increased CRP level has been indicated as a risk factor for atherosclerosis, which results in cardiovascular and cerebrovascular disease (i.e., myocardial infarctions and stroke).[37-39] These findings have led to speculations of a possible relation between the immunopathogenesis of periodontal disease and atherosclerotic diseases (see Chapter 32).[40,41] Recent studies have found a moderate to strong association of the acute-phase protein response to periodontal diseases and the systemic diseases of atherosclerosis.[42-46]

Leukocytes, also known as white blood cells, are distributed throughout the body. Some function as the first line of defense against infectious agents. The granulocytic phagocytic leukocytes (PMNs, or neutrophils) have the primary function to remove infecting agents. Other phagocytic leukocytes such as macrophages function to remove agents as well but also have other important functions. Neutrophils and macrophages act against bacterial and fungal infections.

On the basis of observations of diseases with neutrophil defects, a paradigm developed in which the neutrophil is considered protective and neutrophil abnormalities, for example, in numbers, function, or both, predispose humans to severe periodontal diseases. Neutrophil abnormalities associated with the pathogenesis of periodontal diseases include neutropenias, chemotaxis disorders, reduced intracellular killing, defective degranulation, and defective adherence. Systemic diseases that have such neutrophil disorders and express a heightened risk for periodontal disease include Down syndrome, Chédiak-Higashi syndrome, Papillon-Lefèvre

syndrome, Job syndrome, and diabetes[47-50] (see Chapter 31). Historically, neutrophils and macrophages have been considered the part of the innate system of immunity that keeps gingivitis from progressing to periodontitis. Neutrophils are the first to arrive to an area of infection. They engulf and kill infecting agents. They also contain hydrolytic enzymes (e.g., collagenase and other proteinases) that are released into the surrounding area and cause local tissue damage. Repair, as with any wound area, begins as resolution of the inflammation occurs. Recently, there has been a suggested paradigm shift in the role of the neutrophil in the pathogenesis of periodontal disease.[51,52] Rather than a protective role, it is proposed that neutrophil actions result in local tissue injury and thus have a primary role in the immunopathogenesis of at least some forms of periodontal disease. The basic paradigm shift is that in some cases, PMNs do not exhibit a decrease in function, but rather they become hyperactive and are primed for actions that result in tissue breakdown.[52] The possibility of neutrophil-mediated tissue damage in the periodontal lesion, however, is not a new concept.[53,54] Further understanding of the dual role of neutrophils is an exciting and developing area.

Monocytes, another phagocytic cell, are thought to also play an important role in the immunopathogenesis of periodontal diseases. They are attracted to an area of infection and differentiate into macrophages. They appear after neutrophils and digest dying neutrophils and phagocytize remaining infecting agents. Some appear to be primarily phagocytic (i.e., function to resolve inflammation), whereas some function as antigen-processing cells. Antigen-processing cells engulf infecting agents (e.g., bacteria or bacterial components), process these particles, and present them to lymphocytes. This results in lymphocyte activation and the generation of adaptive immunity. Macrophages also have a dual role similar to the neutrophil in that once activated not only do they protect the host, they also produce substances that are involved in perpetuation of inflammation and result in tissue destruction. These substances are known as cytokines, that is, cell proteins (see discussion later in this chapter). It is evident that if the initial infection of plaque bacteria is to be contained and not progress to periodontitis, macrophages and neutrophils will play an important role in the abrogation of the infection. Conversely, it is also apparent that if the initial infection is not contained and progresses to periodontitis, macrophages and neutrophils do play an important role in the progression of the disease.

Intrinsic protective properties inhibiting initiation and progression of periodontal diseases include the nonspecific activity of innate immunity and other inherent factors. These other components of important protective mechanisms include the mechanical barrier of the epithelium, nonspecific immunoglobulins such as IgA, the washing action of gingival crevicular fluid, and the rapid turnover of periodontal soft tissues.[55] Conversely, there are negative modifying factors that enhance the initiation and progression of periodontal diseases. These negative modifiers include tobacco smoking, diabetes, subgingival or overhanging restorations, psychological stress, and others.[56-61]

FUNCTIONS OF ADAPTIVE IMMUNITY IN PERIODONTAL DISEASES

T Lymphocytes, B Lymphocytes/Plasma Cells, and Macrophages

The mechanisms of innate and adaptive immunity are extensive, overlapping, and redundant. Their roles in the immunopathogenesis of periodontal diseases have been recently reviewed.[6,7] If the functions of innate immunity, including the actions of neutrophils and macrophages, clear the infection then the gingival infection does not progress. If they do not abate the initial infection, an inflammatory infiltrate becomes localized to the connective tissue of the affected area. This infiltrate is composed mainly of lymphocytes and macrophages, with some neutrophils, and reflects an adaptive immune response (see Fig. 5-2). Lymphocytes, macrophages, and other immune cells produce cytokines that drive the immune response to clear the infection. Cytokines are intercellular signals that function to regulate cellular activity, in this case immune function.[62] Interleukins are a subgroup of cytokines that primarily function as intercellular signaling agents between white blood cells. Perhaps the most studied of these substances is interleukin-1 (IL-1). IL-1 was first discovered by a periodontist and named *osteoclast-activating factor* because of its properties in bone cell cultures.[63] Since that nascent report, IL-1 has been established as a primary factor associated with the pathogenesis of periodontal diseases.[1,2,4-6] IL-1 has been localized in gingival fluid and gingival tissues.[64-67] IL-1 stimulates production of other substances, which result in the destruction of periodontal tissues, for example, collagenases and prostaglandin E_2.[1,2,68-70] Macrophages are the major producers of IL-1, and thus were suspected early of playing a primary role in the production of IL-1 and periodontal pathogenesis. Some studies support this concept;[70,71] other studies do not.[72,73] How this adaptive inflammatory response protects the host from infecting microorganisms is complex. The early inflammatory infiltrate is dominated by lymphocytes. These lymphocytes are predominately thymus-derived lymphocytes or T cells.[74-77] Surface markers or antigenic conformations, using surface structures known as cluster determinants (CD), help identify immune cells. T cells have two basic subpopulations: CD4

or helper T cells, and CD8, which are suppressor/cytotoxic T cells. CD4 T cells are further divided into two subsets—Th1 and Th2—based on function. The Th1 subset produces cytokines (e.g., IL-2, interferon-γ), which result in a cell-mediated immune response—that is, a T cell–dominated lesion, while the Th2 subset of CD4 T cells produces cytokines (e.g., IL-4, -5, and -10) that drive an antibody (humoral) immune response, which results in a B cell/plasma cell–dominated lesion. IL-6 produced by lymphocytes and other cells such as macrophages and epithelial cells also plays an important role in the development of a plasma cell–dominated infiltrate. Cytokines and molecules associated with immunopathogenic tissue destruction are presented in Table 5-1. CD8 T cells downregulate the immune response (suppressor activities) or result in the killing of viral-infected cells and cancer cells (cytotoxic activities). Their role in the immunopathogenesis of periodontal disease appears to be a dampening effect of the CD4 T cell responses. T cells also have subsets based on prior exposure to infectious agents. Those that have not had prior exposure are termed *naïve* T cells and are positive for the cell surface marker CD45-RA. Those that have had prior exposure are termed *memory* T cells and are positive for CD45-RO. Memory T cells are considered "primed," which implies a faster response to an infecting agent on subsequent exposures.

Studies of lymphocyte function and phenotypic profiles are dependent on correct disease classification and identification of disease status, that is, active or quiescent. Past studies have used peripheral blood lymphocytes, because they are easily accessible through venipuncture. This should not present a problem if these studies are performed during periods of disease activity, because there is "communication" between the local environment and the periphery during active disease. Current studies often use histolocalization techniques or recovery of immune cells from periodontal tissues that underwent a biopsy. Phenotypic and functional characterization of immune cells associated with forms of periodontal disease have resulted in varying findings. These variations may be caused by a misclassification of the periodontal disease, or perhaps also confounded by degree of disease activity. However, even with these shortcomings assumptions can be made. For example, T cells associated with gingivitis in both adults and children are predominately CD4 T cells.[76,77] Interestingly, CD4 T cells are also predominant in necrotizing ulcerative gingivitis.[78] The inflammatory infiltrate undergoes a phenotypic change with bone marrow–derived lymphocytes or B cells predominating at the expense of T cells when gingivitis progresses to a periodontitis (see Fig. 5-3).[74,75] In addition, there is a decreased CD4/CD8 ratio[79-83] and an increase in memory T cells (CD45RO)[84-86] after this conversion to a periodontitis lesion.

TABLE 5-1   Selected Cytokines and Effector Molecules Associated With Periodontal Tissue Destruction

CYTOKINE/MOLECULE	MAJOR SOURCE	PRINCIPAL ACTIONS
IL-1, TNF-α	Monocyte/macrophage, T cell	• Proinflammatory effects e.g., leukocyte chemotaxis, monocyte/macrophage activation—increased production of IL-1 and PGE_2. • Osteoclast stimulation • Increased MMP production • Activation of T cell
IL-6	T cell, Monocyte/macrophage, fibroblast, epithelial cell	• Proinflammatory effects, e.g., increased production of IL-1, PGE_2, MMP. • Th2 response (B cell differentiation)
IL-8	Epithelial cell	• PMN chemotaxis and transepithelial migration
PGE_2	Monocyte/macrophage, fibroblast	• Osteoclast stimulation • Increased MMP production
MMP-1	Fibroblast, monocyte/macrophage, epithelial cell	• Collagenase
MMP-8	PMN	• Collagenase
IL-2	T cell	• T cell growth and expansion
IL-2, -12, IFN-γ	T cell	• Th1 response (T cell differentiation)
IL-4, -5, -6, -10	T cell	• Th2 response (B cell differentiation)

IFN-γ, Interferon-gamma; IL, interleukin; MMP, matrix metalloproteinase; PGE_2, prostaglandin E_2; PMN, polymorphonuclear leukocyte (neutrophil); Th1, helper T cell 1; Th2, helper T cell 2; TNF-α, tumor necrosis factor-α.

B cells mature and differentiate into plasma cells, which ultimately produce antibodies. If these antibodies are protective, then the infecting organisms are cleared and the infection is abrogated.[6,7] If they fail to protect, the inflammation continues and there is a concomitant increase in loss of periodontal tissue, that is, an advancing lesion of periodontitis. A recent study supports this principle. Antibody response to 40 periodontal bacteria was determined for individuals exhibiting health, gingivitis, or initial periodontitis. No differences in antibody response to the 40 bacterial species were found between the groups.[87] Reports on the nature of the antibody response to periodontal pathogens are diverse.[88-95] As with lymphocyte function and phenotype studies, the correct classification of periodontal disease and identification of disease activity are paramount in the design of antibody response studies. Additional complications include the selection of appropriate antigens such as bacterial cells, sonicates, or specific bacterial components. Given these difficulties, interpretation and application of data from antibody studies may require careful attention.

Early studies comparing disease and nondisease states often turned to statistical significance when comparing antibody response. Since the early 1990s, many researchers have relied on a predetermined definition of positive antibody response. A common definition of positive antibody response is a level at least twice the median response of the control group.[90-92] This is a prudent development because

suspected periodontal pathogens are members of the normal oral flora and they may generate an immune response without disease. Some pathogens also have cross antigenicity with common gut flora. Therefore, it is appropriate to use a threshold such as twice the control group's median value to identify a positive antibody response. By doing so, the background noise of normal antigenic sensitization is eliminated or at least reduced as a confounding factor.

Despite these difficulties in assessing antibody responses, the following generalizations can be made. A strong antibody response to purported periodontal pathogens is often noted in periodontal diseases.[1,6,7] Antibody titers and disease severity commonly express a positive relationship—that is, patients with higher titers have severe disease, especially in patients with chronic periodontitis or localized aggressive periodontitis.[1,6,7] Furthermore, these antibody titers decrease after resolution of periodontal disease.[90,93,94] However, sometimes the antibody response is inadequate either in level (quantitative measure of antibody titer) or avidity (qualitative measure of antibody function). For example, generalized aggressive periodontitis, which exhibits an extremely severe level of clinical disease, is often associated with a low antibody response.[27,92,93] In addition, necrotizing ulcerative gingivitis, in which the clinical disease is severe but limited to the gingiva with little osseous involvement, is also associated with a decreased antibody response.[95]

An adequate host-antibody response is necessary for disease resolution; therefore, antibodies are, for the most part, protective. The limitation of periodontal destruction seen in localized aggressive periodontitis may be due in part to the strong antibody response.[1]

In some cases of chronic periodontitis that have been refractory (i.e., does not respond) to therapy, an inadequate antibody response has been reported.[89,96] In a well controlled study of 32 refractory chronic periodontitis patients, antibody responses to 85 subgingival bacterial species were measured. Although there was a wide range of responses, the mean levels were generally greater than those found in successfully treated or periodontally healthy individuals. In addition, high levels of serum antibodies to specific bacteria (e.g., a *Microbacterium lacticum*–like organism, *Streptococcus oralis*, *Streptococcus constellatus*, *Actinobacillus actinomycetemcomitans* serotype c, and *Haemophilus aphrophilus*) increased the chances of an individual being refractory to therapy.[97]

Taken together it can be argued that specific antibody production results in protection for many patients, but in highly susceptible individuals (e.g., those with generalized aggressive periodontitis) the antibodies produced fail to offer the protection needed for resolution of the infection.[7]

A MODEL FOR THE PROTECTIVE AND DESTRUCTIVE MECHANISMS INVOLVED IN IMMUNOPATHOGENESIS OF PERIODONTAL DISEASES

Interplay of Microbial, Genetic, and Environmental Factors

Immunology research over the last decade has provided an explosion of knowledge in the way that host response intertwines with infectious diseases. Yet many controversies still exist. Models for the immunopathogenic mechanisms of periodontal diseases have been proposed that perhaps reflect the authors' preferences.[3,6,7] Given the complexity and redundancy of the immune system it may not be possible to presently do otherwise. Although neutrophils have usually been considered protective, some evidence suggests that they are damaging. A T cell–dominated lesion is associated with a nonprogressing lesion, and a Th1 response in particular is reported to be protective by some. However, this response has been considered to be damaging by others. Antibodies are generally considered protective, but a plasma cell–dominated lesion is associated with progression of pathogenesis. Is it possible to use this information and attempt to construct a logical model for the immunopathogenesis of periodontal diseases without bias (Fig. 5-4)?

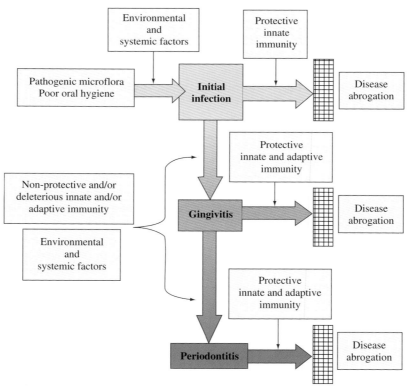

Figure 5-4. A model of periodontal immunopathogenesis. Both innate and adaptive immune responses may promote the immunopathogenic progression or result in disease abrogation. Which path is followed depends on environmental (e.g., smoking) or systemic factors (e.g., genetic bias, presence of certain systemic diseases, stress, and others), or both.

The immunopathogenic mechanisms involved in a disease process are both intriguing and frustrating. Periodontal diseases are a unique group. For the most part, they have a mixed-anaerobic bacterial primary etiology composed of indigenous microflora. The immune response to this infection is extremely complex. Both protective and damaging, the immune response is modified by systemic and local factors such as smoking, genetics, presence of certain systemic diseases, and iatrogenic factors. Our understanding of these processes has greatly progressed.[98] As it continues to evolve, we can expect more opportunities to modulate the host response in our therapeutic approaches and thus better control the deleterious actions of the immune response while selecting for those responses that are protective.[99-101] Current modulators of the immune response include low dose doxycline (Periostat [Collagenex Pharmaceuticals, Newtown, PA]), antiosteoporotic bisphosphonates such as alendronate (Fosamax [Merck Co. Inc, Whitehouse Station, NJ]), nonsteroidal antiinflammatory agents, and hormone replacement therapy. These agents may one day represent the evolutionary beginnings of host modulation therapy.

REFERENCES

1. Ranney RR: Immunologic mechanisms of pathogenesis in periodontal diseases: an assessment, *J Periodont Res* 26:243-254, 1991.

2. Page R: The role of inflammatory mediators in the pathogenesis of periodontal disease, *J Periodont Res* 26:230-242, 1991.

3. Seymour GJ: Importance of the host response in the periodontium, *J Clin Periodontol* 18:421-426, 1991.

4. Genco RJ: Host responses in periodontal diseases: current concepts, *J Periodontol* 63:338-355, 1992.

5. Dennison DK, Van Dyke TE: The acute inflammatory response and the role of phagocytic cells in periodontal health and disease, *Periodontol 2000* 14:54-78, 1997.

6. Offenbacher S: Periodontal diseases: pathogenesis, *Ann Periodontol* 1:821-878, 1996.

7. Gemmell E, Yamazaki K, Seymour GJ: Destructive periodontitis lesions are determined by the nature of the lymphocytic response, *Crit Rev Oral Biol Med* 13:17-34, 2002.

8. Page RC, Schroeder HE: Pathogenesis of inflammatory periodontal disease. A summary of current work, *Lab Invest* 34:235-249, 1976.

9. Payne WA, Page RC, Ogilvie AL, et al: Histopathologic features of the initial and early stages of experimental gingivitis in man, *J Periodont Res* 10:51-64, 1975.

10. Weinmann JP: Progress of gingival inflammation into the supporting structures of the teeth, *J Periodontol* 12:71-82, 1941.

11. Schroeder HE, Lindhe J: Conversion of established gingivitis in the dog into destructive periodontitis, *Arch Oral Biol* 20:775-782, 1975.

12. Hirschfeld L, Wasserman B: A long-term survey of tooth loss in 600 treated periodontal patients, *J Periodontol* 49:225-237, 1978.

13. Brandtzaeg P, Kraus FW: Autoimmunity and periodontal disease, *Odontol Tidsskrift* 73:281-293, 1965.

14. Freedman HL, Listgarten MA, Taichman NS: Electron microscopic features of chronically inflamed human gingiva, *J Periodont Res* 3:313-327, 1968.

15. Nisengard R: Immediate hypersensitivity and periodontal disease, *J Periodontol* 45:344-347, 1974.

16. Asaro JP, Nisengard R, Beutner EH, et al: Experimental periodontal disease. Immediate hypersensitivity, *J Periodontol* 54:23-28, 1983.

17. Ceciliani F, Giordano A, Spagnolo V: The systemic reaction during inflammation: the acute-phase proteins, *Curr Pharm Des* 9:211-223, 2002.

18. Male D: Introduction to the immune system. In Roitt I, Brostoff J, Male D, editors, *Immunology*, ed 6,. St. Louis, 2001, Mosby Year-Book.

19. Morgan BP: Physiology and pathophysiology of complement: progress and trend, *Crit Rev Clin Lab* 32:265-298, 1995.

20. Attstrom R, Laurel AB, Lahsson U, Sjoholm A: Complement factors in gingival crevice material from healthy and inflamed gingiva in humans, *J Periodont Res* 10:19-27, 1975.

21. Schenkein HA, Genco RJ: Gingival fluid and serum in periodontal diseases. II. Evidence for cleavage of complement components C3, C3 proactivator (factor B) and C4 in gingival fluid, *J Periodontol* 48:778-784, 1977.

22. Okada H, Silverman MS: Chemotactic activity in periodontal disease. II. The generation of complement-derived chemotactic factors, *J Periodont Res* 14:147-152, 1979.

23. Okuda K, Takazoe I: Activation of complement by dental plaque, *J Periodont Res* 15:232-239, 1980.

24. Niekrash CE, Patters MR, Lang NP: The relationship of complement cleavage in gingival fluid to periodontal diseases, *J Periodont Res* 19:622-627, 1984.

25. Niekrash CE, Patters MR: Assessment of complement cleavage in gingival fluid in humans with and without periodontal disease, *J Periodont Res* 21:233-242, 1986.

26. Henry CA, Ungchusri T, Charbeneau TD, et al: Relationships of serum opsonins and complement in human experimental gingivitis, *J Periodontol* 58:177-186, 1987.

27. Sjöström K, Darveau R, Page R, et al: Opsonic antibody activity against *Actinobacillus actinomycetemcomitans* in patients with rapidly progressive periodontitis, *Infect Immun* 60:4819-4825, 1992. (Erratum in: *Infect Immun* 61:1167, 1993).

28. Schenkein HA, Fletcher HM, Bodnar M, et al: Increased opsonization of a *prtH*-defective mutant of *Porphyromonas*

gingivalis W83 is caused by reduced degradation of complement-derived opsonins, *J Immunol* 154:5331-5337, 1995.

29. Monefeldt K, Helgeland K, Tollefsen T: In vitro cleavage of serum complement protein C3: a comparison between patients with adult periodontitis and periodontally healthy persons, *J Clin Periodontol* 22:45-51, 1995.

30. Rautemaa R, Meri S: Protection of gingival epithelium against complement-mediated damage by strong expression of the membrane attack complex inhibitor protectin (CD59), *J Dent Res* 75:568-574, 1996.

31. Potempa J, Banbula A, Travis J: Role of bacterial proteinases in matrix destruction and modulation of host responses, *Periodontol 2000* 24:153-192, 2000.

32. Boucher NE Jr, Hanrahan JJ, Kihara FY: Occurrence of C-reactive protein in oral disease, *J Dent Res* 46:624, 1967.

33. Shklair IL, Loving RH, Leberman OF, et al: C-reactive protein and periodontal disease, *J Periodontol* 39:93-95, 1968.

34. Norman ME, Baehni PC, Tsai C-C, et al: Studies of host responses during experimental gingivitis in humans. II. Changes in acute phase reactants, serum immunoglobulins and complement during the development of gingival inflammation, *J Periodont Res* 14:361-369, 1979.

35. Sibraa PD, Reinhardt RA, Dyer JK, et al: Acute-phase protein detection and quantification in gingival crevicular fluid by direct and indirect immunodot, *J Clin Periodontol* 18:101-106, 1991.

36. Pederson ED, Stanke SR, Whitener SJ, et al: Salivary levels of α_2-macroglobulin, α_1-antitrypsin, C-reactive protein, cathepsin G and elastase in humans with or without destructive periodontal disease, *Arch Oral Biol* 40:1151-1155, 1995.

37. Ridker PM, Rifai N, Rose L, et al: Comparison of C-reactive protein and low-density lipoprotein cholesterol levels in the prediction of first cardiovascular events, *N Engl J Med* 347:1557-1565, 2002.

38. Benzaquen LR, Yu H, Rifai N: High sensitivity C-reactive protein: an emerging role in cardiovascular risk assessment, *Crit Rev Clin Lab Sci* 39:459-497, 2002.

39. Wang TJ, Nam B-H, Wilson PWF, et al: Association of C-reactive protein with carotid atherosclerosis in men and women: the Framingham Heart Study, *Arterioscler Thromb Vasc Biol* 22:1662-1667, 2002.

40. Lowe GDO: The relationship between infection, inflammation, and cardiovascular disease: an overview, *Ann Periodontol* 6:1-8, 2001.

41. Di Napoli M, Papa F, Bocola V: Periodontal disease, C-reactive protein, and ischemic stroke, *Arch Intern Med* 161:1234-1235, 2001.

42. Ebersole JL, Cappelli D, Mott G, et al: Systemic manifestations of periodontitis in the non-human primate, *J Periodont Res* 34:358-362, 1999.

43. Slade GD, Offenbacher S, Beck JD, et al: Acute-phase inflammatory response to periodontal disease in the US population, *J Dent Res* 79:49-57, 2000.

44. Wu T, Trevisan M, Genco RJ, et al: Examination of the relation between periodontal health status and cardiovascular risk factors: serum total and high density lipoprotein cholesterol, C-reactive protein, and plasma fibrinogen, *Am J Epidemiol* 151:273-282, 2000.

45. Noack B, Genco RJ, Trevisan M, et al: Periodontal infections contribute to elevated systemic C-reactive protein level, *J Periodontol* 72:1221-1227, 2001.

46. Glurich I, Grossi S, Albini B, et al: Systemic inflammation in cardiovascular and periodontal disease: comparative study, *Clin Diagn Lab Immunol* 9:425-432, 2002.

47. Van Dyke TE, Levine MJ, Al-Hashimi I, et al: Periodontal diseases and impaired neutrophil function, *J Periodont Res* 17:492-494, 1982.

48. Van Dyke TE, Levine MJ, Genco RJ: Neutrophil function and oral disease, *J Oral Pathol* 14:95-120, 1985.

49. Reuland-Bosma W, van Dijk J: Periodontal disease in Down's syndrome: a review, *J Clin Periodontol* 13:64-73, 1986.

50. Waldrop TC, Anderson DC, Hallmon WW, et al: Periodontal manifestations of the heritable Mac-1, LFA-1, deficiency syndrome. Clinical, histopathologic and molecular characteristics, *J Periodontol* 58:400-416, 1987.

51. Kantarci A, Oyaizu K, Van Dyke TE: Neutrophil-mediated tissue injury in periodontal disease pathogenesis: findings from localized aggressive periodontitis, *J Periodontol* 74:66-75, 2003.

52. Van Dyke TE, Serhan CN: Resolution of inflammation: a new paradigm for the pathogenesis of periodontal diseases, *J Dent Res* 82:82-90, 2003.

53. Taichman NS, Tsai C-C, Baehni PC, et al: Interaction of inflammatory cells and oral microorganisms. IV. In vitro release of lysosomal constituents from polymorphonuclear leukocytes exposed to supragingival and subgingival bacterial plaque, *Infect Immun* 16:1013-1023, 1977.

54. McArthur WP, Baehni P, Taichman NS: Interaction of inflammatory cells and oral microorganisms. III. Modulation of rabbit polymorphonuclear leukocyte hydrolase release response to *Actinomyces viscosus* and *Streptococcus mutans* by immunoglobulins and complement, *Infect Immun* 14:1315-1321, 1976.

55. Genco R, Kornman K, Williams R, et al: Consensus report. Periodontal diseases: pathogenesis and microbial factors, *Ann Periodontol* 1:926-932, 1996.

56. Bergström J, Preber H: Tobacco use as a risk factor, *J Periodontol* 65:545-550, 1994.

57. Tonetti MS: Cigarette smoking and periodontal diseases: etiology and management of disease, *Ann Periodontol* 3:88-101, 1998.

58. Soskolne WA, Klinger A: The relationship between periodontal diseases and diabetes: an overview, *Ann Periodontol* 6:91-98, 2001.

59. Lang NP, Kiel RA, Anderhalden K: Clinical and microbiological effects of subgingival restorations with overhanging

or clinically perfect margins, *J Clin Periodontol* 10:563-578, 1983.

60. Breivik T, Thrane PS, Murison R, et al: Emotional stress effects on immunity, gingivitis and periodontitis, *Eur J Oral Sci* 104:327-334, 1996.

61. Moss ME, Beck JD, Kaplan BH, et al: Exploratory case-control analysis of psychosocial factors and adult periodontitis, *J Periodontol* 67:1060-1069, 1996.

62. Okada H, Murakami S: Cytokine expression in periodontal health and disease, *Crit Rev Oral Biol Med* 9:248-266, 1998.

63. Horton JE, Raisz LG, Simmons HA, et al: Bone resorbing activity in supernatant fluid from cultured peripheral blood leukocytes, *Science* 177:793-795, 1972.

64. Hönig J, Rordorf-Adam C, Siegmund C, et al: Increased interleukin-1 beta (IL-1β) concentration in gingival tissue from periodontitis patients, *J Periodont Res* 24:362-367, 1989.

65. Masada MP, Persson R, Kenney JS, et al: Measurement of interleukin-1α and -1β in gingival crevicular fluid: implications for the pathogenesis of periodontal disease, *J Periodont Res* 25:156-163, 1990.

66. Stashenko P, Fujiyoshi P, Obernesser MS, et al: Levels of interleukin 1β in tissue from sites of active periodontal disease, *J Clin Periodontol* 18:548-554, 1991.

67. Wilton JMA, Bampton JLM, Griffiths GS, et al: Interleukin-1 beta (IL-1β) levels in gingival crevicular fluid from adults with previous evidence of destructive periodontitis. A cross sectional study, *J Clin Periodontol* 19:53-57, 1992.

68. Richards D, Rutherford RB: The effects of interleukin 1 on collagenolytic activity and prostaglandin-E secretion by human periodontal-ligament and gingival fibroblast, *Arch Oral Biol* 33:237-243, 1988.

69. Birkedal-Hansen H: Role of cytokines and inflammatory mediators in tissue destruction, *J Periodont Res* 28:500-510, 1993.

70. Offenbacher S, Salvi GE: Induction of prostaglandin release from macrophages by bacterial endotoxin, *Clin Infect Dis* 28:505-513, 1999.

71. Matsuki Y, Yamamoto T, Hara K: Localization of interleukin-1 (IL-1) mRNA-expressing macrophages in human inflamed gingiva and IL-1 activity in gingival crevicular fluid, *J Periodont Res* 28:35-42, 1993.

72. Lo YJ, Liu CM, Wong MY, et al: Interleukin 1beta-secreting cells in inflamed gingival tissue of adult periodontitis patients, *Cytokine* 11:626-633, 1999.

73. Chapple CC, Srivastava M, Hunter N: Failure of macrophage activation in destructive periodontal disease, *J Pathol* 186:281-286, 1998.

74. Seymour GJ, Greenspan JS: The phenotypic characterization of lymphocyte subpopulations in established human periodontal disease, *J Periodont Res* 14:39-46, 1979.

75. Lindhe J, Liljenberg B, Listgarten M: Some microbiological and histopathological features of periodontal disease in man, *J Periodontol* 51:264-269, 1980.

76. Seymour GJ, Crouch MS, Powell RN: The phenotypic characterization of lymphoid cell subpopulations in gingivitis in children, *J Periodont Res* 16:582-592, 1981.

77. Seymour GJ, Gemmell E, Walsh LJ, et al: Immunohistological analysis of experimental gingivitis in humans, *Clin Exp Immunol* 71:132-137, 1988.

78. Rowland RW: Relationship between race and lymphocyte function during acute gingival inflammation, *J Periodont Res* 28:514-516, 1993.

79. Taubman MA, Stoufi ED, Ebersole JL, et al: Phenotypic studies of cells from periodontal disease tissues, *J Periodont Res* 19:587-590, 1984.

80. Stoufi ED, Taubman MA, Ebersole JL, et al: Phenotypic analyses of mononuclear cells recovered from healthy and diseased human periodontal tissues, *J Clin Immunol* 7:235-245, 1987.

81. Cole KL, Seymour GJ, Powell RN: Phenotypic and functional analysis of T cells extracted from chronically inflamed human periodontal tissues, *J Periodontol* 58:569-573, 1987.

82. Kinane DF, Johnston FA, Evans CW: Depressed helper-to-suppressor T-cell ratios in early-onset forms of periodontal disease, *J Periodont Res* 24:161-164, 1989.

83. Okada H, Shimabukuro Y, Kassai Y, et al: The function of gingival lymphocytes on the establishment of human periodontitis, *Adv Dent Res* 2:364-367, 1988.

84. Gemmell E, Feldner B, Seymour GJ: CD45RA and CD45RO positive CD4 cells in human peripheral blood and periodontal disease tissue before and after stimulation with periodontopathic bacteria, *Oral Microbiol Immunol* 7:84-88, 1992.

85. Lundqvist C, Hammarström M-L: T-cell receptor γδ-expressing intraepithelial lymphocytes are present in normal and chronically inflamed human gingiva, *Immunology* 79:38-45, 1993.

86. Yamazaki K, Nakajima T, Aoyagi T, et al: Immunohistological analysis of memory T lymphocytes and activated B lymphocytes in tissues with periodontal disease, *J Periodont Res* 28:324-334, 1993.

87. Tanner ACR, Kent RL Jr, Maiden MF, et al: Serum IgG reactivity to subgingival bacteria in initial periodontitis, gingivitis and healthy subjects, *J Clin Periodontol* 27:473-480, 2000.

88. Ebersole JL, Cappelli D, Holt SC: Periodontal diseases: to protect or not to protect is the question? *Acta Odontol Scand* 59:161-166, 2001.

89. Holbrook WP, Mooney J, Sigurdsson T, et al: Putative periodontal pathogens, antibody titres and avidities to them in a longitudinal study of patients with resistant periodontitis, *Oral Dis* 2:217-223, 1996.

90. Chen HA, Johnson BD, Sims TJ, et al: Humoral immune responses to *Porphyromonas gingivalis* before and following therapy in rapidly progressive periodontitis patients, *J Periodontol* 62:781-791, 1991.

91. Lopatin DE, Blackburn E: Avidity and titer of immunoglobulin G subclasses to *Porphyromonas gingivalis* in adult periodontitis patients, *Oral Microbiol Immunol* 7:332-337, 1992.

92. Whitney C, Ant J, Moncla B, et al: Serum immunoglobulin G antibody to *Porphyromonas gingivalis* in rapidly progressive periodontitis: titer, avidity, and subclass distribution, *Infect Immun* 60:2194-2200, 1992.

93. Johnson V, Johnson BD, Sims TJ, et al: Effects of treatment on antibody titer to *Porphyromonas gingivalis* in gingival crevicular fluid of patients with rapidly progressive periodontitis, *J Periodontol* 64:559-565, 1993.

94. Mooney J, Adonogianaki E, Riggio MP, et al: Initial serum antibody titer to *Porphyromonas gingivalis* influences development of antibody avidity and success of therapy for chronic periodontitis, *Infect Immun* 63:3411-3416, 1995.

95. Rowland RW, Mestecky J, Gunsolley JC, et al: Serum IgG and IgM levels to bacterial antigens in necrotizing ulcerative gingivitis, *J Periodontol* 64:195-201, 1993.

96. Cutler CW, Arnold RR, Schenkein HA: Inhibition of C3 and IgG proteolysis enhances phagocytosis of *Porphyromonas gingivalis*, *J Immunol* 151:7016-7029, 1993.

97. Colombo AP, Sakellari D, Haffajee AD, et al: Serum antibodies reacting with subgingival species in refractory periodontitis subjects, *J Clin Periodontol* 25:596-604, 1998.

98. Page RC: Milestones in periodontal research and the remaining critical issues, *J Periodont Res* 34:331-339, 1999.

99. Kornman KS: Host modulation as a therapeutic strategy in the treatment of periodontal disease, *Clin Infect Dis* 28:520-526, 1999.

100. Paquette DW, Williams RC: Modulation of host inflammatory mediators as a treatment strategy for periodontal diseases, *Periodontol 2000* 24:239-252, 2000.

101. Oringer RJ: Modulation of the host response in periodontal therapy, *J Periodontol* 73:460-470, 2002. (Erratum published in *J Periodontol* 73:684, 2002.)

6

Dental Plaque and Calculus: Microbial Biofilms and Periodontal Diseases

M. Robert Wirthlin, Jr. and Gary C. Armitage

CLINICAL FEATURES

Dental plaques are complex microbial communities that form on virtually all surfaces of the teeth exposed to the bacteria-laden fluids of the mouth. Dental plaques are of considerable clinical importance because they are the primary etiologic agents in the development of dental caries[1,2] and periodontal diseases.[3,4]

Supragingival and Subgingival Plaques

The eruption of teeth into the mouth of an edentulous infant results in the appearance of two unique ecosystems of the oral cavity: portions of the teeth exposed to the supragingival environment and portions exposed to the subgingival environment of the gingival crevice. *Supragingival plaque* can be defined as the community of microorganisms that develops on tooth surfaces coronal to the gingival margin. Important ecologic determinants in the supragingival environment that have major effects on the development of supragingival plaque are the many components of whole saliva and all of the dynamic variables associated with the dietary intake of foods and liquids. *Subgingival plaque* can be defined as the community of microorganisms that develops on tooth surfaces apical to the gingival margin. Before the development of gingivitis, the dimensions of the subgingival ecosystem are quite small because the gingival crevice may only be a few millimeters deep. With the onset of gingivitis and its progression to periodontitis, there is a considerable growth in size of the subgingival compartment. Important ecologic determinants in the subgingival environment that have major effects on the development of subgingival plaque are the many components of gingival crevicular fluid (GCF; e.g., antibodies, complement, serum proteins, neutrophils) that accumulate in the subgingival area as a manifestation of the host's response to the presence of bacteria. In both the supragingival and subgingival environments interactions and competition among different species of bacteria also have a profound effect on the microbial composition of dental plaque.

The clinical appearance of supragingival plaque is highly variable. It can appear as a nearly invisible thin film on the tooth surface (Fig. 6-1) to thick mats of material that completely obscure the tooth surface and cover the gingival margin (Fig. 6-2). Most of the plaque mass is composed of a myriad of microbial clusters surrounded by an adherent matrix of polysaccharides and glycoproteins produced by bacteria within the plaque (Figs. 6-3 and 6-4). Dental plaque is *not* easily dislodged with a water spray or vigorous rinsing. In some patients with particularly poor oral hygiene, an amorphous material composed of bacteria, food particles, debris from desquamated epithelial cells, and neutrophils collects on the surface of supragingival plaque. This loosely adherent debris is sometimes called *materia alba* and can usually be washed away by vigorously rinsing or flushing the area with water. The underlying dental plaque, however, remains in place.

Subgingival dental plaque is difficult to visualize in clinical situations because it is hidden from view within the gingival crevice or periodontal pocket. However, in many cases, it is visible to the unaided eye on extracted teeth. As is the case with supragingival plaque, electron microscopic examination of subgingival plaque clearly shows that it is composed of highly organized masses of

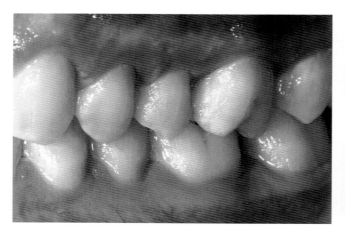

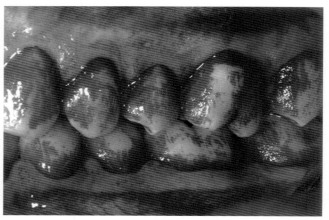

A

B

Figure 6-1. Thin supragingival dental plaque of a 32-year-old man who had not brushed his teeth for 7 days. **A,** Unstained plaque is not readily apparent. **B,** Extent of the plaque becomes apparent when stained with a disclosing solution (i.e., erythrosine dye [FD & C red no. 3]).

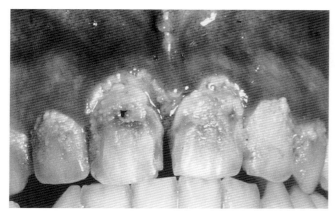

Figure 6-2. Thick supragingival plaque in a 28-year-old man who did not practice oral hygiene procedures at all over several years.

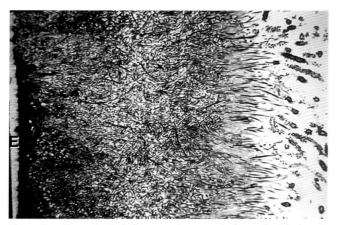

Figure 6-3. Supragingival plaque on the enamel of a tooth with chronic periodontitis. At this site there was a dense, predominantly filamentous bacterial mass adherent to the enamel. **E,** Enamel space. Original magnification × 850. *(Modified from Listgarten M: Structure of the microbial flora associated with periodontal health and disease in man. A light and electron microscopic study, J Periodontol 47:1-18, 1976.)*

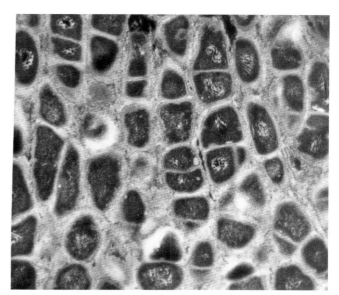

Figure 6-4. Electron micrograph of supragingival plaque showing bacteria and their surrounding polysaccharide and glycoprotein matrix. Original magnification ×13,750.

nities that cause fouling of dental unit waterlines. Supragingival and subgingival dental plaques are classic examples of liquid–solid surface biofilms.[5] Other microbial biofilms of medical importance include those that form on mucous membranes, external surfaces of the eye, artificial heart valves, contaminated prosthetic joints, arteriovenous shunts, endotracheal tubes, dental implants, and indwelling catheters. In addition, biofilms are involved in persistent infections of bone (e.g., osteomyelitis), the biliary tract, prostate (e.g., bacterial prostatitis), and lungs (e.g., cystic fibrosis pneumonia).[6]

Features of Biofilms

Biofilms have several interesting features that serve to protect and enhance the nutritional opportunities for the bacteria that reside within them. Biofilms offer *protection* for resident bacteria by giving them a competitive advantage over free-floating (planktonic) bacteria (Fig. 6-5). Microorganisms of biofilms produce a matrix called the *glycocalyx* that encloses the microbial community and protects it from the potentially harmful effects of the surrounding environment. Many bacteria in the sessile state of a biofilm synthesize extracellular polysaccharides that are generally composed of neutral sugars, amino acids, and some uronic acids. Streptococci make high molecular weight dextrans from glucose and levans from fructose.[7] Gram-negative bacteria make acetylated polymers of uronic acids called alginates that precipitate when exposed to Ca^{2+} in saliva.[8] These slimy coatings keep the bacteria banded together and retain them on the surface, so they are not flushed away by the turbulent action of

bacteria. Many different morphotypes of bacteria are present in subgingival plaque at sites with chronic periodontitis.

DENTAL PLAQUES AS BIOFILMS ON THE TEETH

Biofilms are natural communal aggregations of microorganisms that may form on a wide range of surfaces. They can develop at air–liquid interfaces such as plankton on the sea surface or on algae scum on a mill pond. There are also many liquid–solid surface biofilms such as slimes on rocks in creeks and microbial commu-

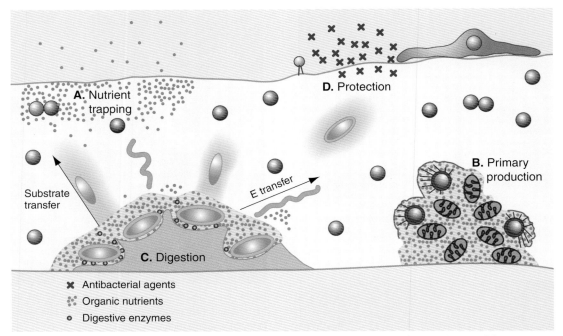

Figure 6-5. Four important features of biofilms are their ability to trap nutrients **(A)**, engage in the primary production of their own nutrients **(B)**, form a digestive consortium **(C)**, and protect bacteria in the biofilm from antibacterial agents or phagocytes **(D)**. *(Redrawn from Costerton JW, Cheng K-J, Geesey GG, et al: Bacterial biofilms in nature and disease, Annu Rev Microbiol 41:435-464, 1987.)*

surrounding fluids (e.g., saliva in the case of supragingival dental plaque biofilms). In addition, the extracellular polysaccharides of the glycocalyx are usually of a high molecular weight and are thereby insoluble. Consequently, biofilms are difficult to remove. Indeed, their removal can often only be achieved by mechanical means (e.g., in the case of dental plaque biofilms by using a toothbrush and dental floss). The necessity for mechanical removal also applies to many other biofilms of medical importance such as biofilm-contaminated artificial joints that often require surgical removal for adequate treatment.[9] The matrix of biofilms also protects bacteria from the effects of antibiotics and antiseptics because these agents cannot easily penetrate the barrier provided by the polysaccharide matrix.[6,10-12]

In addition to its function as a protective barrier, the polysaccharide matrix imparts structure to biofilm communities. Although some biofilms are more highly structured than others, all of them have definite architectural features. For example, in all biofilms, microorganisms are *not* uniformly distributed throughout the biofilm. Instead, there are aggregates of microcolonies with different shapes and sizes dispersed throughout the biofilm. The arrangement of microcolonies within biofilms is partly dependent on the external shear forces from the surrounding environment on the entire biofilm.[13]

The biofilm may start as a patch on the surface, but as it spreads and develops it can take on the form of pillars or mushroom-like columns; thereby channels between the pillars improve the circulation of nutrients and discharge of wastes and toxins.[14,15] In a severely starved biofilm there may be stacks of colonies extending up into the fluid bulk resembling dendrites; whereas in a richly fed dental plaque (e.g., by a high-sucrose diet), a thick and dense biofilm develops.[16]

Microorganisms on the outer surface of biofilms are not as strongly attached or embedded in the matrix and are faster growing than those deep within biofilms. Surface bacteria are susceptible to detachment by predator phagocytes, abrasion, or shear forces of fluid currents. Periodically there may be sloughing of the surface cells. This detachment may serve the community by forming swarms that seed new surfaces for the start of another colony.[17,18]

Biofilms also offer a *nutritional* advantage to bacteria that reside within them.[19] To grow and reproduce bacteria must export enzymes to break up nutrients and then they need to absorb and assimilate the required sugars and amino acids. Microorganisms that are dispersed in a liquid (the planktonic phase) have little chance of encountering nutrients in such an environment and their enzymes are quite diluted. Conversely, biofilm bacteria have a survival advantage by banding together and adhering to a surface, thereby improving their access to nutritional materials (see Fig. 6-5). Biofilms of mixed microorganisms also have the symbiotic benefit of using the products exported by neighbors.

A fascinating feature of biofilms is the wide range of physiologic behavior of bacteria within them. Biofilms provide a vast array of microniches, and the same species of bacteria can behave quite differently depending on their topographic position within the microbial community (e.g., on the surface vs. deep within the biofilm).[14] In addition, bacteria in biofilms communicate with each other through a process known as *quorum sensing*. This process involves the regulation of gene expression in response to changes in the number of bacteria in a given area (i.e., cell density) within a biofilm. When the cell density of microorganisms reaches a certain level, the bacteria release increased amounts of signaling molecules called *autoinducers* that activate gene expression in surrounding bacteria. In general, autoinducers used by gram-negative bacteria are acylated homoserine lactones and those used by gram-positive bacteria are processed oligopeptides.[20] This ability of biofilm bacteria to communicate with one another allows them to coordinate their gene expression and thereby govern or direct the behavior of the entire microbial community. In this context, biofilms appear to act as multicellular units because multiple groups of bacteria demonstrate complex coordinated activities.

Biofilms do not develop as a haphazardly organized community of microorganisms. Their growth and development run through stages that start with *adherence* of bacteria followed by a *lag phase* during which phenotypic shifts occur. Subsequently there is a *rapid growth phase* during which a complex exopolysaccharide is produced. Finally the biofilm reaches a *steady state* or equilibrium of growth during which surface shedding and acquisition of new bacteria may occur.

FORMATION OF DENTAL PLAQUE

Adherence Phase

The initial event in the formation of both supragingival and subgingival dental plaque biofilms is the deposition on the tooth surface of glycoproteins from the oral environment. The thin layer of glycoproteins that are adsorbed to tooth surfaces is called the *acquired pellicle*. Its formation prepares or conditions the intraoral surface and makes it receptive to colonization by specific bacteria in the oral environment. Supragingivally, the principal source of these pellicle-forming glycoproteins is saliva. In subgingival locations, the proteins are derived from GCF. The composition of the acquired pellicle will differ depending to some extent on the physical and chemical characteristics of the surface being coated.[21,22] For example, chemically different glycoprotein coatings (acquired pellicles) form on surfaces of enamel, dentin, cementum, and restorative materials.[23-25] The composition of these

pellicles has a significant effect on the kinds of bacteria that adhere to intraoral surfaces and the microbial components of the biofilms.[26]

Salivary glands produce several types of proteins and peptides that play important roles in the overall ecology of the mouth. Among the many salivary compounds that become incorporated into supragingival-acquired pellicles are the following: mucins, acidic proline-rich proteins (PRPs), histatins, statherin, and cystatins.

Salivary *mucins* are multifunctional molecules that are involved in the formation of the acquired pellicle, lubrication of tooth surfaces to reduce wear, and protection of oral surfaces from dehydration.[27,28] In addition, some mucins play an important role in regulating the interaction of bacteria with mucosal and tooth surfaces.[27,29-31] Secretions from human submandibular and sublingual salivary glands contain a high molecular weight mucin (>1,000 kD), called MUC5B (formerly MG1), and a low molecular weight mucin (150 to 200 kD), called MUC7 (formerly MG2).[32] MUC5B selectively forms heterotropic complexes with many salivary proteins (e.g., histatins, statherin, PRPs) and incorporates them into the acquired pellicle.[32,33] Although it has minimal direct interaction with bacteria, it does attract *Streptococcus sanguis*, *Streptococcus mitis*, and *Actinomyces* spp.[30] MUC7, however, has major interactions with bacteria and is believed to play an important role in their clearance from the oral cavity.[29,30,34-38] It attracts many bacteria including *S. sanguis*, *Streptococcus gordonii*, *Eikenella corrodens*, *Staphylococcus aureus*, and *Pseudomonas aeruginosa*.[29,39] MUC7 has a long protein core with sugar-containing short side chains of varying lengths. At the terminal ends of the sugars there are often sialic acid residues that can bind to receptors on pellicle or on epithelial cells. Neuraminidase produced by certain bacteria in saliva may cleave off the terminal sialic acid, exposing the next molecule in the side chain, which is often galactose.[40,41] *S. sanguis* and *S. mitis*, some of the first bacteria to colonize pellicles, possess adhesins for the sialic acid. Other bacteria such as *Actinomyces viscosus*, *Actinomyces naeslundii*, *Prevotella intermedia*, *E. corrodens*, and *Fusobacterium* spp. have galactosyl adhesins.[42]

Proline-rich proteins (PRPs) are a heterogeneous family of salivary proteins that contain abundant amounts of proline, glutamic acid/glutamine, and glycine. There are three general groups of PRPs: acidic (~16 kD), basic (~6 to 9 kD), and glycosylated (~36 kD).[43] Basic PRPs are found in saliva, as well as in nasal and bronchial secretions. Acidic PRPs are only found in saliva.[30,44] Acidic and glycosylated PRPs are found in newly formed acquired pellicles.[45] Acidic PRPs bind calcium and have a particular affinity for hydroxyapatite of the tooth[45] and are believed to play an important role in the homeostasis of salivary calcium and phosphate levels.[46] The formation of acquired pellicle is a process involving the selective adsorption of many pellicle precursor proteins. Some of these precursor proteins are derived from complex interactions of acidic PRPs with other salivary components such as statherin and histatins.[47]

Statherin is a low molecular weight salivary acidic phosphoprotein found in pellicle that is believed to promote bacterial adhesion to tooth surfaces.[48,49] It is present in human parotid and submandibular saliva and plays a major role in preventing the unwanted and potentially harmful precipitation of calcium and phosphate salts in ducts of salivary glands.[50] At least four statherin variants with slightly different molecular weights are present in saliva.[51]

Histatins are another group of important salivary components that are incorporated into acquired pellicles. The histatin family includes 12 histidine-rich small proteins (or peptides) with potent antifungal properties that are primarily produced by parotid, and to a lesser extent, by submandibular salivary glands.[30,52-56] Some histatins appear to be proteolytic breakdown products of other larger members of the histatin family.[57] Histatin 5 appears to be particularly effective against *Candida albicans* and acts by binding to specific protein receptors on the cell membrane of the organism.[30,52,53] There are also data suggesting that some histatins exert bactericidal effects on certain strains of *Streptococcus mutans*.[58,59] Inhibitory effects on the aggregation, adherence, and protease activity of *Porphyromonas gingivalis* have also been reported.[60-62] It is of interest that salivary histatins have the ability to partially disrupt in vitro biofilms produced by continuous cultures of mixtures of *S. mutans, S. sanguis, Streptococcus salivarius, A. naeslundii, Veillonella parvula, Fusobacterium nucleatum,* and *P. intermedia*.[63]

Cystatins are physiologic inhibitors of cysteine proteinases such as cathepsins B, H, and L, which are potent tissue-degrading enzymes. The cystatin superfamily is divided into three main families. Salivary cystatins belong to "family II" and include acid (S and SA), neutral (SN and D), and basic (C) types.[30] Cystatin C is in most biologic fluids, whereas types S, SA, SN, and D are only found in whole saliva, glandular saliva, and tears. The physiologic function of cystatins is not clear; however, they may play a role in regulating the activity of cysteine proteinases liberated during inflammatory periodontal diseases.[64-67] Partial depletion of some salivary cystatins has been reported in some periodontally diseased patients.[68] Cystatin SA may play a role in pellicle formation[69] and tooth remineralization.[70,71] Although cystatins are constitutive components of saliva, increased levels may be induced by certain foods (e.g., capsaicin, an extract of hot peppers)[72] and may be decreased by taking certain medications (e.g., valproate and phenytoin).[73]

In addition to mucins, PRPs, statherin, histatins, and cystatins, there are many other components of saliva with potent antimicrobial activities that are often incorporated into acquired pellicles. Noteworthy among these are salivary agglutinins,[74] α-amylase,[30,69,75] secretory IgA,[30,69] lysozyme,[30,76] and lactoferrin.[29,75] Clearly, acquired pellicles are complex and diverse mixtures of many biologically active molecules that have a profound influence on the types of bacteria that colonize tooth surfaces.

Pellicle formation starts virtually minutes after a professional scaling and polishing of the teeth. Hydroxyapatite surfaces of teeth carry an overall negative charge that facilitates their interaction with positively charged glycoproteins present in saliva. Although variable, pellicles are usually 1- to 2-μm-thick before they are colonized by bacteria. Within an hour or so, the "pioneer" microorganisms become attached to the pellicle. These first colonists on teeth are generally gram-positive cocci such as *S. sanguis* and *S. gordonii*. The many salivary molecules that have been incorporated into the pellicle have an affinity for proteinaceous ligands, or *adhesins*, on the surface of *S. sanguis* and other pioneer colonizers. Adhesins might be found on fimbriae, pili, and the "O" antigen portion of the saccharide-like part of the endotoxin molecule projecting from cell walls of gram-negative bacteria. Attached to the surface of many streptococci are glucosyl transferases, enzymes that take glucose portions of sucrose molecules and link them in chains by α(1-6) links (dextrans) or α(1-3) links (glucans). The dextran chains may serve as lectins that bind to peptides in the acquired pellicle. The sum of all these "cryptic receptors" (cryptitopes) results in bacterial adherence to oral surfaces.[41]

Lag Phase

The switch from a planktonic phase to a sessile life is thought to result in a phenotypic change in bacteria. There will be a temporary lag in the growth of the newly adherent bacteria as they shift their genetic expression. As a result, changes in mRNA expression and protein profiles occur. Genes involved in polysaccharide synthesis will be promoted, whereas genes involved in flagella production will turn off.[77,78] The phenotypic changes that occur during the lag phase set the trajectory or course for subsequent development of the biofilm.

Rapid Growth Phase

Once the adherent bacteria have shifted their genetic expression they enter a rapid growth phase and begin secreting large amounts of water-insoluble extracellular polysaccharides for the glycocalyx. Gram-negative bacteria participate in the process of matrix production by synthesizing alginates that are acetylated polymers of uronic acids. Precipitation of these alginates occurs when they react with Ca^{2+} in the surrounding environment. In supragingival plaques the amount of exopolysaccharides composed of the dextran, glucan, and levan types are influenced by the sucrose intake of the host. These polymers of glucose and fructose may reach molecular weights of approximately one million. The polysaccharides form a tangled feltlike mesh in which some microorganisms and debris may get trapped. However, most biofilm bacteria adhere by specific molecular interactions of a ligand–substrate nature to the "forest" of protruding molecules. Most of the available information on production of exopolysaccharides of the glycocalyx have been studied during conditions simulating the supragingival environment. Little is known about the matrices of biofilms in subgingival environments.

Growth of microcolonies within the matrix and coaggregation and coadhesion of bacteria increase the thickness of the biofilm.[79] Coaggregation and coadhesion of oral bacteria are important events in the formation and growth of biofilms. *Coaggregation* occurs when bacteria in a suspension (e.g., saliva) adhere to one another to form a clump; *coadhesion* is when free-floating bacteria attach to other bacteria that are already attached to a surface. These associations are not haphazard or random because they involve unique and selective molecular interactions that lead to horizontal and vertical structural stratifications within the biofilm.[23,26] *F. nucleatum* is an excellent "coaggregator" with other bacteria. Indeed, it is a major effector organism that facilitates the colonization of other species.[80-83] For example, all treponemes tested coaggregate with *F. nucleatum,*[82] and it forms important associations with *P. intermedia* and *P. gingivalis.*[80,83] Streptococci are also key members of oral biofilms because they express adhesin arrays on their cell surfaces that facilitate coaggregation with "early" (e.g., *Actinomyces* spp.) and "late" colonizers (e.g., *P. gingivalis, Tannerella forsythensis* [formerly *Bacteroides forsythus*], *Treponema denticola*) of dental plaque.[84-88] The most frequently isolated dental plaque bacteria are those that are good coaggregators such as *F. nucleatum, A. naeslundii,* and *S. sanguis* (Table 6-1).[89] In addition to the effector roles played by streptococci and *F. nucleatum,* numerous other pathogenic and commensal bacteria engage in important associations that affect the microbial composition of plaque biofilms.[90,91]

During the rapid growth phase there is an increase in cell density within the plaque. It is probably during this period of plaque growth when there is a maximum amount of communication among bacteria (i.e., quorum sensing). Quorum sensing, which is triggered by changes in cell density, allows metabolically active bacteria during crowded conditions of the plaque's interior to cooperate with each other in ways that promote survival of the biofilm community.

Steady State

Deep inside the biofilm there are internal transfers of nutrients, and those absorbed from the surface appear to form gradients. Oxygen penetration may be negligible at a depth of only 25 to 30 μm.[92] Within the interior of biofilms bacterial growth may greatly slow or come to a standstill. Static conditions within a biofilm may cause bacteria to shrink into forms unresolvable with a light microscope. The close quarters of the plaque interior may expedite gene sharing through conjugation, plasmid transfer, absorption of DNA from lysed cells, or fusion of mycoplasma-like bacteria without cell walls.[93]

Findings from transmission electron microscopic studies of mature dental plaques are consistent with the view that the interiors of these biofilms exhibit varying degrees of metabolic activity.[94-96] Indeed, as might be expected, bacteria near the surface are morphologically intact, whereas those deep within the plaque mass near the tooth surface show signs of death. For example, deep within the interior of old dental plaques there are many disrupted bacterial cells and "ghost" cell walls devoid of cytoplasm. Near the pellicle, crystals are often observed in the interbacterial matrix that may be the first stages of mineralization to form calculus.[94,95] In the middle portion of mature plaques nearer the surface, there are intact and closely packed bacterial cells. Finally, at the surface of plaques where exposure to turbulent conditions of the mouth is at its greatest, bacteria form cooperative associations such as "corncob" and "bristle-brush" formations.[94-96] Presumably, these associations promote adherence, and therefore survival, of the participating bacteria in the turbulent environment of the oral cavity.

Biofilms in the Subgingival Environment

Supragingival dental plaque at the gingival margin can grow into the gingival crevice and contribute to the development of a subgingival biofilm. Importantly, essentially the entire subgingival niche becomes colonized by bacteria. In a periodontal pocket, there is no unoccupied space (Fig. 6-6). The subgingival environment is quite different from the supragingival microbial niche in many ways. For example, it is bathed in GCF rather than saliva. GCF is an inflammatory exudate rich in proteins and other nutrients and its serum glycoproteins play a key role in the formation of an acquired pellicle analogous to that of saliva in the supragingival environment. After subgingival plaque is removed or disrupted by scaling, a complex flora will develop within 2 to 3 days, which is faster than supragingival plaque.[97]

With the consumption of peptides and amino acids from the GCF, or those from degraded epithelial cells and leukocytes, there is a subgingival accumulation of toxic substances such as volatile fatty acids (e.g., propionate, butyrate, valerate), urea, NH_3, volatile sulfur compounds

TABLE 6-1 Most Numerous Species in Subgingival Samples Associated with Different Periodontal Conditions

HEALTH* (420)	GINGIVITIS† (350)	CHRONIC PERIODONTITIS (3775)	LOCALIZED AGGRESSIVE PERIODONTITIS (1065)	GENERALIZED AGGRESSIVE PERIODONTITIS (1315)
A. naeslundii 19	A. naeslundii 10	A. naeslundii 14	Eubacterium Do6 8	F. nucleatum 8
S. sanguis 11	F. nucleatum 10	F. nucleatum 14	A. naeslundii 7	E. nodatum 8
V. parvula 9	V. parvula 7	S. sanguis 3	F. nucleatum 7	E. timidum 6
F. nucleatum 8	S. sanguis 5	P. micros 3	E. nodatum 6	A. naeslundii 6
S. oralis 5	C. ochracea 5	B. gracilis 3	C. rectus 4	L. uli 6
S. intermedius 3	A. israelii 3	C. concisus 2	V. parvula 4	P. micros 4
Actinomyces serotype 963 3	C. gingivalis 3	E. timidum 2	L. uli 3	Eubacterium Do6 4
P. micros 2	C. sputigena 3	S. oralis 2	S. oralis 3	P. intermedia 3
Streptococcus Do6 2	S. noxia 3	L. uli 2	E. timidum 3	S. intermedius 2
G. morbillorum 2	C. rectus 3	S. sputigena 2	P. micros 3	Streptococcus D39 2
C. ochracea 1	B. gracilis 3	S. intermedius 2	P. oris 2	P. denticola 2
H. segnis 1	P. nigrescens 2	A. odontolyticus 2	F. alocis 2	L. rimae 2
H. parainfluenzae 1	S. oralis 2	L. rimae 2	L. rimae 2	E. brachy 2
S. epidermidis 1	E. brachy 2	E. nodatum 2	Actinomyces serotype 963 2	F. alocis 2
C. gingivalis 1	S. mitis 2	V. parvula 1		P. oris 2
C. rectus 1	E. timidum 2	P. nigrescens 1	P. denticola 2	V. parvula 2
B. gracilis 1	G. morbillorum 1	F. alocis 1	P. anaerobius ID 1	S. noxia 1
A. odontolyticus 1	O. catoniae 1	C. ochracea 1	E. saphenum 1	P. acnes 1
P. acnes 1	P. acnes 1	C. rectus 1	A. odontolyticus 1	P. avidum 1
P. denticola 1	H. segnis 1	P. gingivalis 1	A. actinomycetem-comitans 1	E. saphenum 1
E. timidum 1	C. concisus 1	V. atypia 1	A. meyeri 1	A. israelii 1
Facultative gram-negative rod D24 1	A. odontolyticus 1	A. israelii 1	Prevotella M1 1	C. ochracea 1
S. noxia 1	S. sputigena 1	P. anaerobius ID 1	P. intermedia 1	S. sputigena 1
S. faecium 1	L. buccalis 1	A. generncseriae 1	S. sanguis 1	E. alactolyticum 1
A. meyeri 1	Actinomyces serotype 963 1	E. saphenum 1	E. brachy 1	B. gracilis 1
S. warneri 1	A. meyeri 1	P. anaerobius II 1	B. gracilis 1	C. rectus 1
E. saburreum 1	E. yurii 1	G. morbillorum 1	P. oralis 1	P. nigrescens 1
Leptotrichia D16 1	S. infelix 1	S. infelix 1	C. ochracea 1	P. anaerobius II 1
	S. flueggeii 1	E. alactolyticum 1	P. gingivalis 1	P. anaerobius ID 1
	F. alocis 1	P. denticola 1	S. noxia 1	P. buccae 1
	E. saphenum 1	A. meyeri 1	P. nigrescens 1	A. meyeri 1
	C. curvus 1	S. mutans 1	D. pneumosintes 1	C. curvus 1
	P. oris 1	E. brachy 1	P. anaerobius II 1	S. parvulus 1
	P. micros 1	C. sputigena 1	P. acnes 1	Campylobacter X 1
	L. rimae 1	C. gingivalis 1	A. israelii 1	S. mitis 1
	E. nodatum 1	P. loeschii 1	P. melaninogenica 1	S. parasanguis 1
	Campylobacter X 1	Eubacterium D33 1	S. intermedius 1	D. pneumosintes 1
	V. atypia 1	S. mitis 1	G. morbillorum 1	A. gerencseriae 1
		E. yurii 1		

Modified from Moore WEC, Moore LVH: The bacteria of periodontal diseases, Periodontol 2000 5:66-77, 1994.
Coaggregating bacteria such as Actinomyces naeslundii, Streptococcus sanguis, and Fusobacterium nucleatum are among the most frequently isolated microorganisms in dental plaque. Note their position on the partial list of most numerous species, ranked in order of percentage of isolates taken at random, from subgingival crevices of subjects with different periodontal health conditions. Number in parentheses after each diagnosis is the number of isolates studied. Number after each microorganism is percentage of isolates.
*Sites with Gingival Index = 0 (no clinical inflammation).
†Sites with Gingival Index = 2 (gingival bleeding).

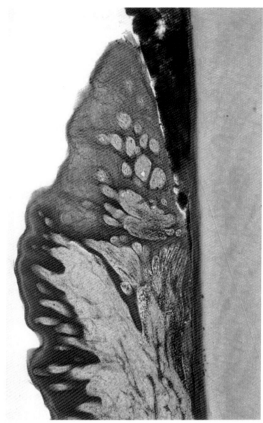

Figure 6-6. Periodontal pocket filled with a subgingival biofilm. There is no unoccupied space in a periodontal pocket. Human dentogingival interface obtained at autopsy from a patient who had chronic periodontitis. Original magnification ×20.

(e.g., H_2S, methyl mercaptan), cadaverine, and putrescine. The pH increases in GCF where dental plaque has grown, increasing from about 6.9 to 8.6. This is associated with putrefaction and production of urea and ammonia.[98] There is also a significant decrease in the oxidation-reduction potential (Eh) as the subgingival biofilm ages. In one study, the average Eh of a healthy gingival sulcus was approximately +74 millivolts (mV), whereas in inflamed periodontal pockets the average Eh was −47 mV.[99] Toxic substances at subgingival sites tend to select for growth of microorganisms such as spirochetes that prefer an environment that has a low Eh and high levels of byproducts from necrotic cells. Dental plaque collected from the gingival crevice and homogenized has been found to be lethal to mammalian cells in culture,[100] or to organ cultures of fetal rat calvaria.[101] The toxicity of the subgingival environment increases with time.

Biofilms Associated With the Crevicular Epithelium

Subgingival plaque that forms on a tooth has its outer surface in close proximity to the soft tissue wall of the gin-

gival crevice or periodontal pocket. This is in sharp contrast to supragingival plaque that has its outer surface exposed to the turbulent movement of fluids such as saliva and dietary liquids. Some bacteria in close contact with the crevicular epithelium have the ability to adhere to these cells. For example, *S. sanguis* has multiple adhesins that allow it to adhere to oral epithelium.[102] Streptococci also can adhere to several host components found in subgingival environments such as fibronectin, fibrinogen, laminin, collagen, actin, and immunoglobulins.[103] Other bacteria found in the subgingival ecosystem also demonstrate the ability to bind to host components. For example, oral treponemes bind to fibronectin[104] and *P. gingivalis* binds to red blood cells, macrophages, fibrinogen, and fibronectin-coated collagen complexes.[105]

Bacterial biofilms that develop on epithelium usually only form monolayers. Turnover and desquamation of crevicular epithelium in a normal state of health usually keep bacteria out of the tissues. However, some bacteria, such as *Actinobacillus actinomycetemcomitans* and *P. gingivalis*, once attached to oral epithelium can become internalized by fusion and endocytosis.[106-109] Having done this they are protected from the immune system and antibiotics and have a most nutritious environment. Epithelial adherence is also part of the process in diseases such as streptococcal sore throat, whooping cough, diphtheria, gonorrhea, and shigellosis.

The spectrum of bacteria associated with the crevicular epithelium is different than the one found in dental plaque on the tooth surface. In one study of samples of curetted crevicular epithelium, the bacterial isolates included 87% cocci and short rods. The top 50% of isolates were *Streptococcus constellatus* (16.4%), *P. gingivalis* (10.4%), *P. intermedia* (8.0%), *Streptococcus morbillorum* (5.0%), *Peptostreptococcus micros* (2.2%), *Bacteroides loeschii* (2.0%), and *Bacteroides melaninogenicus* (6.2%).[110] Notably, these are greater proportions than in dental plaques from teeth (see Table 6-1).

The intercellular spaces of crevicular epithelium are widened in chronically inflamed gingiva, and the migration of neutrophils through the crevicular epithelium from the connective tissue to the crevice leave temporary channels.[111] In addition, the crevicular epithelium is frequently ulcerated in cases of gingivitis and periodontitis. This gives certain bacteria such as *P. gingivalis* access to bind to type IV collagen in basement membranes, which could facilitate its potential invasion of gingival connective tissue.[41,112] However, it is likely that normal host defenses are able to clear such intruders without further damage. A true invasion of tissues should show up as many microcolonies and widespread dissemination. The only evidence of true invasion in periodontal diseases occurs in necrotizing ulcerative gingivitis where treponemes have been found up to 250 μm within vital connective tissue.[113,114]

Motile Bacteria in the Subgingival Ecosystem

Between the subgingival plaque fixed to the pellicle and tooth, and whatever kind of biofilm may have adhered to the pocket epithelium, most of the subgingival microniche is occupied by a mass of bacteria, neutrophils, and sloughed epithelial cells (Fig. 6-7). There is a relation of the percentage of spirochetes in subgingival samples to the percentage of total motile microorganisms.[115,116] The mean number of *T. denticola* at subgingival sites is significantly associated with increased probing depths.[117] In a study using polymerase chain reaction techniques with spirochete-selective primers to detect 16S ribosomal RNA genes, a total of 57 closely related but genetically distinct spirochetes were found in 60 plaque samples from 15 patients. Of the detected treponemes, 10 represented known cultivable and 47 represented uncultivable spirochetes.[118] Importantly, there is a layer of neutrophils between the subgingival plaque and the soft tissue wall of the pocket. These neutrophils are often called the first line of defense against subgingival bacteria.

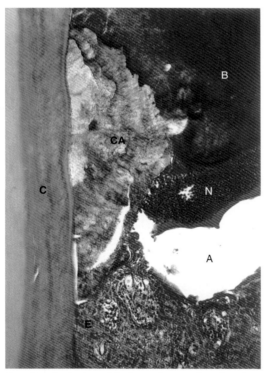

Figure 6-7. Histologic view of the base of a periodontal pocket at a site with chronic periodontitis. On the cementum (C) is a piece of subgingival calculus (CA) that is covered with a plaque biofilm (B). Apical to the plaque is a neutrophil-laden inflammatory exudate (N). Epithelium (E) is in close contact with the apical portion of the calculus. A, Artifactual space due to processing tissue for histologic observation. Human autopsy material. Original magnification ×100.

The subgingival environment is a decidedly hostile location for bacteria. Multiple host defenses such as scavenging phagocytes (e.g., neutrophils), antibodies, and inducible antibacterial substances such as β-defensins from epithelial cells[119,120] are mobilized to thwart the microbial threat presented by subgingival bacteria. Nevertheless, subgingival bacteria are able to survive, and in some cases flourish, as is evidenced by the widespread presence of periodontal diseases in most human populations.

DENTAL CALCULUS

Until the 1960s, the prevalent thinking in dentistry was that dental calculus ("tartar") was the cause of periodontal diseases; that by its roughness it was irritating, and that bacteria then had a secondary influence.[121] However, a series of classic studies on "experimental gingivitis" published from 1965 to 1968 clearly demonstrated the causative relation between dental plaque and gingivitis.[122-125] In addition, the observation that autoclaved human calculus implanted in the peritoneal cavity of guinea pigs resulted in suppurative abscesses was attributed to the presence of heat-stable endotoxin in the calculus.[126] Current thinking is that dental plaque is the precursor of calculus, which is *mineralized plaque*. Calculus is invariably covered with plaque on its surface.[127]

Laboratory studies implicate numerous members of the normal oral flora in mineralization of the dental plaque biofilms to form calculus. Some strains of gram-positive species that will form crystals in vitro when grown in solutions rich in calcium and phosphate include the following: *S. sanguis*, *S. salivarius*, *Bacterionema matruchotii*, *A. naeslundii*, *A. viscosus*, *S. aureus*, *Propionibacterium acnes*, and *Rothia dentocariosa*. Some of the gram-negative bacteria that exhibit this ability include the following: *E. corrodens*, *Veillonella alcalescens*, *P. gingivalis*, *Eubacterium saburreum*, *Haemophilus aphrophilus*, and *Haemophilus segnis*.[127] It is clear that many members of the dental plaque flora possess the ability to calcify during the right conditions. In addition, the observation in germfree rats that mineralized deposits can form on teeth indicates that even the acquired pellicle can calcify.[128,129]

Saliva is the source of the calcium and phosphate necessary for the formation of the minerals of supragingival calculus. Animals that have had the major salivary glands surgically removed do not form calculus.[130] In the case of subgingival calculus, GCF supplies the calcium and phosphate required for calcification of the plaque. X-ray diffraction studies have revealed that there are four different kinds of calcium phosphate crystals in dental calculus: hydroxyapatite $[Ca_{10}(PO_4)_6(OH)_2]$, octacalcium phosphate $[Ca_4H(PO_4)_3 \cdot 2H_2O]$, magnesium whitlockite

$[Ca_9(PO_4)_6 \text{ X } PO_7 \cdot (X = Mg_{11} \cdot F_{11})]$, and brushite $[CaHOP_4 \cdot 2H_2O]$.[131] The earliest crystals form in the interbacterial matrix deep in dental plaque near the pellicle. This area has many degenerated bacteria.

It was once thought that mucin could nucleate the first crystals[132]; however, proteolipids and phospholipids from degenerated bacterial cell walls will nucleate apatite[133] similar to the mineralization process in bone.[134] Calcification of dental plaque is believed to occur by two different mechanisms. The *epitactic mechanism* of formation of calculus mineral occurs by nucleation or crystal seeding of the matrix provided by dental plaque. In the *booster mechanism* there is a local saturation shift of calcium and phosphate caused by a local increase in pH leading to precipitation of mineral.[135] Local increases in pH needed for calcification could be caused by proteolytic activity of plaque bacteria resulting in the release of urea, ammonia, and amines.[136]

On the lingual of the lower anterior teeth and on the facial surfaces of upper molars, near the openings of submandibular and parotid salivary glands, supragingival calculus deposits are usually greater in amount (Fig. 6-8). This is partly because of saliva as a source of calcium and phosphate and partly because of the loss of CO_2 as saliva leaves the ducts causing an upward shift in the local pH.

Brushite is the dominant calcium phosphate mineral in newly formed supragingival calculus.[131,137] Clinically, newly formed calculus is a yellowish-white crumbly deposit that is easily removed.[138] When supragingival calculus ages, the amount of brushite declines as the amounts of magnesium whitlockite, octacalcium phosphate, and hydroxyapatite increase.[131] Subgingival calculus is harder and darker, probably because of the continual presence of calcium and phosphate that allows the crystals to shift with time to octacalcium phosphate and hydroxyapatite.[138] The dark color of subgingival calculus is partly caused by iron heme pigments associated with bleeding of inflamed gingiva (Fig. 6-9).[139]

As calculus ages, the first crystals coalesce into masses of mineralized plaque. In histologic sections, the outlines of bacteria and laminations of successive layers can be observed.[140] Eventually, even the pellicle mineralizes. When this occurs, the calculus becomes difficult to remove because the pellicle is in intimate contact with all of the minute irregularities of the tooth surface.[141] In addition, calculus can be even more firmly attached to the roots of teeth when it becomes mechanically locked in old resorption bays and cemental separations (Fig. 6-10).[142] Sometimes calculus forms at sites of arrested root caries where bacteria have penetrated into the cementum.[143]

Although calculus now has a secondary role in the etiology of periodontal diseases, it has to be dealt with clinically. Calculus promotes the retention of dental plaque

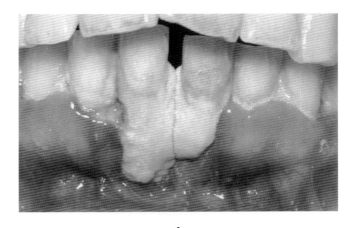

A

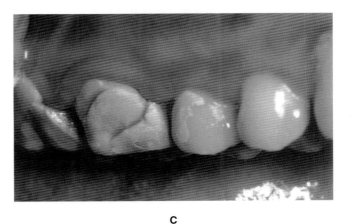

B

C

Figure 6-8. Very heavy deposits of supragingival calculus near the sites where saliva enters the oral cavity through ducts of major salivary glands. Calculus on the facial surfaces of lower incisors in a 35-year-old woman with chronic periodontitis **(A)**; lingual surface of same teeth **(B)**. Heavy deposits on the facial surfaces of upper teeth near the opening of Stensen's duct in a 26-year-old woman with chronic periodontitis **(C)**.

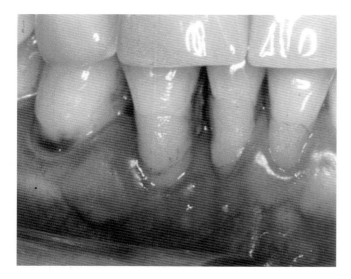

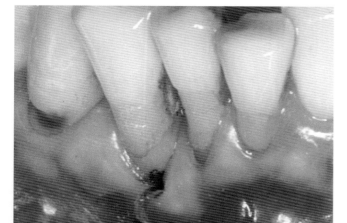

A

B

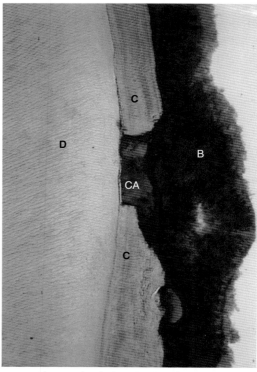

Figure 6-10. Subgingival calculus that has formed on a root with a damaged cemental surface. Extracted tooth from a patient with chronic periodontitis. B, Plaque biofilm; C, cementum; CA, calculus; D, dentin. Original magnification ×95.

Figure 6-9. Subgingival calculus is often brown to black partly because of incorporation of iron heme pigments found in the subgingival environment. Subgingival calculus can occasionally be seen through thin gingival tissue **(A)**. In **B,** the gingiva has been retracted to demonstrate the presence of the dark-colored subgingival calculus.

that calculus is unimportant, but it reaffirms that it is the dental plaque on its surface that is most harmful.

SIGNIFICANCE OF BIOFILMS TO PERIODONTAL DISEASES

Once a biofilm has formed on a tooth, established itself in the gingival sulcus, and developed a flora containing periodontal pathogens, there is little that the host defenses can do to remove the biofilm except by exfoliating the tooth. Indeed, exfoliation of the tooth is frequently the outcome in cases of untreated periodontitis in which the immune and inflammatory response to the biofilm bacteria destroys all of the periodontal attachment.

A patient given instructions in oral hygiene and possessed of motivation can remove dental plaques by physically rubbing the biofilm-coated surfaces with toothbrushes, dental floss, and toothpicks; but it is rare to find someone so skilled and driven who can do this perfectly. The concept of a "detergent and self-cleansing diet" by eating fibrous foods is largely a myth because their consumption has no observable effect on the levels of dental plaque or preventing the development of gingival inflammation.[145]

and may increase the rate of plaque formation. Its porosity can serve as a reservoir for periodontal pathogens and can retain noxious bacterial components such as endotoxin. It has been reported that a junctional epithelium complete with a basal lamina and hemidesmosomes can form on calculus; however, that was in one monkey that had been experimentally treated by toothbrushing, interdental cleansing, and application of an antimicrobial rinse three times a week.[144] This finding does not mean

Water irrigators have been developed in an attempt to reduce the harmful effects of dental plaque biofilms. However, these devices have only met with limited success because dental plaque is resistant to being rinsed away. This resistance is partly because of the high molecular weight dextrans, levans, and glucans produced by gram-positive bacteria and because of the insoluble alginates made by gram-negative microorganisms of plaque. Irrigation of periodontal pockets with water may reduce the percentage of spirochetes between the tooth-borne biofilm and the pocket epithelium, but not significantly.[146] However, irrigation with water has been reported to result in small, but statistically significant, reductions in probing depths and gingival bleeding.[147,148]

Antonie van Leeuwenhoek (1632-1723) was perhaps the first to recognize that biofilms are resistant to the effects of disinfectants. He is reported to have observed with his crude microscopes that vinegar would halt the motion of "animalcules" he had scraped from his teeth and put into a liquid preparation; but when he rinsed his mouth with vinegar it had no effect. He concluded that there was no penetration of vinegar into material between his teeth, and that only surface animalcules were susceptible.[149,150] Biofilm resistance to antimicrobials has been attributed to the following: (1) barrier properties of the glycocalyx matrix, (2) retention of antibiotic-degrading enzymes in the matrix, (3) binding of the negatively charged matrix to cationic antiseptics or repelling negatively charged agents, and (4) inhibition of leukocyte phagocytosis by the indigestible slime. Resistance to antimicrobials might also be caused by *phenotypic changes* in biofilm bacteria such as slow or cessation of growth in response to changes in physiologic conditions. Genetic changes might also occur in the bacteria that makes them no longer susceptible to certain antimicrobials.[151,152]

There are several reasons why tests that evaluate the effectiveness of an antimicrobial agent against bacteria in a planktonic phase are not applicable to bacteria in a biofilm. Traditional laboratory tests of a microorganism's susceptibility to an antimicrobial agent use broth suspensions of 10^5 to 10^7 microorganisms per milliliter to simulate systemic infections of blood, and the result is reported as the minimum inhibitory concentration (MIC). In a biofilm such as dental plaque there are up to 10^{11} bacteria per gram wet weight sequestered in the plaque matrix. Laboratory minimum inhibitory concentration tests may involve exposure to the antimicrobial over a period of several days, whereas contact of a mouthrinse with the biofilm may last only a minute or so. In minimum inhibitory concentration tests, the bacteria are surrounded on all sides by the test agent, whereas only surface bacteria of dental plaque are exposed to the test agent because of the barrier properties of the biofilm matrix. Furthermore, vigorous rinsing with an antimicrobial mouthrinse does not reach subgingival plaque in periodontal pockets. Studies are needed to determine the biofilm-eradicating concentration of an antimicrobial agent.[153]

Acquisition of knowledge of the bacteria that cause periodontal diseases is hampered by problems associated with microbiologic sampling of plaque biofilms. A common method is insertion of two sterile endodontic paper points into the gingival crevice for approximately 10 seconds. This method preferentially collects bacteria and the fluids surrounding them that are readily absorbed by the paper points. Unfortunately, this approach has little hope of obtaining bacteria representative of the biofilm attached to the pellicle and those adhering to the pocket epithelium. Such a sample is not quantified by weight or volume and therefore it is not possible to make accurate estimates of the actual composition of the subgingival flora. Collection of subgingival plaque with curets has a better chance of obtaining a more representative sample. However, it is difficult to place a curet within a pocket such that it collects a sample representative of the entire coronal-to-apical extent of the plaque biofilm.

Once the sample is in the laboratory for cultural analysis, only about 50% of the flora can be grown and identified; the other 50% have such fastidious growth requirements that they are uncultivable. In addition, at the time of sampling it is unknown if the lesion from which the plaque is taken is actively progressing or is in a quiescent stage. Therefore it is likely that studies of the microflora associated with periodontal diseases include a mixture of plaque samples collected from nonprogressing and progressing sites. Consequently, any conclusions regarding cause-and-effect relations between a specific microorganism and periodontal diseases should be viewed with caution. Nevertheless, available data strongly suggest that bacteria such as *P. gingivalis*, *A. actinomycetemcomitans*, and *Tannerella Forsythensis (B. forsythus)* are important periodontal pathogens in susceptible hosts.[154]

CONCLUSION

Dental plaques cause dental caries and most periodontal diseases. Plaque biofilms first appear in the mouth at the time of tooth eruption, forming supragingival plaque as a community of bacteria coronal to the gingival margin. Subgingival plaques form in the gingival crevice apical to the gingival margin. The plaques form, as do most liquid–solid surface biofilms, by going through various stages including microbial *adherence* to acquired pellicles followed by a *lag phase* during which phenotypic shifts occur in the bacteria as they switch from planktonic to a sessile environment. The microorganisms then undergo a *rapid growth phase* during which a complex exopolysaccharide matrix is produced, microcolonies form, and new members are added to the biofilm by coadherence. With time the mature dental plaque biofilm establishes a *steady state* equilibrium with the surrounding environment. Formation of biofilms by oral bacteria offers them a nutritional advantage over other microorganisms and a certain degree of protection from the microbial clearance mechanisms of the oral environment.

Metabolic activities of the bacteria of subgingival plaque biofilms generate a number of toxic substances that are added to by an inflammatory exudate, debris from neutrophils, and deteriorated epithelial cells. These events contribute to the formation of an anaerobic environment with a low Eh that selects for the growth of certain motile and nonmotile bacteria. A number of these microorganisms are able to adhere to the surface of the crevicular epithelium as a biofilm and subsequently become internalized by endocytosis. The crevicular epithelium and other host cells produce proinflammatory cytokines, and the adjacent tissues mount an antibacterial defense including mobilization of neutrophils, macrophages, lymphocytes, and plasma cells. Chronic inflammation caused by the plaque leads to destruction of the periodontal tissues because the body has no means to remove the tooth-borne biofilms.

Dental plaques cannot be easily washed away by vigorous rinsing or water sprays. They also resist disruption by antimicrobial agents that cannot easily penetrate the protective polysaccharide matrix barrier characteristic of biofilms. Therefore, removal of dental plaque requires mechanical intervention such as toothbrushing and flossing. Once plaque becomes mineralized and takes on the form of dental calculus, its removal requires professional interventions such as scaling, root planing, and polishing.

REFERENCES

1. Van Houte J: Role of micro-organisms in caries etiology, *J Dent Res* 73:672-681, 1994.
2. Stenudd C, Nordlund Å, Ryberg M, et al: The association of bacterial adhesion with dental caries, *J Dent Res* 80:2005-2010, 2001.
3. Socransky SS, Haffajee AD, Cugini MA, et al: Microbial complexes in subgingival plaque, *J Clin Periodontol* 25:134-144, 1998.
4. Haffajee AD, Socransky SS: Microbial etiological agents of destructive periodontal disease, *Periodontol 2000* 5:78-111, 1994.
5. Costerton JW, Lewandowski Z: The biofilm lifestyle, *Adv Dent Res* 11:192-195, 1997.
6. Costerton JW, Stewart PS, Greenberg EP: Bacterial biofilms: a common cause of persistent infections, *Science* 284:1318-1322, 1999.
7. Carlsson J: A levansucrase from *Streptococcus mutans*, *Caries Res* 4:97-113, 1970.
8. Sutherland IW: Biosynthesis and composition of gram-negative bacterial extracellular and wall polysaccharides, *Annu Rev Microbiol* 39:243-270, 1985.
9. Carpentier B, Cerf O: Biofilms and their consequences, with particular reference to hygiene in the food industry, *J Appl Bacteriol* 75:499-511, 1993.
10. Socransky SS, Haffajee AD: Dental biofilms: difficult therapeutic targets, *Periodontol 2000* 28:12-55, 2002.
11. Brown MRW, Gilbert P: Sensitivity of biofilms to antimicrobial agents, *J Appl Bacteriol* 74(Suppl):87S-97S, 1993.
12. Xu KD, McFeters GA, Stewart PS: Biofilm resistance to antimicrobial agents, *Microbiology* 146:547-549, 2000.
13. Stoodley P, Dodds I, Boyle JD, et al: Influence of hydrodynamics and nutrients on biofilm structure, *J Appl Microbiol* 85(Suppl):19S-28S, 1999.
14. Costerton JW, Lewandowski Z, DeBeer D, et al: Biofilms, the customized microniche, *J Bacteriol* 176:2137-2142, 1994.
15. Wood SR, Kirkham J, Marsh PD, et al: Architecture of intact human plaque biofilms studied by confocal laser scanning microscopy, *J Dent Res* 79:21-27, 2000.
16. Wimpenny JWT: A unifying hypothesis for the structure of microbial films based on cellular automation models, *FEMS Microbiol Ecol* 22:1-16, 1997.
17. Costerton JW: The etiology and persistence of cryptic bacterial infections: a hypothesis, *Rev Infect Dis* 6(Suppl 3):S608-S616, 1984.
18. Rittman DE: Detachment from biofilms. In Characklis WG, Wilderer PA, editors, *Structure and function of biofilms*, Chichester, 1989, John Wiley & Sons.
19. Bowden GHW, Li YH: Nutritional influences on biofilm development, *Adv Dent Res* 11:81-99, 1997.
20. Miller MB, Bassler BL: Quorum sensing in bacteria, *Annu Rev Microbiol* 55:165-199, 2001.
21. De Jong HP, De Boer P, Busscher HJ, et al: Surface free energy changes of human enamel during pellicle formation: an *in vivo* study, *Caries Res* 18:408-415, 1984.
22. Quirynen M, Marechal M, Busscher HJ, et al: The influence of surface free-energy on planimetric plaque growth in man, *J Dent Res* 68:796-799, 1989.
23. Gibbons RJ: Microbial ecology. Adherent interactions which may affect microbial ecology in the mouth, *J Dent Res* 63:378-385, 1984.
24. Malamud D: Influence of salivary proteins on the fate of oral bacteria. In Mergenhagen SE, Rosan B, editors: *Molecular basis of oral microbial adhesion*, Washington, DC, 1985, American Society for Microbiology.
25. Terpenning M, Bretz W, Lopatin D, et al: Bacterial colonization of saliva and plaque in the elderly, *Clin Infect Dis* 16(Suppl 4):S314-S316, 1993.
26. Whittaker CJ, Klier CM, Kolenbrander PE: Mechanisms of adhesion by oral bacteria, *Annu Rev Microbiol* 50:513-552, 1996.

27. Levine MJ, Reddy MS, Tabak LA, et al: Structural aspects of salivary glycoproteins, *J Dent Res* 66:436-441, 1987.

28. Tabak LA, Levine MJ, Mandel ID, et al: Role of salivary mucins in the protection of the oral cavity, *J Oral Pathol* 11:1-17, 1982.

29. Scannapieco FA: Saliva-bacterium interactions in oral microbial ecology, *Crit Rev Oral Biol Med* 5:203-248, 1994.

30. Schenkels LCPM, Veerman ECI, Nieuw Amerongen AV: Biochemical composition of human saliva in relation to other mucosal fluids, *Crit Rev Oral Biol Med* 6:161-175, 1995.

31. Scannapieco FA, Levine MJ: Salivary mucins and dental plaque formation. In Bowen WH, Tabak LA, editors, *Cariology for the nineties*, Rochester, NY, 1993, University of Rochester.

32. Iontcheva I, Oppenheim FG, Troxler RF: Human salivary mucin MG1 selectively forms heterotropic complexes with amylase, proline-rich proteins, statherin, and histatin, *J Dent Res* 76:734-743, 1997.

33. Iontcheva I, Oppenheim FG, Offner GD, et al: Molecular mapping of statherin- and histatin-binding domains in human salivary MG1 (MUC5B) by the yeast two-hybrid system, *J Dent Res* 79:732-739, 2000.

34. Biesbrock AR, Reddy MS, Levine MJ: Interaction of salivary mucin-secretory IgA complex with mucosal pathogens, *Infect Immun* 59:3492-3497, 1991.

35. Murray PA, Prakobphol A, Lee T, et al: Adherence of oral streptococci to salivary glycoproteins, *Infect Immun* 60:31-38, 1992.

36. Ligtenberg AJM, Walgreen-Weterings E, Veerman ECI, et al: Influence of saliva on aggregation and adherence of *Streptococcus gordonii* HG 222, *Infect Immun* 60:3878-3884, 1992.

37. Groenink J, Ligtenberg AJM, Veerman ECI, et al: Interaction of the salivary low-molecular-weight mucin (MG2) with *Actinobacillus actinomycetemcomitans, Antonie van Leeuwenhoek* 70:79-87, 1996.

38. Hoffman MP, Haidaris CG: Analysis of *Candida albicans* adhesion to salivary mucins. *Infect Immun* 61:1940-1949, 1993.

39. Cohen RE, Levine MJ: Salivary glycoproteins. In Tenovuo JO, editor: *Human saliva: clinical chemistry and microbiology*, Boca Raton, Fla, 1989, CRC Press.

40. Leach SA: A review of the biochemistry of dental plaque. In McHugh WD, editor: *Dental plaque*, Dundee, 1970, E & S Livingstone, Ltd.

41. Gibbons RJ, Hay DI, Childs WC, et al: Role of cryptic receptors (cryptitopes) in bacterial adhesion to oral surfaces, *Arch Oral Biol* 35(Suppl):107S-114S, 1990.

42. Kolenbrander PE, London J: Ecological significance of coaggregation among oral bacteria, *Adv Microb Ecol* 12:183-217, 1992.

43. Bennick A: Salivary proline-rich proteins, *Mol Cell Biochem* 45:83-99, 1982.

44. Sabatini LM, Warner TF, Saitoh E, et al: Tissue distribution of RNAs for cystatins, histatins, statherin, and proline-rich salivary proteins in humans and macaques, *J Dent Res* 68:1138-1145, 1989.

45. Bennick A, Chau G, Goodlin R, et al: The role of human salivary proline-rich proteins in the formation of acquired dental pellicle *in vivo* and their fate after adsorption to the human enamel surface, *Arch Oral Biol* 28:19-27, 1983.

46. Saitoh E, Isemura S, Sanada K: Inhibition of calcium-carbonate precipitation by human salivary proline-rich phosphoproteins, *Arch Oral Biol* 30:641-643, 1985.

47. Yao Y, Lamkin MS, Oppenheim FG: Pellicle precursor protein crosslinking: characterization of an adduct between acidic proline-rich protein (PRP-1) and statherin generated by transglutaminase, *J Dent Res* 79:930-938, 2000.

48. Gibbons RJ, Hay DI: Human salivary acidic proline-rich proteins and statherin promote the attachment of *Actinomyces viscosus* LY7 to apatitic surfaces, *Infect Immun* 56:439-445, 1988.

49. Amano A, Sojar HT, Lee J-Y, et al: Salivary receptors for recombinant fimbrillin of *Porphyromonas gingivalis, Infect Immun* 62:3372-3380, 1994.

50. Hay DI, Smith DJ, Schluckebier SK, et al: Relationship between concentration of human salivary statherin and inhibition of calcium phosphate precipitation in stimulated human parotid saliva, *J Dent Res* 63:857-863, 1984.

51. Jensen JL, Lamkin MS, Troxler RF, et al: Multiple forms of statherin in human salivary secretions, *Arch Oral Biol* 36:529-534, 1991.

52. Tsai H, Bobek LA: Human salivary histatins: promising anti-fungal therapeutic agents, *Crit Rev Oral Biol Med* 9:480-497, 1998.

53. Nikawa H, Jin C, Fukushima H, et al: Antifungal activity of histatin-5 against non-*albicans Candida* species, *Oral Microbiol Immunol* 16:250-252, 2001.

54. Oppenheim FG, Xu T, McMillian FM, et al: Histatins, a novel family of histidine-rich proteins in human parotid secretion. Isolation, characterization, primary structure, and fungistatic effects on *Candida albicans, J Biol Chem* 263:7472-7477, 1988.

55. Xu T, Levitz SM, Diamond RD, et al: Anticandidal activity of major salivary histatins, *Infect Immun* 59:2549-2554, 1991.

56. Jainkittivong A, Johnson DA, Yeh C-K: The relationship between salivary histatin levels and oral yeast carriage, *Oral Microbiol Immunol* 13:181-187, 1998.

57. Xu T, Lal K, Pollock JJ: Histatins 2 and 4 are autoproteolytic degradation products of human parotid saliva, *Oral Microbiol Immunol* 7:127-128, 1992.

58. McKay BJ, Denepitiya L, Iacono VJ, et al: Growth-inhibitory and bactericidal effects of human parotid salivary histidine-rich polypeptides on *Streptococcus mutans, Infect Immun* 44:695-701, 1984.

59. Payne JB, Iacono VJ, Crawford IT, et al: Selective effects of histidine-rich polypeptides on the aggregation and viability of *Streptococcus mutans* and *Streptococcus sanguis*, *Oral Microbiol Immunol* 6:169-176, 1991.

60. Murakami Y, Nagata H, Amano A, et al: Inhibitory effects of human salivary histatins and lysozyme on coaggregation between *Porphyromonas gingivalis* and *Streptococcus mitis*, *Infect Immun* 59:3284-3286, 1991.

61. Murakami Y, Shizukuishi S, Tsunemitsu A, et al: Binding of a histidine-rich peptide to *Porphyromonas gingivalis*, *FEMS Microbiol Lett* 82:253-256, 1991.

62. Imatani T, Kato T, Minaguchi K, et al: Histatin 5 inhibits inflammatory cytokine induction from human gingival fibroblasts by *Porphyromonas gingivalis*, *Oral Microbiol Immunol* 15:378-382, 2000.

63. Helmerhorst EJ, Hodgson R, van't Hof W, et al: The effects of histatin-derived basic antimicrobial peptides on oral biofilms, *J Dent Res* 78:1245-1250, 1999.

64. Henskens YMC, Van der Velden U, Veerman ECI, et al: Protein, albumin and cystatins concentrations in saliva of healthy subjects and of patients with gingivitis and periodontitis, *J Periodont Res* 28:43-48, 1993.

65. Henskens YMC, Veerman ECI, Mantel MS, et al: Cystatins S and C in human whole saliva and in glandular salivas in periodontal health and disease, *J Dent Res* 73:1606-1614, 1994.

66. Henskens YMC, Van den Keijbus PAM, Veerman ECI, et al: Protein composition of whole and parotid saliva in healthy and periodontitis subjects. Determination of cystatins, albumin, amylase and IgA, *J Periodont Res* 31:57-65, 1996.

67. Baron AC, Barrett-Vespone NA, Featherstone JDB: Purification of large quantities of human salivary cystatins S, SA and SN: their interactions with the model cysteine protease papain in a non-inhibitory mode, *Oral Dis* 5:344-353, 1999.

68. Baron AC, Gansky SA, Ryder MI, et al: Cysteine protease inhibitory activity and levels in whole saliva of periodontally diseased patients, *J Periodont Res* 34:437-444, 1999.

69. Al-Hashimi I, Levine MJ: Characterization of in vivo salivary-derived enamel pellicle, *Arch Oral Biol* 34:289-295, 1989.

70. Johnsson M, Richardson CF, Bergey EJ, et al: The effects of human salivary cystatins and statherin on hydroxyapatite crystallization, *Arch Oral Biol* 36:631-636, 1991.

71. Baron AC, DeCarlo AA, Featherstone JDB: Functional aspects of the human salivary cystatins in the oral environment, *Oral Dis* 5:234-240, 1999.

72. Katsukawa H, Ninomiya Y: Capsaicin induces cystatins S-like substances in submandibular saliva of the rat, *J Dent Res* 78:1609-1616, 1999.

73. Henskens YMC, Strooker H, Van den Keijbus PAM, et al: Salivary protein composition in epileptic patients on different medications, *J Oral Pathol Med* 25:360-366, 1996.

74. Boackle RJ, Dutton SL, Fei H, et al: Salivary non-immunoglobulin agglutinin inhibits human leukocyte elastase digestion of acidic proline-rich salivary proteins, *J Dent Res* 80:1550-1554, 2001.

75. Almståhl A, Wikström M, Groenink L: Lactoferrin, amylase and mucin MUC5B and their relation to the oral microflora in hyposalivation of different origins, *Oral Microbiol Immunol* 16:345-352, 2001.

76. Yeh C-K, Dodds MWJ, Zuo P, et al: A population-based study of salivary lysozyme concentrations and candidal counts, *Arch Oral Biol* 42:25-31, 1997.

77. Rice AR, Hamilton MA, Camper AK: Apparent surface associated lag time in growth of primary biofilm cells, *Microb Ecol* 40:8-15, 2000.

78. Sauer K, Camper AK: Characterization of phenotypic changes in *Pseudomonas putida* in response to surface-associated growth, *J Bacteriol* 183:6579-6589, 2001.

79. Costerton JW, Cheng K-J, Geesey GG, et al: Bacterial biofilms in nature and disease, *Annu Rev Microbiol* 41:435-464, 1987.

80. Kolenbrander PE, Anderson RN, Moore LVH: Coaggregation of *Fusobacterium nucleatum*, *Selenomonas flueggei*, *Selenomonas infelix*, *Selenomonas noxia*, and *Selenomonas sputigena* with strains from 11 genera of oral bacteria, *Infect Immun* 57:3194-3203, 1989.

81. Kinder SA, Holt SC: Characterization of coaggregation between *Bacteroides gingivalis* T22 and *Fusobacterium nucleatum* T18, *Infect Immun* 57:3425-3433, 1989.

82. Kolenbrander PE, Parrish KD, Andersen RN, et al: Intergeneric coaggregation of oral *Treponema* spp. with *Fusobacterium* spp. and intrageneric coaggregation among *Fusobacterium* spp., *Infect Immun* 63:4584-4588, 1995.

83. Bradshaw DJ, Marsh PD, Watson GK, et al: Role of *Fusobacterium nucleatum* and coaggregation in anaerobe survival in planktonic and biofilm oral microbial communities during aeration, *Infect Immun* 66:4729-4732, 1998.

84. Kolenbrander PE, Williams BL: Lactose-reversible coaggregation between oral actinomyces and *Streptococcus sanguis*, *Infect Immun* 33:95-102, 1981.

85. Jenkinson HF, Lamont RJ: Streptococcal adhesion and colonization, *Crit Rev Oral Biol Med* 8:175-200, 1997.

86. Lamont RJ, Hersey SG, Rosan B: Characterization of the adherence of *Porphyromonas gingivalis* to oral streptococci, *Oral Microbiol Immunol* 7:193-197, 1992.

87. Lamont RJ, Bevan CA, Gil S, et al: Involvement of *Porphyromonas gingivalis* fimbriae in adherence to *Streptococcus gordonii*, *Oral Microbiol Immunol* 8:272-276, 1993.

88. Lamont RJ, Demuth DR, Davis CA, et al: Salivary-agglutinin-mediated adherence of *Streptococcus mutans* to early plaque bacteria, *Infect Immun* 59:3446-3450, 1991.

89. Moore WEC, Moore LVH: The bacteria of periodontal diseases, *Periodontol 2000* 5:66-77, 1994.

90. Goulbourne PA, Ellen RP: Evidence that *Porphyromonas (Bacteroides) gingivalis* fimbriae function in adhesion to *Actinomyces viscosus, J Bacteriol* 173:5266-5274, 1991.

91. Yao EX, Lamont RJ, Leu SP, et al: Interbacterial binding among strains of pathogenic and commensal oral bacterial species, *Oral Microbiol Immunol* 11:35-41, 1996.

92. Wimpenny JWT, Coombs JP: Penetration of oxygen into bacterial colonies, *J Gen Microbiol* 129:1239-1242, 1983.

93. Roberts AP, Pratten J, Wilson M, et al: Transfer of a conjugative transposon, Tn5397 in a model oral biofilm, *FEMS Microbiol Lett* 177:63-66, 1999.

94. Listgarten MA, Mayo HE, Tremblay R: Development of dental plaque on epoxy resin crowns in man. A light and electron microscopic study, *J Periodontol* 46:10-26, 1975.

95. Listgarten MA: Structure of the microbial flora associated with periodontal health and disease in man. A light and electron microscopic study, *J Periodontol* 47:1-18, 1976.

96. Westergaard J, Frandsen A, Slots J: Ultrastructure of the subgingival microflora in juvenile periodontitis, *Scand J Dent Res* 86:421-429, 1978.

97. Salkind A, Oshrain HI, Mandel ID: Bacterial aspects of developing supragingival and subgingival plaque, *J Periodontol* 42:706-708, 1971.

98. Bickel M, Cimasoni G: The pH of human crevicular fluid measured by a new microanalytical technique, *J Periodont Res* 20:35-40, 1985.

99. Kenney EB, Ash MM Jr: Oxidation reduction potential of developing plaque, periodontal pockets and gingival sulci, *J Periodontol* 40:630-633, 1969.

100. Baboolal R, Mlinek A, Powell RN: A study of the effects of gingival plaque extracts on cells cultured in vitro, *J Periodont Res* 5:248-254, 1970.

101. Larjava H: Effect of human dental bacterial plaque extract on the connective tissue of *in-vitro* cultured fetal rat calvaria, *Arch Oral Biol* 28:371-374, 1983.

102. Hasty DL, Ofek I, Courtney HS, et al: Multiple adhesins of streptococci, *Infect Immun* 60:2147-2152, 1992.

103. Jenkinson HF: Cell surface protein receptors in oral streptococci, *FEMS Microbiol Lett* 121:133-140, 1994.

104. Dawson JR, Ellen RP: Tip-oriented adherence of *Treponema denticola* to fibronectin, *Infect Immun* 58:3924-3928, 1990.

105. Hamada S, Amano A, Kimura S, et al: The importance of fimbriae in the virulence and ecology of some oral bacteria, *Oral Microbiol Immunol* 13:129-138, 1998.

106. Lamont RJ, Chan A, Belton CM, et al: *Porphyromonas gingivalis* invasion of gingival epithelial cells, *Infect Immun* 63:3878-3885, 1995.

107. Madianos PN, Papapanou PN, Nannmark U, et al: *Porphyromonas gingivalis* FDC381 multiplies and persists within human oral epithelial cells in vitro, *Infect Immun* 64:660-664, 1996.

108. Meyer DH, Lippmann JE, Fives-Taylor PM: Invasion of epithelial cells by *Actinobacillus actinomycetemcomitans*: a dynamic, multistep process, *Infect Immun* 64:2988-2997, 1996.

109. Rudney JD, Chen R, Sedgewick GJ: Intracellular *Actinobacillus actinomycetemcomitans* and *Porphyromonas gingivalis* in buccal epithelial cells collected from human subjects, *Infect Immun* 69:2700-2707, 2001.

110. Dzink JL, Gibbons RJ, Childs WC, et al: The predominant cultivable microbiota of crevicular epithelial cells, *Oral Microbiol Immunol* 4:1-5, 1989.

111. Saglie R, Newman MG, Carranza FA Jr, et al: Bacterial invasion of gingiva in advanced periodontitis in humans, *J Periodontol* 53:217-222, 1982.

112. Naito Y, Gibbons RJ: Attachment of *Bacteroides gingivalis* to collagenous substrata, *J Dent Res* 67:1075-1080, 1988.

113. Listgarten MA: Electron microscopic observations on the bacterial flora of acute necrotizing ulcerative gingivitis, *J Periodontol* 36:328-339, 1965.

114. Listgarten MA: Pathogenesis of periodontitis, *J Clin Periodontol* 13:418-425, 1986.

115. Listgarten MA, Levin S: Positive correlation between the proportions of subgingival spirochetes and motile bacteria and susceptibility of human subjects to periodontal deterioration, *J Clin Periodontol* 8:122-138, 1981.

116. Armitage GC, Dickinson WR, Jenderseck RS, et al: Relationship between the percentage of subgingival spirochetes and the severity of periodontal disease, *J Periodontol* 53:550-556, 1982.

117. Simonson LG, Goodman CH, Bial JJ, et al: Quantiative relationship of *Treponema denticola* to severity of periodontal disease, *Infect Immun* 56:726-728, 1988.

118. Dewhirst FE, Tamer MA, Ericson RE, et al: The diversity of periodontal spirochetes by 16S rRNA analysis, *Oral Microbiol Immunol* 15:196-202, 2000.

119. Weinberg A, Krisanaprakornkit S, Dale DA: Epithelial antimicrobial peptides: review and significance for oral application, *Crit Rev Oral Biol Med* 9:399-414, 1998.

120. Krisanaprakornkit S, Weinberg A, Perez CN, et al: Expression of the peptide antibiotic human β-defensin 1 in cultured gingival epithelial cells and gingival tissue, *Infect Immun* 66:4222-4228, 1998.

121. Mandel ID, Gaffar A: Calculus revisited. A review, *J Clin Periodontol* 13:249-257, 1986.

122. Löe H, Theilade E, Jensen SB: Experimental gingivitis in man, *J Periodontol* 36:177-187, 1965.

123. Theilade E, Wright WH, Jensen SB, et al: Experimental gingivitis in man. II. Longitudinal clinical and bacteriological investigation, *J Periodont Res* 1:1-13, 1966.

124. Löe H, Theilade E, Jensen SB, et al: Experimental gingivitis in man. III. The influence of antibiotics on gingival plaque development, *J Periodont Res* 2:282-289, 1967.

125. Jensen SB, Löe H, Schiött CR, et al: Experimental gingivitis in man. IV. Vancomycin induced changes in bacterial plaque composition as related to the development of gingival inflammation, *J Periodont Res* 3:284-293, 1968.

126. Allen DL, Kerr DA: Tissue response in the guinea pig to sterile and non-sterile calculus, *J Periodontol* 36:121-126, 1965.

127. Sidaway DA: A microbiological study of dental calculus. II. The in vitro calcification of microorganisms from dental calculus, *J Periodont Res* 13:360-366, 1978.

128. Glas J-E, Krasse B: Biophysical studies on dental calculus from germfree and conventional rats, *Acta Odontol Scand* 20:127-134, 1962.

129. Gustafsson B, Krasse B: Dental calculus in germfree rats, *Acta Odontol Scand* 20:135-142, 1962.

130. Kakehashi S, Baer PN, White C: Studies on experimental calculus formation in the rat. VII. Effect of selective desalivation of the major salivary glands, *J Periodontol* 35:467-469, 1964.

131. Schroeder HE: *Formation and inhibition of dental calculus*, Berne, 1969, Hans Huber Publishers.

132. Draus FJ, Tarbet WJ, Miklos FL: Salivary enzymes and calculus formation, *J Periodont Res* 3:232-235, 1968.

133. Ennever J, Vogel JJ, Boyan-Salyers B, et al: Characterization of calculus matrix calcification nucleator, *J Dent Res* 58:619-623, 1979.

134. Mandel ID: Histochemical and biochemical aspects of calculus formation, *Periodontics* 1:43-52, 1963.

135. Mukherjee S: Formation and prevention of supra-gingival calculus, *J Periodont Res* 3(Suppl 2):1-35, 1968.

136. Driessens FCM, Borggreven JMPM, Verbeeck RMH, et al: On the physicochemistry of plaque calcification and the phase composition of dental calculus, *J Periodont Res* 20:329-336, 1985.

137. Boyan-Salyers BD, Vogel JJ, Ennever J: Pre-apatitic mineral deposition in *Bacterionema matruchotii*, *J Dent Res* 57:291-295, 1978.

138. Forsberg A, Lagergren C, Lönnerblad T: Dental calculus. A biophysical study, *Oral Surg Oral Med Oral Pathol* 13:1050-1060, 1960.

139. Leung SW, Jensen AT: Factors controlling the deposition of calculus, *Int Dent J* 8:613-626, 1958.

140. Selvig KA: Attachment of plaque and calculus to tooth surfaces, *J Periodont Res* 5:8-18, 1970.

141. Zander HA: The attachment of calculus to root surfaces, *J Periodontol* 24:16-19, 1953.

142. Moskow BS: Calculus attachment in cemental separations, *J Periodontol* 40:125-130, 1969.

143. Kopczyk RA, Conroy CW: The attachment of calculus to root planed surfaces, *Periodontics* 6:78-83, 1968.

144. Listgarten MA, Ellegaard B: Electron microscopic evidence of a cellular attachment between junctional epithelium and dental calculus, *J Periodont Res* 8:143-150, 1973.

145. Lindhe J, Wicén P-O: The effects on the gingivae of chewing fibrous foods, *J Periodont Res* 4:193-201, 1969.

146. Drisko CL, White CL, Killoy WJ, et al: Comparison of dark-field microscopy and a flagella stain for monitoring the effect of a Water-Pik® on bacterial motility, *J Periodontol* 58:381-386, 1987.

147. Newman MG, Cattabriga M, Etienne D, et al: Effectiveness of adjunctive irrigation in early periodontitis: multicenter evaluation, *J Periodontol* 65:224-229, 1994.

148. Cutler CW, Stanford TW, Abraham C, et al: Clinical benefits of oral irrigation for periodontitis are related to reduction of pro-inflammatory cytokine levels and plaque, *J Clin Periodontol* 27:134-141, 2000.

149. Bibel DJ: The discovery of the oral flora—a 300-year retrospective, *J Am Dent Assoc* 107:569-570, 1983.

150. Slavkin HC: Biofilms, microbial ecology and Antoni van Leeuwenhoek, *J Am Dent Assoc* 128:492-495, 1997.

151. Hoyle BD, Costerton JW: Bacterial resistance to antibiotics: the role of biofilms, *Prog Drug Res* 37:91-105, 1991.

152. Nichols WW: Susceptibility of biofilms to toxic compounds. In Characklis WG, Wilderer PA, editors, *Structure and function of biofilms*, Chichester, 1989, John Wiley & Sons.

153. Anwar H, Strap JL, Costerton JW: Eradication of biofilm cells of *Staphylococcus aureus* with tobramycin and cephalexin, *Can J Microbiol* 38:618-625, 1992.

154. Genco R, Kornman K, Williams R, et al: Consensus report. Periodontal diseases: pathogenesis and microbial factors, *Ann Periodontol* 1:926-932, 1996.

7

Local Contributing Factors

Henry Greenwell, Gary C. Armitage, and Brian L. Mealey

ANATOMIC CONTRIBUTING FACTORS
Proximal Contact Relation
Cervical Enamel Projections and Enamel Pearls
Intermediate Bifurcation Ridge
Root Anatomy
Cemental Tears
Accessory Canals
Root Proximity
Adjacent Teeth

RESTORATIVE CONTRIBUTING FACTORS
Overhanging Restorations
Margin Location
Crown Contours
Pontic Form
Restorative Materials

ORTHODONTIC CONTRIBUTING FACTORS
Crowding, Malalignment, and Malocclusion

HABITS AS CONTRIBUTING FACTORS
Toothbrush and Floss Trauma
Mouth Breathing and Tongue Thrust
Factitial Injuries

This chapter focuses on local factors that contribute to periodontal diseases but are not themselves etiologic factors. These factors tend to accelerate the progression of disease, often in a localized area, and sometimes in a dentition minimally affected by periodontitis. For the clinician, the most important step is to recognize the presence of a contributing factor and to understand its effect on diagnosis, prognosis, and treatment. For example, the presence of a contributing factor that is difficult or impossible to modify may cause the prognosis of a tooth to be downgraded or may change the treatment recommendation from periodontal surgery to extraction. If a contributing factor goes unrecognized, then crown and bridge therapy might be unwisely recommended for a tooth with a very questionable prognosis. Conversely, the presence of a readily modifiable contributing factor may improve the prognosis of the tooth, because elimination of the contributing factor would be expected to be associated with improved periodontal status. To provide the best possible treatment for patients, it is important that all factors affecting the outcome of treatment be recognized and appropriately considered in formulating a treatment plan. The contributing factors discussed later are not a complete listing, but do encompass those the clinician may routinely encounter in a complete examination of the periodontium.

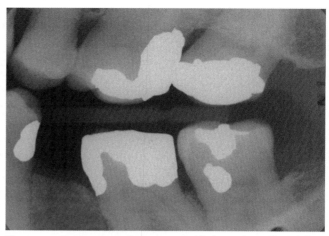

Figure 7-1. Open contact between mandibular molars allowed food impaction. This situation may increase the risk for bone loss and attachment loss. (*Courtesy of Dr. David Adams, University of Louisville, Louisville, Ky.*)

ANATOMIC CONTRIBUTING FACTORS

Proximal Contact Relation

Open interproximal contacts or uneven marginal ridge relations are factors that may predispose to food impaction. Food impaction is defined as the forceful wedging of food into the interproximal space by occlusal forces.[1] It can lead to inflammation, bone loss, and attachment loss (Fig. 7-1). Research has shown that not every open contact or uneven marginal ridge leads to food impaction.[2,3] Interproximal areas with wide open contacts that are easily cleansable may be as healthy as those with a proper contact relation. Loose contacts, in contrast, are most likely to result in food impaction.[3] Food impaction can be prevented by establishing proper contact and marginal ridge relations when interproximal areas require a restoration. If open contacts and uneven marginal ridges are widespread in the mouth, orthodontic therapy may be considered.

In patients affected by periodontal destruction and recession, the interproximal embrasure is often open and prone to collect food particles. Pressure from the tongue and facial soft tissues direct food into these spaces, resulting in what has come to be known as lateral food impaction. Rather than forceful wedging, this is often interproximal food collection. Because the food is loosely collected, and not impacted, it is easily removed. To pre-

vent increased inflammation and periodontal destruction patients should be trained to use interproximal cleaning devices, such as brushes, wedges, or toothpicks, that will eliminate food collected during mastication.

Cervical Enamel Projections and Enamel Pearls

Cervical enamel projections (CEPs) occur primarily on molars where amelogenesis has failed to halt before root formation. They appear as narrow wedge-shaped extensions of enamel pointing from the cementoenamel junction (CEJ) toward the furcation area.[4-11] These projections occur most frequently on mandibular molars, approximately 30% of the time, and are found on maxillary molars with about half that frequency.[4,5,9] They are much more likely to occur on second than on first molars and on buccal rather than lingual, mesial, or distal surfaces. CEPs have been classified into three grades (Fig. 7-2)[4]:

Grade 1: A distinct change in the CEJ pointing toward the furcation.

Grade 2: The CEP approaches, but does not enter, the furcation.

Grade 3: The CEP extends into the furcation.

The clinical significance of CEPs is that they are plaque retentive and can predispose to furcation involvement. Research has shown that 90% of isolated furcation involvements are associated with CEPs.[4] This means that a lone furcation involvement in a patient who otherwise has minimal periodontal destruction should prompt the clinician to examine for the presence of a CEP.

Treatment of CEPs is generally directed by the periodontal treatment required for the affected tooth. If no bone or attachment loss is associated with a CEP, which is often the case for Grade 1 and sometimes Grade 2

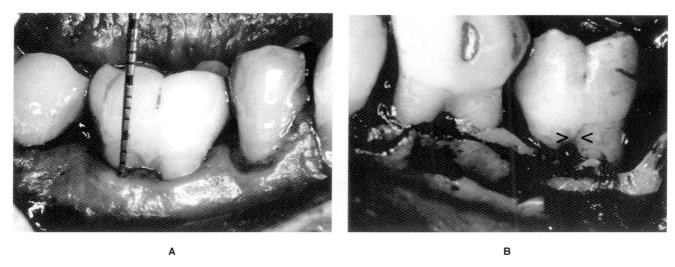

A   B

Figure 7-2. A, Grade 2 cervical enamel projection on tooth #30. Enamel projection approaches but does not enter the furcation. **B,** Grade 3 cervical enamel projection on tooth #18. Enamel projection extends into the furcation proper and is a contributing factor to attachment loss and bone loss in the furcation region.

CEPs, there is usually no treatment required for the CEP. If bone loss and attachment loss are present in the furcation with a CEP, the CEP may need to be removed. This is particularly true if regenerative periodontal surgery is planned, because new connective tissue attachment will not form on enamel. In cases in which the enamel is thin, the CEP can be removed with a diamond bur or finishing bur. When the enamel is thicker, complete removal with a bur may be attempted, but the clinician must take care not to expose the pulp. If the CEP is removed on a vital tooth, the patient should be warned of possible thermal sensitivity, especially if the affected root surface will be in a supragingival location after therapy.

Enamel pearls are most common in the furcation region, particularly on third molars (Fig. 7-3). They range in size from very small to quite large. When small, they may be removed as a part of periodontal therapy. However, larger enamel pearls have underlying dentin and even possible pulpal extensions and should be removed cautiously.

Intermediate Bifurcation Ridge

The intermediate bifurcation ridge is a convex excrescence of cementum that runs longitudinally between the mesial and distal roots of a mandibular molar.[11-13] It may be located at the midpoint between the buccal and lingual surfaces of the area of root division or it may be located in

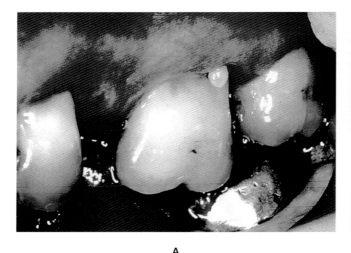

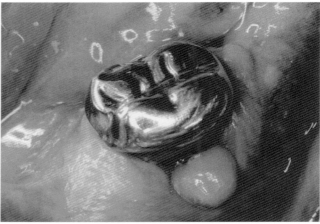

A   B

Figure 7-3. A, Small enamel pearl visible at gingival margin on tooth #14. **B,** Large enamel pearl on the lingual aspect of tooth #31.

a more lateral position. These ridges are found more frequently on first molars. The significance of this formation is the irregular contours it creates that make plaque and calculus removal more difficult. Inadequate plaque and calculus removal can lead to failure of furcation treatment, especially regenerative therapy.

Root Anatomy

Palatogingival groove

The palatogingival groove, frequently termed the *palatoradicular groove*, often begins at the cingulum and extends apically for a variable distance (Figs. 7-4 and 7-5).[14-16] When the groove extends onto the root, which occurs about 50% of the time, pocketing and attachment loss may occur.[16] These grooves are found on up to 6% of maxillary lateral incisors and up to 3% of central incisors, although some have reported a less frequent occurrence.[16-18] They are most commonly found in the midroot area but may extend to the distal or mesial area. The groove may be shallow or may be seen as a deep invagination of the root surface. Pocketing of maxillary incisors, especially isolated, deep pocketing, should prompt an examination for this plaque-retentive root anomaly. If the palatogingival groove is associated with bone loss and attachment loss, the clinician may attempt to remove the groove through odontoplasty or to reduce its depth to minimize plaque retention.

Attachment area

The amount of root available for periodontal attachment has been termed the *attachment area*.[19-23] For maxillary first molars, the root trunk contributes 32% of the attachment area, whereas the mesial, distal, and palatal roots contribute 25%, 19%, and 24%, respectively.[21] For mandibular first molars, the root trunk contributes 31% of the attachment area, whereas the mesial and distal roots contribute 37% and 32%, respectively.[22] Studies of attachment area point out that when the tooth has 50% bone loss there is considerably greater than 50% loss of attachment area.[19,23] This phenomenon is easily conceptualized if the root is thought of as an inverted pyramid. Although this is an exaggerated example, it clearly points out that the greatest attachment area is found at the pyramid base, analogous to the root trunk, and that the least attachment area is at the pyramid apex, which is analogous to the root apex. Thus there is substantially more attachment area in the coronal half of the root than in the apical half. These numbers are particularly useful when evaluating teeth for root resection procedures; however, it must be remembered that these are mean values and should only be used as a guideline during clinical evaluation. If a tooth has a blunted or shortened root or roots, the attachment area is decreased. This may contribute to the presence of mobility when bone loss occurs. A tooth with 5 mm of bone loss measured from the CEJ, having a total root length of 10 mm, may have greater mobility than a tooth with a root length of 15 mm having a similar degree of bone loss.

Root trunk length

The root trunk is the portion of the root between the CEJ and the point of root division.[24-26] It contributes about 30% of the attachment of molar roots, whereas the individual roots make up the remaining 70%.[26] Teeth with short root trunks are more likely to have a furcation involvement when only minimal attachment loss has occurred. In this sense, a longer root trunk length is a favorable anatomic feature. However, once periodontal destruction has resulted in furcation involvement, the presence of a long root trunk may complicate therapy. Teeth with long root trunks are not good candidates for root resection because there is a reduced amount of attachment area apical to root division. Root resection is also more technically difficult on molars with long root trunks. Often root grooves are found on the root trunk and occur about 50% to 60% of the time for first molars and more than 90% of the time for second molars.[26] These grooves favor plaque accumulation and can predispose to furcation involvement.

Interroot separation

The amount of root separation is usually greater for first molars than for second molars.[27] Mean buccal and lingual root separation is from 2 to 3 mm, whereas mesial and distal roots are separated by 4 to 4.5 mm. Wide separation, seen in maxillary mesial and distal furcations, is less responsive to regeneration of furcation bone than the smaller dimension associated with buccal or lingual

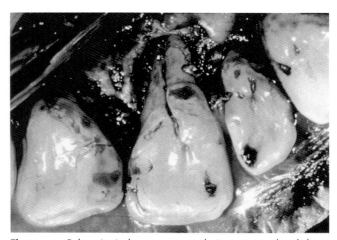

Figure 7-4. Palatogingival groove on tooth #9 associated with bone loss and attachment loss.

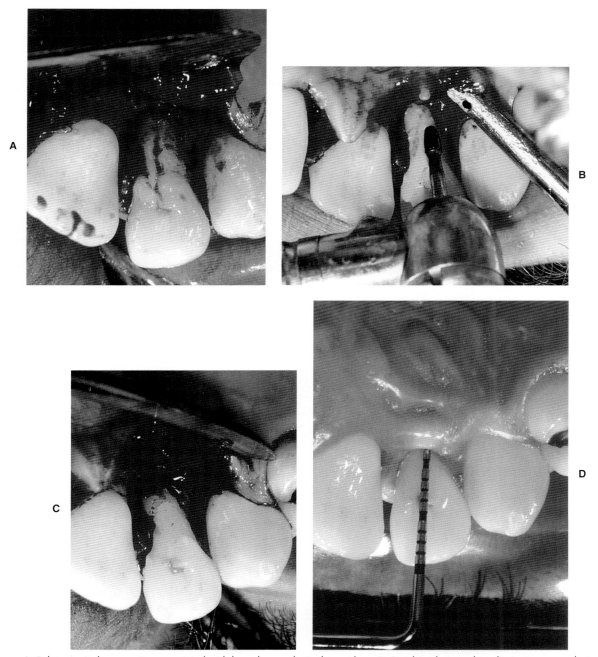

Figure 7-5. **A,** Palatogingival groove #10 associated with bone loss and attachment loss. **B,** Finishing bur used to eliminate groove during surgery. **C,** Palatogingival groove eliminated, with elimination of niche for plaque formation. **D,** A 4-month postoperative probing shows only 3 mm probing depth, with significant attachment gain.

furcations. However, there is a clinical impression that minimal root separation may lead to more rapid bone loss and may also be more difficult to regenerate. Critical dimensions for regeneration based on the amount of inter-root separation have not been established at this time.

Root fusion

Fused roots occur in about 30% of molars, with more maxillary molars affected than mandibular, 35% versus 24% according to one report.[28] The third molar is affected more than the second molar, whereas the first molar rarely has fused roots. The order of frequency of molar fusion by tooth type was maxillary third molar (89%), mandibular third molar (52%), maxillary second molar (52%), mandibular second molar (45%), maxillary first molars (8%), and mandibular first molars (3%). Females

exhibit about 5% more fused molars than males. These numbers are derived from American patients of European ancestry, and percentages may vary among different ethnic groups.[28,29]

Cemental Tears

A cemental tear is a piece of detached cementum, often with some dentin, that may remain attached to periodontal ligament fibers. The tear can be induced by occlusal trauma or other forms of acute trauma, and may appear as a radiopaque fragment in the periodontal ligament space. It can lead to rapid periodontal bone loss and produce a vertical bony defect (Fig. 7-6). When there is rapid periodontal bone loss at an isolated site, a cemental tear should be considered in the differential diagnosis.[30] Treatment of the cemental tear often involves surgical

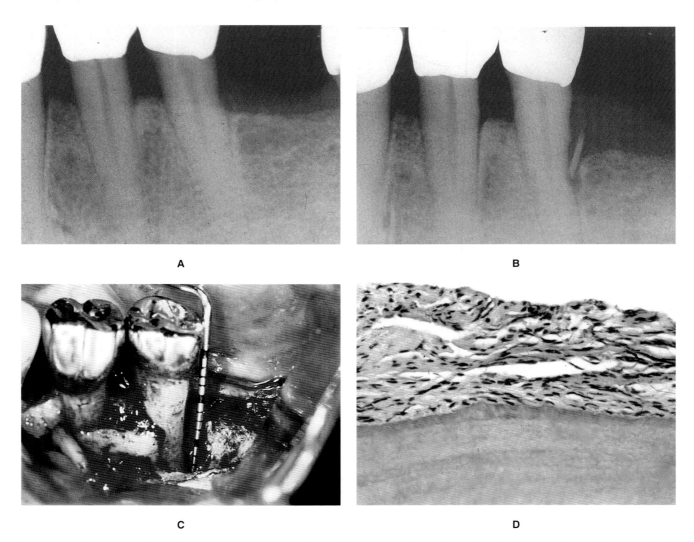

Figure 7-6. A, Radiograph of lower left quadrant before cemental tear. **B,** Radiograph of tooth #20 with visible foreign body on distal aspect. **C,** Flap reflection showing degree of destruction #20D. Foreign body was removed and submitted for histologic examination. **D,** Specimen shows dentin and overlying layer of cementum, with inserting periodontal ligament fibers. The diagnosis was a cemental tear (although dentin was also involved).

debridement, removal of cementum/dentin fragments, and attempted regenerative therapy.

Accessory Canals

Lateral or accessory canals may furnish a communication between the pulp chamber or canal and the periodontal ligament (Fig. 7-7).[31-33] Pulpal necrosis could contribute to the formation of a periodontal defect through an accessory canal (see Chapter 30). Or, conversely, a periodontal lesion could lead to pulpal inflammation or necrosis. Accessory canals occur in approximately 25% to 50% of molars and tend to occur more frequently in first molars than in second molars. Periodontal lesions, particularly

isolated lesions associated with endodontically involved teeth, should be evaluated to determine if an accessory canal is a contributing factor. In cases of a nonvital tooth, adequate root canal therapy is required if the tooth is to be retained and treated periodontally.

Root Proximity

Some clinicians believe that close approximation of tooth roots, with an accompanying thin interproximal septum, leads to an increased risk for periodontal destruction (Fig. 7-8).[34] The crowns of these teeth, especially anterior teeth, are very closely approximated and may have long interproximal contacts, and minimal or no embrasure space,

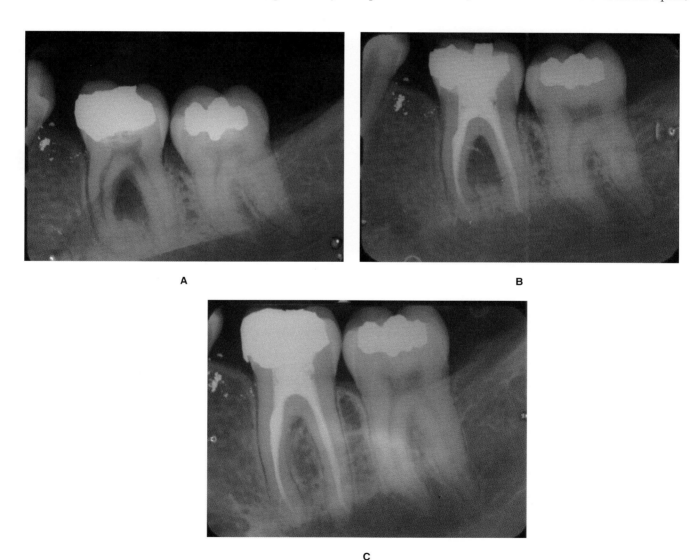

A **B** **C**

Figure 7-7. **A,** Radiographs of an isolated furcation invasion on tooth #19 in an otherwise healthy mouth. Tooth #19 was nonvital. Probing through the sulcus did not communicate with the furcation lesion. **B,** Endodontic treatment was performed, and an accessory canal is clearly visible on the distal aspect of the mesial root. **C,** One-year postendodontic therapy follow-up radiograph shows complete healing of the furcation defect. No periodontal therapy was indicated or provided. (*Courtesy of Dr. Stephen J. Clark, University of Louisville, Louisville, Ky.*)

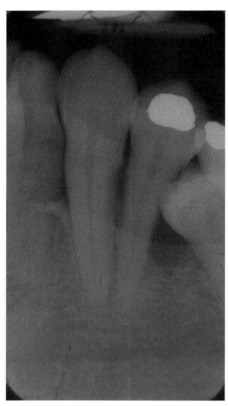

Figure 7-8. Radiograph of root proximity between 27 and 28 associated with horizontal bone loss. (*Courtesy of Dr. Brenton Lahey, University of Louisville, Louisville, Ky.*)

which makes plaque removal difficult. Treatments such as orthodontics, tooth preparation, or selective extraction have been proposed. Some studies have reported that a thin interproximal septum is not more susceptible to bone loss, whereas other studies have associated a wide interproximal septum with vertical bone loss and thin septa with horizontal bone loss.[35-37] Prophylactic treatment of root proximity is probably not indicated, but each clinical situation should be carefully evaluated and treatment provided when needed to prevent additional bone loss.

Adjacent Teeth

There has been concern that retention of a periodontally "hopeless" tooth, or a periodontally compromised tooth, may have a detrimental effect on an adjacent periodontally healthy tooth. Studies have shown that if the compromised tooth receives appropriate periodontal treatment, then attachment levels on the healthy tooth will be unaffected.[38,39] Conversely, if the compromised tooth remains untreated, then attachment levels on the healthy tooth may be adversely affected, and extraction may be of benefit.[40,41] When both teeth are periodontally compromised extraction will have the most pronounced effect on adjacent sites with deeper probing depths.[41]

Adjacent third molars are of particular concern in patients with periodontitis. Frequently, the area between the second and third molar is difficult for the patient, and the professional, to adequately clean, making it difficult to arrest bone and attachment loss in this inaccessible area. Some believe prophylactic extraction of third molars is justified to prevent this and other problems.[42,43] Removal of the third molar, however, also poses some risk for bone and attachment loss on the distal of the second molar, particularly with difficult extractions, or when the distal bone is thin.[42,43] Studies suggest that this loss may be minimal.[44,45] Each case must be considered individually and the benefits and risks carefully evaluated. In addition to periodontitis, other reasons to recommend third molar extraction include cystic changes, root resorption, lack of space, pericoronitis, caries, or anticipated irradiation therapy.[42,43,46,47] It has been suggested that the best time for extraction of third molars is in the late teenage years, before the complete formation of third molar roots, which is usually before the occurrence of periodontitis, but at a time when osseous healing is optimal.[42,43]

RESTORATIVE CONTRIBUTING FACTORS

Overhanging Restorations

Dental restorations with overhanging or open margins create plaque-retentive areas that can increase gingival inflammation, bone loss, and attachment loss.[48-50] In general, more attachment loss is associated with large overhangs than with small ones.[51] Overhangs that extend apically to a position close to the marginal bone are more likely to induce bone loss and attachment loss than overhangs that do not extend as far apically. Overhanging restorations act to extend the sphere of influence of plaque apically. Overhang removal improves gingival conditions and helps prevent attachment loss (Fig. 7-9).[52] Removal should be accomplished in the initial phase of periodontal therapy when possible.[52] Overhangs may also be removed during surgery or by replacement of the defective restoration. When surgery is indicated, the best final restoration may be achieved after completion of surgery, when the restorative dentist has the best access and visibility. Overhangs may be removed with curettes, sonic or ultrasonic scalers, chisels, diamond or finishing burs, or other appropriate instrumentation.[53,54]

Overhanging restorative margins have also been reported to qualitatively alter the composition of the subgingival microflora.[55] In the presence of overhanging restorations, the levels of bacteria associated with chronic periodontitis increase (e.g., anaerobes and black-pigmented *Bacteroides* species). Removal of the overhanging margin reverses this change and promotes the return of a microflora associated with periodontal health.[55]

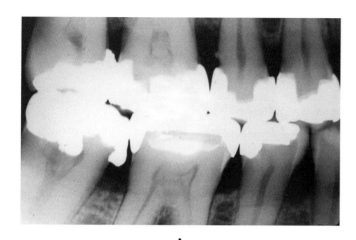

A

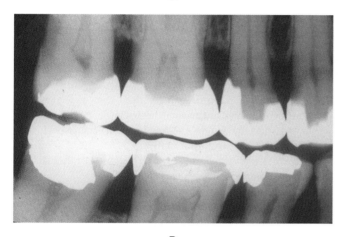

B

Figure 7-9. A, Radiograph showing the presence of several overhanging restorations before scaling and root planing. Subgingival instrumentation included removal of the overhangs. **B,** Radiograph taken 6 months after overhang removal.

Margin Location

The marginal fit of a restoration is the key to its compatibility with the periodontal attachment structures. The periodontal attachment, progressing coronally from the osseous crest, consists of about 1 mm of gingival connective tissue and about 1 mm of junctional epithelium.[56] Coronal to the attachment structures is a gingival sulcus that is usually 2 to 3 mm in depth. In general, the average value of the biologic width (attachment zone for junctional epithelium and connective tissue) is approximately 2 mm. In addition, a dimension of 1 to 2 mm must be allowed between the base of the sulcus and the crown margin, composing a total dimension of at least 3 to 4 mm. If the restoration does not leave room for these normal anatomic features, a chronic, unaesthetic, marginal inflammation results. This inflammation, often manifesting as a circumferential dull blue or deep red marginal halo, may cause persistent bleeding or

discomfort. Initially, the inflammatory process may produce swelling of the soft tissue, but over time it can lead to recession and exposure of the restoration margin. Inflammation caused by violation of biologic width can be resolved with periodontal surgery to establish an adequate 3 to 4 mm distance between the prospective restoration margin and bone, followed by replacement of the improperly designed restoration. In the maxillary anterior region, this surgery may result in an esthetic compromise because biologic width must be reestablished by removal of bone, which will lead to a more apically located gingival margin and will produce "longer" teeth.

All restorative margins located apical to the gingival margin should be within the confines of the gingival sulcus and are termed *intracrevicular* margins.[57] The term *intracrevicular* implies knowledge of biologic width, determination of the attachment location, then placement of the restoration margin at least 1 mm coronal to the attachment. The term *subgingival margin* implies that the restoration margin was merely placed apical to the gingival margin without regard to the attachment location, without an attempt to keep the margin within the gingival sulcus, and most likely in violation of biologic width. The periodontal attachment is more coronally located interproximally than on the facial and lingual surfaces. Thus the tooth preparation should conform to the shape of the attachment, which generally runs in a line parallel to the CEJ around the circumference of the tooth. A preparation that is at the same level circumferentially, particularly on anterior teeth, will most likely violate interproximal biologic width. Studies show that compatibility with the periodontium is best established by margins located either supragingivally or at the level of the gingival margin.[58-61] In the maxillary anterior, esthetic considerations preclude the use of a supragingival margin, but close attention to the concept of biologic width, and use of intracrevicular margins, will promote the best possible gingival esthetics and periodontal health.

Crown Contours

In general, flat buccal and lingual crown contours that follow the root surface contour are more compatible with periodontal health than those that reproduce, or accentuate, the cervical bulge.[62-67] This bulge tends to accumulate plaque and promote gingival inflammation. In the maxillary anterior where facial contours cannot be flattened for esthetic reasons the flat contour is preserved within the sulcus, whereas normal contours and embrasures are established coronal to the gingival margin. This is referred to as establishing a zero-degree emergence angle.

Interproximally overcontoured restorations that close the embrasure and crowd out the papilla make cleaning difficult and lead to gingival inflammation. Establishment of a proper, open embrasure and flat or convex interproximal surface is critical to gingival and papillary health.[63]

Furcation invasion associated with poor crown contours requires a change in restoration design to prevent plaque accumulation and further loss of bone and attachment in the furcation. During tooth preparation the tooth structure coronal to the furcation is grooved.[67] This prevents the restoration coronal to the furcation from bulging over the furcation entrance area and creating an area that favors plaque accumulation. The deep grooves in the furcation area may substantially narrow the crown of the tooth and should be wide enough in the mesial-distal dimension to ensure a gradual contour that will be easily cleansable.

Pontic Form

From a periodontal standpoint, pontics should be esthetic and cleansable.[68-71] As with full coverage restorations, the contours and embrasures should be properly designed. In addition, a pontic should have a ridge-facing (intaglio) surface that is convex and easily cleaned. In general, three types of pontics fulfill these requirements: (1) ovate, (2) modified ridge-lap, and (3) sanitary. The ridge-lap pontic, which straddles the ridge much like a saddle, has a concave ridge-facing surface that cannot be cleaned and should not be used (Fig. 7-10).

The ovate pontic, which is tapered, may lightly contact the ridge in the posterior. In the maxillary anterior, for esthetic reasons, the ridge-facing portion is slightly embedded in the gingival tissue. As the pontic emerges from the gingival tissue it gives the natural appearance of a tooth emerging from the gingival sulcus. This pontic is preferred in esthetic areas when a suitable ridge is present. The modified ridge-lap pontic is also esthetic and may be used in anterior or posterior sites. The sanitary pontic, which does not contact the ridge, has minimal effect on the soft tissues, as long as there is adequate opening under the pontic to facilitate cleaning. Because its ridge-facing surface is far from the edentulous ridge, it is not used in esthetic regions.

Restorative Materials

In general, most restorative materials such as amalgam, composite, glass ionomer, gold, and porcelain are compatible with gingival tissues.[72-75] Allergy to a restorative material can, however, create periodontal problems. Rapid bone loss has been associated with nickel allergy.[76] Allergy to alloys with high nickel content should be considered in the differential diagnosis of unusual bone loss associated with new restorations.

ORTHODONTIC CONTRIBUTING FACTORS

Crowding, Malalignment, and Malocclusion

Crowded or malaligned teeth can be more difficult to clean than properly aligned teeth. In general, studies show a detrimental effect on the periodontium, although some studies have reported no effect.[77-82] This conflict in the literature demonstrates that the effect is not pronounced or even necessarily detectable. Malocclusion, as determined by Angle's Classification, has no significant relation to periodontal status.[83] Also, there seems to be little relation between vertical overbite or horizontal overjet and periodontal status.[81,82]

Orthodontic elastics may become embedded in the gingival sulcus or pocket and, if undetected, can create periodontal problems ranging from severe bone loss to unintended extraction of a tooth.[84-87] Although these problems are rare, they need to be recognized and the elastic removed at the earliest possible time to minimize the severe, often rapid, damage that can occur.

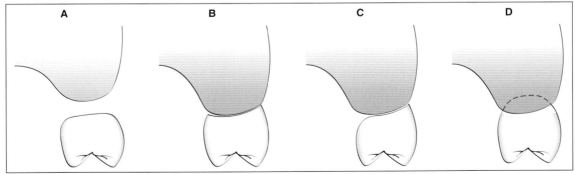

Figure 7-10. Different pontic designs. **A,** Sanitary pontic design places the convex ridge-facing (intaglio) surface of pontic 3mm or more away from the tissue surface; **B,** Ridge-lap pontic has concave intaglio surface straddling the ridge and is difficult to clean adequately with floss; **C,** Modified ridge-lap pontic has slightly concave intaglio surface on the facial aspect, but the lingual aspect is convex, allowing better access for plaque removal than with the ridge-lap pontic; **D,** Ovate pontic has a completely convex intaglio surface that extends into a prepared region of the soft tissue. Dental floss is able to pass in all dimensions between the intaglio surface of the pontic and the adjacent tissue surface. This pontic design is most often used in esthetic regions of the mouth, where patient access for flossing is favorable.

HABITS AS CONTRIBUTING FACTORS

Toothbrush and Floss Trauma

The toothbrush may cause damage to dental soft and hard tissues (Fig. 7-11). A new toothbrush, and especially a hard toothbrush, can abrade epithelium and leave painful ulcerations on the gingiva.[88] Thin marginal gin-

giva that is abraded away can lead to gingival recession and exposure of the root surface.[89] The tooth surface, usually the root surface, can be abraded away by improper toothbrushing technique, especially with a hard toothbrush.[89,90] The abrasives in toothpaste may contribute significantly to this process.[91] The defect usually manifests as v-shaped notches at the level of the CEJ. Patients with this problem should be advised to use a soft toothbrush, a minimally abrasive toothpaste, and should avoid use of a horizontal, back and forth toothbrushing motion.

Flossing can also cause damage to dental hard and soft tissues (Fig. 7-12). Flossing clefts may be produced when floss is forcefully snapped through the contact point so that it cuts into the gingiva.[92] Also an aggressive up and down cleaning motion can produce a similar injury. Sawing of the floss against the tooth using a back and forth motion can, over a period of time, cut into the tooth and create a groove.[93] Asking the patient to demonstrate their flossing technique often will reveal exactly how the injury was created and, at the same time, allow the clinician to demonstrate the technique they should avoid using.

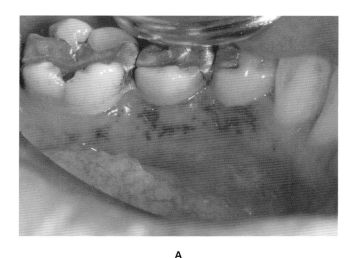

A

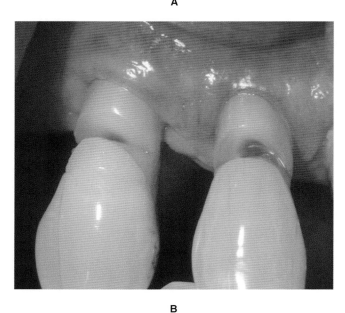

B

Figure 7-11. **A,** Gingival trauma caused by overzealous toothbrushing on the lingual aspect of the lower premolars. Patient was a 26-year-old woman with generalized moderate periodontitis who had been given plaque control instructions by her dentist at the previous visit. **B,** Severe cervical abrasion on the facial root surfaces of the upper canine and lateral incisor. The patient was a 54-year-old woman who had used a hard toothbrush and vigorously "scrubbed" her teeth for more than 30 years.

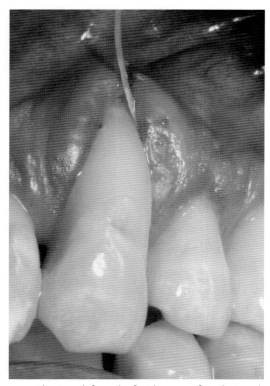

Figure 7-12. Flossing cleft on the facial aspect of tooth #11. Floss was directed apically by patient, creating a gingival cleft over the mid-root. (*Courtesy of Dr. William W. Hallmon, Baylor College of Dentistry, Dallas, Tex.*)

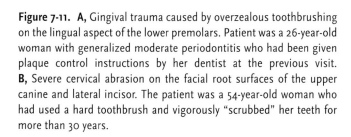

Mouth Breathing and Tongue Thrust

Mouth breathing can dehydrate the gingival tissues and increase susceptibility to inflammation.[94,95] These patients may or may not have increased levels of dental plaque. In some cases gingival enlargement may also occur. Excellent plaque control and professional cleaning should be recommended, although these measures may not completely resolve the gingival inflammation.

Tongue thrusting is often associated with an anterior open bite (Fig. 7-13).[96] During swallowing the tongue is thrust forward against the teeth instead of being placed against the palate. When the amount of pressure against the teeth is great it can lead to tooth mobility and cause increased spacing of the anterior teeth. This problem is difficult to treat but must be recognized in the diagnostic phase as a potentially destructive contributing factor.

Factitial Injuries

Self-inflicted or factitial injuries can be difficult to diagnose because the presentation is often unusual. These injuries are produced in a variety of ways including pricking the gingiva with a fingernail, by fingernail biting and embedding of fingernail fragments, with knives, and by using toothpicks or other oral hygiene devices (Figs. 7-14 and 7-15).[97-100] In most cases, once the mechanism of injury is identified, the patient can be instructed to avoid the injurious behavior. If the habit or behavior is associated with certain emotional or psychological problems, referral for psychiatric evaluation and treatment may be warranted.

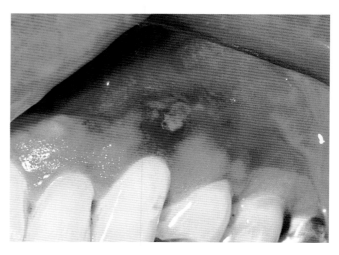

A

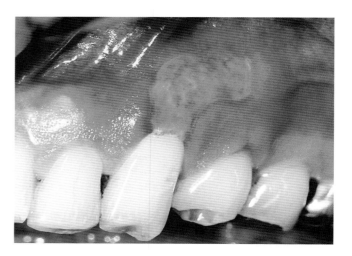

B

Figure 7-15. A, Self-inflicted injury to the gingiva and alveolar mucosa on the facial surface of a lower cuspid in a 58-year-old man. Initially, the patient injured the site with a toothbrush and to "help the area heal" applied 3% H_2O_2 to the site 4 to 5 times a day over a 3-week period. **B,** The patient was instructed to stop this regimen and 1 week later the lesion had begun to resolve

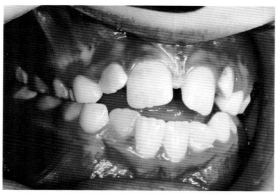

Figure 7-13. Anterior open bite with anterior tongue thrust on swallowing. (*Courtesy of Dr. Annibal Silveira, University of Louisville, Louisville, Ky.*)

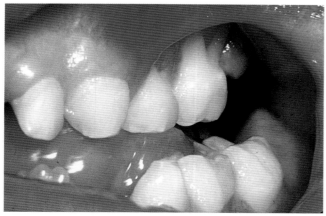

Figure 7-14. Self-inflicted (factitial) gingival recession on the facial surfaces of the primary first and second molars in a 6-year-old boy. The child was upset by the divorce of his parents and developed the nervous habit of scratching his gingiva in the area with his fingernails.

REFERENCES

1. Hirschfeld I: Food impaction, *J Am Dent Assoc* 17:1504, 1930.
2. Kepic TJ, O'Leary TJ: Role of marginal ridge relationship as an etiologic factor in periodontal disease, *J Periodontol* 49:570, 1978.
3. Hancock EB, Mayo CV, Schwab RR, Wirthlin MR: Influence of interdental contacts on periodontal status, *J Periodontol* 51:445, 1980.
4. Masters DH, Hoskins SW: Projection of cervical enamel into molar furcations, *J Periodontol* 35:49, 1964.
5. Lieb A, Berdon J, Sabes W: Furcation involvements correlated with enamel projections from the cementoenamel junction, *J Periodontol* 38:330, 1967.
6. Bissada NF, Abdelmalek RG: Incidence of cervical enamel projections and its relationship to furcation involvement in Egyptian skulls, *J Periodontol* 44:583, 1973.
7. Tsatsas B, Mandi F, Kerani S: Cervical enamel projections in the molar teeth, *J Periodontol* 44:312, 1973.
8. Swan RH, Hurt WC: Cervical enamel projections as an etiologic factor in furcation involvement, *J Am Dent Assoc* 93:342, 1976.
9. Grewe JM, Meskin LH, Miller T: Cervical enamel projections: prevalence, location, and extent; with associated periodontal implications, *J Periodontol* 36:460, 1965.
10. Moskow B, Canut P: Studies on root enamel. (I). Some historical notes on cervical enamel projections, *J Clin Periodontol* 17:29, 1990.
11. Hou GL, Tsai CC: Cervical enamel projection and intermediate bifurcational ridge correlated with molar furcation involvements, *J Periodontol* 68:687, 1997.
12. Everett FG, Jump E, Holder T, Williams S: The intermediate bifurcational ridge: a study of the morphology of the bifurcation of the lower first molar, *J Dent Res* 37:162, 1958.
13. Everett FG: Bifurcation involvement, *Oregon State Dent J* 28:2, 1959.
14. Lee KW, Lee EC, Poon KY: Palatogingival grooves in the maxillary incisors, *Br Dent J* 124:14, 1968.
15. Everett FG, Kramer GM: The disto-lingual groove in the maxillary lateral incisor: a periodontal hazard, *J Periodontol* 43:352, 1972.
16. Kogon SL: The prevalence, location, and conformation of palatoradicular grooves in maxillary incisors, *J Periodontol* 57:231, 1986.
17. Withers J, Brunsvold M, Killoy W, Rahe A: The relationship of palatogingival grooves to localized periodontal disease, *J Periodontol* 52:41, 1981.
18. Hou GL, Tsai CC: Relationship between palato-radicular grooves and localized periodontitis, *J Clin Periodontol* 20:678, 1993.
19. Levy A, Wright W: The relationship between attachment height and attachment area of teeth using a digitizer and a digital computer, *J Periodontol* 49:483, 1978.
20. Anderson RW, McGarrah HE, Lamb RD, Eick JD: Root surface measurements of mandibular molars using stereophotogrammetry, *J Am Dent Assoc* 107:613, 1983.
21. Hermann DH, Gher ME, Dunlap RM, Pelleu GB: The potential attachment area of the maxillary first molar, *J Periodontol* 54:431, 1983.
22. Dunlap RM, Gher ME: Root surface measurements of the mandibular first molar, *J Clin Periodontol* 56:234, 1985.
23. Gher ME, Dunlap RM: Linear variation of the root surface area of the maxillary first molar, *J Periodontol* 56:39, 1985.
24. Larato D: Some anatomical factors related to furcation involvement, *J Periodontol* 46:608, 1975.
25. Hou GL, Tsai CC: Types and dimensions of root trunk correlating with diagnosis of molar furcation involvements, *J Clin Periodontol* 24:129, 1997.
26. Kerns DG, Greenwell H, Wittwer JW, et al: Root trunk dimensions of 5 different tooth types, *Int J Periodontics Restorative Dent* 19:82, 1999.
27. Ward C, Greenwell H, Wittwer JW, Drisko C: Furcation depth and interroot separation dimensions for 5 different tooth types, *Int J Periodontics Restorative Dent* 19:251, 1999.
28. Ross IF, Evanchik PA: Root fusion in molars: incidence and sex linkage, *J Periodontol* 52:663, 1981.
29. Hou GL, Tsai CC, Huang JS: Relationship between molar root fusion and localized periodontitis, *J Periodontol* 68:313, 1997.
30. Haney JM, Leknes KN, Lie T, et al: Cemental tear related to rapid periodontal breakdown: a case report, *J Periodontol* 63:220, 1992.
31. Vertucci FJ, Williams RG: Furcation canals in the human mandibular first molars, *Oral Surg Oral Med Oral Pathol* 38:308, 1974.
32. Guttman JL: Prevalence, location, and patency of accessory canals in the furcation region of permanent molars, *J Periodontol* 49:21, 1978.
33. Vertucci FJ, Anthony RL: A scanning electron microscopic investigation of accessory foramina in the furcation and pulp chamber floor of molar teeth, *Oral Surg Oral Med Oral Pathol* 62:319, 1986.
34. Kramer GM: A consideration of root proximity, *Int J Periodontics Restorative Dent* 7:9, 1987.
35. Heins P, Thomas R, Newton J: The relationship of interradicular width and alveolar bone loss, *J Periodontol* 59:73, 1988.
36. Artun J, Kokich VG, Osterberg SK: Long term effect of root proximity on periodontal health after orthodontic treatment, *Am J Orthod Dentofacial Orthop* 91:125, 1987.
37. Tal H: Relationship between the interproximal distance of roots and the prevalence of intrabony pockets, *J Periodontol* 55:604, 1984.
38. DeVore CH, Beck FM, Horton JE: Retained "hopeless" teeth. Effects on the proximal periodontium of adjacent teeth, *J Periodontol* 59:647, 1988.

39. Wojik MS, DeVore CH, Beck FM, Horton JE: Retained "hopeless" teeth: lack of effect periodontally treated teeth have on the proximal periodontium of adjacent teeth 8-years later, *J Periodontol* 63:663, 1992.

40. Machtei EE, Zubery Y, Yehuda AB, Soskolne WA: Proximal bone loss adjacent to periodontally hopeless teeth with and without extraction, *J Periodontol* 60:512, 1989.

41. Grassi M, Tellenbach R, Lang NP: Periodontal conditions of teeth adjacent to extraction sites, *J Clin Periodontol* 14:334, 1987.

42. Ash MM: Third molars as periodontal problems, *Dent Clin North Am* 51:51, 1964.

43. Fielding A, Douglass A, Whitley R: Reasons for early removal of impacted third molars, *Clin Prev Dent* 6:19, 1981.

44. Osborne W, Snyder A, Tempel T: Attachment levels and crevicular depths at distal of mandibular second molars following removal of adjacent third molars, *J Periodontol* 53:93, 1983.

45. Chin Quee T, Gosselin D, Millar E, Stamm J: Surgical removal of fully impacted mandibular third molars, *J Periodontol* 56:625, 1985.

46. Stanley H, Alattar M, Collett W, et al: Pathological sequelae of neglected impacted third molars, *J Oral Pathol* 17:113, 1988.

47. Nemcovsky CE, Libfeld H, Zubery Y: Effect of non-erupted 3rd molars on distal roots and supporting structures of approximal teeth. A radiographic survey of 202 cases, *J Clin Periodontol* 23:810, 1996.

48. Gilmore N, Sheiham A: Overhanging dental restorations in periodontal disease, *J Periodontol* 42:8, 1971.

49. Highfield J, Powell R: Effects of removal of posterior overhanging metallic margins of restorations upon the periodontal tissues, *J Clin Periodontol* 5:169, 1978.

50. Hakkarainen K, Ainamo J: Influence of overhanging posterior tooth restorations on alveolar bone heights in adults, *J Clin Periodontol* 7:114, 1980.

51. Jeffcoat MK, Howell TH: Alveolar bone destruction due to overhanging amalgams in periodontal disease, *J Periodontol* 51:599, 1980.

52. Rodriguez-Ferrer H, Strahan J, Newman H: Effect on gingival health of removing overhanging margins of interproximal subgingival amalgam restorations, *J Clin Periodontol* 7:457, 1980.

53. Vale J, Caffesse R: Removal of amalgam overhangs—a profilometric and scanning electron microscopic evaluation, *J Periodontol* 50:245, 1979.

54. Brunsvold MA, Lane JJ: The prevalence of overhanging dental restorations and their relationship to periodontal disease, *J Clin Periodontol* 17:67, 1990.

55. Lang NP, Kiel RA, Anderhalden K: Clinical and microbiological effects of subgingival restorations with overhanging or clinically perfect margins, *J Clin Periodontol* 10:563, 1983.

56. Gargiulo AW, Wentz FM, Orban B: Dimensions and relations of the dentogingival junction in humans, *J Periodontol* 32:261, 1961.

57. Nevins M, Skurow HM: The intracrevicular restorative margin, the biologic width, and the maintenance of the gingival margin, *Int J Periodontics Restorative Dent* 4:31, 1984.

58. Marcum J: The effect of crown margin depth upon gingival tissue, *J Prosthet Dent* 17:497, 1967.

59. Löe H: Reactions of the marginal periodontal tissues to restorative procedures, *Int Dent J* 18:759, 1968.

60. Silness J: Periodontal conditions in patients treated with dental bridges. II. The influence of full or partial crowns on plaque accumulation, development of gingivitis and pocket formation, *J Periodont Res* 5:219, 1970.

61. Silness J: Periodontal conditions in patients treated with dental bridges. III. The relationship between the location of the crown margin and periodontal condition, *J Periodont Res* 5:225, 1970.

62. Morris M: Artificial crown contours and gingival health, *J Prosthet Dent* 12:1146, 1962.

63. Wheeler RC: Complete crown form and the periodontium, *J Prosthet Dent* 11:722, 1962.

64. Yuodelis R, Weaver J, Sapkos S: Facial and lingual contours of artificial complete crown restorations and their effects on the periodontium, *J Prosthet Dent* 29:61, 1973.

65. Parkinson CF: Excessive crown contours facilitate endemic plaque niches, *J Prosthet Dent* 35:424, 1976.

66. Sackett B, Gildenhuys R: The effect of axial crown overcontour on adolescents, *J Periodontol* 47:320, 1976.

67. Becker CM, Kaldahl WB: Current theories of crown contour, margin placement, and pontic design, *J Prosthet Dent* 45:268, 1981.

68. Stein RS: Pontic residual ridge relationships: a research report, *J Prosthet Dent* 16:251, 1966.

69. Podshadley AG: Gingival response to pontics, *J Prosthet Dent* 19:51, 1968.

70. Silness J: Periodontal conditions in patients treated with dental bridges. IV. The relationship between the pontic and the periodontal condition of the abutment teeth, *J Periodont Res* 9:50, 1974.

71. Silness J, Gustavsen F, Mangersnes K: The relationship between pontic hygiene and mucosal inflammation in fixed bridge recipients, *J Periodont Res* 17:434, 1982.

72. Hadavi F, Caffesse RG, Charbeneau GT: A study of the gingival response to polished and unpolished amalgam restorations, *J Can Dent Assoc* 52:211, 1986.

73. Van Dijken JW, Sjostrom S, Wing K: The effect of different types of composite resin fillings on marginal gingiva, *J Clin Periodontol* 14:185, 1987.

74. Adamczyk E, Spiechowicz E: Plaque accumulation on crowns made of various materials, *Int J Prosthodont* 3:285, 1990.

75. van Dijken JW, Sjostrom S: The effect of glass ionomer cement and composite resin fillings on marginal gingiva, *J Clin Periodontol* 18:200, 1991.

76. Lamster IB, Kalfus DI, Steigerwald PJ, Chasens AI: Rapid loss of alveolar bone associated with nonprecious alloy crowns in two patients with nickel hypersensitivity, *J Periodontol* 58:486, 1987.

77. Geiger AM, Wasserman BH, Turgeon LR: Relationship of occlusion and periodontal disease. Part VIII. Relationship of crowding and spacing to periodontal destruction and gingival inflammation, *J Periodontol* 45:43, 1974.

78. Ingervall B, Jacobsson U, Nyman S: A clinical study of the relationship between crowding of teeth, plaque and gingival condition, *J Clin Periodontol* 4:214, 1977.

79. Jensen B, Solow B: Alveolar bone loss and crowding in adult periodontal patients, *Community Dent Oral Epidemiol* 17:47, 1989.

80. Griffiths GS, Addy M: Effects of malalignment of teeth in the anterior segments on plaque accumulation, *J Clin Periodontol* 8:481, 1981.

81. Silness J, Roynstrand T: Relationship between alignment conditions of teeth in anterior segments and dental health, *J Clin Periodontol* 12:312, 1985.

82. Buckley LA: The relationship between malocclusion, gingival inflammation, plaque and calculus, *J Periodontol* 52:35, 1981.

83. Geiger AM, Wasserman BH, Thompson RH Jr, Turgeon LR: Relationship of occlusion and periodontal disease. Part V. Relation of classification of occlusion to periodontal status and gingival inflammation, *J Periodontol* 43:554, 1972.

84. Kwapis BW, Knox JE: Extrusion of teeth by elastics: report of two cases, *J Am Dent Assoc* 84:629, 1972.

85. Zager NI, Barnett ML: Severe bone loss in a child initiated by multiple orthodontic rubber bands: case report, *J Periodontol* 45:701, 1974.

86. Zilberman Y, Shteyer A, Azaz B: Iatrogenic exfoliation of teeth by the incorrect use of orthodontic elastic bands, *J Am Dent Assoc* 93:89, 1976.

87. Vandersall DC, Varble DL: The missing orthodontic elastic band, a periodontic orthodontic dilemma, *J Am Dent Assoc* 97:661, 1978.

88. Pattison G: Self-inflicted gingival injuries: literature review and case report, *J Periodontol* 54:299, 1983.

89. Sognnaes RF: Periodontal significance of intraoral frictional ablation, *J West Soc Periodontol* 25:112, 1977.

90. Harte DB, Manley RS: Effect of toothbrush variables on wear of dentin produced by four abrasives, *J Dent Res* 54:993, 1975.

91. Sangnes G: Traumatization of teeth and gingiva related to habitual tooth cleaning procedures, *J Clin Periodontol* 3:94, 1976.

92. Hallmon WW, Waldrop TC, Houston GD, Hawkins BF: Flossing clefts-clinical and histologic observations, *J Periodontol* 57:501, 1986.

93. Everett FG: Abrasion through the use of dental floss, *J Periodontol* 24:186, 1953.

94. Jacobsen L: Mouthbreathing and gingivitis, *J Periodont Res* 8:269, 1973.

95. Wagaiyu EG, Ashley FP: Mouth breathing, lip seal and upper lip coverage and their relationship with gingival inflammations, *J Clin Periodontol* 18:698, 1991.

96. Moyers R: Tongue problems and malocclusion, *Dent Clin North Am* 8:529, 1964.

97. Hasler JF, Schultz WF: Factitial gingival traumatism, *J Periodontol* 39:362, 1968.

98. Stewart DJ: Minor self-inflicted injuries to the gingiva, *J Clin Periodontol* 3:128, 1976.

99. Austin G, Mesa M, Lambert C: The Keyes technique and self-inflicted injuries: three case reports, *J Periodontol* 56:537, 1985.

100. Krejci CB: Self-inflicted gingival injury due to habitual fingernail biting, *J Periodontol* 71:1029, 2000.

PART

II

PERIODONTAL EVALUATION, TREATMENT PLANNING, AND NONSURGICAL THERAPY

Brian L. Mealey and Louis F. Rose

8 Clinical Periodontal Examination

Gary C. Armitage

An oral examination should not be considered complete unless it includes an assessment of the patient's periodontal status. Information collected during a clinical periodontal examination is essential for determining the diagnosis and prognosis of a patient's dentition and for formulating a treatment plan. A thorough periodontal examination includes assessment of potential etiologic factors, the extent of gingival inflammation, and the amount of damage to periodontal structures, as well as an appraisal of factors that may affect the success of therapeutic intervention. To be considered clinically competent, all dentists must master the skills necessary to perform a complete periodontal examination.

ASSESSMENT OF ETIOLOGIC FACTORS

In the past several decades it has been well established that periodontal diseases are mixed infections associated with relatively specific groups of bacteria.[1-3] Consequently, during a periodontal examination it is necessary to assess the patient's current level of plaque control and to identify local conditions that might promote the colonization of teeth by periodontopathic bacteria. For example, notation should be made of dental restorations with overhanging subgingival margins, because they are difficult to clean and can enhance the proliferation of certain periodontal pathogens.[4] Similarly, any situation that makes daily plaque removal difficult, such as crowded or malaligned teeth, furcation involvements, and poorly contoured restorations, should be recorded.

Even the clinical absence of heavy plaque deposits can be of significance and should be noted. For example, in some periodontal infections, such as localized aggressive periodontitis, massive periodontal damage and considerable infection can exist with only slight amounts of clinically visible plaque. Indeed, a characteristic of some sites harboring high percentages of *Actinobacillus actinomycetemcomitans*, *Porphyromonas gingivalis*, or certain other gram-negative bacteria is *not* to exhibit thick deposits of plaque and calculus.

RECOGNITION OF GINGIVAL INFLAMMATION

Recognition of gingival inflammation is a basic skill required to detect infected periodontal tissues. When periodontal pathogens colonize subgingival sites in sufficient numbers, the host mounts an inflammatory response that can be observed clinically. In general, infected sites exhibit one or more of four common signs of gingival inflammation: color change, edema (swelling), bleeding on gentle probing, and gingival crevicular fluid (GCF) or exudate (Figs. 8-1 and 8-2).

Inflamed gingival tissues can exhibit a wide range of color changes. Most of the changes, however, are various

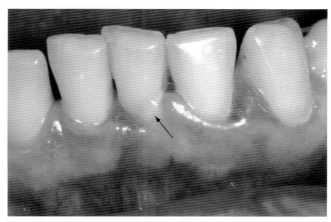

Figure 8-1. Clinical signs of inflammation in a 55-year-old woman with chronic periodontitis. Gingival swelling and color change are particularly noticeable in interproximal areas. Purulent exudate (*arrow*) can be seen on the distal half of the left central incisor.

hues of red. The redness is primarily caused by an increased blood supply to the inflamed site. The best way to detect inflammatory color change is to compare the color of the gingival margin with the color of the adjacent attached gingiva (Fig. 8-3). In other words, one compares the area that is nearest the subgingival flora (and thereby inflamed) with the area least likely to be inflamed.[5]

Gingival swelling or edema is a common feature of inflamed gingival tissues. Edematous gingival enlargement is caused by accumulation of fluids in the inflamed gingival connective tissue. The fluid is primarily serum that has emerged from blood vessels with increased permeability because of local inflammation. Recognition of gingival edema is easy when it is marked. However, it is valuable to recognize this sign of inflammation before it becomes strikingly obvious.[5]

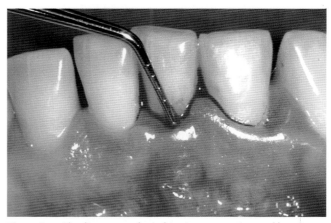

Figure 8-2. Bleeding on gentle probing in same patient and location as shown in Figure 8-1.

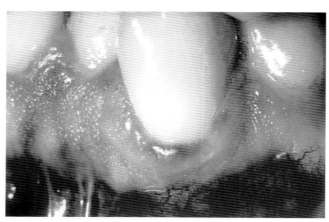

Figure 8-3. Gingival color change (redness) of marginal gingiva of a lower left canine. Inflammatory change can be detected by comparing the color of the gingival margin with that of adjacent attached gingiva. *(From Parr RW, Green E, Ratcliff PA, et al: Recognizing periodontal disease, San Francisco, 1978, Praxis Publishing.)*

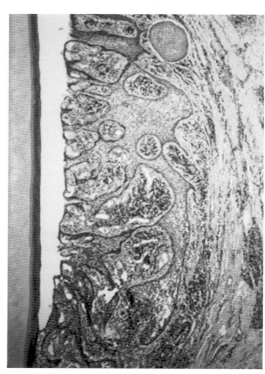

Figure 8-4. Photomicrograph of thin, microulcerated epithelial lining of the soft tissue wall of an infected pocket. Such sites readily bleed when gently probed. Original magnification ×16.

In its earliest stages, gingival edema is usually confined to the first few millimeters of the gingival margin and involves changes in contour, form, texture, and consistency. Healthy sites generally have knife-edged gingival margins, and the surrounding tissues are firm and resilient. The gingiva fits snugly against the tooth. Edematous sites, in contrast, usually have rounded gingival margins, and the adjacent tissues are somewhat enlarged and puffy. The gingiva does not fit tightly against the tooth. Detection of small amounts of gingival edema takes practice and requires that the clinician have a clear knowledge what healthy gingiva looks like. Fortunately, gingival edema is frequently found in association with one or more of the other signs of inflammation, thereby making its recognition easier.

In clinical practice, bleeding on gentle probing is a relatively objective sign of gingival inflammation. Subjective decisions necessary for the detection of gingival redness or edema are not required, because bleeding is either present or absent. Inflamed gingival tissues bleed when gently probed in cases in which the epithelial lining of an infected pocket has become quite thin or has microulcerations (Fig. 8-4). This histologic change in the pocket wall is a frequent occurrence in both gingivitis and periodontitis. Gentle manipulation of an intact epithelial lining of a healthy gingival sulcus with a blunt instrument, such as a periodontal probe, does not elicit bleeding. Bleeding on probing also does not occur at sites when there is a trivial amount of inflammation and where microulcerations of the pocket wall have not yet developed. Hence bleeding on probing is a simple and rapid way to identify inflamed sites.

In addition to the presence of inflammation, bleeding on probing can also be caused by a variety of factors such as multiple or repeated probe insertions at a single site in a short period of time.[6] This probably occurs because of inadvertent trauma to the pocket wall. It is, of course, possible to induce gingival bleeding when too much probing force is used during the examination procedure. It has been reported that if an insertion force greater than 0.25 N is used, bleeding frequently occurs at healthy sites because of trauma to the soft tissue wall of the gingival sulcus.[7] In such cases, the presence of bleeding on probing would lead to the false conclusion that the gingival tissues are inflamed. It should be emphasized that periodontal probing, as a general rule, is a painless procedure. Therefore, one indication that too much probing force is being used is when patients experience pain during the examination procedure. However, a few patients with low pain thresholds may experience pain during periodontal probing even when minimal insertion forces are used.

There are many clinical situations wherein an underlying infection in deep pockets can be "hidden" by deceptively healthy looking gingiva. Bleeding on probing can be particularly useful in identifying such sites, because it can detect inflammation at the base of periodontal pockets that would otherwise be masked from view. For example, the marginal gingival tissues in smokers often appear pink and firm, even when significant periodontal destruction has occurred. However, probing to the base of the pocket may elicit bleeding, indicating the presence of submarginal inflammation.

In addition to its value as a sign of inflammation, the presence or absence of bleeding on probing is associated with the risk for the progression of periodontitis. For example, in treated patients on a periodontal maintenance/recall program, the continual absence of bleeding on probing is an excellent predictor of periodontal stability.[8-10] Data also show that at a single examination, the mere presence of bleeding from a site is not strongly related to the progression of periodontitis.[8-10] However, on the basis of a meta-analysis, sites that exhibit bleeding on probing visit after visit during a maintenance program are approximately at a threefold greater risk for progression than sites that only occasionally bleed.[11]

The last major sign of gingival inflammation is the presence of GCF that oozes from the pocket orifice. The fluid is produced by the inflamed soft tissue wall of the pocket and may range from a clear serous liquid to highly viscous pus (i.e., purulent exudate). GCF is primarily composed of inflammatory cells (mostly polymorphonuclear neutrophilic leukocytes) and serum proteins. In addition, the fluid contains bacteria, tissue breakdown products, enzymes, antibodies, complement, and a wide variety of inflammatory mediators.[11] The amount and rate of fluid production at a given site are highly variable and are, in a very general way, related to the severity of inflammation.

Three basic methods can be used for the detection of GCF. The first method involves isolating a site, drying it with an air syringe, and inserting a small filter paper strip into the crevice or pocket for approximately 60 seconds. The strip is then removed from the site and placed in an electronic device (i.e., Periotron [Harco Electronics, Winnipeg, MB, Canada]) that indirectly measures the volume of fluid absorbed by the strip.[12-14] This method is particularly valuable as a research tool, because small amounts of gingival fluid can be detected and measured objectively. However, it has limited value in clinical practice because the amount of gingival fluid provides no diagnostic or prognostic information. It does not distinguish between sites with gingivitis or periodontitis and cannot identify progressing lesions. Nevertheless, in the future it may be possible to detect, or even predict, important clinical events such as the progression of periodontitis. On the basis of preliminary experiments, several authors suggest that certain components of GCF may serve as risk markers for the progression of periodontitis.[11] Indeed, more than 45 different GCF components representing tissue breakdown products, host-derived enzymes, and inflammatory mediators have been currently examined. Most notably among these components are alkaline phosphatase,[15] dipeptidyl peptidase,[16] certain

matrix metalloproteinases,[15,17] glycosaminoglycans,[18] and bone-specific pyridinoline cross-links.[19] It should be emphasized that none of these GCF components has been completely validated as a marker for the progression of periodontitis.

The second way to detect crevicular fluid simply involves isolating and drying a site and waiting for visible amounts of fluid to collect at the pocket orifice. This method is not particularly useful in clinical situations because sites that produce visible quantities of crevicular fluid also usually exhibit one or more of the other signs of inflammation.

In the third method, digital pressure is applied to the gingiva overlying the approximate base of the pocket and the clinician's finger is moved coronally. This forces visible quantities of the exudate out of the pocket. This is the best way to determine if purulent exudate (a form of crevicular fluid) is being produced at a given site.

CLINICAL ASSESSMENT OF DAMAGE TO PERIODONTAL STRUCTURES

Two of the main purposes of a periodontal examination are to systematically record (1) probing depths (PDs) and (2) clinical attachment level (CAL) around each tooth. Periodontal pockets are pathologically deepened gingival sulci that develop at infected sites and are conceptually important because they represent the subgingival habitats for periodontopathic bacteria.[20] PD is the distance from the gingival margin to the base of the probeable crevice. CAL is the distance from the cementoenamel junction (CEJ) to the base of the probeable crevice. When the CEJ is not detectable or is missing because of the presence of a dental restoration, the CAL cannot be measured. In such cases, another fixed landmark such as the margin of a restoration or an incisal/occlusal edge of a tooth can be used to obtain a measurement called the relative attachment level. This is the distance from a fixed landmark, other than the CEJ, to the base of the probeable crevice. Attachment loss readings, such as the CAL or relative attachment level, are important because they are the best assessment of how much damage has occurred to the periodontal apparatus.

Because a pocket can develop at any point around a tooth, its entire circumference must be probed. Probing involves "stepping" a calibrated periodontal probe around the tooth and recording the deepest point at each of six tooth surfaces: distofacial, facial, mesiofacial, distolingual, lingual, and mesiolingual (Fig. 8-5). As a general rule, a probe reading that falls between two calibrated marks on the probe should be *rounded upward* to the next highest millimeter. Thus if the probe penetrates far enough to cover the 3 mm mark, it should be recorded as 4 mm.[5]

Periodontal probing should be done gently. Ordinarily, patients should not experience discomfort from the

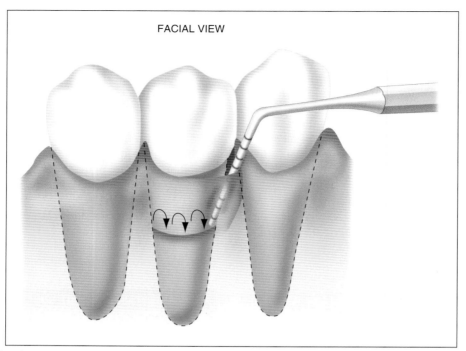

FACIAL VIEW

Figure 8-5. Periodontal probing involves "stepping" a calibrated probe around the tooth.

procedure. As the probe is inserted into the pocket and moved apically along the root surface, a piece of subgingival calculus may be encountered. In such cases, the probe is gently teased past the calculus and moved apically until "soft" resistance from the tissues at the base of the probeable pocket is encountered. With a little practice, most examiners can readily determine when the soft tissue at the base of the lesion is reached.

At most locations an attempt should be made to probe parallel to the long axis of the tooth. Exaggerated probe angulations can lead to spuriously high PD readings. A notable exception to this rule is when probing interproximal areas where it is necessary to angle the probe slightly so that the site directly under the contact point can be reached. Care should be taken to probe the area under the contact from both lingual and facial aspects, because deep pockets frequently develop in this location (Fig. 8-6).

Measurement and recording of PDs and CAL readings should be recorded at regular periods during the care of patients. Most practitioners record PD and CAL measurements at the following stages: (1) the baseline or first visit, (2) approximately 1 month after completion of initial anti-infective therapy (i.e., oral hygiene instructions and scaling and root planing), (3) some time after the healing phase if periodontal surgery has been necessary, and (4) at various intervals during the life of the periodontal maintenance program. The specific reasons PD and CAL measurements are taken periodically during the care of patients are summarized in Table 8-1. Many of these

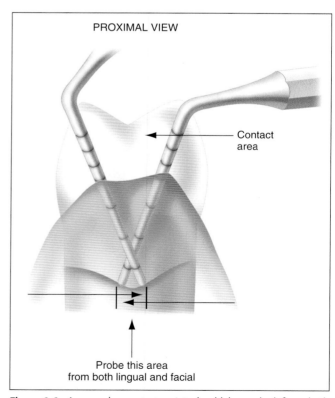

PROXIMAL VIEW

Contact area

Probe this area from both lingual and facial

Figure 8-6. Area under contact point should be probed from both facial and lingual aspects, because deep pockets frequently develop in this location.

TABLE 8-1	Reasons Probing Depth and Clinical Attachment Level Measurements Are Recorded During the Various Stages of Periodontal Therapy
STAGE OF THERAPY	**REASONS FOR RECORDING THE MEASUREMENTS**
Baseline or initial visit	PD measurements provide an assessment of the location and extent of potential habitats of infecting bacteria. CAL measurements provide an overall assessment of the location and extent of damage to periodontal tissues.
After completion of antiinfective therapy (~1 month after scaling root planing)	PD measurements provide an assessment of how effective therapy has been in achieving pocket closure (i.e., probing depth reduction, downsizing of microbial habitat). If the infection has been controlled and the patient is ready for placement in a maintenance/recall program, CAL measurements provide a baseline for future comparisons.
After healing phase, if periodontal surgery has been performed	PD measurements provide an assessment of how effective surgery has been in reducing probing depths (i.e., downsizing of microbial habitat). If the patient is ready for placement in a maintenance/recall program, CAL measurements provide a baseline for future comparisons.
Maintenance/recall program	PD measurements provide an assessment of any recurrence of probing depths (i.e., recurrence of habitat for infecting bacteria). CAL measurements provide an assessment of how effective the recall program has been in stabilizing the remaining level of the periodontal attachment apparatus.

CAL, Clinical attachment level; PD, probing depth.

reasons are related to how effective treatment has been in reducing the habitat of infecting periodontal pathogens (i.e., reduction in depth of periodontal pockets).

Some practitioners do not record CAL readings at the initial examination but wait until the patient is ready to enter the maintenance phase of therapy. The two main reasons behind this approach are that many changes occur in CAL readings as a result of therapy and that the readings are easier to obtain once plaque and calculus have been removed and the inflammation has been controlled. Other practitioners prefer to record CAL readings at the initial examination because it gives them site-by-site baseline assessments of the amount of damage before treatment. Comparison of the baseline CAL measurements with those recorded after treatment provide an assessment of how effective treatment has been in resolving the amount of periodontal damage.

CAL measurements taken at two different times are the best way to determine if progression of periodontitis has occurred.[21] Collection of these readings can be difficult and time-consuming because it requires that one locate the CEJ as the landmark from which measurements are taken. This can be particularly difficult if there has been minimal gingival recession and the gingival margin is located coronal to the CEJ. In such cases, the position of the CEJ must be estimated by feeling for it with the probe tip. If there has been enough recession, the gingival margin will be located somewhere on the root and the CEJ will be in full view, thereby making CAL measurements easier to obtain. The time and trouble required to collect CAL measurements are worth the effort, because these readings serve as a baseline for future comparisons during the maintenance phase of therapy. Using only PD measurements to determine periodontal status may result in misdiagnosis. The gingival margin, from which the PD is measured, is subject to change in position. For example, gingival inflammation and swelling can "enlarge" the marginal tissues, resulting in a gingival margin position coronal to its usual noninflamed position. Conversely, recession may move the gingival margin position apical to the CEJ (Fig. 8-7). Hence a measurement using a fixed reference point (the CEJ) is desirable for monitoring patients over long periods.

The gingival margin position may be recorded as a positive number when the marginal gingiva is apical to the CEJ (recession), or as a negative number if the gingival margin is coronal to the CEJ. Once the PD is determined, the clinical attachment level is calculated as the PD plus the gingival margin-to-CEJ measurement. For example, if a site has 2 mm of recession and a PD of 5 mm, the CAL is 7 mm (2 mm + 5 mm). Conversely, if the gingival margin is located 2 mm coronal to the CEJ, and a 5-mm PD is present, the CAL is 3 mm (-2 mm + 5 mm). In some cases, the gingival margin will be located at the CEJ, in which case the PD and CAL are the same.

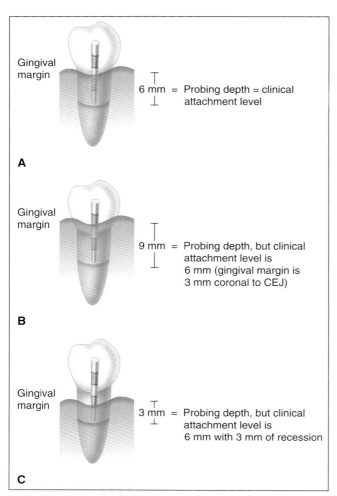

Gingival margin

6 mm = Probing depth = clinical attachment level

A

Gingival margin

9 mm = Probing depth, but clinical attachment level is 6 mm (gingival margin is 3 mm coronal to CEJ)

B

Gingival margin

3 mm = Probing depth, but clinical attachment level is 6 mm with 3 mm of recession

C

Figure 8-7. Probing depth and clinical attachment level. **A,** Gingival margin is at cementoenamel junction (CEJ). **B,** Gingival margin is coronal to the CEJ (gingival swelling). **C,** Gingival margin is apical to the CEJ (gingival recession).

FACTORS THAT MAY AFFECT SUCCESS OF THERAPEUTIC INTERVENTION

Reliability and Reproducibility of Periodontal Probing

Without question, properly used periodontal probes currently are the best way to measure PDs and CAL during clinical examinations. However, periodontal probing has several drawbacks when it is used to monitor periodontal status longitudinally. From one visit to the next, it is difficult to duplicate precisely the insertion force and to reproduce the site and angulation of probe insertion. Because of these technical problems, when consecutive readings of PD are taken at a given site, it is generally expected that the PD measurements may vary by up to 1 mm as a function of the limited sensitivity of this system of measurement.[11,22]

In addition, it has been established that the extent of probe penetration is influenced by the inflammatory status of the tissues.[11,23-26] In most instances when healthy tissues are examined, the probe tip stops coronal to the apical termination of the junctional epithelium (Fig. 8-8), whereas at inflamed sites the probe tip frequently passes apical to this point (Fig. 8-9). The depth of probe penetration partially depends on the extent to which the gingival connective tissue has been lysed or infiltrated by inflammatory cells. In other words, intact connective tissue underlying the crevicular epithelium is an important factor resisting probe penetration.

This has important implications regarding how measurements taken with periodontal probes are interpreted. Because probes rarely stop at the exact location of the most apical cells of the junctional epithelium, probing measurements are clearly not precise assessments of the actual level of the connective tissue attachment. Probing overestimates connective tissue attachment loss at inflamed sites and underestimates it at non-inflamed sites. Consequently, gains in clinical attachment as a result of treatment are not necessarily because of the formation of a new connective tissue attachment,[25] rather, changes in CAL after treatment may be because of reduced tissue penetration of the probe as inflammation is reduced. Despite these problems, properly used periodontal probes provide critically important information regarding the periodontal status of patients. Measurements obtained with periodontal probes are the best way to assess damage caused by periodontal infections and are essential for longitudinally monitoring the response to treatment.

In an attempt to overcome some of the technical problems associated with conventional manual periodontal probes, numerous electronic periodontal probes have been developed that permit probe insertion with a controlled force.[11] The controlled-force probe that has received the most widespread use is the Florida Probe (Florida Probe Co., Gainesville, FL). This computer-linked device has an in vitro resolution of 0.1 mm and is capable of recording PDs and relative attachment levels.[27-33] A modified version of the Florida Probe has been developed that can automatically detect the CEJ, and therefore is theoretically capable of making CAL measurements easier to obtain.[34] Comparative reproducibility data from multiple studies do not show any major differences between conventional and various types of controlled-force probes.[35-42] Clinical measurements obtained with conventional manual probes are consistently greater than those obtained with controlled-force probes.[36-39,43-45] One of the possible reasons for this is the reduced tactile sensitivity associated with the use of controlled-force probes. This is especially true in patients with untreated periodontitis for whom the

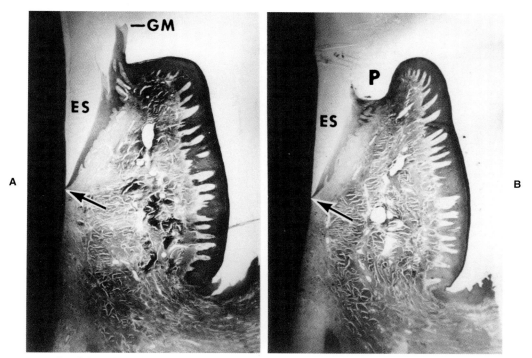

Figure 8-8. Photomicrographs of clinically healthy facial gingiva of a lower incisor from a beagle dog. **A,** Site without periodontal probe. **B,** Adjacent site with probe. End of transparent plastic probe (*P*) is located coronal to the apical termination of junctional epithelium (*arrows*). ES, Enamel space; GM, gingival margin. Original magnification ×30. *(From Armitage GC, Svanberg GK, Löe H: Microscopic evaluation of clinical measurements of connective tissue attachment levels, J Clin Periodontol 4:173-190, 1977. ©1977 Munksgaard International Publishers, Ltd., Copenhagen, Denmark.)*

presence of subgingival calculus can interfere with probe insertion. With conventional probes it is generally easier for the operator to manipulate the probe tip past subgingival calculus deposits. A definite advantage of computer-linked probes is that they can automatically record probe readings. Some systems even allow voice-activated data entry.[46] The usefulness of controlled-force probes in day-to-day clinical practice has not yet been demonstrated.[11] One possible reason for the lack of widespread acceptance of controlled-force electronic probes by practitioners might be increased patient discomfort when the devices are used, particularly around the anterior teeth. During probing with conventional manual probes, the operator can rapidly decrease the insertion force if the patient shows any early signs of discomfort. With controlled-force probes, this patient-dentist feedback is not possible because the probe is inserted into the pocket in one motion and with a fixed or predetermined force.

Assessment of Furcation Involvement

When periodontal infections occur around multirooted teeth, destruction of the soft tissue and bone in the furcation area is frequently observed. Infection in these areas presents a considerable therapeutic problem, because furcations are difficult for both the patient and the therapist to clean. The type of treatment for furcation involvement is highly dependent on the extent to which the periodontal infection has destroyed tissues in the area. Therefore, for treatment planning purposes, it is important during a periodontal examination to assess the extent of furcation involvement. One of the best ways to detect furcation openings is with a curved instrument such as an explorer or a furcation probe (Fig. 8-10). A simple and useful classification system for assessing the severity of furcation involvements is as follows:[47]

Class I: Beginning involvement. The tissue destruction should not extend more than 2 mm (or not more than one third of the tooth width) into the furcation.

Class II: Cul-de-sac involvement. The tissue destruction extends deeper than 2 mm (or more than one third of the tooth width) into the furcation but does not completely pass from one furcation opening (e.g., facial) to the next (e.g, lingual).

Class III: Through-and-through involvement. The tissue destruction extends throughout the entire length of the furcation, so that an instrument can

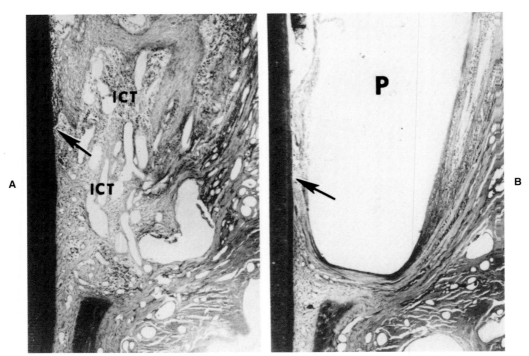

Figure 8-9. Photomicrographs of facial gingiva of a lower premolar in a beagle dog with periodontitis. **A,** Site without periodontal probe. Note extensive inflamed connective tissue (*ICT*) and epithelial proliferation. **B,** Adjacent site with probe. Transparent plastic probe (*P*) has gone past the apical termination of junctional epithelium (arrows). Probe tip is in contact with connective tissue near the alveolar crest. (X75). *(From Armitage GC, Svanberg GK, Löe H: Microscopic evaluation of clinical measurements of connective tissue attachment levels, J Clin Periodontol 4:173-190, 1977. ©1977 Munksgaard International Publishers, Ltd., Copenhagen, Denmark.)*

be passed between the roots and emerge on the other side of the tooth.

Potential Mucogingival Problems

During a periodontal examination, notation is usually made of sites that have a narrow zone of attached gingiva. The boundary between keratinized attached gingiva and nonkeratinized alveolar mucosa is readily visible in most patients; it is called the mucogingival junction (Fig. 8-11). In general, sites with less than 1 or 2 mm of keratinized gingiva are usually noted and charted because some patients have difficulty in comfortably cleaning these areas. A toothbrush can usually be passed over keratinized gingiva without discomfort, whereas brushing of nonkeratinized alveolar mucosa can be painful. As a result, some patients avoid cleaning sites with little or no keratinized gingiva and plaque-induced disease develops. It should be emphasized, however, that many patients with a "narrow" zone of keratinized or attached gingiva can maintain these areas quite well and require no therapeutic intervention other than routine professionally administered cleaning.[48] In any event, it is advisable to record sites with potential mucogingival problems for treatment planning and monitoring purposes.

Assessment of Tooth Mobility

Because one of the major causes of increased tooth mobility is the loss of alveolar support secondary to periodontal infections, it is important that abnormal tooth mobility be recorded as part of a complete periodontal examination. Although longitudinal assessment of CAL is a superior method of determining the progression of periodontitis, increasing tooth mobility over time suggests that some deterioration may be occurring. In addition, tooth hypermobility may have some prognostic significance.[49] A simple classification system for recording tooth mobility is as follows:

Class I: The tooth can be moved less than 1 mm in a buccolingual or mesiodistal direction.

Class II: The tooth can be moved 1 mm or more in a buccolingual or mesiodistal direction but does not exhibit abnormal mobility in an occlusoapical direction.

Class III: The tooth can be moved 1 mm or more in both buccolingual or mesiodistal *and* occlusoapical directions.

Notably, increased tooth mobility may have a variety of causes unrelated to periodontal infections. For example, hypermobility is commonly observed when teeth are under extremely heavy functional loads, for a time after orthodontic movement, and when teeth have extensive periapical disease (i.e., endodontic lesions).

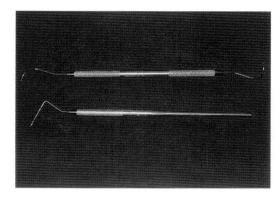

A

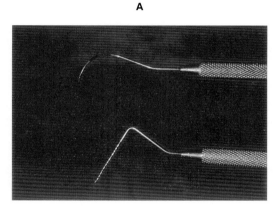

B

Figure 8-10. A and **B,** Examples of probing instruments. Straight periodontal probe with 1-mm markings (UNC 15 probe [Hu-Friedy Manufacturing Co., Chicago, IL]) is used for determining probing depth and clinical attachment levels. Curved probe with 3-mm markings is used for determining furcation classification.

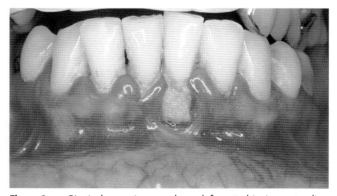

Figure 8-11. Gingival recession on a lower left central incisor extending well past the mucogingival junction into alveolar mucosa in a 42-year-old man. Note the heavy deposits of plaque and calculus on the root surface. The patient avoided cleaning the site because the alveolar mucosa was tender when brushed.

It is important to remember that all teeth are mobile to some extent because they are separated from bone by the periodontal ligament. However, with practice it is relatively easy to determine abnormal tooth mobility. To test for tooth mobility, the clinician may place a finger on the lingual surface and gently push on the facial surface with the handle of an instrument such as a probe or mouth mirror. Usually, using an adjacent nonmoving tooth as a reference point, one can feel and see movement (Fig. 8-12). Some clinicians prefer to test for tooth mobility by using the handles of two instruments and alternating the gentle pushing action between the facial and lingual surfaces of the tooth (Fig. 8-13). In this case, detection of abnormal mobility relies on visual assessment of tooth displacement facially and lingually. The mesiodistal mobility is difficult to assess in teeth with interproximal contacts. However, mesiodistal mobility should be examined whenever possible, such as terminal teeth and teeth adjacent to an edentulous area or diastema.

Basics of Periodontal Charting

A periodontal chart should be uncomplicated, easy to read, and contain all of the basic information required for determining the patient's periodontal diagnosis, prognosis, and treatment plan. In addition, it should provide a permanent record that can be used to evaluate longitudinally the response to therapy.

Before therapy, essential information to be recorded on a periodontal chart should include PD and clinical attachment level readings for six sites around each tooth, the amount of gingival recession on a site-by-site basis, furcation involvement, mobility, potential mucogingival problems, malalignment or crowding of teeth, defective restorations, and any other observations that may influence decisions relating to the diagnosis, prognosis, and treatment plan. An overall appraisal of the severity of inflammation, level of plaque control, and amount of supragingival and subgingival calculus is desirable. Conceptually, the periodontal chart represents a database from which the extent of damage can be assessed and probable etiologic factors can be identified.

On completion of periodontal therapy, before placing the patient on a maintenance/recall program, the periodontal examination should be repeated. The primary purposes of this examination are the following: (1) to determine how successful the treatment was in controlling the etiologic factors and arresting the disease, and (2) to provide a basis for future comparisons as the patient proceeds through the maintenance program. It is important that CAL readings be taken during this and subsequent examinations because such measurements are the most reliable way to determine if progression of disease is occurring over time.

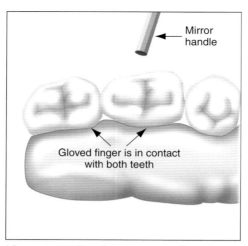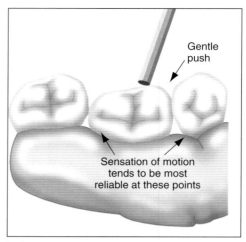

Figure 8-12. Method for testing tooth mobility using a rigid instrument and a finger.

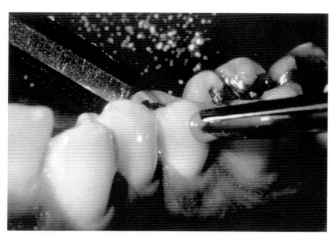

Figure 8-13. Handles of two instruments used to check tooth mobility.

REFERENCES

1. Socransky SS, Haffajee AD, Cugini MA, et al: Microbial complexes in subgingival plaque, *J Clin Periodontol* 25:134-144, 1998.
2. Haffajee AD, Socransky SS: Microbial etiological agents of destructive periodontal disease, *Periodontol 2000* 5:78-111, 1994.
3. Socransky SS, Haffajee AD: Dental biofilms: difficult therapeutic targets, *Periodontol 2000* 28:12-55, 2002.
4. Lang NP, Kiel RA, Anderhalden K: Clinical and microbiological effects of subgingival restorations with overhanging or clinically perfect margins, *J Clin Periodontol* 10:563-578, 1983.
5. Parr RW, Green E, Ratcliff PA, et al: *Recognizing periodontal disease*, San Francisco, 1978, Praxis Publishing.
6. van der Weijden GA, Timmerman MF, Saxton CA, et al: Intra-/inter-examiner reproducibility study of gingival bleeding, *J Periodont Res* 29:236-241, 1994.
7. Karayiannis A, Lang NP, Joss A, Nyman S: Bleeding on probing as it relates to probing pressure and gingival health in patients with a reduced but healthy periodontium. A clinical study, *J Clin Periodontol* 19:471-475, 1992.
8. Lang NP, Joss A, Orsanic T, et al: Bleeding on probing. A predictor for the progression of periodontal disease? *J Clin Periodontol* 13:590-596, 1986.
9. Lang NP, Adler R, Joss A, Nyman S: Absence of bleeding on probing. An indicator of periodontal stability, *J Clin Periodontol* 17:714-721, 1990.
10. Kaldahl WB, Kalkwarf KL, Patil KD, Molvar MP: Relationship of gingival bleeding, gingival suppuration, and supragingival plaque to attachment loss, *J Periodontol* 61:347-351, 1990.
11. Armitage GC: Periodontal diseases: diagnosis, *Ann Periodontol* 1:37-215, 1996.
12. Tsuchida K, Hara K: Clinical significance of gingival fluid measurement by Periotron, *J Periodontol* 52:697-700, 1981.
13. Bickel M, Ciamsoni G: Reliability of volume measurements with the new Periotron® 6000, *J Periodont Res* 19:313-316, 1984.
14. Stewart JE, Chritenson PD, Maeder LA, Palmer MA: Reliability of filter-paper sampling of gingival crevicular fluid for volume determination using the Periotron, *J Periodont Res* 28:227-230, 1993.
15. Nakashima K, Giannopoulou C, Andersen E, et al: A longitudinal study of various crevicular fluid components as markers of periodontal disease activity, *J Clin Periodontol* 23:832-838, 1996.
16. Eley BM, Cox SW: Correlation between gingival crevicular fluid dipeptidyl peptidase II and IV activity and periodontal attachment loss. A 2-year longitudinal study in chronic periodontitis patients, *Oral Dis* 1:201-213, 1995.

17. Alpagot T, Bell C, Lundergan W, et al: Longitudinal evaluation of GCF MMP-3 and TIMP-1 levels as prognostic factors for progression of periodontitis, *J Clin Periodontol* 28:353-359, 2001.

18. Waddington RJ, Langley MS, Guida L, et al: Relationship of sulphated glycosaminoglycans in human gingival crevicular fluid with active periodontal disease, *J Periodont Res* 31:168-170, 1996.

19. Giannobile WV, Lynch SE, Denmark RG, et al: Crevicular fluid osteocalcin and pyridinoline cross-linked carboxyterminal telopeptide of type I collagen (ICTP) as markers of rapid bone turnover in periodontitis. A pilot study in beagle dogs, *J Clin Periodontol* 22:903-910, 1995.

20. Armitage GC: Clinical evaluation of periodontal diseases, *Periodontol 2000* 7:39-53, 1995.

21. Goodson JM: Clinical measurements of periodontitis, *J Clin Periodontol* 13:446-455, 1986.

22. Glavind L, Löe H: Errors in the clinical assessment of periodontal destruction, *J Periodont Res* 2:180-184, 1967.

23. Armitage GC, Svanberg GK, Löe H: Microscopic evaluation of clinical measurements of connective tissue attachment levels, *J Clin Periodontol* 4:173-190, 1977.

24. Robinson PJ, Vitek RM: The relationship between gingival inflammation and resistance to probe penetration, *J Periodont Res* 14:239-243, 1979.

25. Fowler C, Garrett S, Crigger M, Egelberg J: Histologic probe position in treated and untreated human periodontal tissues, *J Clin Periodontol* 9:373-385, 1982.

26. Tessier J-F, Ellen RP, Birek P, et al: Relationship between periodontal probing velocity and gingival inflammation in human subjects, *J Clin Periodontol* 20:41-48, 1993.

27. Gibbs CH, Hirschfeld JW, Lee JG, et al: Description and clinical evaluation of a new computerized periodontal probe—the Florida Probe, *J Clin Periodontol* 15:137-144, 1988.

28. Magnusson I, Fuller WW, Heins PJ, et al: Correlation between electronic and visual readings of pocket depths with a newly developed constant force probe, *J Clin Periodontol* 15:180-184, 1988.

29. Magnusson I, Clark WB, Marks RG, et al: Attachment level measurements with a constant force electronic probe, *J Clin Periodontol* 15:185-188, 1988.

30. Marks RG, Low SB, Taylor M, et al: Reproducibility of attachment level measurements with two models of the Florida Probe, *J Clin Periodontol* 18:780-784, 1991.

31. Yang MCK, Marks RG, Magnusson I, et al: Reproducibility of an electronic probe in relative attachment level measurements, *J Clin Periodontol* 19:541-548, 1992.

32. Clark WB, Yang MCK, Magnusson I: Measuring clinical attachment: reproducibility of relative measurements with an electronic probe, *J Periodontol* 63:831-838, 1992.

33. Clark WB, Magnusson I, Namgung YY, Yang MCK: The strategy and advantage in use of an electronic probe for attachment measurement, *Adv Dent Res* 7:152-157, 1993.

34. Preshaw PM, Kupp L, Hefti AF, Mariotti A: Measurement of clinical attachment levels using a constant-force periodontal probe modified to detect the cementoenamel junction, *J Clin Periodontol* 26:434-440, 1999.

35. Kalkwarf KL, Kaldahl WB, Patil KD: Comparison of manual and pressure-controlled periodontal probing, *J Periodontol* 57:467-471, 1986.

36. Galgut PN, Waite IM: A comparison between measurements made with a conventional periodontal pocket probe, an electronic pressure probe and measurements made at surgery, *Int Dent J* 40:333-338, 1990.

37. Osborn J, Stoltenberg J, Huso B, et al: Comparison of measurement variability using a standard and constant force periodontal probe, *J Periodontol* 61:497-503, 1990.

38. Osborn J, Stoltenberg J, Huso B, et al: Comparison of measurement variability in subjects with moderate periodontitis using a conventional and constant force periodontal probe, *J Periodontol* 63:283-289, 1993.

39. Quirynen M, Callens A, van Steenberghe D, Nys M: Clinical evaluation of a constant force electronic probe, *J Periodontol* 64:35-39, 1993.

40. Mullally BH, Linden GJ: Comparative reproducibility of proximal probing depth using electronic pressure-controlled and hand probing, *J Clin Periodontol* 21:284-288, 1994.

41. Tupta-Veselicky L, Famili P, Ceravolo FJ, Zullo T: A clinical study of an electronic constant force periodontal probe, *J Periodontol* 65:616-622, 1994.

42. Wang S-F, Leknes KN, Zimmerman GJ, et al: Reproducibility of periodontal probing using a conventional manual and automated force-controlled electronic probe, *J Periodontol* 66:38-46, 1995.

43. Rams TE, Slots J: Comparison of two pressure-sensitive periodontal probes and a manual periodontal probe in shallow and deep pockets, *Int J Periodontics Restorative Dent* 13:521-529, 1993.

44. Perry DA, Taggart EJ, Leung A, Newbrun E: Comparison of a conventional probe with electronic and manual pressure-regulated probes, *J Periodontol* 65:908-913, 1994.

45. Hull PS, Clerehugh V, Ghassemi-Aval A: An assessment of the validity of a constant force electronic probe in measuring probing depths, *J Periodontol* 66:848-851, 1995.

46. Mintzer RE, Derdivanis JP: Automated periodontal probing and recording. In Yukna RA, Newman MG, Williams RC, editors: *Current opinion in periodontology*, Philadelphia, 1993, Current Science.

47. Ramfjord SP, Ash MM Jr: *Periodontology and periodontics*, Philadelphia, 1979, WB Saunders.

48. Kennedy JE, Bird WC, Palcanis KG, Dorfman HS: A longitudinal evaluation of varying widths of attached gingiva, *J Clin Periodontol* 12:667-675, 1985.

49. Fleszar TJ, Knowles JW, Morrison EC, et al: Tooth mobility and periodontal therapy, *J Clin Periodontol* 7:495-505, 1980.

9 Radiography for the Periodontal Examination

Dale A. Miles and Mark V. Thomas

Although they are only two-dimensional representations of three-dimensional structures, radiographic images of the hard periodontal tissues are an essential, useful, and indispensable diagnostic adjunct to the clinical periodontal examination. The clinical and the radiographic examinations complement each other, and both should be used for an accurate assessment of the patient's periodontal status. Without the radiographic images, the clinician could not effectively evaluate alveolar crestal bone architecture. Other estimates of crown-to-root ratio, possible vertical defects, and the amount of horizontal bone loss also would be impossible.

Using digital imaging techniques and electronic image processing, the clinician can even "quantify" bone loss or gain by using digital image subtraction techniques. This chapter discusses the need for radiographic images, the desirable image characteristics for optimum hard tissue assessment, the techniques available, digital imaging techniques, and possible future trends for periodontal radiographic imaging.

IMAGE REQUIREMENTS

Unlike imaging for dental caries, which demands high-contrast images, the periodontal image demands different image characteristics. For one thing, the image should have a longer scale of contrast—that is, to be able to show many more shades of gray than the caries image. Subtle bone changes at the alveolar crest, demonstration of calculus deposits, and the extent of horizontal bone loss are sometimes lost in a high-contrast image. Vertical-, rather than horizontal-oriented, bitewings often are preferred and demand different image detector placement. Figure 9-1 shows the difference between a cavity-detecting radiographic image and one used for periodontal assessment. Figure 9-2 shows two scales of contrast, one with few grays and one with many.

Unfortunately, most x-ray generators currently sold have fixed kV (kilovoltage) settings (usually 70 kV) that preferentially produce high-contrast images for caries detection. Fortunately, the newer image receptors, such as storage phosphor plates and solid-state detectors (CCD or CMOS), discussed later in this chapter may help the clinician to compensate for this shortcoming. Figure 9-3 shows before and after views of a digital image subjected to electronic image processing to enhance periodontally induced disease changes.

In the periodontal assessment, there is a critical need for ideal image geometry to reflect the most accurate horizontal bone levels. Properly positioned bitewing and periapical radiographs for this task require a paralleling technique using appropriate positioning devices. The paralleling technique further requires the image receptor to be positioned away from the teeth, especially in

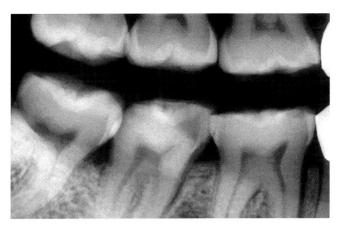

A

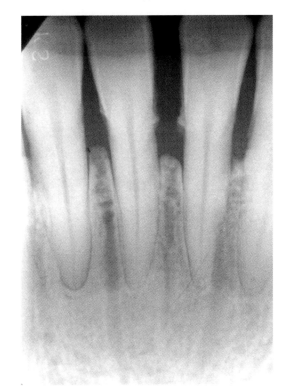

B

Figure 9-1. A, High-contrast x-ray image used for detecting interproximal carious lesions. **B,** X-ray film with a longer gray scale contrast for detecting early bone loss at the alveolar crest.

the maxillary arch, so that the arch curvature and shape does not orient the film or image receptor improperly. Figure 9-4 shows what happens when a maxillary image receptor is placed too close to the teeth. These errors, called "foreshortening" and "elongation," can lead to distortion of the true bone levels. This is much more common in

Long scale (many grays, high kV technique)

Short scale (black and white, low kV technique)

Figure 9-2. A long scale of contrast (top) reveals many shades of gray. A short scale of contrast (bottom) reveals only blacks and whites.

the "bisecting-angle" technique than with the paralleling technique.

The accurate assessment of "bone height" is essential to successful periodontal disease management. Unfortunately, there are many technical errors attributable to radiographic image acquisition that can affect the appearance of the bony structures, and thus the clinician's assessment. "Radiographic bone height" may be different from "actual bone height" because of vertical angulation errors present in poorly positioned films. Radiography is only "shadow casting," and the operator can cast the "shadow" of the bone higher on the radiographic image than is truly present. This is especially true of periapical as opposed to bitewing images. Exposure geometry is extremely important and, if not

compensated for, can lead to serious errors in radiographic interpretation and, consequently, diagnosis. Ritchey and Orban[1] studied the effect of varying exposure geometry on the radiographic appearance of bony defects in dried specimens. Radiographic images at various vertical angulations provided radically different views of the defects. By varying vertical angulation from a baseline of 0 degrees (right angle to the long axis of the tooth) to ±25 degrees, for example, significant furcal radiolucencies could be made to appear larger or to disappear entirely.

SELECTION CRITERIA

Although it should not be controversial, the use of radiographic selection criteria for prescribing medically necessary radiographs has engendered some debate in the dental professional community. **Simply put, no radiograph should be exposed on a patient without performing a thorough, clinical examination first to determine how many images and what types of images are needed for a particular patient.** Thus, it is the clinical examination that determines the number, type, and location of radiographs to be taken. The radiographs are "selected" on the basis of needs dictated by the clinical examination.

The complete periodontal examination will most often require both bitewing radiographs and selected periapical radiographs of the remaining teeth. In many cases, the patient will have a full dentition, therefore the periapical

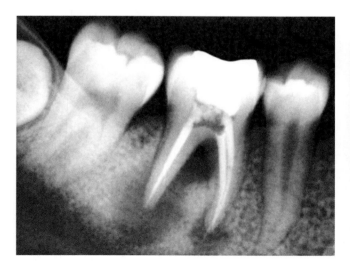
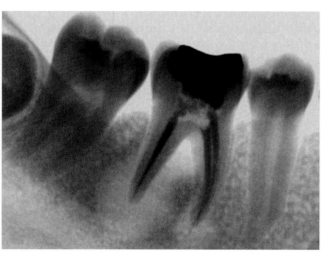

A　　　　　　　　　　　　**B**

Figure 9-3. A, This image shows what appears to be significant bone loss in the furcation area of the first molar. However, when subjected to image processing **(B),** there is more bone apparent in the region as shown by the reverse contrast tool and gray scale information filling most of the "defect."

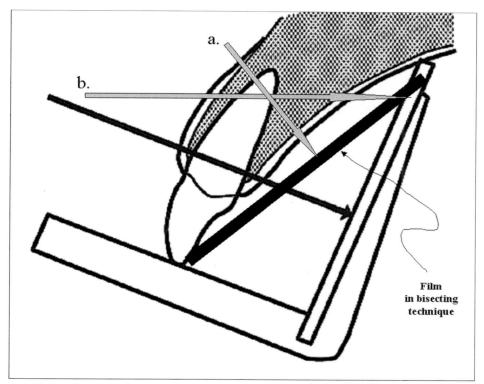

Figure 9-4. If the receptor (film) is placed too close to the teeth, the tooth length will be too short (foreshortening) if the central x-ray beam comes in too steeply, as depicted by the arrow marked *a*, or too long (elongation) if the central x-ray beam comes in too shallow, as depicted by the arrow marked *b*. The receptor (film) needs to be placed farther away from the teeth, against the vertical portion of the film holder.

"coverage" might require as many as 18 to 20 images, conventional (film-based) or perhaps digital (Fig. 9-5). Although intraoral films are generally preferred over panoramic surveys, some investigators have reported close correlation between clinical examination results and bone levels on panoramic films.[2] Indeed, some investigators suggest that panoramic surveys of high quality may be satisfactory if supplemented with intraoral films in selected areas.[3,4]

In addition to periapical radiographs, properly positioned and exposed bitewing radiographs (horizontal or vertical) are considered mandatory in the periodontal

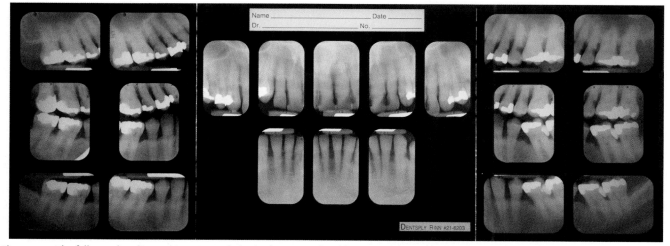

Figure 9-5. The full-mouth radiographic series includes both periapical and bitewing radiographs. The teeth and periodontal structures are visible in their entirety.

"hard-tissue" assessment for most patients, because of the characteristics outlined below:

1. The alveolar crest height is as accurately depicted as possible.
2. The relation of the cementoenamel junction (CEJ) to the alveolar crest can be accurately determined.
3. The presence of vertical bony defects can be demonstrated more precisely than with periapical images.
4. Early crestal bone loss in the posterior dentition can be found more readily than with periapical images.

Using an appropriate combination of bitewing and periapical radiographs, the clinician can create a complete and accurate picture of the bony changes related to periodontitis for patient treatment planning and disease management. Using individualized selection criteria, judicious prescription for and careful exposure of the necessary images is made only *after* a thorough clinical examination and review of the patient history.

RADIOGRAPHIC IMAGE TYPES AND TECHNIQUES

There are three basic intraoral radiographic techniques to consider for assessment of the bone status in patients with clinical features of periodontitis. This discussion is limited to features of the images created using these techniques, rather than the techniques themselves. (Refer to contemporary textbooks on oral and maxillofacial radiology for explanation of the actual positioning techniques.) The standard techniques for radiographic assessment of the patient with suspected periodontal bone loss are:

1. Horizontal bitewing
2. Vertical bitewing
3. Periapical

Horizontal Bitewing Technique

Bitewing radiographs are probably the most important images for establishing the true radiographic picture of the alveolar bone height in most patients with periodontal disease. With the teeth in a close approximation of their normal occlusion, the angulation used (positive 7 to 10 degrees) is favorable to projecting the image of both the maxillary and mandibular posterior teeth in their most parallel orientation. Well positioned, well exposed, horizontal bitewings will give excellent image geometry and will result in the most accurate diagnostic images of the teeth and crestal bone (Fig. 9-6). Horizontal bitewings are usually ordered when the patient has suspected "mild to moderate" horizontal bone loss, as determined by the clinical examination.

If properly positioned, the clinician should expect to see:

1. Superimposition of the buccal and lingual/palatal cusps

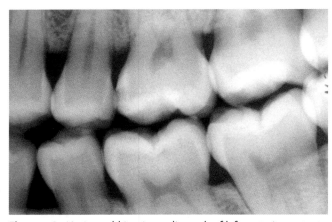

Figure 9-6. Horizontal bitewing radiograph of left posterior sextants. Note that the bony crest is visible in both arches, but it is close to the edge of the film between the mandibular premolars. The root trunks of the molar teeth are not entirely visible.

2. A sharp or well-defined alveolar crestal margin
3. No horizontal "overlap" between adjacent teeth (i.e., "open" interproximal spaces without overlap in the contact areas)

Vertical Bitewing Technique

Vertical bitewings are useful if the patient has demonstrated deep probing depths on clinical examination and the clinician expects the patient to have moderate to severe horizontal bone loss. Some clinicians prefer vertical bitewings over horizontal bitewings for the majority of patients with any signs of alveolar bone loss.

The operator should be cautioned about two potential problems during image acquisition. The first is that the image receptor (film) oriented vertically will impinge more readily on the palatal curvature because of the increased height of the receptor (film). This is especially true if the patient has a relatively shallow palatal vault. This impingement may lead to image distortion. The second is that vertical orientation reduces the image information in an anterior–posterior dimension because the receptor is narrower in the horizontal direction in this orientation. Thus, there may be an additional vertical image required for complete coverage of the structures being examined. Figure 9-7 shows examples of vertical bitewing radiographs.

Periapical Technique

Periapical radiographs make excellent supplemental images for periodontal bone level determination and are essential for assessing the crown-to-root ratio, root morphology, periodontal ligament spaces, and periapical status. The two types of images discussed, bitewing and periapical, are complementary and both image sets most likely will be

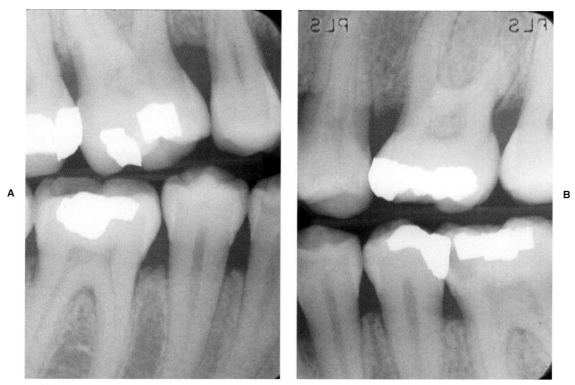

Figure 9-7. Vertical bitewing radiographs of the right **(A)** and left **(B)** posterior regions. Note that a greater amount of alveolar bone is visible compared with the horizontal bitewing shown in Figure 9-6. The root trunks of the molar teeth are visible in their entirety. However, because the film is oriented vertically, there is less visibility anteroposteriorly. Thus, an additional vertical bitewing would be needed on each side to see all the posterior teeth.

necessary for patients with periodontal problems. However, applying selection criteria principles, periapical images are not mandatory on every patient. The patient with simple gingivitis and no evidence of attachment loss may not require periapical images. If the bitewing images are properly exposed and assessed, they will indicate the need for prescribing additional periapical radiographs in many cases. That being said, bitewing images are unable to provide information that may be critical to diagnosis and treatment planning, such as the position of important anatomic structures (e.g., mandibular nerve, floor of the maxillary sinus) and the presence or absence of periapical lesions. If such information is needed, the selection criteria would dictate that the clinician order the appropriate periapical radiographs.

RADIOGRAPHIC INTERPRETATION AS APPLIED TO THE PERIODONTAL PATIENT

Use and Limitations

It is not possible to render a definitive periodontal diagnosis by means of a radiograph.[5] For example, consider the patient with advanced periodontitis who has had a good clinical response to adequate and appropriate therapy. The patient may well have minimal probing depths, but the radiographic bone levels will likely remain largely unchanged after treatment. It will be impossible to determine whether that individual requires further treatment by examining posttreatment radiographs alone. Conversely, serial radiographs taken at baseline (pretreatment) and at subsequent appointments may reveal ongoing bone loss and, therefore, will be indispensable, but only in the context of supplementing the findings from the clinical examination.

Another obvious example is the endodontically involved mandibular molar that reveals radiolucency in the furcation region. Probing may reveal no increase in probing depth or clinical attachment loss—that is, there has been no apical migration of the epithelial attachment and the sulcus is not continuous with the furcation area. This is strictly an endodontic problem unless and until the sulcus becomes continuous with the furcation (see Chapter 30). Nevertheless, the radiographic image may mimic the appearance of significant furcation involvement caused by periodontal destruction.

The caveat needs to be borne in mind then that the radiographic appearance may be deceptive in that

(1) bone loss may be more advanced than indicated by the radiograph, (2) a radiograph taken at one point in time says nothing about disease activity or progress, but only represents a history of tissue destruction, and (3) radiographs cannot be used as a surrogate measure of probing depth (or any aspect of the clinical examination). Despite these limitations, however, radiographs are absolutely necessary in the proper diagnosis and treatment of periodontitis. There is much information that can be obtained *only* from radiographs[5,6]: root length and morphology, root trunk dimensions, crown-to-root ratio, an approximate idea of bone destruction, coronal extent of the interdental septum, some sense of the bony topography, and anatomic structures that may be of interest when planning therapy (e.g., mental foramen, mandibular canal, maxillary sinus, nasal cavity). Similarly, there are a number of parameters that cannot be assessed using conventional radiography[5,6]: periodontal probing depth or attachment levels, morphology of bony defects (although this may be suggested), soft-to-hard tissue relation, tooth mobility, and bony topography on the buccal and lingual surfaces of the teeth.[7]

Interdental Septum and Crestal Lamina Dura

One of the areas of chief interest in the periodontal examination is the interdental septum. The interdental sep-

tum, or septal bone, is located between the roots of adjacent teeth. It is therefore more clearly visualized than bone that is located on the buccal or lingual aspect of the tooth (the latter being partially obscured by the superimposed image of the root). The shape of the interdental septum is a function of the morphology of the contiguous teeth. Teeth that are quite convex on the approximating surfaces (i.e., "cup-shaped") will give rise to a wider interdental space in the mesiodistal dimension. This will result in flatter, broader septa of larger mesiodistal width. Teeth that present with a flatter, less convex interproximal profile will tend to produce narrower interdental spaces. This results in formation of a "septal peak" and is most commonly seen in the anterior regions. Loss of this architecture results in "blunting" or loss of septal height and may indicate early periodontitis (although evidence of clinical attachment loss will precede radiographically evident bone loss). Figure 9-8 shows early and more advanced blunting of the septal crests.

The normal shape of the crowns of the posterior teeth gives rise to a relatively flat alveolar crest and this, in turn, results in a rather flat interdental image on the bitewing radiograph. The thin, radiopaque line at the top of the crest, which is continuous with the lamina dura adjacent to the periodontal ligament (PDL), is known as the crestal

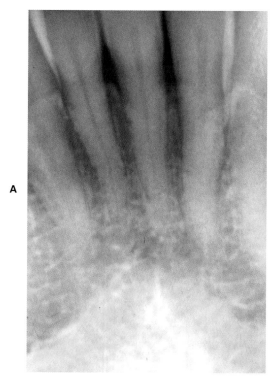
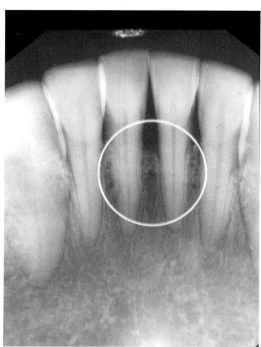

Figure 9-8. A, Early loss of the septal peak between the mandibular incisors. **B,** More advanced loss of the septal peak. As bone loss occurs, the clinician can see that the distance between the alveolar crest and the cementoenamel junction increases.

lamina dura (Fig. 9-9). It has been suggested that loss of the crestal lamina dura may correspond to periodontal disease activity. However, failure to visualize the crestal lamina dura with conventional imaging may occur in a high percentage of interproximal sites, and thus may be regarded as within normal limits.[8] Greenstein and co-workers[9] report that the crestal lamina dura is not significantly related to any of a number of clinical periodontal parameters. While the *absence* of the crestal lamina is not indicative of current or impending disease activity, there is evidence to suggest that the *presence* of a crestal lamina dura may be associated with clinical stability.[8] Increased

density of the crestal lamina dura has been reported after successful periodontal therapy.[10] Normally, the alveolar crest meets the lamina dura at a right angle. However, when teeth are tipped, the appearance of the crestal lamina may mimic a vertical bone defect. **Because of the improper vertical angulation or orientation of the tipped tooth, the CEJ is positioned inferiorly relative to the adjacent tooth. This creates the impression of a vertical bony defect when in reality there is no bony defect.** A similar "CEJ discrepancy" can occur as a simple anatomic variation from normal. Some people have a mesial tilt to the posterior teeth that can result in the appearance of vertical defects adjacent to the mesial surfaces of multiple teeth. Figure 9-9 provides for an explanation of this phenomenon. Ritchey and Orban[11] report that lines drawn between the adjacent CEJs should parallel the crestal lamina dura, and this simple test will readily distinguish true vertical defects from "pseudo-defects" caused by tooth angulation.

Radiographic Evidence of Bone Loss

A number of investigators, using dried jaw specimens, have determined that significant amounts of bone must be removed before bone loss is visible on conventional radiographs. Ortman and co-workers[12] used dried specimens with artificially created bone defects and report that radiographic examination tends to underestimate the artificial bone loss when 30% or less of the bone was removed. Bender and Seltzer[13] found that mandibular lesions created with a bur were not visible until some cortical bone was removed. Ramadan and Mitchell[14] determined that significant amounts of bone removal in their dried specimens did not consistently produce changes in the radiographic images.

In clinical studies on actual patients, most investigators have found that radiographic images tend to underestimate bone loss as compared with clinical measurements.[15-20] The amount by which this loss is underestimated has been variously reported as 1.2,[21] 1.3,[18] and 2.3 mm.[17] This is important for the clinician to keep in mind, because the radiographic examination is likely to give a "best case scenario." Treatment plans, therefore, should account for the potential to find more significant bone loss during surgical therapy. In one recent study, radiographic images significantly underestimated bone levels when compared with direct measurements made during surgery.[22] Some workers also have reported that this tendency is more pronounced in untreated than treated sites.[18] Lastly, it has been shown that clinical changes (i.e., clinical attachment loss) precede radiographic changes.[23]

One of the primary problems in radiographic examination is the lack of consistency among serial radiographs taken under normal clinical conditions.[24] Relatively small changes in film positioning can result in large changes

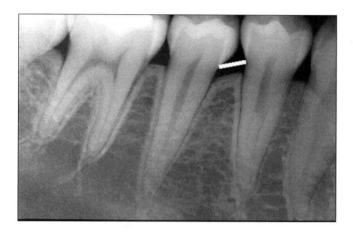

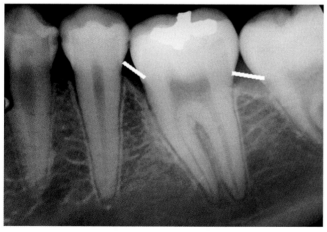

Figure 9-9. The crestal lamina dura is apparent between the premolar and molars in these radiographs. In each radiograph, if a line is drawn from the cementoenamel junction (CEJ) of one tooth to the CEJ of the adjacent tooth, and that line parallels the alveolar crest, then there is no true vertical bone defect. The "apparent" vertical defect is really caused by tooth angulation/inclination. If a measurement is made from the CEJ to the crest of bone at each tooth surface, the measurement is approximately 1.5 to 2.0 mm, indicating that the crestal bone is at a normal height. This patient therefore has no bone loss and no vertical bony defects.

in bone appearance. Lesions can appear or disappear. Generally, changes in bone height have been determined by comparing the distance from the CEJ to the alveolar crest at two different time points (e.g., before and after some type of treatment). If a certain amount of loss is detected, then the label of "bone loss" can be affixed. Given the variations in consistency, various thresholds of bone loss have been described, ranging from greater than 1 mm to greater than 3 mm.[25,26]

The lack of consistency is not to suggest that the radiograph is useless or ineffective in the diagnosis of periodontal disease. Although clinical attachment loss is often more advanced than would be indicated by the radiograph, the latter is often a good approximation of the former. Prichard[6] suggests that the radiograph should be a "critic" of the clinical examination, and further cautions that if there is a pronounced lack of congruity between what is seen radiographically and the results of the clinical examination, then a reason must be sought so that these conflicting data can be reconciled. An example might be a patient with good home care and a history of previous periodontal therapy. Periodontal probing reveals minimal probing depths with little recession. The radiographs, however, reveal significant horizontal bone loss. The most obvious reason for this seeming anomaly is the presence of a long junctional epithelial attachment subsequent to the previous periodontal intervention. In this case, *repair* took place and health was restored, but complete *regeneration* of the attachment apparatus, including the alveolar bone, did not occur. The opposite condition may also be observed. For example, a patient presents for routine examination and a 10-mm pocket is detected on the distolingual aspect of the mandibular right second molar; however, there is no radiographic evidence of a bone defect at this site. Again, there is a simple explanation: the dense (i.e., radiopaque) buccal and lingual cortical plates in this molar region are superimposed on the defect image, thereby preventing it from being seen on the radiograph. In the event of such inconsistency between clinical and radiographic examinations, however, it is prudent to reexamine the site (or sites) clinically to ensure that pathology has not been overlooked.

Patterns of Bone Loss and Defect Morphology

A distinction often is made between "horizontal" bone loss and "vertical" bone loss. Horizontal bone loss is the symmetric loss of bone on both the mesial and distal surfaces of contiguous teeth such that the bony architecture appears to be rather flat. This is in contrast to vertical bone defects, which have a funnel-shaped appearance and plunge apically on one tooth surface, whereas there is little or no bone loss on the contiguous tooth surface (Fig. 9-10).

One variant of this pattern is the so-called hemiseptal defect in which significant bone loss has occurred on the

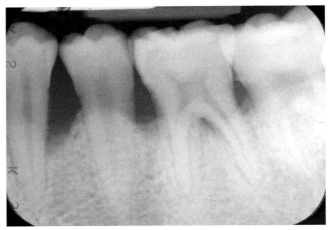

Figure 9-10. Periapical radiograph of lower left posterior sextant showing multiple vertical defects. The most prominent is on the distal aspect of tooth #21. Note the more coronal position of the bony crest on the mesial of tooth #20 compared with the distal of #21. This radiograph also demonstrates radiographic suggestion of calculus on the mesial of tooth #18, mesial of #19, and distal of #21. A radiolucent area suggestive of bone loss also is noted in the furcation of tooth #19.

proximal surface of one tooth, to the extent that both buccal and lingual cortical plates have been destroyed, but the bone level on the adjacent tooth surface is at a relatively normal level (or at least has not experienced the same degree of loss).[6] Thus, roughly one half of the interdental septum is lost, giving rise to the term *hemiseptal*. These defects (also known as "one-wall" defects because they have only one bony wall facing the involved tooth surface) are among the most challenging to treat. (See Chapter 23.)

The most common type of periodontal osseous defect is the two-walled interdental crater, which is located between adjacent posterior teeth. (See Chapter 23.) The walls referred to represent the buccal and lingual *bony* walls. The presence of buccal and lingual bony walls, with their cortical bone intact, often prevents these defects from being clearly visualized by conventional radiography. The three-walled defect is the type of bony defect most amenable to regeneration. Like the two-walled crater, this defect may be difficult to visualize on the radiograph, because the buccal and lingual walls remain intact and obscure the radiographic image of the defect.

When the clinician examines a radiographic series of the entire mouth, some patterns of bone loss are strongly suggestive of certain disease entities. Recognition of patterns of bone loss is valuable in establishing a diagnosis and formulating a treatment plan. For example, in determining whether a diagnosis of generalized or localized disease will be made, the radiographs may be of significant value. This is particularly true of localized aggressive periodontitis (previously referred to as "localized juvenile periodontitis")[27] (see Chapter 2). This clinical entity is essentially defined by involvement of some or all of the first molars and incisors, with little involvement of other teeth.

Periodontal Ligament Space

The periodontal ligament space often can be discerned on routine radiographs as a thin radiolucent line interposed between the root and the radiopaque line that outlines the root. This radiopaque line (which is not consistently visible in all projections) is the image of the cribriform plate or alveolar bone proper. This radiographic image is known as the *lamina dura*, which is continuous with the *crestal* lamina dura (discussed earlier), which is the radiopaque line at the most superior aspect of the interdental septum (see Fig. 9-9). The width of the PDL has been considered important in the diagnosis of various conditions, including occlusal trauma (see Chapter 29). However, the PDL width varies with varying tube/film geometry and exposure conditions and with root morphology.[28] Thus, it has not been demonstrated that PDL width can be measured consistently and reliably with conventional radiographs. Nonetheless, various authorities have suggested that a widened PDL space is suggestive of occlusal trauma.[29] Specifically, occlusal trauma may be manifested as a widening of the PDL space or may present as a funneling of the coronal aspect of the PDL space. Widening of the periodontal ligament space also is seen in vertical root fractures,[30,31] in progressive systemic sclerosis (scleroderma),[32-34] and occasionally as a manifestation of periapical pathology.

Furcation Defects

Loss of bone in the furcation areas of molar teeth may occur as a result of periodontitis, endodontic infection, root perforation during dental procedures, or occlusal trauma. These changes are most readily seen in the mandibular molar region. Because most mandibular molars have only two roots, one mesial and one distal, any loss of bone where the roots meet the crown is normally detected easily (see Figs. 9-10 and 9-11). There is a radiolucent appearance in the furcation, and the clinician often can follow the bone level from the interproximal areas to the furcation.

Because most maxillary molars have three roots, early change in their furcation areas are more difficult to assess. Bone loss in the facial furcation may occasionally be detected on radiographs, but the superimposition of the palatal root makes such detection difficult. Defects occurring between the mesiobuccal and palatal roots and between the distobuccal and palatal roots often are easier

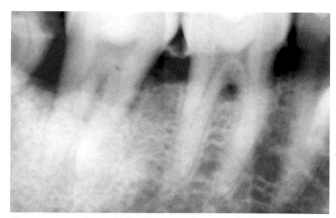

Figure 9-11. Radiograph demonstrates distinct radiolucency in the furcation region of the mandibular first molar, suggestive of furcal bone loss. Note also the appearance of heavy calculus deposits. The roots of the first molar are relatively divergent, whereas the roots of the second molar are in close proximity.

to detect radiographically. Lesions involving these mesial and distal furcations often are manifested by the presence of furcation "arrows"[35] (Fig. 9-12). Approximately 30% to 55% of grade 2 or 3 furcation involvements have a furcation arrow present on the radiograph. Thus, although the furcation arrow is a useful tool to complement the clinical examination, it should not be relied on as a lone diagnostic tool to detect mesial and distal maxillary molar furcation defects, because many furcations with bone loss do not demonstrate a furcation arrow. Conversely, the presence of the furcation arrow had a high degree of specificity (relatively few false-positives)—that is, furcation areas without bone loss rarely showed a furcation arrow on the radiograph.

Tests with a high specificity often are clinically useful.[36] In such a test, the results are almost always *negative* (e.g., no furcation arrow present on the radiograph) when the condition being assessed (e.g., furcation involvement) is *absent*. If a furcation arrow is *present* on the radiograph, there is a high likelihood that a furcation involvement is *present*. This is of particular interest in the case of the mesial and distal maxillary molar furcations, which are difficult to evaluate clinically because of their interproximal location. Therefore, it is suggested that the clinician compare the radiographic appearance of the maxillary molars with the clinical findings. If furcation arrows are present, but the examination reveals no furcation involvement, it may be prudent to reevaluate those sites clinically.

Root Morphology

The radiograph is the only method, short of direct observation, of visualizing the morphology of the roots. There

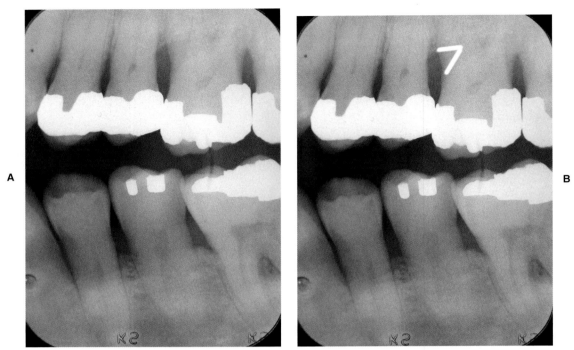

Figure 9-12. Loss of bone in the mesial and distal furcations of maxillary molars may present as a "furcation arrow" **(A)** such as that seen in this vertical bitewing radiograph. **B,** The arrow is simply a triangular region shaped like an arrowhead, with its tip pointing directly into the furcation opening on the mesial aspect of the maxillary first molar. These radiographs also suggest loss of bone in the mandibular first molar furcation.

are a number of radiographic parameters that may be of clinical significance, including the length of the root trunk, root length, root divergence/convergence, root resorption, and root shape. The most fundamental dimension of interest is the length of the root, both in absolute terms and relative to the apicocoronal dimension of the crown. The ratio between the two is the so-called crown-to-root ratio. Radiographs also can reveal root resorption, either idiopathic or as a result of orthodontic tooth movement. Root resorption deprives the tooth of support just as periodontitis does. Clinically significant root resorption may jeopardize the prognosis of affected teeth. This is particularly true when resorption occurs in a setting of previous attachment loss. For this reason, it is suggested that adult orthodontic patients receive a pretreatment radiographic series and periodic films throughout treatment to detect such changes.

The root trunk is of particular interest in periodontal disease and treatment. The root trunk is the dimension from the CEJ to the furcal entrance. Teeth with short root trunks may have earlier furcation invasion and may be less amenable to osseous resective surgery and crown lengthening (because these techniques may result in iatrogenic furcation defects) (see Chapter 23). Conversely, teeth with unusually long root trunks (i.e., those with a taurodont appearance) may be difficult or impossible to treat once the furcation is invaded, because of its apical position.

Roots of multirooted teeth often diverge or become more separated as they course apically (see Fig. 9-11). Sometimes, however, they will converge or come closer together. This is more common for second molars than for first molars. This root convergence may complicate furcation therapy, because access is limited. Root resection is made more complicated by convergence. Extremely divergent roots may present difficulties in extraction, often requiring resection before extraction of the tooth.

Radiographic examination may reveal other root anomalies such as gemination or fusion,[37] root dilacerations, and additional roots that would not generally be present on certain teeth, such as a third root on mandibular molars or double-rooted mandibular premolars. Such root anatomy may impact periodontal therapy and should be noted during the examination and diagnostic phases of periodontal treatment.

Calculus

Clinically significant calculus deposits often are seen on routine radiographic examination (see Figs. 9-11 and 9-13). However, the radiograph is not a sensitive indicator of calculus. Buchanan and co-workers[38] report that radiographic evaluation of calculus did not correlate well with its presence. Although the false-positive rate was only 7.5%, the sensitivity (i.e., the proportion of sites with calculus that also have radiographic

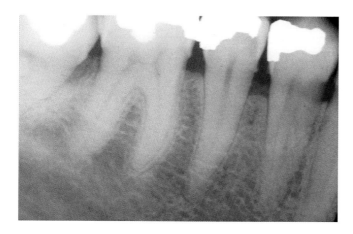

A

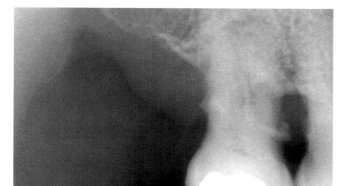

B

Figure 9-13. A, Small "spurs" of calculus at the cementoenamel junction of each of the mandibular posterior teeth are revealed. **B,** Demonstration of much heavier calculus deposits surrounding the circumference of the maxillary molar.

evidence of calculus) was poor at 44%. These authors conclude that conventional radiography is not a very discriminating method of calculus detection.[38] When any radiographic subgingival calculus is observed, it is usually indicative of very heavy deposits. The clinician should not interpret the absence of radiographic calculus as indicative of an absence of calculus clinically, because most subgingival calculus deposits will not be present radiographically.

DIGITAL IMAGING AND PERIODONTAL BONE LOSS

Many clinicians are adopting digital x-ray systems to replace conventional film-based images. It is likely that this conversion to digital systems will continue in the future, as it has in medicine. Every image acquired digit-

ally in medicine is changed or processed to extract features about the disease process under consideration. In fact, manufacturers of these medical systems often produce software algorithms for particular diseases—for example, a computer program is required to optimize the image for breast calcifications or lung nodules. These two imaging programs would require very different processing software because breast calcifications are small and scattered, whereas lung nodules are larger and more diffuse. The breast calcification detection would require a program with far greater contrast resolution than the lung lesion.

Because periodontal bone change can be subtle, digital subtraction radiography (DSR) techniques (software algorithms) have been developed. Unfortunately, their use is not commonplace so their cost remains high. But they represent one of the few areas in all of dentistry where dentists can quantify disease change, even at very early stages.[39]

In the DSR technique, a second image is taken at some point after the initial image. The images are then compared after normalization and image alignment. The elements that remained unchanged are "subtracted" from the two images and the remaining image information is displayed. Using pseudocolorization techniques, only the areas that changed are visible to the dentist.[40] Positive and negative changes will be shown and these areas of change measured to calculate the percent differences. Figure 9-14 shows a typical subtraction image. An early technical challenge in DSR was the requirement that the consecutive images be closely aligned for an accurate comparison to be made. This was accomplished using custom stents and other devices that made the technique less practical for clinical use. Recent technologic enhancements have enabled compensation for imprecision in placement, thereby allowing for the accurate "superimposition" of the images, which is required for DSR.[39] This has made DSR much easier, and it is widely used in periodontal research. However, the technique is still not commonly used by clinicians.

Continued advances in this field will undoubtedly result in DSR protocols and instrumentation that are less technique-sensitive, while providing robust diagnostic data.[41] One promise of this technology is the ability to detect very early changes in bone level.[42] This would enable early interventions that may be both more cost-effective and less invasive than treatment performed at a later date, when the periodontal destruction is more advanced. Another application is the evaluation of regenerative therapies such as guided tissue regeneration and bone grafting. Early results have been encouraging, but more work is needed in this field.[43,44] Jeffcoat and Reddy[45] also have demonstrated that DSR can be useful in evaluating periimplant bone changes.

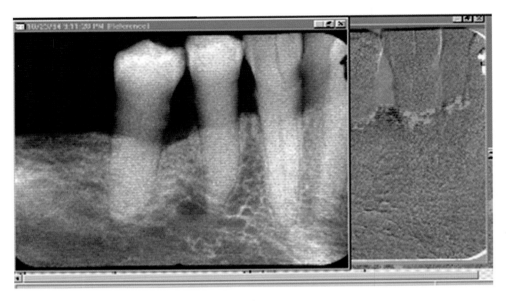

A

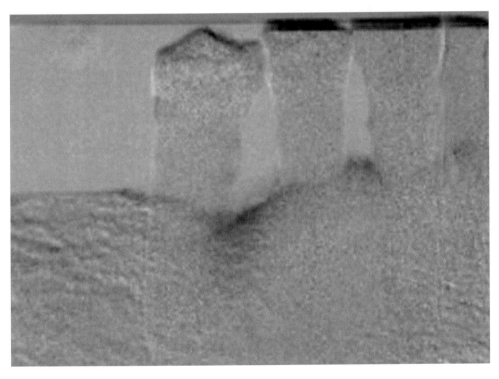

B

Figure 9-14. Digital subtraction radiographic (DSR) technique used to assess the effects of periodontal therapy in area of teeth #27 to #29. The radiograph on the left **(A)** is subjected to color enhancement (right) to show areas with increased bone density in red and areas of decreased bone density in green. DSR measures changes in bone density over time. **B,** The unenhanced DSR image shows areas of increased bone density as dark areas in the interdental bony crest region between teeth #27 and #28, and #28 and #29. Subtle changes in bone density are more difficult to see without color enhancement algorithms.

Continued

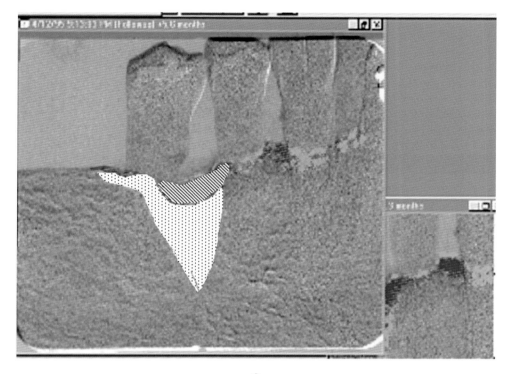

C

Figure 9-14. cont'd. C, Other enhancement techniques can be formulated to show areas of significant change (e.g., hash-marked area at bony crest between teeth #28 and #29 showed most intense gain in bone density; whereas the dotted region extending further apically between teeth #28 and #29 showed less intense change, with mixed gain/loss in bone density). (Adapted from Newman M, Takei H, Carranza F: *Carranza's clinical periodontology*, ed 9, Philadelphia, 2002, WB Saunders.)

PRESURGICAL PLANNING

Radiographs are indispensable as presurgical planning aids. Before surgical intervention, it is necessary to know the location of vital structures that may be in proximity to the surgical site. This is true in periodontal surgical procedures and even more applicable in the surgical placement of dental implants (see Chapter 26). Many implant protocols call for a certain minimal space (e.g., 2 mm) between the apical extent of the osteotomy site and any vital structure, such as the mandibular canal. Such an allowance is necessary, because the implant drills usually have beveled points that extend beyond the depth of the actual implant insertion. Because this type of surgery often involves placing implants in relatively close proximity to such structures, it is necessary to know the vertical and horizontal magnification of the radiographic image. For example, the panoramic radiographic image often is used in planning implant surgery. These images have a certain clinically significant degree of magnification and this must be compensated for to avoid surgical misadventure. Most implant manufacturers supply clear plastic templates with images of their implants at various magnification levels to aid in the treatment planning process.

In addition to knowledge about the location of structures such as the maxillary sinus and mandibular canal, certain imaging techniques provide information regarding bone density. Computed tomography (CT) produces images made up of individual units known as *voxels*. The density of the image is measured in *Hounsfield units*, named for the inventor of CT: Sir Godfrey Hounsfield. Water has a Hounsfield value of 0 and is the standard for comparison. It is possible to relate the density of the CT image in Hounsfield units to the density of the bone.[46] This information is valuable in assessing the suitability of a site for dental implant placement and also may have implications for decisions concerning the timing of implant loading and decisions regarding what type of implant surface would be preferred for a given site. Although it is beyond the scope of this chapter to consider these techniques in detail, a diagnostic wax up and stent are usually required, with some sort of radiopaque marker to indicate the proposed site of the planned implant fixture.[47] (See Chapter 26.) Cross-sectional images often are valuable during the diagnostic phase of implant therapy, and CT is one technique many clinicians prefer, especially when multiple implants are to be placed. Linear and spiral tomography also are available for cross-sectional imaging, and they often are preferred when only one or a few implants are to be placed. Although tomography is not always required in implant treatment planning, it is a great aid in situations in which conventional radiographic images do not provide sufficient information.

CONCLUSION

The radiograph and clinical periodontal examination complement one another. Neither is sufficient by itself, but together they can provide a sound foundation for diagnosis and treatment planning. Despite certain limitations, the conventional dental radiograph is an indispensable adjunct in diagnosis and treatment planning. While acknowledging the value of diagnostic imaging, it is wise to remember its limitations and to take these into account during the treatment planning process. It is likely that continued improvements in imaging technology will improve the clinical use of radiographic imaging and permit earlier and more accurate visualization of relatively small changes in bone topography.[48,49]

REFERENCES

1. Ritchey TR, Orban BJ: Three-dimensional roentgenographic interpretation in periodontal diagnosis, *J Periodontol* 31:275-282, 1960.
2. Walsh TF, al-Hokail OS, Fosam EB: The relationship of bone loss observed on panoramic radiographs with clinical periodontal screening, *J Clin Periodontol* 24:153-157, 1997.
3. Akesson L, Rohlin M, Hakansson J et al: Comparison between panoramic and posterior bitewing radiography in the diagnosis of periodontal bone loss, *J Dent* 17:266-271, 1989.
4. Akesson L, Rohlin M, Hakansson J: Marginal bone in periodontal disease: an evaluation of image quality in panoramic and intra-oral radiography, *Dentomaxillofac Radiol* 18:105-112, 1989.
5. Prichard JF: Interpretation of radiographs in periodontics, *Int J Periodontics Restorative Dent* 3:8-39, 1983.
6. Prichard JF: *Advanced periodontal disease: surgical and prosthetic management*, ed 2, Philadelphia, 1972, WB Saunders.
7. Rees TD, Biggs NL, Collings CK: Radiographic interpretation of periodontal osseous lesions, *Oral Surg Oral Med Oral Pathol* 32:141-153, 1971.
8. Rams TE, Listgarten MA, Slots J: Utility of radiographic crestal lamina dura for predicting periodontitis disease-activity, *J Clin Periodontol* 21:571-576, 1994.
9. Greenstein G, Polson A, Iker H, Meitner S: Associations between crestal lamina dura and periodontal status, *J Periodontol* 52:362-366, 1981.
10. Dubrez B, Graf JM, Vuagnat P, Cimasoni G: Increase of interproximal bone density after subgingival instrumentation: a quantitative radiographical study, *J Periodontol* 61:725-731, 1990.
11. Ritchey TR, Orban BJ: Crests of the interdental alveolar septa, *J Periodontol* 24:17, 1953.
12. Ortman LF, McHenry K, Hausmann E: Relationship between alveolar bone measured by 125I absorptiometry with analysis of standardized radiographs: 2. Bjorn technique, *J Periodontol* 53:311-314, 1982.
13. Bender I, Seltzer D: Roentgenographic and direct observation of experimental lesions in bone, *J Am Dent Assoc* 62:152-160, 1961.
14. Ramadan A, Mitchell D: Roentgenographic study of experimental bone destruction, *Oral Surg Oral Med Oral Pathol* 15:934-943, 1962.
15. Suomi JD, Plumbo J, Barbano JP: A comparative study of radiographs and pocket measurements in periodontal disease evaluation, *J Periodontol* 39:311-315, 1968.
16. Eickholz P, Benn DK, Staehle HJ: Radiographic evaluation of bone regeneration following periodontal surgery with or without expanded polytetrafluoroethylene barriers, *J Periodontol* 67:379-385, 1996.
17. Akesson L, Hakansson J, Rohlin M: Comparison of panoramic and intraoral radiography and pocket probing for the measurement of the marginal bone level, *J Clin Periodontol* 19:326-332, 1992.
18. Tonetti MS, Pini Prato G, Williams RC, Cortellini P: Periodontal regeneration of human infrabony defects. III. Diagnostic strategies to detect bone gain, *J Periodontol* 64:269-277, 1993.
19. Shrout MK, Hildebolt CF, Vannier MW: The effect of alignment errors on bitewing-based bone loss measurements, *J Clin Periodontol* 18:708-712, 1991.
20. Hausmann E: A contemporary perspective on techniques for the clinical assessment of alveolar bone, *J Periodontol* 61:149-156, 1990.
21. Eickholz P, Kim TS, Benn DK, Staehle HJ: Validity of radiographic measurement of interproximal bone loss, *Oral Surg Oral Med Oral Pathol Oral Radiol Endod* 85:99-106, 1998.
22. Eickholz P, Hausmann E: Accuracy of radiographic assessment of interproximal bone loss in intrabony defects using linear measurements, *Eur J Oral Sci* 108:70-73, 2000.
23. Goodson JM, Haffajee AD, Socransky SS: The relationship between attachment level loss and alveolar bone loss, *J Clin Periodontol* 11:348-359, 1984.
24. Benn DK: A review of the reliability of radiographic measurements in estimating alveolar bone changes, *J Clin Periodontol* 17:14-21, 1990.
25. Hugoson A, Rylander H: Longitudinal study of periodontal status in individuals aged 15 years in 1973 and 20 years in 1978 in Jonkoping, Sweden, *Community Dent Oral Epidemiol* 10:37-42, 1982.

26. Latcham NL, Powell RN, Jago JD et al: A radiographic study of chronic periodontitis in 15 year old Queensland children, *J Clin Periodontol* 10:37-45, 1983.

27. Tonetti MS, Mombelli A: Early-onset periodontitis, *Ann Periodontol* 4:39-53, 1999.

28. van der Linden LW, van Aken J: The periodontal ligament in the roentgenogram, *J Periodontol* 41:243-248, 1970.

29. Carranza FA, Takei H: Radiographic aids in the diagnosis of periodontal disease. In Newman M, Takei H, Carranza FA, editors, *Carranza's clinical periodontology*, ed 9, Philadelphia, 2002, WB Saunders.

30. Testori T, Badino M, Castagnola M: Vertical root fractures in endodontically treated teeth: a clinical survey of 36 cases, *J Endod* 19:87-91, 1993.

31. Bergenholtz G, Hasselgren G: Endodontics and periodontics. In Lindhe J, Karring T, Lang NP, editors, *Clinical periodontology and implant dentistry*, ed 3, Copenhagen, 1997, Munksgaard.

32. Janssens X, Herman L, Mielants H et al: Disease manifestations of progressive systemic sclerosis: sensitivity and specificity, *Clin Rheumatol* 6:532-538, 1987.

33. Robbins JW, Craig RM, Jr, Correll RW: Symmetrical widening of the periodontal ligament space in a patient with multiple systemic problems, *J Am Dent Assoc* 113:307-308, 1986.

34. Alexandridis C, White SC: Periodontal ligament changes in patients with progressive systemic sclerosis, *Oral Surg Oral Med Oral Pathol* 58:113-118, 1984.

35. Hardekopf JD, Dunlap RM, Ahl DR, Pelleu GB Jr: The "furcation arrow." A reliable radiographic image?, *J Periodontol* 58:258-261, 1987.

36. Sackett D, Strauss S, Richardson W et al: *Evidence-based medicine: how to practice and teach EBM*, Edinburgh, 2000, Churchill Livingstone.

37. Trebilcock CE, Mealey BL, Dickson SS: Multidisciplinary restoration of fused maxillary incisors: a case report, *Pract Periodontics Aesthet Dent* 7:47-53; quiz 54, 1995.

38. Buchanan SA, Jenderseck RS, Granet MA et al: Radiographic detection of dental calculus. *J Periodontol* 58:747-751, 1987.

39. Jeffcoat MK, Reddy MS, Webber RL et al: Extraoral control of geometry for digital subtraction radiography, *J Periodont Res* 22:396-402, 1987.

40. Reddy MS, Bruch JM, Jeffcoat MK, Williams RC: Contrast enhancement as an aid to interpretation in digital subtraction radiography, *Oral Surg Oral Med Oral Pathol* 71:763-769, 1991.

41. Nummikoski PV, Steffensen B, Hamilton K, Dove SB: Clinical validation of a new subtraction radiography technique for periodontal bone loss detection, *J Periodontol* 71:598-605, 2000.

42. Griffiths GS, Bragger U, Fourmousis I, Sterne JA: Use of an internal standard in subtraction radiography to assess initial periodontal bone changes, *Dentomaxillofac Radiol* 25:76-81, 1996.

43. Christgau M, Wenzel A, Hiller KA, Schmalz G: Quantitative digital subtraction radiography for assessment of bone density changes following periodontal guided tissue regeneration, *Dentomaxillofac Radiol* 25:25-33, 1996.

44. Wenzel A, Warrer K, Karring T: Digital subtraction radiography in assessing bone changes in periodontal defects following guided tissue regeneration, *J Clin Periodontol* 19:208-213, 1992.

45. Jeffcoat MK, Reddy MS: Digital subtraction radiography for longitudinal assessment of peri-implant bone change: method and validation, *Adv Dent Res* 7:196-201, 1993.

46. Kircos LT, Misch CE: Diagnostic and imaging techniques. In Misch CE, editor, *Contemporary implant dentistry*, St. Louis, 1999, Mosby, pp 73-87.

47. Rosenfeld AL, Mecall RA: Using computerized tomography to develop realistic treatment objectives for the implant team. In Nevins M, Mellonig JT, Fiorellini JP, editors, *Implant therapy: clinical approaches and evidence of success*, Chicago, 1998, Quintessence.

48. Chai UDO, Ludlow JB, Tyndall DA, Webber RL: Detection of simulated periodontal bone gain by digital subtraction radiography with tuned-aperture computed tomography. The effect of angular disparity, *Dentomaxillofac Radiol* 30:92-97, 2001.

49. Jeffcoat MK, Wang IC, Reddy MS: Radiographic diagnosis in periodontics, *Periodontol 2000* 7:54-68, 1995.

10 The Electronic Patient Record

Paul R. Rhodes

The field of periodontology is rapidly evolving. Information management is becoming an area of "critical mass" for many dental practices, including those actively involved in periodontal therapy. The ability to accurately gather, analyze, and share dental data has become a key to the success of the practice. This chapter deals with the components and functionality of a computer-based oral health record and the significant enhancements it offers over traditional paper-based records.

The Electronic Patient Record (EPR) for dentistry is seen by many to be a component of the overall EPR for all of healthcare.[1-8] As research during the last decade has shown how periodontal health and disease can affect other systemic conditions, it is essential that this component relation exists between the dental record and the medical record (Fig. 10-1). Such a component model for the EPR was introduced in 1991 by the Institute of Medicine and was further elucidated for dentistry by Abbey.[1] The EPR can be much more than a substitute for the traditional paper-based patient record. The EPR can take the clinical practice of health care into a new paradigm.[9-12]

The traditional paper-based clinical record is static documentation of the history of observations and events related to a patient while under dental care. In addition to written notes, it commonly contains film-based radiographs and photographs (prints or transparencies) documenting oral conditions or treatments. It is an inanimate, unresponsive document. Its value is dependent on the extent and accuracy of the information it contains, its legibility (when hand-written), and the reader's ability to interpret various symbols, codes, or acronyms used by the writer. Moreover, its value is based on the knowledge of the reader in relation to his or her ability to interpret the information contained in this record and ability to draw appropriate conclusions from it (i.e., diagnoses, treatment needed, relative outcome of treatment performed). The record itself cannot perform any function on the data it contains. In the digital information age, a paper- and film-based record is described as being "static or dead."

On the other hand, an electronic clinical record can be dynamic. It not only is a repository of information, but it also has the potential for providing vital functionality in the areas of chronic care patient management, decision support, and outcomes evaluation. If one were to give the EPR a personality, it could be described as an expert colleague, a patient educator, a risk manager, a patient project coordinator, and with the proper ancillary image capturing tools, a clinical intraoral and radiographic imaging manager. Depending on how the software has been designed, it could do the following:

- Standardize clinical data
- Speed up the entry of information
- Encourage the entry of more comprehensive information
- Result in greater legibility of information
- Provide easier and faster access to information
- Facilitate the sharing of information
- Allow for greater security and privacy of information
- Display information in several ways, including both graphical and textual
- Enhance the capture and use of clinical images
- Provide new ways to analyze information
- Incorporate forms of artificial intelligence to enhance the accuracy of diagnosis, assessment of treatment outcomes, and management of chronic care

STANDARDIZATION OF TERMINOLOGY USED IN PERIODONTAL RECORDS

The use of paper-based periodontal records traditionally has been associated with a lack of standardization of the data parameters collected and the terminology and abbreviations used in clinical record-keeping. A review of commercially available paper periodontal charts reveals that some offer specific fields for pocket measurement; a few offer specific fields for other parameters of examination data such as gingival recession, gingival width, furcation classifications, tooth mobility, bleeding or suppuration points, and attachment level or attachment loss. Few include terms for various signs or symptoms that are commonly observed during examination. Most narrative note entry is done by the generation of hand-written text with the terminology being at the writer's discretion.

Electronic clinical records have been used in various areas of medical and nursing care and are undergoing

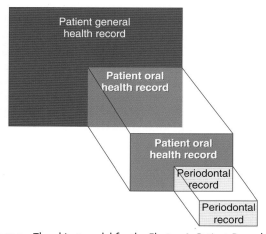

Figure 10-1. The object model for the Electronic Patient Record (EPR) in which the periodontal record is a section inside of the Oral Health Record, which in turn is a section in the overall Electronic Patient Health Record.

rapid development and implementation.[12] A significant factor in the development of EPRs is the use of standardized terminology. Standardization in medical terminology has been developed much more than in dentistry. In the mid-19th century, English physicians started the development of a standardized terminology and code set to document causes of death. This code set, known as the I.C.D. system, has undergone 10 updates since it was first published more than a century ago. Its content has been expanded to include not just disease names but also clinical conditions (findings, signs, symptoms). The periodontal terminology in the most recent I.C.D. does not include the currently accepted diagnostic terminology developed by the American Academy of Periodontology and is limited in the number of terms representative of the various clinical findings that can be observed during periodontal examination.

Approximately 40 years ago, the College of American Pathology started organizing a similar set of codes and nomenclature, first used by pathologists and then expanded into other areas of medicine. This code set has been organized into a digital database format that makes its use more valuable both in terms of rapid and more accurate data collection, but even more important in relation to data analysis. Because of its expansion, organization, and digital format, this coding system, known as *SNOMED* or the *Standardized NOmenclature for MEDicine*, is coming into greater acceptance as a nomenclature system for medicine.

Although terminology in dentistry has been partially defined in various textbooks, up until recently there has been no accepted comprehensive nomenclature system for dentistry. Standardization of nomenclature in dentistry has focused only on the development of codes, terms, and definitions for treatment procedures. The official resource for this in the United States is the American Dental Association's "Current Procedural Terminology." Several dental specialty academies, including the American Academy of Periodontology, have developed standardized glossaries of terminology that in addition to nomenclature for treatment procedures also include terminology for conditions and diagnoses. These glossaries have been used by the American Dental Association to develop a more comprehensive nomenclature system for dentistry. This dental nomenclature set, known as *SNODENT*, has been incorporated into the *SNOMED* system.

Terms included in *SNOMED* and *SNODENT* consist of diagnostic terms and terms describing symptoms, clinical signs and findings, radiographic observations and related test findings—this group of terms is known as *conditions*. A diagnostic term is defined as a "family name" for a specific unique set of conditions (i.e., "children"). For example, pocket depth, not associated with loss of alveolar bone but seen in conjunction with signs of inflammation and a variety of changes to the periodontal soft tissues and the presence of bacterial plaque, would be a family of conditions that would suggest a diagnosis of Plaque-Related Gingivitis.

The use of standardized terminology in a clinical record enhances the understanding of what has transpired during the course of a patient's care. In addition, its use is essential to the analysis of global information for the purpose of assessing the outcomes of care and what constitutes quality care. That information can lead to better diagnostic decisions and treatment planning. Furthermore, it can provide a basis for designing into the digital record forms of artificial intelligence to further assist the dental care provider in making more accurate diagnostic decisions.

Therefore, periodontal clinical charting software that includes specific fields for the documentation of a greater variety of examination parameters and that includes a rich glossary of standardized terms can be a significant enhancement to periodontal records not found in the paper-based chart.

SPEED UP ENTRY OF INFORMATION

Neither handwriting nor typing are rapid ways of creating textual information when compared with computer-based mechanisms such as the use of the mouse, light pen, touch screen technology, or voice recognition for data entry. Properly designed software can provide for data entry as fast as the user can speak or think. Specialized devices such as electronic periodontal probes can also facilitate the entry of some quantifiable parameters of periodontal examination data. The rapid capture of clinical images and their incorporation into the digital record make obsolete the classic paper chart of tooth outlines for drawing icons representative of existing dental care or conditions. The time needed to draw on a paper-based tooth graphic the missing teeth, the types and outlines of various restorations present in the mouth, the malpositioning of teeth (tipped teeth, extruded teeth, teeth in buccoversion or linguoversion), the presence of diastemata, and other such data could be much greater than that required for an assistant to take digital images of the occlusal, facial, and lingual views of the maxilla and mandible. The accuracy of these images obviously would be much greater than any hand drawn representations on a paper-based tooth graphic.

ENCOURAGE ENTRY OF MORE COMPREHENSIVE INFORMATION

Generally, clinical dental charts are lacking in adequate detail to support the treatment suggested, as well as detail about the treatment that has been provided. Dental records often do not include a diagnosis; they are commonly limited to documentation of problems (conditions) and treatments. Frequently, proper peer review or legal action for the purposes of resolving patient complaints is hampered by the lack of critical information in the patient's record. This can result in unnecessary settlements because there is not enough information to support either the dentist's actions or the lack of compliance by the patient. Time is a critical factor in day-to-day practice. Therefore, clinical software designed to speed up the entry of data and narrative notes could encourage the inclusion of greater detail in the clinical periodontal patient record.[13]

GREATER LEGIBILITY OF INFORMATION

Obviously, text viewed on a display screen is far more legible than much of the handwritten documentation that has been common in the paper-based dental chart. Handwriting done in a hurried manner or the use of acronyms that are not commonly accepted can be difficult for others to interpret. For example, in the team approach to management of the partially edentulous patient with periodontal disease and altered occlusion, there are often multiple providers. In addition to the primary care dentist and hygienist, specialists in periodontics, orthodontics, and prosthodontics also could become part of the patient's team of therapists. In this team approach to patient management, legibility of records and detailed content of clinical information are most important.

EASIER AND FASTER ACCESS TO CLINICAL INFORMATION

With networked computers and comprehensive digital information software throughout a clinical care facility, there is no need to move around a manila folder. In the author's survey of more than 30 practices, it has been estimated that in the average, full-time, solo dental practice, the staff spends an average of more than 1000 hours per year pulling and filing paper charts and searching for lost charts. With all administrative and clinical information accessible to view on the display screen at any workstation on the network, there is no need to pull or file charts. With clinical information stored in databases the ability to search these databases can result in faster access to specific topics or items of interest. Properly designed clinical software will use the power of information compiled in a well designed database to facilitate searching and analysis of specific items of information. This allows practitioners to do things with clinical information that they have not been able to do with the traditional paper-based chart, because of the time (and cost) that would be involved.

EASIER AND FASTER SHARING OF CLINICAL INFORMATION IN THE TEAM APPROACH TO CARE

With modems or broadband access to telecommunications systems, clinical data can be shared with others in distant facilities for the purpose of consultation or for the purpose of team development and coordination of a complex multidisciplinary treatment plan.[14,15] Properly designed systems will maintain the privacy of this patient information by not allowing persons without login IDs and passwords to access the practice's network, as well as by encryption of data that is being accessed or shared through telecommunications channels.[16,17] This protection of privacy of healthcare records has been legislated in the United States and in several other countries.

PROVIDE NEW WAYS OF ANALYZING CLINICAL INFORMATION

The paper-based chart has always been a static, historical document. Only the viewer can cognitively manipulate or analyze the content of the clinical record. The computer-based clinical record can be a vital participant in the process of clinical decision making and clinical outcomes analysis. By taking textual or numeric information and rearranging it or converting it to a graphic display, the viewer can more easily interpret the data. Expert systems can be developed so that the software can suggest pathways toward a diagnosis or use rule-based decision support systems to assist the practitioner in making the most accurate diagnosis.[18]

Some paper-based clinical records for endodontic and periodontal examination already store and display information in the form of a *grid*. The spreadsheet is a computer graphic format that facilitates the viewing of multiple parameters of data by specific site. For example, all of the parameters may be listed in horizontal rows and the tooth sites appear in vertical columns, allowing the examiner to view all of the parameters of data for a specific tooth or site in one column. Multiple examination data sets can be graphically displayed to analyze site- and parameter-specific changes over time. Many of the decisions made in managing chronic care are made on the basis of changes to parameters over time. Furthermore, software can be designed to participate in the decision-making process by the incorporation of expert systems such as rule-based decision support or neural networking. Software using these types of expert systems has already started to develop in other areas of health care.

The digital radiographic image is an excellent example of applying computer tools to view an image in a way that cannot be done in film-based radiography. The ability to reassign gray scale values to pixels in a digital radiographic image—similar to how we adjust brightness and contrast on our television—can allow the human eye to recognize subtle changes that may be missed in the static film image. The dentist diagnosing radiographs is commonly viewing tissues with four different levels of density: enamel, dentin, cortical bone and cancellous bone. A single film exposed at one dose of radiation cannot provide optimal conditions for all of these various densities, whereas the reassignment of gray scale values in a digitized image can provide that enhancement, thus improving the recognition of anomalies or pathologic changes by the examiner.

PROVIDE NEW WAYS OF NETWORKED DIAGNOSIS OF MULTIDISCIPLINARY PROBLEMS

Traditionally, when the primary care practice has referred a patient for specialty care, such care has been diagnosed and treated by a specialist, with little or no input from others, and when therapy has succeeded in resolving a specific subset of the patient's conditions, the patient is then returned to the primary care practice for continuation of care or referral to the next specialist. This segmented approach to care might be adequate for a patient with simple problems, but in patients with multiple problems of periodontal disease, partial edentulism, malocclusion, and dental esthetics, newer strategies call for the team of treating dentists to codiagnose and codevelop a comprehensive treatment plan. This network model for team diagnosis and planning relies on the integration of data from all team members before

development of a comprehensive plan of care. Key to the success of this team approach to both diagnosis and treatment is the need to have continuous communication among all members of the treatment team. As implant restorative services increase, a need for such dynamic communication becomes quite apparent because it is common for the patient to be treated in phases, going back and forth between the surgeon and the restorative dentist. Through use of modern telecommunications channels, the EPR can greatly increase the effectiveness of such an approach to care (Fig. 10-2).

OUTCOMES ANALYSIS OF CLINICAL DATA

Storing clinical information in the form of a database, using standardized terms and collecting more detailed information, can be of significant value by providing an economic method of performing outcomes analysis. Various fields of medicine have used clinical outcomes analysis to answer the questions of which treatment modality is best for the health and well being of the patient, as well as the most cost effective. Studies using such clinical databases have examined numerous clinical, economic, and patient-centered outcomes of various therapeutic approaches to managing systemic diseases. Similar clinical outcomes analysis data for oral health can easily be gathered using computer-based dental records. Such analyses add to the evidence base for various dental treatment approaches.

The organization of clinical information in a database is important to facilitating analysis of clinical outcomes.

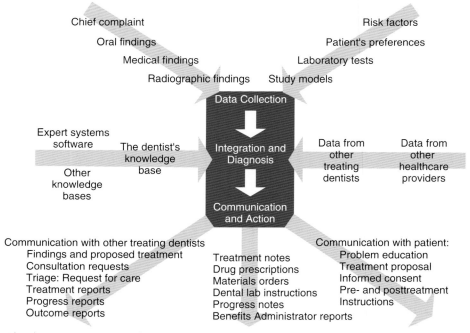

Figure 10-2. The Electronic Patient Record (EPR) can enhance data gathering, organization, processing, and communications.

In its simplest form, clinical outcomes should ask the question: did the treatment provided resolve or improve the clinical conditions that the patient had before treatment? The obvious subdivisions of information that can be generated from this question would be "Conditions" and "Treatments." In addition, one can interject a commonly used term: Diagnoses. This term as a noun, not a verb, is *a family name given to a specific set of conditions (family members).*

Conditions

Conditions are inclusive of chief complaints; signs; symptoms; clinical, radiographic, and laboratory test findings; or observations. This family of terms is also commonly referred to as *subjective and objective clinical findings.*

Diagnoses

Diagnoses are terms applied to a specific set of conditions observed and documented during the examination of the patient. A diagnostic term is only valid if it relates to a unique set of conditions. At least one condition must exist in a set of conditions that makes it unique from other condition sets to support a unique diagnostic term. Furthermore, a diagnostic term should suggest a specific list of potential treatments that could be applied to resolve this set of conditions.

Treatment Procedures

Treatment procedures are already well defined, because most dental fees are procedure based. The selection of procedures to treat a patient's conditions can be facilitated by the act of making a diagnosis first.

In 1993, the Informatics Committee of the American Academy of Periodontology identified 210 Conditions relevant to periodontics, 34 Diagnoses, and 144 Treatment Procedures. The committee then went on to take each diagnostic term and identify which of the 210 conditions might be associated with a specific diagnostic term. It then identified which of the 144 treatments might be considered in treating a patient with each specific diagnosis. This information provides the basis for focusing the decision process, which can be built into EPR software (Fig. 10-3). The scheme shown in Figure 10-3 is a simplified example of *rule-based decision support.* This can be programmed into software to assist the examining dentist in more accurately diagnosing and treatment planning a patient's conditions set.

About 90% of dental practices in the United States use computer-based digital information management for accounting and billing. The capture or conversion of radiographic images along with the digitization of intraoral color images captured with digital or analog video cameras also has shown significant adoption in the last decade. It is

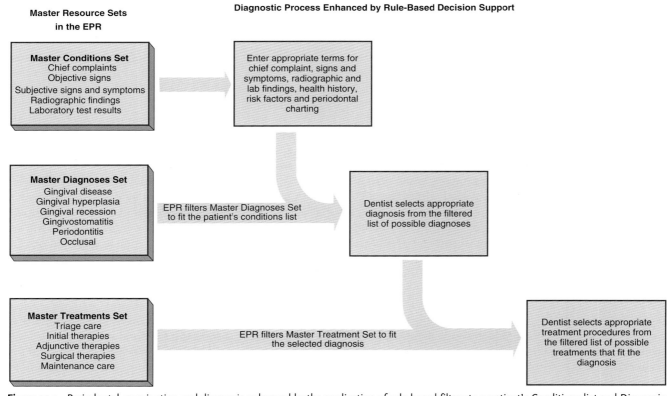

Figure 10-3. Periodontal examination and diagnosis enhanced by the application of rule-based filters to a patient's Conditions list and Diagnosis.

natural that the final conversion from paper (and film) to digital information management in dentistry will be digital systems for the digital entry and management of examination data, treatment narratives, and progress notes.

DIGITAL IMAGING AS PART OF THE ELECTRONIC PATIENT RECORD

Digital radiography was first introduced to dentistry in 1989. Currently, there are at least 16 manufacturers of digital dental radiographic systems worldwide. A survey in 2002 suggested that 14% of dental practices have converted to using digital radiography. Digital systems have been shown to produce radiographic images of diagnostic quality, with reduced radiation to the patient and with greater dynamic range (margin of error in exposure settings). Digital imaging has unique advantages over film-based imaging. Dental imaging usually involves looking at hard tissues of a considerable range of density: enamel, dentin, cortical bone, and cancellous bone. Being static, a film-based image cannot optimally disclose all information on such a wide range of densities. As mentioned earlier, software can be used to enhance the examiner's ability to visualize details in digital images by brightening or darkening the image, by increasing or decreasing contrast, by zooming or enlarging the image, and by applying "smoothing" routines to sharpen the image, to mention a few. Filling a 15" or 17" monitor with one periapical image affords a dramatic increase in the examiner's ability to see detail that might otherwise be overlooked in a traditional dental film-sized image.

Digital radiography can be divided into two major sectors: direct and indirect. Indirect digital radiography involves the initial capture of a radiographic image on film, which, after chemical processing, is converted to a digital image through the use of a flatbed scanner fitted with a transparency adaptor. This does not eliminate the need for a darkroom and the use of processing chemicals, and it includes a secondary processing task—converting the analog film–based image to a digital computer–based image. Although this is a complex process, it does afford the ability to use software to enhance the image once it is digitized.

Direct "wired" digital radiography involves the initial capture of an image by a solid-state silicon chip—either a wired Charged Couple Device (CCD) or Complimentary Metal Oxide Semiconductor (CMOS). Both of these technologies were invented in the late 1960s and have been used for image capture in video cameras and more recently in digital cameras. CCD semiconductors produce diagnostic quality radiographic images. Currently, there does not appear to be any compelling reason to suggest that CMOS is better than CCD technology for dental radiography. Both of these systems produce an image on the screen within a few seconds and totally eliminate "processing" and the

associated work and costs associated with darkrooms and processing chemicals. The cassettes that house the semiconductor sensors and their related components (microcontroller, random access memory chip) are relatively bulky, the overall size of the cassette being much larger than the area of the image captured by the semiconductor. The large size of the cassette (related to the area of image capture) and its thickness present challenges to its intraoral placement for proper image capture and alignment with the x-ray generator tube. The cassettes are attached through a cable to an adjacent computer with a special video capture board (frame grabber board). Because of these design features, they require different holders for stabilizing the imaging cassette during x-ray exposure.

Direct "wireless" digital radiography involves the initial capture of an image by Photostimulable Phosphor (PSP) technology. These thin plates closely resemble conventional dental x-ray film in overall size and thickness and therefore do not require the mastering of new techniques, as called for with intraoral placement of the bulkier cabled sensors. Therefore, they are more easily adaptable to the process of producing periapical and vertical bitewing images in a classic standard full-mouth series of radiographs. They consist of a thin plate coated on one side with "phosphors" that when excited by x-radiation undergo changes that are stored on the plate (temporarily). After removal from the mouth, each plate must be placed into a special scanner where they are made to fluoresce by a laser. The resultant image is captured in digital form by a computer attached to this scanner. This digital processing of the phosphor plate usually takes 1 to 5 minutes depending on the number and size of imaging plates being processed. After each use, the stored imaging information on a used plate can be "erased" allowing for the imaging plate to be used again. These plates are durable, but care must be taken in their handling to minimize scratching of the phosphor layer, which may affect subsequent images.

Digital radiographic imaging has been most widely used in relation to endodontic diagnosis and treatment. Similarly, the easy capture and ability to rapidly view periapical radiographs can be of strategic use during creation of an osteotomy site for endosseous implant placement, similar to how the endodontist or general dentist will use radiographs during canal preparation and obturation. The use of intraoperative digital radiography during the surgical placement of dental implants can markedly improve the proper fixture placement.

In addition to the above intraoral imaging devices, there are digital panoramic systems available from at least a half dozen manufacturers worldwide. Coupled with newer panoramic x-ray machines that incorporate systems to improve head positioning and mechanisms for reducing distortion, magnification, and superimposition of the spinal image over orofacial structures, these systems can produce imaging useful in the recognition and analysis of periodontal- and implant-related conditions and temporomandibular joint disorders. Although the "gold standard" for periodontal radiologic diagnosis in the past has been the full-mouth series of periapical and bitewing radiographs, it has been suggested that a modern digital panoramic coupled with a digital vertical bitewing series may be a reasonable alternative in many patients.

CLINICAL IMAGES (PHOTOGRAPHY)

In the past, light-sensitive oral imaging predominantly has been based on the use of 35 mm single lens reflex (SLR) film-based cameras modified for oral macrophotography. The past decade has seen the emergence of the intraoral video "cameras on a wand." It has been estimated that approximately 30% of dental practices have implemented use of this means of intraoral color imaging, mostly for patient education. Oral imaging can be more than a patient education tool. It can be a strategic part of the EPR and can assist in documenting the patient's presenting problems or conditions, how they were treated, and what the outcome of care has produced. With an increasing emphasis on consideration of esthetic changes to the periodontium, this form of oral imaging is key to proper diagnosis and evaluation of treatment outcomes. The quality of digital cameras has increased significantly. Digital cameras in the range of 3 to 6 megapixels, modified for oral macrophotography, are capable of producing images greater in quality than most intraoral video "cameras on a wand" and nearly equal to the granularity of processed transparency film. Many of these cameras are light in weight and small enough to be used with one-handed operation, making photographic image capture during dental treatment more attractive and convenient. These cameras capture images on a "card" that is easily removed from the camera and placed into a "reader" attached to a computer that the computer "sees" as another "hard disk" displaying the image files. The images also may be directly downloaded to a computer hard drive. These images can be copied and pasted into the patient's EPR or enhanced and stored in image management software. They can be sent to other treating dentists as part of examination or treatment reports, thus facilitating information sharing during the team approach to care. They also can be shared with the patient, thus enhancing their understanding, appreciation, and involvement in their own care. They also enhance the detail of information, which can provide a better basis for risk management.

LEGALITY OF THE ELECTRONIC PATIENT RECORD

Legislation exists throughout the United States and several other countries validating the use of electronic healthcare records. Legal precedent validating the use of electronic healthcare records in professional liability court actions in the United States dates back to the early 1990s.

A significant factor limiting the defense of a dentist in allegations of professional liability is the lack of information in the patient's chart. The standardization, legibility, and ease of data entry can make a significant difference in the volume and detail of information contained in the patient's electronic dental record. The ease with which electronic records can be copied and stored in escrow accounts provides a method of defense against the allegation that the defendant/dentist may have tampered with the patient's record and added information after the commencement of legal action. The escrowed copies, not being accessible by the defendant, can be used to disprove this allegation.

One of the high priority legal responsibilities of dental care practices is to maintain patient records in a secure environment. Paper-based records are vulnerable to fire, earthquake, and other forms of natural disaster, as well as water damage, a not uncommon property loss incident in dental offices. The periodic copying of EPRs is recommended, with their off-site storage in an escrowing service, bank vault, or similar secure environment. This type of record copying is not practical with paper-based records because of the time, space, and cost factors involved. With current digital technologies for backup, several thousand patient records can be backed up in a few minutes on media with a cost of only a few dollars or less.

Legislation is in place in the United States, Canada, and some European countries calling for the protection of privacy for information contained in patients' healthcare records. Patient charts in hospitals and other healthcare facilities must be kept in secure rooms or locked file cabinets. Charts cannot be left out on desks or counters when not currently being used by clinical staff. Although this level of security is not currently mandated in the dental care environment, it is possible that it will be required in the near future. If patient records exist only on the computer network in a dental practice, their security becomes much easier.[17,18] When clinical staff are not using the computer or are away from their desk, they would log off of the computer, thus blocking unauthorized access to the computer network. If the practice network is connected to the "outside" by modem or broadband telecommunications, secure "firewalls" can be installed to protect against unauthorized access to the practice's databases.

In conclusion, security and privacy of patient clinical information when using digital information systems can be much greater than in traditional paper-based information management.

THE IMPACT OF TELECOMMUNICATIONS ON DENTAL PRACTICE MODELS

As dental technologies become more complex, there is the potential for more dental care delivery to involve a team approach.[14] Patients with advanced periodontal problems frequently have associated problems of partial edentulism, malocclusion, or pulpal pathology, which can be most effectively treated by a team of various dental specialists working with the primary care dentist and hygienist. To successfully carry out such complex treatment calls for effective communication and coordination between the team members. The "paper chase" and "telephone tag" are common frustrations or impediments to effective communication in the traditional paper-based information world. The sharing of information facilitated by various digital options can increase the effectiveness of communications between care providers and the patient.

There is an emerging trend for dental practices to develop websites on the Internet to supply information on dental health, to provide a means of making appointments with the practice, to fill out forms online, to access preoperative and postoperative instructions for specific dental procedures, and to receive answers to common questions frequently asked by patients. This web-based dental practice information provides more effective patient communication and reduces the paperwork burden that office staff experience.[19]

Secure electronic mail (e-mail) can be used to share information between team care providers.[20] This must incorporate encryption when patient data are being shared to protect the privacy of patient information.

A virtual private network can be set up for practices with multiple office locations, all being served by a common "server" computer accessible from any of the practice's locations, thus eliminating the need to transport charts from one location to another. A virtual private network could be set up between a group of individual practices incorporating multiple generalists and a variety of dental specialists in a "Virtual Dental Group." This group could share certain common administrative functions, thus making use of an "economy-of-scale" approach to reducing administrative costs, whereas in other ways maintaining much of the autonomy commensurate with traditional solo practice. Such a network could provide a secure method of easily sharing patient information when participating in the team approach to care. It is feasible to think that the EPR software in such a group practice would allow each participating care provider access to enter and to use data for patients being treated by the various dentists. This model of practice would allow a group of dentists to form a business alliance, which could offer significant advantages to both patients and care providers.

Currently, more than 90% of periodontal practices use computer-based information management for practice administration, and 10% to 20% of practices use it for clinical information management. To start a practice today using only paper-based information management would be like starting a practice in 1970 without having a telephone, typewriter, air turbine handpiece, or x-ray machine. The EPR is an emerging phenomenon that offers great promise to the practice of dentistry, and periodontal health records are a key component of the EPR.

REFERENCES

1. Abbey LM: Computer based decision support: the substrate for dental practice in the 21st century, *J Dent Educ* 55(4):262-263, 1991.
2. Rhodes PR: The computer-based oral health record: exploring a new paradigm, *J Calif Dent Assoc* 22(11):29-33, 1994.
3. Rhodes PR: The computer-based oral health record, *J Dent Educ* 60(1):14-18, 1996.
4. Benn DK, Kostewicz SH, Dankel DD et al: Designing an electronic patient record with multiple real time decision support modules for managing diseases, *Proc AMIA Symp* p 1168, 2000.
5. Schleyer T, Spallek H: Dental informatics. A cornerstone for dental practice, *J Am Dent Assoc* 132:605-613, 2001.
6. Atkinson JC, Zeller GG, Shah C: Electronic patient records for dental school clinics: more than paperless systems, *J Dent Educ* 66(5):634-642, 2003.
7. Bates DW, Ebell M, Gotlieb E et al: A proposal for electronic medical records in US primary care, *J Am Med Inform Assoc* 10(1):1-11, 2003.
8. Bauer JC, Brown WT: The digital transformation of oral health care. Teledentistry and electronic commerce, *J Am Dent Assoc* 132:204-209, 2001.
9. Delrose DC, Steinberg RW: The clinical significance of the digital patient record, *J Am Dent Assoc* 131(Suppl):57S-60S, 2000.
10. Peterson LC, Cobb DS, Reynolds DC: ICOHR: intelligent computer based oral health record, *Medinfo* 8(Pt 2):1709, 1995.
11. Sharkey SE, Murison JM: Towards a general computer-based dental record system, *Int J Biomed Comput* 4(4):271, 1973.
12. Buller-Close K, Schriger DL, Baraff LJ: Heterogeneous effect of an emergency department expert charting system, *Ann Emerg Med* 41:644-652, 2003.
13. Berthelsen CL, Stilley KR: Automated personal health inventory for dentistry: a pilot study, *J Am Dent Assoc* 131:59-66, 2000.
14. Schleyer T, Eisner J: The computer-based oral health record: an essential tool for cross-provider quality management, *J Calif Dent Assoc* 22(11):57-58,60-61,63-64, 1994.

15. Suddick RP: The dental clinical workstation and the computer-based patient record, *NY State Dent J* 61(8):36-41, 1995.

16. Day J: Cyberinfo: privacy and personal health data in cyberspace. *J Contemp Dent Pract* 1(4):87-96, 2000.

17. Day J: Privacy and personal health data in cyberspace, *J Contemp Dent Pract* 2(1):45-56, 2001.

18. Wagner IV, Schneider W: Computer based decision support in dentistry, *J Dent Educ* 55(4):263-267, 1991.

19. Schleyer TK, Dasari VR: Computer-based oral health records on the World Wide Web, *Quintessence Int* 30(7):451-460, 1999.

20. Younai FS, Messadi DV: E-mail-based oral medicine consultation, *J Calif Dent Assoc* 28(2):144-151, 2000.

11

Formulating a Periodontal Diagnosis and Prognosis

Mark V. Thomas and Brian L. Mealey

DIAGNOSIS: THE RATIONALE

Diagnosis is derived from the Greek *gnosis* ("to know") and *dia* ("through"). In clinical practice, diagnosis usually consists of the act of classification—that is, assigning a name to a given patient's illness. Early in the practice of medicine, physicians were more or less limited to naming the diseases of their patients and offering crude estimates of the likely course of the disease (i.e., the *prognosis*). Therapeutic interventions were limited, and those that were available were often unreliable and dangerous. However, the very act of identifying a condition probably afforded the patient some comfort.

CLINICAL UTILITY

To have clinical use, the act of formulating a diagnosis should tell something about the likely course of the disease and help guide selection of treatment modalities. If all periodontal conditions had the same prognosis and required the same treatment, there would be no reason for diagnosis beyond simply establishing the presence of periodontal disease. However, this has not proven to be the case. Periodontal diseases are the result of complex interactions between the host and the periodontal microflora. This interaction gives rise to a variety of clinical entities. The clinical expression of the disease seen is a function of the *differential susceptibility* of the host combined with the *composition* of the microflora. Although there are many similarities among the various forms of periodontal diseases, there are also significant differences that must be taken into account when formulating diagnoses and treatment plans.

The goal of periodontal diagnosis, therefore, is to classify periodontal diseases in some biologically meaningful way that will aid in the selection of the most optimal therapeutic modality and will help to develop a realistic prognosis. These therapeutic options are the subject of the remainder of this book. In this chapter, we consider the formulation of a diagnosis and prognosis and how they are used in clinical care.

RESEARCH UTILITY

Diagnostic classification is also an important component of periodontal research. It is necessary to classify periodontal diseases on the basis of objective criteria into valid and distinct categories so that patterns of disease within populations can be assessed and various treatments evaluated. Among other applications, this permits public health organizations and dental educators to make manpower projections that can be used to determine dental school class size and other factors. Accurate diagnosis is needed so that similar cases may be grouped together when evaluating new interventions and studying the pathogenesis or natural history of periodontal disease. The *heterogeneity* of periodontal diseases and the difficulty of developing a classification scheme based on etiology have complicated clinical epidemiology and interventional research efforts.

The type of disease assessment used by epidemiologists and other investigators often differs somewhat from that used in clinical practice. The epidemiologist often uses diagnostic *indexes* that assign scores to patients based on their overall periodontal condition. An index is usually based on an abbreviated assessment known as a screening examination. An example of such an index is the Community Periodontal Index of Treatment Needs, or CPITN. Such examinations permit screening relatively large numbers of individuals quickly, often in less than ideal settings (e.g., school gymnasiums). The resultant score is correlated, to a greater or lesser extent, to conventional diagnostic categories. Occasionally, such indexes are adapted for limited use in clinical practice. The CPITN, for example, is used by some clinicians as the Periodontal Screening and Recording (PSR) examination (see Chapter 18), although its original purpose was to provide a means of assessing periodontal manpower needs.[1] Generally, such indexes tend to underestimate the extent and severity of disease and are generally not used in the assessment of individual patients in clinical practice.

ADMINISTRATIVE UTILITY

Diagnosis also has administrative use, although this is secondary to the reasons stated earlier. In the United States and many other developed nations, many patients' dental needs are covered by third parties such as dental insurance carriers or government entities. Before claims are paid, third party payers will commonly wish to see the diagnosis and, possibly, supporting information such as probing charts and radiographs. This information permits the insurance carrier to assess the appropriateness of care (at least according to the guidelines used by the third party). Another important form of administrative use is for communication between clinicians (e.g., a referring general dentist and a specialist periodontist). For example, it is important for both parties to mean the same thing when they use the term *gingivitis* or *periodontal abscess*.

DIAGNOSIS: THE BIOLOGICAL BASIS

Disease Classification

The first step in the systematic study of natural phenomena is classification. Classification schemes are man-made constructs that facilitate the study of such phenomena.

One of the early efforts at scientific classification was Linnaeus' plan to categorize plant and animal life. Linnaean taxonomy organized organisms in a systematic manner on the basis of readily observable characteristics. Rational taxonomy accelerated progress in biology. Similarly, early efforts to catalogue human disease were similarly instrumental in enhancing early medical research.

When we name something, we give it a certain reality. We call this process *reification*, which means that we make an abstract concept (a group of different cases of a similar condition) tangible or real. When we speak of *gingivitis*, for example, this brings to mind an image of an individual with bleeding and inflamed gingival tissues. However, gingivitis does not occur as an abstract entity. Gingivitis always occurs in a specific individual patient at a specific point in time. Thus, the disease, gingivitis, is superimposed on an individual, with a unique set of oral hygiene habits, host response, and bacterial flora. In a real sense then, each case of gingivitis is unique. Gingivitis, for example, predictably develops within 21 days if hygiene is withheld. This was demonstrated in the 1960s in a series of now classic experiments.[2] Later work confirmed these early findings, but found a rather large degree of individual variation in the extent and severity of the gingivitis that developed.[3] This underscores that individual cases of gingivitis (or any medical or dental condition) may vary somewhat from the textbook example, because of inherent biological variability of the host or flora. This concept of individual variation is important in understanding human disease.

In some cases, our current level of understanding allows us to distinguish between similar conditions with differing etiologic factors. For example, in an individual infected with HIV, the commensal yeast, *Candida albicans*, may cause an erythematous lesion that resembles regular gingivitis (*linear gingival erythema*, or LGE).[4] LGE may be (and often is) superimposed on preexisting gingivitis. However, LGE is more difficult to treat than normal, "garden variety" gingivitis, and thus it is useful to distinguish between the two.

In other cases, our current level of understanding does not allow us to make such distinctions. For example, consider the case of a 22-year-old college student that presents for routine treatment at the university dental clinic. She has relatively good brushing habits, but flosses only occasionally. Examination reveals mild interproximal bleeding on probing. The diagnosis is plaque-induced gingivitis. Contrast this with the case of another 22-year-old student with similar oral hygiene habits. In the second case, however, the bleeding is profuse even with the slightest provocation. We will classify both diseases as gingivitis, although we have no good method of distinguishing the latter, more florid case from the first, milder case (unless there is some recognized modifying factor

such as pregnancy). Sometimes we may identify systemic conditions such as pregnancy or diabetes that may account, in part, for the clinical presentation. However, in most cases, we cannot ascribe the differences in clinical presentation to any specific component of the flora or host response.

Thus, a distinction must be made between the abstract concept of a disease entity (e.g., gingivitis) and the actual condition as it applies to a specific patient. There are two schools of thought with regard to disease classification. *Ontologists* (ontology being the branch of metaphysics that deals with the nature of being) emphasize *the disease* as an abstract category. They would tend to emphasize the similarities among all cases of gingivitis. Conversely, the *physiological* approach emphasizes *the individual's illness*, with all of the ramifications this implies. In other words, the physiologic approach would tend to describe a given patient's gingival inflammation, but in the particular context of that individual patient's general health, home care status, cultural beliefs and expectations (e.g., avoidance of the dentist except when oral pain occurs), and economic state (e.g., she is a single mother with three small children and cannot easily afford dental care). In simpler terms, ontologists prefer to consider the *general concept of a disease*, whereas physiologists prefer to consider the *particular case of illness* in a specific patient.

Biology and Diagnosis

Knowing the names of the schools of thought of biology and diagnosis is not important in clinical practice. What is important is to understand that both points of view have some validity and clinical use. They are simply different perspectives and are not mutually exclusive. If we are to study diseases in some systematic fashion, we must be able to organize diseases into logical categories on the basis of objective criteria (consistent with the ontologic view). Conversely, we must not lose sight of the idea that each disease occurs in an individual, and treatment must be tailored to the individual's circumstances (the physiologic perspective). This is particularly true during reevaluation of response to therapy. If the response to adequate and appropriate therapy* is suboptimal, then it may be necessary to revise the diagnosis. For this reason, the

---

*Use of the term *adequate and appropriate therapy* is applied in a very specific sense in this chapter. This phrase implies that the response to treatment is meaningful only if the intervention chosen is appropriate to the disease state and that it is competently performed. Obviously, coronal polishing with a rubber cup, no matter how well done, is unlikely to have a significant impact on severe periodontitis. Similarly, scaling and root planing, if done by a first-year dental student with inadequate instruments and very little time allotted, is likely to be less effective than the same treatment provided by an experienced operator with adequate resources. For comparisons of the treatment response to be meaningful, the treatment provided must meet the accepted standard of care.

primary diagnosis is sometimes referred to as the *presumptive diagnosis*. Response to therapy will be determined by the choice of therapy and how well it was delivered. Therapy is usually directed toward reduction or elimination of an etiologic agent (e.g., periodontal pathogens) or, occasionally, neutralizing the effects of the agent by strengthening or modifying the host (e.g., fluoride, smoking cessation).

To be useful, a classification scheme should possess both clinical utility and biological plausibility. Clinical utility implies that a particular diagnosis will dictate or suggest possible treatment options and the likely course of the disease. Clinical utility of diagnosis can be seen as a natural consequence of a scheme based on causality. A nondental example is the patient with an ulcer that proves to be primary syphilis. Such a diagnosis will dictate the choice of antibiotic and will trigger certain public health surveillance protocols. Not all ulcers will have similar treatment and public health implications; indeed, most will not. However, the cause, consequences, and communicability of syphilis dictate the treatment plan. In addition to the implications for treatment of the individual patient, a rational classification scheme aids the epidemiologist who desires to learn more about the risk factors that predispose to a disease and to the clinical researcher who wishes to test the effectiveness of various therapeutic interventions.

A biologically plausible classification scheme should permit the clinician to distinguish between conditions that may have similar clinical presentations but different etiologies. This would be of particular interest if the two target disorders required different treatment strategies. Such a scheme presupposes the existence of a robust understanding of the pathogenesis and etiology of the target disorders, as well as the existence of tests that can differentiate between them. In the case of many bacterial diseases, such as syphilis, meningitis, and tuberculosis, such tests exist. In the case of periodontitis, such tests could conceivably be based on a combination of etiologic agents (e.g., microbial assays) and host factors (e.g., genetic predisposition to disease).

Currently, however, most periodontal diagnosis is done by mechanically measuring the historical record of disease that has already occurred in the form of attachment loss. Although a consideration of diagnostic methods is beyond the scope of this chapter, it is obvious that the historical record of past disease activity, although important, does not indicate whether the disease is actively progressing (unless two measurements are taken at different points in time and compared).

Evaluating Diagnostic Tests

Uncertainty is inherent in the formulation of a diagnosis and in the interpretation of all diagnostic tests, regardless of sophistication. In a sense, every time a patient sees a dentist or physician, a miniature scientific experiment is conducted. The scientist/clinician performs various tests and examinations and, after examining the data, places a diagnostic label on the patient (or the patient's illness). This is analogous to formulating a scientific hypothesis concerning the nature of the illness. The diagnosis may or may not be correct, just as a scientific hypothesis may or may not be correct. Just as the scientist performs experiments to determine the validity of the hypothesis, the clinician performs therapeutic interventions, the response to which will confirm or refute the initial diagnosis.

Diagnosis, like scientific hypothesis, involves some uncertainty. For any given diagnostic test under a specific set of circumstances, there will be a certain probability that the results will be accurate or valid. Thus, there is always a chance that the test will identify someone as having the target disorder that does not really have the disorder; this is known as a false-positive result. There is also a chance that a patient who does have the disorder will be incorrectly identified as being disease-free; this is known as a false-negative result.

We can calculate *the probability that a diseased individual will have a positive test*; this is known as *sensitivity*. A test with high sensitivity will have few false negative results—that is, it will identify most of those who truly have the target disorder. Unfortunately, tests that are very sensitive often have a high rate of false-positive results. *The probability that an individual without disease will actually test negative is known as specificity*. A test with high specificity will have a very low rate of false-positive results. Almost all of those who test positive will actually have the disease. However, tests with high specificity will often fail to identify some individuals with the disease. Instead, they will be falsely labeled as healthy; these are known as false-negative results. Sensitivity and specificity often have a reciprocal relation. Tests with high sensitivity often have low specificity and vice versa. A test with high specificity would result in few false-negative results; it is highly *specific* for those who actually have the disease. Table 11-1 shows a device known as a "2 × 2 contingency table" or matrix that is commonly used to aid in evaluating diagnostic tests (and in other forms of epidemiologic research).

In Table 11-1, the sensitivity of a given test may be calculated as a/a + c—that is, the denominator is the number of patients who truly have the disease (a + c), whereas the numerator is the number of patients *with disease* who also had a positive test result (a). Stated simply, the sensitivity is the likelihood that a patient *with* disease will have a *positive* test result. Conversely, the specificity of a given test may be calculated as d/b + d—that is, the denominator is the number of patients who do *not* have the disease (b + d), whereas the numerator is the number of patients *without* disease who also had a *negative* test

TABLE 11-1	Sensitivity, Specificity, Positive Predictive Value, and Negative Predictive Value of Diagnostic Tests	
	TRUE DISEASE STATUS (AS DEMONSTRATED BY "GOLD STANDARD" TEST)	
TEST RESULT	**DISEASE PRESENT**	**DISEASE ABSENT**
Positive	a (true positive)	b (false positive)
Negative	c (false negative)	d (true negative)
Total	a + c	b + d

result (d). Stated simply, the specificity is the likelihood that an individual *without disease* will have a *negative* test result.

An extreme dental example may help illustrate these concepts. Assume that we are conducting a study and wish to recruit individuals with periodontitis. We decide to include only those individuals with circumferential probing depth in excess of 8 mm, combined with suppuration, on at least five teeth. This would be a *highly specific* test for periodontitis; it is likely that all individuals with those clinical findings would truly have periodontitis. However, the *sensitivity* would be very low. Of the entire universe of individuals with periodontitis, few would present with findings as extreme as those listed above. Therefore, there would be many false-negative results—that is, many individuals with periodontitis would be falsely diagnosed as without disease. Many individuals with less severe forms of the disease would be misdiagnosed.

The tradeoff between specificity and sensitivity can be seen clearly in the assessment of disease activity. Periodontal disease activity is usually measured in terms of attachment loss. The difficulty is in deciding what level of observed attachment loss will be accepted as actually representing true attachment loss—that is, at what *threshold value* will you state that "disease activity has occurred." It might seem logical to pick a low value, such as 1 mm. The only problem with this approach is that probing error, inflammation, and a host of other factors make probing errors of 1 mm common. This presents a conundrum to research investigators and clinicians alike in assessing disease activity. If the threshold is set too low (at 1 mm, for example), many sites will be included that have not truly lost attachment. The test will have high sensitivity in that it will pick up most cases of true attachment loss, but it will not be very specific because it will include some sites that did not actually lose attachment. As the threshold is increased to 2 or 3 mm, the number of false-positive results will decrease—that is, increasing the accepted threshold for attachment loss will increase the specificity, but will decrease the sensitivity.

A related concept is predictive value. Predictive value is actually of more use to the clinician. Positive predictive value (PPV; often referred to as *predictive value positive* or *predictive value +*) is the *probability that an individual who tests positive actually has the disease*. As might be expected, negative predictive value is the *probability that an individual who tests negative does not have the disease*. In Table 11-1, the PPV would be calculated as a/a + b—that is, the denominator is the total number of patients who have a positive test result (a + b), whereas the numerator is the number of patients *with a positive test* who also truly have the disease (a). Stated simply, the PPV is the likelihood that a patient with a *positive* test actually *does* have the disease. Conversely, the negative predictive value would be calculated as d/(c + d)—that is, the denominator is the total number of patients with a negative test (c + d), whereas the numerator is the number of patients *with a negative* test who are truly *without disease* (d). The negative predictive value of a test is the likelihood that a person with a *negative* test is actually *without disease*. A somewhat related concept is the *likelihood ratio*. This is the ratio between the likelihood of a positive test if one has the target disorder divided by the likelihood of a positive test if one does not have the disorder. The concept is actually somewhat more complex in that one often specifies the pretest probability of a target disorder. (The likelihood ratio concept is discussed at length in most evidence-based medicine texts.[5,6])

DIAGNOSIS: THE PROCESS

Data Collection

Although the examination process is discussed in detail elsewhere in this book (see Chapter 8), it is worthwhile to touch on a few points. Accurate data collection must precede diagnosis. The quality of the diagnosis cannot exceed the quality of the data on which the diagnosis is based. Inaccurate or incomplete probing information, failure to record mobility, or poorly exposed radiographs will compromise the diagnostic process and result in suboptimal care. Some studies have demonstrated that adequate information on periodontal status is often missing from charts in general dental offices. McFall and colleagues[7] report finding a periodontal diagnosis in only 16.3% of approximately 2500 charts audited. Heins and colleagues[8] report that 62% of general dental offices in Florida performed a complete periodontal probing for new patients. It can be inferred that the periodontal diagnosis was missing or inaccurate for approximately 40% of the new patients, because complete probing is required to make such a diagnosis.

Data collection is facilitated by a systematic approach to the patient. Organization and structured examination protocols help to ensure that no aspect of the patient's status is overlooked. Various structured examination forms or computer programs may help to ensure that the data collection process is complete by encouraging the recording assistant to prompt the examiner for information. The medium for recording examination findings may be a physical entity, such as paper, or may be computerized (see Chapter 10). Software programs are readily available in which the assistant enters the information directly into a database. This aids in subsequent data analysis or tracking trends, computing percentage of bleeding sites, and other tasks. Regardless of the medium used to record the data, it must be easy to compare probing depths and attachment levels over time because *changes* or *trends* in attachment level are often as or more important than the *absolute values*. On completion of the examination, it is helpful to have a form that outlines all of the information collected during the examination.

A distinction is made between a *comprehensive periodontal examination* and a *limited or focused examination* in which only a specific problem is addressed. It may be permissible to perform a limited examination in certain circumstances (e.g., an acute condition). However, in those cases, the patient should receive a comprehensive examination and assessment as soon as it is practical after resolution of the acute problem.

Presumptive Diagnosis

In diagnosing health and disease states, the clinician never knows that the diagnosis is correct with 100% certainty. The goal is to limit uncertainty, Nevertheless, much of medicine and dentistry consists of making decisions with only incomplete information. This is even more relevant for chronic diseases such as diabetes, atherosclerosis, and periodontitis. Chronic diseases are often multifactorial—that is, the result of many factors, both endogenous (e.g., genetic factors) or exogenous (e.g., periodontal pathogens). It is often impossible to know all the factors contributing to the patient's condition. Thus, it is likely that some contributing or modifying factors are omitted when formulating diagnoses. Indeed, it is likely

that when examining a group of patients diagnosed with *aggressive periodontitis*, we may, in reality, be looking at several different diseases that we are not able to differentiate at this point in our understanding.[9]

Because the diagnostic process is not infallible, the clinician must be prepared to change the diagnosis based on the response to therapy. Thus, if a patient presents with a condition that normally responds predictably to treatment (e.g., plaque-induced gingivitis), but the patient does not respond to adequate and appropriate therapy, then the original diagnosis may have been incorrect or incomplete. As noted earlier, this is the reason that some may consider the initial or pretreatment diagnosis as the *presumptive diagnosis*, which is subject to change based on response to treatment.

For example, certain patients infected with HIV have a form of gingival inflammation that may resemble plaque-induced gingivitis, but the patient does not respond well to conventional therapy (LGE). Gingivitis usually responds quickly to treatment, and a suboptimal response to adequate and appropriate therapy can suggest that there may be systemic factors at work, or that the patient's home care may be inadequate (the latter being far more common than the former).

The real point, however, is that our diagnoses are, of necessity, *presumptive* and subject to change. We must reassess the patient after initial therapy and at each maintenance appointment. Assessment, or diagnosis, is an ongoing process because the patient's periodontal and systemic conditions are not static but dynamic and subject to change. For this reason, assessment must be an integral part of each maintenance visit and sufficient time must be allowed for it.

Disease Activity and Diagnosis

Central to the concept of evidence-based dentistry is the predication of diagnostic tests on solid, scientifically valid evidence. The field of periodontology has been hampered by the concept of *disease activity* as it relates to diagnosis. In the context of periodontology, disease activity is defined as the loss of clinical attachment caused by periodontitis. There are no currently available, practical methods to tell whether a site or patient is about to lose attachment, although there is knowledge of some risk factors that increase the likelihood that such loss will occur. Instead, we must rely on the historical record of attachment loss that has already occurred: clinical or radiographic evidence of attachment loss. This is somewhat analogous to a burglar alarm that is activated after the thieves have made their getaway.

The reasons for this lack of knowledge are manifold. It is partly the result of the complexity of the disease process and partly a result of what epidemiologists call *misclassification*. Misclassification has been defined as *the erroneous classification of an individual, a value, or an attribute into a category other than that to which it should be assigned.* It is likely that what we call "periodontitis" is really a group of diseases with similar clinical manifestations, but differing somewhat in etiology.

This incomplete knowledge of etiologic agents may or may not make a difference in determining therapeutic outcomes. Assume that there are two individuals with generalized chronic periodontitis of moderate severity. Then further assume that one case is primarily caused by the presence of bacteria A, B, and C, whereas the other patient's disease is largely caused by a complex consisting of bacteria B, D, and E. Scaling and root planing is performed on both patients and both respond well to treatment. In these cases, it made no difference that somewhat different bacteria were responsible for the observed disease. Mechanical disruption of the biofilm was sufficient, in both cases, to arrest the disease. This is largely true of periodontal infections caused by different bacteria. It is known that periodontal diseases respond well to currently used periodontal interventions. This has been the consistent finding from outcomes studies over many years. We can thus infer that periodontal infections of somewhat differing etiology *usually* respond well to therapy, despite differences in the actual flora responsible for the disease. *Usually* is the key word in this statement, however.

Some subsets of patients do not respond well to normal periodontal therapy. This is more likely to be the case when there is an unidentified or unchangeable systemic component. Such cases were previously placed in a diagnostic category known as *refractory periodontitis*. Fortunately, this is a rare phenomenon, and the disease category "refractory periodontitis" is no longer in the accepted classification system because multiple disease categories may demonstrate less than favorable results after treatment (see Chapter 2). Again, note that failure to use appropriate therapy or perform it well also may cause the treatment to fail. Such a failure merely reflects an inappropriate choice of therapy or performance failure, which must be distinguished from the rare phenomenon of true refractory disease. Similarly, the failure to treat a case until most teeth are without bony support will greatly alter the prognosis. Pretreatment disease severity plays a significant role in determining response to therapy.

DIAGNOSIS OF PERIODONTAL HEALTH STATUS

Health

The most elementary distinction to be made during periodontal diagnosis is the differentiation between health, gingivitis, and periodontitis; however, this is not quite as clearcut as it might seem. *Periodontal health* may be defined as a state in which the tissues are free from inflammation. Therefore, an 18-year-old individual with no probing depths greater than 3 mm, no bleeding on probing, no recession, no mobility, and no color changes would be considered to be in a state of periodontal health. No active treatment is required. The patient will receive only primary preventive care.

What about the case of a 60-year-old individual with no probing depths greater than 3 mm, no bleeding on probing, no color changes, minimal mobility, but significant recession? This patient has a history of periodontal disease, for which she was treated surgically, with subsequent recession. Despite the recession, which we assume to be nonprogressive, this patient is also in a state of health. However, she has demonstrated susceptibility to periodontal disease and, for that reason, merits a more aggressive maintenance regimen and will require ongoing assessment of periodontal status.

How do we apply these concepts of health in the care of our patients? The clinician must tailor the maintenance interval to the patient's current clinical status and history of disease (see Chapter 15). Therefore, an individual with no history of periodontal disease or caries might be seen every 6 months or even yearly, if home care was acceptable. Conversely, an individual with a history of significant periodontal attachment loss that has been successfully treated and maintained is likely to be maintained at 3- or 4-month intervals, with careful monitoring of periodontal status at these visits.

Gingivitis

Gingivitis is simply an inflammatory process confined to the gingival tissues. It is most often caused by a relatively nonspecific accumulation of plaque and is usually reversible. The most common form of gingivitis is *plaque-induced gingivitis* and it is easily treated. Studies have demonstrated conclusively that establishing good home care, in the absence of plaque-retentive areas such as calculus and overhanging restorations, is sufficient to establish gingival health.[2] Gingivitis develops within a short period (e.g., 10 to 20 days) when normal plaque control is suspended. This consequence appears to be universal, although there is some individual variation.[3] There are other forms of gingivitis, such as those seen in various systemic conditions. These variants generally do not respond as well to standard treatment regimens (these regimens are discussed in detail in other sections of this text).

The essential components of therapy for gingivitis include instruction in home care, correction of plaque-retentive areas such as calculus and overhanging restorations, and reevaluation. The reevaluation, although often omitted in cases of gingivitis, is identical to that performed after treatment of periodontitis. An examination is performed to assess the commonly measured parameters of periodontal status, such as probing depth, bleeding on probing, and changes in color and consistency. If health is attained, the patient is placed on a regular maintenance interval. If not, a cause for the suboptimal response is sought.

It was formerly believed that untreated gingivitis would inevitably result in periodontitis, but this is not accurate. Although it is likely that all periodontitis begins as gingivitis, not all cases of gingivitis lead to periodontitis, even in the absence of personal plaque control or professional treatment. This was demonstrated in longitudinal studies of Sri Lankan tea workers who lacked access to professional dental care or oral hygiene aids.[10] During the study, the majority (89%) of workers experienced periodontitis as manifested by interproximal attachment loss and tooth loss. However, 11% did not progress beyond gingivitis despite a total lack of hygiene and dental care. This is an example of the concept of differential susceptibility, which has significant impact on prognosis and risk assessment.

A special case is the patient with gingivitis who has had a significant history of successfully treated periodontitis. We refer to this as gingivitis in a setting of a reduced periodontium. This individual has a demonstrated susceptibility to periodontitis and should be presumed to be at increased risk for further attachment loss. The general plan would be the same as discussed earlier for gingivitis, but this individual would normally be seen at more frequent intervals (e.g., 3 or 4 months) for maintenance visits. Further deterioration in attachment levels would lead to a diagnosis of periodontitis and would result in a return to active treatment.

There is another special case of gingivitis that merits discussion. This is sometimes seen when the biologic width is encroached on during crown preparation (see Chapters 21, 23, and 27)—that is, the crown margins are carried too far apically so that the margin ends in or near the supraalveolar connective tissue. This often occurs in the maxillary anterior region, because the restoration margin is often prepared evenly around the tooth, rather than following the rise and fall of the cementoenamel junction in the interproximal space. The inflamed tissue in those instances may be confined to the interdental papilla. This normally results in the formation of a periodontal pocket, but sometimes only gingivitis is noted at the site. The tissue appears red and edematous and bleeds profusely on probing. Probing these areas is often quite painful, which is uncharacteristic of gingivitis. Plaque control alone or in combination with professional cleaning is unlikely to resolve these areas of gingivitis. Instead, resolution of the biologic width problem is required through surgical and restorative treatment.

Periodontitis

In some cases, inflammation may not remain confined to the gingiva, but may involve the attachment apparatus: cementum, periodontal ligament, alveolar bone, and related tissues. There are a group of diseases that begin as gingivitis, but progress to destroy the bone and connective tissues that support the tooth. They are collectively known as *periodontitis*. The *sine qua non* of periodontitis is *inflammation combined with loss of attachment*. In periodontitis, the connective tissue attachment is destroyed and the junctional epithelium proliferates apically down the root. This results in clinically detectable loss of attachment. If no recession occurs and the gingival margin remains in its original position, then the sulcus deepens. The pathologically deepened sulcus is referred to as a *periodontal pocket*. As noted previously, this period during which connective tissue attachment is lost is referred to as *disease activity*. Notably, if the gingival tissue recedes apace with the bone loss, then recession occurs and this may result in a clinical situation in which there is attachment loss, but no significant increase in pocket depth. (See Chapters 1 and 8 and below for a more detailed discussion.)

Periodontitis is, of course, caused by an interaction between bacteria and the host defenses. Most diseases of microbial origin are classified with regard to the causative agent. We, therefore, distinguish trichomoniasis (caused by the parasitic protozoan *Trichomonas vaginalis*) from another sexually transmitted disease, gonorrhea (caused by the gram-negative bacterium *Neisseria gonorrhea*). Although both may have similar clinical presentations, there are diagnostic tests that allow the clinician to make the diagnosis with certainty. This is important because the therapeutic regimens are quite different.

It would seem logical to similarly classify periodontal diseases according to etiology. Such a classification scheme could serve as a guide to selecting an appropriate therapeutic modality. Attempts have been made to correlate the wide array of host and microbial factors that produce the clinical expression of disease, but this goal has proven elusive. In practice, treatment decisions are rarely based on the identification of periodontal pathogens. Indeed, the use of microbial assays to identify the periodontal pathogens present in a given case is only infrequently performed.

This may seem odd, given that most periodontal diseases are caused by the interaction of bacteria with the host. However, it has been demonstrated that patients with similar clinical presentations may have quite different bacterial flora; conversely, patients with similar subgingival flora may have quite different clinical presentations. It is often said that bacteria are *necessary but not sufficient* to cause periodontitis—that is, periodontal pathogens must be present, but their presence does not imply that the occurrence of periodontitis is inevitable (see Chapters 3 and 4). The implication is that host factors or other risk factors are of equal, if not greater, importance. A clear example of this may be found in the Erie County study, an epidemiologic investigation of the association of various risk factors with periodontitis.[11,12] These investigators found smoking to be a more important risk factor than the presence of certain periodontal pathogens.

Chronic diseases, such as diabetes, cardiovascular disease, and periodontitis, are multifactorial, involving a complex interplay between host and environmental factors. There are undoubtedly genetic components to the host response, some of which have been identified and most of which have not (see Chapter 3). The complex interaction of these variables has made it difficult to catalogue periodontal diseases on the basis of bacterial etiology and other factors. The application of sophisticated analytic tools such as cluster analysis has shed some light on these relations, but more work is clearly needed before such information will have clinical use.[13-15] The science of epidemiology has played a critical role in the identification of risk factors, but such studies are expensive and time-consuming and must involve sufficient numbers of subjects. However, additional research will be necessary if causality is to be established and the relative importance of various risk factors further clarified. The ability to distinguish between disease states having similar clinical presentation but differing etiologies may become more important if the association between periodontal infection and certain systemic diseases is confirmed (see Chapter 32).

Classification of Periodontal Diseases and Conditions

The current classification system of the American Academy of Periodontology was the result of an international conference of experts held in 1999. Broadly viewed, the current scheme organizes periodontal diseases into the following groups (which are covered in detail in Chapter 2):

- Gingival diseases
- Chronic periodontitis
- Aggressive periodontitis
- Necrotizing periodontal diseases
- Abscesses of the periodontium
- Periodontitis associated with endodontic lesions
- Developmental or acquired deformities and conditions

Classification systems other than that promulgated by the American Academy of Periodontology exist, such as the International Classification of Diseases (ICD) published by the World Health Organization. The latest iteration is the ICD-10. There is a specialty version available, known as the ICD-DA, which applies to dentistry and stomatology.[16] These schemes are important internationally and from a public health perspective,

but are rarely (if ever) used in clinical practice in the United States.

The goal of periodontal disease classification is a biologically based scheme that possesses clinical utility and is able to provide clinically useful distinctions between diseases that have similar clinical presentations. Such a scheme will aid in the treatment of patients and will facilitate research into the epidemiology, causes, and treatment of periodontal disease. Disease classification should not be viewed as static, but rather a dynamic work in progress, subject to change. As our understanding of the disease process changes, further changes in classification can be anticipated.

Conceptual Basis of Disease Classification

Periodontal diseases could conceivably be classified on the basis of clinical presentation, etiology, or genetic predisposition.[9] A syndromic classification groups diseases on the basis of symptoms and signs—that is, by the clinical presentation. It is fair to say that most of the American Academy of Periodontology classification system is based on syndromic criteria. Classification by etiology or predisposition would seem to be more biologically meaningful and possibly more relevant to therapeutic decision making. This is particularly true of diseases of microbial origin, such as periodontitis. Unfortunately, it is not currently possible to construct such a scheme, because of gaps in our knowledge of the disease processes.

Specific Components of a Periodontal Diagnosis: Disease Type, Extent, and Severity

A periodontal diagnosis consists of three components: disease type, extent, and severity. The disease type will generally be based on the classification system recommended by the American Academy of Periodontology (see earlier and in Chapter 2).

The primary distinction is between chronic and aggressive forms of periodontitis. The presumptive diagnosis of aggressive periodontitis is made on the basis of several features, including the relative lack of local factors sufficient to explain the extent and severity of the disease observed. Other criteria seen in aggressive periodontitis include: patients are otherwise clinically healthy, rapid attachment loss, familial aggregation, the occasional presence of certain pathogens, the occasional presence of a hyperresponsive macrophage phenotype, and other host defense abnormalities. Note that the some of these features suggest the possibility of a genetic component.

The clinical presentation of aggressive forms of the disease is in contrast to chronic periodontitis for which the clinical presentation is consistent with the local factors present. In other words, in chronic periodontitis, plaque and calculus are usually visibly present and the tissue is often inflamed, although this may be masked by smoking. Previously, age was considered important in distinguishing aggressive periodontitis from chronic periodontitis; indeed, aggressive forms were collectively referred to as early-onset periodontitis. In the latest classification this distinction has been removed, although it is clinically useful to bear in mind that generalized disease of significant severity is uncommonly seen in young patients. Aggressive forms of the disease have a somewhat less predictable response to therapy and may require closer follow up after active therapy.

Extent of disease distinguishes between localized and generalized disease patterns (see Chapter 2). In general, the disease is considered to be localized if less than 30% of sites are affected, whereas generalized disease affects more than 30% of sites. This is often a useful distinction. In cases where only an isolated defect is seen, this may hold clues as to the cause of the problem. Consider, for example, a patient in previously good dental health who has an 8-mm pocket on the facial aspect of a maxillary premolar. The tooth has a large cast restoration, post-and-core, and has been treated endodontically. There is no other evidence of periodontal disease present. The localized nature of this problem strongly suggests a nonperiodontal etiology, such as a vertical root fracture or root perforation (Fig. 11-1). Consider the same situation, but this time the patient has numerous generalized probing depths of this magnitude. In the latter case, it likely that the patient has periodontitis, whereas in the former case, it is likely that there is a specific nonperiodontal etiology. The treatment plan for these two individuals will differ radically, and more diagnostic information may well be required in the first case, including the possible need for exploratory surgery.

Thus, the distinction between localized and generalized disease speaks generally to an important concept in diagnosis: Are there sufficient factors present to explain the disease extent and severity? If the disease is quite localized, then there may be some strong local factor such as a fractured root, overhanging restoration, or violation of biologic width that may explain the local disease. Periodontitis is often said to be a *site-specific* disease, in that one site on a tooth may be affected whereas another is not. Despite this assertion, there is evidence that susceptibility to periodontitis occurs on a subject level—that is, the entire mouth is at risk in susceptible individuals. Given the importance of the host response, this makes perfect sense. A similar host response is likely to be operant in all areas of the mouth. This offers one rationale why full-mouth bleeding scores and mean probing depths may be more predictive of breakdown somewhere in the mouth than single-site scores are predictive for the future attachment loss in an individual site (see Prognosis: The Rationale and Biological Basis). Therefore, when very local destruction is seen, particularly in a setting of generalized periodontal health, local causes should be sought.

The severity of periodontitis is often categorized as being slight or early, moderate, or advanced.[17] Slight periodontitis exists when a site has a clinical attachment level of 1 to 2 mm. When a clinical attachment level of 3 to 4 mm is present, the disease as categorized as moderate, whereas severe disease exists with attachment levels of 5 mm or more.

The Relationship between Treated Disease, Probing Depth, Attachment Level, Recession, and Diagnosis

The relation between probing depth, recession, and attachment loss often proves confusing to student dentists and may warrant a brief discussion, because it is central to the concept of periodontal diagnosis. If there has been no recession, and there is no gingival enlargement or significant gingival edema (i.e., no pseudopockets), and there has been no previous periodontal treatment performed, then diagnosis is relatively straightforward.

Given the situation described above, we may then conclude that a state of periodontal health exists if there are no pockets greater than 3 mm and no signs of inflammation such as changes in color or consistency, swelling, or bleeding on gentle probing. If, however, there are no pockets greater than 3 mm, but *there is inflammation present* in the form of bleeding or color changes, then the patient may be diagnosed with plaque-induced gingivitis, particularly if plaque is observed at the gingival margin. If there are pockets measuring greater than 3 mm, accompanied by signs of inflammation and clinical attachment loss, then periodontitis can be reliably diagnosed.

Now let us add some of the qualifiers listed above and see what happens. Recession commonly occurs on the labial of anterior teeth and premolars, but can occur on other surfaces. Because the root surface is normally the site of the insertion of Sharpey's fibers of the periodontal ligament, the

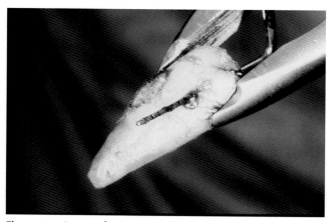

Figure 11-1. Root perforation created during post preparation. Patient had localized periodontitis isolated to this single tooth.

presence of recession always implies *de facto* evidence of attachment loss. However, recession is not always the result of periodontitis, but is often the result of mechanical trauma such as overzealous brushing, particularly in the setting of thin labial tissue. With that in mind, consider some cases that may clearly demonstrate these concepts.

Case 1: The patient is a 19-year-old student who seeks routine care in the clinic of the College of Dentistry. On examination, you note 2 mm of recession on the labial aspect of teeth #6 and #11. There is more than 3 mm of attached gingiva remaining in the area. The patient is unsure how long the recession has been present, but her orthodontist had remarked on it several years ago. There are no probing depths measuring greater than 3 mm, and there is no evidence of inflammation. What is the diagnosis? Clearly, the patient has attachment loss. The recession is indicative of that. But her tissue appears healthy, with no bleeding, good home care, and minimal probing depth. What is the diagnosis? What treatment is needed?

Analysis: This patient appears to be relatively stable from a periodontal standpoint. The recession is probably because of thin tissue overlying the prominent canines and is more likely caused by mechanical trauma from brushing than by inflammatory periodontal disease. Nevertheless, it should be documented and followed, because treatment of progressive recession is often warranted. The patient should, of course, be instructed in atraumatic home care techniques so as not to exacerbate the condition. The primary point, however, is that this individual is probably not at risk for periodontitis, barring the occurrence of an additional risk factor such as smoking.

Case 2: The patient is a 42-year-old man assigned to you at the beginning of your fourth year in dental school. He has been a patient at the school for many years, during which time he has been treated for periodontitis. Examination reveals good home care, minimal bleeding on probing, probing depths measuring 1 to 4 mm, and generalized gingival recession, especially in the posterior sextants. The recession ranges from 2 to 4 mm. Review of his past periodontal charting reveals little or no change in either his recession or his probing depths over the last few years. Review of radiographs taken at various intervals also suggest clinical stability. He is an ex-smoker; his medical history is otherwise noncontributory. What is your diagnosis? What treatment will you recommend?

Analysis: The recession is obviously a result of his previous periodontal disease, his therapy, or a combination of both. The probing depths are unchanged, bearing in mind that 1 mm changes are within the range of measurement error, particularly with multiple operators conducting the examination, as would be the case in a dental school setting. This patient is probably stable, although he has demonstrated susceptibility to periodontal disease and, therefore, must be followed closely for signs of recurrence.

Case 3: The patient discussed earlier (Case 2) is placed under your care and does well. He is seen on a 3-month maintenance regimen. At his most recent maintenance appointment, you note that he exhibits relatively widespread bleeding (65% of sites), although probing depth remains essentially unchanged. What is your diagnosis? What treatment will you recommend?

Analysis: The increased bleeding certainly is indicative of inflammation. Does this mean that the patient has periodontitis (inflammation plus loss of attachment)? Or does he have gingivitis superimposed on a preexisting periodontitis that is no longer active? This is admittedly confusing to the student dentist, but this is the sort of situation often encountered in practice. On one hand, probing depth is essentially unchanged; on the other hand, inflammation is certainly present. The diagnosis, according to the current classification system, would be gingivitis in the setting of a reduced periodontium. In other words, the classification takes into account the previous attachment loss, but still classifies the problem as one of gingival inflammation. This seems reasonable, because a number of studies indicate that attachment loss is infrequent in patients receiving maintenance therapy.

Case 4: The patient in Cases 2 and 3 returns yet again for a maintenance visit. This time, the findings are as before, with the added problem that 9 of the 120 sites in his mouth show increased probing depth, with increases ranging from 1 to 2 mm. Recession is unchanged. What is your diagnosis now? What treatment options might you consider?

Analysis: This situation is much different than Cases 2 and 3. This seems to be true attachment loss in the presence of inflammation—recession is unchanged but probing depths have increased. We should assume that the patient has entered a period of disease activity, on the basis of relatively clearcut evidence. Are there any possible mitigating circumstances that would lead us to a false conclusion in this regard? One possibility that should always suggest itself is measurement error. Although this may be reduced somewhat if only one operator is performing all examinations, it is nevertheless possible. However, the finding of increased probing depth at several sites, combined with inflammation, certainly suggests disease activity. As noted earlier, there is no current gold standard for predicting disease activity other than the historical record of attachment loss that has already occurred. The increased attachment loss strongly suggests that professional intervention is warranted.

Overview of the Treatment Planning Process

After arriving at a diagnosis, the clinician must use this information to formulate a treatment plan and prognosis. More than one prognosis may be projected, on the basis of therapeutic options, including the baseline option of "no treatment." The manner in which the diagnosis and prognosis inform the treatment planning process is considered later in this chapter, following a discussion of prognosis.

PROGNOSIS: THE RATIONALE AND BIOLOGICAL BASIS

Formulating a prognosis is the art of clinical forecasting. The prognosis is a forecast of the probable course and final outcome of a disease. It is the basis on which the clinician makes recommendations and is a key factor in aiding the patient in choosing a course of treatment. It would be preferable to rely exclusively on an evidence-based model for all of our decision making, including establishing a prognosis. There are, however, gaps in our knowledge that preclude this. Periodontal prognosis, therefore, remains somewhat subjective because of our incomplete understanding of disease processes. Despite these limitations, there is much that is known about periodontal disease progression. This knowledge, incomplete though it is, should inform our treatment planning processes.

Prognosis and Causality

Prognosis rests on the related concepts of *causality* and *risk*. These topics are discussed in detail in Chapter 3, but will be reviewed briefly in this chapter in the context of determining a prognosis. Establishing causality and assessing risk lie within the realm of clinical epidemiology and use the scientific and statistical tools of that field.[18] The establishment of causality involves identification of the agents that are responsible for causing a target disorder. Some years ago, the epidemiologist Sir Austin Bradford Hill enumerated several criteria that help establish causality[19] including the following:

- Strength of the association: The stronger the relationship, the greater the likelihood that the relationship is causal. The relationship between smoking and periodontal disease is quite strong, thus suggesting true causality.
- Dose–response relationship: This strongly suggests causality, but does not conclusively demonstrate it because of the potential effect of confounders (see later). Again, many studies have reported a dose–response effect with regard to severity of periodontal disease and amount of tobacco consumption.
- Temporality: The cause must precede the effect. Some types of epidemiologic studies (e.g., cross-sectional) are unable to demonstrate this, by virtue of their design. Temporality is best demonstrated in a longitudinal (cohort) study.
- Consistency: If several studies show essentially the same results, this strengthens the case for causality. Again, smoking is a useful example because almost all studies have reported a positive association between smoking and periodontitis.

Causality is usually suggested initially by cross-sectional epidemiologic studies and confirmed by prospective cohort studies and by interventional studies in which the presumptive etiologic agent is eliminated or neutralized. Such interventional studies are known as clinical trials. A number of such trials have compared treatment outcomes after various modalities of periodontal therapy. A hierarchy of evidence can be established, with the highest level being the randomized controlled trial in which individuals are randomly assigned to one of two or more treatment modalities. If the study is well designed and has a large enough number of subjects, good information regarding treatment efficacy and, by extension, etiologic factors will be gained. Other sources of evidence include case–control studies, case series from private practice settings, and single case reports.

Uncontrolled observations, such as case series and anecdotal case reports, although of some value, lack the validity necessary to inform clinical judgments in practice. The details regarding the characteristics, strengths, and weaknesses of the various types of epidemiologic studies may be found in a standard textbook of epidemiology.[20,21] Finding the best evidence and basing treatment decisions on such evidence is the goal of *evidence-based healthcare*.[6] The best evidence often consists of results derived from a number of randomized clinical trials. Such a synopsis of results is called a *systematic review* or *metaanalysis* (which has somewhat more specific statistical implications). All healthcare disciplines are moving toward evidence-based systems in which treatment decisions are based on valid outcomes research. Ideally, such an approach will improve outcomes and allow for more rational decision making.

Risk assessment consists of weighing the relative strengths of all risk factors present in an effort to quantitate the risk for development of a disorder. The term *exposure* is often used in epidemiology to refer to contact with or proximity to an etiologic agent. For example, smoking is an exposure associated with increased risk for development of lung cancer.

A number of factors are associated with increased risk for periodontitis, the most obvious of which are bacteria. It is well established that bacteria are necessary, but not sufficient, to cause periodontitis. According to the currently accepted model of periodontal disease, the presence of bacteria is required to initiate and sustain the disease process. Presumably, if a person was born into a germ-free environment and isolated from all organisms indefinitely, there would be no chance of periodontitis developing. This concept has been validated by studies of germ-free or so-called gnotobiotic animals.

Despite this, the presence of bacteria, even those strongly implicated in the pathogenesis of periodontitis, is not sufficient to cause periodontitis in all individuals who harbor them. For example, it is well established that some individuals carry periodontal pathogens such as *Porphyromonas gingivalis* in the subgingival microflora, yet do not exhibit significant disease activity (i.e., attachment loss). What is the explanation for this? Periodontitis is a chronic disease. Chronic diseases such as diabetes and atherosclerosis are often multifactorial, having both precipitating etiologic agents such as bacteria and predisposing factors that increase the likelihood or risk of the target disease developing. It has been stated that a "chronic disease can be defined as a disease that has a prolonged course, that does not resolve spontaneously, and for which a complete cure is rarely achieved."[22] Although the question as to whether periodontitis may be cured or only controlled may not be resolved, the multifactorial nature of periodontal pathogenesis seems beyond dispute.[23] Although bacteria are the precipitating cause of periodontitis, there are many predisposing causes that contribute to the disease process. These risk factors increase the likelihood that periodontitis will develop in an individual. This is analogous to the situation seen in other chronic diseases. For example, lung cancer does not develop in all smokers, but smoking greatly increases the probability that it will.

The Relationship between Prognosis and Risk

Predisposing factors may be called *effect modifiers, modifying factors,* or *risk factors.* The *Dictionary of Epidemiology* defines *risk factor* as "an aspect of personal behavior or lifestyle, an environmental exposure, or an inborn or inherited characteristic, that, on the basis of epidemiologic evidence, is known to be associated with health-related conditions considered important to prevent."[24] This term is often used imprecisely, sometimes referring to an actual etiologic agent such as periodontal pathogens, and at other times used to describe factors that contribute to susceptibility, such as smoking or diabetes. The most common usage in the dental literature implies that the risk factor is directly involved in the pathogenesis, although the International Epidemiological Association makes no such distinction, as noted in the definition above.[24]

The terms *risk indicator* or *risk marker* imply that the factor, although associated with increased risk for disease development, is not necessarily causal in the strictest sense. Such factors merely *predispose* an individual to disease, thereby increasing the risk for development of the disorder and may therefore be thought of as predisposing factors. Other factors may be associated with increased risk, but only because they are associated with yet another factor that increases risk. This may sometimes be the case with race and susceptibility to various diseases, including periodontitis. In the case of some ethnic groups, it may not be race per se that causes increased risk, but the fact that a greater percentage of some races are economically disadvantaged. The economic disparities may be the actual cause of the increased susceptibility. It is a key epidemiologic concept that *association does not necessarily imply causality.*

The presence of a risk factor increases the probability of disease development and may present a possible target for therapeutic or preventive interventions. Some risk factors and indicators are modifiable in that they may be eliminated or otherwise neutralized to reduce the risk for development of the disorder. For example, smoking cessation may improve the periodontal prognosis of a young woman with early periodontitis. Some factors are intrinsic, such as genetic predisposition, and may not be amenable to modification. This concept has clinical use, because an individual with an intrinsic, nonmodifiable risk factor will remain at increased risk even after successful treatment. It is likely that such an individual will require more intensive surveillance and maintenance therapy to prevent disease recurrence.

When all these various risk factors and indicators are considered together, it is theoretically possible to assess the degree of risk for periodontitis developing in a given individual or group. This process is known as *risk assessment* and its relation to prognosis should be evident. Unfortunately, not all risk factors and indicators for periodontitis are known, and those that are known are difficult to quantitate. The role of smoking, one of the most important risk factors, was virtually ignored for most of the last century. It was only during the 1990s that its true significance became apparent. Many members of the subgingival microflora have not been identified or cultivated. We are only beginning to unlock the secrets of the human genome, which will undoubtedly shed additional light on genetic predisposition. It is this incomplete state of our science that led Prichard to state more than 30 years ago that prognosis "is an art based on a science."[25] The statement is still true, although our knowledge has increased substantially since that time. The goal of periodontal research is to reduce the amount of art required by increasing the amount of scientifically valid, clinically relevant information that is available. This process is the foundation of evidence-based medicine and is directly related to concepts of causality and risk.

Establishing causality is central to modern biomedical science, because it involves the identification of the agents responsible for disease. This, in turn, suggests possible preventive and therapeutic interventions. Causality is also related to prognosis in a most direct way. Treatment of many diseases involves removal of the true offending or causal agent (or at least reducing its impact).

To the extent that this can be done, the treatment will be effective and the prognosis good. To the extent that the actual agent is not identified or cannot be reduced or eliminated, suboptimal outcomes may be expected and the prognosis will, in those cases, be less favorable.

Occasionally, it is questioned whether pretreatment risk and posttreatment prognosis represent the same phenomenon. Are the same factors responsible for disease recurrence as for initiating the disease in the first place? In other words, are the factors that first triggered the disease likely to cause or contribute to a treatment failure (and, therefore, a poor prognosis)? It seems plausible that the risk factors or etiologic agents that initiated and sustained the disease process in the first instance would similarly act to cause a recurrence after treatment, assuming that they have not been eliminated or neutralized by treatment. However, there have been reports suggesting that the factors that initiate disease are not necessarily the same as those that cause disease progression.[26] In any event, the clinical value of determining causality lies in the ability to suggest specific preventive or therapeutic interventions that may be used to reduce or eliminate the causal agents.

Lung cancer is a useful example. The pioneering work of Doll and Hill[27,28] established smoking as the primary cause of lung cancer. These findings, in turn, suggested that smoking cessation might be effective in reducing the incidence of lung cancer. It also suggested that patients who were treated successfully for this disease would be at increased risk if they did not quit smoking, compared with those who successfully quit. It is biologically plausible that most risk factors would, if present after treatment, continue to predispose the recurrence of disease. A corollary is that risk factors that cannot be modified, such as genetic predisposition, would continue to constitute a risk even after treatment and that the subset of patients possessing such a risk factor would merit more careful observation. This point is examined later in this chapter as part of the discussion of genetic predisposition to periodontitis.

Outcomes

Another critical factor relating to prognosis is that of *outcomes*. Outcomes are "all the possible results that may stem from exposure to a causal factor, or from preventive or therapeutic interventions; all identified changes in health status arising as a consequence of the handling of a health problem."[24] In a research study, outcomes that are measured or observed are known as *variables*. The *independent variable* is said to exert an influence or cause variation in the *dependent* or *response variable*. If lung cancer is being studied, the incidence of lung cancer may be the dependent variable and smoking the independent variable.

Continuing the lung cancer example, one outcome of interest might be disease recurrence. A question that

would have to be answered is: How do we define disease recurrence? Would a suspicious spot on a chest radiograph be sufficient? Or would we require a more meaningful outcome, such as death from lung cancer? The outcome chosen is important. There are different types of outcomes. A distinction is often made between *true* and *surrogate* outcomes.[29] A true end-point or outcome would "reflect unequivocal evidence of tangible benefit to the patient."[29] In periodontology, a *true* outcome would be loss of a tooth, because this has real consequences for the patient. A *surrogate* outcome would be attachment loss, which, if untreated, is assumed to eventually result in the loss of the tooth. A patient does not usually know if attachment loss has progressed, and probably does not care. Patients care about outcomes that are meaningful to them, such as tooth loss or esthetic compromise.

It is important that surrogate outcomes can be related in some meaningful way to real outcomes. It may seem intuitively obvious that an increase in attachment loss may lead to tooth loss. Certainly, if the attachment loss continued indefinitely, tooth loss would be the ultimate result. But there is an alternative scenario. Imagine that attachment loss progressed to a point short of the apex and then ceased entirely. This may be unlikely, but it is possible. In such a case, attachment loss would not be related positively to tooth mortality. Longitudinal studies are required to relate surrogate outcomes to real outcomes. Because most studies of periodontal outcomes use attachment loss as the outcome of interest, it is important that attachment loss be related to the "real world" outcome of tooth mortality. Such validation recently has been demonstrated. Hujoel and colleagues,[29] using data from a large cohort of 565 Norwegian men, found that attachment loss of moderate severity was associated with increased risk for tooth loss. For example, sites that experienced 3 mm or more attachment loss had a 270% increase in tooth mortality.[30] In the following section, factors used to predict attachment loss and, by extension, tooth loss are examined. This act of prediction is a key component of establishing a prognosis.

CLINICAL APPLICATIONS

Levels of Prognosis: Tooth and Arch

Prognoses may be formulated at different levels. For example, we may speak of the prognosis of an individual tooth, an arch, or the entire dentition. These are somewhat arbitrary categories. For example, if there are only two teeth remaining in an arch, the prognoses of these two teeth will, of necessity, determine the prognosis of the entire arch. Therefore, the number of remaining teeth, although not considered a classical risk factor, often plays a practical role in limiting treatment options. The prognosis of individual teeth is often a function of how much attachment loss has been sustained, local factors such as furcation lesions, and systemic factors such as smoking. It also will be affected by the restorative treatment plan. For example, a high degree of predictability may be required if a tooth is to be used as an abutment for a multiunit fixed partial denture.

In complex cases, one arch may be significantly worse than the other. This may be termed the *limiting arch* because it may exert a disproportionate influence on the treatment plan. The classical example of the limiting arch concept, at least in the preimplant era, was the hopeless mandibular arch opposed by a relatively full complement of salvageable maxillary teeth. Many clinicians believed that a mandibular denture opposed by upper natural teeth would result in rapid loss of alveolar bone in the mandibular arch, the so-called combination syndrome. It was common in such cases to advise removal of the maxillary teeth and the mandibular. This has changed somewhat, because of the predictability of implant-borne restorations. Indeed, the impact of implants on the treatment planning process has been profound (see Chapter 26).

Another useful distinction is that between long- and short-term prognoses. Although somewhat arbitrary, short-term usually refers to a period of 5 years or less, whereas long-term usually refers to a period longer than 5 years. Generally, accuracy diminishes with increasing timeframe of the forecast. Prognoses are often most meaningful when comparing various forms of treatment. Patient and clinician may both be interested in a *differential prognosis* depending on which of two therapies is chosen. Interventions may differ significantly in terms of cost, morbidity, and esthetic outcomes. In such cases, the differential prognosis would be an important consideration in the decision-making process.

Levels of Prognosis: Systemic or Global Prognosis

At first glance, it might seem logical to assume that the prognosis for the entire dentition might be equivalent to the sums of the prognoses of the individual teeth. However, this is not the case. There is evidence that the clinical picture presented by the entire mouth is a more important overall predictor than information related to an individual site. This may best be demonstrated by example. In a widely cited article, Lang and colleagues[31,32] report that bleeding on probing was not a good predictor of attachment loss. Assuming that these results have external validity—that is, can be generalized to the entire "universe" of periodontal patients—it could be assumed that bleeding on probing is not extremely important. In other words, bleeding on probing is not a particularly good predictor of attachment loss at the *site level*.

A different picture emerges, however, if the whole-mouth bleeding score is examined—that is, if mean values from each patient are examined at the *patient* or *subject level*. As explained below, there is some evidence that although the presence of bleeding is not a good predictor of impending attachment loss at the site level, the whole-mouth mean bleeding score may be somewhat meaningful on the subject level. When the bleeding score of the entire mouth is increased, some investigators have reported that it is more likely that attachment will be lost somewhere in the mouth, although not necessarily at an individual bleeding site.[33] Similar observations have been made regarding pocket depths persisting after treatment.[34-36] This is consistent with a disease that is heavily influenced by the host defenses, particularly because these would be presumed to be more or less constant at all sites. Individual risk factors are examined later along with their contributions to periodontal disease progression.

IMPACT OF INDIVIDUAL RISK FACTORS ON PERIODONTAL PROGNOSIS

Systemic Risk Factors

Smoking

Smoking is a major risk factor for development of periodontitis, as well as modifying treatment response (see Chapter 34). This relation was clarified during the 1990s. Before then, the role of smoking was not understood. Currently, smoking is considered a major risk factor for periodontitis. It was recently reported, for example, that heavy smokers were almost three times more likely to lose teeth after periodontal therapy than nonsmokers.[37] The same investigators reported that the combined effects of smoking and a genetic risk factor were so strong that, when present, none of the traditional risk factors added to the risk assessment. Smoking is presumed to act at the subject level, although there is also some evidence of a local effect. It has been reported, for example, that smoking increases attachment loss in the maxillary lingual and mandibular anterior regions.[38] McGuire and Nunn,[39-42] in a study of periodontal patients in a private practice, assigned initial prognoses to teeth and observed patients over time to determine which factors were good risk predictors; tooth loss was the outcome of interest, rather than surrogate variables. They reported that smoking decreased the likelihood of an improved prognosis after treatment by 60% compared with nonsmokers.

Genetic predisposition

Twin studies and other evidence support the concept that heredity plays a large role in periodontal susceptibility, accounting for perhaps as much as 50% of the risk for chronic periodontitis[43] (see Chapter 3). This relation persisted, even after correcting for confounding variables such as smoking. The exact nature of this relation had remained somewhat elusive until recently. In 1997, Kornman and colleagues[44] described a genetic polymorphism at the genes that code for the production of the proinflammatory cytokine interleukin-1 (IL-1), which was associated with increased risk for periodontal attachment loss. The presence of this genotype results in the individual's macrophages producing more of the proinflammatory cytokine IL-1 when stimulated by agents such as lipopolysaccharide from gram-negative bacteria. This polymorphism is found in approximately 30% of the white population, but in much lower percentages in other racial groups. Such racial differences may help to explain some of the differences in risk for periodontal diseases among populations and may play a role in establishing a prognosis for patients from various racial groups. This is not to say that a prognosis should be assigned on the basis of a racial category. Rather, the chance that the IL-1 genotype might play a role in disease pathogenesis and might be a factor in establishing a prognosis is greater in a population of white patients in which the prevalence of the genotype is around 30% than it is in a Chinese-American population in which the prevalence of the genotype is less than 3%.[45]

McGuire and Nunn[37,40] found that individuals possessing this IL-1 gene polymorphism are about 2.7 times more likely to lose teeth than those without the genotype. The risk is increased by 7.7-fold in genotype-positive individuals who are also long-time heavy smokers. The genotype is acting as an *effect modifier* of the smoking, and the nature of the interaction is multiplicative rather than additive—that is, the observed effect is greater than the sums of the two factors acting independently. Therefore, the clinician might rationally assign a less favorable overall prognosis for a patient who was both a heavy smoker and had the IL-1 genotype than for a patient who neither smoked nor had the genotype. Notably, there are no longitudinal studies demonstrating an increased incidence of attachment over time in people with the IL-1 genotype, compared with those without the genotype. This example is used simply to demonstrate how genetic risk factors might play a role in determining the prognosis.

The IL-1 genotype and other potential genetic risk markers act at the subject level. Although it is true that nothing can be done to alter the individual's genetic makeup, other than through gene therapy, it is possible that certain compensatory therapies (e.g., ranging from host modulation to more frequent maintenance intervals) may be used to offset genetic risk factors at the mechanistic level. These approaches require more research before any such conclusions can be made.

Age

Age is a risk factor for periodontitis in the sense that virtually all studies have found that older age groups show greater periodontal destruction than younger age cohorts. This is true regarding prevalence, extent, and severity.[11,12] The extent and severity of periodontal attachment loss increase with age, because of the cumulative effect of a lifetime of bacterial–host interactions. The destruction seen at any point in time is the sum of all preceding episodes of attachment loss. All other factors being equal, the older individual is at increased risk for development of periodontal disease and, if present, is at risk for greater extent and severity. This is intuitively obvious. There is an additional explanation for the increased prevalence of periodontitis in older age cohorts: the increased presence of plaque-retentive restorations.[46]

That older individuals are more likely to have experienced periodontal destruction in the past is of minimal relevance to establishing a prognosis for the future. Rather, the clinician is mainly concerned with whether age itself increases the risk for progressive periodontal destruction over time. If so, then a less favorable prognosis might be given to a 70-year-old patient than would be given to a 40-year-old patient with a similar level of destruction. Most studies have shown no increased risk for progressive disease on the basis of age,[46] although one study in Japanese subjects did show more disease progression in older individuals.[47]

Age is often cited as a factor in determining posttreatment prognosis for reasons that are the inverse of those listed above. This is best shown by example. Imagine two nonsmoking individuals with identical clinical findings of moderate to advanced chronic periodontitis, with similar extent and severity of probing depth, attachment loss, and mobility, but different ages. One patient is 35 years old and the other is 65 years old. It is often stated that the prognosis is better for the older of the two subjects. The rationale for this is that it took the older individual longer to reach the current state of health or disease, which implies a relatively greater degree of resistance. In addition, the younger individual will be required to maintain his or her dentition for many more years than the older individual. Although the short-term prognosis may be similar, the long-term prognosis may be deemed better for the older person. There seems to be little experimental evidence to support this claim, although it is biologically plausible. An additional question worth asking is whether age modifies the response to therapy. It is conceivable, for example, that certain regenerative procedures may not work as well in older individuals. However, there is little evidence that older people respond either less favorably or more favorably to most modalities of therapy. Definitive answers to this question must await additional research.

Race

Racial differences in periodontal disease prevalence seem to be largely because of socioeconomic factors. However, race and ethnicity do play a role in disease susceptibility in certain chronic diseases. This is exemplified by the propensity of the Pima Indians to develop type 2 diabetes. There are distinct racial differences in the host immunoinflammatory response to periodontal pathogens that may provide some explanation for the greater prevalence of this disease in these populations. However, current evidence does not provide a basis for assigning prognostic categories simply on the basis of race. Definitive answers will have to await studies that involve diverse populations.

Sex

Male individuals tend to have more periodontal disease than female individuals, and the disease tends to be more severe when it does occur. Although men, as a group, use dental services less than women and tend to have poorer home care, the increase in periodontal disease persists after correcting for these factors.[12,48] It has been speculated that this may be because of hormonal influences, and the bone-sparing effect of estrogen has been cited as an example.[48] As with race, not enough is known about the influence of sex on progression of periodontal diseases or response to periodontal therapy to alter prognostication significantly on the basis of sex.

Systemic diseases and conditions

Periodontal tissues are influenced by the systemic state of the host. Not surprisingly, a number of systemic influences are associated with increased risk for development of periodontitis (see Chapter 31). Among these are the common diseases diabetes mellitus and osteoporosis. Poorly controlled diabetes, in particular, is a significant risk factor for increased prevalence, extent, and severity of periodontal attachment loss.[49] Any condition that causes a suppression of the host defenses also can predispose to periodontal disease, including HIV/AIDS, neutrophil defects, and similar conditions. Psychosocial factors such as stress also have been implicated as risk factors. Nutritional factors have been somewhat neglected, but recent evidence suggests that low intake of certain nutrients such as calcium and vitamin C also may confer some risk. Systemic conditions should definitely be considered in formulating a periodontal prognosis. For example, the clinician might assign a less favorable overall prognosis to a patient with poorly controlled diabetes and high financial stress levels than to a systemically healthy patient with a similar degree of periodontal destruction, especially if the clinician and patient cannot effect changes in diabetic control or stress levels.

Local Risk Factors

Gingival inflammation

Gingival inflammation is one of the most common periodontal findings. The presence of inflammation is most often defined by the clinical finding of bleeding on gentle probing, but gingival redness or erythema occasionally has been used. These are rather nonspecific indicators of gingival inflammation that may represent simple, reversible gingivitis, or may be associated with destructive periodontitis. A number of studies have attempted to find an association between gingival inflammation and attachment loss, at either the site or subject level. However, one important factor complicates the interpretation of these data. Smoking is a risk factor for periodontitis. Oddly enough, smoking also has a suppressive effect on gingival bleeding, probably mediated through an effect on the microvasculature. Smoking is thus a third variable that has an effect on the target disorder (periodontitis or attachment loss) and on the clinical finding of gingival bleeding. A factor that is related in this fashion both to the exposure and the outcome of interest is known as a *confounder* or *confounding variable*. The effect of this confounder would most likely be to make bleeding on probing a less reliable predictor of attachment loss (i.e., weaken the association) in a patient who smokes.

Site level analyses. Most investigators have found little correlation between bleeding on probing at a given site and subsequent attachment loss at that site. Bleeding on probing has been shown to be of low PPV and limited specificity.[31,32] Thus, the use of bleeding on probing at a site as a prognostic variable and a predictor of future disease would result in a high number of false-positive results; many sites that did bleed on probing would not demonstrate progressive destruction. Conversely, the *absence* of bleeding on probing has been shown to be an excellent predictor of clinical stability.[32] About 98% of clinically stable sites did not bleed when probed. Thus, when assigning a prognosis for a given tooth, the absence of bleeding on probing over several appointments could indicate an improved prognosis compared with a tooth with similar levels of periodontal destruction that bled repeatedly on probing.

Subject level analysis. Does the general gingival bleeding status throughout the mouth help the clinician assign a prognosis? If the host response is really an important factor in determining susceptibility to periodontal disease, then it is plausible that average bleeding scores that reflect the inflammatory state throughout the mouth may be of value. The evidence is mixed in this regard. Some investigators have reported modest associations between full-mouth bleeding scores and risk for attachment loss. Joss and colleagues[33] report that more than 60% of sites losing at least 2 mm of attachment were found in a subset of patients with bleeding scores of 30% or greater. Other investigators, however, have found no relation between whole-mouth average bleeding scores and future periodontal disease progression.[36] The general level of bleeding on probing may provide the clinician with input on the overall prognosis for the patient because it would be considered an overall assessment of gingival inflammation, but prognosis for individual sites or teeth is likely more related to bleeding or lack of bleeding at those specific sites or teeth.

Suppuration

Suppuration is considered by some clinicians to be a particularly "bad omen." However, there is little evidence that this is true.[36,50-52] Most studies fail to demonstrate an increased risk for progressive destruction at sites having suppuration.[36] Suppuration should be considered in a way similar to bleeding on probing; namely, if widely present throughout the mouth, it should be considered in the overall prognosis as a general indicator of the overall level of periodontal inflammation.

Compliance with maintenance recommendations

Patients who have been treated for periodontitis require regular maintenance to prevent disease recurrence (see Chapter 15). Although the interval must be tailored to the individual patient, such visits are normally scheduled at 3- or 4-month intervals. This requires an ongoing commitment on the part of the patient. The degree to which a patient follows such therapeutic recommendations is known as *compliance*. Compliance is a major issue in periodontal therapy, as it is in the treatment of all chronic diseases, and compliance must be considered in formulating a prognosis. A number of studies have shown that good compliance is associated with better periodontal outcomes, including less tooth loss. In formulating a prognosis, the clinician examines the patient's history of compliance with dental visits and recommended care. Those with a poor history of compliance may be given a less favorable initial prognosis than those who are have been compliant. The clinician also must consider the potential for improvement in compliance. For many patients, the dentist does not have a treatment history. In these cases, many clinicians assume that the patient will comply with maintenance when assigning an initial prognosis, and then adjust that prognosis accordingly as treatment progresses, on the basis of the demonstrated patient compliance.

Plaque and calculus

Bacteria are necessary for the development of periodontitis and gingivitis. Plaque is unquestionably related to the development of gingivitis in a very direct manner. The same cannot be said of periodontitis. Numerous studies demonstrate that meticulous plaque removal will normally prevent the development of periodontal disease, but several longitudinal studies describe a more tenuous relation between plaque levels and periodontal attachment loss. Generally, most studies have shown either no or weak correlation with plaque and future attachment loss at the site level.[51,52] (See Chapter 13 for a complete discussion of this relation.)

Persistent deep pockets

It is plausible to presume that increased pocket depth persisting after therapy would be a risk factor for future attachment loss. Deep pockets are more apt to harbor periodontal pathogens and are harder for the patient and therapist to maintain.[53] Deeper pockets are generally associated with an increased percentage of histologically inflamed tissue,[54] and this is validated by the related finding that deeper pockets are more likely to exhibit bleeding on probing.[53] It is conceivable that such pockets might serve as a reservoir for periodontal pathogens, which could put the deep site at risk (site level effect) or serve to reinfect other sites (subject level effect). It has been shown that the source of bacteria that repopulate sites after treatment is generally derived from the patient's own flora.[55] Surgical pocket reduction can lead to a profound shift in the subgingival microbiota toward that associated with health, which may be a key to maintaining periodontal stability.[56] The importance of persistent deep pockets as possible bacterial reservoirs is indirectly suggested by evidence that persistent deep pockets have an adverse effect on regenerative outcomes.[57] This knowledge may result in the dentist assigning a less favorable posttreatment prognosis in a patient with persistent deep pockets who has had regenerative surgical therapy than for a patient with shallow probing depths after treatment.

There is also direct evidence from longitudinal studies suggesting that the percentage of deep sites may be a more important indicator of risk at the subject rather than site level.[34-36] In a study of 271 Japanese subjects, greater mean probing depths and prior attachment loss were strong predictors of future attachment loss during a 12-month period.[47] Most of the rationale for multiple deep pockets as a subject level risk factor has been based on the assumption that such sites could act as bacterial reservoirs and serve to reinfect other sites. However, it is also conceivable that patients with a number of persistent deep probing sites are simply more susceptible to disease because of an aberrant host defense mechanism. The presence of numerous deep pockets after therapy may likewise indicate a patient whose response to therapy has been less favorable and who may be at greater risk for future periodontal destruction. Such a patient might be assigned a less favorable prognosis.

Amount of remaining attachment

The amount of attachment remaining is of prognostic significance for one obvious reason. If a tooth has little remaining attachment, then a relatively small amount of continued attachment loss may cause the loss of the tooth. If a large amount of attachment remains, then much more disease activity would be required to cause the loss of the tooth. Therefore, in general, a tooth or a dentition with severe attachment loss will have a less favorable prognosis than one with minimal attachment loss.

Mobility and related factors

The relation between tooth mobility and prognosis is controversial because conflicting evidence exists. In a 10-year longitudinal study, mobility at baseline was associated with increased bone loss over time.[58] In a series of long-term studies, Fleszar and colleagues[59] showed better healing responses after periodontal treatment in firm rather than mobile teeth. Mobility also has been associated with less favorable results after regenerative surgical therapy[60] and with increased risk for tooth loss during maintenance.[42] Not all investigators have confirmed an association between mobility and periodontal disease progression or unfavorable responses to treatment. For example, Rosling and coworkers[61] found that mobility had no effect on treatment outcomes.

Miscellaneous factors

A number of anatomic factors may predispose to attachment loss (see Chapter 7). These include plaque-retentive features such as furcation lesions, grooves, root fractures, areas of cemental hypoplasia, cervical enamel projections, and others. Restorative factors such as overhanging restorations and violations of biologic width also may predispose to periodontal destruction. In formulating a prognosis, the dentist must consider both the impact of these factors on existing disease and the dentist's ability to eliminate those factors as part of the treatment plan. The ability to minimize or eliminate such factors directly affects the prognosis. For example, if a tooth has an overhang that can be eliminated, the prognosis is likely very favorable. Conversely, if a tooth has a root fracture, which cannot be eliminated, the prognosis is likely to be poor or hopeless.

Multirooted teeth with existing furcation involvements generally have a less favorable prognosis than teeth with intact furcations. This is because furcation regions are difficult to access for personal or professional debridement. Numerous long-term studies show that furcation-involved molars are lost more commonly than single-rooted teeth or multirooted teeth without furcation involvement.[62-64] Likewise, multirooted teeth with short root trunks that predispose to furcation involvement after minimal attachment loss often have a less favorable prognosis than single-rooted teeth or multirooted teeth with long root trunks.

APPLICATION OF DIAGNOSIS AND PROGNOSIS TO PERIODONTAL DECISION ANALYSIS

It is readily apparent that formulating a prognosis is far from an exact science. The series of articles by McGuire and McGuire and Nunn clearly illuminate the shortcomings of our current knowledge in this area.[39-42] These investigators describe the results of a long-term study of 100 treated periodontal patients followed for 15 years in a private practice environment. All subjects received similar treatment by the same periodontist. They were initially diagnosed with chronic, generalized moderate to advanced adult periodontitis. Teeth were assigned to one of five prognosis groups. Assignment of prognosis was done immediately after active therapy and at 5- and 8-years after active therapy using the prognostic categories found in Box 11-1. Teeth assigned a good prognosis initially tended to remain good for the duration of the study. If the

---

Box 11-1   Prognostic Categories

Good prognosis: Teeth with a good prognosis have one or both of the following characteristics: adequate remaining periodontal support and ease of maintenance.

Fair prognosis: Teeth with a fair prognosis have one or both of the following characteristics: attachment loss to the point that the tooth cannot be considered to have a good prognosis and presence of a Class I furcation lesion (with the caveat that the furcation is believed to be maintainable).

Poor prognosis: Teeth with a poor prognosis exhibit one or both of the following characteristics: moderate attachment loss with Class I or Class II furcation lesions (that can presumably be maintained, but with difficulty).

Questionable prognosis: Teeth with a questionable prognosis exhibit one or more of the following characteristics: severe attachment loss resulting in a poor crown-to-root ratio; poor root form; root proximity; Class II or III furcation lesions (not amenable to maintenance); and mobility of 2+ or greater.

Hopeless prognosis: Inadequate attachment to maintain the tooth in health, comfort, and function. In such cases, extraction is recommended.

From McGuire MK: Prognosis versus actual outcome: a long-term survey of 100 treated periodontal patients under maintenance care, J Periodontol 62:51-58, 1991.

teeth were assigned to any other category, however, the predictive value was poor. Clearly, many of the commonly used clinical parameters proved ineffective in predicting the outcome for teeth other than those with a good prognosis. Although teeth with a poor prognosis were lost at a greater rate than those with a good prognosis, extreme variation was noted in survival times. At 5 or 8 years, prognoses for posterior teeth were no better than a coin toss. Prognoses for single-rooted teeth tended to be more accurate. The authors found that certain clinical parameters had somewhat more validity: probing depth, mobility, furcation involvement, percentage of bone loss, parafunctional habit without an occlusal guard, and smoking. The authors concluded that the current method of assigning prognosis does not take into account the concept of differential susceptibility.

To at least partially account for susceptibility, McQuire and Nunn tested the IL-1 genotype as well as "heavy smoking" as effect modifiers. Of the patients in the study, 38% were positive for the genotype, but this subset of patients accounted for almost 60% of the tooth loss. Patients positive for the genotype were 2.7 times more likely to lose teeth after therapy. Heavy smoking (defined as $\geq$20 pack-years) was another significant risk factor for tooth loss, increasing the risk by 2.9 times. The combination of heavy smoking and IL-1 genotype resulted in a 7.7-fold increased risk for tooth loss.

The implications of McGuire and Nunn's work are significant. At the very least, they underscore the importance of smoking cessation as part of every treatment plan and quantitate the risk in terms of a real variable—tooth loss. The study also reveals some reasonably predictive risk factors in nonsmoking individuals: furcation lesions, mobility, probing depth, percentage of bone loss, and poor crown/root ratio. When determining the prognosis for a nonsmoking patient, these factors assume greater importance. In a smoker, the effect of smoking overshadows the other factors, a fact that should be considered during the treatment planning process.

A SUGGESTED DIAGNOSTIC PROTOCOL

- The first step in formulating a diagnosis and prognosis is accurate and complete data collection. This necessitates a comprehensive examination. If an acute condition is present (e.g., necrotizing ulcerative gingivitis, periodontal abscess), that problem should be addressed before proceeding to the comprehensive examination and treatment plan.
- Data collection is followed by assignment of a presumptive diagnosis, using the American Academy of Periodontology classification system (see Chapter 2). The components of the diagnosis are disease type, extent, and severity, as noted earlier.

- Next, prognoses for individual teeth should be assigned, using criteria shown in Box 11-2 (but remembering that some of these criteria may be imperfect).
- After assignment of individual prognoses, questionable or hopeless teeth can be deleted from the arch diagrams. This sometimes suggests possible prosthetic schemes. A prognosis can then be assigned to each arch.
- After tooth and arch prognoses have been assigned, a global or full-mouth assessment should be performed and a whole-dentition prognosis given. Depending on the clinical circumstances, this may also affect the individual tooth prognoses. This is particularly true in the case of a strong risk factor, such as smoking (Box 11-3).
- The treatment plan in most cases of periodontitis will begin with initial nonsurgical therapy (Box 11-4). In most cases, it is desirable to defer final decisions regarding surgical intervention and tooth extraction until the reevaluation. This is particularly true when removal of a tooth will necessitate a provisional restoration. There are many circumstances, however, in which badly involved teeth are removed at the time of scaling and root planing.

Box 11-2 **Prognostic Factors: Tooth Level**

Mobility
Amount of remaining attachment
Probing depth
Bone loss
Presence/absence/severity of furcation lesions
Crown-to-root ratio
Endodontic status
Caries

Box 11-3 **Prognostic Factors: Subject (Patient) Level**

Age
Smoking
Diabetes (degree of control important) or other
  systemic diseases
Overall degree of bone loss, attachment loss
Number of residual deep pockets after therapy
Percentage or number of bleeding sites after therapy
Genetic predisposition
Compliance with home care
Compliance with maintenance
Number and position of remaining teeth
Patient desires
Economic factors

Box 11-4	**Normal Sequence of Periodontal Therapy**

1. Systemic phase (evaluation of overall patient health, consultation as indicated)
2. Initial therapy (antiinfective therapy)
   a. Emergency treatment
   b. Extraction of hopeless teeth
   c. Restorative and endodontic therapy
   d. Oral hygiene assessment and instruction
   e. Debridement (scaling/root planing)
   f. Adjunctive treatment (e.g., occlusal therapy, antibiotic therapy, host modulation, minor tooth movement, provisional splinting, as indicated)
3. Reevaluation
4. Surgical therapy (if indicated)
5. Postsurgical reevaluation and assessment of revised prognosis
6. Definitive restorative therapy, including orthodontic tooth movement, if indicated
7. Maintenance therapy

- A formal reevaluation of treatment response should usually occur 6 to 8 weeks after nonsurgical debridement. At that time, tissues should be assessed for signs of inflammation and for changes in probing depth and clinical attachment. Although some additional improvement may occur over a period of several months, most of the improvement is seen within 2 months after therapy. At the time of the reevaluation, the original presumptive diagnosis is subject to validation or revision. In particular, if the disease fails to respond to adequate and appropriate therapy, then the diagnosis may need to be changed. If the response is consistent with pretreatment expectations, the original diagnosis will be confirmed. Likewise, response to initial therapy, or lack of response, may alter the prognosis.
- If the response is generally good, then the patient may be placed on maintenance (i.e., appointed for regularly scheduled assessment and debridement appointments).
- If the response is generally good, but some problem areas remain, then additional therapy will be recommended. This may take the form of enhanced nonsurgical therapy such as the addition of local delivery antimicrobial agents to mechanical debridement, or surgery.
- If the response is generally poor, then a cause should be sought. This may be as simple as poor home care, although systemic factors should be considered.
- After active therapy, whether that be entirely nonsurgical or a combination of nonsurgical and surgical treatment, a posttreatment reevaluation should be performed. The exact timing of this reevaluation depends on the nature of the periodontal therapy provided. Many clinicians

wait longer to reevaluate the patient if regenerative surgical therapy was used than if a nonregenerative approach was used. At the time of this posttreatment reevaluation, the clinician should again determine the prognosis for the patient at the tooth, arch, and dentition levels. The findings at this posttreatment reevaluation, and the prognoses rendered, will serve as the new baseline for the patient as he or she moves into the maintenance phase.

CLINICAL APPLICATIONS

Below are some clinical examples that illustrate the application of the concepts discussed in this chapter.

Case 1: The patient is a 58-year-old woman who reported for initial examination in the 1980s. She was referred for evaluation of her remaining lower teeth (Fig. 11-2). She was having a good deal of difficulty with them, because they were quite loose and her partial denture no longer fit well. She consulted a dentist who had suggested removal of the remaining teeth and replacement with an implant-borne prosthesis. Although the patient was interested in this, she was unable to afford the combined fees of the surgeon and prosthodontist. She had been told that her jaw was resorbed too severely to allow her to wear a conventional denture. She was wearing a maxillary complete denture, which she tolerated well. The patient was very concerned with and attentive to her appearance. The medical history was noncontributory, except for a history of smoking. The patient had been a relatively heavy smoker, but quit several years earlier. Examination revealed evidence of widespread periodontal destruction on the remaining teeth. Probing depth ranged from 1 to 9 mm, with most interproximal sites probing greater than 6 mm. Most teeth exhibited mobility of grade 2. Tooth #30 was not mobile, but did have a Class III furcation lesion. Recession was generalized and severe. The supragingival hygiene was surprisingly good, but there were heavy deposits of subgingival calculus present. Other examination findings were unremarkable.

Analysis: The diagnosis given at the time (in the late 1980s) was generalized severe adult periodontitis (equivalent classification today would be generalized severe chronic periodontitis). Most teeth had a highly questionable initial prognosis, simply because of the limited amount of remaining attachment. The mandibular arch likewise had a questionable prognosis. The one nonmobile tooth (#30) had a Class III furcation lesion. Because there were so few remaining teeth, treatment options were limited. Implants were rejected by the patient because of financial constraints. There were several positive factors, however. The patient had quit smoking, although the full impact of this was not generally

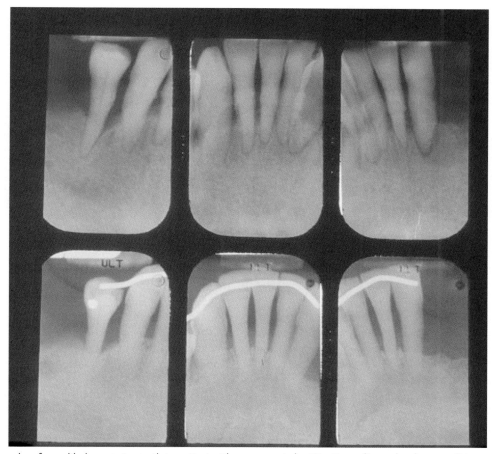

Figure 11-2. Radiographs of mandibular anterior teeth in patient with severe periodontitis. Top radiographs show condition at initial examination. Bottom radiographs show condition 20 years later, after successful periodontal treatment and maintenance. Teeth have been splinted with fixed intracoronal splint.

appreciated at that time. With the exception of her teeth, this patient was well groomed and seemed motivated to save or delay the loss of her teeth. She was prepared to spend time and money toward this end, if the total outlay were within her budget. The overall prognosis for the lower arch seemed hopeless, given the few remaining teeth and their relative lack of attachment and mobility. This was related to the patient, who was adamant about retaining the mandibular teeth for as long as possible. She realized that these teeth would eventually be lost, but felt that delaying their loss would be an acceptable use of her resources.

Given the patient's wishes and the lack of other acceptable alternatives (because she had absolutely ruled out the use of implants), the following treatment plan was proposed and accepted. The patient agreed to have the teeth splinted using an intracoronal splint consisting of heavy orthodontic wire bonded in a slot cut into the enamel. Splinting would consist of two segments (teeth #21 to #27 and #29 to #30). After splinting, scaling and root planing

were to be performed, together with oral hygiene instruction and assessment. No teeth were to be extracted.

If there was a reasonably good response to mechanical debridement noted at the time of reevaluation, a "swing-lock" partial denture was to be fabricated (Figs. 11-3 and 11-4). Although this prosthetic design is rarely used today, it does have some advantages, including the ability to add teeth (if lost), the ability to engage significant undercuts without expensive cast restorations, and relatively low cost (in comparison with other alternatives). The patient was warned that the treatment plan would, at best, allow her to retain her teeth for a few years. She agreed to the treatment plan as presented. Active treatment was completed uneventfully. Her posttreatment prognosis was still questionable because of the severity of attachment loss, although the decreased mobility from splinting and her excellent oral hygiene were positive factors. She was originally seen at 2-month intervals for maintenance, which was eventually lengthened to 4-month intervals. Her hygiene remained exemplary and consisted of three

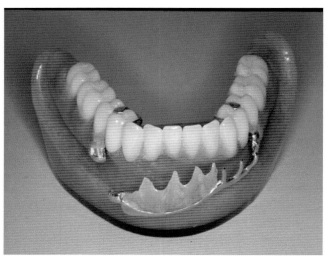

Figure 11-3. Mandibular swing-lock removable partial denture fabricated to stabilize remaining teeth and replace missing teeth.

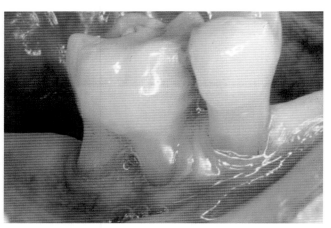

Figure 11-5. Excellent soft tissue health around teeth #29 and #30 twenty years after active therapy. Tooth #30 still had Class III furcation invasion, but bone and attachment levels were stable.

components: manual brushing, an interproximal brush, and a wooden toothpick in a plastic holder. Almost 20 years after therapy, the patient continued to do well (Fig. 11-2). She lost no teeth and received only nonsurgical therapy. Probing depths ranged from 1 to 4 mm and there was minimal bleeding on probing. The furcation lesion was still patent, but had not progressed. Tissue health is good, as can be noted in postoperative photographs (Figs. 11-5 and 11-6).

Posttreatment analysis: In retrospect, this case confirms several concepts regarding prognosis. The first is the observation that any prognosis other than good has relatively little predictive value. The individual teeth and the mandibular arch as a whole were given a questionable prognosis at the initiation of treatment and again at the posttreatment reevaluation; yet, these teeth were still present more than 20 years later. The second concept is the impor-

tance of smoking as a risk factor. Although it is impossible to know with certainty, it is likely that smoking cessation played a role in the exceptional treatment response. Mobility, as a risk factor, was neutralized by means of splinting. This case is a reminder that some patients with severe bone loss, attachment loss, and tooth mobility can be treated successfully with a combination of splinting and periodontal therapy.[65] Although the role of hygiene is less straightforward, this patient's exceptional home care likely contributed to the response seen, as did her compliance with maintenance recommendations. Lastly, all the teeth, except for #30, were single-rooted. Single-rooted teeth usually have a better prognosis than do teeth with furcation lesions.[62-64] With regard to tooth #30, however, a number of studies suggest that teeth with furcation lesions can sometimes be maintained for long periods with relatively simple interventions.[66,67]

Case 2: At the time of referral, the patient was 33 years old. She had received periodontal treatment during her

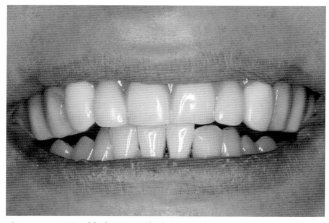

Figure 11-4. Mandibular swing-lock removable partial denture in place opposing a maxillary complete denture.

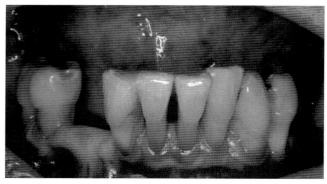

Figure 11-6. Excellent soft tissue health in stable mandibular anterior region.

20s, which consisted of four quadrants of surgery. She was being seen at regular intervals for maintenance, but continued to lose bone and clinical attachment and sought a second opinion after the loss of her maxillary incisors. The medical history was significant for a smoking history of 15 pack-years. Probing depths ranged from 2 to 10 mm. Significant mobility was noted; tooth #3 depressible. Home care was good. There was minimal bleeding on probing. The diagnosis at the initial examination in 1990 was generalized rapidly progressive periodontitis of advanced severity (using the current classification system, the diagnosis would be generalized severe aggressive periodontitis), modified by smoking and occlusal trauma. Representative pretreatment radiographs are shown in Figures 11-7 through 11-9. The initial prognosis for the entire dentition was poor, as was the prognosis for maxillary and mandibular arches individually. The initial prognosis for the individual teeth shown in Figures 11-7 through 11-9 were as follows: hopeless: #3; questionable: #2, #12, #14, and #15; poor: #13, #23 to #27; fair: #4 to #6, #11, #22, and #27.

Treatment recommendations included initial therapy followed by a reevaluation and smoking cessation. The patient quit smoking and underwent scaling and root planing of all teeth, combined with systemic antibiotic therapy. Tooth #3 was extracted. She had a positive treatment response, and a second phase of treatment was recommended. Because a number of teeth had a questionable prognosis, it was decided to have the teeth prepared for a heat-cured, long-lasting provisional fixed partial denture for the maxillary arch. This could be removed at the time of surgery to allow better access to defects. It was also felt that this would be less traumatic to the tissues after surgery than would a temporary acrylic

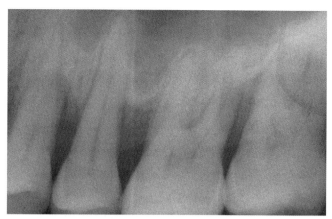

Figure 11-8. Radiograph of maxillary left posterior sextant showing severe bone loss at baseline examination in patient with severe generalized aggressive periodontitis.

resin removable partial denture. Provisionalization was completed and surgery was subsequently performed in all areas, using a modified Widman approach combined, in some areas, with osseous autografts. The patient tolerated the procedures well and had a good response in terms of

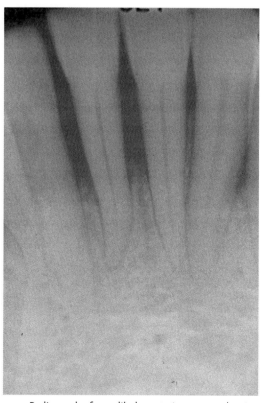

Figure 11-9. Radiograph of mandibular anterior sextant showing severe bone loss at baseline examination in patient with severe generalized aggressive periodontitis.

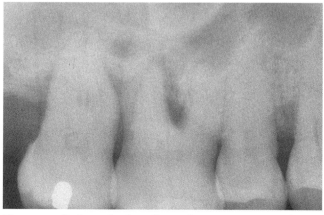

Figure 11-7. Radiograph of maxillary right posterior sextant showing severe bone loss at baseline examination in patient with severe generalized aggressive periodontitis.

probing depth reduction and clinical attachment gain. She was placed on 2-month maintenance. At the posttreatment reevaluation, the positive response resulted in an improved prognosis. The entire dentition was given a fair prognosis, as were the individual arches. Individual teeth seen in Figures 11-10 through 11-13 were given the following prognoses: poor: #15; fair: #2, #5, #14, #24; good: #4, #6, #11 to #13, #22, #23, and #25 to #27.

After she demonstrated several months of clinical stability, the definitive prosthesis was fabricated. Telescoping copings were placed on most of the remaining maxillary teeth (Fig. 11-14). An impression was taken and a restoration was fabricated that incorporated features of both fixed and removable prostheses (Fig. 11-15). The copings were milled precisely so that the restoration was held in place by friction only—it was not cemented and was removed nightly using a crown puller.

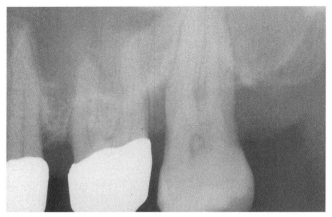

Figure 11-12. Posttreatment radiograph of teeth #13 to #15. Tooth #15 still has poor prognosis.

Posttreatment analysis: This patient exhibited a high degree of susceptibility to periodontal disease, as shown by both the severity of tissue destruction at an early age and her failure to respond to therapy during her 20s.

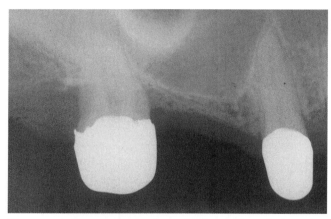

Figure 11-10. Posttreatment radiograph of teeth #2 to #4 in patient originally diagnosed with severe generalized aggressive periodontitis. Excellent response to therapy resulted in improved posttreatment prognosis.

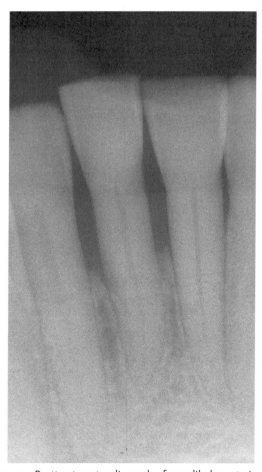

Figure 11-13. Posttreatment radiograph of mandibular anterior teeth. Note improvement in bone levels.

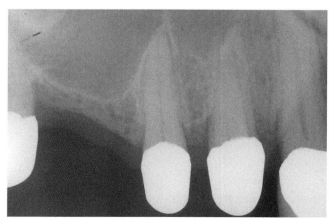

Figure 11-11. Posttreatment radiograph of teeth #4 to #6.

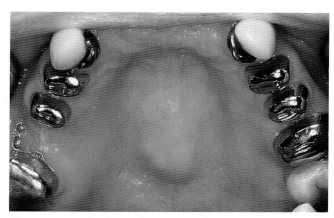

Figure 11-14. Occlusal view of cast copings that retain the maxillary partial denture. Teeth remained stable over the 10-year period after active therapy.

Smoking may have played a large role, because it has been shown to cause suboptimal treatment outcomes. This patient quit smoking during initial therapy, and thereby improved her prognosis. Although it is not known to what extent her bruxism may have contributed to her disease, she wore a series of occlusal guards since completion of therapy. Her hygiene and compliance with maintenance was excellent. Tissue health was excellent and attachment levels and probing depths remained stable for more than 10 years. Radiographic appearance was also suggestive of clinical stability (Figs. 11-10 through 11-13). As with the preceding case, Case 2 seems to exemplify many of the points made by McGuire and Nunn.[39-42] Both cases underscore the effectiveness of adequate and appropriate therapy, as well as the general inaccuracy of initial prognostic categorization. In this latter case, the initial prognosis would have suggested the eventual loss of the remaining teeth. However, the patient responded very well to therapy. The posttreatment prognosis was much more accurate in predicting her eventual outcome. This is usually expected because the clinician has had a chance to evaluate the patient's response to periodontal therapy in the short-term, and that response may provide a clue as to the long-term response and stability.

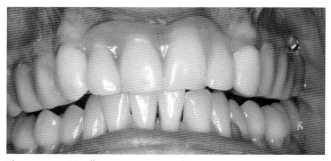

Figure 11-15. Maxillary restoration in place.

THE FUTURE

It is likely that additional risk factors for periodontal diseases will be identified. In particular, additional genetic markers are likely to be identified that confer risk for periodontal disease. One of the major challenges will be the analysis and application of this information in the formulation of a diagnosis, prognosis, and treatment plan for the individual patient.[68] The use of computerized analytical instruments may help in this regard. Persson and colleagues[69] have developed a computerized risk assessment tool for periodontal patients called the Periodontal Risk Calculator, or PRC. These investigators report that the "risk scores determined using the PRC are accurate and valid predictors of future periodontal deterioration, as measured by actual alveolar bone loss and tooth loss over a period of 15 years." Such tools may provide improved prognostic abilities in the future. Similarly, evaluation of products in gingival crevicular fluid may one day provide more accurate assessments of the risk for disease initiation and progression (see Chapters 3 and 5).

Clearly, more work needs to be done in the area of periodontal diagnosis and risk assessment. The clinical and research communities both require reliable, practical, and reproducible methods that will allow the assessment of disease activity. Current diagnostic and classification schemes provide a good deal of guidance in the treatment of periodontal conditions. Despite the heterogeneity of conditions, a large number of outcomes studies suggest that periodontal treatment, based on these imperfect classification schemes, is effective. As we learn more about the nature and causes of these complex diseases, however, we will be able to target certain high-risk individuals and sites with greater sophistication and precision.

REFERENCES

1. Ainamo J, Barmes D, Beagrie G et al: Development of the World Health Organization (WHO) community periodontal index of treatment needs (CPITN), *Int Dent J* 32:281-291, 1982.
2. Loe H, Theilade E, Jensen SB: Experimental gingivitis in man, *J Periodontol* 36:177-187, 1965.
3. Van der Weijden GA, Timmerman MF, Danser MM et al: Effect of pre-experimental maintenance care duration on the development of gingivitis in a partial mouth experimental gingivitis model, *J Periodont Res* 29:168-173, 1994.
4. Grbic JT, Mitchell-Lewis DA, Fine JB et al: The relationship of candidiasis to linear gingival erythema in HIV-infected homosexual men and parenteral drug users, *J Periodontol* 66:30-37, 1995.
5. Jaeschke R, Guyatt G, Lijmer J: Diagnostic tests. In Guyatt G, Rennie D, editors: *Users' guide to the medical literature*, Chicago, 2002, American Medical Association Press, pp 187-217.

6. Sackett D, Strauss S, Richardson W et al: *Evidence-based medicine: how to practice and teach EBM*, Edinburgh, UK, 2000, Churchill Livingstone.

7. McFall WT Jr, Bader JD, Rozier RG, Ramsey D: Presence of periodontal data in patient records of general practitioners, *J Periodontol* 59:445-449, 1988.

8. Heins PJ, Fuller WW, Fries SE: Periodontal probe use in general practice in Florida, *J Am Dent Assoc* 119:147-150, 1989.

9. Tonetti MS, Mombelli A: Early-onset periodontitis, *Ann Periodontol* 4:39-53, 1999.

10. Loe H, Anerud A, Boysen H, Morrison E: Natural history of periodontal disease in man. Rapid, moderate and no loss of attachment in Sri Lankan laborers 14 to 46 years of age, *J Clin Periodontol* 13:431-445, 1986.

11. Grossi SG, Zambon JJ, Ho AW et al: Assessment of risk for periodontal disease. I. Risk indicators for attachment loss, *J Periodontol* 65:260-267, 1994.

12. Grossi SG, Genco RJ, Machtei EE et al: Assessment of risk for periodontal disease. II. Risk indicators for alveolar bone loss, *J Periodontol* 66:23-29, 1995.

13. Kornman KS, Newman MG, Alvarado R et al: Clinical and microbiological patterns of adults with periodontitis, *J Periodontol* 62:634-642, 1991.

14. Socransky SS, Haffajee AD, Cugini MA et al: Microbial complexes in subgingival plaque, *J Clin Periodontol* 25:134-144, 1998.

15. Socransky SS, Smith C, Haffajee AD: Subgingival microbial profiles in refractory periodontal disease, *J Clin Periodontol* 29:260-268, 2002.

16. World Health Organization: *Application of the international classification of diseases to dentistry and stomatology*, Geneva, 1995, World Health Organization.

17. Armitage GC: Development of a classification system for periodontal diseases and conditions, *Ann Periodontol* 4:1-6, 1999.

18. Elwood M: *Critical appraisal of epidemiological studies and clinical trials*, New York, 1988, Oxford University Press.

19. Hill AB: *Principles of medical statistics*, New York, 1971, Oxford University Press.

20. Gordis L: *Epidemiology*, ed 2, Philadelphia, 2000, WB Saunders.

21. Lilienfeld DE, Stolley PD: *Foundations of epidemiology*, ed 3, New York, 1994, Oxford University Press.

22. Marks JS, McKenna MT, Taylor WR: Current issues and challenges in chronic disease control. In Brownson RC, Remington PL, Davis JR, editors: *Chronic disease epidemiology and control*, Washington, DC, 1998, American Public Health Association, pp 1-26.

23. Greenstein G: Periodontal diseases are curable, *J Periodontol* 73:950-953, 2002.

24. Last JM: *A dictionary of epidemiology*, ed 4, Oxford, 2001, Oxford University Press.

25. Prichard JF: *Advanced periodontal disease: surgical and prosthetic management*, ed 2, Philadelphia, 1972, WB Saunders.

26. Beck JD, Koch GG, Offenbacher S: Incidence of attachment loss over 3 years in older adults—new and progressing lesions, *Community Dent Oral Epidemiol* 23:291-296, 1995.

27. Doll R, Hill AB: Smoking and carcinoma of the lung: preliminary report, *BMJ* 2:739-748, 1950.

28. Doll R, Hill AB: Mortality of British doctors in relation to smoking: observations on coronary thrombosis, *Natl Cancer Inst Monogr* 19:205-268, 1966.

29. Hujoel PP, DeRouen TA: A survey of endpoint characteristics in periodontal clinical trials published 1988-1992, and implications for future studies, *J Clin Periodontol* 22:397-407, 1995.

30. Hujoel PP, Loe H, Anerud A et al: The informativeness of attachment loss on tooth mortality, *J Periodontol* 70:44-48, 1999.

31. Lang NP, Joss A, Orsanic T et al: Bleeding on probing. A predictor for the progression of periodontal disease? *J Clin Periodontol* 13:590-596, 1986.

32. Lang NP, Adler R, Joss A, Nyman S: Absence of bleeding on probing. An indicator of periodontal stability, *J Clin Periodontol* 17:714-721, 1990.

33. Joss A, Adler R, Lang NP: Bleeding on probing. A parameter for monitoring periodontal conditions in clinical practice, *J Clin Periodontol* 21:402-408, 1994.

34. Rams TE, Listgarten MA, Slots J: Efficacy of CPITN sextant scores for detection of periodontitis disease activity, *J Clin Periodontol* 23:355-361, 1996.

35. Rams TE, Listgarten MA, Slots J: Utility of 5 major putative periodontal pathogens and selected clinical parameters to predict periodontal breakdown in patients on maintenance care, *J Clin Periodontol* 23:346-354, 1996.

36. Claffey N, Egelberg J: Clinical indicators of probing attachment loss following initial periodontal treatment in advanced periodontitis patients, *J Clin Periodontol* 22:690-696, 1995.

37. McGuire MK, Nunn ME: Prognosis versus actual outcome. IV. The effectiveness of clinical parameters and IL-1 genotype in accurately predicting prognoses and tooth survival, *J Periodontol* 70:49-56, 1999.

38. Haffajee AD, Socransky SS: Relationship of cigarette smoking to attachment level profiles, *J Clin Periodontol* 28:283-295, 2001.

39. McGuire MK: Prognosis versus actual outcome: a long-term survey of 100 treated periodontal patients under maintenance care, *J Periodontol* 62:51-58, 1991.

40. McGuire MK: Prognosis vs outcome: predicting tooth survival, *Compend Contin Educ Dent* 21:217-220, 222, 224, 230, 2000.

41. McGuire MK, Nunn ME: Prognosis versus actual outcome. II. The effectiveness of clinical parameters in developing an accurate prognosis, *J Periodontol* 67:658-665, 1996.

42. McGuire MK, Nunn ME: Prognosis versus actual outcome. III. The effectiveness of clinical parameters in accurately predicting tooth survival, *J Periodontol* 67:666-674, 1996.

43. Michalowicz BS, Diehl SR, Gunsolley JC et al: Evidence of a substantial genetic basis for risk of adult periodontitis, *J Periodontol* 71:1699-1707, 2000.

44. Kornman KS, Crane A, Wang HY et al: The interleukin-1 genotype as a severity factor in adult periodontal disease, *J Clin Periodontol* 24:72-77, 1997.

45. Armitage GC, Wu Y, Wang HY et al: Low prevalence of a periodontitis-associated interleukin-1 composite genotype in individuals of Chinese heritage, *J Periodontol* 71:164-171, 2000.

46. Axelsson P: *Diagnosis and risk prediction of periodontal diseases*, Vol 3, Chicago, 2000, Quintessence.

47. Haffajee AD, Socransky SS, Lindhe J et al: Clinical risk indicators for periodontal attachment loss, *J Clin Periodontol* 18:117-125, 1991.

48. Genco RJ: Risk factors for periodontal disease. In Rose LF, Genco RJ, Mealey BL, Cohen DW, editors: *Periodontal medicine*, Hamilton, Ontario, 2000, B.C. Decker, pp 11-33.

49. Mealey BL: Diabetes mellitus. In Rose LF, Genco RJ, Mealey BL, Cohen DW, editors: *Periodontal medicine*, Hamilton, Ontario, 2000, B.C. Decker, pp 121-150.

50. Kaldahl WB, Kalkwarf KL, Patil KD, Molvar MP: Evaluation of gingival suppuration and supragingival plaque following 4 modalities of periodontal therapy, *J Clin Periodontol* 17:642-649, 1990.

51. Kaldahl WB, Kalkwarf KL, Patil KD, Molvar MP: Relationship of gingival bleeding, gingival suppuration, and supragingival plaque to attachment loss, *J Periodontol* 61:347-351, 1990.

52. Haffajee AD, Socransky SS, Goodson JM: Clinical parameters as predictors of destructive periodontal disease activity, *J Clin Periodontol* 10:257-265, 1983.

53. Greenstein G: Contemporary interpretation of probing depth assessments: diagnostic and therapeutic implications. A literature review, *J Periodontol* 68:1194-1205, 1997.

54. Harper DS, Robinson PJ: Correlation of histometric, microbial, and clinical indicators of periodontal disease status before and after root planing, *J Clin Periodontol* 14:190-196, 1987.

55. von Troil-Linden B, Saarela M, Matto J et al: Source of suspected periodontal pathogens re-emerging after periodontal treatment, *J Clin Periodontol* 23:601-607, 1996.

56. Levy RM, Giannobile WV, Feres M et al: The effect of apically repositioned flap surgery on clinical parameters and the composition of the subgingival microbiota: 12-month data, *Int J Periodontics Restorative Dent* 22:209-219, 2002.

57. Nowzari H, Slots J: Microbiologic and clinical study of polytetrafluoroethylene membranes for guided bone regeneration around implants, *Int J Oral Maxillofac Implants* 10:67-73, 1995.

58. Nieri M, Muzzi L, Cattabriga M et al: The prognostic value of several periodontal factors measured as radiographic bone level variation: a 10-year retrospective multilevel analysis of treated and maintained periodontal patients, *J Periodontol* 73:1485-1493, 2002.

59. Fleszar TJ, Knowles JW, Morrison EC et al: Tooth mobility and periodontal therapy, *J Clin Periodontol* 7:495-505, 1980.

60. Cortellini P, Tonetti MS, Lang NP et al: The simplified papilla preservation flap in the regenerative treatment of deep intrabony defects: clinical outcomes and postoperative morbidity, *J Periodontol* 72:1702-1712, 2001.

61. Rosling B, Nyman S, Lindhe J: The effect of systematic plaque control on bone regeneration in infrabony pockets, *J Clin Periodontol* 3:38-53, 1976.

62. Hirschfeld L, Wasserman B: A long-term survey of tooth loss in 600 treated periodontal patients, *J Periodontol* 49:225-237, 1978.

63. McFall WT Jr: Tooth loss in 100 treated patients with periodontal disease. A long-term study, *J Periodontol* 53:539-549, 1982.

64. Goldman MJ, Ross, IF, Goteiner D: Effect of periodontal therapy on patients maintained for 15 years or longer. A retrospective study, *J Periodontol* 57:347-353, 1986.

65. Lindhe J, Nyman S: The role of occlusion in periodontal disease and the biological rationale for splinting in treatment of periodontitis, *Oral Sci Rev* 10:11-43, 1977.

66. Carnevale G, Pontoriero R, Lindhe J: Treatment of furcation-involved teeth. In Lindhe J, Karring T, Lang NP, editors: *Clinical periodontology and implant dentistry*, Oxford, UK, 2003, Blackwell Munksgaard, pp 705-730.

67. Hamp SE, Nyman S, Lindhe J: Periodontal treatment of multirooted teeth. Results after 5 years *J Clin Periodontol* 2:126-135, 1975.

68. Position paper: diagnosis of periodontal diseases. American Academy of Periodontology, *J Periodontol* 74:1237-1247, 2003.

69. Persson GR, Mancl LA, Martin J, Page RC: Assessing periodontal disease risk: a comparison of clinicians' assessment versus a computerized tool, *J Am Dent Assoc* 134:575-582, 2003.

12 Acute Periodontal Conditions

David G. Kerns

Acute periodontal conditions encompass a number of different pathologic lesions that may affect the periodontium. These pathoses often present diagnostic problems for the clinician. Most acute lesions have a rapid onset and are accompanied by pain. Acute lesions often include periodontal abscesses, gingival abscesses, periapical abscesses, pericoronitis, necrotizing ulcerative gingivitis, and necrotizing ulcerative periodontitis. Rees[1] reported that patients with other acute oral conditions such as herpetic gingivostomatitis, aphthous stomatitis, and desquamative lesions may also present for treatment.

When an abscess is confined to the marginal gingiva, it is often termed a *gingival abscess.*[2,3] Gingival abscesses usually occur in a previously disease-free site and are confined to the marginal gingiva or interdental papilla (Figs. 12-1 and 12-2). The lesion is localized, painful, and rapidly expanding, usually manifesting as an acute inflammatory response to a foreign body (toothbrush bristle or piece of food) forced into the gingival tissue. Initially, it will appear as a red swollen area with a smooth, shiny surface. Within the first 24 to 48 hours, the site is usually fluctuant and pointed and will express seropurulent exudate through a surface orifice. If left untreated, it will usually rupture spontaneously. Histologically, the gingival abscess appears as a purulent lesion in connective tissue surrounded by diffuse infiltration of polymorphonuclear leukocytes, edema, and vascular enlargement.

Periodontal abscesses have been recognized as a distinct clinical entity since the latter part of the 19th century. The International Conference on Research in the Biology of Periodontal Disease in 1977 defined a periodontal abscess as "an acute, destructive process in the periodontium resulting in localized collections of pus communicating with the oral cavity through the gingival sulcus or other periodontal sites and not arising from the tooth pulp."[4] Although reference is often made to a chronic form,[5] chronic periodontal abscesses may be indistinguishable

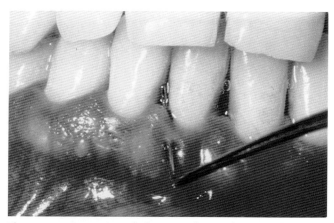

Figure 12-2. Same gingival abscess with a probe inserted into the draining abscess and exiting the gingival sulcus on the distal facial of the mandibular incisor.

from lesions of chronic periodontitis, even when a sinus tract is present.

Despite their long historical recognition, periodontal abscesses often present a challenge in terms of diagnosis, etiology, treatment, and prognosis. An accurate diagnosis and effective treatment must be given immediately. The dentist must therefore have established an effective treatment program based on recognition of the clinical symptoms, an accurate differential diagnosis, and an understanding of the etiologic factors.

CLINICAL FEATURES

The periodontal abscess is often associated with a preexisting periodontal pocket. Some acute periodontal abscesses are found with impaction of foreign objects—frequently seeds, corn kernels, or nut husks lodged in the gingival sulcus or pocket. As long as the pocket communicates with the oral cavity, infectious material within the pocket can drain. If the orifice of the pocket becomes occluded by impaction of a foreign object or by healing, purulent material within the pocket cannot drain. The infectious material then accumulates within the occluded pocket, resulting in many of the clinical symptoms discussed here.

The most common symptom is pain. The patient is often oblivious to most of the accompanying symptoms until pain becomes evident. Gingival, or mucosal swelling, or both, are usually seen in the site of pain. Swelling may vary from a small enlargement of the gingival unit to a diffuse swelling involving the gingiva, alveolar mucosa, and oral mucosa and may extend to the face and neck. The affected tissues will be red to reddish blue. The swelling and associated changes are usually adjacent to the tooth affected (Fig. 12-3). Occasionally the affected tooth may be one or two teeth distant from the swelling

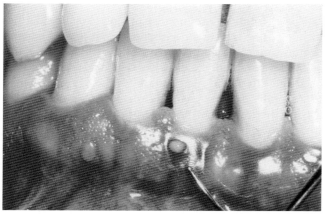

Figure 12-1. Gingival abscess on facial of mandibular central incisor demonstrating pus.

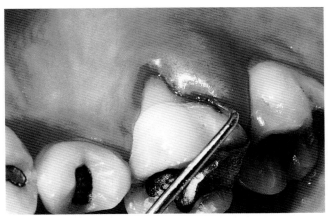

Figure 12-3. Periodontal abscess on the palatal aspect of a maxillary right first molar with a periodontal probe in place demonstrating deep probing depth, with gingival enlargement and discoloration.

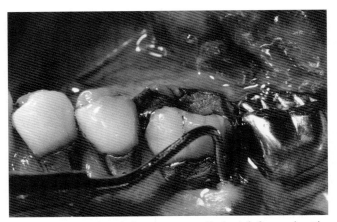

Figure 12-4. Periodontal abscess on mandibular left first molar. The tooth tests vital and has a 12-mm probing depth.

and color changes. The tooth or teeth affected by a periodontal abscess are usually tender on chewing and sensitive to percussion. Frequently the tooth is mobile and may even extrude from the alveolar socket and feel "high" to the occlusion. Occasionally the abscess may already be draining through one or more sinus tracts into the oral cavity. Purulent exudate can often be noted in the periodontal pocket around the affected tooth. Regional lymphadenopathy and occasionally slight increase of body temperature may accompany periodontal abscesses.

Dental radiographs are helpful in confirming the diagnosis. They frequently reveal a radiolucent area along the lateral aspect of the tooth involved. It is possible, however, if the abscess is located on the facial or lingual surfaces of the tooth that the radiograph will not reveal its presence.

ETIOLOGY

A periodontal abscess is a bacterial infection involving the periodontal tissues. Both environmental and microbiologic factors play an important role in the development, progression, and treatment of the infection.

Environmental Factors

In most cases, the periodontal abscess occurs in a preexisting periodontal pocket. The pocket is therefore a major factor in the etiology of the abscess. In both spontaneous remission and remission through partial treatment, healing occurs primarily at the coronal aspect of the pocket. The epithelial tissues can reattach to the root of the tooth, whereas bacteria and debris remain in the apical aspect of the pocket. With the coronal portion of the pocket occluded, drainage is impaired and an abscess may result (Fig. 12-4). The deeper, narrower, or more tortuous the pocket, the more likely the abscess is to occur after partial healing.

Other local factors may set the stage for abscess formation. When foreign material such as a popcorn husk, impacted food, or even a toothbrush bristle is forced into the gingival tissue or occludes the pocket orifice, bacteria can proliferate, leading to an abscess. If this foreign material remains in the pocket, a bacterial infection may occur, and a gingival or periodontal abscess can result. A periodontal abscess can also occur with improper use of oral irrigating devices that introduce bacteria into the tissues or subsequent to a scaling session when a piece of calculus becomes dislodged and remains in the pocket.

Microbiologic Factors

About forty-five years ago, Ludwig[6] studied the microbiota of suppurative periodontal abscesses. He considered the abscess to be a mixed infection including such microorganisms as *Streptococcus viridans*, *Staphylococcus albus*, nonhemolytic streptococci, *Neisseria*, diphtheroids, and *Escherichia coli*. As late as 1977,[7-9] *S. viridans* was still considered the predominant microorganism; these studies used aerobic culturing techniques.

These findings are not surprising considering the technology at that time. Sampling most often included healthy and diseased sites, as well as supragingival and subgingival microorganisms. These pooled samples often obscured differences. Laboratory technology was unable to cultivate oxygen-sensitive microorganisms, thereby leaving the impression that the primary etiologic agents were aerobic microorganisms.[10]

Studies using continuous anaerobic culture techniques have shown anaerobes to be important in periodontal abscesses. For example, Newman and Sims[10] found the microflora of periodontal abscesses to be predominantly gram-negative (66.2%) and anaerobic (65.2%), in contrast to the gram-positive (71.0%) and facultative (78.3%) microflora in healthy sites. They reported that the microorganisms most commonly found in periodontal abscesses were *Bacteroides melaninogenicus* subspecies, *Fusobacterium* species, "vibrio-corroders," *Capnocytophaga* species, *Peptococcus* species, and *Peptostreptococcus* species. van Winkelhoff and colleagues[11] found *Bacteroides gingivalis* (known today as *Porphyromonas gingivalis*) and *Bacteroides intermedius* (known today as *Prevotella intermedia*) in all of the periodontal abscesses they cultured. DeWitt and coworkers[12] noted the presence of bacteria and fungi in the connective tissue wall of 100% of the periodontal abscesses they studied. Hence bacterial invasion of ulcerated and necrotic tissues observed was by predominantly gram-negative bacteria. The presence of fungi resembling *Candida* species in these periodontal abscesses was also observed. *Candida albicans* has also been found in abscesses of lung, heart, kidney, brain, and other organ systems. Because *Candida* is often a secondary invader in areas of preexisting infection, these organisms may play a role in the progression of the abscess.

Slots and Listgarten[13] have focused attention on *Actinobacillus actinomycetemcomitans, Porphyromonas gingivalis,* and *Prevotella intermedia* as prominent periodontal pathogens. Spirochetes have also been reported to be present in significant numbers in periodontal abscesses when using darkfield microscopy.[14] *Fusobacterium nucleatum, Campylobacter rectus,* and *Capnocytophaga* species have also been reported in the literature to be found in periodontal abscesses.[15-17] More recently, Hafström and associates[18] reported that *P. gingivalis* and *P. intermedia* were involved in 90% of the periodontal abscesses in their study. Using enzyme-linked immunosorbent assay methodology, the IgG antibody levels in patient sera against antigens of homologous bacterial strains remained constant for the 6-month duration of the study. The disappearance of *P. gingivalis* from abscess sites after therapy seems to implicate this microorganism with periodontal abscess formation. Herrera and colleagues[19] report that 62% of the abscesses in their study occurred in patients who had not received periodontal treatment. Molars accounted for 69% of the abscesses seen in 29 patients, and 90% of the patients in their study reported pain. They also report high prevalence rates of *F. nucleatum, Peptostreptococcus micros, P. gingivalis, P. intermedia, and Bacteroides forsythus* (known today as *Tannerella forsythensis*). Overall, studies indicate that the microorganisms found in periodontal abscesses are similar to those found in chronic periodontitis sites with deep probing depths.

DIFFERENTIAL DIAGNOSIS

Periodontal abscesses usually occur as a result of a preexisting periodontitis.[20,21] Gray and colleagues[22] reported in a retrospective study that periodontal abscesses were the third most frequent cause of an emergent dental visit (up to 14%). They also reported that 13.5% of patients under-

going periodontal therapy had periodontal abscesses, and 59.7% of patients diagnosed yet not treated for periodontal disease had periodontal abscesses. These authors found that teeth most frequently involved with abscess formation were maxillary second molars, which accounted for 17% of periodontal abscesses.

Signs and symptoms of a periodontal abscess, such as pain, swelling, color changes, mobility, extrusion, purulence, sinus tract formation, lymphadenopathy, fever, and radiolucency, are not always present, and they are not unique to this lesion. Drainage of pus may occur during probing or spontaneously. Periodontal abscesses do not always drain on the same surface of the tooth as that where the etiologic agent resides. Because other dental infections and conditions share some of these symptoms, it is mandatory to make a differential diagnosis so that correct treatment procedures may be used.

Periapical Abscess

Periapical abscess is the most perplexing abscess because it shares many of the symptoms of a periodontal abscess. Radiographically, a radiolucency often appears at the apex of the offending tooth. However, in an early periapical abscess, there may be no radiographic changes evident.

A lack of pulpal vitality and the presence of deep carious lesions, deep restorations, and crowns are helpful when a periapical abscess is suspected, but they are not specific to this disorder. Although a periapical abscess is always associated with a nonvital tooth, a periodontal abscess may also occur on a nonvital tooth. Pain on palpation of the soft tissue at the apex of the tooth can be evidence of periapical infection. (The periodontal abscess usually occurs in a preexisting pocket.) Probing will often identify a communication between the gingival margin and the abscess area.

Pain itself may be the most helpful symptom in differentiating between a periapical and a periodontal abscess. In a periapical abscess, the pain is sharp, intermittent, severe, and diffuse. The patient may not be able to locate the offending tooth. In contrast, in a periodontal abscess, the pain is dull, constant, and less severe but localized. The patient can easily identify the affected tooth. Pain on percussion is very severe in a periapical abscess. Although a periodontal abscess exhibits pain after percussion, it is less severe. This severe reaction to percussion is considered by many experienced clinicians to be pathognomonic of pulpal infection.

Acute Pulpitis

Acute pulpitis lacks most of the symptoms of a periodontal abscess except pain. The pain is diffuse, like that of a periapical abscess, and may affect the entire side of the face. It is common for the patient to have pain in the opposite arch. The pain can be affected by thermal changes. Teeth that exhibit only acute pulpitis do not have associated soft tissue swelling or purulent drainage because the pulp is vital.

Incomplete Tooth Fracture

A cracked tooth often poses a diagnostic dilemma for the dentist. The patient has very real symptoms, but clinically the fracture is often difficult to detect. Endodontically treated teeth are especially prone to vertical fractures. The most common symptoms are pain or sensitivity on biting and sensitivity to cold. Heat seldom causes discomfort. Pressure on individual cusps may elicit the pain. Having the patient bite on a rubber wheel or rubber anesthetic stopper can help localize the problem. Although occlusal adjustment will temporarily eliminate the pain, the tooth is better treated with a restoration providing cuspal protection. If the fracture extends into the root, there is often colonization by microorganisms through the fracture line into the periodontal ligament, resulting in a persistent periodontal abscess or a deep, narrow, draining periodontal pocket along the fracture line.

Pericoronitis

This is a local accumulation of exudate within the overlying gingival flap surrounding the crown of a partially erupted tooth. The gingival tissue appears red and swollen. The infection may spread posteriorly into the oropharyngeal area and medially to the base of the tongue. Regional lymph nodes may be involved. Patients often relate the symptom of dysphagia (difficulty swallowing). Some patients may even experience fever, leukocytosis, malaise, and dehydration. The mandibular third molars are most frequently involved.

Periodontal Cyst

The radiographic appearance of a periodontal cyst is a well defined oval radiolucency on the lateral surface of the root. It has a predilection for the mandibular canine and premolar region but can also occur at other locations. If periodontitis extends apically to a preexisting periodontal cyst, the cyst may become infected and clinically indistinguishable from a lateral periodontal abscess.

Osteomyelitis

Osteomyelitis is a serious infection of the bone and bone marrow that tends to spread. It has a rapid onset, with pain being the only symptom, and is initially without radiographic evidence. Rapid diffuse bone destruction may occur within a few days, extending a significant distance from the original site of infection. The radiographic picture then may show an indistinct trabeculation and disappearance of the lamina dura. As this infection increases, lymphadenopathy, fever, and malaise are common symptoms.

Manifestation of Systemic Diseases

Any time that the host defense mechanism of a patient is significantly decreased, such as chronic lymphocytic leukemia (Fig. 12-5, *A*), an existing periodontitis can develop into one or several periodontal abscesses. Systemic disease should be suspected in any patient with multiple abscesses or with repeated recurrences of periodontal abscesses. Diabetes mellitus is the most

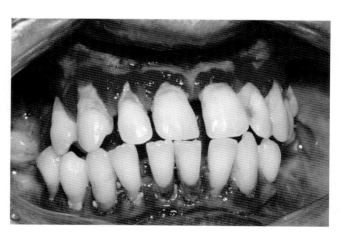

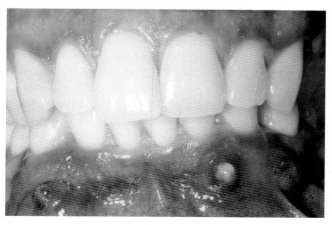

A   B

Figure 12-5. **A,** A 44-year-old white man with chronic lymphocytic leukemia, demonstrating diffuse gingival involvement. **B,** A 38-year-old black man with multiple periodontal abscesses (mandibular left second premolar, mandibular left canine, and mandibular right canine). The patient had undiagnosed diabetes.

common systemic disease that presents with periodontal abscesses (Fig. 12-5, *B*). Patients with diabetes mellitus often have decreased host resistance caused by impaired cellular immunity, decreased leukocyte chemotaxis, or phagocytosis (see Chapter 31). These patients often have vascular changes and altered collagen metabolism that may affect their ability to manage periodontal abscess formation.[23]

Systemic Antibiotic Therapy

Systemic antibiotic therapy has been suggested in some studies as a possible trigger mechanism for multiple periodontal abscess formation in some patients.[24,25] These studies indicate that systemic administration of antibiotics for nonoral infections in patients with untreated periodontal disease may lead to superinfection with opportunistic organisms resulting in periodontal abscess formation.

TREATMENT

Periodontal abscesses most often present as a painful emergency. The patient should be treated immediately to relieve pain and resolve the infection, which left untreated may spread and lead to severe, irreversible periodontal attachment loss. After a thorough clinical examination, the symptoms are assessed and a differential diagnosis is reviewed to eliminate unlikely diagnoses. Pulp vitality testing is critical. Additional observations, radiographs, and clinical tests will hopefully narrow the choices to a single diagnosis. Familiarity with all aspects of a periodontal abscess enables the dentist to make the diagnosis rather rapidly. It should be noted that in most clinics treating a broad range of dental patients, about 85% of toothaches are pulpal in origin and about 15% are because of periodontal abscesses. This percentage will vary markedly, however, according to the nature of the population served.

Treatment of the periodontal abscess should include drainage through an incision or through the gingival crevice or pocket orifice, as well as the use of antimicrobial agents when appropriate.

Repair Potential

Although a periodontal abscess usually results in considerable bone loss during its acute phase, in turn, this lesion has an excellent potential for repair after adequate treatment. The dentist should, therefore, consider treatment of the acutely affected tooth, even though there seems to be little remaining periodontal support, because remarkable regeneration of lost periodontal attachment may occur. The location and shape of the osseous destruction, as well as its degree of activity, appear to affect the prognosis of the periodontal abscess. Nabers and coworkers[26] noted that acute abscesses repaired more completely than similar chronic lesions. They also concluded that narrow infrabony lesions had a better repair potential than wide lesions without bony walls.

Earlier methods of treatment[27] recommended that the abscess be incised and drained to reduce the acute phase and that the chronic phase be corrected by periodontal flaps and osseous correction. In view of the improved repair potential of an acute abscess, it would seem more logical now to definitively treat during the acute phase. The selection of treatment methods should always consider this repair potential.

Closed Approach

Incision and drainage are often best obtained through the pocket orifice. Although drainage may be accomplished by directly incising into the surface of the fluctuant abscess, root planing is still required. After adequate local anesthesia, the pocket is opened with a sharp curette to the depth of the abscess. Immediate drainage and hemorrhage are often obtained. The root surface is then thoroughly root planed to remove plaque and calculus deposits. During this root planing the occluded pocket is further opened and drainage is enhanced. Thorough irrigation with sterile saline, 0.1% povidone-iodine or 3% hydrogen peroxide, may aid in debridement and elimination of bacteria. In the absence of systemic symptoms, antibiotic therapy is seldom necessary. If, however, the patient has lymphadenopathy, fever, or malaise, systemic antibiotics should be considered.

Open-Flap Approach

The dentist should attempt to maximize the repair potential of the periodontal abscess by definitively treating the abscess during the acute phase. This requires that in addition to establishing drainage, the diseased root surface must be free of all deposits. In some instances, full access to the diseased root may be best obtained with a full-thickness mucoperiosteal flap on both the facial and the lingual surfaces with sufficient reflection to completely visualize the infected root surface. The initial internal beveled incision can be made intrasulcularly or close to the gingival margin to preserve as much keratinized gingiva as possible. This incision should be continued laterally to allow for flap displacement for adequate visualization and access. If necessary for access, vertical incisions can be made over intact alveolar bone at the line angles of the adjacent uninvolved teeth.

The attached gingival tissue can be reflected with a blunt tissue elevator. The reflection should be adequate to thoroughly visualize the entire infected root surface. With the aid of good light (the use of fiber optics is ideal) and sharp curettes, all visible bacterial deposits, both hard and soft, must be planed from the root surface that has been exposed to a preexisting periodontal pocket. The exposed bone can also be carefully débrided to remove soft tissue from the osseous defect. Thorough irrigation is absolutely required.

After root planing, the flaps are replaced and sutured. The patient should rinse with a plaque inhibitor such as chlorhexidine twice a day for at least 1 week.

Use of Antibiotics

The goal of the open-flap approach is to maximize healing and to gain new attachment or regeneration of the periodontal tissues to the previously diseased root surface. If systemic signs or symptoms are present or antibiotics are considered necessary for other reasons, it is desirable to give the patient a systemic antibiotic that is appropriate to treat the acute infection.

On the basis of early aerobic microbiologic studies, penicillin became the systemic therapy of choice. However, Goldberg[28] cultured periapical and periodontal infections and found that 26% of those infecting bacteria were resistant to penicillin. He also noted a high number of gram-negative rods that were resistant to the antibiotics tested.

The best method to determine the appropriate antibiotic is to obtain a sample of the pus or abscess fluid, culture, and test for sensitivity. Because the causative microorganisms are usually anaerobic, anaerobic culturing should be requested in addition to aerobic culturing. While waiting for the result of culture and sensitivity testing, it is prudent to begin antibiotic therapy, selecting a systemic antibiotic that usually satisfies treatment goals. Penicillins are frequently used as the drug of choice. A common regimen, for example, is 500 mg Penicillin VK every 6 hours for 7 days. Tetracycline hydrochloride is a relatively safe, broad-spectrum antibiotic that concentrates in the gingival crevicular fluid at a level two to four times that in serum.[29] Tetracycline usually reaches those microorganisms thought to cause the abscess, as well as those thought to cause periodontitis.[30] Many clinicians still prescribe a treatment program of 250 mg tetracycline four times a day for 10 days. Others prefer doxycycline because it can be given in a 100-mg dose only once or twice a day. Other common antibiotic regimens reported in the literature for treatment of periodontal abscesses include: 500 mg azithromycin as a single dose on the first day, then 250 mg once daily for 3 days); 500/125 mg amoxicillin/clavulanate, once every 8 hours for 8 days; 500 mg metronidazole every 8 hours for 10 days; or, 150 to 300 mg clindamycin three times a day for 7 days.[19] Once the results of the culture and sensitivity testing are known, the appropriate antibiotic can be selected and prescribed, if the bacteria are not sensitive to the original drug chosen by the clinician. Because most periodontal abscesses respond well to mechanical debridement (closed or open) without adjunctive antibiotics, the role of systemic antibiotics in the treatment of periodontal abscesses remains controversial.

COMPLICATIONS AND POSTOPERATIVE CARE

Occasionally a periodontal abscess will spread to involve other facial tissues, resulting in a cellulitis. Cellulitis may result in serious systemic symptoms, endanger the airway, or threaten a cavernous sinus infection. In these severe and generalized cases, an aggressive treatment regimen with penicillin is preferred until the results of culture and sensitivity testing are obtained.

Postoperative care is important for the successful treatment of a periodontal abscess. The patient should be seen within 1 to 2 days of initial treatment and again at weekly intervals if necessary to evaluate resolution of the abscess. The area should be thoroughly débrided and all calculus, plaque, and stain should be removed. Because periodontal abscesses most often occur in patients with periodontitis, a full examination of the patient for evidence of periodontal disease is appropriate 1 or 2 weeks after the abscess has healed. If periodontitis is diagnosed, then a treatment plan should be formulated to allow for definitive treatment of the abscess area if necessary.

Some clinicians have suggested recurrent periodontal abscess as a just cause for deeming a tooth hopeless.[31] It has also been reported as the main reason for extraction in patients undergoing the maintenance phase of therapy.[32] McLeod and colleagues[21] report in a retrospective study that 45% of teeth that experienced a periodontal abscess during maintenance were extracted.

NECROTIZING PERIODONTAL DISEASES

Necrotizing ulcerative gingivitis (NUG) is an acute gingival disease that often recurs and may affect the deeper periodontal structures. MacCarthy and Claffey[33] termed these cases *necrotizing ulcerative periodontitis* (NUP) when teeth experienced loss of attachment. Williams and coworkers[34] stated that further progression of the disease past the mucogingival junction is termed *necrotizing stomatitis*. Novak[35] recommended that NUG and NUP be classified together under the category necrotizing periodontal diseases on the basis of clinical characteristics. In the past the disease has been known by names such as cheilokake, Vincent's infection, trench mouth, ulcerative stomatitis of soldiers, ulceromembranous gingivitis, and acute necrotizing ulcerative gingivitis (ANUG). More severe forms have been termed *cancrum oris*[36] or *noma*.[37]

NUG is an inflammatory disease that ulcerates and necroses the papillae and gingival margins. The papillae become necrotic and ulcerated and give a characteristic punched-out or eroded appearance. This appearance is readily detectable. A yellowish or gray–white film of sloughing tissue termed *pseudomembrane* covers the papillae. The film consists of fibrin, necrotic tissue, leukocytes, erythrocytes, and bacteria. Removing the film causes bleeding and exposure of ulcerated tissue. Under the pseudomembrane is an area of intense erythema.

The lesions are often painful and cause patients to seek dental treatment. Pain is the hallmark of NUG and NUP. The early lesions are seen interproximally. These patients often have a pronounced fetid odor. The classic presentation is that of pain, interproximal necrosis, and bleeding.

Histologically, lesions of NUG appear as four distinct zones.[38] Beginning at the tooth/root surface and progressing into the gingival tissues, the first layer is the bacterial zone, which is composed of many bacteria and spirochetes. The next layer is the band of polymorphonuclear neutrophils. The third layer is the zone of tissue necrosis, which is dominated by spirochetes. At the deepest level of the lesion (250 μm), the zone of spirochete infiltration is observed, demonstrating the spirochete's ability to penetrate deep into gingival tissues. More recent studies found that rods constitute approximately 43% of the bacterial samples in NUG patients, followed by 29% cocci, and 28% spirochetes.[39] Eight different forms of spirochetes have been associated with NUG, as has the periodontal pathogen *P. intermedia*.[40]

Several factors have been identified in the literature that seem to play a role in the onset of the disease. These include poor oral hygiene and existing gingivitis, stress, and smoking.[41-43] Bacterial plaque, poor oral hygiene and preexisting gingivitis have all been held as common risk factors for NUG.[44] Barnes and colleagues[45] report that 87% of the patients with NUG had poor oral hygiene compared with 40% of control subjects.

Decreased host resistance is a common factor found in patients with NUG. Malnutrition has frequently been reported in the dental literature to be associated with NUG and noma.[36,46] (See Chapter 31.) Malnutrition and dehydration depress leukocyte function in any disease and further contribute to debilitation. T-lymphocyte helper/suppressor ratios are reported to be inverted in patients with NUG.[47]

Researchers have linked emotional stress as a contributing factor in NUG.[42,43,46] Formicola[48] reported that patients with a dominant personality trait had a positive correlation with NUG, whereas there is a negative correlation between NUG and the personality trait of abasement. Dominant personalities are not able to maintain personal control of situations such as examination periods in college or basic training and wartime situations in the military. This may account for an even greater stress level in such individuals. Adrenocortical steroid activity is increased during periods of stress. The urinary output of 17-hydroxycorticosteroids in patients with NUG may be elevated.[42] Increased levels of 17-hydroxycorticosteroids occur during episodes of NUG, followed by a decrease when NUG is no longer active.[49]

Smoking has been reported as a predisposing factor to NUG/NUP for many years. A high prevalence of heavy smokers is often found in studies of NUG populations.[41] Studies have also documented a role of smoking in chronic periodontitis and altered periodontal wound healing.[50,51] The relation between tobacco habits and NUG/NUP appears to be complex. Studies have yet to show conclusive evidence that smoking adversely affects the periodontium by altering the bacterial flora. However, smoking has been shown to depress T-cell and polymorphonuclear leukocyte functions.

Lymphocyte and polymorphonuclear leukocyte function in patients with NUG demonstrate significant reduction in chemotaxis and phagocytosis.[52] Up to 91% of patients with NUG may have a neutrophil chemotactic defect.[53] Systemic diseases, which impair immunity, predispose patients to NUG and NUP. This is why patients with HIV or leukemia often exhibit necrotizing periodontal diseases (see Chapter 31).

Incidence/Prevalence

Barnes and colleagues[45] report that NUG and NUP are diseases primarily found in young adult populations. Most studies report the mean age of patients with NUG to be in their early 20s. However, necrotizing periodontal diseases may be found at any age in the presence of systemic disease, malnutrition, or blood disorders. The incidence and prevalence rates of necrotizing periodontal diseases are 0.01% in the general population.[54] Among college-age students, the incidence rate is approximately 3%.[41] Among military service members, the rate of incidence ranges from 0.19% to 2%.[43,45,46] Enwonwu[47] report an incidence rate of 15% in an underprivileged African population. A previous history of necrotizing periodontal disease increases the risk for recurrent episodes, with incidence rates ranging from 16% to 33%.[55,56]

Therapy

Pain is usually the symptom that causes most patients with necrotizing periodontal disease to seek dental treatment. Some patients report severe pain, whereas others report less discomfort in the areas of necrosis. Unless there is evidence of systemic involvement, most NUG and NUP cases can be successfully treated with debridement through scaling and root planing (Fig. 12-6, *A* and *B*). Patients often experience discomfort with instrumentation and many patients with NUG and NUP will require topical or local anesthesia. Both ultrasonic and hand instrumentation have been used to treat necrotizing diseases.

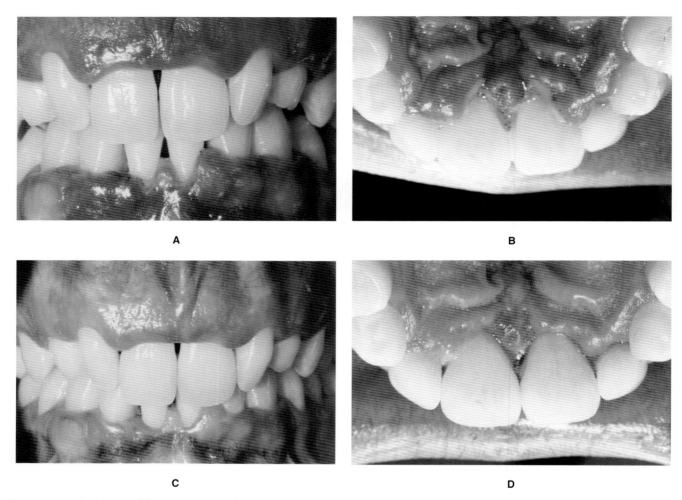

Figure 12-6. A, Initial view of the anterior gingival tissues in a 22-year-old white female smoker with necrotizing ulcerative gingivitis. **B**, Palatal view of the same patient. **C**, Facial view of the same patient, 2 days after initial scaling and cessation of smoking. **D**, Palatal view of the same patient, 2 days after initial scaling and cessation of smoking.

Ultrasonic instrumentation will aid in visual inspection and lavage of the areas of necrosis. The aim of therapy is to eliminate suspected microorganisms and to prevent the ongoing tissue necrosis from spreading laterally and apically. Toothbrushing the treated areas will be uncomfortable for most patients. Toothbrushing should be limited to removal of surface debris using a very soft brush. Therefore, patients may be instructed to use chemotherapeutics such as hydrogen peroxide (3%) with equal parts of warm water every 2 to 3 hours or twice daily rinses of chlorhexidine. These mouthrinses do not penetrate subgingivally, so their effects are limited to the marginal tissues.[57,58] Patients should be informed to avoid tobacco and alcohol products. They should also limit their physical activities for the next few days and make sure they have adequate intake of nutritional food and fluids. Clinical improvement is rapidly seen in patients that receive mechanical debridement.

The patient should be instructed to return in 1 to 2 days for follow-up (Fig. 12-6, C and D). The gingival margins will often be red, but without a pseudomembrane covering. The patient may be gently débrided again and given the same oral hygiene instructions as at the initial visit. A subsequent visit should be scheduled and the patient should receive a scaling and further treatment if needed. Most patients will feel much better after the first 4 to 6 days. Patients with systemic involvement have been prescribed any of the following: metronidazole, penicillin, or tetracycline. Topical antibiotics have proved to be of little value in treatment of NUG and NUP (Fig. 12-7).

After healing of the acute lesions, some areas may still need to be treated because of residual soft tissue crater formations, which are plaque retentive. These sites often require surgical correction. As with any surgery, the patient's individual medical and dental history should be reviewed and evaluated to see if the patient is a surgical candidate.

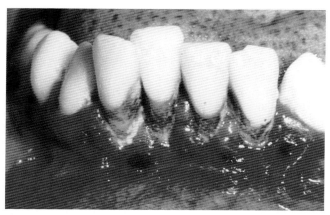

Figure 12-7. A 32-year-old black patient diagnosed with HIV. Appearance at initial dental examination after referral from physician. Clinical diagnosis of necrotizing ulcerative periodontitis.

HERPETIC GINGIVOSTOMATITIS

Herpes simplex (HSV) is a herpes virus infection that is classically divided into two types: type 1 and type 2 (see Chapter 31). Type 1 (HSV-1) typically develops above the waist and is found in or around the oral cavity. Type 2 (HSV-2) generally is found in genital areas. By the time an individual reaches middle age, about 70% will have been infected with HSV-1, but the majority of infections are subclinical in nature (90%). Herpes infections are transmitted by physical contact and typically arise in early childhood, but occasionally are seen in adults.

Patients with the primary clinical infection present with a distinct intraoral ulcerative pattern. Primary herpetic gingivostomatitis is the most common viral infection that affects gingival tissue. The incubation period of the virus is 10 to 14 days. The classic initial presentation is that of fever and lymphadenopathy, followed within a couple of days by diffuse involvement of the gingival tissues and oral mucosa (Fig. 12-8, *A* and *B*). The gingiva will demonstrate intense gingivitis and pain. The free gingival margins on the facial and lingual surfaces will often display ulcerations. This is in contrast to NUG, which primarily affects interdental regions. Fragile vesicles soon develop on any intraoral mucosal surface and then rapidly ulcerate. The ulcers tend to be a few millimeters in diameter, but frequently coalesce. From time to time, the lesions may resemble aphthous stomatitis, but fever and presence of ulcerations on bound mucosa (gingiva) help rule out that diagnosis.

After the primary infection, HSV-1 or -2 is often found residing quiescently in the trigeminal ganglion in a latent form. Various stimuli are implicated in reactivation including trauma, illness, emotional stress, and ultraviolet radiation.[59,60] Recurrent lesions typically occur on or near the vermillion border of the lips (herpes labialis), but recurrent oral lesions are found only in bound down gingival or palatal tissues.

Primary herpetic gingivostomatitis often mimics severe gingivitis, NUG, erythema multiforme, and vesiculobullous disease. Antiviral treatment with acyclovir or similar agents, if initiated within the first 3 days of onset, may shorten the duration of symptoms. Other medications prescribed for treatment of herpes infections include famciclovir and valacyclovir. Famciclovir may decrease the prevalence of latent infection with HSV-1.

Herpes Zoster

Reactivation of a primary infection such as varicella or chickenpox normally affects ganglia in the thoracic region. Occasionally it affects branches of the trigeminal ganglion and causes intraoral and facial herpes zoster (see Chapter 31). Oral lesions typically appear on the palatal tissue and are unilateral. They appear as numerous small

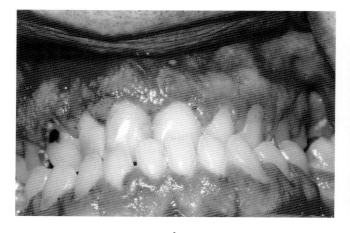

A

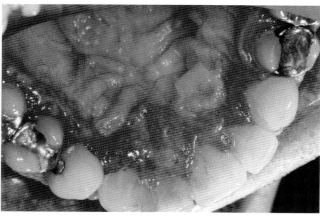

B

Figure 12-8. **A**, A 51-year-old white man with primary herpetic gingivostomatitis. **B**, Palatal view of same patient.

vesicles or ulcerations and have an intense erythematous halo.[61] The lesions are painful but heal in a few days. Palliative treatment includes a soft diet, adequate hydration, rest, and gentle oral hygiene aided by chlorhexidine rinses. Systemic antiviral therapy is generally indicated to reduce the clinical severity of the infection and to prevent postherpetic neuralgia.

PERICORONITIS

Pericoronitis or operculitis is an inflammation of gingival tissue around the crown of a tooth. Pericoronitis is often a painful condition that drives a patient to seek dental treatment. The patient relates a clinical picture of a foul taste and soreness on opening the jaws. The overlying tissue (operculum) is often very red, swollen, and exquisitely tender (Fig. 12-9). The patient relates pain that radiates to the ear and throat areas. The cheek may be swollen in severe cases and regional lymphadenopathy is not uncommon. The patient may also present with fever, malaise, dehydration, and leukocytosis. Pericoronitis is most often associated with an incompletely erupted mandibular third molar in an early adult patient. It can also occur on any tooth during the course of tooth eruption. The treatment of pericoronitis depends on the systemic conditions, inflammation severity, and whether the tooth is retained. If the operculum is symptom-free, the patient should be scheduled for a surgical procedure to remove the excess tissue as a preventive measure, if the tooth is to be retained. The affected tooth may be extracted, if indicated.

If the operculum is symptomatic, the area should first be irrigated with warm water to remove debris and any drainage. The underside of the flap/operculum can be swabbed with an antiseptic such as chlorhexidine. Antibiotics are often prescribed, particularly if any systemic involvement is suspected. If the operculum is

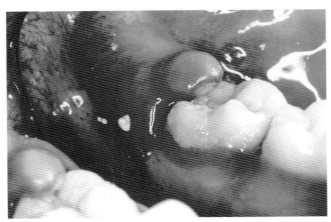

Figure 12-9. Pericoronitis in a 25-year-old white man. (*Courtesy of Dr. Tom Stanford, Baylor College of Medicine, Dallas, TX.*)

fluctuant and swollen, an incision and drainage may be required. The patient should be followed closely if an incision and drainage is performed. The infection may spread posteriorly into the oropharyngeal spaces and medially under the base of the tongue, making swallowing difficult and causing respiratory embarrassment. Peritonsillar abscess, cellulitis, and Ludwig's angina are infrequent, but serious potential sequelae of an acute episode of pericoronitis.

Once the acute situation has abated, a decision must be made whether to retain the offending tooth. If further eruption into good occlusal function is likely, the tooth may be retained. If not, the tooth should be removed.

APHTHOUS STOMATITIS

Aphthous ulcerations are recurring lesions of the oral cavity and are classified into three categories: minor, major, and herpetiform. About 80% of the cases are the minor form. Minor aphthae are almost exclusively found on nonkeratinized movable mucosa and demonstrate a fibrinopurulent membrane surrounded by a red halo. Most lesions are less than 1 cm in diameter, are painful, and heal without scarring the tissue. Many patients have one to five lesions when an episode arises. The lesions heal in 10 to 14 days. The recurring episodes are extremely variable.

The etiology of minor aphthae is unknown, but it seems to be linked to both the humoral and cell-mediated immune systems. Heredity, stress, local trauma, vitamin deficiencies, and food allergies have been suspected. L-form *streptococci*, reactivation of varicella zoster virus, and cytomegalovirus have all been suspected as trigger mechanisms. Patients with increased keratinization of the oral mucosa such as found in smokers seem to have a lower incidence of aphthae outbreaks.

Topical steroid elixirs and gels appear to be the most effective treatment of the lesions. Chlorhexidine rinses have been used with varying degrees of success. Chlorhexidine seems to be most useful when used early in the course of the lesion.

Major aphthae are recurrent ulcerations and appear similar to minor aphthae, except that they tend to be much larger and take longer to heal. About 10% of all aphthous ulcers are major aphthae. Patients typically have 1 to 10 lesions that vary in size from one to several centimeters in diameter (Fig. 12-10). These lesions may take up to 6 weeks to heal. Therefore, many patients with major aphthae are rarely without a lesion because of rapid recurrence and long healing periods. Topical corticosteroids are often not effective treatments of these lesions. Greater potency steroids administered intralesionally or systemically are often required to treat major aphthous ulcers. Thalidomide is sometimes used in severe cases of major aphthae despite its potential teratogenic effects.

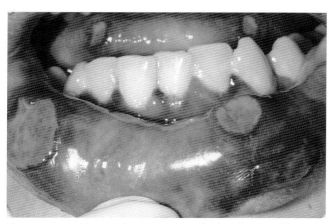

Figure 12-10. Major aphthae in 27-year-old white female soldier who received orders sending her into a war zone 3 days before oral examination.

Herpetiform aphthous ulcers account for about 10% of aphthous stomatitis cases. The ulcers are similar in appearance to minor aphthae, but they tend to be smaller and occur in greater numbers. The lesions are typically less than 2 mm in size. Patients may have 10 to 100 lesions present in the oral cavity at any given time. These lesions tend to be extremely painful and often cluster or coalesce. Any mucosal surface may be involved. The cause is unknown. As with all aphthous ulcerations, other conditions need to be evaluated in a differential diagnosis such as: Crohn's disease, Behçet's disease, blood dyscrasia, and nutritional deficiencies. Topical steroid elixirs and gels are the treatment of choice for their palliative effect and temporary remission. There is no permanent cure.

MUCOCUTANEOUS DISORDERS

Any mucocutaneous disorder may present as an acute gingival condition and should be considered in a differential diagnosis. These diseases may also involve other intraoral areas or extraoral sites such as the genitalia, skin, or internal organs. A detailed discussion of these lesions is beyond the scope of this chapter; however, they are discussed in detail in Chapter 35. Some disorders that may elicit gingival lesions include the following: lichen planus, mucous membrane pemphigoid, pemphigus, lupus erythematosus, or psoriasis.

REFERENCES

1. Rees TD: Adjunctive therapy. In *Proceedings of the World Workshop in Clinical Periodontics*, Chicago, 1989, American Academy of Periodontology, pp 32-34.
2. McFall WT: The periodontal abscess, *JNC Dent Soc* 47:34, 1964.
3. O'Brien TI: Diagnosis and treatment of periodontal and gingival abscesses, *J Ont Dent Assoc* 47:16, 1970.
4. Ranney RR: Pathogenesis of periodontal disease: position report and review of literature. International Conference on Research in the Biology of Periodontal Disease, Chicago, 1977.
5. Grant DA, Stern IB, Everett EO: *Orban's periodontics*, ed 4, St. Louis, 1972, Mosby.
6. Ludwig TO: An investigation of the oral flora of suppurative oral swellings, *Aust Dent* 12:259, 1957.
7. Merchant NE: Infections related to the jaws, *Practitioner* 209:679, 1972.
8. Moore IR, Russell C: Bacteriological investigation of dental abscesses, *Dent Pract Dent Rec* 22:390, 1972.
9. Epstein S, Scopp IW: Antibiotics and the intraoral abscess, *J Periodontol* 48:236-238, 1977.
10. Newman MO, Sims TN: The predominant cultivable microbiota of the periodontal abscess, *J Periodontol* 50:350, 1978.
11. van Winkelhoff AJ, Carlee AW, de Graaff J: Bacteroides endodontalis and other black-pigmented Bacteroides species in odontogenic abscesses, *Infect Immun* 49:494, 1985.
12. DeWitt GV, Cobb CM, Killoy WJ: The acute periodontal abscess: microbial penetration of the soft tissue wall, *Int J Periodontics Restorative Dent* 5:39, 1985.
13. Slots J, Listgarten MA: Bacteroides gingivalis, Bacteroides intermedius and Actinobacillus actinomycetemcomitans in human periodontal diseases, *J Clin Periodontol* 15(2):85-93, 1988.
14. Trope M, Tronstad L, Rosenberg ES, Listgarten M: Darkfield microscopy as a diagnostic aid in differentiating exudates from endodontic and periodontal abscesses, *J Endod* 14:35-38, 1988.
15. van Winkelhoff AJ, van Steenbergen TJM, de Graff J: The role of black-pigmented *Bacteroides* in human oral infections, *J Clin Periodontol* 15:145-155, 1988.
16. Kulkarni GV, Lee WK, Aitken A, et al: A randomized, placebo-controlled trial of doxycycline: effect on the microflora of recurrent periodontitis lesions in high risk patients, *J Periodontol* 62:197-202, 1991.
17. Aitken S, Birek P, Kulkarni GV, et al: Serial doxycycline and metronidazole in prevention of recurrent periodontitis in high-risk patients, *J Periodontol* 63:87-92, 1992.
18. Hafström CA, Wikström MB, Renvert SN, Dahlén GG: Effect of treatment on some periodontopathogens and their antibody levels in periodontal abscesses, *J Periodontol* 65:1022-1028, 1994.
19. Herrera D, Roldán S, González I, Sanz M: The periodontal abscess (1). Clinical and microbiological findings. *J Clin Periodontol* 27:387-394, 2000.
20. Ahl DR, Hilgeman JL, Synder JD: Periodontal emergencies, *Dent Clin North Am* 30:459-472, 1986.
21. McLeod DE, Lainson PA, Spivey JD: Tooth loss due to periodontal abscesses: a retrospective study, *J Periodontol* 68:963-966, 1997.

22. Gray JL, Flanary DB, Newell DH: The prevalence of periodontal abscess, *J Indiana Dent Assoc* 73:18-23, 1994.

23. Lalla E, Lamster IB, Schmidt AM: Enhanced interaction of advanced glycation end products with their cellular receptor RAGE: implications for the pathogenesis of accelerated periodontal disease in diabetes, *Ann Periodontol* 3:13-19, 1998.

24. Topoll HH, Lange DE, Müller RF: Multiple periodontal abscesses after systemic antibiotic therapy, *J Clin Periodontol* 17:268-272, 1990.

25. Helovuo H, Hakkarainen K, Paunio K: Changes in the prevalence of subgingival enteric rods, staphylococci and yeasts after treatment with penicillin and erythromycin, *Oral Microbiol Immunol* 8:75-79, 1993.

26. Nabers JM, Meador HL, Nabers CL, O'Leary TJ: Chronology, an important factor in the repair of osseous defects, *Periodontics* 2:304, 1964.

27. Trott IR: The acute periodontal abscess, *J Can Dent Assoc* 25:601, 1959.

28. Goldberg MH: The changing biologic nature of acute dental infection, *J Am Dent Assoc* 80:1048, 1970.

29. Gordon M, Walker CB, Murphy JC, et al: Tetracycline: levels achievable in gingival crevice fluid and in vitro effect on subgingival organisms. I. Concentrations in crevicular fluid after repeated doses, *J Periodontol* 52:609, 1981.

30. Walker CB, Gordon JM, McQuilkin SJ, et al: Tetracycline: levels achievable in gingival crevice fluid and in vitro effect on subgingival organisms. II. Susceptibilities of periodontal bacteria, *J Periodontol* 52:1513, 1981.

31. Becker W, Becker BE, Berg LE: Periodontal treatments without maintenance. A retrospective study in 44 patients, *J Periodontol* 55:505-509, 1984.

32. Chace R Sr, Low SB: Survival characteristics of periodontally-involved teeth: a 40-year study, *J Periodontol* 64:701-705, 1993.

33. MacCarthy D, Claffey N: Acute necrotizing ulcerative gingivitis is associated with attachment loss, *J Clin Periodontol* 18:776-779, 1991.

34. Williams CA, Winkler JR, Grassi M, Murray PA: HIV-associated periodontitis complicated by necrotizing stomatitis, *Oral Surg Oral Med Oral Pathol* 69:351-355, 1990.

35. Novak MJ: Necrotizing ulcerative periodontitis, *Ann Periodontol* 4:74-77, 1999.

36. Emslie RD: Cancrum oris, *Dent Prac* 13:481-495, 1963.

37. MacDonald JB, Sutton RM, Knoll ML, et al: The pathogenic components of an experimental fusospirochetal infection, *J Infect Dis* 98:15-20, 1956.

38. Listgarten MA: Electron microscopic observations of the bacterial flora of acute necrotizing ulcerative gingivitis, *J Periodontol* 36:328, 1965.

39. Falkler WA, Martin S, Vincent J, et al: A clinical, demographic and microbiological study of ANUG patients in an urban dental school, *J Clin Periodontol* 14:307-314, 1987.

40. Rowland RW, Mestecky J, Gunsolley JC, Cogen RB: Serum IgG and IgM levels to bacterial antigens in necrotizing ulcerative gingivitis, *J Periodontol* 64:195-201, 1993.

41. Melnick SL, Roseman JM, Engel D, Cogen RB: Epidemiology of acute necrotizing ulcerative gingivitis, *Epidemiol Rev* 10:191-211, 1988.

42. Shannon I, Kilgoe W, O'Leary T: Stress as a predisposing factor in necrotizing ulcerative gingivitis, *J Periodontol* 40:240-242, 1969.

43. Shields WD: Acute necrotizing ulcerative gingivitis: a study of some of the contributing factors and their validity in an army population, *J Periodontol* 48:346-349, 1977.

44. Schluger S: Necrotic ulcerative gingivitis in the army: incidence, communicability and treatment, *J Am Dent Assoc* 38:174-183, 1949.

45. Barnes GP, Bowles WF, Carter HG: Acute necrotizing gingivitis: a survey of 218 cases, *J Periodontol* 44:35-42, 1973.

46. Pindborg JJ: The epidemiology of ulceromembranous gingivitis showing the influence of service in the Armed Forces, *Paradontology* 10:114-118, 1956.

47. Enwonwu CO: Cellular and molecular effects of malnutrition and their relevance to periodontal diseases, *J Clin Periodontol* 21:643-657, 1994.

48. Formicola A, Witte E, Curran P: A study of personality traits and acute necrotizing ulcerative gingivitis. *J Periodontol* 41:36-38, 1970.

49. Maupin CC, Bell WB: The relationship of 17-hydroxycorticosteroid to acute necrotizing ulcerative gingivitis. *J Periodontol* 46:721-722, 1975.

50. Haber J, Wattles J, Crowley M, et al: Evidence for cigarette smoking, bacterial pathogens, and periodontal status. *J Periodontol* 64:16-23, 1993.

51. Ah MK, Johnson GK, Kaldahl WB, et al: The effect of smoking on the response to periodontal therapy. *J Clin Periodontol* 21:91-97, 1994.

52. Cogen R, Stevens JAW, Cohen-Cole S, et al: Leukocyte function in the etiology of acute necrotizing ulcerative gingivitis. *J Periodontol* 54:402-407, 1983.

53. Claffey N, Russell R, Shanley D: Peripheral blood phagocyte function in acute necrotizing ulcerative gingivitis. *J Periodont Res* 21:288-297, 1986.

54. Skack M, Zabrodsky S, Mrklas L: A study of the effect of age and season on the incidence of ulcerative gingivitis. *J Periodont Res* 5:187-190, 1970.

55. Jiminez LM, Baer PM: Necrotizing ulcerative gingivitis in children, a nine year clinical study. *J Periodontol* 46:715-720, 1975.

56. Giddon DB, Zacklin JS, Goldhabert P: Acute necrotizing ulcerative gingivitis in college students. *J Am Dent Assoc* 68:381-386, 1964.

57. Wennström J, Lindhe J: Effect of hydrogen peroxide on developing plaque and gingivitis in man, *J Clin Periodontol* 6:115-130, 1979.

58. Gjermo P: Chlorhexidine in dental practice, *J Clin Periodontol* 1:143-152, 1974.

59. Sculley P: Orofacial herpes simplex virus infection: current concepts on the epidemiology, pathogenesis and treatments and disorders in which the virus may be implicated, *Oral Surg Oral Med Oral Pathol* 68:701-718, 1989.

60. Bergstom T, Lycke E: Neuroinvasion by herpes simplex virus. An *in vitro* model for characterization of neurovirulent strains, *J Gen Virol* 71:405-410, 1990.

61. Eisenburg E: Intraoral isolated herpes zoster, *Oral Surg Oral Med Oral Pathol* 45:214-219, 1978.

13 Oral Physiotherapy

Mark V. Thomas

Home care, oral hygiene, oral physiotherapy, personal oral hygiene, and personal plaque control are all terms that have been used to describe those methods used by the patient to remove plaque. A distinction is made between personal oral hygiene (performed by the patient) and professional debridement (performed by the dentist or hygienist). This chapter deals with various aspects of personal oral hygiene. The biologic rationale for plaque control is examined, followed by a review of devices and techniques currently in use. The chapter concludes with a consideration of sociobehavioral factors, adverse effects of hygiene procedures, and future directions for research. There are a number of recent reviews that deal with plaque control. The interested reader is directed to these for additional information.[1-4]

Periodontal disease is largely preventable. Like many chronic diseases, behavioral or lifestyle choices play a significant role in the pathogenesis of periodontitis. Of course, there are many risk factors involved in periodontal disease expression: the subgingival flora, genetic predisposition, stress, and systemic disease. Some of these risk factors, such as genetic predisposition, cannot be modified. Others, such as oral hygiene practices, are amenable to change. As shown later in this chapter, the relation between oral hygiene and periodontal disease is more complex than might be thought. Adequate home care remains, however, one of the foundations of periodontal health and therapy.

BIOLOGIC RATIONALE FOR PERSONAL PLAQUE CONTROL

Plaque control is only one of many variables that determine an individual's periodontal status. However, it is one of the risk factors most amenable to change. The term *plaque* is rather nonspecific. Plaque may be supragingival or subgingival and may be adherent or nonadherent to tooth or tissue.[3] In addition, the microbial composition of plaque varies from person to person and from site to site within the same mouth. Oral hygiene, as used in this chapter, refers largely to efforts to remove the supragingival plaque.

Supragingival plaque is the etiologic agent of gingivitis. In a series of classic experiments conducted in the 1960s, oral hygiene was suspended in a group of dental students.[5,6] All of the subjects rapidly formed supragingival plaque, and gingivitis developed within 2 to 3 weeks. When oral hygiene was resumed, the condition was reversed and health was reestablished. This confirmed supragingival plaque as the etiologic agent of gingivitis. Subsequent work has validated these findings, although some workers have reported significant individual variation in the extent to which gingivitis developed.[7]

The flora responsible for gingivitis is relatively nonspecific. As the plaque matures and becomes thicker, the composition of the flora shifts from gram-positive facultative organisms to an increasingly gram-negative anaerobic flora. This shift is aided by a slight swelling of the gingival margin that renders the subgingival environment more anaerobic and more hospitable to obligate anaerobes. The subsequent inflammation results in a protein-rich exudate that is required by many of these asaccharolytic organisms as carbon and energy sources.[8]

There is evidence that accumulation of supragingival plaque may affect the composition of the subgingival microbiota, particularly in pockets probing less than 6 mm.[9-11] Plaque forms more quickly in sites of gingival inflammation.[12-14] This may be because the inflammatory exudate seen in gingivitis is more conducive to supporting the growth of fastidious periodontal pathogens, given its protein-rich nature. Acceptable plaque control has been shown to cause a reduction in histologic inflammation, even in the absence of subgingival debridement.[15] However, these effects may be minimal in deeper pockets.

What are the implications of supragingival plaque in the development and progression of periodontitis? Although not all cases of gingivitis progress to periodontitis, gingivitis is normally a necessary intermediate step in the development of periodontitis. In a classic longitudinal study of Sri Lankan tea workers who had no dental care and poor oral hygiene, periodontitis occurred in 89% of subjects with chronic gingivitis.[16] Because gingivitis can be prevented or reversed by a combination of personal and professional care, it seems logical to infer that periodontitis may be similarly prevented by adherence to a regimen of personal oral hygiene and routine professional care.

Despite the plausibility of this assertion, the exact relation between supragingival plaque and periodontitis has proven to be somewhat more complex. On one hand, research has demonstrated that good plaque control is effective in preventing periodontal disease and halting its progress when combined with professional therapy.[17] However, epidemiologic studies have not always found such a clearcut relation between plaque levels and periodontal status, and some have found that supragingival plaque is not a significant risk factor for periodontitis.[18,19]

A number of studies have examined the effect of inadequate plaque control on therapeutic outcomes and found that periodontal therapy is relatively ineffective in the absence of adequate home care.[20-22] In fact, studies of various periodontal surgical techniques have generally shown that the most important determinant of improvement in periodontal status is not the type of surgical technique used, but the level of patient plaque control and the willingness of patients to comply with a periodontal maintenance regimen.[23,24] Plaque control is particularly important immediately after periodontal surgical therapy. Better outcomes have been reported when patients demonstrate excellent plaque control in the 6 months after surgery compared with patients whose plaque control is poor during this period.[25] The quality of plaque removal may be a major factor in determining disease recurrence in patients treated for periodontitis.[26] Patients with poor plaque control tend to lose attachment, whereas those with effective home care are generally stable, with proper maintenance. In one study of patients who had received surgical treatment for severe periodontitis but no structured recall system, the responsibility for oral cleanliness was left with the patients.[27] At 4 years after surgery, patients with poor plaque control had worse outcomes than patients with better hygiene.

Conversely, it should also be noted that plaque control without professional therapy is of limited effectiveness in treating periodontal disease.[4,28,29] For example, Cercek and colleagues[28] conducted a three-phase study that examined the relative effects of oral hygiene and subgingival debridement on periodontal status in a group of patients with generalized chronic periodontitis. During the first and second phases, patients used only personal plaque control measures (i.e., toothbrush, floss, and interdental cleaners). During the third phase, the patients also received professional subgingival debridement in addition to their home care regimen. Most of the clinical improvement that occurred was seen only after the professional subgingival debridement.

The relation between oral hygiene practices and disease progression reflects a complex interplay between exogenous risk factors and host defenses. The identification of risk factors is currently the focus of major research initiatives (see Chapter 3). Determining risk factors will eventually allow the clinician to target those individuals at greatest risk, allowing for more effective use of resources and avoiding overtreatment or undertreatment. It is likely that some of the above contradictions can be explained by the *differential susceptibility* of individuals. A medical example of differential susceptibility is tuberculosis. It is estimated that active tuberculosis will eventually develop in approximately 10% of those infected with *Mycobacterium tuberculosis*.[30] Whether active disease develops depends largely on host factors.

The concept of differential susceptibility is also true of periodontitis, as shown by the findings of Loe and colleagues[16] in their study of Sri Lankan tea workers. The study population had little or no access to dental care and oral hygiene was universally poor. As might be expected, many of the subjects lost teeth because of the ravages of periodontal disease. However, 11% exhibited no disease progression beyond gingivitis, even in the complete absence of personal or professional plaque control. Thus,

although supragingival plaque is an important, modifiable risk factor for periodontitis, it is clearly not the only risk factor.

Clinical Application

How can we apply this information to clinical practice? It is likely that some individuals are more susceptible than others to periodontal attachment loss. In some cases, we can identify individuals who are at increased risk for attachment loss, on the basis of our current state of knowledge—for example, the patient who smokes or who has poorly controlled diabetes mellitus. In the absence of good predictors for periodontal disease, however, it would seem prudent to stress the importance of proper plaque control and proceed on the assumption that home care is an important determinant of periodontal health for many patients. The preponderance of the evidence would suggest that satisfactory treatment outcomes are most likely when professional debridement is accompanied by regular plaque removal by the patient.

Proper oral hygiene may seem a mundane and unexciting topic in a specialty that has embraced implantology, regenerative therapy, and molecular biology. Pedestrian it may be, but it is often one of the most important determinants of treatment success or failure.

HOME CARE TECHNIQUES

The goal of oral hygiene is the physical and chemical disruption of the biofilm on a frequent basis. A variety of devices and techniques have been used in this pursuit, from the simple toothbrush and home irrigation systems to sophisticated electromechanical devices.

Toothbrushing

Evidence exists that the ancient Chinese used toothbrushes as early as the fifteenth century AD. Toothbrushing is probably the most fundamental and common oral hygiene practice. There are several questions that are reasonable to ask regarding brushing:

- Are there any significant differences between various brush designs?
- Do electromechanical brushes (EMBs) offer any advantages?
- How often should the toothbrush be replaced?
- What method of brushing is superior?
- What is the effect of brushing frequency on gingival inflammation?
- What are the shortcomings of studies in this area and what are desirable directions for future research?

Manual toothbrushes

Over the years, manufacturers have offered a bewildering array of toothbrushes, some well designed, others less so.

For the most part, studies that have compared manual brushes have found relatively little difference among designs.[31-33] It has often been asserted that a brush should have bristles with rounded tips that are soft enough to prevent damage to the teeth and gingiva, but beyond these general statements there has been little scientific evidence to differentiate the various types of manual brushes.

More recently, manufacturers have been innovative in developing unique brush designs (Figs. 13-1 and 13-2). These innovations have largely involved variations in handle shape and orientation of the bristles. Some of these designs have been shown to be more effective than older toothbrush designs in short-term studies,[34-36] whereas others have not confirmed an enhanced effectiveness.[36,37] Currently, it is safe to assume that the differences among manual brushes are likely to be insignificant compared with the parameters of time spent brushing, frequency of use, and operator dexterity. However, it is quite possible that a given patient may have better results with one particular toothbrush. This underscores an important point in the practical application of this information to patient care: the oral hygiene regimen should be tailored to the individual. Efforts to adopt a "one size fits all" approach are not likely to be successful.

The entire field of toothbrush design has been so active that it is difficult to attempt more than a general survey of design features. Brushes generally differ with regard to head size, bristle characteristics, and handle design (see Figs. 13-1 and 13-2). Older brushes had natural bristles of porcine origin. Most modern brushes use nylon bristles, which are of solid monofilament construction. The desired diameter of the bristles is often stated to be around 0.007 inch, a dimension promoted many years ago by Bass, a physician and former dean of the Tulane College of Medicine who developed an interest in oral hygiene. A comparison of two brushes with 0.007- and 0.008-inch diameter bristles found similar effectiveness between brushes.[38] There is some evidence that rounded bristles are less damaging than those with cut ends.[39] Similarly, hard or stiff bristles are more damaging than softer bristles.[40]

What is the useful life of an average toothbrush? Several studies have examined this question, but the results are somewhat contradictory. A short-term study in dental students found that replacement of the brushes every 2 weeks improved plaque removal, although this had no effect on gingival inflammation.[41] These results were consistent with other investigators' findings that new brushes performed better than old, matted brushes.[42] These investigators suggested that brushes be discarded at the first signs of matting. Contrary to these findings, others have reported that 3-month-old brushes performed as well as new brushes, and that toothbrush wear was unrelated to plaque removal efficiency.[43]

As with so many other facets of oral hygiene, we lack the necessary information to make evidence-based recommendations regarding the useful life of toothbrushes. Furthermore, it is likely that different brushes, being of different designs and made from various materials, would exhibit differences in longevity, so that results from a study of brand A toothbrushes could not readily be extrapolated to brands B and C. It is unlikely that relatively new brushes will be *worse* than older brushes, so perhaps a 3-month replacement schedule is a reasonable recommendation. Some commercially available brushes have bristles that change color after a certain amount of use, which serves as a reminder to the patient that it is time to replace the brush.

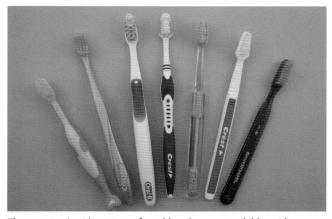

Figure 13-1. A wide variety of toothbrushes are available, with numerous different bristle designs. (*Courtesy Dr. David Hardison and Ms. Amy Simmons.*)

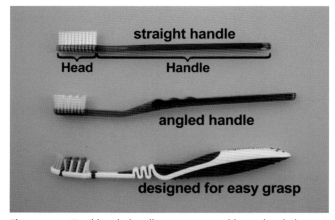

Figure 13-2. Toothbrush handles are as variable as head designs. (*Courtesy Dr. David Hardison and Ms. Amy Simmons.*)

Manual brushing techniques

Over the years, many toothbrushing techniques have been advocated. The actual technique used is not as important as the result. If a patient can do a good job removing plaque without damage to the teeth and gingival tissues, then there is no reason to suggest a change. If, however, a patient needs improvement in plaque control, the technique should be reassessed. The oral hygiene regimen must be tailored to the individual patient's circumstances. Special patients such as young children, the elderly, and patients with neuromuscular conditions may benefit from specialized techniques or devices such as electric brushes or large-handled manual brushes. In extreme cases, caregivers may have to assist with or actually perform basic oral hygiene measures.

Toothbrushing techniques can be grouped by the type of stroke used. Some of the more common methods described below include:

- Bass and horizontal scrub techniques (Figs. 13-3 and 13-4)
- Charters technique (Fig. 13-5)
- Roll technique (Fig. 13-6)

The Bass method emphasizes sulcular brushing and, for this reason, has long been popular among periodontists.[44] In this method, the bristles are angled toward the gingival margin at a 45-degree angle and gently introduced into the sulcus (see Fig. 13-3). The brush is then moved in a short vibratory stroke (see Fig. 13-4). This penetration of the bristle into the sulcus has the goal of disrupting subgingival plaque, and studies have shown a sulcular penetration of approximately 1 mm using this technique.[45] Presumably, this would be the limit of direct plaque disruption by the brush. Using a horizontal scrub

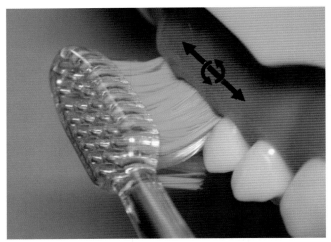

Figure 13-4. The Bass brushing technique. The bristles are moved in a short vibratory stroke that has a circular pattern. (*Courtesy Dr. David Hardison and Ms. Amy Simmons.*)

motion may be viewed as a modification of the Bass technique. The bristles are positioned in a similar 45-degree relation to the sulcus, but the brush is moved back and forth in a scrubbing motion rather than in short, circular vibratory strokes.

In the Charters technique, the bristles are perpendicular to the long axis of the teeth[46] (see Fig. 13-5). The bristles are then gently forced into the interproximal embrasures, which causes some deflection of the bristles toward the occlusal surfaces of the teeth. The side of the bristles eventually rests on the surface of the gingiva, unlike the Bass method in which the bristle tip enters the sulcus. The Charters method was supposedly good for gingival

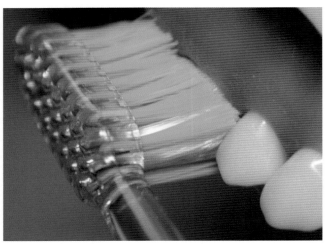

Figure 13-3. The Bass brushing technique. The bristles are angled into the sulcus at a 45-degree angle. (*Courtesy Dr. David Hardison and Ms. Amy Simmons.*)

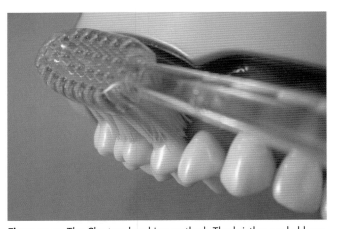

Figure 13-5. The Charters brushing method. The bristles are held perpendicular to the long axis of the teeth and are forced into the interproximal spaces. The bristles of the brush deflect toward the occlusal surface (opposite to the Bass method in which bristles are directed into the sulcus). (*Courtesy Dr. David Hardison and Ms. Amy Simmons.*)

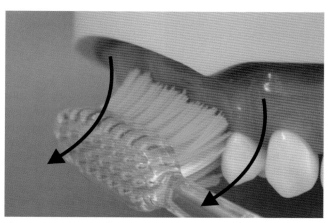

Figure 13-6. The modified Stillman or "roll" technique. The bristles are angled into the sulcus at a 45-degree angle and overlap onto the facial gingiva. The head of the brush is then "rolled" so that the bristles move occlusally. (*Courtesy Dr. David Hardison and Ms. Amy Simmons.*)

massage and was alleged to be indicated in cases of advanced periodontitis when the interdental embrasures are relatively open. It can be argued, however, that one of the various interdental brushes might be more effective in this application. The Charters method also has been recommended for use in the postsurgical healing phase, to prevent damage to the immature attachment apparatus.

In the roll technique, the bristles are placed against the teeth as in the Bass method, but instead of vibrating the bristles, the head is rotated so that the bristles eventually are pointed toward the occlusal surfaces, in a sort of "rolling" motion. The modified Stillman technique is similar to the roll technique, except that the bristle ends are placed both into the sulcus and onto the marginal gingiva before the rolling motion is started[47] (see Fig. 13-6). This brushing stroke is sometimes suggested for use after periodontal plastic surgery to treat gingival recession. The rolling motion is used to "guide" the healing tissues coronally.

In the horizontal "scrub-brush" technique, the brush is moved in a back-and-forth motion, suggestive of a scrub brush. This is a commonly used technique by patients because it gives a sense of vigorous cleansing. Unfortunately, this technique may result in effective plaque removal from the most convex regions of the tooth, but may be ineffective in removing plaque from the line angles and interproximal surfaces. It is sometimes suggested that the horizontal scrub technique, especially when combined with a hard-bristled brush, may result in gingival trauma leading to recession, although convincing evidence is lacking.

In general, three concepts must be stressed regardless of the technique used. First, adequate time must be set aside for brushing. For most patients, it is best to time

their brushing sessions. Various EMBs incorporate a timer, which may be useful in this regard. Second, brushing must be systematic so as not to miss any surfaces. Most patients find it better to brush in the same sequence each time because this ensures that all areas will be adequately covered. Third, no method of manual brushing is sufficient to remove interdental plaque; therefore, the use of one or another of the various interdental aids is required. An important aspect of all oral hygiene methods is habit. For most patients, it may be desirable that these techniques are done at the same time and in the same manner each day. Unfortunately, with the busy, stressful lives of many, this may be difficult.

In the 1970s, a number of studies compared the various methods of brushing, with most reporting no significant difference in plaque removal. This is probably the primary reason that this area is currently a low research priority, with relatively few recent studies appearing in the literature. Because the available evidence does not permit clear distinctions between methods on the basis of efficacy, it would seem reasonable to begin with a standard technique such as the Bass method for most patients. If an individual patient is unable to do a good job with the recommended method, then other techniques may be suggested. It is not so much the method that is important, however, as it is the thoroughness with which it is done. This therapeutic equivalence may not extend to powered brushes, however. There is convincing evidence that some EMBs may offer real, if modest, advantages over manual brushing.

Electromechanical toothbrushes

The first electric brushes became commercially available in the 1960s. These early designs were not particularly effective and resembled conventional manual toothbrushes both in appearance and movement of the brush head. The current generation of electric brushes may be marked by the appearance of the RotaDent and Interplak (Rotadent: Professional Dental Technologies; Batesville, AR; Interplak: Conair; Stamford, CT) in the 1980s. These new brushes are more reliable and sophisticated than their predecessors and have become popular among dentists and patients. In this review, the term *electromechanical brush* (EMB) refers to those brushes that use a powered brush head. This term may be preferable to *electric brush* in that it more clearly describes the common design feature of these brushes, namely a mechanical device powered by electricity.

What sorts of caveats apply to research in this area? There are several difficulties inherent in comparing brushes. One is the novelty effect. Study subjects may be impressed with the novelty or technology of an EMB and may initially use it more diligently than the manual brush. Unfortunately, however, this enthusiasm may be short-lived. Therefore, it is recommended that such studies be conducted for a sufficiently long period (i.e., 6 months) to allow for the novelty to "wear off." Second is the "Hawthorne effect," which occurs when research subjects behave differently *because they realize that they are being observed.* Thus, the very act of studying the subjects alters their behavior. Long-term studies are less likely to be influenced by this effect. Studies involving EMBs should compare the powered brush to a positive control such as a manual brush. Examiners should be blinded so they are unaware of what device the subject is using. Lastly, EMBs differ greatly in design. Therefore, proof of efficacy of one brush cannot be extrapolated to other EMBs.

How effective are EMBs? Effectiveness in this regard may be related to either plaque removal or reduction of gingival inflammation. One would assume that these are positively related, but this is not always the case (see later). Many studies have shown a similar effectiveness between manual brushes and EMBs, whereas others have shown EMBs to be superior. The cost of EMBs is clearly higher than manual brushes; therefore, the cost effectiveness of EMBs must be considered for each individual patient. One area in which most EMBs appear to be superior to manual brushes is in the amount of time required to remove plaque. A number of studies suggest that many EMBs remove plaque at a faster rate than do manual brushes. Perhaps more important than the speed of plaque removal, several EMBs are equipped with timers that provide a standard time for brushing. For example, some EMBs have a timer that begins when the brush is activated and runs for 2 minutes, at which point the timer produces an audible sound letting the patient know the 2-minute period has expired. Because most patients brush for only a short time at each session, this feature can be quite helpful. A recent study compared one such EMB with manual brushing: 66% of EMB users brushed for 2 minutes versus only 17% of those using a manual brush.[48] Several studies have reported that EMBs were more effective than manual brushes in removing stain.[32,49,50]

Of equal or greater importance, research has shown that various EMBs are often more effective in removal of interproximal plaque than manual brushes.[51] Thus, EMBs may offer a clear advantage for patients who do not floss regularly. In a systematic review of studies comparing EMBs and manual brushes, the reviewers concluded that an oscillating electric brush offered modest improvements in reducing plaque and gingivitis.[52,53]

With regard to individual brands of EMBs, the following brushes have been shown to be superior to manual brushing, at least in some studies: the Rotadent (round head, rotary action), Interplak (counter-rotational tufts on rectangular brush head), Braun Oral-B (several variations;

all have round head that oscillates [Braun GmbH; Kronberg, Germany]), and Sonicare (high-frequency "vibrating" bristles on conventional-appearing brush head [Philips Oral Healthcare Inc.; Snoqualmie, WA]).

In conclusion, the new generation of EMBs appears to be more effective in plaque removal than manual brushing. This is particularly true in interproximal areas. Most studies have shown that EMBs remove plaque more rapidly than manual brushes. Despite this improved efficacy, it appears that EMBs are unlikely to cause clinically significant tooth abrasion or recession when used in the proper manner. Careful professional instruction is required if the individual is to receive the full benefit of the brush. Because the novelty factor is sometimes responsible for short-term improvements in home care that may not be sustained in the long term, the clinician must constantly reemphasize the need for consistent oral hygiene. EMBs are not necessary for all patients, because many patients perform adequate oral hygiene with a manual brush in combination with floss or interdental cleaning aids. These devices are worth considering mainly for those patients who need extra help with plaque control.

Interdental Cleaning Aids

The interdental embrasure offers a protected sanctuary for plaque to accumulate undisturbed. Manual toothbrushing does not generally have much of an effect on interdental plaque and gingivitis. In a study of 119 adults, Graves and colleagues[54] found that brushing reduced gingival bleeding by 35%, whereas the combination of brushing and floss reduced bleeding by 67%. Most patients do not floss daily as recommended, and those who do not floss have more plaque and calculus accumulation than those who do.[55] Therefore, it is necessary to augment toothbrushing with special interdental cleaning aids. The choice of aids depends largely on the size and shape of the interdental embrasure and the degree to which soft tissue fills the space.

Dental floss

The most common interdental cleaning aid is dental floss. Dental floss is available in a variety of different sizes and configurations. Originally, the choice was limited to waxed and unwaxed floss. The purpose of the wax was ostensibly to make flossing between tight contacts easier. Waxed and unwaxed floss are equally effective in removing plaque.[56] Floss made with expanded polytetrafluoroethylene (ePTFE), which also improves access in tight contacts, has been shown to be equivalent to unwaxed floss as well.[57] Waerhaug[58] reported that floss was effective at removal of subgingival interproximal plaque up to a depth of 2 mm. Superfloss (Oral B Laboratories, the Gillette Company; Boston, MA) is a type of floss consisting of a terminal segment of stiff plastic that is used for inserting it beneath fixed partial dentures and through tight embrasures. The remainder is composed of a foamlike material that has more bulk than regular floss. Superfloss is generally more useful under bridges and in areas with more open embrasures. Floss threaders are often required to permit introduction of floss under fixed prostheses and orthodontic appliances. Studies have shown little or no difference among various types of floss.[56,57,59] For some patients the use of "floss aids" may allow easier management of the floss. These are used as an option to wrapping of the floss around the fingers. Although these devices do not appear to improve effectiveness of plaque removal, some patients may prefer them to using their fingers.[60]

A piece of floss about 12 to 15 inches in length should be wrapped around the fingers. Some patients may benefit from tying the ends of a length of floss to form a circle, which may be grasped more easily. The floss is generally wrapped around the middle finger of each hand so that the index fingers can be used to guide the floss (Fig. 13-7). The floss is introduced into an interproximal space by gently moving it buccolingually in a "sawing" motion. The floss should not be allowed to snap through the contact, because this may damage the papilla. Once introduced into the embrasure, the floss should be pressed firmly against the proximal surface of one of the contiguous teeth in a C-configuration and then moved along the tooth in an apicocoronal direction (see Fig. 13-7). The patient should be encouraged to develop a routine that he or she can use each time flossing is performed. Beginning with the same interproximal space each time, and progressing through all subsequent interproximal spaces in a

standard order may help to ensure that all surfaces are contacted with floss on each occasion.

If the floss becomes shredded, or if it is difficult to introduce through the contact, there may be a defective restoration, calculus, or some other problem. The cause of shredding should be determined and corrected. Conversely, flossing may also reveal a loose or open contact, which may require restoration. It is important to explain clearly to the patient that the purpose of flossing is not to remove food debris, but to contact the interproximal surface of each tooth with multiple up and down flossing strokes so that plaque can be removed thoroughly.

In the case of fixed partial dentures, floss cannot be passed through the interdental contact, because this is closed. Instead, a device known as a *floss threader* (Fig. 13-8) should be used to thread the floss under the bridge. The end of the floss threader is passed under the pontic or fixed partial denture connector from the facial aspect (Fig. 13-9). The floss is passed through the "eye" of the floss threader. The end of the threader is grasped with the fingers and the remainder of the floss threader is pulled through to the lingual while the opposite hand grasps the two ends of the floss from the facial aspect (Fig. 13-10). Releasing one end of the floss and holding the other, the threader is pulled the rest of the way through to the lingual, carrying the free end of the floss along with it. In this fashion, one end of the floss is grasped from the facial aspect, and the free end is then grasped from the lingual (Fig. 13-11). The floss can then be used to clean the intaglio surface (tissue side) of the pontic and the interproximal tooth surfaces facing the edentulous space using the C-shaped fashion and apicocoronal motion described earlier (Fig. 13-12).

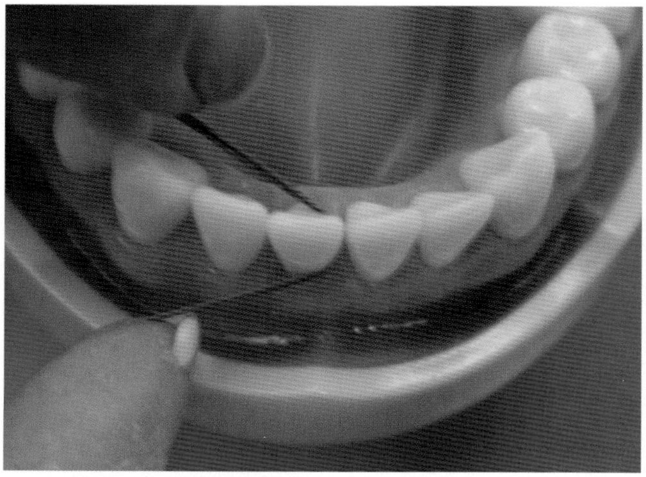

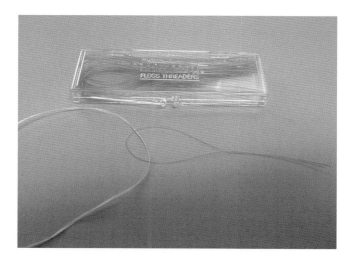

Figure 13-7. The floss is guided into each interproximal space and then curved in a C-shape around each tooth surface. The floss is moved in multiple apicocoronal strokes to remove tooth-adherent plaque. (*Courtesy Dr. David Hardison and Ms. Amy Simmons.*)

Figure 13-8. The floss threader has an "eye" loop at one end, into which the dental floss is passed. (*Courtesy Dr. David Hardison and Ms. Amy Simmons.*)

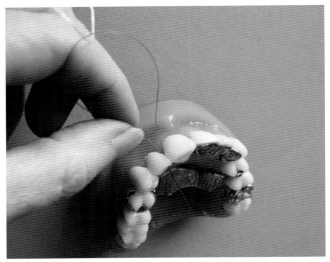

Figure 13-9. The end of the floss threader is passed into the embrasure space between the retainer and the pontic. (*Courtesy Dr. David Hardison and Ms. Amy Simmons.*)

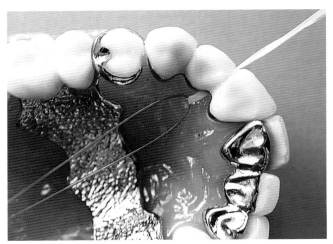

Figure 13-10. The floss is inserted through the "eye" loop and the threader is passed through to the lingual. (*Courtesy Dr. David Hardison and Ms. Amy Simmons.*)

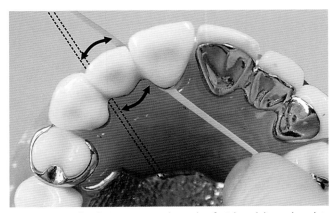

Figure 13-11. The floss is grasped on the facial and lingual and is passed along the intaglio surface of the pontic. (*Courtesy Dr. David Hardison and Ms. Amy Simmons.*)

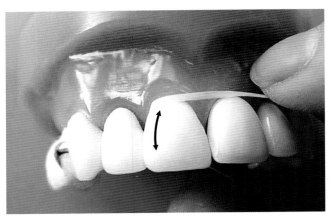

Figure 13-12. The floss is moved apicocoronally along the interproximal surfaces of the abutment teeth. (*Courtesy Dr. David Hardison and Ms. Amy Simmons.*)

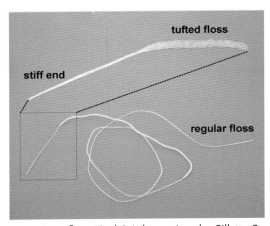

Figure 13-13. Superfloss (Oral B Laboratories, the Gillette Company; Boston, MA) has three portions: a rigid end, a spongy tufted region, and a region similar to dental floss. (*Courtesy Dr. David Hardison and Ms. Amy Simmons.*)

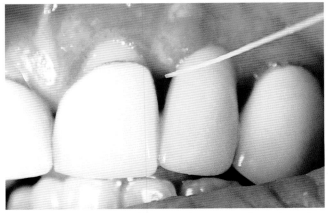

Figure 13-14. The rigid end of the Superfloss is passed into the embrasure space between the retainer and the pontic. (*Courtesy Dr. David Hardison and Ms. Amy Simmons.*)

An alternative to the floss threader is Superfloss, a type of floss that incorporates a rigid plastic portion that can be introduced under fixed bridges (Fig. 13-13). Distal to the rigid plastic portion is a spongy region that is ideal for plaque removal. The terminal portion of Superfloss is similar to standard dental floss. Superfloss is generally easier to use than floss threaders. The rigid portion is passed into the embrasure space between the retainer and the pontic and pulled through to the lingual aspect (Fig. 13-14). The spongy region is then used in an apico-coronal stroke along the interproximal surfaces of the abutment teeth and along the intaglio surface of the pontic (Fig. 13-15).

Floss holders

A number of devices are commercially available to assist patients who have difficulty flossing. These are primarily plastic handles that hold the floss in such a way as to serve as "substitute fingers" (Figs. 13-16 and 13-17). Some patients benefit from these devices, especially those who have difficulty with manual dexterity, but they can be difficult to use initially. The floss is gently "sawed" through the interdental contact in the manner shown earlier, and once past the contact, the floss is held against each interproximal surface and moved apicocoronally. One problem with some of these devices is the difficulty in keeping the floss taut enough to allow the floss to pass easily through the contact. The floss must continually be advanced and tightened.

Automated interdental cleaners

There is at least one automated interdental cleaning device on the market: the Braun Interclean (Braun

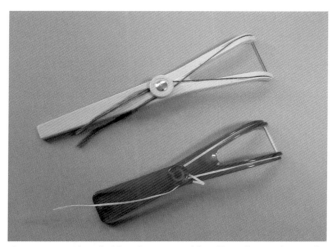

Figure 13-16. Floss holders have a rigid handle with a "yoke" at the end, over which dental floss is stretched. The patient holds the handle and passes the floss into each interproximal space. (*Courtesy Dr. David Hardison and Ms. Amy Simmons.*)

GmbH; Kronberg, Germany). This device removes interproximal plaque by means of rotating monofilaments. Several short-term studies have reported that the device is as effective as finger flossing.[61-63]

Toothpicks and woodsticks

The toothpicks and woodsticks group of interproximal aids includes conventional round or flat toothpicks, in addition to triangular toothpicks designed for interdental cleaning, such as the Stim-U-Dent (Johnson & Johnson;

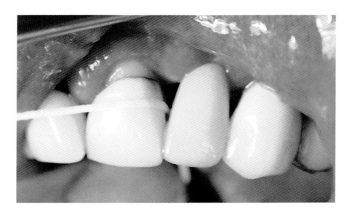

Figure 13-15. The Superfloss is then curved into a C-shape and moved apicocoronally along the interproximal surfaces of the abutment teeth. It is also used to clean the intaglio surface of the pontic. (*Courtesy Dr. David Hardison and Ms. Amy Simmons.*)

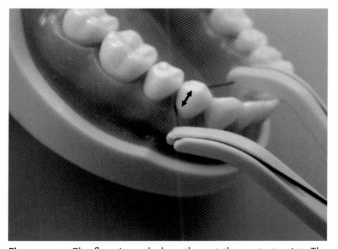

Figure 13-17. The floss is worked gently past the contact point. The handle can then be moved mesially and distally to bring the floss into contact with the interproximal tooth surfaces. (*Courtesy Dr. David Hardison and Ms. Amy Simmons.*)

New Brunswick, NJ) (Fig. 13-18). It has been suggested that these aids are better for situations in which there is a slightly receded interdental papilla. One study demonstrated the superiority of Stim-U-Dents to brushing alone, but there was no comparison to dental floss.[64] Wolffe[65] found no difference in efficacy of plaque removal when comparing a triangular woodstick, dental floss, and a single-tufted brush in a group of patients with open interdental embrasures. Some studies have found a round toothpick to be inferior to either a triangular toothpick or dental floss.[66] The triangular woodstick is an effective aid, but it is somewhat difficult to use in the posterior regions because the triangular cross-sectional design must pass into the embrasure space at a specific angle. A variation on the toothpick theme is a plastic handle designed to hold a round toothpick that has been broken off. This device is commercially available as the Perio-Aid (Marquis Dental Manufacturing; Aurora, CO) and is similar to floss in its effectiveness[28] (Figs. 13-19 and 13-20).

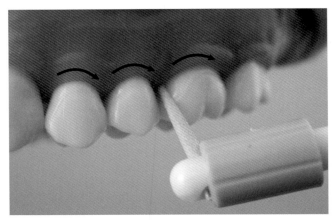

Figure 13-20. The end of the toothpick can be passed along the gingival margin and into the interproximal spaces. (*Courtesy Dr. David Hardison and Ms. Amy Simmons.*)

Interdental brushes

A variety of interdental brushes are commercially available (Figs. 13-21 and 13-22). Most of these consist of two components: a handle and a small, replaceable brush head. The brush heads are conical or cylindrical in shape. These brushes are best used in open embrasures with low papillary height where the brush can fit easily in the available space without causing trauma to the papilla. Some of the heads have a metal wire "backbone" that can prove uncomfortable for those individuals with root sensitivity, whereas other heads have a plastic-coated "backbone" that may reduce sensitivity. The angle of the handle permits use in posterior areas, although patients require careful instruction in the use of these devices. A number of studies have demonstrated that the interdental brush is superior to floss and

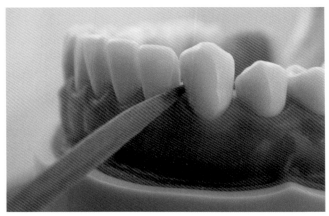

Figure 13-18. A wooden interdental cleaner with a triangular cross section. (*Courtesy Dr. David Hardison and Ms. Amy Simmons.*)

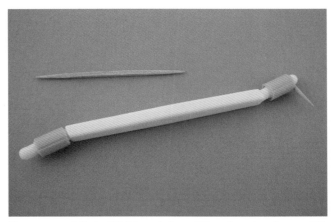

Figure 13-19. A Perio-Aid (Marquis Dental Manufacturing; Aurora, CO) consists of a holder for a round toothpick. (*Courtesy Dr. David Hardison and Ms. Amy Simmons.*)

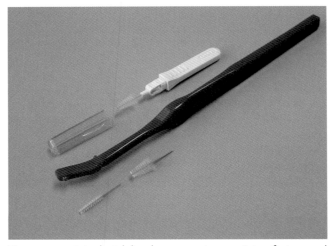

Figure 13-21. Interdental brushes come in a variety of sizes and shapes. (*Courtesy Dr. David Hardison and Ms. Amy Simmons.*)

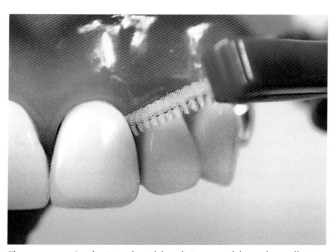

Figure 13-22. As the interdental brush is passed buccolingually into and out of the interdental space, the bristles clean the tooth surfaces. (*Courtesy Dr. David Hardison and Ms. Amy Simmons.*)

triangular woodsticks in cases where the embrasure is open enough to permit their use.[67-69] Therefore, these devices are probably the instrument of choice for cleaning open embrasures.

FREQUENCY OF PLAQUE REMOVAL

There is a lack of clarity regarding the appropriate frequency of plaque removal for the prevention of gingivitis. Some studies show that plaque removal every 48 hours is effective at preventing gingivitis.[70,71] However, these studies used dental students and faculty as subjects, a population likely to be more adept and thorough with plaque removal. Thus, the results may not be readily transferable to other patient groups—that is, such studies may lack *external validity*. Once gingival inflammation is established, there is some evidence that plaque may form more rapidly at inflamed than uninflamed sites.[12-14] Therefore, results on brushing frequency might be quite different for a group of patients with disease as opposed to a group with good gingival health at baseline. It is unlikely that the average patient removes supragingival plaque completely when performing oral hygiene. To suggest that doing so only once every other day will be sufficient to prevent gingival inflammation is unlikely to lead to success. Lacking the type of rigorous evidence that would permit an unequivocal answer to this question, it would seem that the usual recommendation to brush twice daily and use interdental cleaning aids at least once daily is reasonable. It is likely that the thoroughness and duration of the oral hygiene session, rather than the frequency, are the critical factors.

CHEMICAL PLAQUE CONTROL

A variety of topical antiseptic agents are commercially available as mouthrinses to aid in plaque control. The most common generally are part of one of the following categories: bisbiguanides, essential oils, metallic ions, quaternary ammonium compounds, sanguinarine, and triclosan. Some of these agents also have been used in oral irrigating devices. These topically applied antigingivitis agents are reviewed in Chapter 16.

In addition to agents that prevent plaque accumulation and gingivitis, chemical agents are available to inhibit formation of supragingival calculus. Supragingival calculus represents mineralized dental plaque, and the surface of the calculus is covered with a layer of unmineralized plaque. Supragingival calculus is composed of several calcium-containing minerals, including brushite, octacalcium phosphate, hydroxyapatite, and whitlockite. The predominant mineral in the superficial layer is octacalcium phosphate, whereas hydroxyapatite predominates in the deeper layers. The exact mechanism by which calculus forms has not been elucidated, but it seems to involve intracellular calcification of degenerating bacteria within the plaque mass. Chemical anticalculus agents aim to reduce calculus formation by adhesion to developing calculus crystals, thereby inhibiting further crystal growth. Pyrophosphates and zinc-containing compounds have been shown to have anticalculus effects. Newer agents, such as hexametaphosphate, are also the subject of clinical investigation.[72] Toothpastes containing 2% zinc chloride have been shown to significantly reduce calculus formation, but the taste is unacceptable.[73] Lower concentrations of zinc salts are more palatable, but are not as effective. Dentifrices containing triclosan and a copolymer can reduce supragingival calculus by up to 36% compared with a fluoride-containing control paste.[74]

HOME IRRIGATION IN THE TREATMENT OF PERIODONTAL DISEASE

Irrigation has been a source of controversy within the specialty of periodontology. This stems in part from conflicting reports in the literature and their interpretation. A wide variety of agents have been used, along with various methods of introducing them. The latter have ranged from commercially available pulsating water jets, such as the Waterpik (Waterpik Technologies, Inc.; Newport Beach, CA), to simple irrigating syringes equipped with blunt or side-port cannulas. Irrigation often has been compared as a monotherapy to standard therapies, when irrigation is, in reality, an adjunct designed to complement or enhance other home care methods.[75] The following discussion is limited to patient-performed irrigation as a component of a home care regimen, as opposed to professional irrigation performed at the time of debridement.

Supragingival Irrigation and Gingivitis

Supragingival irrigation has been used as a strategy to disrupt supragingival plaque, the etiologic agent of plaque-induced gingivitis. It has been reported that a pulsating stream of water is better than a continuous flow.[76] The continuous stream is alleged to compress the tissues and prevent the "drainage" of sulcular contents, whereas the pulsating jet compresses the tissue only intermittently, allowing for flushing of the dislodged bacteria during the decompression phase. The clinical effects seen are presumably caused by disruption of the biofilm, flushing of inflammatory mediators, or both.

Early studies suggest few or no additional advantages when irrigation is added to a standard home care regimen, but more recent research has shown some benefits. The benefits are generally greater when an antiseptic agent is used as an irrigant, rather than water. In one study, supragingival irrigation resulted in a 50% decrease in gingivitis even when professional debridement was not performed.[77] In many studies of irrigation, greater decreases are seen in gingivitis than in plaque scores.[78,79] The reasons for this paradox have not been explained.

Subgingival Irrigation and Periodontitis

In the treatment or prevention of gingivitis, it is sufficient to disrupt the supragingival plaque. In the treatment of periodontitis, however, it seems plausible that the agent must penetrate subgingivally. This would likely be true whether the effect was mediated by a chemotherapeutic action or simply the physical disruption of the biofilm caused by the irrigant jet. Most investigators report that supragingival irrigation is not able to penetrate more than 3 mm subgingivally.[80] This is not a universal finding, however. For example, significant reductions in bacteria at a depth of 5 to 6 mm apical to the gingival margin have been seen when an irrigating device (Waterpik) was held perpendicular to the tooth.[81] These authors attributed this to deflection of the water into the pocket after striking the tooth, and suggested that this "hydrokinetic" action was responsible for disrupting the plaque.

Tips have been developed for oral irrigators that are designed to be directed into the periodontal pocket. Using such a tip (Pik Pocket: Waterpik Technologies, Inc.; Newport Beach, CA), irrigating solution can be delivered to a depth of 90% of pockets 6 mm or less.[82] Penetration is reduced to about two thirds of the depth in pockets 7 mm or greater. Some investigators report that a cannula (or blunt-ended needle) gives greater pocket penetration than a standard supragingival tip.[78] Although important,

the degree of penetration is somewhat difficult to assess experimentally because of a variety of methodologic problems. This makes interpretation of the penetration studies difficult. Of more immediate importance to clinicians is the effect of irrigation on various clinical parameters.

A number of agents have been used as subgingival irrigants in the treatment of periodontitis, including stannous fluoride, tetracycline, and various antiseptic mouthrinses. Some of these have proven to have increased efficacy over water, whereas others have not. Since none of these agents has substantivity in a periodontal pocket because of the constant flow of crevicular fluid, their use has been questioned. In addition, use of an antiseptic as an irrigant increases the cost to the patient, when compared with water.

There is some evidence that home irrigation may be capable of reducing inflammatory mediators. Several studies have demonstrated that subgingival irrigation with water in patients with chronic periodontitis improved periodontal status and reduced crevicular fluid inflammatory mediators such as interleukin-1, reactive oxygen species, and prostaglandin E_2 better than scaling and root planing alone[83] or oral hygiene alone.[84]

Irrigation and Dental Implants

Few studies have examined the potential benefits of irrigation around dental implants. Felo and colleagues[85] compared maintenance of periimplant mucosal health using either a regimen of subgingival irrigation with 0.06% chlorhexidine or rinsing with 0.12% chlorhexidine and found that irrigation resulted in less periimplant mucosal inflammation. More research is needed in this area before evidence-based clinical recommendations can be made.

Clinical Application

The best candidates for home irrigation may be those patients who do not do well with other hygiene aids, particularly because of local factors such as orthodontic appliances[86] or intermaxillary fixation.[87] Burch and colleagues[88] reported that the use of an oral irrigator significantly reduced gingival inflammation and plaque in a group of 47 adult orthodontic patients. Other potential applications include patients in whom surgery is indicated but cannot be performed because of medical, behavioral, or financial constraints. If home irrigation is recommended after surgery, it should be deferred for at least 1 month.[76] In the case of regenerative surgery, it is likely that delaying resumption of irrigation for about 6 months would seem prudent, but there is no experimental evidence on which to base such recommendations. Although the topic is discussed later in this chapter (see Adverse Effects of Hygiene Measures), there is evidence that irrigation may cause bacteremias and is, therefore, not recommended in patients for whom this would constitute a risk (e.g., those at increased risk for endocarditis).

AGENTS FOR HYPERSENSITIVITY AND ROOT CARIES

Root Caries

Root caries is a significant complication of periodontal disease. A study of employed adults reported the prevalence of decayed or filled root surfaces to be 71% in the 75- to 79-year-old cohort and 54% in the 60- to 64-year-old age group.[89] Clearly, caries is a significant public health problem. The lesions of root caries are often in areas that are difficult to restore and maintain. If nonrestorable, these lesions can cause tooth loss even if the periodontal disease process has been successfully arrested.

Root caries, like coronal caries, requires a triad of factors: a susceptible host, fermentable carbohydrates, and suitable microflora. Despite some similarities, however, the process of root caries differs from coronal caries. Dentin and cementum are demineralized more easily than enamel; the pH required for dissolution is 6.0 to 6.5, which is less acidic than that required for coronal caries.[90] Major risk factors for root caries include suboptimal fluoride exposure, recently exposed root surfaces, xerostomia, cariogenic microflora (e.g., lactobacilli and mutans streptococci), frequent consumption of fermentable carbohydrates, and poor plaque control.[91] The presence of more than one of these factors may greatly increase the risk for development of root caries lesions. Using this information, it may be possible to identify patients at increased risk for root caries and then target them accordingly.

Significant root exposure may occur immediately after some types of periodontal surgery. Because of root debridement during surgery, it is also possible that there will be a relatively low concentration of fluoride on the exposed root surface. These factors, particularly if combined with medication- or age-related xerostomia, may predispose the patient to significant root caries and may warrant institution of a formal caries reduction protocol.

Root caries can be arrested by meticulous home care and frequent application of fluoride.[92-94] The oral hygiene component is critical—with poor home care, fluoride is likely to be ineffective.[95] Supporting these findings is the observation that buccal root caries, being more accessible for plaque removal, are more likely to be converted into inactive lesions than distal caries, which are much more difficult to clean.[96] Dietary analysis and reduction of fermentable carbohydrates is of significant value. During the treatment planning process, a history of root caries may cause the therapist to modify the treatment plan. Surgical procedures that cause exposure of root surfaces may be avoided or deferred. It also may be prudent to recommend fluoride treatment of newly exposed root surfaces after a suitable period of postsurgical healing.

Dentinal Hypersensitivity

Dentinal hypersensitivity refers to the phenomenon in which exposed root surfaces are sensitive to tactile, thermal, or chemical/osmotic stimuli. This condition is more frequently seen on buccal surfaces, in patients with a high level of hygiene. It may be caused by toothbrush abrasion and recession caused by traumatic brushing, resective periodontal surgery, and repeated professional instrumentation. A number of theories have been advanced to explain the phenomenon of dentinal hypersensitivity, but none has been universally accepted. The most widely held is the hydrodynamic theory, which states that sensitivity is a result of fluid movement within the dentinal tubules.[97] A number of agents have been used, primarily in toothpastes, to reduce sensitivity. Many of these are thought to act by occluding the open orifices of the dentinal tubules. Agents that have been used include strontium chloride, potassium nitrate, potassium citrate, formaldehyde, and various fluoride preparations. Although some patients undoubtedly derive great benefit from desensitizing agents, there is contradictory evidence for their efficacy. A comprehensive systematic review concluded there was no strong evidence supporting the efficacy of these products.[98] More research is clearly needed on this condition and its treatment.

ORAL HYGIENE INSTRUCTION AND HEALTH PROMOTION

Oral hygiene instruction is an example of a more general concept known as *health promotion*. Health promotion collectively refers to those activities that are carried out for the express purpose of improving the health of a group, but the concept may be applied to the efforts of an individual practice. Health promotion draws on clinical and biologic disciplines, as well as social sciences such as psychology, sociology, and economics.

A number of investigators have studied various methods of oral hygiene instruction, including personal one-on-one instruction and other self-instructional approaches. Most investigators have found self-instructional methods using booklets and video presentations to be similarly effective as personal instruction.[99-101] With regard to the amount of time spent on home care instruction, Soderholm and colleagues found that a two-visit program was as effective as a five-visit program in the short-term and that 30-minute appointments were no more effective than 15-minute appointments.[102]

Regardless of the method used, a formal plaque reduction protocol should be part of all dental practices. It may be necessary to tailor the protocol to the particular practice. An orthodontic practice will face different challenges than a periodontal or general practice. It is important that such a program be evidence-based and there should be a mechanism to ensure that the program is functioning as intended. The program should include different approaches that will be able to accommodate a wide range of patient behaviors, from the compliant patient who willingly follows instructions to the patient with erratic compliance.

COMPLIANCE AND PATIENT MOTIVATION

Compliance has been defined as the degree to which a patient follows a regimen prescribed by a healthcare practitioner. It is closely related to the concept of adherence, which can be defined as the degree to which a patient continues an agreed-on course of therapy. Obviously, this concept has application in all branches of medicine and dentistry. The term *agreed-on* implies the formation of a therapeutic alliance between the patient and practitioner. Such an alliance is implicit in all forms of healthcare practice, but is particularly important in the treatment of chronic diseases that are often the result of lifestyle choices. Ideally, this alliance would be formed before disease is present, with the goal of preventing disease occurrence. This primary prevention model is one that dentistry has long emphasized with great success. There are, however, other levels of prevention that are used when disease has already occurred.

Levels of Prevention

The public health literature identifies three levels of prevention: primary, secondary, and tertiary.[103] Primary prevention includes *health promotion* and *health protection* strategies. Health promotion can be defined as the "process of enabling people to increase control over and improve their health."[104] This would include activities such as health education, maintenance of a healthy lifestyle, and health screening. Health protection, however, centers on things such as immunizations, personal hygiene, and proper nutritional intake. Secondary prevention has as its goal diagnosis and treatment of disease at an early stage—for example, the treatment of gingivitis or early periodontitis. Tertiary prevention focuses on limiting disability and promoting rehabilitation. A dental example of tertiary prevention would be extensive periodontal and implant surgery to correct the ravages of tooth loss and periodontal disease.

Applying these constructs to dentistry, instruction and feedback concerning oral hygiene in the absence of dental disease can be viewed as an example of primary pre-

vention. But oral hygiene is important in all phases of dentistry; therefore, plaque control measures are also part of secondary prevention in an individual with early disease such as gingivitis, or as part of tertiary prevention in an individual who has received oral rehabilitation (e.g., regenerative therapy in advanced periodontitis).

The Special Challenge of Chronic Disease

Obviously, it is easier and more cost-effective to prevent chronic disease (primary prevention) than it is to treat the ravages of disease after they have occurred (tertiary prevention). These concepts were irrelevant until several decades ago. In the first decade of the twentieth century, the leading causes of death in the United States were infectious diseases such as tuberculosis, influenza, and pneumonia. By the end of the century, the leading causes of death were chronic diseases related to lifestyle and behavioral factors, such as heart disease, stroke, and cancer.

It is important to appreciate that most dental disease is preventable by easily practiced home care procedures and simple interventions. That there remains much untreated, but preventable, dental disease in the United States, even among those who have received instruction in proper oral hygiene procedures, underscores the primacy of sociobehavioral factors in dental disease. The emerging field of health psychology has as its goal to identify and study those psychological factors that influence health and health-related behaviors.

A *biopsychosocial model* of illness is developing as contrasted with the earlier *biomedical model*. The biomedical model is a mechanistic construct that focuses on disease mechanisms at the molecular, cellular, or organ level, whereas the biopsychosocial model considers the patient as an individual, including psychological, social, behavioral, and biologic factors. Given the complexity of these psychosocial factors, it is not surprising that studying them is difficult. In the area of periodontal disease, the importance of biopsychosocial risk factors cannot be overemphasized. In a recent review of periodontal risk factors, many were related to patient behaviors or psychological state (e.g., coping behaviors and stressful life events, oral hygiene practices, and smoking).[105] The difficulty in quantifying many of these factors has hampered efforts to relate their presence to disease.

A number of models have been proposed to facilitate understanding of these behavioral factors. The ultimate goal is, of course, the application of sociobehavioral research in the service of improving the dental health of the individual and population. Although none of these models has proven entirely satisfactory, it is important to become familiar with their basic tenets. Early theories were *behavior-centered learning theories* such as operant conditioning, in which desired behavior is rewarded (behavior modification). An application of this model is provided by Iwata and Becksfort,[106] who found that reducing fees if patients improved their hygiene reinforced the desired hygiene behavior for up to 6 months.

The *social/cognitive* models are more complex and include the *health belief model*. The health belief model represents a theoretical foundation for health education and promotion. The health belief model is based on the theory that an individual's beliefs about health practices will influence health-related behavior, including compliance with recommendations. The model can be used to plan health education activities and as a predictor of health-related behaviors. For example, to the extent that patients do not perceive dental disease to be either likely or of immediate importance, they are less likely to engage in oral health-related behaviors, such as flossing and regular maintenance visits. Many periodontal academicians have advocated an approach in which the patient is educated about the periodontal disease process and its consequences. These strategies are based on the health belief model in that the goal is to change the beliefs to achieve compliance with recommended treatment regimens.

Although this logical transfer of information concerning the health benefits of proper oral hygiene may be quite effective in many patients, it is likely to be ineffective in others to whom the prospect of periodontal disease may seem remote and nonthreatening. For example, it has been suggested that the demonstration of a patient's subgingival flora by phase contrast microscopy may be effective in improving home care by increasing the level of awareness of the bacterial flora. Although this seems logical and has been suggested as a motivational strategy, patients who viewed their own flora microscopically have been shown to have plaque and gingivitis scores similar to patients who did not.[107]

Other strategies may involve an appeal based on social factors, as opposed to appeals based on disease or health. The appearance and health of the face and mouth are important components of physical beauty and contribute to self-esteem and self-image. As such, oral cleanliness has important social and sexual implications, and these may be more powerful motivators to patients than appeals to physical health, particularly if the health risks seem remote and unlikely. There is also evidence that toothbrushing patterns are part of a broader array of lifestyle choices and behaviors.[108] Whatever strategies are employed, it is important that patients understand the importance of oral cleanliness and health in maintaining systemic well being. (See Chapter 32.)

There is a good deal of information concerning compliance in the dental literature. Unfortunately, much of it is of a negative nature. Compliance with treatment recommendations is generally poor, particularly in chronic diseases in which the threat is not immediate or life threatening.[109-112] Even when survival is at stake, many patients find compliance difficult, as seen by the number of individuals who continue to smoke despite knowledge of the health consequences. Compliance with oral hygiene recommendations is generally poor, particularly with regard to interdental cleaning aids. Compliance with flossing is particularly bad. Patients often find flossing difficult. Unfortunately, periodontal disease affects interproximal sites disproportionately, and it is these sites that often exhibit significant amounts of plaque. The most optimistic studies report that rates of compliance with toothbrushing regimens are less than 50%; other studies show it to be an even smaller rate. In studies focusing on the use of interproximal cleaning aids, compliance is poorer still.

In one study of compliance with recommended maintenance, Wilson and colleagues[112] were able to decrease noncompliance by 50% in a private periodontal practice by implementing several changes. In a somewhat modified form, these changes are listed below, along with specific suggestions as to how they might be applied in an oral hygiene protocol:

- Simplify the protocol (few oral hygiene devices)
- Accommodate the patient's preferences (tailor the regimen to the patient; if someone has repeatedly refused to floss, perhaps recommend interdental woodsticks)
- Send reminders (cards sent to patients to remind them of oral hygiene commitments; signs that can be placed in the bathroom to serve as a gentle reminder to floss, and so on)
- Keep records of compliance (chart plaque and bleeding and give patient a written copy of the current score, the target score, and the score at last visit)
- Provide positive reinforcement (praise progress; start with "small wins" and try for incremental improvement)
- Identify potential noncompliers and modify treatment as needed (avoiding surgery in patients with poor plaque control)

In summary, the sociobehavioral determinants of oral hygiene behaviors are obviously complex and incompletely understood. It is unlikely that simplistic, one-dimensional models will prove useful. Instead, more complex models are being developed that take into account the various factors that influence patient behavior. Such a model is the *new century model of oral health promotion* suggested by Inglehart and Tedesco.[113] They recommend a comprehensive approach that considers patient's feelings and affect, cognitive factors such as dental health beliefs, past or current health-related behavior, and the patient's current life situation. Inglehart and Tedesco[113] have advanced a more comprehensive perspective than previous models. Their new century model is certainly more consistent with the biopsychosocial model. This approach may have significant implications for patient care, health promotion, and dental education.

Currently, the application of these sociobehavioral concepts to the actual practice of dentistry is difficult. Translational studies are needed to test the clinical application of these models within the context of the everyday practice of dentistry. What is clear, however, is the need for a therapeutic alliance between patient and therapist, with shared responsibility for the outcome.

ASSESSMENT OF HOME CARE

Assessment of the effectiveness of patient plaque control is an ongoing process, beginning at the initial evaluation and continuing throughout therapy, including maintenance. Home care can be assessed using a variety of methods. First, the teeth can simply be inspected visually for the presence or absence of plaque. This is the least effective method, because plaque may be difficult to see. Second, plaque can be made visible through the use of a *disclosing solution*. Disclosing solution is available in either liquid or tablet form. The liquid can be applied to the teeth using a cotton-tipped applicator or the patient may rinse with the material for a few seconds and then expectorate. The tablets are chewed and dissolved in saliva, which is then swished in the mouth and expectorated. The liquid may offer some advantages in that the operator can ensure that all surfaces are adequately covered. The red disclosing agents have one disadvantage: the solution may temporarily stain the lips and gingiva. Lip balm or petroleum jelly may minimize staining of the lips, which some patients find objectionable. Contact with clothing should be avoided, because the stain is difficult to remove.

Regardless of how the plaque is visualized, some provision must be made for measuring the amount of plaque present. Various indexes have been developed for this purpose. Such indexes can serve two purposes: (1) for use in monitoring a patient's progress (e.g., for assessing whether home care is sufficient to permit surgical intervention), or (2) as a patient motivation tool. In general, a simple plaque index is preferable. One widely used index is the O'Leary plaque index.[114] Disclosing solution is used, and the percentage of sites with visible plaque is calculated. A useful (if somewhat arbitrary) target may be no more than 20% of surfaces with visible plaque. A modification of the O'Leary plaque index is preferred by some clinicians, in which the percentage of surfaces with plaque is subtracted from 100. This gives the percentage of *plaque-free* surfaces. Some patients prefer trying to achieve a score of 100% with this modified O'Leary plaque index, rather than trying to achieve a score of 0% with the original index.

Strategies for Improving Home Care Performance

The first step in addressing insufficient home care is to determine the cause of the problem. There are, essentially, three possibilities:

1. The patient knows what to do, but is unable to perform (lacks dexterity)
2. The patient does not know what to do (lacks knowledge)
3. The patient knows what to do, is able to do it, but simply doesn't comply with the regimen (lacks motivation)

To define the problem, it is necessary to observe the patient in the performance of the recommended procedures. This can best be done in a room with a wall-mounted mirror, similar to that found in a home bathroom. It is difficult for some patients to perform hygiene procedures while seated in a dental chair, with a mirror in one hand and the brush in the other. This observational step, often omitted, is essential. Without observation, there is no way to structure an intervention that will be effective.

Case 1: On observation, this patient is seen to lack the ability to use the brush effectively. She does not position the brush correctly. She is primarily using floss to remove food from between the teeth instead of using it in a manner that will remove plaque. For whatever reason, the patient does not understand what she must do to remove plaque. Reinstruction is indicated. If continued efforts at instruction and feedback are ineffective, an alternative might be considered, such as another brushing technique or an EMB.

Case 2: This patient has rather poor home care, which has persisted after instruction in proper technique. On observation, she is enthusiastic, but her efforts seem clumsy and ineffective. This appears to be because of a lack of dexterity, which is probably a consequence of her long-standing and severe rheumatoid arthritis. It will probably be best to find an alternative method (e.g., an EMB) that will enhance her efforts. It may also be necessary to see her more frequently for maintenance.

Case 3: This patient understands the recommended procedures well. This is not surprising, for he has received the instructions numerous times. On observation, there is no doubt that he has the requisite dexterity. Indeed, he claims to be performing the procedures twice daily at home, but this is belied by his high plaque and bleeding sores. What seems to be missing is the motivation or self-discipline necessary to maintain a satisfactory level of hygiene. The key is to focus on the problem: the presence of unacceptable amounts of plaque and the associated biologic response to the plaque, such as bleeding on probing. The therapist who is willing to work with such patients will sometimes be rewarded. Given the high level of noncompliance documented in the research literature, it is unrealistic to dismiss patients who do not meet our hygiene targets. If continued efforts at reinforcement fail, there are ways in which the patient can still be helped, as seen later in this chapter.

Although it is necessary to give all patients honest feedback on their plaque control efforts, it is also important to reward positive performance and not to harbor unrealistic expectations. If the therapeutic alliance is to endure for many years, it must be built on trust and mutual respect. It is necessary that candid feedback be tempered by positive reinforcement, so that the patient will not dread each maintenance visit. Striking a balance here can be challenging. In some cases, despite the best efforts of the therapist, the patient is simply not going to achieve the levels of home care desired. In such cases, it is necessary to use compensatory strategies (while still trying to motivate the patient).

COMPENSATING FOR POOR ORAL HYGIENE

We have seen that compliance is a significant issue in periodontal therapy. Given the literature on compliance, it is a certainty that the clinician will see patients who do not follow instructions regarding home care. Perhaps more accurately, clinicians will have many patients who follow instructions *incompletely*. Probably the most common example is the patient who does not floss, despite receiving instructions and multiple admonitions to do so. Does this lack of compliance doom these patients to treatment failure? Not necessarily. There are several strategies that might partially compensate for poor oral hygiene.

The novelty of a new device such as an EMB will often result in improvement, at least in the short term. The EMB also has the advantage of better interproximal plaque removal. This is important because the interproximal region is the area most frequently neglected by patients. A similar strategy may be to suggest an alternative interdental aid. Some patients who have difficulty with floss (and many do) will readily accept other interdental aids, such as Stim-U-Dents. The conscientious use of such an aid might result in an acceptable level of plaque removal.

Oral hygiene may be less important in determining outcomes than adherence to professional maintenance.[115] This may be because of the primacy of subgingival debridement vis-à-vis supragingival home care. One intervention, then, would be an increase in the frequency of maintenance visits. Another strategy might be to use various adjunctive aids that may provide incremental benefits, such as antimicrobial mouthrinses. It must be borne in mind that these strategies also require compliance, however.

Many patients who smoke also have less than ideal home care, and smoking in and of itself is a major risk factor for periodontitis. The clinician should strongly and positively encourage the noncompliant patient to quit smoking. If the risk factor of smoking is removed, this can result in a nonsmoking, noncompliant patient, which is preferable and probably easier to maintain. Smoking cessation should, of course, be part of every periodontal treatment plan for patients who use tobacco (see Chapter 34).

Another strategy for dealing with noncompliance may be to modify the treatment plan. It may be wise to delay or avoid surgery in a patient with poor home care. Such patients may be better managed by nonsurgical means including initial therapy followed by frequent maintenance. This type of patient also may benefit from adjunctive topical antigingivitis agents such as rinses.

In the final analysis, we cannot entirely compensate for lack of proper home care on the part of the patient. Nevertheless, there are strategies that may help to limit or circumvent the effects of noncompliance.

ADVERSE EFFECTS OF ORAL HYGIENE AIDS

No therapeutic intervention is without adverse effects, including oral hygiene practices. Tooth abrasion and gingival recession are both alleged to be caused by traumatic brushing. It is difficult to study this phenomenon because of several confounding variables.

Tooth Abrasion

Evidence implicating the toothbrush in cases of abrasion comes primarily from *in vitro* studies, case reports, and cross-sectional studies. Some studies have implicated a horizontal scrubbing stroke as a more important risk factor for tooth abrasion than bristle stiffness. Other studies have indicated that abrasive toothpastes are the primary cause of tooth abrasion (see Chapter 21). There is some evidence that EMBs may be less likely to cause abrasion, possibly because less force is applied to these brushes.[116,117]

Gingival Recession

Gingival recession is the result of an interaction between precipitating factors, such as trauma to the gingival tissues, and predisposing factors, such as a thin tissue complex. Gingival recession, particularly that occurring on the buccal surface, is often presumed to be the result of toothbrush trauma. It seems logical to assume that the thin gingival biotype might be more easily traumatized (see Chapter 21). There is evidence suggesting that thin tissue is more prone to recession.[118,119] In addition to thin marginal soft tissues, buccal recession also has been associated with the presence of a narrow zone of attached gingiva and labioverted or prominent roots.[120] Teeth that have been moved orthodontically may, in some circumstances, be more susceptible to recession, particularly if they have been moved through the labial cortical bone.

The method of brushing has been implicated in gingival recession, as have stiff bristles, frequency of brushing, abrasive toothpaste, and cut (rather than rounded) bristle ends. It is well established that gingival trauma, such as ulcers, can be caused by improper brushing. Repeated trauma can eventually lead to recession. It is useful to consider, however, that gingival recession also can be the result of destructive periodontal disease. In their study of Sri Lankan tea workers and Norwegian academicians, Loe and colleagues[121] suggested that recession was seen at both ends of the hygiene spectrum—when hygiene was aggressive and when it was insufficient.

The clinical application of this information would involve identifying patients at risk and planning interventions such as alternative brushing techniques. High-risk patients would include those with evidence of toothbrush trauma, labially positioned teeth, thin alveolar housing, and minimal width and thickness of gingiva. Such patients may be at risk for development of recession defects, particularly if these factors are combined with planned orthodontic treatment that may cause labial displacement of teeth. In such cases, it would seem worthwhile to inform the patient of the risk and modify the hygiene regimen to minimize trauma. In particular, a very soft brush or an EMB would seem indicated.

Gingival clefts are sometimes caused by overzealous or improper flossing (see Chapter 7). Other interdental aids, such as triangular woodsticks and toothpicks also can cause damage if used incorrectly or overzealously. The patient must be taught to use these devices in an atraumatic fashion. It is best for the clinician to observe patients in the dental office as they use these devices to ensure that they have learned the proper technique.

Possible Adverse Effects of Home Irrigation

A number of investigators have examined the effect of pulsating water jet devices on gingiva and mucosa and most have concluded there is little risk for tissue damage when such devices are used according to manufacturer's instructions.[76] In one investigation, the use of an irrigator at 60 psi in untreated periodontal pockets created no more tissue damage than was found in the "no irrigation" control group.[81] There is some question as to whether irrigation causes bacteremias. Some investigators have reported no bacteremia after irrigation, whereas others have reported that this does occur. Because this could have implications for individuals at risk for endocarditis, some authorities have recommended that the devices not be used by individuals at risk.[122]

Oral Hygiene after Regenerative Procedures

Thorough plaque removal may enhance the results of regenerative surgical therapy and may help provide stability to the gains in clinical attachment achieved.[123,124]

In the immediate postoperative period, plaque control is accomplished by means of chemotherapeutic agents such as chlorhexidine gluconate rinses, and mechanical plaque removal is generally avoided. Some tissue maturation should occur before resumption of normal oral hygiene. Critical to the regenerative outcome is wound stability and the preservation of the delicate fibrin linkage that forms on the root surface. The presence of this fibrin clot may prevent the downgrowth of the epithelium, thereby permitting regeneration of the attachment apparatus. (See Chapter 25.) Overzealous plaque removal, whether professional or personal, may be deleterious to the healing process and should be avoided. Unfortunately, there is a lack of controlled studies on which to base clinical decisions. It is often recommended that professional subgingival debridement and probing be avoided for 6 months after regenerative surgery, but little is said about the resumption of oral hygiene measures.[125] This is clearly an area that requires additional research.

DIRECTIONS FOR FURTHER RESEARCH

The relation between supragingival plaque, the subgingival microbiota, and periodontitis needs to be clarified. It is likely that the somewhat contradictory research findings can be explained by the concept of differential susceptibility between patients. In the coming years, risk assessment techniques may be developed that will find application in clinical practice. Such tools will enable the clinician to assign patients to differential risk categories, with implications for treatment planning and prognosis. High-risk individuals can be targeted for more intensive interventions, whereas low-risk individuals will receive less intense therapy.

Plaque control and frequent maintenance will be much more critical in the susceptible patient than in the individual who is relatively resistant to periodontitis. Strategies that allow the clinician to identify sites and individuals at risk for attachment loss would permit targeted therapy and avoidance of overtreatment or undertreatment.

It is also likely that the dental care industry will continue to produce different designs of both manual brushes and EMBs to maintain or to achieve a market share advantage. It is unlikely that sufficient funding will be available to permit the academic research community to conduct the sort of long-term studies that would allow evidence-based distinctions to be made among the different designs. Because the evidence suggests at least a rough equivalence of brushes and techniques, it would seem that a more fruitful area for academic research would be the development of practical and effective health promotion strategies to help patients become more compliant. It is also possible that future emphasis may be directed toward simplified home care regimens that are practical and easily implemented. For the foreseeable future, it is likely that plaque control will continue to be an important aspect of therapy and an important determinant of success.

REFERENCES

1. Ciancio SG: Chemical agents: plaque control, calculus reduction and treatment of dentinal hypersensitivity, *Periodontol 2000* 8:75-86, 1995.

2. Ciancio S: *Mechanical and chemical supragingival plaque control*, vol 8, Copenhagen, 1995, Munksgaard.

3. Shibly O, Rifai S, Zambon JJ: Supragingival dental plaque in the etiology of oral diseases, *Periodontol 2000* 8:42-59, 1995.

4. Corbet EF, Davies WI: The role of supragingival plaque in the control of progressive periodontal disease. A review, *J Clin Periodontol* 20:307-313, 1993.

5. Loe H, Theilade E, Jensen SB: Experimental gingivitis in man, *J Periodontol* 36:177-187, 1965.

6. Theilade E, Wright WH, Jensen SB, Loe H: Experimental gingivitis in man. II. A longitudinal clinical and bacteriological investigation, *J Periodont Res* 1:1-13, 1966.

7. Van der Weijden GA, Timmerman MF, Danser MM et al: Effect of pre-experimental maintenance care duration on the development of gingivitis in a partial mouth experimental gingivitis model, *J Periodont Res* 29:168-173, 1994.

8. Banbula A, Bugno M, Goldstein J et al: Emerging family of proline-specific peptidases of Porphyromonas gingivalis: purification and characterization of serine dipeptidyl peptidase, a structural and functional homologue of mammalian prolyl dipeptidyl peptidase IV. *Infect Immun* 68:1176-1182, 2000.

9. Dahlen G, Lindhe J, Sato K et al: The effect of supragingival plaque control on the subgingival microbiota in subjects with periodontal disease. *J Clin Periodontol* 19:802-809, 1992.

10. Hellstrom MK, Ramberg P, Krok L, Lindhe J: The effect of supragingival plaque control on the subgingival microflora in human periodontitis, *J Clin Periodontol* 23:934-940, 1996.

11. Katsanoulas T, Renee I, Attstrom R: The effect of supragingival plaque control on the composition of the subgingival flora in periodontal pockets, *J Clin Periodontol* 19:760-765, 1992.

12. Daly CG, Highfield JE: Effect of localized experimental gingivitis on early supragingival plaque accumulation, *J Clin Periodontol* 23:160-164, 1996.

13. Ramberg P, Lindhe J, Dahlen G, Volpe AR: The influence of gingival inflammation on de novo plaque formation, *J Clin Periodontol* 21:51-56, 1994.

14. Ramberg P, Axelsson P, Lindhe J: Plaque formation at healthy and inflamed gingival sites in young individuals, *J Clin Periodontol* 22:85-88, 1995.

15. Bouwsma O, Caton J, Polson A, Espeland M: Effect of personal oral hygiene on bleeding interdental gingiva. Histologic changes, *J Periodontol* 59:80-86, 1988.

16. Loe H, Anerud A, Boysen H, Morrison E: Natural history of periodontal disease in man. Rapid, moderate and no loss of attachment in Sri Lankan laborers 14 to 46 years of age, *J Clin Periodontol* 13:431-445, 1986.

17. Axelsson P, Lindhe J: Effect of controlled oral hygiene procedures on caries and periodontal disease in adults, *J Clin Periodontol* 5:133-151, 1978.

18. Grossi SG, Zambon JJ, Ho AW et al: Assessment of risk for periodontal disease. I. Risk indicators for attachment loss, *J Periodontol* 65:260-267, 1994.

19. Grossi SG, Genco RJ, Machtei EE et al: Assessment of risk for periodontal disease. II. Risk indicators for alveolar bone loss, *J Periodontol* 66:23-29, 1995.

20. Kaldahl WB, Kalkwarf KL, Patil KD et al: Long-term evaluation of periodontal therapy: I. Response to 4 therapeutic modalities, *J Periodontol* 67:93-102, 1996.

21. Kaldahl WB, Kalkwarf KL, Patil KD et al: Long-term evaluation of periodontal therapy: II. Incidence of sites breaking down, *J Periodontol* 67:103-108, 1996.

22. Sbordone L, Ramaglia L, Gulletta E, Iacono V: Recolonization of the subgingival microflora after scaling and root planing in human periodontitis, *J Periodontol* 61:579-584, 1990.

23. DeVore CH, Duckworth JE, Beck FM et al: Bone loss following periodontal therapy in subjects without frequent periodontal maintenance, *J Periodontol* 57:354-359, 1986.

24. Nyman S, Lindhe J, Rosling B: Periodontal surgery in plaque-infected dentitions, *J Clin Periodontol* 4:240-249, 1977.

25. Westfelt E, Nyman S, Socransky S, Lindhe J: Significance of frequency of professional tooth cleaning for healing following periodontal surgery, *J Clin Periodontol* 10:148-156, 1983.

26. Lindhe J, Westfelt E, Nyman S et al: Long-term effect of surgical/non-surgical treatment of periodontal disease, *J Clin Periodontol* 11:448-458, 1984.

27. Raeste AM, Kilpinen E: Clinical and radiographic long-term study of teeth with periodontal destruction treated by a modified flap operation, *J Clin Periodontol* 8:415-423, 1981.

28. Cercek JF, Kiger RD, Garrett S, Egelberg J: Relative effects of plaque control and instrumentation on the clinical parameters of human periodontal disease, *J Clin Periodontol* 10:46-56, 1983.

29. Loos B, Claffey N, Crigger M: Effects of oral hygiene measures on clinical and microbiological parameters of periodontal disease, *J Clin Periodontol* 15:211-216, 1988.

30. Raviglione MC, O'Brien RJ: Tuberculosis. In Braunwald E, Fauci AS, Kasper DL, Hauser SL, Longo DL, Jameson JL, editors: *Harrison's principles of internal medicine*, New York, 2001, McGraw-Hill, pp 1024-1035.

31. Claydon N, Addy M: Comparative single-use plaque removal by toothbrushes of different designs, *J Clin Periodontol* 23:1112-1116, 1996.

32. Grossman E, Cronin M, Dembling W, Proskin H: A comparative clinical study of extrinsic tooth stain removal with two electric toothbrushes [Braun D7 and D9] and a manual brush, *Am J Dent* 9(Spec No):S25-29, 1996.

33. Reardon RC, Cronin M, Balbo F et al: Four clinical studies comparing the efficacy of flat-trim and multi-level trim commercial toothbrushes, *J Clin Dent* 4:101-105, 1993.

34. Benson BJ, Henyon G, Grossman E: Clinical plaque removal efficacy of three toothbrushes, *J Clin Dent* 4:21-25, 1993.

35. Sharma NC, Galustians J, McCool JJ et al: The clinical effects on plaque and gingivitis over three-month's use of four complex-design manual toothbrushes, *J Clin Dent* 5:114-118, 1994.

36. Sharma NC, Galustians J, Rustogi KN et al: Comparative plaque removal efficacy of three toothbrushes in two independent clinical studies, *J Clin Dent* 3:C13-C20, 1994.

37. Grossman E, Dembling W, Walley DR: Two long-term clinical studies comparing the plaque removal and gingivitis reduction efficacy of the Oral-B Advantage Plaque Remover to five manual toothbrushes, *J Clin Dent* 5:46-53, 1994.

38. Beatty CF, Fallon PA, Marshall DD: Comparative analysis of the plaque removal ability of .007 and .008 toothbrush bristles, *Clin Prev Dent* 12:22-27, 1990.

39. Breitenmoser J, Mormann W, Muhlemann HR: Damaging effects of toothbrush bristle end form on gingiva, *J Periodontol* 50:212-216, 1979.

40. Khocht A, Simon G, Person P, Denepitiya JL: Gingival recession in relation to history of hard toothbrush use, *J Periodontol* 64:900-905, 1993.

41. Glaze PM, Wade AB: Toothbrush age and wear as it relates to plaque control, *J Clin Periodontol* 13:52-56, 1986.

42. Kreifeldt JG, Hill PH, Calisti LJ: A systematic study of the plaque removal efficiency of worn toothbrushes, *J Dent Res* 59:2047-2055, 1980.

43. Tan E, Daly C: Comparison of new and 3-month-old toothbrushes in plaque removal, *J Clin Periodontol* 29:645-650, 2002.

44. Bass CC: The optimum characteristics of toothbrushes for personal oral hygiene, *Dental Items of Interest* 70:696, 1948.

45. Waerhaug J: Effect of toothbrushing on subgingival plaque formation, *J Periodontol* 52:30-34, 1981.

46. Charters W: Proper home care of the mouth, *J Periodontol* 19:136-137, 1948.

47. Stillman PR: A philosophy of the treatment of periodontal disease, *Dent Digest* 38:314, 1932.

48. Dentino AR, Derderian G, Wolf MA et al: Six-month comparison of powered versus manual toothbrushing for safety and efficacy in the absence of professional instruction in mechanical plaque control, *J Periodontol* 73:770-778, 2002.

49. McInnes C, Johnson B, Emling RC, Yankell SL: Clinical and computer-assisted evaluations of the stain removal ability of the Sonicare electronic toothbrush, *J Clin Dent* 5:13-18, 1994.

50. Moran JM, Addy M, Newcombe RG: A comparative study of stain removal with two electric toothbrushes and a manual brush, *J Clin Dent* 6:188-193, 1995.

51. Tritten CB, Armitage GC: Comparison of a sonic and a manual toothbrush for efficacy in supragingival plaque removal and reduction of gingivitis, *J Clin Periodontol* 23:641-648, 1996.

52. Heanue M, Deacon SA, Deery C, Robinson PG et al: Manual versus powered toothbrushing for oral health, *Cochrane Database Syst Rev* CD002281, 2003.

53. Neiderman R: Manual versus powered toothbrushes. The Cochrane review, *J Am Dent Assoc* 134:1240-1244, 2003.

54. Graves RC, Disney JA, Stamm JW: Comparative effectiveness of flossing and brushing in reducing interproximal bleeding, *J Periodontol* 60:243-247, 1989.

55. Lang WP, Farghaly MM, Ronis DL: The relation of preventive dental behaviors to periodontal health status, *J Clin Periodontol* 21:194-198, 1994.

56. Lamberts DM, Wunderlich RC, Caffesse RG: The effect of waxed and unwaxed dental floss on gingival health. Part I. Plaque removal and gingival response, *J Periodontol* 53:393-396, 1982.

57. Ciancio SG, Shibly O, Farber GA: Clinical evaluation of the effect of two types of dental floss on plaque and gingival health, *Clin Prev Dent* 14:14-18, 1992.

58. Waerhaug J: Healing of the dento-epithelial junction following the use of dental floss, *J Clin Periodontol* 8:144-150, 1981.

59. Wunderlich RC, Lamberts DM, Caffesse RG: The effect of waxed and unwaxed dental floss on gingival health. Part II. Crevicular fluid flow and gingival bleeding, *J Periodontol* 53:397-400, 1982.

60. Carter-Hanson C, Gadbury-Amyot C, Killoy W: Comparison of the plaque removal efficacy of a new flossing aid (Quik Floss) to finger flossing, *J Clin Periodontol* 23:873-878, 1996.

61. Cronin M, Dembling W: An investigation of the efficacy and safety of a new electric interdental plaque remover for the reduction of interproximal plaque and gingivitis, *J Clin Dent* 7:74-77, 1996.

62. Cronin M, Dembling W, Warren P: The safety and efficacy of gingival massage with an electric interdental cleaning device, *J Clin Dent* 8:130-133, 1997.

63. Gordon JM, Frascella JA, Reardon RC: A clinical study of the safety and efficacy of a novel electric interdental cleaning device, *J Clin Dent* 7:70-73, 1996.

64. Barton J, Abelson D: The clinical efficacy of wooden interdental cleaners in gingivitis reduction, *Clin Prev Dent* 9:17-20, 1987.

65. Wolffe GN: An evaluation of proximal surface cleansing agents, *J Clin Periodontol* 3:148-156, 1976.

66. Bergenholtz A, Bjorne A, Vikstrom B: The plaque-removing ability of some common interdental aids. An intraindividual study, *J Clin Periodontol* 1:160-165, 1974.

67. Bergenholtz A, Olsson A: Efficacy of plaque-removal using interdental brushes and waxed dental floss, *Scand J Dent Res* 92:198-203, 1984.

68. Gjermo P, Flotra L: The effect of different methods of interdental cleaning, *J Periodont Res* 5:230-236, 1970.

69. Kiger RD, Nylund K, Feller RP: A comparison of proximal plaque removal using floss and interdental brushes, *J Clin Periodontol* 18:681-684, 1991.

70. Lang NP, Cumming BR, Loe H: Toothbrushing frequency as it relates to plaque development and gingival health, *J Periodontol* 44:396-405, 1973.

71. Kelner RM, Wohl BR, Deasy MJ, Formicola AJ: Gingival inflammation as related to frequency of plaque removal, *J Periodontol* 45:303-307, 1974.

72. White DJ, Cox ER, Suszcynskymeister EM, Baig AA: In vitro studies of the anticalculus efficacy of a sodium hexametaphosphate whitening dentifrice, *J Clin Dent* 13:33-37, 2002.

73. Rustogi KN, Volpe AR, Petrone ME: A clinical comparison of two anticalculus dentifrices, *Compend Contin Educ Dent* 9:78-79, 1988.

74. Lobene RR, Battista GW, Petrone DM et al: Clinical efficacy of an anticalculus fluoride dentifrice containing triclosan and a copolymer: a 6-month study, *Am J Dent* 4:83-85, 1991.

75. Newman HN: Periodontal pocket irrigation as adjunctive treatment, *Curr Opin Periodontol* 4:41-50, 1997.

76. Rethman M, Greenstein G: Oral irrigation in the treatment of periodontal diseases, *Curr Opin Periodontol* 99-110, 1994.

77. Ciancio SG, Mather ML, Zambon JJ, Reynolds HS: Effect of a chemotherapeutic agent delivered by an oral irrigation device on plaque, gingivitis, and subgingival microflora, *J Periodontol* 60:310-315, 1989.

78. Boyd RL, Hollander BN, Eakle WS: Comparison of a subgingivally placed cannula oral irrigator tip with a supragingivally placed standard irrigator tip, *J Clin Periodontol* 19:340-344, 1992.

79. Flemmig TF, Newman MG, Doherty FM et al: Supragingival irrigation with 0.06% chlorhexidine in naturally occurring gingivitis. I. 6 month clinical observations, *J Periodontol* 61:112-117, 1990.

80. Greenstein G: Supragingival and subgingival irrigation: practical application in the treatment of periodontal diseases, *Compend Contin Educ Dent* 13:1098, 1102, 1104 passim, 1992.

81. Cobb CM, Rodgers RL, Killoy WJ: Ultrastructural examination of human periodontal pockets following the use of an oral irrigation device in vivo, *J Periodontol* 59:155-163, 1988.

82. Braun RE, Ciancio SG: Subgingival delivery by an oral irrigation device, *J Periodontol* 63:469-472, 1992.

83. Al-Mubarak S, Ciancio S, Aljada A et al: Comparative evaluation of adjunctive oral irrigation in diabetics, *J Clin Periodontol* 29:295-300, 2002.

84. Cutler CW, Stanford TW, Abraham C et al: Clinical benefits of oral irrigation for periodontitis are related to reduction of pro-inflammatory cytokine levels and plaque, *J Clin Periodontol* 27:134-143, 2000.

85. Felo A, Shibly O, Ciancio SG et al: Effects of subgingival chlorhexidine irrigation on peri-implant maintenance, *Am J Dent* 10:107-110, 1997.

86. Attarzadeh F: Water irrigating devices for the orthodontic patient, *Int J Orthod* 28:17-22, 1990.

87. Phelps-Sandall BA, Oxford SJ: Effectiveness of oral hygiene techniques on plaque and gingivitis in patients placed in intermaxillary fixation, *Oral Surg Oral Med Oral Pathol* 56:487-490, 1983.

88. Burch JG, Lanese R, Ngan P: A two-month study of the effects of oral irrigation and automatic toothbrush use in an adult orthodontic population with fixed appliances, *Am J Orthod Dentofacial Orthop* 106:121-126, 1994.

89. Miller AJ, Brunelle JA, Carlos JP et al: Oral health of United States adults: the National Survey of Oral Health in U.S. Employed Adults and Seniors, 1985-1986: National Findings. Bethesda, Md, 1987, U.S. Dept. of Health and Human Services, Public Health Service, National Institutes of Health.

90. Hoppenbrouwers PM, Driessens FC, Borggreven JM: The mineral solubility of human tooth roots, *Arch Oral Biol* 32:319-322, 1987.

91. Eliasson S, Krasse B, Soremark R: Root caries. A consensus conference statement, *Swed Dent J* 16:21-25, 1992.

92. Billings RJ, Brown LR, Kaster AG: Contemporary treatment strategies for root surface dental caries, *Gerodontics* 1:20-27, 1985.

93. Nyvad B, Fejerskov O: Active root surface caries converted into inactive caries as a response to oral hygiene, *Scand J Dent Res* 94:281-284, 1986.

94. Nyvad B, Kilian M: Microflora associated with experimental root surface caries in humans, *Infect Immun* 58:1628-1633, 1990.

95. Rolla G, Ogaard B, Cruz Rde A: Topical application of fluorides on teeth. New concepts of mechanisms of interaction, *J Clin Periodontol* 20:105-108, 1993.

96. Emilson CG, Ravald N, Birkhed D: Effects of a 12-month prophylactic programme on selected oral bacterial populations on root surfaces with active and inactive carious lesions, *Caries Res* 27:195-200, 1993.

97. Addy M, West N: Etiology, mechanisms, and management of dentine hypersensitivity, *Curr Opin Periodontol* 71-77, 1994.

98. Poulsen S, Errboe M, Hovgaard O, Worthington HW: Potassium nitrate toothpaste for dentine hypersensitivity, *Cochrane Database Syst Rev* CD001476, 2001.

99. Glavind L, Christensen H, Pedersen E et al: Oral hygiene instruction in general dental practice by means of self-teaching manuals, *J Clin Periodontol* 12:27-34, 1985.

100. Glavind L, Zeuner E, Attstrom R: Oral hygiene instruction of adults by means of a self-instructional manual, *J Clin Periodontol* 8:165-176, 1981.

101. Lim LP, Davies WI, Yuen KW, Ma MH: Comparison of modes of oral hygiene instruction in improving gingival health, *J Clin Periodontol* 23:693-697, 1996.

102. Soderholm G, Nobreus N, Attstrom R, Egelberg J: Teaching plaque control. I. A five-visit versus a two-visit program, *J Clin Periodontol* 9:203-213, 1982.

103. Timmreck TC: *An introduction to epidemiology*, ed 3, Sudbury, MA, 2002, Jones & Bartlett.

104. Last JM: *A dictionary of epidemiology*, ed 4, Oxford, 2001, Oxford University Press.

105. Genco RJ: Risk factors for periodontal disease. In Rose LF, Genco RJ, Mealey BL, Cohen DW, editors: *Periodontal medicine*, Hamilton, Ontario, 2000, B.C. Decker, pp 11-33.

106. Iwata BA, Becksfort CM: Behavioral research in preventive dentistry: educational and contingency management approaches to the problem of patient compliance, *J Appl Behav Anal* 14:111-120, 1981.

107. Tedesco LA, Christersson LA, Albino JE, Genco RJ: Using phase-contrast microscopy to change oral health beliefs and behaviors, *Clin Prev Dent* 7:26-30, 1985.

108. Macgregor ID, Balding J, Regis D: Toothbrushing schedule, motivation and 'lifestyle' behaviours in 7,770 young adolescents, *Community Dent Health* 13:232-237, 1996.

109. Wilson TG Jr: Compliance. A review of the literature with possible applications to periodontics, *J Periodontol* 58:706-714, 1987.

110. Wilson TG Jr: Compliance and its role in periodontal therapy, *Periodontol 2000* 12:16-23, 1996.

111. Wilson TG Jr: How patient compliance to suggested oral hygiene and maintenance affect periodontal therapy, *Dent Clin North Am* 42:389-403, 1998.

112. Wilson TG Jr, Hale S, Temple R: The results of efforts to improve compliance with supportive periodontal treatment in a private practice, *J Periodontol* 64:311-314, 1993.

113. Inglehart M, Tedesco LA: Behavioral research related to oral hygiene practices: a new century model of oral health promotion, *Periodontol 2000* 8:15-23, 1995.

114. O'Leary TJ, Drake RB, Naylor JE: The plaque control record, *J Periodontol* 43:38, 1972.

115. Ramfjord SP, Morrison EC, Burgett FG et al: Oral hygiene and maintenance of periodontal support, *J Periodontol* 53:26-30, 1982.

116. McLey L, Boyd RL, Sarker S: Clinical and laboratory evaluation of powered electric toothbrushes: laboratory determination of relative abrasion of three powered toothbrushes, *J Clin Dent* 8:76-80, 1997.

117. van der Weijden GA, Timmerman MF, Reijerse E et al: Toothbrushing force in relation to plaque removal, *J Clin Periodontol* 23:724-729, 1996.

118. Olsson M, Lindhe J: Periodontal characteristics in individuals with varying form of the upper central incisors, *J Clin Periodontol* 18:78-82, 1991.

119. Olsson M, Lindhe J, Marinello CP: On the relationship between crown form and clinical features of the gingiva in adolescents, *J Clin Periodontol* 20:570-577, 1993.

120. Kallestal C, Uhlin S: Buccal attachment loss in Swedish adolescents, *J Clin Periodontol* 19:485-491, 1992.

121. Loe H, Anerud A, Boysen H: The natural history of periodontal disease in man: prevalence, severity, and extent of gingival recession, *J Periodontol* 63:489-495, 1992.

122. Page RC, Offenbacher S, Schroeder HE et al: Advances in the pathogenesis of periodontitis: summary of developments, clinical implications and future directions, *Periodontol 2000* 14:216-248, 1997.

123. Cortellini P, Pini-Prato G, Tonetti M: Periodontal regeneration of human infrabony defects (V). Effect of oral hygiene on long-term stability, *J Clin Periodontol* 21:606-610, 1994.

124. Tonetti MS, Pini-Prato G, Cortellini P: Factors affecting the healing response of intrabony defects following guided tissue regeneration and access flap surgery, *J Clin Periodontol* 23:548-556, 1996.

125. Slots J, MacDonald ES, Nowzari H: Infectious aspects of periodontal regeneration, *Periodontol 2000* 19:164-172, 1999.

14 Nonsurgical Therapy

Jacqueline M. Plemons and Becky DeSpain Eden

The goal of periodontal therapy is to eliminate disease and restore the periodontium to a state of health, which includes comfort, function, and esthetics that can be maintained adequately by both the patient and dental professional. Nonsurgical therapy aims to control the bacterial challenge characteristic of gingivitis and periodontitis while addressing local risk factors and minimizing the potential impact of systemic factors. Alteration or elimination of putative periodontal pathogens and resolution of inflammation are paramount objectives of nonsurgical therapy, creating an environment conducive to periodontal health and decreasing the likelihood of disease progression. The term nonsurgical therapy includes the use of oral hygiene self-care, periodontal instrumentation, and chemotherapeutic agents to prevent, arrest, or eliminate periodontal disease. This chapter deals primarily with periodontal instrumentation and its role in nonsurgical therapy.

RATIONALE AND EVIDENCE

Instrumentation performed as a part of nonsurgical therapy is aimed directly at changing the prevalence of certain periodontal pathogens or reducing the levels of these microorganisms. Whether by direct removal of pathogenic organisms and their byproducts or removal of contributing factors such as calculus and overhanging restorations, the goal is to decrease the quantity of organisms below a critical mass and alter the composition of the remaining bacterial flora to one associated with health. Thus equilibrium between the remaining bacterial plaque and host response can be reached, resulting in a clinical state of periodontal health.

Scaling and root planing and subgingival debridement have long been established as effective treatment modalities in the management of periodontal disease. Subgingival instrumentation results in a significant reduction of gram-negative anaerobic organisms and encourages repopulation with gram-positive cocci and rods associated with health. Levels of spirochetes, motile microbes, and specific periodontal pathogens such as *Porphyromonas gingivalis*, *Prevotella intermedia*, and *Actinobacillus actinomycetemcomitans*, as well as *Bacteroides* species, are significantly reduced after scaling and root planing.[1-5] Reduction in inflammatory cytokines that are responsible for tissue damage observed in gingivitis and periodontitis occurs subsequent to shifts in microbial composition.[6] These microbial changes are most likely transient in nature, and periodic scaling and root planing must be performed to sustain positive results.[7,8]

Changes in the microflora after scaling and root planing are accompanied by concomitant changes in clinical measurements of periodontal health. Decreased bleeding on probing that may approach 45% in areas with initial probing depths of 4.0 to 6.5 mm is evidence that inflammation is reduced.[9] Changes in probing depth and attachment levels after scaling and root planing vary depending on initial measurements and generally reflect the combination of a gain in clinical attachment and resolution of edema or shrinkage (recession). Areas of initial probing depth of 1 to 3 mm experience a mean probing depth reduction of 0.03 mm and loss of attachment of 0.34 mm, whereas areas of 4 to 6 mm initial probing depth demonstrate a 1.29 mm mean reduction in probing depth and 0.55 mm mean gain in attachment. Similar measurements for areas of initial probing depth of 7 mm or greater include 2.16 mm mean reduction in probing depth and 1.19 mm mean gain in attachment.[10]

CHALLENGES AND LIMITATIONS

Scaling and root planing are demanding clinical procedures that require time and skill. Complete removal of plaque and calculus from root surfaces, especially within deep pockets, is unrealistic and rarely attained. In pockets with initial probing depth of 5 mm or greater, clinicians have been shown to inadequately débride roots 65% of the time.[11] Taken together, studies evaluating residual calculus after periodontal instrumentation with or without surgical access exhibit 11% to 85% residual calculus.[12-16] Areas most prone to demonstrating residual deposits after scaling and root planing are furcations, line angles, the cementoenamel junction, and root concavities. Despite these significant clinical challenges, thorough instrumentation remains paramount to the success of periodontal therapy.

Although the production of a smooth, glassy root surface is often used as an end-point during periodontal instrumentation, its absolute necessity for successful therapy is unclear.[17-19] Complete removal of cementum in an attempt to eliminate endotoxin adherent to the root surface is unnecessary and may result in hypersensitivity.[20-22]

Scaling and root planing significantly reduce the level of periodontal pathogens. However, sustained eradication of certain organisms has proven to be a challenge. The ability of organisms such as *Actinobacillus actinomycetemcomitans* to invade the soft tissues of the periodontium has been associated with the potential for recolonization and a poorer clinical response, especially in patients with aggressive periodontitis.[23,24]

Several studies have compared the effectiveness of different treatment modalities used in the management of patients with periodontitis.[25-29] Although many studies report no significant differences in clinical results between nonsurgical and surgical therapy, care must be taken in the evaluation of these studies. Differences in research design, including method of instrumentation (time spent and skill of the clinician) and evaluation of data (lack of sufficient statistical power in the analysis of deep pockets), complicate clinical application.[30] Access required for regenerative periodontal therapy is achieved only with the use of a surgical approach. Nonetheless, nonsurgical therapy remains a definitive therapeutic approach to the management of patients with mild to moderate chronic periodontitis and as an initial phase of treatment for patients expected to require surgical intervention.[31,32]

TREATMENT PLANNING AND SEQUENCE

Treatment planning during nonsurgical periodontal therapy begins with the development of an oral hygiene self-care program designed specifically to meet the needs of each individual patient. This plan may include various oral hygiene aids to assist in supragingival plaque removal (see Chapter 13), as well as counseling regarding disease risk factors such as smoking. Episodes of periodontal debridement are planned to eliminate or disrupt bacterial plaque and byproducts such as endotoxin and to remove calculus from the coronal surfaces, roots, and within periodontal pockets. Periodontal instrumentation is often planned to occur in multiple appointments concentrating on affected sites in one or two quadrants at a single visit. For patients with severe inflammation and gross deposits, full-mouth debridement may be planned to establish initial healing, followed by more definitive periodontal instrumentation. Recent information suggests that multiple episodes of full-mouth debridement or disinfection performed within a close time period (24 hours) may reduce potential reservoirs of cross-infection and may result in a favorable clinical response.[33-36] Most patients will require local anesthesia to allow thorough instrumentation of deeper or more inflamed sites. Plaque control is reassessed during episodes of periodontal debridement and local risk factors such as overhanging restorations are eliminated.

EVALUATION OF RESULTS

The end-point of nonsurgical therapy is a return to periodontal health. Healing after periodontal debridement usually is assessed during a reevaluation appointment scheduled 4 to 6 weeks after treatment. Periodontal charting is performed, as well as an evaluation of oral self-care effectiveness. The benefits expected after periodontal debridement include reduction of clinical inflammation (erythema, edema, and bleeding on probing), microbial shifts to a less pathogenic bacterial flora, reduction of probing depth, and gain of clinical attachment. Healing after scaling and root planing results in the formation of a long junctional epithelium that is consistent with periodontal health in the presence of good oral self-care. Factors that may reduce the effectiveness of periodontal

debridement and alter the healing response include anatomic factors such as root concavities and furcations, presence of deep pockets, inadequate personal plaque control, presence of systemic risk factors, and variability in the clinician's skill. Patients who demonstrate clinical stability at the reevaluation appointment are placed on a program of supportive periodontal care, whereas patients with areas that demonstrate residual inflammation may require alternative therapeutic intervention, including the use of pharmacotherapeutics, additional debridement, or periodontal surgery.[37]

MANUAL INSTRUMENTATION

Because the success of nonsurgical periodontal therapy largely depends on the technical skill of the clinician providing treatment, complete knowledge and understanding of periodontal instruments, their design and maintenance, and technique principles for their use are necessary.

Instrument Design

The architectural principles of form and function also apply to dental instruments. The clinician's comprehension of instrument design facilitates effective and efficient nonsurgical therapy. Familiarity with instrument design is the foundation for maintenance and sharpening of instruments and provides the clinician with a basis on which to evaluate new instruments and to make sensible instrument purchases.

Figure 14-1 depicts the three parts of a dental instrument: the *handle, shank*, and *working end*. The handle makes up the bulk of the instrument. Therefore, instrument weight is the most important consideration of the handle.

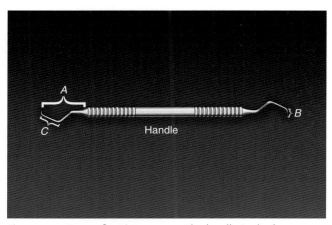

Figure 14-1. Parts of an instrument. The handle is the largest part of an instrument. A, The shank joins the handle to (*B*) the working end. *C*, Terminal shank is the last part of the shank closest to the working end.

Metal instruments typically have hollow handles to reduce weight, which in turn decreases the pressure needed to control the instrument and increases tactile sensitivity. The instrument handles displayed in Figure 14-2 vary in size from 5 to 1o mm. Those larger than a standard pencil size were once considered too heavy, until lighter weight handles made of composite material became available. These larger, lightweight instruments have increased in popularity because they contribute to efficiency of the clinician. *Knurling*—the texture, ribbing, or scoring applied in a myriad of patterns to handles—prevents slipping and improves control of the instrument.

The shank connects the working end of the instrument to the handle. The last section of the shank adjacent to the working end is known as the *terminal shank*, an important designation used in principles of instrumentation. Two characteristics of the shank, length and curvature, determine access to a particular area of the mouth. The overall length of the shank, the distance from the handle to the working end, is uniform among instruments, as seen in Figure 14-3. A length of 30 to 40 mm is ideal, providing appropriate leverage for most dental procedures. The distance from the first bend in the shank to the working end is the *functional length* (Fig. 14-4), which varies between instruments. A longer functional shank is needed when access to the treatment area is limited—that is, select an instrument with a long functional shaft for a longer clinical crown, deeper periodontal pockets, or posterior tooth surfaces.

Instrument shanks can be classified as *straight, curved,* or *contraangled*, as shown in Figure 14-5. The functional shank of a straight instrument lies in the same plane as the long axis of the handle. These instruments are used

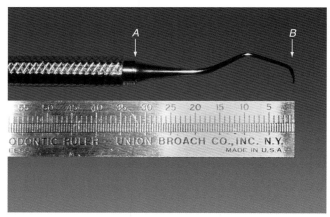

Figure 14-3. Instrument shank length. The overall shank length of an instrument is the distance from (*A*) the junction of the handle and shank to (*B*) the working end.

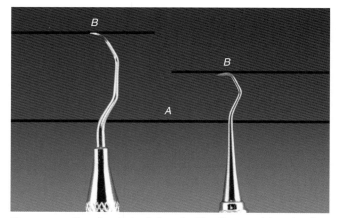

Figure 14-4. Functional shank length. The functional length of an instrument shank is the distance from (*A*) the first bend in the shank nearest the handle to (*B*) the working end.

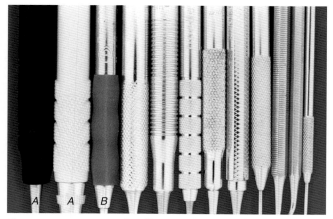

Figure 14-2. Instrument handles. Handle designs vary widely with sizes ranging from 5 to 1o mm in diameter. *A*, Handles made of lightweight composite. *B*, Inset for comfort. Remaining handles are metal. Note the knurling or texturing added to improve the grasp and control of the instrument.

in areas of the mouth where access is unrestricted, such as anterior teeth. A curved or angled instrument has a bend in the functional shank that deviates from the handle axis in one direction only. Curved instruments are more versatile—that is, more adaptable to both posterior and anterior teeth. A contraangled instrument has two bends in the functional shank in opposite directions. These instruments are specifically designed for surfaces with limited access, including distal surfaces of posterior teeth and deep periodontal pockets.

The design of the shank also influences the function of an instrument. The diameter of the shank, compared in Figure 14-6, determines the strength of the instrument. A thicker shank is stronger, and hence necessary for removal of heavy calculus deposits. A manufacturer may add metal to the shank to increase the strength of an instrument, labeling this feature with a "P" (prophylaxis)

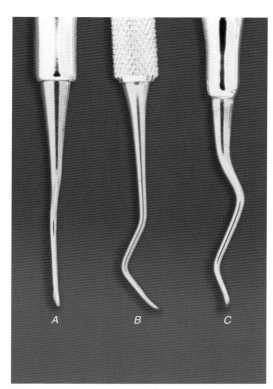

Figure 14-5. Instrument shank design. Three instrument shank designs are available: (*A*) straight, (*B*) curved, and (*C*) contraangled.

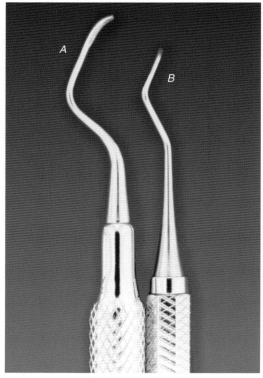

Figure 14-6. Diameter of the instrument shank. *A*, Curette with a thicker shank used for calculus removal. *B*, Curette with a thinner shank, more suitable for removing light deposits and root planing.

or "R" (rigid) in the instrument name. Conversely, the flexibility of the shank is a product of length and diameter. Flexing of the shank relieves force applied to the instrument during scaling and root planing, the advantage of which is protecting the root surface from damage. Instruments with thin or flexible shanks are preferable for root planing.

Periodontal instruments are available with *paired* working ends that are mirror images to adapt to opposing tooth surfaces, *double-ended* with two dissimilar working ends, or *single-ended* with only one working end on a handle. Because they improve economy of motion and are less expensive, double-ended and paired instruments are more desirable. *Balance*, a critical feature of an instrument, is defined as the working end of the instrument centered with the long axis of the handle and shank (a balanced instrument is shown in Fig. 14-7). An instrument that does not have balance feels awkward and harder to control during use.

The working end, called the *blade* on some instruments, is the functioning part of the instrument. An exact nomenclature describes specific regions of the working end (Figs. 14-8 and 14-9). The last third of the working end is the *tip*, whereas the termination of the working end is the *toe*. The *heel* is the first portion of the working end, closest to the shank. The *face* of the instrument is the surface between the two cutting edges. Opposite of the face is the *back* of the instrument. The region of the working end between the face and back is the *lateral surface*. The *cutting edge* of an instrument is the line formed by the convergence of the face and the lateral surface. The angle produced by the intersection of the face and lateral surface is the *internal angle*. The internal angle is uniform among scaling instruments, ranging from 70 to 80 degrees.

The shape and contour of the working end is unique for each instrument type. The instruments used

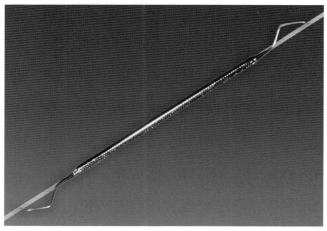

Figure 14-7. Balance. A balanced instrument has the working end centered over the long axis of the handle.

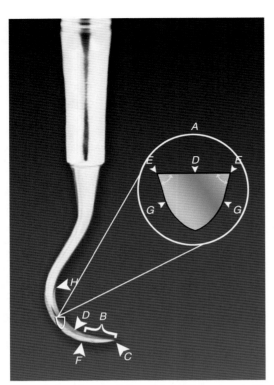

Figure 14-8. Design characteristics of the sickle scaler. *A,* Triangular cross section of the sickle scaler. *B,* Tip, last third of the working end. *C,* Toe, which is *pointed. D,* Face. *E,* Cutting edge. *F,* Back. *G,* Lateral surface. *H,* Heel. Internal angle, 70 to 80 degrees.

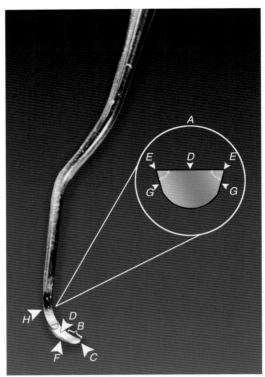

Figure 14-9. Design characteristics of the curette. *A,* Semicircular cross section of the curette. *B,* Tip, last third of the working end. *C,* Toe, which is *rounded. D,* Face. *E,* Cutting edge. *F,* Back. *G,* Lateral surface. *H,* Heel.

in nonsurgical periodontal therapy include periodontal probes, explorers, sickle scalers, curettes, and periodontal files.

The *periodontal probe* is used during patient assessment to examine and evaluate the periodontium. It has a long, thin, rod-shaped end distinguished by millimeter markings that are used to measure periodontal structures. In cross section, a probe can be either round or flat, with a blunt toe. The length and angles of the probe vary widely, as do the measurements marked on the probe (Fig. 14-10). Some are color-coded to enhance visibility of the measurements. The periodontal probe is used to measure the depth of the sulcus or pocket, to identify bleeding areas of the sulcular epithelium, to locate the mucogingival junction, and to measure keratinized gingiva or oral lesions.

An *explorer* has a thin, flexible, wirelike working end that is circular in cross section and tapers to a sharp point; examples of the wide variety of explorers available are shown in Figure 14-11. The explorer is used during patient assessment to detect lesions of tooth structure, to evaluate the topography of a tooth surface, to determine the need for deposit removal, to locate subgingival calculus, and to evaluate treatment.

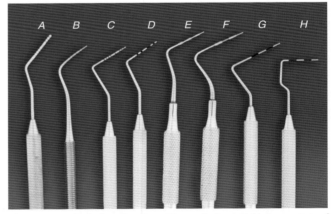

Figure 14-10. Periodontal probes. The probe is available in a variety of shapes, lengths, angles, and measurements. *A,* Goldman-Fox; *(B)* Williams; *(C)* Michigan O; *(D)* #10; *(E)* #2 12; *(F)* #4; *(G)* #10; *(H)* #NT2 probes. Note the color coding on probes *D* through *H,* which enhances visibility of markings.

The *sickle scaler* is designed for removing supragingival calculus. Sickle scalers are triangular in cross section— that is, they have two straight cutting edges and a pointed toe (see Fig. 14-8). Note that the back of a sickle is a line,

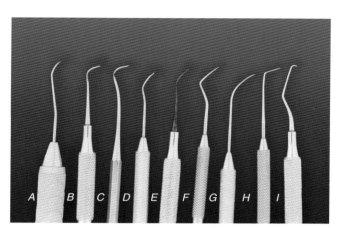

Figure 14-11. Explorers. An explorer is available to suit the preferences of any clinician or to adapt to any tooth surface topography. (A) #17; (B) #6; (C) #3A; (D) Classic #2; (E) #3ML; (F) #2; (G) #3 "pig-tail"; (H) #3CH "Cow horn"; (I) ODU 11/12 explorers.

which is often fairly sharp, and can damage soft tissue if the instrument is used subgingivally. The notable feature of a sickle scaler is the strength furnished by the design. This characteristic is a distinct disadvantage when scaling root surfaces (vs. enamel surfaces) which may be easily scored or gouged by an instrument. Figure 14-12 shows the two types of sickle scalers, curved and straight, as well as sickle scalers designed for use in the anterior and posterior regions of the mouth, with a straight shank and a curved shank, respectively.

The *curette* is designed for subgingival instrumentation but is the most versatile periodontal instrument. It also can be used for supragingival calculus and stain removal, fine scaling, root planing, and tissue curettage.

Figure 14-9 depicts the unique characteristics of the curette, which is semicircular in cross section. This shape creates a curved back that is compatible with the soft tissue during subgingival instrumentation. A curette has two parallel cutting edges that converge in a rounded toe; the two curette types are compared in Figure 14-13. The *universal curette,* so named because a paired instrument adapts to all four tooth surfaces, has two straight cutting edges and a face angled at 90 degrees to the terminal shank; Figure 14-14 displays examples of universal curettes.

The face of an *area-specific curette* is offset or tilted at a 60- to 70-degree angle to the terminal shank, which further enhances biologic compatibility and makes the

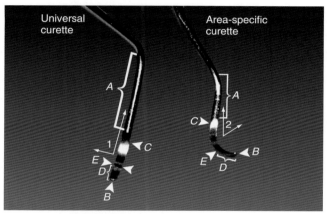

Figure 14-13. Comparison of a universal curette to an area-specific curette. *A,* Terminal shank. *B,* Toe. *C,* Heel. *D,* Tip. *E,* Cutting edge. *1,* The angle formed by the terminal shank and the face of a universal curette is 90 degrees. *2,* The angle formed by the terminal shank and the face of an area-specific curette is 60 to 70 degrees.

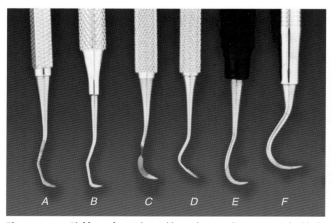

Figure 14-12. Sickle scalers. The sickle scaler may have a straight blade as (A) #31/32T and (B) J3, or a curved blade as (C) #204, (D) #204S, (E) H6/H7, and (F) U15. The sickles with straight shanks (B, E, F) are used in the anterior regions, whereas those with curved shanks (A, C, D) are designed for the posterior.

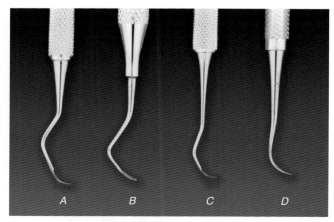

Figure 14-14. Universal curettes. These universal curettes are double-ended and can be used throughout the dentition. A, 4R/4L; (B) McCall 13/14S; (C) Columbia 13/14; (D) Younger-Good 7/8 curettes.

instrument easier to use subgingivally. The working end of an area-specific curette curves in two planes, the only instrument with a curved cutting edge that facilitates adaptation to curved tooth surfaces. Only one cutting edge of this instrument is usable, therefore each working end adapts to just one of the four tooth surfaces. The cutting edge used in instrumentation is the lower edge (i.e., the longer outer curved edge to the left; see Fig. 14-9). The inside edge is not used and is machined off by the manufacturer. Figure 14-15 shows a series of area-specific curettes originally designed before 1940 by Dr. Clayton Gracey. Each one of the Gracey curettes is intended for a specific region of the dentition, although many can be applied correctly in multiple areas, decreasing the number of instruments needed per patient.

The challenges of subgingival instrumentation are numerous. Clinicians continually search for better ways and enhanced instruments to improve outcomes. Many have designed new instruments or modified existing ones. Standard instruments carry the name of the designer or their institution, such as Gracey or Columbia curettes. Figure 14-16 demonstrates recent modifications of an area-specific curette for specific situations. The usual Gracey 1/2 is shown along with one that has 3 mm added to the terminal shank for deep periodontal pockets and another with a working end shortened by half, which is designed for narrow pockets.

The *file* (Fig. 14-17) is a specialized instrument used for crushing and removing calculus deposits located in deep, narrow periodontal pockets where instruments with longer or wider working ends do not reach. A file has multiple parallel cutting edges, generally three to five, arranged on a working end that is continuous with the terminal shank. The working end is a small oval or rectangular base on which the cutting edges are mounted.

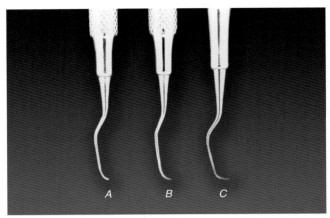

Figure 14-16. Modifications of an instrument. Each of the three instruments is a Gracey 1/2. *B*, Conventional design. *A*, The working end is shortened by half the regular length, whereas the working end (*C*) has been lengthened for supragingival calculus removal.

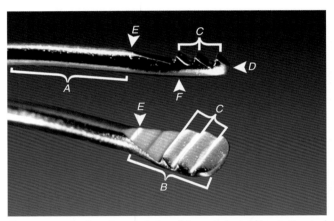

Figure 14-17. Design characteristics of the periodontal file. *A*, Terminal shank. *B*, Working end. *C*, Cutting edges. *D*, Toe. *E*, Heel. *F*, Back.

Multiple working ends with different angles are needed to adapt to the four tooth surfaces. The file can easily damage a root surface because of its heavy design, and the clinician should use one judiciously. Improved design of ultrasonic scaling inserts has reduced the use of files to a few unusual circumstances.

The mouth mirror has multiple uses in dental procedures, including indirect vision, reflection of light to improve visibility, and retraction of the lips, cheeks, and tongue. It also may be used for transillumination, directing light through a structure to enhance inspection, which is especially helpful for identifying calculus deposits on proximal surfaces of anterior teeth.

The clinician holds the mirror in the nondominant hand, opposite the working instruments. The mirror hand is stabilized on the patient's dentition with a finger

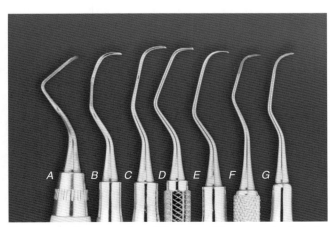

Figure 14-15. Gracey curettes. This series of Gracey curettes includes (*A*) 17/18; (*B*) 13/14; (*C*) 11/12; (*D*) 7/8; (*E*) 5/6; (*F*) 3/4; (*G*) 1/2.

rest to avoid resting the mirror on the gingival or other soft tissue. Contact with the teeth when inserting or removing the mirror from the mouth can be prevented by turning the mirror until it is parallel with the occlusal plane. When retracting the lips and cheeks, avoid placing pressure on the labial commissures by pulling the cheeks away from the dentition, rather than back toward the posterior teeth. Fogging of the mirror can be avoided by warming it to body temperature by placing it against the buccal mucosa.

PATIENT AND CLINICIAN POSITIONING

Periodontal procedures often require extended treatment time. Comfortable positions that both the patient and clinician can maintain with minimal physical stress and a modest degree of relaxation facilitate successful outcomes of periodontal care.

The clinician must develop the habit of using an operating position that yields immediate comfort, reduced fatigue, and long-term musculoskeletal health.[38] Figure 14-18 presents the desirable seated position for the clinician. The operator's stool is adjusted to knee height so that when seated, the clinician's feet are flat on the floor with the thighs approximately parallel to the floor. During treatment, body weight is supported on the stool and the clinician places the feet at least shoulder width apart to maintain balance. The back and neck are straight. The dental chair is adjusted so that the patient's head is at the level of the clinician's elbow, which allows the clinician to keep the shoulders in a natural, relaxed position, helping to prevent work-related neck and shoulder pain.[39,40] In addition, the clinician should keep the head erect over the spine and maintain an operating distance of at least 14 inches from the patient's face.

The patient is placed in a reclining or supine position during dental care. The back of the dental chair is reclined to an angle of no more than 10 degrees to the floor. The legs and feet of the patient are raised to about the same level as the head. During treatment, the clinician directs the patient to turn the head either toward or away from the clinician to center the treatment area in the dental light beam. More importantly, this position protects the patient's airway during dental procedures. The patient's head position is adjusted slightly upward or downward for the arch treated. For instrumentation of maxillary teeth the patient is asked to raise or tilt the chin up so that the occlusal plane is nearly perpendicular to the floor. For mandibular teeth, either the patient's head is tilted down toward the chest or the back of the chair is raised slightly so that the occlusal plane is almost parallel with the floor. The direction of the dental light is different for each arch. Initially, the light beam is directed on the patient's neck area and then the lamp is rotated slowly up to the oral

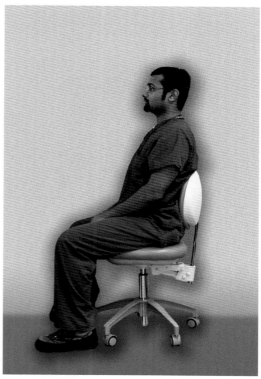

Figure 14-18. The clinician's position. The height of the operator's stool is adjusted so that the thighs are parallel to the floor, with the feet flat on the floor and apart about a shoulder's width. The back and neck are straight with the head erect.

cavity—a 45-degree angle to the floor to illuminate the maxillary arch and a 90-degree angle to the floor to illuminate the mandibular arch.

The dentition is divided into sextants to organize and to manage assessment, treatment, and evaluation procedures efficiently. Each sextant has a facial and lingual aspect, which are mirror images. A specific clinician position, patient head orientation, and precise instrumentation apply to each of the twelve regions. The clinician's position relative to the patient is described by the positions on a clock face (Fig. 14-19). Figures 14-20 through 14-23 provide a map and the details for positioning for each treatment area.

PRINCIPLES OF INSTRUMENTATION

A set of general principles widely recognized in the profession guide the use of instruments in nonsurgical periodontal therapy. The novice clinician follows these principles closely until clinical experience provides the judgment and confidence to modify them for personal preferences or special circumstances, or to achieve a particular outcome.

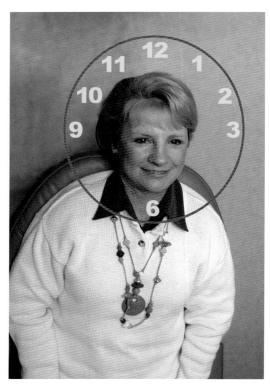

Figure 14-19. Clinician positioning relative to the patient. The clinician's position around the patient during treatment, denoted like time on the face of a clock face. The patient's chin is at 6 o'clock. The right-handed clinician sits between 9 and 12 o'clock. The left-handed clinician sits on the opposite side, from 12 to 3 o'clock.

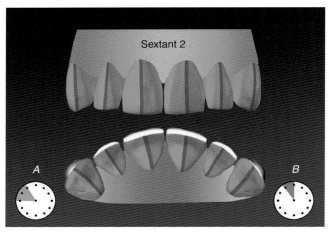

Figure 14-21. Positioning for sextant 2. Dividing facial and lingual surfaces at the midline, *green* portions are toward the clinician and *blue* portions are away from the clinician during treatment. For surfaces toward the clinician, the patient's head is turned away with the chin tilted upward. *A*, The clinician is in the region from 9 and 11 o'clock. For surfaces away from the clinician, the patient's head is turned toward the clinician and the chin tilted upward. *B*, The clinician is in the 11 to 12 o'clock region.

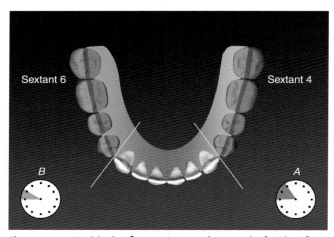

Figure 14-22. Positioning for sextants 4 and 6. For the facial surfaces in sextant 4 and the lingual surfaces in sextant 6 (in *blue*), the patient's head is turned toward the clinician with the chin tilted down. *A*, The clinician is seated in the 9 to 11 o'clock region. For lingual surfaces in sextant 4 and the facial surfaces in sextant 6 (in *green*), the patient's head is turned away from the clinician with the chin tilted upward. *B*, The clinician is seated in the 9 to 10 o'clock region.

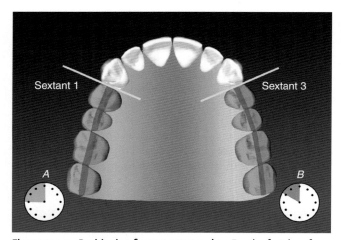

Figure 14-20. Positioning for sextants 1 and 3. For the facial surfaces in sextant 1 and the lingual surfaces in sextant 3 (in *green*), the patient's head is turned away from the clinician with the head tilted upward. *A*, The clinician is in the region from 9 to 12 o'clock. For lingual surfaces in sextant 1 and the facial surfaces in sextant 3 (in *blue*), the patient's head is turned toward the clinician with the chin tilted upward. *B*, The clinician is in the 10 to 12 o'clock region.

The *modified pen grasp* (Fig. 14-24) is used to hold instruments during most nonsurgical dental procedures. This grasp allows maximum control of the instrument, creates the range of motion for instrumentation, enhances tactile sensitivity, and decreases clinician fatigue.

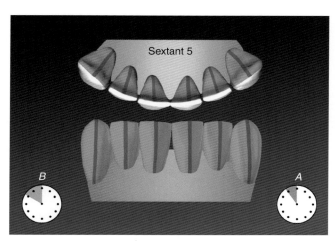

Figure 14-23. Positioning for sextant 5. Dividing facial and lingual surfaces at the midline, *green* portions are toward the clinician and *blue* portions are away from the clinician during treatment. For surfaces away from the clinician, the patient's head is turned toward the clinician with the chin tilted down. *A,* The clinician is in the region between 11 and 12 o'clock. For surfaces toward the clinician, the patient's head is turned away with the chin tilted down. *B,* The clinician is in the region from 10 to 12 o'clock.

To execute the modified pen grasp, place the index finger (or forefinger) and thumb opposite of each other near the junction of the handle and shank. The index finger and thumb hold the instrument, allowing the clinician to maneuver it around the tooth during instrumentation. Place the middle finger on the shank to stabilize the instrument. The middle finger receives tactile stimuli from the working end during instrumentation. The pads of the fingers should touch the instrument because this

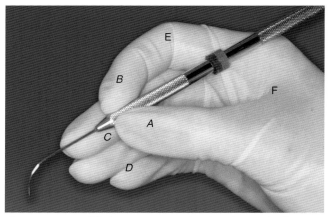

Figure 14-24. Modified pen grasp. *A,* Thumb and (*B*) index finger on the handle close to the junction with the shank. *C,* Pad of middle finger rests on the shank. *D,* Ring finger and fourth finger touching, curved, and relaxed. The handle will rest in the region from *E* to *F.*

region has the most nerve receptors. The third or ring finger supports the hand during procedures. Although the fourth finger serves no function in the grasp, all four fingers touch so that the hand functions as a unit during instrumentation. The instrument handle rests in the region between the second joint of the forefinger and the "V" formed by the thumb and index finger. Finally, the fingers stay curved and relaxed to expand the range of motion, increase tactile sensitivity, and prevent clinician fatigue.

A scaling instrument operates as a lever, with the third finger (the ring finger) serving as a *fulcrum* and as a stabilizing point for the hand. A fulcrum is the point on which the lever pivots. In periodontal instrumentation, the fulcrum allows the instrument to function. The work of the instrument is cleaving or prying deposits from the tooth surface. Furthermore, the fulcrum provides stability and control of the instrument to prevent injury or trauma to the surrounding tissues and to assure the patient of the clinician's steadiness.

The ideal location for the fulcrum is on the dentition, which is an *intraoral fulcrum.* The third finger (ring finger) during periodontal instrumentation serves as both a rest for the hand and a fulcrum for the instrument. A clinician attains the greatest stability by placing the fulcrum close to the working area, generally on the same arch and in the same quadrant. A fulcrum established on an occlusal or incisal surface or in the embrasure gives better control than one placed on a flat tooth surface, which can be slippery. Avoid placing a fulcrum on mobile or prosthetic teeth because little security is provided and the pressure may cause discomfort to the patient. The instrumentation hand position for maxillary teeth that allows the clinician to pivot on the fulcrum is sometimes described as "palm up," with the palm of the hand facing the occlusal plane. In contrast, turn the hand "palm down" to instrument mandibular teeth.

An *extraoral fulcrum* may be necessary or desirable in some situations—for example, missing or mobile teeth, temporomandibular joint disorder, or a patient's limited ability to open. To apply an extraoral fulcrum as shown in Figure 14-25, use either the palm or back of the hand rather than a single point to reduce the pressure on the patient's soft tissue. When using an extraoral fulcrum, the clinician should concentrate on moving the hand as a unit.

A *substitute fulcrum* is another option when encountering difficulty with an intraoral fulcrum. As shown in Figure 14-26, the index finger of the nonoperating hand is placed either in the vestibule near the treatment area or on the occlusal surfaces of adjacent teeth. The fulcrum is then established on that finger, rather than on the dentition. Leverage is usually better with a substitute fulcrum compared with an extraoral fulcrum because the distance from the pivot to the working end is shorter.

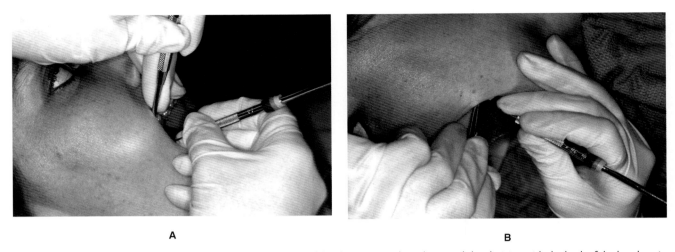

Figure 14-25. Extraoral fulcrum. A, An extraoral fulcrum for areas of the dentition on the side toward the clinician with the back of the hand against the face. **B,** An extraoral fulcrum for areas of the mouth on the side away from the clinician, with the palm cupping the chin.

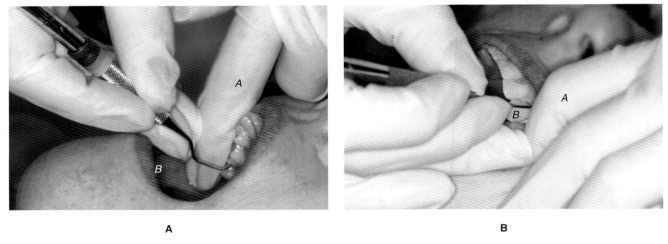

Figure 14-26. Substitute fulcrum. A, A finger of the nonoperating hand (*A*) placed on the occlusal surfaces of the teeth in the region to serve as a stable area on which the fulcrum finger (*B*) can rest. **B,** A finger of the nonoperating hand (*A*) placed in the vestibule to serve as a stable area on which the fulcrum finger (*B*) can rest.

Once the clinician masters the concepts of the modified pen grasp and the fulcrum, the remaining principles of instrumentation pertain to applying the working end of the instrument to the individual tooth surface. To begin with, the correct end of the instrument must be identified. Figure 14-27 illustrates that the clinician recognizes the correct end by holding the instrument with the toe pointed into the interproximal and looking for parallelism of the terminal shank and the proximal surface. When the wrong end is chosen, the terminal shank will be perpendicular to the proximal surface.

Adaptation refers to the relation of the working end to the tooth surface. The primary goal of adaptation is to keep the instrument tip in continuous contact with the surface during each successive instrument stroke. To accomplish this, the tip must be adapted to the varying contours of each surface, as well as to periodontal structures, by rolling the handle between the index finger and thumb. The instrument tip must be in continual contact with the tooth surface around the circumference of the tooth. Each stroke overlaps the previous one to ensure complete coverage of the surface. If the instrument is not adequately rolled around the line angle, the tip projects away from the root surface and into the gingival tissue, causing trauma. An improperly adapted tip may cause the clinician to miss deposits on the root surface, especially in any root depressions or grooves.

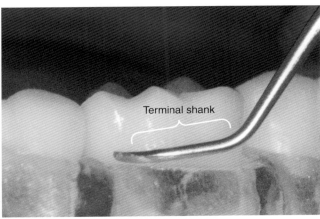

A   **B**

Figure 14-27. Identifying the correct working end of the instrument. A, With the toe of the instrument directed into the interproximal space, the terminal portion of the shank is parallel to the long axis of the tooth. **B,** If using the wrong end of the instrument, the terminal shank is perpendicular to the long axis of the tooth, even though the toe is directed toward the interproximal space.

Knowledge of dental anatomy, particularly root anatomy, is essential to proper instrument adaptation. Longitudinal depressions are common on proximal root surfaces. The furcations of multirooted teeth and the depressions leading from the cementoenamel junction to the furca are among the most difficult areas to instrument. Figure 14-28, which shows a curette adapted to a proximal root surface of a premolar, demonstrates the challenge posed in these procedures. When the tip is not visible during subgingival instrumentation, the clinician uses the position of the terminal shank as a visual cue to judge the working end.

Angulation describes the relation of the face of the instrument tip and the tooth surface (see Fig. 14-28).

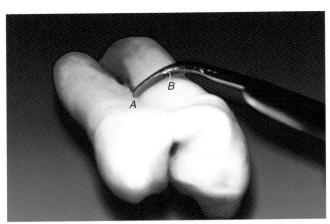

Figure 14-28. Curette adapted to root surface. *A,* Furcations and depressions of multirooted teeth are some of the most difficult areas to instrument. *B,* Angulation, the relation of the face of the blade to the tooth surface, in this case, is approximately 60 degrees.

Moving the instrument toward or away from the tooth surface by pivoting on the fulcrum modifies angulation. Proper angulation of an instrument during the stroke, also called *working angulation,* is greater than 45 degrees and less than 90 degrees. The ideal angle for scaling is approximately 88 degrees. For root planing strokes, angulation ranges from 80 to 45 degrees, gradually reduced as the surface becomes smoother. When the face is parallel to the tooth surface, angulation is 0 degree or *closed.* Closed angulation is acceptable for exploratory strokes used to locate calculus deposits with an instrument; it is also appropriate for initial insertion of the instrument into the periodontal pocket. However, using angulation of less than 40 degrees to remove deposits is futile at best and may result in producing a burnished deposit that is quite difficult to remove. Angulation is described as *open* when the face is 90 degrees or greater to the tooth surface. Open angulation can gouge the root surface and places the opposite (nonworking) cutting edge against the pocket wall where it can traumatize tissue. Figure 14-29 compares the variations in angulation of the working end.

The clinician also must rely on the position of the terminal shank to judge proper angulation because the face cannot be seen during scaling and root planing procedures. The visual cue of the terminal shank for angulation is the degree of parallelism with the tooth surface. Figure 14-30 compares the possible relations between the terminal shank and the tooth surface, and the angulation each represents.

Activation is the motion of the hand pivoting on the fulcrum that produces an instrument stroke. The clinician activates an instrument with wrist-arm motions that roll from the fulcrum finger (Fig. 14-31). Rotary wrist motion

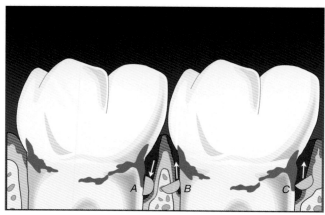

Figure 14-29. Angulation. The angle of the face of the instrument to the tooth surface is either (A) closed, nearing 0 degree; (B) open, greater than 90 degrees; or (C) working, more than 45 degrees but less than 90 degrees.

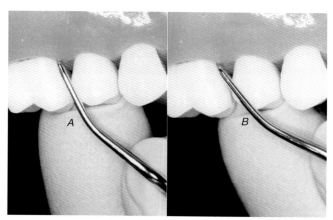

Figure 14-30. Terminal shank position as a visual cue to angulation. When the face of the instrument is not visible (subgingival), the terminal shank position with the tooth surface is used to determine angulation. A, Terminal shank is parallel to mesial surface, indicating correct angulation. B, Terminal shank is not parallel, indicating angulation of more than 90 degrees.

involves rotating the forearm to turn the instrument on the fulcrum in much the same way as one turns a doorknob. Wrist flexion is movement of the hand at the wrist as done in waving or painting with a brush. Fingers alone are not used to activate the instrument stroke because finger movements use smaller, less powerful muscles, produce a limited range of motion, and do not engage the fulcrum.

The pressure exerted against the fulcrum is a critical component of activation. If too little pressure is used, leverage is compromised. Use of heavy pressure results in patient discomfort and clinician fatigue. The clinician generally applies moderate pressure on the fulcrum

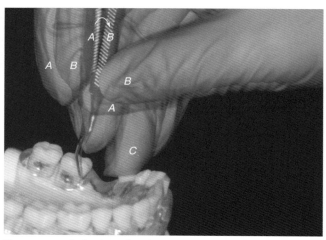

Figure 14-31. Activation of an instrument. A, Hand and instrument position at the beginning of a stroke and (B) as the stroke is completed. The instrument is activated with wrist-forearm rotation pivoting on the (C) fulcrum. Note that the position of fingers in the grasp does not change because no finger motion is used.

during activation, adjusting it as needed according to the treatment.

The *stroke* is the single movement in one direction of an instrument that carries out the function of the instrument. During the stroke, force is transmitted to the working end from pivoting on the fulcrum, which is referred to as *lateral pressure*. The clinician modifies lateral pressure according to the procedure. Short, forceful strokes are used to cleave a ledge or larger deposit of calculus. Removal of softer calculus or stain requires less force and slightly longer strokes. Root planing strokes use significantly less lateral pressure to minimize the amount of root structure removed. Instrument strokes are defined and described in several other ways.

Instrument strokes classified by task or function are exploratory, scaling and root planing. An *exploratory stroke* is movement of an instrument for detection of deposits or identification of structures. This examining or feeling stroke uses a light grasp and light lateral pressure so that vibrations and other tactile stimuli are transmitted from the working end to the fingers. *Scaling* is the removal of plaque, calculus, and stain from crown and root surfaces of teeth.[41] A scaling stroke uses a firm grasp and moderate to moderately heavy lateral pressure, depending on the extent of calculus. *Root planing* is removal of plaque, residual calculus, and contaminated surface root structure until the tooth surface is compatible with gingival health. Root planing strokes use decreasing lateral pressure and increasing stroke length as the surface becomes smoother.

The direction of instrument stroke is designated by relation to the long axis of the tooth. Figure 14-32 shows

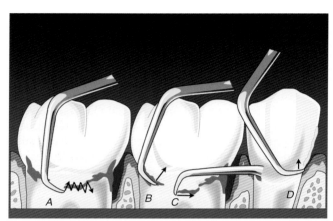

Figure 14-32. Direction of instrument strokes. *A,* Walking stroke used for detection of calculus. Tip moves apically and coronally with slight spacing between strokes. *B,* Oblique stroke. *C,* Horizontal stroke, perpendicular to the long axis of the tooth. When the stroke is longer and continues around the line angles, it is a circumferential stroke. *D,* Vertical stroke, parallel to the long axis of the tooth.

vertical, oblique, horizontal, and circumferential strokes. Horizontal strokes are directed toward tissue and are reserved for procedures using light pressure or maximum control of the instrument. Scaling, which involves greater lateral pressure, usually uses vertical and oblique strokes. Instrument strokes also may be described as pull, push, and walking. A pull stroke moves the instrument coronally away from the gingiva. Push strokes, which move the instrument apically toward the gingiva, are rarely used in periodontal procedures because of the risk for soft tissue

injury. A walking stroke (also diagramed in Fig. 14-32) moves the instrument in both directions with little distance between each stroke. Typically, a clinician uses a walking stroke with the periodontal probe and the explorer.

Each stroke during instrumentation should overlap the previous one to ensure that no portion of the tooth surface is missed. Moreover, effective instrument strokes must cover the tooth surface completely from the junctional epithelium to the gingival margin. For this reason, insertion is another important element of adaptation. The goal of insertion is to ensure that the instrument tip reaches the most apical portion of the sulcus or periodontal pocket. To reach the base of the pocket, the toe of the instrument is inserted first and then lightly pushed toward the bottom of the pocket until contact with soft tissue. Proper insertion is often described as "leading with the tip" because of this process. Another way to describe insertion is by orientation of the tip in relation to the apex of the tooth. Correct tip position is designated as apically directed—that is, the instrument tip is angled slightly toward the base of the pocket. Incorrect tip direction allows the back of the instrument to touch the junctional epithelium first, with the instrument tip pointed up and away from the base of the pocket, which transmits the same sensation of reaching a tissue barrier to the grasp fingers. With the working end under the free gingiva, the clinician must rely on visual cues from the terminal shank to determine the orientation of the tip (Fig. 14-33). The terminal shank is parallel with the long axis of the tooth when the instrument tip is accurately positioned. Figure 14-33 also demonstrates the importance of tip

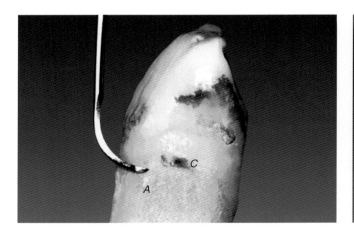

A

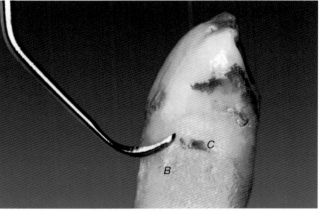

B

Figure 14-33. Terminal shank position as a visual cue to orientation of the tip. **A,** When the terminal shank is parallel to the long axis of the tooth, the tip is directed apically. In this position, the tip will encounter the calculus deposit (*C*) as it moves toward the midline of the proximal surface. **B,** When the terminal shank is not parallel to the long axis of the tooth, the tip is improperly oriented. Note that the calculus deposit (*C*) likely will be missed with the instrument stroke.

position in detection and removal of calculus. Proper tip direction is critical for complete deposit removal.

THE PROCESS OF NONSURGICAL PERIODONTAL THERAPY

The clinician is prepared to undertake initial periodontal therapy with an understanding of the principles for use of periodontal instruments. Following is one strategy for implementing instrumentation. Determine the region of the dentition that is to be treated and position the patient appropriately. Review the condition of the periodontium in the selected region using the patient's dental chart and the periodontal probe. If conditions indicate, start with subgingival debridement procedures using either powered or manual instruments. Once debridement is completed, the clinician undertakes more definitive treatment of each tooth, surface by surface. To begin, use an exploratory stroke with either an explorer or a curette to locate remaining calculus. When a deposit is discovered, place the tip of an area-specific or universal curette on the outermost edge, tighten the grasp, establish the cutting edge at an 88-degree angle to the surface, apply appropriate pressure to the fulcrum and activate a scaling stroke to dislodge the deposit. Continue successive overlapping strokes along the remainder of the deposit until no obvious calculus is detectable on this surface. At this point, residual calculus, altered cementum, and attached plaque should be removed from the entire surface with an area-specific curette using root planing strokes, reduced angulation, and less lateral pressure. The clinician must be thorough during this phase of instrumentation but also cautious not to over instrument. Go to the next surface, repeating the process until the entire tooth has been treated. Evaluate the surface initially for smoothness with an explorer. Irrigate the pocket thoroughly and compress the tissue for 15 to 30 seconds to stop bleeding. Finally, assess the immediate tissue response, identifying continued bleeding, remaining epithelial tissue tags, and change in color. The ultimate evaluation of successful treatment occurs after a 4- to 6-week period to allow inflammation to resolve and healing to occur.

During instrumentation, the clinician maintains a mental image of the expected contours of the tooth surface, interprets tactile sensations transmitted through the instrument, and uses visual cues from the terminal instrument shank while moving the instrument around the circumference of the tooth inside the periodontal pocket. The process actually is as difficult as the description makes it sound. Development of the skills to accomplish effective scaling and root planing requires time, diligence, persistence, patience, and concentration.

POWERED MECHANICAL INSTRUMENTATION

Powered scalers have been available for use as a part of nonsurgical periodontal therapy for many years. Initially advocated for the removal of gross supragingival calculus, powered scalers appealed to clinicians because of the speed of deposit removal and reduced clinician fatigue. Several reports indicate that the use of powered scalers for subgingival instrumentation produces similar results as hand instrumentation with regard to deposit removal and healing.[42-47] A distinct advantage associated with the use of powered instrumentation is the reduced time needed to produce equivalent clinical results.[44-49] Tip penetration approaches the apical portion of periodontal pockets with powered instrumentation[50] and may be improved with the use of small-diameter, extended shank tips.[51,52] In areas with anatomic challenges, such as Class II and III furcations, ultrasonic instrumentation may be superior to hand instrumentation.[53]

Sonic and Ultrasonic Scalers

Powered instruments used for periodontal debridement can be classified into two groups on the basis of their operating frequencies: sonic and ultrasonic. Sonic scalers operate at a relatively low frequency of 3000 to 8000 cycles per second and are driven by compressed air from the dental unit. A rotor system is activated to vibrate the tip that is within the audible range for patients. The stroke pattern of sonic scalers is elliptical to orbital, and all surfaces of the tip may be adapted to root surfaces. Ultrasonic scalers can be further categorized into magnetostrictive and piezoelectric, on the basis of the mechanism used to convert the electrical current used for energy to activate the tips. Magnetostrictive ultrasonics operate inaudibly and transfer electrical energy to metal stacks made of nickel–iron alloy or to a ferrous rod (Fig. 14-34). Electrical energy applied to the magnetostrictive insert changes its shape resulting in vibrations. The tip vibrates in an elliptical to orbital motion at 18,000 to 42,000 kHz (cycles per second). As a result, all surfaces of the tip may be useful in debridement. Piezoelectric scalers (Fig. 14-35) also are inaudible, operating within a range of 24,000 to 45,000 kHz. This type of powered scaler uses electrical energy to activate crystals within the handpiece to vibrate the tip. In contrast to the magnetostrictive scalers, the motion of the tip is linear in nature resulting in activation of mainly the lateral surfaces of the tip.

Ultrasonic scalers may be tuned manually or automatically. Both types have controls to adjust power and water, whereas the manually tuned units require adjustments for fluctuations in frequency. The power setting determines the length of the stroke and is generally kept to a low or medium setting for patient comfort. The water

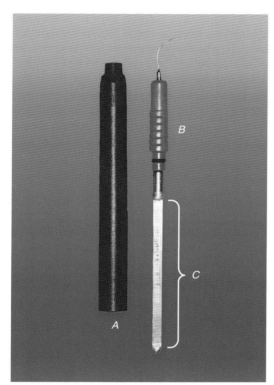

Figure 14-34. Magnetostrictive ultrasonic handpiece. *A*, The handpiece, which is hollow, attaches to the unit by way of water tubing and detaches for sterilization. *B*, The tip is carried on a removable insert. *C*, The metal stack to which energy is transmitted to move the tip.

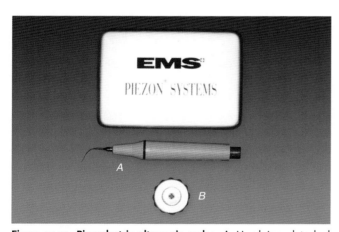

Figure 14-35. Piezoelectric ultrasonic scaler. *A*, Handpiece detached from the unit. *B*, Wrench for attaching and removing tips from the handpiece. The handpiece detaches from the water tubing for sterilization. The tip attaches directly to the handpiece.

flow is essential to dissipate the heat produced by the vibration of the tip. Although most disruption and removal of subgingival deposits is accomplished through the vibration of the oscillating tip, the water spray produced

by the use of sonic and ultrasonic instruments also plays an important role in debridement. The water creates a lavage effect, as well as acoustical streaming, acoustic turbulence, and cavitation.[54] Cavitation results from the implosion of bubbles created as water passes through the handpiece producing shock waves that may alter or kill bacteria. Acoustic turbulence and acoustical streaming occur when water exits the tip creating an agitating effect or unidirectional flow that is deleterious to periodontal pathogens.

Sonic and Ultrasonic Tips

Various tips are available for use with sonic and ultrasonics scalers. Sonic scalers have a limited selection of tips attached to the handpiece with a special instrument. Tips for sonic scalers possess straight shanks with relatively large diameters and are provided in a sickle-shaped, universal, or an extended-length periodontal tip (Fig. 14-36). Ultrasonic scalers offer a wider variety of tips ranging from a large-diameter, straight universal tip (Fig. 14-37) for supragingival calculus removal to a thin, smaller diameter straight, right, or left tip for subgingival instrumentation (Fig. 14-38). Tips for magnetostrictive ultrasonic scalers have internal or external water delivery, whereas all piezoelectric ultrasonic scaler tips have internal water delivery. Ultrasonic tips vary in size and shape for a variety of uses and tooth surfaces. Tips will shorten in length because of wear and should be examined periodically for replacement. In addition, the metal stacks in magnetostrictive ultrasonic tips should closely approximate each other without separation or splaying.

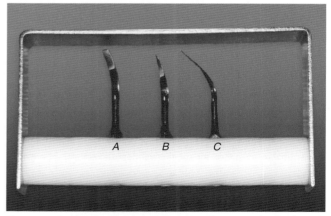

Figure 14-36. Tips for the sonic scaler. Tips have straight shanks with a somewhat wide diameter. *A*, Broad-tipped universal designed for removing supragingival calculus and stain from facial and lingual surfaces. *B*, Sickle-shaped tip designed for deposit removal on proximal surfaces. *C*, Extended-length periodontal tip designed with a narrow tip for subgingival scaling.

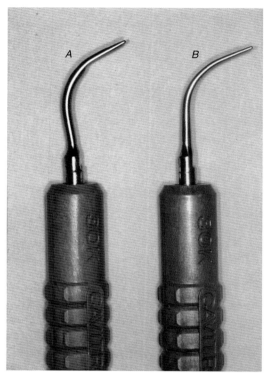

Figure 14-37. Inserts for ultrasonic scaler. *A*, Straight universal tip designed for supragingival deposit removal. *B*, Straight tip designed for subgingival deposit removal, with longer, thinner tip.

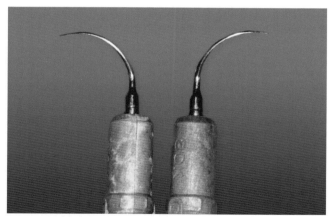

Figure 14-38. Paired inserts for ultrasonic scaler. Right and left tips are mirror images, designed for subgingival deposit removal on proximal surfaces.

Technique

The clinician position remains identical for powered mechanical instrumentation as described previously for manual instrumentation. The handpiece is held in a pen or modified pen grasp with light pressure allowing for optimal vibration of the tip. An intraoral or extraoral fulcrum is critical for control during instrumentation. Proper insertion requires the tip to be placed parallel to the root surface being instrumented to prevent damage to the root surface or adjacent soft tissue (Fig. 14-39). If the tip is angled in toward the root surface, the root will be gouged. If the tip is angled out toward the pocket or sulcus lining, soft tissue damage will occur. Continuous movement in an overall coronal–apical direction is accomplished with overlapping strokes that may be vertical, oblique, or horizontal. When using right and left tips with offset angulations, care must be taken to ensure correct insert selection. For instrumentation of interproximal areas, the tip should be placed parallel with the root surface being instrumented as previously described (Fig. 14-40). For instrumentation of facial or lingual

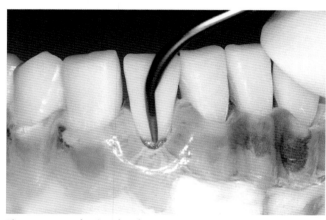

Figure 14-39. Adapting the ultrasonic tip. The tip of the insert, shown here on an anterior facial surface, is parallel with the tooth surface during instrumentation for access and to protect the tooth and gingival tissue.

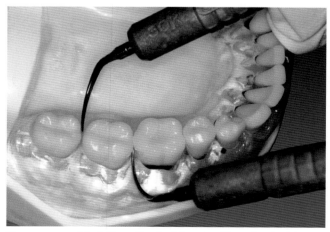

Figure 14-40. Adaptation of paired inserts. Tips of paired inserts adapt to contralateral tooth surfaces. Note that the tips are parallel to the proximal surfaces.

surfaces, the tip should be inserted so that the convex working surface of the tip is in contact with the root. Inappropriate positioning with the concave surface against the root may result in gouging or damage to the root surface. Constant movement with an appropriately adapted tip with minimal lateral pressure produces optimal results with little or no damage.

Contraindications

Contraindications to powered instrumentation include both dental and medical concerns. Dental concerns are site specific and include instrumentation in areas of demineralization that may result in extensive removal of tooth structure and subsequent hypersensitivity. In addition, it is possible that the use of powered instrumentation may adversely affect the marginal integrity of certain restorations. Powered instrumentation is contraindicated in patients with dental implants, except with the use of special tips designed to prevent damage to the implant surface (Fig. 14-41). Medical contraindications include patients with cardiac pacemakers, especially those placed before the mid-1980s that are subject to electromagnetic interference from ultrasonic devices. Patients with significant respiratory problems may be intolerant to aerosol

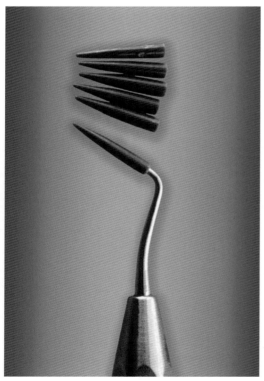

Figure 14-41. Ultrasonic tips for implants. Tips that are specially designed to protect the implant surface from the pitting and scratching that a conventional tip produces.

production during powered instrumentation despite the use of high volume evacuation. Patients with infectious diseases that may be transmitted through aerosol production are also poor candidates for powered debridement.

POLISHING

Traditionally, polishing of exposed tooth surfaces with a soft rubber cup and abrasive follows scaling and root planing. The primary objective of polishing is the removal of extrinsic stain and supragingival plaque. The rationale for this procedure includes improving the appearance of the dentition, demonstrating a standard of oral cleanliness for the patient to attain on a daily basis, and motivating the patient to improve plaque control, as well as the belief that the outcome of a quality periodontal service should be a plaque-free mouth. However, the therapeutic benefit of polishing is uncertain, because plaque re-forms within 24 hours.

A number of side effects associated with polishing have been documented. Because polishing involves the use of an abrasive, a microscopic amount of tooth structure is lost during the process.[55] For this reason, polishing may not be appropriate for the patient at risk for caries because the outer tooth surface is protected by exposure to fluoride. Such a loss of tooth structure also may be significant as it accumulates over a lifetime from repeated polishing. Abrasion of the tooth surface occurs at a much faster rate when it involves carious or demineralized enamel or root structure, which is about half as calcified as enamel.[56,57] Therefore, routine polishing is contraindicated on decalcified enamel and exposed root surfaces.

After polishing, tooth surfaces actually may be rougher because the abrasives used in prophylaxis pastes are harder than those in dentifrices used daily by the patient. Indeed, scratches made during polishing are visible with magnification. Absence of plaque and stain then should preclude polishing. Likewise, many restorative materials may be easily damaged by abrasives and should not be polished.

The abrasive particles in prophylaxis pastes can enter gingival tissue without an intact epithelial barrier, a frequent result of periodontal instrumentation. Delayed healing or a foreign body reaction may result. For this reason, polishing is often delayed after nonsurgical periodontal procedures until gingival healing has occurred.

Finally, aerosol and splatter formed during polishing procedures pose a challenge to infection control. The clinician should consider this when planning treatment for a patient with compromised health or for a patient at high risk for infectious disease.

Use of appropriate methods neutralizes some of the disadvantages of polishing. Operating the slow-speed handpiece at less than 20,000 revolutions per minute decreases abrasion. Lower speed also prohibits excessive heat caused by friction that can damage the pulp. To decrease heat production and the rate of abrasion, apply only slight intermittent pressure during polishing, just enough to flare the rubber cup to adapt to the tooth surface. Fine particle size in abrasives or polishing paste removes the least amount of tooth structure. Use caution to keep the rotating cup away from the gingival margin where it can abrade and burn the tissue.

Selective polishing is a treatment approach that prevents such complications and side effects. Using this philosophy, polishing is reserved for only those teeth with obvious stain remaining after scaling and is limited to intact enamel surfaces. In other words, polishing is not automatically implemented but is provided for those patients with a specific need. If necessary, stain can be removed with manual instruments and plaque can be removed with toothbrushing.

Figure 14-42 demonstrates application of the rubber cup to the tooth surface. After distributing a small amount of prophylaxis paste over the tooth surfaces in a working area, the rotating rubber cup is moved away from the gingiva and across the tooth surface in a systematic way. Irrigate completed areas periodically to rinse away the polishing preparation and keep the field clear. After the procedure, use dental floss to remove any remaining abrasive particles from between the teeth.

An automated polishing method, sometimes called air-powder polishing or jet polishing, has been available for the past three decades. This method uses finely powdered sodium bicarbonate as the abrasive, which is delivered under pressure through the narrow nozzle of a specialized handpiece surrounded by a mist of warm water. The resulting slurry is propelled against the tooth surface to remove plaque and extrinsic stain by mechanical abrasion. The advantage is a remarkably thorough process of deposit removal accomplished in minimal time, although no long-term effect on oral health status has been shown.[58,59] The abrasive is quite fine and, despite the pressure of application, results in minimal loss of enamel when used according to the manufacturer's directions. However, significant loss of root structure may occur even with careful use. For patients with gingival recession who elect stain removal for esthetic reasons, air-powder polishing removes less tooth structure than manual instruments.[60]

The disadvantages of air-powder polishing include the creation of a significant aerosol, epithelial abrasion when applied too close to the gingival margin, a salty taste, and a mild stinging sensation in other areas of the mouth caused by the deflected spray. Air-powder polishing is contraindicated for patients on a sodium-restricted diet, for patients with respiratory illness, for patients who wear contact lenses, on composite restorations, around the margins of cast restorations, and on demineralized enamel.[61-63]

Using proper technique with this polishing method minimizes side effects and prevents patient injury. The handpiece is held with a modified pen grasp but a fulcrum is not essential because no pressure is required during a stroke. The tip is positioned 4 to 5 mm away from the tooth surface and is kept in constant motion using circular, brushlike strokes directed at the middle third of the anatomic crown. The spray is directed at an 80-degree angle to facial and lingual surfaces of posterior teeth and at a 60-degree angle for anterior teeth (Fig. 14-43). A 90-degree angle is used only on occlusal surfaces.

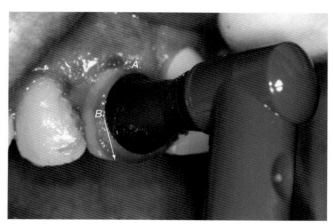

Figure 14-42. Rubber cup polishing. *A,* The apical (gingival) edge of the rubber cup flared to reach the cervical area without traumatizing the marginal gingiva. *B,* The movement of the rubber cup is away from the gingiva.

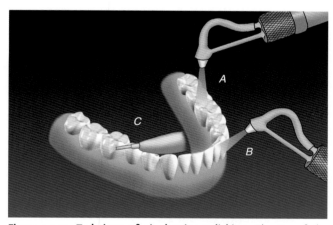

Figure 14-43. Technique of air-abrasive polishing. The tip of the polishing device is held 4 to 5 mm from the tooth and moved continuously. The spray is directed (*A*) at a 90-degree angle to occlusal surfaces, (*B*) 60 degrees to facial and lingual surfaces of anterior teeth, and (*C*) 80 degrees to facial and lingual surfaces of posterior teeth.

Polishing has limited benefit for periodontal health and potential adverse consequences. The clinician should explain the effects of this practice to the patient and discuss its use instead of reflexively proceeding. Promoting oral self-care may be a better investment of the clinician's time and effort.

INSTRUMENT SHARPENING

Sharp periodontal instruments are fundamental to successful nonsurgical procedures.[64,65] A clinician may precisely detect calculus on tooth surfaces and perfectly apply principles of instrumentation but will fail to thoroughly remove the deposit if the instrument is dull. Sharp instruments remove calculus more completely with fewer strokes, create smoother root surfaces, improve tactile sensitivity, require less lateral pressure, increase control of strokes, and reduce clinician fatigue.

The cutting edge of a periodontal instrument is formed by the intersection of the face and the lateral surface of the working end. This intersection of two planes is a line, which by definition has no width. This knifelike edge dulls or flattens to a rounded surface during scaling and root planing. Consequently, sharpening of instruments is an integral component of nonsurgical periodontal therapy, necessary both before and during patient treatment.

The goal of instrument sharpening is to recreate a sharp edge while maintaining the original shape of the instrument. Sharpening is accomplished by the removal of metal along the lateral surface with a sharpening stone to restore the cutting edge to a sharp line. The primary objective is to maintain the 60- to 70-degree internal angle of the blade (see Figs. 14-8 and 14-9).

A number of sharpening devices have been developed, but the simplest, most efficient, and cost-effective method for manual scaling instruments remains manual sharpening with a stone. The armamentarium for this procedure (Fig. 14-44) includes a flat stone, a cylindrical or conical stone, a lubricant for the stone, sterile gauze to clean debris from the working end after sharpening, magnification to observe the cutting edge, a plastic test stick to evaluate sharpness, and a source of adequate lighting, usually the dental lamp.

Instrument sharpness can be evaluated in one of two ways. The first method is to inspect the working end with the aid of magnification and bright illumination. A sharp instrument reflects light along the cutting edge. Light does not reflect from a dull cutting edge because the surface is a flat plane. The other method is to test the cutting edge using working angulation against an acrylic or plastic rod. A sharp instrument sticks or catches when using light pressure.

Several types of stones are available for dental instrument sharpening—for example, natural mineral stones,

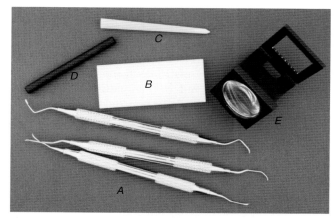

Figure 14-44. Armamentarium for instrument sharpening. *A*, Sterile instruments. *B*, Flat sharpening stone. *C*, Conical sharpening stone. *D*, Plastic sharpening test stick. *E*, Magnification. Also needed, an appropriate lubricant for the stone, a wipe for the instrument, and a bright, direct source of light.

such as the hard Arkansas stone, and manufactured stones like the ruby or ceramic stone (Fig. 14-45). Natural stones must be lubricated with oil before sharpening to prevent metal particles from embedding the surface. Artificial stones are made of hard substances containing abrasive particles, which include aluminum oxide, silicon dioxide, diamond, or carborundum. These stones are lubricated with water to reduce frictional heat that may alter the instrument's metal. Sharpening stones are available in different grades of abrasiveness. Fine stones are preferred because less metal is removed from the instrument during sharpening. Medium grit stones are used only to recontour instruments.

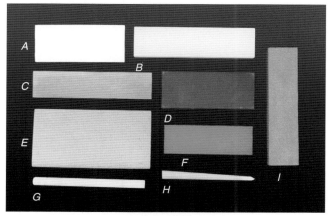

Figure 14-45. Sharpening stones. *A*, Ceramic; (*B*) synthetic aluminum oxide; (*C*) Arkansas hard; (*D*) carborundum stone; (*E*) Arkansas wedge shaped; (*F*) India oil stone (medium grit); (*G*) ceramic cylindrical; (*H*) Arkansas conical; (*I*) India oil stone (fine grit) sharpening stones.

Two approaches are possible for manual sharpening, the moving stone–stationary instrument method or the moving instrument–stationary stone method. The basic principles of sharpening are the same regardless of the method used. Both the instrument and the sharpening stone must be stabilized to maintain precise angles and the shape of the working end during the process. Figure 14-46 shows the palm grasp used to control the instrument and the firm grasp of the stone needed to move it evenly along the instrument. To attain even greater stability during sharpening, the clinician should rest the forearms against a fixed surface such as a cabinet or brace elbows against the body to steady the arms.

Figures 14-47 and 14-48 illustrate the application of the sharpening stone to the blade of a sickle scaler and a universal curette. The face of the blade is held so that it is parallel with the floor. Then the stone is aligned with the lateral surface to create a supplementary angle of 100 to 110 degrees to the internal angle. This angle is easily established by finding first a 90-degree angle and then rotating the stone 10 to 20 degrees. This concept is illustrated in the diagrams with the aid of an imaginary clock face. Twelve o'clock is located on the terminal

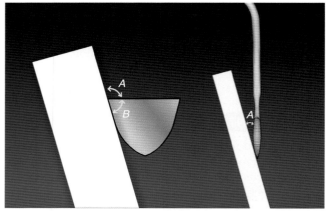

Figure 14-47. Sharpening technique for the sickle scaler. The angle (*A*) formed by the face of the blade with the surface of the sharpening stone is 100 to 110 degrees. This angle maintains the internal angle of the blade (*B*), which is 70 to 80 degrees. *A* and *B* are supplementary angles, totaling 180 degrees. Both cutting edges must be sharpened on the sickle scaler.

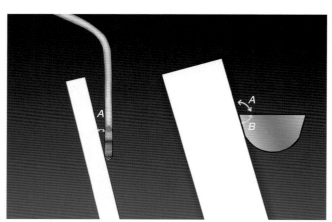

Figure 14-48. Sharpening technique for the curette. The angle (*A*) formed by the face of the blade with the surface of the sharpening stone is 100 to 110 degrees. This angle maintains the internal angle of the blade (*B*), which is 70 to 80 degrees. *A* and *B* are supplementary angles, totaling 180 degrees. Both cutting edges must be sharpened on the universal curette. The tip of the instrument should remain rounded.

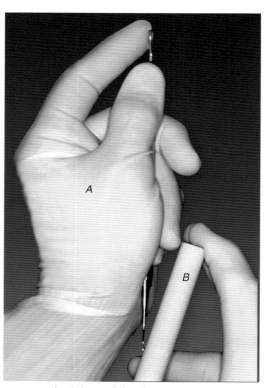

Figure 14-46. Maintaining stability during sharpening. To maintain control during sharpening, (*A*) the instrument is held with the palm grasp. *B*, The stone is held firmly at both ends so that it does not move unevenly during sharpening strokes.

shank, which is perpendicular to the face, and the stone is angled to either 11 or 1 o'clock, depending on which edge is being sharpened.

The stone is moved up and down with short strokes and light pressure to reduce the lateral surface until a knifelike edge is reproduced. Formation of a wire edge, defined as tiny bits of metal projecting from the cutting edge, is prevented by ending with a downward stroke of the stone. If a wire edge is detected after sharpening, it is removed with a cylindrical or conical stone (Fig. 14-49). The stone is placed in full contact with the face and both

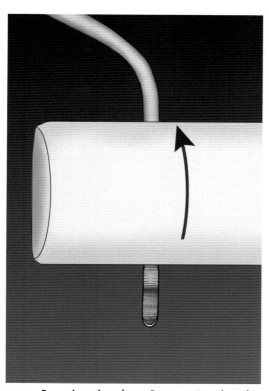

Figure 14-49. Removing wire edges. Remove wire edges that sometimes form along the cutting edge during sharpening with a cylindrical or conical stone. The entire face and both cutting edges must contact the stone to preserve the contour of the blade. The stone is rotated toward the terminal shank while moving along the length of the blade.

cutting edges. Using light pressure, the stone is rotated toward the heel while being moved toward the toe of the instrument. One or two such strokes are sufficient to abrade the wire edge.

Begin sharpening by placing the stone near the heel of the working end and move it toward the toe. Because the blade curves or tapers toward the toe, the stone can engage only a segment of the cutting edge at a time (see Figs. 14-47 and 14-48). Figure 14-50 depicts the many positions of the sharpening stone as it is adapted uniformly along the full length of the cutting edge to preserve the contour of the cutting edge. For the sickle scaler, this means maintaining the pointed toe as shown in Figure 14-47. Retaining the rounded toe of the curette is somewhat more challenging. Note that sharpening strokes shown in Figure 14-50 extend completely around the toe to the opposite edge. In addition, the toe of a curette has a 45-degree bevel that must be conserved. Figure 14-50 shows both the bevel of the curette toe and the 135-degree angle of the stone necessary to maintain both the toe and the bevel. The area-specific curette has only one cutting edge to sharpen, but the extremely curved cutting edge presents difficulty (Fig. 14-50). Many

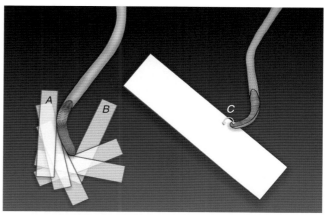

Figure 14-50. Sharpening the area-specific curette. Only the single cutting edge of an area-specific curette is sharpened, as shown on the left. Sharpening strokes begin (*A*) at the heel and continue along the curved cutting edge around (*B*) the toe. To maintain (*C*) the 45-degree bevel of the toe of the curette, the angle of the face to the stone is adjusted to 135 degrees.

narrow strokes of the straight stone are needed to retain the shape of the cutting edge.

Abrading the face of the instrument with a round stone could achieve a sharp edge, but this method weakens the instrument and can result in a broken tip instrument when scaling pressure is applied. Figure 14-51 illustrates how removing metal from the face of a sickle scaler or a curette reduces the dimension of the blade in the same

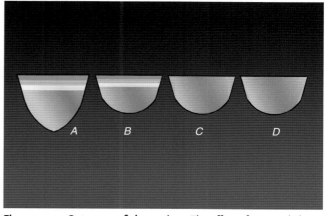

Figure 14-51. Outcomes of sharpening. The effect of repeated sharpening of the face of (*A*) the sickle scaler and (*B*) a curette. Metal removed weakens the instrument. *C*, Instrument sharpened with the stone at a 90-degree angle to the face, increasing the internal angle so that proper angulation is difficult to achieve and complete calculus removal will be difficult. *D*, Instrument sharpened with an angle of greater than 110 degrees, creating an acute internal angle that may scratch or gouge the tooth surface and will dull rapidly during use.

direction as force is applied during instrumentation. The drawing also shows the effects of improper sharpening. When the stone is applied to the face at an angle less than 100 degrees, the internal angle created is increased. The effect is similar to using a dull instrument. Deposit removal is more difficult and the natural reaction of the clinician is to increase lateral pressure. Calculus is more likely to be burnished than dislodged by the instrument. When the stone is applied to the lateral surface of the blade at an angle greater than 110 degrees, the internal angle is reduced to less than 60 degrees. This more acute angle may penetrate the root surface, producing a rougher surface. Furthermore, this angle dulls easily during instrumentation, shortening the lifespan of the instrument.

Sharpening is the primary cause of instrument wear; therefore, any scaling instrument has limited usefulness. With each sharpening, the width of the working end is reduced. As the blade narrows, strength of the instrument decreases and breaking the tip is more likely. Some clinicians use multiples of the same curette, selecting a different working end width depending on the task. For example, newer curettes may be used for initial deposit removal and narrower curettes may be used for root planing. Before patient treatment, the condition of the instruments should be assessed to determine if the instrument is suitable for the amount, tenacity, and location of the deposit to be removed.

Sharpening skills, like instrumentation skills, develop with practice. Both are essential to quality initial periodontal therapy.

Acknowledgments

The authors thank and recognize Patti Haskins, Computer Graphics Specialist, Media Resources, Baylor College of Dentistry, TAMUS Health Science Center, for her contributions. Patti tweaked our photographs, amended our mistakes, and put our ideas into a visual form, making this a much better work than it would have been without her. Patti worked with us graciously and cheerfully for more than half a year while she underwent surgery, chemotherapy, and radiation treatments in a courageous battle against breast cancer. We appreciate and admire her good humor, talent, and patience and wish her God speed on the road to recovery.

REFERENCES

1. Doungudomdacha S, Rawlinson A, Walsh TF, Douglas CW: Effect of non-surgical periodontal treatment on clinical parameters and the numbers of Porphyromonas gingivalis, Prevotella intermedia and Actinobacillus actinomycetemcomitans at adult periodontitis sites, *J Clin Periodontol* 28:437-445, 2001.
2. Cugini MA, Haffajee AD, Smith C et al: The effect of scaling and root planing on the clinical and microbiological parameters of periodontal diseases: 12-month results, *J Clin Periodontol* 27:30-36, 2000.
3. Haffajee AD, Cugini MA, Dibart S et al: The effect of SRP on the clinical and microbiological parameters of periodontal diseases, *J Clin Periodontol* 24:324-334, 1997.
4. Renvert S, Wikstrom M, Dahlen G et al: Effect of root debridement on the elimination of Actinobacillus actinomycetemcomitans and Bacteroides gingivalis from periodontal pockets, *J Clin Periodontol* 17:345-350, 1990.
5. Mousques T, Listgarten MA, Phillips RW: Effect of scaling and root planing on the composition of the human subgingival microbial flora, *J Periodont Res* 15:144-151, 1980.
6. Tuter G, Kurtis B, Serdar M: Effects of phase I periodontal treatment on gingival crevicular fluid levels of matrix metalloproteinase-1 and tissue inhibitor of metalloproteinase-1, *J Periodontol* 73:487-493, 2002.
7. Lowenguth RA, Greenstein G: Clinical and microbiological response to nonsurgical mechanical periodontal therapy, *Periodontol 2000* 9:14-22, 1995.
8. Shiloah J, Patters MR: Repopulation of periodontal pockets by microbial pathogens in the absence of supportive therapy, *J Periodontol* 67:130-139, 1996.
9. Cobb CM: Clinical significance of non-surgical periodontal therapy: an evidence-based perspective of scaling and root planing, *J Clin Periodontol* 29(Suppl 2):6-16, 2002.
10. Cobb CM: Non-surgical pocket therapy: mechanical, *Ann Periodontol* 1(1):443-490, 1996.
11. Caffesse RG, Sweeney PL, Smith BA: Scaling and root planing with and without periodontal flap surgery, *J Clin Periodontol* 13:205-210, 1986.
12. Sherman PR, Hutchens LH Jr, Jewson LG: The effectiveness of subgingival scaling and root planing. II. Clinical responses related to residual calculus, *J Periodontol* 61:9-15, 1990.
13. Drisko CH: Initial preparation: anti-infective therapy, *Alpha Omegan* 93(4):43-50, 2000.
14. Fleischer HC, Mellonig JT, Brayer WK et al: Scaling and root planing efficacy in multirooted teeth, *J Periodontol* 60:402-409, 1989.
15. Buchanan SA, Robertson PB: Calculus removal by scaling/root planing with and without surgical access, *J Periodontol* 58:159-163, 1987.
16. Rabbani GM, Ash MM Jr, Caffesse RG: The effectiveness of subgingival scaling and root planing in calculus removal, *J Periodontol* 52:119-123, 1981.
17. Oberholzer R, Rateitschak KH: Root cleaning or root smoothing. An in vivo study, *J Clin Periodontol* 23:326-330, 1996.
18. Khatiblou FA, Ghodssi A: Root surface smoothness or roughness in periodontal treatment. A clinical study, *J Periodontol* 54:365-367, 1983.

19. Rosenberg RM, Ash MM Jr: The effect of root roughness on plaque accumulation and gingival inflammation, *J Periodontol* 45:146-150, 1974.

20. Drisko CL, Cochran DL, Blieden T et al: Position paper: sonic and ultrasonic scalers in periodontics. Research, Science and Therapy Committee of the American Academy of Periodontology, *J Periodontol* 71:1792-1801, 2000.

21. Nyman S, Westfelt E, Sarhed G, Karring T: Role of "diseased" root cementum in healing following treatment of periodontal disease. A clinical study, *J Clin Periodontol* 15:464-468, 1988.

22. Nyman S, Sarhed G, Ericsson I et al: Role of "diseased" root cementum in healing following treatment of periodontal disease. An experimental study in the dog, *J Periodont Res* 21:496-503, 1986.

23. Mombelli A, Schmid B, Rutar A, Lang NP: Persistence patterns of Porphyromonas gingivalis, Prevotella intermedia/nigrescens, and Actinobacillus actinomyetemcomitans after mechanical therapy of periodontal disease, *J Periodontol* 71:14-21, 2000.

24. Rodenburg JP, Van Winkelhoff AJ, Winkel EG et al: Occurrence of Bacteroides gingivalis, Bacteroides intermedius and Actinobacillus actinomycetemcomitans in severe periodontitis in relation to age and treatment history, *J Clin Periodontol* 17:392-399, 1990.

25. Becker W, Becker BE, Caffesse R et al: A longitudinal study comparing scaling, osseous surgery, and modified Widman procedures: results after 5 years, *J Periodontol* 72:1675-1684, 2001.

26. Becker W, Becker BE, Ochsenbein C et al: A longitudinal study comparing scaling, osseous surgery and modified Widman procedures. Results after one year, *J Periodontol* 59:351-365, 1988.

27. Kaldahl WB, Kalkwarf KL, Patil KD et al: Long-term evaluation of periodontal therapy: I. Response to 4 therapeutic modalities, *J Periodontol* 67:93-102, 1996.

28. Kaldahl WB, Kalkwarf KL, Patil KD et al: Evaluation of four modalities of periodontal therapy. Mean probing depth, probing attachment level and recession changes, *J Periodontol* 59:783-793, 1988.

29. Ramfjord SP, Caffesse RG, Morrison EC et al: 4 modalities of periodontal treatment compared over 5 years, *J Clin Periodontol* 14:445-452, 1987.

30. Greenstein G, Rethman MP: Advantages and limitations of nonsurgical periodontal therapy in the management of chronic periodontitis, *Alpha Omegan* 93(4):34-42, 2000.

31. Greenstein G: Nonsurgical periodontal therapy in 2000: a literature review, *J Am Dent Assoc* 131:1580-1592, 2000.

32. Greenstein G: Periodontal response to mechanical nonsurgical therapy: a review, *J Periodontol* 63:118-130, 1992.

33. Greenstein G: Full-mouth therapy versus individual quadrant root planing: a critical commentary, *J Periodontol* 73:797-812, 2002.

34. De Soete M, Mongardini C, Peuwels M et al: One-stage full-mouth disinfection. Long-term microbiological results analyzed by checkerboard DNA-DNA hybridization, *J Periodontol* 72:374-382, 2001.

35. Mongardini C, van Steenberghe D, Dekeyser C, Quirynen M: One stage full- versus partial-mouth disinfection in the treatment of chronic adult or generalized early-onset periodontitis. I. Long-term clinical observations, *J Periodontol* 70:632-645, 1999.

36. Vandekerckhove BN, Bollen CM, Dekeyser C et al: Full- versus partial-mouth disinfection in the treatment of periodontal infections. Long-term clinical observations of a pilot study, *J Periodontol* 67:1251-1259, 1996.

37. Drisko CH: Nonsurgical periodontal therapy, *Periodontol 2000* 25:77-88, 2001.

38. Hardage JL, Gildersleeve JR, Rugh JD: Clinical work posture for the dentist: an electromyographic study, *J Am Dent Assoc* 107:937-939, 1983.

39. Oberg T, Karsznia A, Sandsjo L, Kadefors R: Work load, fatigue, and pause patterns in clinical dental hygiene, *J Dent Hyg* 69(5):223-229, 1995.

40. Akesson I, Hansson GA, Balogh I et al: Quantifying work load in neck, shoulders and wrists in female dentists, *Int Arch Occup Environ Health* 69:461-474, 1997.

41. *Glossary of periodontal terms*, ed 4, Chicago, 2001, American Academy of Periodontolgy.

42. Beuchat M, Busslinger A, Schmidlin PR et al: Clinical comparison of the effectiveness of novel sonic instruments and curettes for periodontal debridement after 2 months, *J Clin Periodontol* 28:1145-1150, 2001.

43. Boretti G, Zappa U, Graf H, Case D: Short-term effects of phase I therapy on crevicular cell populations, *J Periodontol* 66:235-240, 1995.

44. Laurell L, Pettersson B: Periodontal healing after treatment with either the Titan-S sonic scaler or hand instruments, *Swed Dent J* 12(5):187-192, 1988.

45. Badersten A, Nilveus R, Egelberg J: Effect of nonsurgical periodontal therapy. III. Single versus repeated instrumentation, *J Clin Periodontol* 11:114-124, 1984.

46. Badersten A, Nilveus R, Egelberg J: Effect of nonsurgical periodontal therapy. I. Moderately advanced periodontitis, *J Clin Periodontol* 8:57-72, 1981.

47. Torfason T, Kiger R, Selvig KA, Egelberg J: Clinical improvement of gingival conditions following ultrasonic versus hand instrumentation of periodontal pockets, *J Clin Periodontol* 6:165-176, 1979.

48. Drisko CH, Lewis LH: Ultrasonic instruments and antimicrobial agents in supportive periodontal treatment and retreatment of recurrent or refractory periodontitis, *Periodontol 2000* 12:90-115, 1996.

49. Copulos TA, Low SB, Walker CB et al: Comparative analysis between a modified ultrasonic tip and hand instruments on clinical parameters of periodontal disease, *J Periodontol* 64:694-700, 1993.

50. Clifford LR, Needleman IG, Chan YK: Comparison of periodontal pocket penetration by conventional and microultrasonic inserts, *J Clin Periodontol* 26:124-130, 1999.

51. Dragoo MR: A clinical evaluation of hand and ultrasonic instruments on subgingival debridement. 1. With unmodified and modified ultrasonic inserts, *Int J Periodontics Restorative Dent* 12:310-323, 1992.

52. Stambaugh RV, Dragoo M, Smith DM, Carasali L: The limits of subgingival scaling, *Int J Periodontics Restorative Dent* 1:30-41, 1981.

53. Leon LE, Vogel RI: A comparison of the effectiveness of hand scaling and ultrasonic debridement in furcations as evaluated by differential dark-field microscopy, *J Periodontol* 58:86-94, 1987.

54. Drisko CH: Root instrumentation. Power-driven versus manual scalers, which one? *Dent Clin North Am* 42:229-244, 1998.

55. Tinanoff N, Wei SH, Parkins FM: Effect of a pumice prophylaxis on fluoride uptake in tooth enamel, *J Am Dent Assoc* 88:384-389, 1974.

56. Stookey GK: In vitro estimates of enamel and dentin abrasion associated with a prophylaxis, *J Dent Res* 57:36, 1978.

57. Zuniga MA, Caldwell RC: Pastes on normal and "white-spot" enamel. The effect of fluoride-containing prophylaxis, *ASDC J Dent Child* 36:345-349, 1969.

58. Weaks LM, Lescher NB, Barnes CM, Holroyd SV: Clinical evaluation of the Prophy-Jet as an instrument for routine removal of tooth stain and plaque, *J Periodontol* 55:486-488, 1984.

59. DeSpain B, Nobis R: A comparison of rubber cup polishing and air polishing, *J Dent Res* 66:1084, 1987.

60. Berkstein S, Reiff RL, McKinney JF, Killoy WJ: Supragingival root surface removal during maintenance procedures utilizing an air-powder abrasive system or hand scaling. An in vitro study, *J Periodontol* 58:327-330, 1987.

61. Eliades GC, Tzoutzas JG, Vougiouklakis GJ: Surface alterations on dental restorative materials subjected to an air-powder abrasive instrument, *J Prosthet Dent* 65(1):27-33, 1991.

62. Barnes CM, Russell CM, Gerbo LR et al: Effects of an air-powder polishing system on orthodontically bracketed and banded teeth, *Am J Orthod Dentofacial Orthop* 97(1):74-81, 1990.

63. Cooley RL, Lubow RM, Patrissi GA: The effect of an air-powder abrasive instrument on composite resin, *J Am Dent Assoc* 112:362-364, 1986.

64. Pattison GL, Pattison AM: *Periodontal instrumentation*, ed 2, Norwalk, CT, 1991, Appleton & Lange.

65. Nield-Gehrig JS: *Fundamentals of periodontal instrumentation*, ed 4, Philadelphia, 2000, Lippincott Williams & Wilkins.

15

Periodontal and Dental Implant Maintenance

John W. Rapley

PERIODONTAL MAINTENANCE

The goal of periodontal maintenance therapy is to prevent or minimize the reoccurrence and progression of periodontal disease in periodontally treated patients. Other goals include the prevention or reduction in tooth loss and the diagnosis and treatment of other disease conditions found in the oral cavity.[1] The maintenance phase has long been described as the cornerstone of successful periodontal therapy.

Success of Periodontal Therapy

The effectiveness of periodontal treatment either with or without maintenance is seen in a comparison of three studies done by the same investigators on patients with similar levels of periodontal disease (Table 15-1). In the first study of untreated disease, the adjusted average of tooth loss per patient was 0.36 per year in a group of patients who were evaluated but did not receive any periodontal treatment.[2] The second group of patients that were periodontally treated but not maintained experienced a tooth loss rate of 0.22 teeth per year.[3] The third group of patients were periodontally treated and also maintained, with the result of 0.11 tooth loss per year for each patient.[4] Comparing these three studies illustrates that periodontal therapy is successful, and the addition of an adequate maintenance program enhances treatment success.[2-5]

Success of Periodontal Maintenance

Several long-term retrospective maintenance studies have classified a patient's response to therapy according to the number of teeth lost during the study period. In all of these studies, patients received regular periodontal maintenance appointments and therapy; however, the response to therapy varied among patients. In the three studies referenced in Table 15-2,[6-8] patients were placed into the well maintained group if they lost up to 3 teeth, and it should be noted that the majority of patients (62% to 83%) were in this category. The second group of patients (12.5% to

TABLE 15-1   Success of Periodontal Therapy

TREATMENT CATEGORY	NUMBER OF PATIENTS	AVERAGE TIME OF FOLLOW-UP	TOOTH LOSS PER YEAR*
Untreated periodontal disease[2]	30	3.7 yr	0.36
Treated periodontal disease, but no maintenance[3]	44	5.25 yr	0.22
Treated with maintenance[4]	95	6.5 yr	0.11

Tooth loss data are adjusted by excluding teeth with an initially hopeless prognosis.

TABLE 15-2   Success of Periodontal Treatment and Maintenance

AUTHOR	AVERAGE LENGTH OF STUDY (yr)	CATEGORY	PATIENTS IN EACH CATEGORY (%)	PATIENTS IN EACH CATEGORY/ PATIENTS IN STUDY (n)	AVERAGE TOOTH LOSS PER PATIENT OVER ENTIRE STUDY PERIOD
Hirschfeld and Wasserman (1978)[6]	22	WM	83.2	499/600	0.68
		DH	12.6	76/600	5.7
		EDH	4.2	25/600	13.3
McFall (1982)[7]	19	WM	77.0	77/100	0.68
		DH	15.0	15/100	6.1
		EDH	8.0	8/100	14.4
Goldman and colleagues (1986)[8]	22.2	WM	62.0	131/211	2.0
		DH	28.0	59/211	5.8
		EDH	10.0	21/211	14.2

DH, Downhill group (patients lost between 4 and 9 teeth); EDH, extreme downhill group (patients lost between 10 and 23 teeth); WM, well maintained group (patients lost between 0 and 3 teeth).

28%) lost between 4 and 9 teeth and was referred to as the downhill group. The final group (4% to 10%) lost between 10 and 23 teeth per patient and was referred to as the extreme downhill group. This last group was unresponsive to therapy and continued to experience progressive periodontal disease until a large number of their teeth were extracted; this group also can be categorized as refractory patients. It can be noted that the majority of teeth lost in these studies were lost by a relatively small total number of patients. The overall tooth loss in the studies ranged from 8% to 13.5%; however, the loss of furcated teeth was a substantially greater percentage of 31% to 57%. These and other studies illustrate the increased risk and problems in maintaining furcated teeth because of the initial disease severity, problems in furcation treatment, and difficulty of maintenance procedures in these teeth.[6-10]

Maintenance therapy with good plaque control has been shown to be a key factor in treatment success regardless of the surgical modality. Two key studies evaluated five different surgical techniques that were completed by the same group of clinicians on two patient groups with similar levels of disease. One group received frequent maintenance and demonstrated adequate plaque control, whereas the other group received no maintenance and had inadequate plaque control over the 2 years of the investigations. The maintenance group had excellent gingival health with minimal probing depths, whereas the group that did not receive maintenance had continued progression of periodontitis. These studies demonstrated that all surgical treatment modalities were successful in the presence of excellent plaque control and maintenance, and all were unsuccessful in the absence of maintenance and adequate plaque control.[11,12] Other maintenance studies done by different clinicians have shown that maintenance is a key factor in the success of a variety of periodontal therapy techniques.[13-22]

Maintenance Interval

Various methods of determining maintenance intervals have been investigated.[23] The 3-month interval is the most frequently used, but can be shortened or lengthened based on an individual patient's clinical parameters and needs.[24] The 3-month rationale is based on the time required for bacterial repopulation of the subgingival environment after mechanical debridement[25] and multiple studies that have shown clinical success with this interval. As previously noted, a continued level of good individual oral hygiene is critical to maintain periodontal health.[26-30] However, other studies have shown that patients with recurrent gingivitis who are compliant with their 3-month maintenance appointments maintained their attachment level regardless of the severity of the recurrent gingivitis.[31,32] A regular schedule of periodontal maintenance thus appears critical to sustaining health.

Maintenance Compliance

Patient compliance with maintenance programs is an ongoing problem in dental practices, and various strategies for improvement have been investigated. In an 8-year retrospective analysis of 961 patients, one private periodontal practice reported that only 16% of patients completely complied with their recommended maintenance schedule. In this same study, 49% of the patients were erratic compliers, whereas 34% never reported for any maintenance therapy. In a follow-up study done in the same practice, efforts were made to increase the compliance rate by telephone and mailing reminders, and by attempting to accommodate patients' schedules in setting up their dental appointments. These efforts doubled the size of the complete compliance group from 16% to 32%, whereas the erratic compliers group stayed basically the same.[33,34] The authors of these studies reported on the tooth loss in a subset of the compliant and the erratic groups and noted that all tooth loss had occurred in the erratic group.[35] Other studies have shown slightly different but still consistently poor rates for compliance with periodontal maintenance.[36-40] Reasons for noncompliance have been varied and include fear, cost of therapy,[41] type of treatment received,[42] lack of patient motivation, and smoking,[40] with no single reason being identified. Many studies have noted that if patients are going to discontinue their maintenance, they generally stop reporting for treatment within the first year after active therapy.[38-40]

Maintenance Procedures

The patient's maintenance appointment[43] in many aspects mirrors the diagnosis appointment in that the clinical parameters of health and disease are monitored (Box 15-1):

1. An update of the medical and dental health history is completed with special interest given to any oral manifestation of a systemic disease.[44] For example, uncontrolled or undiagnosed diabetes mellitus may present with multiple periodontal abscesses, and these patients may have experienced a significant amount of periodontal destruction from this systemic disorder. Patients with immunosuppression (such as patients undergoing chemotherapy or patients with HIV/AIDS) may have significant changes in their periodontal status that may mirror their immune competency and necessitate alterations in their maintenance interval or procedures. Severe progression of disease in a short time should warrant thorough investigation by the therapist and possible referral to a physician for evaluation of any systemic condition. If the patient is a smoker, then smoking cessation programs should be recommended and emphasized again because of the deleterious effects of smoking on the periodontium.

2. An extraoral and intraoral examination is completed to monitor any oral conditions that may have been

Box 15-1	**Procedures Performed During Periodontal Maintenance**

Maintenance Procedures	Time Spent
Patient greeting	8.50 min
Medical and dental history	1.12 min
Periodontal assessment	3.25 min
Plaque index	3.04 min
Oral hygiene review	4.20 min
Polishing and flossing	10.9 min
Ultrasonic instrumentation	6.83 min
Hand instrumentation and sharpening	10.05 min
Assessment of caries/restorative	1.00 min
Chemical therapy	1.50 min
Fluoride rinse	1.00 min
Patient dismissal and reappointment	1.00 min
Total	**52.61 min**

Modified from Schallhorn R, Snider L: Periodontal maintenance therapy, J Am Dent Assoc 103: 227-231, 1981).

present and unresolved during therapy, and to detect any abnormalities that may have arisen since the last maintenance visit.

3. A periodontal examination includes an evaluation of the probing depths, bleeding on probing, mobility, the health of the gingival tissues, amount of additional recession, furcation involvement, mobility, and incidence of suppuration. Determining the percentage of sites with bleeding on probing can be helpful, and repeated site-specific bleeding on probing may indicate an individual area of periodontal breakdown.[45-47] An increase in the total percentage of bleeding sites may indicate the need for a shortened maintenance interval and therapeutic intervention.[46] The presence of suppuration is also a significant clinical parameter and the area should be evaluated for treatment.[48,49] Any desired microbial monitoring can be accomplished at this stage of the appointment.[50] The therapist is continually reevaluating the success of the periodontal therapy and determining future maintenance procedures with the assessment of these clinical parameters.

4. Periodic vertical bitewing radiographs are taken to monitor for any radiographic bone loss or caries; these radiographs are compared with previous radiographs. During maintenance therapy, a full mouth series of radiographs may be beneficial approximately every 5 years to be able to accomplish a complete radiographic evaluation. If general periodontal deterioration is noted from the clinical parameters, then radiographs can be ordered at any appointment. Conversely, if the patient maintains excellent periodontal stability, a full-mouth series of radiographs may not be needed every 5 years.

5. A plaque assessment using disclosing solution can indicate areas that the patient consistently misses in their daily hygiene regimen and may indicate a needed change in patient hygiene techniques or instrumentation. Patients frequently need reinforcement of instruction and motivation to continue diligent oral hygiene.[51] An overall increase in gingival inflammation with a generalized increase in the bleeding index may indicate continual poor patient oral hygiene efficiency. A significant increase in the bleeding index with an acceptable plaque index at the maintenance appointment may indicate the patient performed adequate oral hygiene for only the few days immediately before the appointment.

6. Debridement procedures including scaling, root planing, and polishing vary depending on the clinical parameters and any presence of deteriorating sites. If significant deposits of subgingival calculus are detected, this may indicate a need for nonsurgical retreatment of selected areas. If multiple sites are found to need additional scaling and root planing, the patient may need to be reappointed for additional treatment because the actual time for debridement during a maintenance visit is limited (see Box 15-1). In some instances, a locally delivered antimicrobial agent may be indicated (see Chapter 16).[52] Topical fluoride treatment for caries prevention is often indicated. Caries and restoration assessments are accomplished at every appointment because exposed root surfaces resulting from periodontal disease can be at risk for root caries.[51,53]

7. Retreatment of selected areas.

Retreatment During Maintenance

During the maintenance visit, areas of periodontal breakdown may be indicated by increasing probing depths, increased attachment loss, an increase in bleeding on probing, radiographic bone loss, or progressing mobility.[54,55] Treatment schema vary depending on the findings as follows:

1. If the cause of the generalized breakdown is poor patient plaque control, then surgical therapy should be delayed until nonsurgical therapy is reaccomplished and an adequate plaque control level is maintained by the patient.

2. Retreatment of a single failing site will generally include scaling and root planing, with or without local drug delivery (see Chapter 16). If the area has not responded by the next maintenance appointment, localized surgical therapy may be necessary.[56,57]

3. If health of multiple adjacent sites is not improving, surgical therapy in the area often is indicated.

4. If there is a generalized loss of attachment detected, a thorough analysis for any possible systemic disease should be accomplished. At this retreatment, systemic antibiotics may be considered as an adjunct to the

scaling and root planing of the affected areas (see Chapter 17), with reevaluation for any possible surgical intervention.

5. If increasing mobility is detected, a thorough occlusal evaluation should be completed to determine if any occlusal adjustment is necessary.

Periodontal Maintenance: A Rationale for Therapy

The following conclusions can be made concerning periodontal maintenance:

1. The goals of periodontal and maintenance therapies are identical: a healthy, comfortable, esthetic, and functional dentition with stable probing depths.

2. Studies have demonstrated that periodontal therapy is successful for most patients over extended periods.

3. Long-term maintenance studies have shown the importance and success of maintenance therapy.

4. The maintenance interval is normally 3 months but is individualized for each patient.

5. Compliance by patients with maintenance schedules is erratic. Efforts should be made by the clinician to emphasize the importance of maintenance and to facilitate appointment scheduling for the patient.

6. The maintenance appointment consists of data collection and the reevaluation of all clinical parameters.

7. Retreatment is needed at times and is considered a part of the maintenance phase of periodontal therapy.

DENTAL IMPLANT MAINTENANCE

Periimplant Tissues

The periodontal attachment consists of a junctional epithelium mediated by hemidesmosomes with insertion of connective tissue fibers into the cementum (see Chapter 1). Similarly, the attachment of the periimplant tissues is by a junctional epithelium mediated through a basal lamina and hemidesmosomes[58] (see Chapter 26). This attachment has been consistently demonstrated with various implant materials and in different animal models.[59-62] However, in contrast to the periodontal attachment, there is not a connective tissue fiber insertion to the implant surface. Instead, there is a connective tissue "cuff" that in is close approximation to the epithelial attachment that surrounds the implant.[63,64] It has been noted that there may be a similar and consistent "biologic width" associated with implants, one with a less variable connective tissue cuff than the junctional epithelial attachment component.[65] The periimplant tissue connective tissue fibers begin at the bone level and run parallel with the abutment surface. The percentage of both parallel and perpendicular collagen fibers varies depending on the tissue type, with keratinized tissue having more perpendicular fibers. There are also vascular differences between the periodontal and periimplant tissues, and a significant difference is the presence of fewer blood vessels in the periimplant mucosa.[66]

These differences of a lack of connective tissue fiber insertion and decreased vascular supply may lead to a greater susceptibility to plaque-induced inflammation. This has been demonstrated in animal models using ligatures for plaque accumulation, resulting in a more pronounced periimplant lesion with increased bone loss, progression of the lesion into the bone marrow, and increased inflammatory infiltrate.[67,68] The increased susceptibility to plaque-induced inflammation appears to be similar regardless of the type, coating, or design of the implant.[69]

Implant Microbiology

The microflora of a healthy implant site and a periodontally healthy site are comparable. Both microfloras consist predominantly of gram-positive, aerobic, nonmotile bacteria with a high percentage of cocci and few spirochetes.[70-72] In addition, the microflora of a periimplantitis site is similar to the microflora of a periodontally diseased site.[73,74] There is a shift to gram-negative, anaerobic, and motile bacteria,[75,76] with the detection of pathogens such as *Prevotella intermedia* and *Porphyromonas gingivalis*[77,78] (see Chapter 4). Similarly, increased plaque accumulation leads to subsequent inflammation[79] resulting in increased periimplant probing depths, similar to the process occurring around teeth.[73] Similar rates of plaque formation and succession have been found for both implants and teeth.[80,81] The phenomenon of reinfection has been described around implants in the partially edentulous individual, with bacteria being seeded from the subgingival environment around teeth to the periimplant sulcus or pocket.[78,82-84] This reinfection has been demonstrated as early as 14 to 28 days after a second-stage surgical implant procedure, when the abutment is connected to the implant.[85] Thus the periodontal status of an individual can profoundly influence the periimplant health.[86]

Clinical Parameters Assessed During Maintenance

Implant probing

The method of periimplant probing may be affected by the type of implant restoration. When a titanium surface, such as an abutment surface, is present within the periimplant sulcus, probing should be performed using a plastic probe to prevent surface alterations. Alterations of the surface could lead to pitting corrosion in the chloride-containing body fluids, but repassivation by an oxide layer prevents corrosion.[87] Conversely, if a gold or other metal restoration, or a porcelain restoration is placed to the fixture level, resulting in the presence of no titanium within the periimplant sulcus, use of a metal probe is appropriate. A metal probe is no more likely to damage such an implant-retained restoration as it would be to damage a similar restoration on a tooth.

The type and thickness of the tissue that surrounds the implant affects periimplant probing depths. A keratinized periimplant tissue margin is usually associated with shallow depths, whereas alveolar mucosa is generally associated with deeper probing depths.[87] There has been some debate on the value of periimplant probing depth measurements, because some individuals feel that without a connective tissue fiber insertion into the implant surface the probe may penetrate the inflamed epithelial attachment into the subadjacent connective tissue.[88] Other authors have found probing to be a reliable indicator for attachment loss around implants when the periimplant tissue is relatively healthy gingiva[89,90] and have concluded that a change in periimplant probing depth can be a valid assessment of tissue health status.[88,91,92] It is also recommended that probing should include the measurement of attachment levels relative to a fixed reference point on the abutment or prosthesis.[93] Accurate periimplant probing may be difficult in some implant designs because of the presence of exposed implant threads, which may stop the probe and prevent accurate probe tip placement. The design of the restoration may also hinder probe placement. If the restoration emerges off of the implant at the level of the fixture table and takes on the shape of a tooth, the crown contours may prevent probe placement along a path parallel with the implant axis. For example, a 7-mm-wide restoration emerging off of a 4-mm implant platform will have a very convex emergence profile, preventing placement of a probe in the sulcus directly along the side of the implant. These variables may result in improper assessment of relative attachment levels.

Bleeding on probing is used as a clinical parameter in the dentate individual, but controversy exists as to its importance in the periimplant tissue. Investigators have found that some tissue without histologic signs of inflammation clinically demonstrated bleeding on probing. This may represent a traumatic wounding of the tissue and may not be a valid sign of true inflammatory tissue changes.[73] However, other investigators have shown a positive correlation between periimplant bleeding on probing and histologic signs of inflammation.[92] Periimplant probing was recommended to monitor implant health in both the 1978 and 1988 National Institutes of Health (NIH) Implant Consensus Development statements.[94,95]

Implant radiology

Radiographic interpretation of periimplant bone levels has been shown to be a valuable measure of implant health.[89,90,94,96,97] The inability to assess accurate probing depths because of some implant designs and possible subtle changes in implant mobility increases the value of the radiograph as a diagnostic tool. The panoramic radiograph with poor resolution capabilities cannot detect minor or subtle changes in the periimplant hard tissues but can be used as a screening radiograph.[98] Subsequent periapical radiographs may be required to assess individual areas of bone loss.[96] Normal bone density surrounding implants have been described as having horizontal perifixtural trabeculations related to the implant surface and radiating from the implant surface.[97] Stereoscopic radiographs of two additional exposures taken at 6 and 12 degrees in horizontal angulation may aid in the radiographic confirmation of osseous defects.[99] The NIH Consensus Development Conference[94] produced guidelines for radiographic evaluation of various types of implants, but it did not indicate what findings indicated a possible onset of implant failure.

Exposure time is determined so that the internal mechanical structure of the fixture is visible.[97] Paralleling film holders are often used,[100] but may be impractical, depending on implant and restoration design and the patient's anatomy. Disposable grid overlays may be used to correct magnification errors in measurements.[101] Accurate intraoral radiographs may be difficult to obtain because of anatomic limitations. For example, in a severely resorbed mandible with a resulting shallow vestibule, the correct apical film placement for a diagnostic radiograph is difficult.[100] In addition, a parallel image–film relation in an individual with a significantly resorbed maxilla is also often difficult or impossible to obtain.

Radiographs are recommended to be taken at the time of fixture placement, abutment insertion, and prosthesis insertion. Follow-up radiographs are generally taken 6 months after insertion of the restoration, and then annually thereafter. If no complications are detected radiographically or clinically, then the interval could be lengthened to 2 years.[102] In the future, digital subtraction may be a sensitive noninvasive method of assessing subtle density changes in the periimplant tissue.[103-105]

Tissue health

Several studies have investigated the difference in clinical parameters found with different tissue types in the implant collar region. In some studies, a keratinized tissue collar resulted in less attachment loss and less recession than a nonkeratinized tissue collar,[106-109] whereas other studies found minimal differences among tissue types.[107-114] The connective tissue cuff may also be affected by the mobility of the periimplant tissue. The overall conclusion is that the presence of a specific type of periimplant tissue may not be as critical as the oral hygiene proficiency. Thus the periimplant tissue should be examined just as the periodontal tissue for changes in color, contour, and consistency, and appropriate treatment should be initiated if disease activity is detected.

Crevicular fluid

The periimplant crevicular fluid is similar to the periodontal crevicular fluid[115] and can be monitored for disease activity.[116,117] Enzymes that have been investigated include aryl-sulfatase, aspartate aminotransferase, beta-glucuronidase, elastase, myeloperoxidase, and neutral protease. There are no conclusive data to support routine crevicular fluid analysis as a diagnostic tool for periimplant disease.

Mobility and occlusion

Implant mobility is difficult to assess and is not a normal finding. However, because mobility may indicate implant failure, it is important that it is evaluated by the clinician. A screw-retained prosthesis may need to be removed to assess individual implant mobility. When implants are splinted through a restoration, determination of mobility for any one implant usually requires removal of the restoration. Commercial products are available to assess mobility and the changes in mobility during maintenance.[118,119] The occlusion should also be evaluated at every maintenance appointment and any loose or fractured screws or other signs of occlusal disharmonies should be identified and corrected, because occlusal overload may cause rapid and substantial periimplant bone loss.[120]

Maintenance Procedures Performed by the Patient

The oral hygiene devices or techniques that are effective in a dentate patient's home care regimen are also effective in the implant patient's home care. The principal aid is the soft bristled toothbrush, which may include both manual and electromechanical toothbrushes (see Chapter 13). Patients may find smaller diameter toothbrush heads to be beneficial in areas of difficult access. When single tooth implants are present, they can generally be cleaned just like teeth—with a toothbrush and dental floss. Conversely, when restorations are attached to multiple implants in a splinted fashion, or when hybrid-type prostheses are present, oral hygiene can become much more difficult for the patient (Figs 15-1 through 15-4).

Interproximal plaque can be removed using floss, yarn, nylon "floss" products, or other products that can be manipulated under or around prostheses or abutments for adequate access (see Figs. 15-1 and 15-2, and Chapter 13). The interdental brush with a plastic-coated wire hub is effective to access most interproximal areas and may prove to be the most efficient for interproximal plaque removal especially in areas of difficult access (see Fig. 15-3). Gauze strips can be easily used to clean under posterior cantilever areas using a "shoeshine" technique

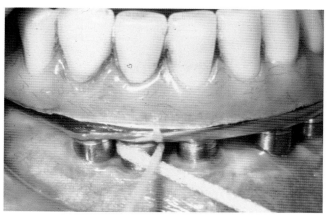

Figure 15-1. Use of yarn to remove interproximal plaque from an implant abutment. In a patient with a hybrid prosthesis, the prosthesis is attached to multiple dental implants through transmucosal titanium abutments. Another excellent device for this purpose is Superfloss (see Chapter 13). Use of metal instruments on such abutments may cause damage to the titanium surface.

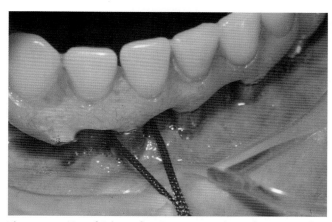

Figure 15-2. Use of "plastic floss" to remove plaque from an implant abutment.

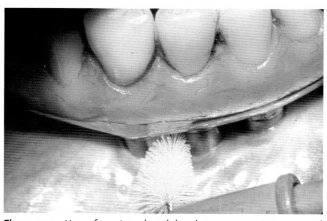

Figure 15-3. Use of an interdental brush to remove interproximal plaque from an implant abutment.

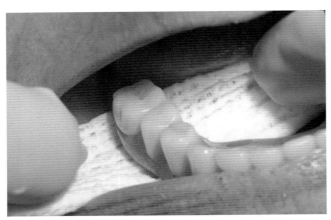

Figure 15-4. Use of gauze pads to remove plaque from the posterior cantilever areas of a implant prosthesis.

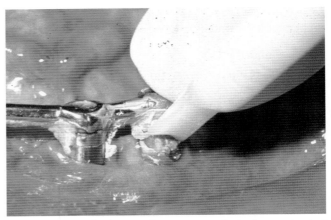

Figure 15-5. Use of a plastic scaler to remove calculus from an implant prosthesis. This scaler design is only appropriate when the abutment is exposed coronal to the gingival margin. It could not be used effectively for subgingival debridement.

(see Fig. 15-4). These home care aids have been consistently found not to alter the implant abutment surface and can be safe and effective for daily use.[121-124] A smooth implant surface will form less plaque than a rough surface on a comparable implant.[125] Regular use of antimicrobial mouthrinses can decrease supragingival plaque formation and may provide a significant long-term benefit.[126,127]

Therapist Instrumentation

The recommended instrumentation for implant debridement includes plastic, nylon, or special alloy instruments that will not alter the implant surface[121,122,124] (Fig. 15-5). These instruments come in a variety of designs and materials, and although they may not cause surface alterations, they may not have the same efficiency for easy and complete calculus removal compared with metal instruments used for teeth. A rubber cup with or without flour of pumice may remove surface alterations and improve the surface (Fig. 15-6). The air-powder abrasive system has been shown to have minimal effect if any on the implant surface, and thus may be a valuable aid in plaque and stain removal if used correctly.[128,129] However, excessive and prolonged exposure times can cause surface alterations that may be significant[130] (Fig. 15-7). The instruments that have shown to be detrimental to the implant surface causing significant and profound alterations include metal scalers or curettes, ultrasonic scalers using metal tips of various designs, and sonic scalers with metal tips[121,122,131-133] (Fig. 15-8). Sonic or ultrasonic scalers that use a plastic cap over the metal tip have been shown to be both safe and effective[134,135] (Fig. 15-9).

If the implant-retained restoration is made of gold or another nontitanium metal or of porcelain, a guideline for debridement can be followed that is similar to probing. That is, gentle use of metal instruments in a manner

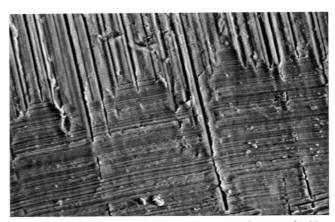

Figure 15-6. Scanning electron photomicrograph after use of rubber cup with flour of pumice at slow speed for 5 minutes (original magnification × 655). Instrumented area is at the bottom, where surface appears to have decreased roughness.

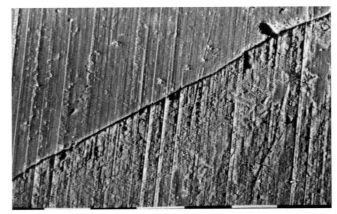

Figure 15-7. Scanning electron photomicrograph after use of an air-powder abrasive for 5 minutes (original magnification × 170). Instrumented area is at the bottom.

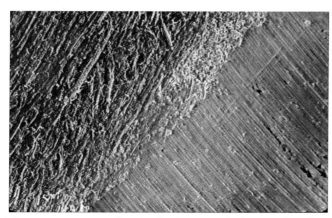

Figure 15-8. Scanning electron photomicrograph after use of an ultrasonic for 30 seconds (original magnification × 85). Instrumented area is at the left and is clearly roughened compared with the machined surface to the right.

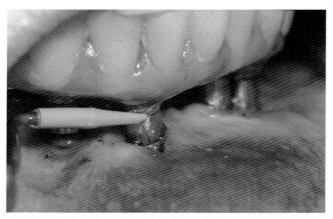

Figure 15-9. Use of a sonic scaler with a plastic sleeve on the tip for removal of plaque and calculus from an implant abutment and prosthesis. The plastic sleeve protects the titanium abutment surface.

similar to that used for periodontal maintenance on teeth with similar restorations is appropriate. Clinicians must be aware of the type of restoration present and the presence or absence of titanium surfaces in the periimplant sulcus.

Implant Maintenance: A Rationale for Therapy

The keys to maintaining periimplant health are:

1. Proper and regular evaluation of implant health using clinical and radiographic techniques
2. Assessment of occlusal forces and occlusal stability over time
3. Proper plaque control by the patient using whatever mechanical aids each individual patient requires; this depends on the type of implant and the type of implant restoration present

4. Thorough removal of bacterial plaque and calculus using techniques that do not damage the implant, the abutment, or the restoration.

REFERENCES

1. The American Academy of Periodontology: Supportive periodontal therapy (AAP Position Paper), *J Periodontol* 69:502-506, 1998.
2. Becker W, Berg L, Becker B: Untreated periodontal disease: a longitudinal study, *J Periodontol* 50:234-244, 1979.
3. Becker W, Becker B, Berg L: Periodontal treatment without maintenance. A retrospective study in 44 patients, *J Periodontol* 55:505-509 1984.
4. Becker W, Berg L, Becker B: The long-term evaluation of periodontal treatment and maintenance in 95 patients, *Int J Periodontics Restorative Dent* 4:55-71, 1984.
5. Kocker T, Konig J, Dzierzon U et al: Disease progression in periodontally treated and untreated patients. A retrospective study, *J Clin Periodontol* 27:866-872, 2000.
6. Hirschfeld L, Wasserman B: A long term survey of tooth loss in 600 treated periodontal patients, *J Periodontol* 49:225-237, 1978.
7. McFall W: Tooth loss in 100 treated patients with periodontal disease. A long term study, *J Periodontol* 53:539-549, 1982.
8. Goldman M, Ross I, Goteiner D: Effect of periodontal therapy on patients maintained for 15 years or longer. A retrospective study, *J Periodontol* 57:347-353, 1986.
9. Wood W, Greco GW, McFall W: Tooth loss in patients with moderate periodontitis after treatment and long-term maintenance care, *J Periodontal* 60:516-520, 1989.
10. McLeod D, Lainson P, Spivey J: The effectiveness of periodontal treatment as measured by tooth loss, *J Am Dent Assoc* 128:316-325, 1997.
11. Rosling B, Nyman S, Lindhe J, Jern B: The healing potential of the periodontal tissue following different techniques of periodontal surgery in plaque-free dentitions: a 2-year study, *J Clin Periodontol* 3:233-250, 1976.
12. Nyman S, Lindhe J, Rosling B: Periodontal surgery in plaque-infected dentitions, *J Clin Periodontol* 4:240-249, 1977.
13. Knowles J, Burgett F, Morrison E et al: Comparison of results following three modalities of periodontal therapy related to tooth type and initial pocket depth, *J Clin Periodontol* 7:32-47, 1980.
14. Hill R, Ramfjord S, Morrison E et al: Four types of periodontal treatment compared over two years, *J Periodontol* 52:655-662, 1981.
15. Knowles J, Burgett F, Nissle R et al: Results of periodontal treatment related to pocket depth and attachment level. Eight years, *J Periodontol* 50:225-233, 1979.
16. Pihlstrom B, McHugh R, Olophant T, Ortiz-Campos C: Comparison of surgical and non-surgical treatment of

periodontal disease. A review of current studies and additional results after 6 1/2 years, *J Clin Periodontol* 10:524-541, 1983.

17. Lindhe J, Westfelt E, Nyman S et al: Long-term effect of surgical/non-surgical treatment of periodontal disease, *J Clin Periodontol* 11:448-458, 1984.

18. Nabers C, Stalker W, Esparza D et al: Tooth loss in 1535 treated periodontal patients, *J Periodontol* 59:297-300, 1988.

19. Meador H, Lane J, Suddick R: The long-term effectiveness of periodontal therapy in a clinical practice, *J Periodontol* 56:253-258, 1985.

20. Becker W, Becker B, Ochsenbein C et al: A longitudinal study comparing scaling, osseous surgery and modified Widman procedures. Results after one year, *J Periodontol* 59:351-365, 1988.

21. Kaldahl W, Kalkwarf K, Patil K et al: Evaluation of four modalities of periodontal therapy, *J Periodontol* 59:783-793, 1988.

22. Ramfjord S, Caffesse R, Morrison E et al: Four modalities of periodontal treatment compared over five years, *J Clin Periodontol* 14:445-452, 1987.

23. Listgarten M, Sulllivan P, George C et al: Comparative longitudinal study of two methods of scheduling maintenance visits: 4-year data, *J Clin Periodontol* 16:105-115, 1989.

24. Echeverria J, Mandau C, Guerrero A: Supportive care after active periodontal treatment. A review, *J Clin Periodontol* 23:898-905, 1996.

25. Mousques T, Listgarten M, Phillips R: Effect of scaling and root planing on the composition of the human subgingival microbial flora, *J Periodont Res* 15:144-151, 1980.

26. Westfelt E, Nyman S, Socransky S, Lindhe J: Significance of frequency of professional tooth cleaning for healing following periodontal surgery, *J Clin Periodontol* 10:148-156, 1983.

27. Lindhe J, Nyman S: Long-term maintenance of patients treated for advanced periodontal disease, *J Clin Periodontol* 11:504-514, 1984.

28. Nyman S, Rosling B, Lindhe J: Effect of professional tooth cleaning on healing after periodontal surgery, *J Clin Periodontol* 2:80-86, 1975.

29. Rosling B, Nyman S, Lindhe J: The effect of systematic plaque control on bone regeneration in infrabony pockets, *J Clin Periodontol* 3:38-53, 1976.

30. Lindhe J, Westfelt E, Nyman S et al: Healing following surgical/non-surgical treatment of periodontal disease. A clinical study, *J Clin Periodontol* 9:115-128, 1982.

31. Ramfjord S, Morrison E, Burgett F et al: Oral hygiene and maintenance of periodontal support, *J Periodontol* 53:26-30, 1982.

32. Morrison E, Ramfjord S, Burgett F et al: The significance of gingivitis during the maintenance phase of periodontal treatment, *J Periodontol* 53:31-34, 1982.

33. Wilson T, Glover M, Schoen J et al: Compliance with maintenance therapy in a private periodontal practice, *J Periodontol* 55:468-473, 1984.

34. Wilson T, Hale S, Temple R: The results of efforts to improve compliance with supportive periodontal treatment in private practice, *J Periodontol* 64:311-314, 1993.

35. Wilson J, Glover M, Malik A, et al: Tooth loss in maintenance patients in a private periodontal practice, *J Periodontol* 58:231-235, 1987.

36. Anneken C, Treinen J, Willershausen B: Patients compliance in periodontal therapy: a retrospective investigation on the basis of a clinical group, *Eur J Med Res* 6:75-82, 2001.

37. Schmidt J, Morrison E, Kerry G, Caffesse R: Patient compliance with suggested maintenance recall in a private periodontal practice, *J Periodontol* 61:316-317, 1990.

38. Demetriou N, Tsami-Pandi A, Parashis A: Compliance with supportive periodontal treatment in private periodontal practice. A 14 year study, *J Periodontol* 66:145-149, 1994.

39. Novaes A, Novaes A Jr, Moraes N: Compliance with supportive therapy, *J Periodontol* 67:213-216, 1996.

40. Mendoza A, Newcomb G, Nixon K: Compliance with supportive periodontal therapy, *J Periodontol* 62:731-736, 1991.

41. Wilson T: Compliance. A review of the literature with possible applications to periodontics, *J Periodontol* 58:706-714, 1987.

42. Novaes A Jr, de Lima F, Novaes A: Compliance with supportive periodontal therapy and its relation to the bleeding index, *J Periodontol* 67:976-980, 1996.

43. Schallhorn R, Snider L: Periodontal maintenance therapy, *J Am Dent Assoc* 103:227-231, 1981.

44. Hancock E, Newell D: Preventive strategies and supportive treatment, *Periodontol 2000* 25:59-76, 2001.

45. Kalkwarf K, Kaldahl W, Patil K, Molvar M: Evaluation of gingival bleeding following four types of periodontal therapy, *J Clin Periodontol* 16:601-608, 1989.

46. Lang N, Joss A, Orsanic T et al: Bleeding on probing. A predictor for the progression of periodontal disease? *J Clin Periodontol* 13:590-596, 1986.

47. Lang N, Adler R, Joss A, Nyman S: Absence of bleeding on probing. An indicator of periodontal stability, *J Clin Periodontol* 17:714-721, 1990.

48. Chaves E, Caffesse R, Stults D: Diagnostic discrimination of bleeding and exudate during maintenance periodontal therapy, *J Dent Res* 65:227, 1986 (abstract).

49. McLeod D, Lainson P, Spivey J: Tooth loss due to periodontal abscess: a retrospective study, *J Periodontol* 68:963-966, 1997.

50. Listgarten M, Slots J, Rosenberg J et al: Clinical and microbiological characteristics of treated periodontitis patients on maintenance, *J Periodontol* 60:452-459, 1989.

51. Shick R: Maintenance phase of periodontal therapy, *J Periodontol* 52:576-583, 1981.

52. Slots J, Jorgensen M: Efficient antimicrobial treatment in periodontal maintenance care, *J Am Dent Assoc* 131: 1293-1304, 2000.

53. Axelsson P, Lindhe J, Nystrom B: On the prevention of caries and periodontal disease: results of a 15-year longitudinal study in adults, *J Clin Periodontol* 18:182-189, 1991.

54. Chance R: Retreatment in periodontal practice, *J Periodontol* 48:410-412, 1977.

55. Rateitschak K: Failure of periodontal treatment, *Quintessence Int* 25:449-457, 1994.

56. Ramfjord S: Maintenance care for treated periodontitis patients, *J Clin Periodontol* 14:433-437, 1987.

57. Kaldahl W, Kalkwarf K, Patil K et al: Long term evaluation of periodontal therapy. II: Incidence of sites breaking down, *J Periodontol* 67:103-108, 1996.

58. Listgarten MA, Lang NP, Schroeder HE, Schroeder A: Periodontal tissues and their counterparts around endosseous implants, *Clin Oral Impl Res* 2:1-19, 1991.

59. McKinney RV, Steflik DE, Koth DL: Evidence for a junctional epithelial attachment to ceramic dental implant: a transmission electron microscopic study, *J Periodontol* 56:579-591, 1985.

60. James RA, Kelln E: A histopathological report on the nature of the epithelium and underlying connective tissue which surround oral implants, *J Biomed Mater Res* 5:373-382, 1974.

61. Hansson F-A, Albrektsson T, Branemark P-I: Structural aspects of the interface between tissue and titanium implants, *J Prosthet Dent* 50:108-113, 1983.

62. Swope EM, James JA: A longitudinal study on hemidesmosome formation at the dental implant-tissue interface, *J Oral Implantol* 9:412-422, 1981.

63. Berglundh T, Lindhe J, Ericsson I et al: The soft tissue barrier at implants and teeth, *Clin Oral Implants Res* 2:81-90, 1991.

64. Ruggeri A, Franchi M, Marini N et al: Supracrestal circular collagen fiber network around osseointegrated nonsubmerged titanium implants, *Clin Oral Implants Res* 3:169-175, 1992.

65. Cochran DL, Hermann JS, Schenk RK et al: Biologic width around titanium implants. A histometric analysis of the implanto-gingival junction around unloaded and loaded nonsubmerged implants in the canine mandible, *J Periodontol* 68:186-198, 1997.

66. Berglundh T, Lindhe J, Jonsson K, Ericsson I: The topography of the vascular systems in the periodontal and peri-implant tissues in the dog, *J Clin Periodontol* 21:189-193, 1994.

67. Lindhe J, Berglundh T, Ericsson I et al: Experimental breakdown of peri-implant and periodontal tissues, *Clin Oral Implants Res* 3:9-16, 1992.

68. Berglundh T, Lindhe J, Marinello C et al: Soft tissue reaction to de novo plaque formation on implants and teeth. An experimental study in the dog, *Clin Oral Implants Res* 3:1-8, 1992.

69. Tillmanns HW, Hermann JS, Cagna DR et al: Evaluation of three different dental implants in ligature-induced peri-implantitis in the beagle dog. Part I. Clinical evaluation, *Int J Oral Maxillofac Implants* 12:611-620, 1997.

70. Lekholm U: Osseointegrated implants in clinical practice, *J Oral Implantol* 12:357-364, 1986.

71. Rams TE, Robert TW, Tatum H, Keyes P: The subgingival microbial flora associated with human dental implants, *J Prosthet Dent* 51:529-534, 1984.

72. Mombelli A, Buser D, Lang NP: Colonization of osseointegrated titanium implants in edentulous patients. Early results, *Oral Microbiol Immunol* 3:133-120, 1988.

73. Lekholm U, Ericsson I, Adell R, Slots J: The condition of the soft tissues at the tooth and fixture abutment supporting fixed bridges, *J Clin Periodontol* 13:558-562, 1986.

74. Apse P, Allen RP, Overall CM, Zarb GA: Microbiota and crevicular fluid collagenase activity in osseointegrated dental implant sulcus: a comparison of sites in edentulous and partially edentulous patients, *J Periodont Res* 24:96-105, 1989.

75. George K, Zafiropoulous K, Murat Y et al: Clinical and microbiological status of osseointegrated implants, *J Periodontol* 65:766-770, 1994.

76. Salcetti J, Moriarty JD, Cooper LF et al: The clinical, microbial, and host response characteristics of the failing implant, *Int J Oral Maxillofac Implants* 12:35-42, 1997.

77. Becker W, Becker BE, Newman MG, Nyman S: Clinical and microbiological findings that may contribute to dental implant failure, *Int J Oral Maxillofac Implants* 5:31-38, 1990.

78. Quirynen M, Listgarten M: The distribution of bacterial morphotypes around natural teeth and titanium implants ad modum Branemark, *Clin Oral Implants Res* 1:8-12, 1990.

79. Abrahamsson I, Berglundh T, Lindhe J: Soft tissue response to plaque formation at different implant systems. A comparative study in the dog, *Clin Oral Implants Res* 9:73-79, 1998.

80. Gatewood RR, Cobb CM, Killoy WJ: Microbial colonization on natural tooth structure compared with smooth and plasma sprayed dental implant surfaces, *Clin Oral Implants Res* 4:53-64, 1993.

81. Nakazato G, Tsuchiya H, Sato M, Yamauchi M: In vivo plaque formation on implant materials, *Int J Oral Maxillofac Implants* 4:321-326, 1989.

82. Mombelli A, Marxer M, Gaberthuel T et al: The microbiota of osseointegrated implants in patients with a history of periodontal disease, *J Clin Periodontol* 22:124-130, 1995.

83. Gouvousis J, Sindhusake D, Yeung S: Cross infection from periodontitis sites to failing implant sites in the same mouth, *Int J Oral Maxillofac Implants* 12:666-673, 1997.

84. Papaioannou W, Quirynen M, van Steenberghe D: The influence of periodontitis on the subgingival flora around implants in partially edentulous patients, *Clin Oral Implants Res* 7:405-409, 1996.

85. Koka S, Razzoog ME, Bloem TJ, Syed S: Microbial colonization of dental implants in partially edentulous subjects, *J Prosthet Dent* 70:141-144, 1993.

86. Bragger U, Burgin WB, Hammerle CH, Lang NP: Associations between clinical parameters assessed around implants and teeth, *Clin Oral Implants Res* 8:412-421, 1997.

87. van Steenberghe D: Periodontal aspects of osseointegrated oral implants modum Branemark, *Dent Clin North Am* 32:355-370, 1988.

88. Lang NP, Wetzel AC, Stich H, Caffesse RG: Histologic probe penetration in healthy and inflamed peri-implant tissues, *Clin Oral Implants Res* 5:191-201, 1994.

89. Adell R, Lekholm U, Branemark P-I, Lindhe J: Marginal tissue reactions at osseointegrated titanium fixtures, *Swed Dent J Suppl* 28:175-182, 1985.

90. Quirynen M, van Steenberghe D, Jacobs R et al: The reliability of pocket probing around screw-type implants, *Clin Oral Implants Res* 2:186-192, 1991.

91. Adell R, Lekholm U, Rockler B, Branemark PI: A 15-year study of osseointegrated implants in the treatment of the edentulous jaw, *Int J Oral Surg* 10:387-416, 1981.

92. Lekholm U, Adell R, Lindhe J et al: Marginal tissue reactions at osseointegrated titanium fixtures (II). A cross-sectional study, *Int J Oral Surg* 15:53-61, 1986.

93. Newman MG, Flemmig TF: Periodontal considerations of implants and implant associated microbiota, *J Dent Educ* 52:737-744, 1988.

94. Schnitman P, Shulman L, editors: *Dental implants: benefit and risk*, NIH-Harvard Consensus Development Conference, NIH publ no. 81-1531, 1978.

95. National Institute for Dental Research (Sponsor)/ Loe H (Director): National Institutes of Health Consensus Development Conference Statement on Dental Implants, Bethesda, MD, June 13-15, 1988.

96. Wie H, Larheim TA, Karlsen K: Evaluation of endosseous implant abutments as a base for fixed prosthetic appliances. A preliminary clinical study, *J Oral Rehabil* 6:353-363, 1979.

97. Strid KG: Radiographic results. In Branemark P-I, Zarb GA, Albrektsson T, editors: *Tissue-integrated prostheses: osseointegration in clinical dentistry*, Chicago, 1985, Quintessence Publishing, pp 187-209.

98. Friedland B: The clinical evaluation of dental implants: a review of the literature, with emphasis on the radiographic aspects, *Oral Implantol* 13:101-111, 1987.

99. Hollender L, Rockler B: Radiographic evaluation of osseointegrated implants of the jaws, *Dentomaxillofac Radiol* 9:91-95, 1980.

100. Cox JF: Radiographic evaluation of tissue-integrated prostheses. In van Steenberghe D, Albrektsson T, Branemark P-I et al, editors: *Tissue-integration in oral and maxillo-facial reconstruction*, Amsterdam, 1986, Excerpta Medica, pp 278-286.

101. Larheim TA, Wie H, Tvieto L, Effen S: Method for radiographic assessment of alveolar bone level at endosseous implants and abutment teeth, *Scand J Dent Res* 87:146-154, 1979.

102. Albrektsson T, Zarb G, Worthington P, Eriksson AR: The long term efficacy of currently used dental implants: a review and proposed criteria of success, *Int J Oral Maxillofac Implants* 1:11-25, 1986.

103. Bragger U, Burgin MS, Lang NP, Buser D: Assessment of changes in peri-implant bone density, *Int J Oral Maxillofac Implants* 6:160-166, 1991.

104. Jeffcoat MK, Reddy MS, van den Berg HR, Bertens E: Quantitative digital subtraction radiography for the assessment of peri-implant bone change, *Clin Oral Implants Res* 3:22-27, 1992.

105. Reddy MS, Mayfield-Donahoo TL, Jeffcoat MK: A semi-automated computer assisted method for measuring bone loss adjacent to bone implants, *Clin Oral Implants Res* 3:28-31, 1992.

106. Hanisch O, Cortella CA, Boskovic MM et al: Experimental peri-implant tissue breakdown around hydroxyapatite-coated implants, *J Periodontol* 68:59-66, 1997.

107. Warrer K, Buser D, Lang NP, Karring T: Plaque-induced peri-implantitis in the presence or absence of keratinized mucosa. An experimental study in monkeys, *Clin Oral Implants Res* 6:131-138, 1995.

108. Artzi Z, Tal H, Moses O, Kozlovsky A: Mucosal considerations for osseointegrated implants, *J Prosthet Dent* 70:427-432, 1993.

109. Block MS, Kent JN: Factors associated with soft- and hard-tissue compromise of endosseous implants, *J Oral Maxillofac Surg* 48:1153-1160, 1990.

110. Strub JR, Gaberhuel TW, Grunder U: The role of attached gingiva in the health of peri-implant tissue in dogs. Part I. Clinical findings, *Int J Periodontics Restorative Dent* 11:317-333, 1991.

111. Mericske-Stern R, Steinlin-Schaffner T, Marti P, Geering AH: Peri-implant mucosal aspects of ITI implants supporting overdentures. A five-year longitudinal study, *Clin Oral Implants Res* 5:9-18, 1994.

112. Wennstrom J, Bengazi F, Lekholm U: The influence of the masticatory mucosa on the peri-implant soft tissue condition, *Clin Oral Implants Res* 5:1-8, 1994.

113. Krekeler G, Schilli W, Diemer J: Should the exit of the artificial abutment tooth be positioned in the region of the attached gingiva? *Int J Oral Surg* 14:504-508, 1985.

114. Apse P, Zarb G, Schmitt A, Lewis D: The longitudinal effectiveness of osseointegrated dental implants. The Toronto study: peri-implant mucosal response, *Int J Periodontics Restorative Dent* 11(2):94-111, 1991.

115. Adonogianaki E, Mooney J, Wennstrom JL et al: Acute-phase proteins and immunoglobulin-G against Porphyromonas

gingivalis in peri-implant crevicular fluid: a comparison with gingival crevicular fluid, *Clin Oral Impants Res* 6:14-23, 1995.

116. Eley BM, Cox SW, Watson RM: Protease activities in peri-implant sulcus fluid from patients with permucosal osseointegrated dental implants. Correlation with clinical parameters, *Clin Oral Implants Res* 2:62-70, 1991.

117. Paolantonio M, De Placido G, Tumini V et al: Aspartate aminotransferase activity in crevicular fluid from dental implants, *J Periodontol* 71:1151-1157, 2000.

118. Teerlinck J, Quirynen M, Darius P, van Steenberghe D: Periotest: an objective clinical diagnosis of bone apposition toward implants, *Int J Oral Maxillofac Implants* 6:55-61, 1991.

119. Truhlar R, Morris H, Ochi S: Stability of the bone-implant complex. Results of longitudinal testing to 60 months with the Periotest device on endosseous dental implants, *Ann Periodontol* 5:42-55, 2000.

120. Miyata T, Kovayashi Y, Araki H et al: The influence of controlled occlusal overload on peri-implant tissue: a histologic study in monkeys, *Int J Oral Maxillofac Implants* 13:677-683, 1998.

121. Rapley J, Swan R, Hallmon W, Mills M: The surface characteristics produced by various oral hygiene instruments and materials on titanium implant abutments, *Int J Oral Maxillofac Implants* 5:47-52, 1990.

122. Thomson-Neal D, Evans G, Meffert R: Effects of various prophylactic treatments on titanium, sapphire, and hydroxyapatite-coated implants: an SEM study, *Int J Periodontics Restorative Dent* 4:301-311, 1989.

123. Hallmon WW, Waldrop TC, Meffert RM, Wade BW: A comparative study of the effects of metallic, nonmetallic, and sonic instrumentation on titanium abutment surfaces. *Int J Oral Maxillofac Implants* 11:96-100, 1996.

124. Orton G, Steele D, Wolinsky L: The dental professional's role in monitoring and maintenance of tissue-integrated prostheses, *Int J Oral Maxillofac Implants* 4:305-310, 1989.

125. Quirynen M, van der Mei H, Bollen C et al: An in vivo study of the influence of the surface roughness of implants

on the microbiology of supra- and subgingival plaque, *J Dent Res* 72:1304-1309, 1993.

126. Ciancio S, Lauciello F, Shibly O et al: The effect of an antiseptic mouthrinse on implant maintenance: plaque and peri-implant gingival tissue, *J Periodontol* 66:962-965, 1995.

127. Burchard W, Cobb C, Drisko C, Killoy W: The effects of chlorhexidine and stannous fluoride on fibroblast attachment to different implant surfaces, *Int J Oral Maxillofac Implants* 6:418-426, 1991.

128. Barnes C, Fleming L, Mueninghoff L: An SEM evaluation of the in-vitro effects of an air-abrasive system on various implant surfaces, *Int J Oral Maxillofac Implants* 6:463-469, 1991.

129. Parham P, Cobb C, French A et al: Effects of an air-powder abrasive system on plasma-sprayed titanium implant surfaces: an in vitro evaluation, *J Oral Implantol* 15:78-86, 1989.

130. Chairay J, Boulekbache J, Jean A et al: Scanning electron microscopic evaluation of the effects of an air-abrasive system on dental implants: a comparative in vitro study between machined and plasma-sprayed titanium surfaces, *J Periodontol* 68:1215-1222, 1997.

131. Fox S, Moriarty J, Kusy R: The effects of scaling a titanium implant surface with metal and plastic instruments: an in vitro study, *J Periodontol* 61:485-490, 1990.

132. Meschenmoser A, d'Hoedt B, Meyle J et al: Effects of various hygiene procedures on the surface characteristics of titanium abutments, *J Periodontol* 67:229-235, 1996.

133. Matarasso S, Quaremba G, Goraggio F et al: Maintenance of implants: an in vitro study of titanium implant surface modifications subsequent to the application of different prophylaxis procedures, *Clin Oral Implants Res* 7:64-72, 1996.

134. Gantes, B, Nelveus R: The effects of different hygiene instruments on titanium: SEM observations, *Int J Periodontics Restorative Dent* 11:225-239, 1991.

135. Bailey G, Gardner J, Day M, Kovanda B: Implant surface alterations from a nonmetallic ultrasonic tip, *J West Soc Periodontol* 46:69-73, 1998.

16 Locally Acting Oral Chemotherapeutic Agents

Margaret Hill and Regan L. Moore

ROLE OF CHEMOTHERAPEUTIC AGENTS AS ADJUNCTS TO PERIODONTAL THERAPY

The concept of using chemicals to treat conditions in the mouth has been a widely accepted part of dental practice for hundreds of years. The father of modern dentistry, Pierre Fauchard, advocated both mechanical and chemical treatment of the diseased periodontium.[1] Periodontal diseases are infections that elicit an immune response resulting in the loss of the supporting structures of the teeth.[2] The primary goal of treating these inflammatory diseases—gingivitis and periodontitis—is the removal of supragingival and subgingival bacteria.[3]

Supragingival plaque is accessible to the patient and can be effectively disrupted or removed during tooth brushing and use of interproximal cleaning devices. When combined with regular professional care, mechanical plaque removal has been shown to be effective in preventing or reversing the signs and symptoms of gingivitis including erythema, edema, and bleeding on probing.[4] However, when patients are unable to adequately perform plaque removal by ordinary mechanical means, the use of chemotherapeutic agents as an adjunct to mechanical therapy may be warranted.[5]

Treatment of periodontitis is aimed at the pathogenic gram-negative anaerobic organisms living subgingivally in a complex organized bacterial microcosm called biofilm (see Chapter 6). The bacteria living in this biofilm work together in ways that result in destruction of tissues subgingivally. They produce proteolytic enzymes and toxins, and stimulate the immune response resulting in destruction of the periodontal supporting tissues.[6] Mechanical disruption of this subgingival biofilm is the goal of scaling and root planing and is usually very effective in treating periodontitis.[7] However, scaling and root planing does not always remove all the subgingival microorganisms,[8] and additional treatment may be needed to achieve complete resolution of the periodontal infection. Local delivery of antimicrobial agents directly into the subgingival environment offers an adjunctive treatment option, especially in patients who are not good candidates for more complex and invasive treatment such as resective or regenerative surgery. Chemotherapeutic agents can be delivered topically to the exposed surfaces of teeth and gingiva through dentifrices, gels, mouthrinses, and supragingival irrigants. Most of these systems are designed for home use for the treatment of gingivitis, whereas others aimed at treating periodontitis require professional application. This chapter focuses on those topically applied chemotherapeutic agents that are active against plaque and gingivitis, as well as site-specific local drug delivery systems that are placed subgingivally by a dental professional for the treatment of periodontitis.

TOPICALLY APPLIED ANTIGINGIVITIS AGENTS

Oral antimicrobial agents have been used in a variety of formulations with varying success over the years in the treatment of gingivitis (Table 16-1). They are generally effective in reducing plaque and gingivitis but have little effect on periodontitis, unless they are delivered subgingivally. The ideal antimicrobial is one that can be delivered to the diseased area in an effective form and remains for a sufficient amount of time to accomplish the desired results without the development of resistant bacterial strains or damage to oral tissues. In addition, these products should be cost-effective and pleasant to use.[9] Other desirable characteristics of chemotherapeutic agents include low toxicity, high potency, good permeability, intrinsic efficacy, and substantivity.[10] The American Dental Association grants the Seal of Acceptance for treatment of gingivitis to products that reduce plaque and demonstrate effective reduction of gingival inflammation over a period of at least 6 months without adverse side effects.

Baking Soda, Salt, and Hydrogen Peroxide

Baking soda, salt, and hydrogen peroxide were touted as a treatment for periodontal diseases when used as part of Keyes's technique. Scaling and root planing were combined with a system of home care using a paste of baking soda, salt, and hydrogen peroxide as a dentifrice and irrigation with a saturated salt solution. Microbiologic monitoring was also performed, and tetracycline hydrochloride, a broad-spectrum antibiotic, was administered orally when phase-contrast microscopy evaluation of the subgingival plaque revealed increased levels of spirochetes and other motile bacteria.[11] Studies comparing Keyes's technique to conventional treatment showed no statistically significant differences in clinical effectiveness; hence the technique is not recommended by most practitioners today.[12]

Chlorhexidine

Chlorhexidine gluconate has been widely investigated as a topically applied antibacterial agent and has worldwide acceptance as an effective antiplaque and antigingivitis agent. Chlorhexidine is considered the "gold standard" to which all other topical antimicrobial mouthrinses are compared.[13] It is a cationic bisbiguanide that acts by rupturing cell membranes. Chlorhexidine exhibits the quality of *substantivity*, which is the ability of an agent to adhere to soft and hard tissues and then be released over time, allowing antimicrobial activity to continue over 6 hours or more. It has been found to be safe and effective when used as a mouthrinse, but undesirable side effects of staining, calculus formation, and taste alteration make chlorhexidine less useful for long-term topical treatment.[14]

Chlorhexidine mouthrinse is available as a 0.12% solution in the United States and as a 0.2% solution

TABLE 16-1   Comparison of Topically Applied Antigingivitis Agents

AUTHOR	AGENT	DECREASE IN GINGIVITIS (%)	DECREASE IN PLAQUE SCORES (%)	VEHICLE	MECHANISM OF ACTION
Grossman and colleagues (1986)[16] Banting and colleagues (1989)[17]	Chlorhexidine	45	50-55	Mouthrinse	Cell wall lysis, precipitation of cytoplasm
Lamster and colleagues (1983)[24] Gordon and colleagues (1985)[25]	Essential oils	29	25	Mouthrinse	Cell wall disruption, inhibition of enzyme production
Beiswanger and colleagues (1995)[46]	Stannous fluoride	19	None	Dentifrice	Alteration of cellular aggregation and metabolism
Cubells and colleagues (1991)[51]	Triclosan and copolymer	20	25	Dentifrice	Nonionic germicide
Lobene and colleagues (1977)[34]	Cetylpyridinium chloride	24	14	Mouthrinse	Cell wall rupture

outside of the United States. Studies have shown there are no significant differences in the antimicrobial effects or the clinical efficacy when comparisons are made between these two concentrations.[15] Studies of the 0.12% chlorhexidine formulation show 50% to 55% reductions in plaque and reductions in gingivitis up to 45%.[16,17] Chlorhexidine is used as a 15-ml rinse for 30 seconds twice daily. Patients should be advised to allow at least 30 minutes to lapse between use of a dentifrice and rinsing with chlorhexidine. Interactions of chlorhexidine with sodium lauryl sulfate and fluoride contained in the dentifrice may reduce its effectiveness.[18] Wound healing is enhanced when chlorhexidine rinses are used before extractions[19] and after scaling and root planing or periodontal surgery.[20] It is also beneficial as a prerinse in reducing the salivary bacterial load by approximately 90%, thus minimizing the aerosol contamination associated with many dental procedures.[21]

Essential Oils

Chemotherapeutic agents containing essential oils have been used for oral care for many years; Listerine (Pfizer; New York, NY) is the oldest of these products and contains thymol, eucalyptol, menthol, and methylsalicylate. The mechanism of action of essential oils appears to be by cell wall disruption and inhibition of bacterial enzymes.[22] Studies using essential oil mouthrinses have evaluated their effectiveness before intraoral procedures that produce aerosols. Use of a preprocedural rinse resulted in a 94.1% reduction in bacteria collected from aerosols produced by ultrasonic scalers.[23] Studies of Listerine as an antiseptic oral rinse have shown plaque reduction and gingivitis reduction up to 34% when used twice per day after brushing.[24,25] The vehicle for the oral rinse contains 21.6% to 26.9% alcohol depending on the formulation, and may impart a burning sensation, especially in patients with tissue sensitivity to alcohol. Caution should also be used with patients who are recovering from alcohol dependency and recommendations for use of oral products containing alcohol should be avoided.

Povidone Iodine

Povidone iodine is classified as an iodophor, created by adding polyvinyl-pyrrolidone to elemental iodine. It is a water-soluble antimicrobial and is effective against many types of microorganisms, including bacteria, viruses, and fungi.[26] Povidone iodine has been used for many years as a presurgical scrub for skin disinfection. Use of a dilute povidone iodine solution has been studied as a preprocedural rinse and was found to decrease streptococci in saliva when used in a 5% solution applied for 30 seconds; bacterial levels did not rebound after 90 minutes.[27] It has been studied as a mouthrinse and as an irrigant in various dilutions, and the results have found povidone iodine to be comparable with other chemotherapeutic agents.[28] When used in combination with hydrogen peroxide as a mouthrinse, a significant reduction in papillary bleeding scores was observed.[29] When topically applied in conjunction with basic nonsurgical therapy and maintenance of patients with advanced periodontitis, the positive outcome of mechanical therapy was improved by the use of povidone iodine over a 13-year period.[30] There is some concern about chronic, daily use of povidone iodine because there is a possibility of development of iodine toxicity with prolonged use.[31] Patient sensitivity to iodine should be assessed before use, and patients with known allergies to povidone iodine or shellfish, thyroid dysfunction, or women who are pregnant or lactating should be excluded from use.[32] Povidone iodine can temporarily stain teeth and soft tissues, but the tooth staining can be removed through prophylaxis.

Quaternary Ammonium Compounds

The most common formulations of quaternary ammonium compounds are cetylpyridinium chloride used alone (Cepacol: Combe; White Plains, NY) or in combination with domiphen bromide (Scope: Procter and Gamble; Cincinnati, OH). They are cationic surface active agents that act by rupturing cell walls. This group of compounds binds to oral tissues, but releases rapidly, limiting substantivity, and ultimately effectiveness.[33] A 6-month study using cetylpyridinium chloride showed a 14% reduction in plaque and a 24% reduction in gingivitis.[34]

Sanguinarine

Sanguinarine is an herbal alkaloid extract from the plant *Sanguinaria canadensis* or bloodroot. It has been studied in both dentifrice and mouthrinse formulations, and it is often augmented with zinc chloride. The most effective combination seems to use both the dentifrice and the mouthrinse in combination. Six-month studies showed plaque reductions of 17% to 42% and gingivitis reduction of 18% to 57%.[35-37] In other studies using the dentifrice only, differences between control and experimental groups were not significant.[38,39]

Sodium Hypochlorite

Sodium hypochlorite (bleach) has been used as an endodontic irrigant for years and was one of the first locally delivered antimicrobials used in treatment of periodontitis, when a concentrated solution of sodium hypochlorite, called antiformin, was used to irrigate subgingivally.[40] It is an effective agent against bacteria, viruses, and fungi, and has the advantages of ease of access and low cost. Odor, need for fresh solutions, some corrosive effects on metals, and bleaching if spilled on surfaces are disadvantages to use.[41] It has been studied as a subgingival irrigant alone and with citric acid,[42,43] and in a study on extracted teeth, it was found to decrease endo-

toxin adherence more than water.[44] Sodium hypochlorite is rarely used in periodontics today.

Stannous Fluoride

Stannous fluoride has been used as an anticaries agent for years, and received the first American Dental Association Seal of Acceptance in 1960 for the prevention of tooth decay in dentifrice. Studies have shown that stannous fluoride also exhibits effects on plaque and gingivitis, probably related to the presence of the tin ion.[45] Six-month studies of stannous fluoride dentifrices showed significant reductions in gingivitis but were not accompanied by a decrease in plaque scores.[46,47] Stannous fluoride has also been studied as a professionally applied subgingival irrigant[48,49] and has shown limited benefits. Stannous fluoride is also available in a gel formulation.

Triclosan

Triclosan has been used as a topical antimicrobial agent in many types of products, including soaps and antiperspirants. It is a bisphenol with broad-spectrum antimicrobial activity and has been incorporated into several different types of oral products.[50] Triclosan has been combined with zinc citrate for additional antiplaque and anticalculus effects, added to a copolymer of polyvinylmethyl and maleic acid to increase substantivity and provide some anticalculus properties, and combined with pyrophosphates to add anticalculus benefits.[14] Triclosan with copolymer has been studied in a dentifrice formulation and showed a 20% reduction in gingivitis and a 25% reduction in plaque formation.[51]

LOCAL DRUG DELIVERY SYSTEMS

Local or controlled delivery systems represent a variety of products that combine agents with vectors or devices that can be placed directly into the periodontally diseased pocket. "Controlled" implies that the carrier material releases the active ingredient over time at a constant concentration. These controlled release drug delivery devices are capable of releasing high concentrations of antibiotics into the pocket for up to 14 days at fractions of the total dose required for systemic administration.[52] The basic premise is that concentrated amounts of active medications can be delivered to the precise site of the disease process with minimal systemic uptake of the medication. Compared with systemically delivered drugs, the side effects and drug interactions are mostly nonexistent with locally delivered sustained released antimicrobial agents.

Indications and Contraindications for Locally Delivered Drugs

If preventive care combined with conventional professional treatment is sufficient to control periodontal disease progression, then no further treatment is needed, except for maintenance care at an appropriate interval. When localized diseased sites do not respond to initial oral hygiene and scaling and root planing treatments, or when localized diseased sites are present in an otherwise stable maintenance patient, local drug delivery systems may be indicated. Local drug delivery systems are useful as adjuncts to conventional mechanical therapy because they offer other options for patients who exhibit need for additional treatment but for some reason may not be candidates for more invasive therapy, such as resective or regenerative surgical procedures. Locally delivered drugs are not intended for use in place of mechanical therapy, or as therapy for aggressive forms of periodontitis that may require systemic antibiotics to eradicate the disease. Other treatment alternatives may be indicated instead of locally delivered drugs if multiple sites are nonresponsive. Use of local delivery devices in patients who are allergic to any component of the system is contraindicated, as is their use in the pregnant or lactating patient.[53]

Clinical Significance

Interpretation of results from clinical studies of controlled delivery systems has been debated, and statistical versus clinical significance has been an issue that has gained more attention as the number of controlled clinical trials testing these products has increased.[54] As emphasis has been placed on using an evidence-based approach to improve clinical treatment decisions, there is more demand to provide both types of information as results are reported.[55] Statistical significance is defined as the probability that the results of the study are not merely because of chance. Clinical significance is a highly subjective issue and may vary from clinician to clinician. Although each clinical treatment situation is unique and requires careful consideration of options, there are some guidelines that have been recommended to aid in the interpretation of results when considering treatment options.[54] A suggested level of change to denote clinical significance is improvement of 2 mm or more in probing depth or in clinical attachment levels.[54] All of the local delivery agents that are currently available for use in the United States have exhibited improvement of 2 mm or more in probing depth or attachment levels at approximately 30% to 40% of sites treated in multicenter randomized controlled clinical trials (Table 16-2). However, mean changes in probing pocket depths and gains in clinical attachment for all treated sites are modest and range from 0.95 to 1.90 mm depending on the agent and the particular clinical trial. It is difficult to predict which patients will have a good response to local drug delivery; however, the drugs listed in Table 16-2 have been shown to significantly reduce probing pocket depths and bleeding on probing when used in conjunction with scaling and root planing. In some reports, these agents have been used as a

monotherapy. Some studies report other adjunctive effects including gains in clinical attachment. Few studies report any adverse effects from using these locally delivered drugs.

Delivery Devices

The first attempts at controlled subgingival delivery used tetracycline in a hollow cellulose fiber. Other early devices that were used for subgingival delivery include dialysis tubing, gels, acrylic strips, and ethylcellulose strips. The first product that gained U.S. Food and Drug Administration approval is an ethyl vinyl acetate fiber containing 25% tetracycline hydrochloride.[56] Other devices that are currently in use include a biodegradable film of hydrolyzed gelatin, a liquid biodegradable polymer system that hardens on subgingival placement, and a bioabsorbable microencapsulated microsphere, in addition to other systems available in countries outside the United States.

A number of agents and systems have been tested, but products that have gained acceptance by the U.S. Food and Drug Administration are tetracycline fibers (Actisite:Alza Corp.; Palo Alto, CA), chlorhexidine chip (PerioChip: Dexcel Pharma; Edison, NJ), doxycycline gel (Atridox: Atrix Laboratories; Fort Collins, CO), and minocycline microspheres (Arestin: Orapharma; Warminster, PA). Several other products are available in other countries including metronidazole gel (Elyzol: Dumex; Copenhagen, Denmark), minocycline gel (Dentomycin: Lederlee Dental Division; Gosport, Hampshire, U.K.), and minocycline ointment (Periocline; Japan). All products have been tested in conjunction with scaling and root planing in 9- to 12-month multicenter clinical trials. In all cases, the locally delivered drugs shown in Table 16-2 were applied at least 2 to 3 times to pockets that were 5 mm or greater in depth, and that bled on probing during the 9-month trials. The cost-effectiveness of using the chlorhexidine chip has been evaluated in moderate to advanced periodontitis cases. Results of this study suggest that treatment with chlorhexidine chips may be a slightly more expensive alternative to surgical therapy.[57]

Subgingivally Applied Agents

Tetracycline fibers

Tetracycline fibers (Actisite) consist of a woven tube made of the polymer ethylene vinyl acetate saturated with 25% tetracycline hydrochloride. They are marketed as a 23-cm length of 0.5 mm diameter fiber and contain 12.7 mg tetracycline hydrochloride. The flexible fiber is placed in an overlapping pattern into the periodontal pocket until it fills the pocket 1 mm apical to the gingival margin (Fig. 16-1, A and B). A serrated cord packing instrument is helpful in fiber placement. The gingival margin is then sealed with isocyanoacrylate. The placement of the cord does not in itself require anesthesia, but thorough root debridement is always required before placement of the

Table 16-2   Comparison of Local Drug Delivery in Studies Treating More Than 100 Subjects

Author	Delivery Device	Subjects (n)	SRP Alone Probing Depth Change	SRP plus Device Probing Depth Change	Sites ≥2 mm Gain SRP Plus Device
Goodson and colleagues (1991)[61]	Tetracycline fiber	107	0.67 mm	1.02 mm (drug only)	Not reported
Newman and colleagues 1994[62]	Tetracycline fiber	105	1.08 mm	1.81 mm	Not reported
Drisko and colleagues 1995[63]	Tetracycline fiber	116	1.1 mm	1.0 mm	Not reported
Jeffcoat and colleagues 1998[65]	Chlorhexidine gel (chip)	443	0.64 mm	0.95 mm	19%*
Soskolne and colleagues 1997[66]	Chlorhexidine gel (chip)	118	1.30 mm	1.50 mm	35%*
Garrett and colleagues 1999[69]	Doxycycline gel	411	1.08 mm	1.30 mm (drug only)	38%* (drug only)
Wennstrom and colleagues 2001[70]	Doxycycline gel	105	1.30 mm	1.50 mm	52%*
Williams and colleagues 2001[71]	Minocycline microspheres	728	1.08 mm	1.32 mm	42%*
Ainamo and colleagues 1992[72]	Metronidazole gel	206	1.30 mm	1.50 mm (drug only)	Not reported
van Steenburghe and colleagues 1999[77]	Minocycline ointment	103	1.20 mm	1.90 mm	Not reported

Available in United States.
SRP, Scaling and root planing.

fiber. Postoperative instructions require the patient to not brush or floss the specific area, and the patient is asked to rinse twice daily with chlorhexidine for 2 weeks with the fiber in place and 1 week after removal.[58]

Tetracycline fibers release bactericidal concentrations of tetracycline (>1300 μg/ml) steadily up to 10 days.[59] Multiple studies compare the fiber in many treatment configurations to scaling and root planing alone, to placebo fiber, to no treatment, to fiber plus scaling and root planing, as active treatment, and as maintenance treatment.[60-63] In general these studies showed improvement in all treatment groups, with reductions in probing depths, bleeding on probing, periodontal pathogens, and gains in clinical attachment levels. Tetracycline fibers are rarely used today.

Chlorhexidine chip

The chlorhexidine chip (PerioChip) incorporates 2.5 mg chlorhexidine gluconate into a biodegradable film of hydrolyzed gelatin. It is 0.35 mm in thickness and 4 × 5 mm in height/width (Fig. 16-2, *A*). The chip is self-retentive on contact with moisture, therefore no adhesives or dressings are needed. The chip has only been tested in conjunction with scaling and root planing and is placed immediately after the completion of scaling and root planing. The PerioChip has been reformulated to enable storage

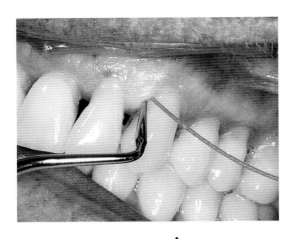

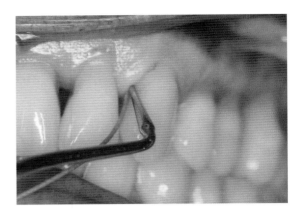

A   B

Figure 16-1. A, Actisite fiber is placed into a 7-mm pocket on the mesial surface of tooth #11. **B,** The fiber is overlapped until it the pocket is filled within 1 mm of the gingival margin.

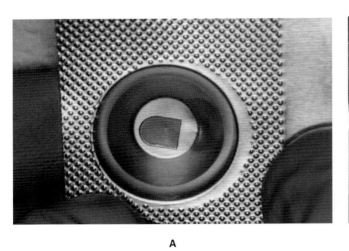

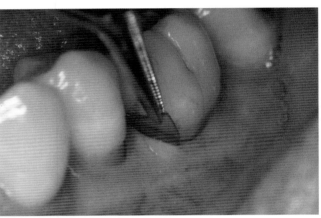

A   B

Figure 16-2. A, The PerioChip is a biodegradable film of hydrolyzed gelatin 0.35 mm in thickness and 4 × 5 mm, containing 2.5 mg chlorhexidine gluconate. **B,** The PerioChip is inserted into a 6-mm pocket on the mesial surface of tooth #19.

at room temperature, and the handling characteristics have improved, eliminating the tendency of the chip to stick to instruments and tissues during placement. Using cotton forceps to grasp the chip, it is inserted into the pocket (Fig. 16-2, *B*). Keeping the chip and the surrounding tissues dry is also helpful, but not as critical as it was with the previous formulation. The dimensions of the chip prevent placement into small, tortuous pockets, so placement into pockets of less than 5 mm may be difficult and is not recommended. Some subjects have reported a slightly uncomfortable burning sensation with chip placement. Since the chip biodegrades, no postoperative appointment for removal is necessary. The patient is instructed not to brush or floss the area for 7 days and twice daily chlorhexidine rinses may be recommended for 2 weeks after placement.[58]

Chlorhexidine is released from the chip in a peak concentration (2007 μg/ml) at 2 hours after placement and progressively decreases over 9 days (mean = 57 μg/ml).[64] Investigations comparing the chlorhexidine chip combined with scaling and root planing to scaling and root planing alone found that the combined therapy resulted in a statistically significant improvement in probing depths and attachment levels over scaling alone.[65-67]

Doxycycline gel

Doxycycline gel (Atridox) is a liquid biodegradable polymer that hardens after a few minutes following exposure to the fluid in the periodontal pocket. Bioassays have detected levels in gingival fluid of approximately 250 μg/ml doxycycline hyclate at the end of 7 days in the pocket.[68] Atridox comes in two syringes that are coupled together before use and mixed by moving the contents of the syringes back and forth for 100 cycles (Fig. 16-3, A). The delivery syringe is attached to a 23-gauge blunt cannula and the material is injected into the periodontal pocket (Fig. 16-3, B and C). This product is also available premixed in a single syringe. Any overflow material is gently packed in the pocket with a cord packing instrument or the back of a curet. Periodontal dressing or adhesive may aid retention but are not necessary if the patient can avoid brushing, flossing, or eating in the treated area for a minimum of 7 days. Because the material is biodegradable, no additional appointments for removal are required and the patient is instructed to remove any residual material with their tooth brush and dental floss at the end of 1 week.[58] Two large, multicenter trials showed sites treated with the doxycycline polymer alone compared with scaling and root planing alone were equivalent.[69] Another study compared the effectiveness of doxycycline gel with scaling and root planing to

doxycycline gel with full-mouth ultrasonic debridement. Both techniques showed gains in clinical attachment levels and decreases in probing depths.[70] Although the doxycycline gel was studied and approved as a monotherapy by the U.S. Food and Drug Administration, it is normally used as an adjunctive therapy at the time of scaling and root planing or maintenance procedures.[53] Use of the doxycycline gel alone would not result in removal of any calculus present on the root surface.

Minocycline microspheres

Minocycline microspheres (Arestin) consist of the antibiotic minocycline hydrochloride microencapsulated in a bioabsorbable polymer of polyglycolide-co-dl lactide. This system is designed for use as an adjunctive treatment with scaling and root planing. The microspheres are dispensed subgingivally using a disposable plastic cartridge (containing 1 mg of minocycline on a stainless steel handle (Fig. 16-4, A) by inserting the tip to the base

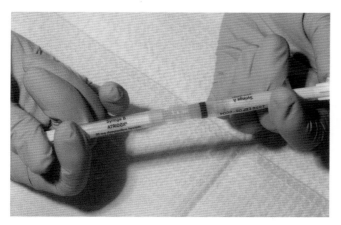

A

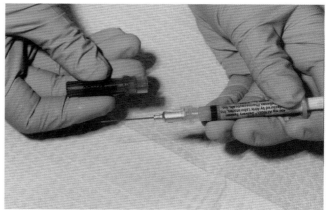

B

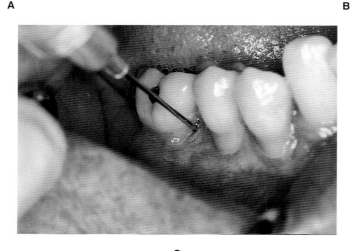

C

Figure 16-3. **A,** Atridox in two syringes that are coupled together for mixing. Atridox also comes in a single syringe, premixed formulation. **B,** After mixing, the delivery syringe is attached to a blunt cannula. **C,** Atridox is placed into a 7-mm pocket on the mesial surface of tooth #30.

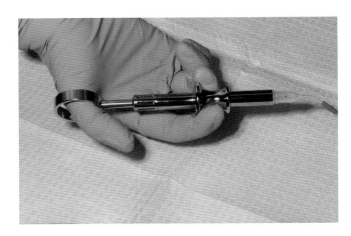

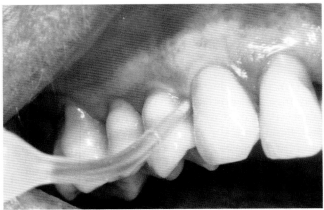

A

B

Figure 16-4. A, Arestin is applied using an autoclavable stainless steel handle with disposable plastic cartridges containing one dose per cartridge (1 mg minocycline). **B,** Arestin is placed into a 6-mm pocket on the mesial surface of tooth #5.

of the periodontal pocket and applying the material while withdrawing the tip (Fig. 16-4, *B*). The material is bioadhesive on contact with moisture and does not require additional adhesives or periodontal dressings to hold it in place subgingivally. The patient should be instructed to avoid brushing for 12 hours, with no interproximal cleaning for 10 days. No additional appointments are needed for removal of the material because it is bioabsorbable. The minocycline microspheres maintain therapeutic drug concentrations for 14 days. A 9-month study comparing scaling and root planing alone, scaling and root planing plus minocycline microspheres, and scaling and root planing plus the carrier microspheres without minocycline showed a greater therapeutic effect of the scaling and root planing plus minocycline microspheres compared with the other treatment modalities.[71]

Metronidazole gel

Metronidazole gel contains 25% metronidazole in a glyceryl mono-oleate and sesame oil base and is applied to the pocket using a syringe with a blunt cannula. This agent is not currently available in the United States. It is easy to place but may require multiple applications to achieve desirable results. Studies using metronidazole gel as a monotherapy show similar results compared with scaling and root planing.[72,73] When metronidazole gel was used in studies with two other adjunctive treatments to scaling and root planing and compared with scaling and root planing alone, all treatments improved over 6 months with no significant differences among treatment groups.[74,75]

Minocycline ointment and gel

Minocycline ointment contains 2% minocycline hydrochloride and is applied using a syringe with blunt cannula. This agent is not currently available in the United States.

A 2% minocycline gel has also been used in several studies. In a multicenter study of patients with moderate to severe periodontitis, results of treatment with minocycline ointment combined with scaling and root planing was found to be statistically significant when compared with treatment with a vehicle control with scaling and root planing.[76,77] When subgingivally applied minocycline gel was used as one of three adjunctive treatments to scaling and root planing compared with scaling and root planing alone, all treatments showed improvement with no significant differences among groups.[74,75]

CONCLUSION

Use of locally acting chemotherapeutic agents can be a valuable adjunct to conventional mechanical therapeutic modalities. Topically applied agents such as dentifrices and mouthrinses are useful in controlling gingivitis in patients who cannot perform adequate home care with mechanical oral hygiene. Agents such as triclosan are now a component part of commercially available dentifrices and are in widespread use. In patients with periodontitis, locally delivered drugs placed subgingivally are particularly valuable in treatment of patients who have localized sites of 5 mm or more that bleed on probing and that are not responsive to primary therapy, including oral hygiene and scaling and root planing. Locally delivered drugs can have limited positive effects in deeper pockets for patients who are not good candidates for periodontal surgery. Subgingivally applied local drug delivery systems in conjunction with scaling and root planing may also be a viable treatment option for maintenance patients who develop localized areas of recurrent periodontitis. Although research seems to indicate that clinical parameters such as decrease in pocket depth and attachment level gain are minimal after the adjunctive use of locally delivered drugs compared with the changes that are seen with scaling and root planing alone, the value of these adjunctive therapies must be clinically evaluated on an individual basis. Individual sites may demonstrate larger or smaller changes, which are not readily evident when clinical calculations are based on full-mouth treatment. A recent comprehensive meta-analysis demonstrated a statistically significant improvement in probing depth reduction (minocycline microspheres) and clinical attachment gain (chlorhexidine chip and doxycycline gel) when these products were used as adjuncts to scaling and root planing.[78] Further studies are needed to continue testing the available devices to define conditions for optimal use. Other drugs and delivery systems may be found that will provide alternative options for treating periodontal diseases in all types of patients, including the increasingly complex medically compromised individuals who present unique challenges in all phases of care.

REFERENCES

1. Ring ME: *Dentistry. An illustrated history*, St. Louis, 1985, CV Mosby.
2. Haffajee Ad, Socransky SS: Microbial and etiologic agents of destructive periodontal diseases, *Periodontology 2000* 5:78-111, 1994.
3. Lindhe J, Nyman S: The effect of plaque control and surgical pocket elimination on the establishment and maintenance of periodontal health. A longitudinal study of periodontal therapy in cases of advanced disease, *J Clin Periodontol* 2:67-79, 1975.
4. Axelsson P, Lindhe J, Nystrom B: On the prevention of caries and periodontal disease. Results of a 15 year longitudinal study in adults, *J Clin Periodontol* 18:182-189, 1991.
5. Hancock EB: Prevention, *Ann Periodontol* 1:223-249, 1996.
6. Dahan M, Nawrocki B, Elkaïm R et al: Expression of matrix metalloproteinases in healthy and diseased human gingiva, *J Clin Periodontol* 28:128-136, 2001.
7. Cobb CM: Non-surgical pocket therapy: mechanical, *Ann Periodontol* 1:443-490, 1996.
8. Haffajee AD, Cugini MA, Dibart S et al: The effect of SRP on the clinical and microbiological parameters of periodontal diseases, *J Clin Periodontol* 24:324-334, 1997.
9. van der Ouderaa FJG: Anti-plaque agents. Rationale and prospects for prevention of gingivitis and periodontal disease, *J Clin Periodontol* 18:447-454, 1991.
10. Goodson JM: Pharmacokinetic principles controlling efficacy of oral therapy, *J Dent Res* 68:1625-1632, 1989.
11. Keyes PH, Wright WE, Howard SA: The use of phase-contrast microscopy and chemotherapy in the diagnosis and treatment of periodontal lesions—an initial report (I), *Quintessence Int* 9:51-56, 1978.
12. Greenwell H, Bissada NF: A dispassionate scientific analysis of Keyes' technique, *Int J Periodontics Restorative Dent* 5:64-75, 1985.
13. Lang NP, Brecx MC: Chlorhexidine digluconate—an agent for chemical plaque control and prevention of gingival inflammation, *J Periodont Res* 21(suppl):74-89, 1986.
14. American Academy of Periodontology: Chemical agents for control of plaque and gingivitis. Committee on Research, Science and Therapy. Position Paper, Chicago, 1994, The Academy.
15. Quirynen M, Avontroodt P, Peeters W et al: Effect of different chlorhexidine formulations in mouthrinses on de novo plaque formation, *J Clin Periodontol* 28:1127-1136, 2001.
16. Grossman E, Reiter G, Sturzenberger OP et al: Six-month study on the effects of a chlorhexidine mouthrinse on gingivitis in adults, *J Periodont Res* 21:33, 1986.
17. Banting D, Bosma M, Bollmer B: Clinical effectiveness of a 0.12% chlorhexidine mouthrinse over two years, *J Dent Res* 68:1716, 1989.
18. Barkvoll R, Rolla G, Svendsen AK: Interaction between chlorhexidine digluconate and sodium lauryl sulfate in vivo, *J Clin Periodontol* 16:593, 1989.
19. Hermesch CB, Hilton TJ, Biesbrock AR et al: Perioperative use of 0.12% chlorhexidine gluconate for the prevention of alveolar osteitis: efficacy and risk factor analysis, *Oral Surg Oral Med Oral Pathol Oral Radiol Endod* 85:381-387, 1998.
20. Beiswanger BB, Mallat ME, Jackson RD et al: Clinical effects of a 0.12% chlorhexidine rinse as an adjunct to scaling and root planing, *J Clin Dent* 3:33-38, 1992.
21. Ciancio S: Expanded and future uses of mouthrinses, *J Am Dent Assoc* 125(Suppl 2):29S-32S, 1994.
22. Scheie AAA: Modes of action of currently known chemical antiplaque agents other than chlorhexidine, *J Dent Res* 68:1609, 1989.
23. Fine DH, Mendieta C, Barnett ML et al: Efficacy of preprocedural rinsing with an antiseptic in reducing viable bacteria in dental aerosols, *J Periodontol* 63:821-824, 1992.
24. Lamster IB, Alfano MC, Seiger MC et al: The effect of Listerine antiseptic on reduction of existing plaque and gingivitis, *Clin Prev Dent* 5:12, 1983.
25. Gordon JM, Lamster IB, Seiger MC: Efficacy of Listerine antiseptic in inhibiting the development of plaque and gingivitis, *J Clin Periodontol* 12:697, 1985.
26. Quirynen M, Teughels W, De Soete M et al: Topical antiseptics and antibiotics in the initial therapy of chronic adult periodontitis: microbiological aspects, *Periodontol 2000* 28:72-90, 2002.
27. Rahn R: Review presentation on povidone-iodine antisepsis in the oral cavity, *Postgrad Med J* 69:S4-S9, 1993.
28. Greenstein G: Povidone-iodone's effects and role in the management of periodontal diseases: a review, *J Periodontol* 70:1397-1405, 1999.
29. Clark WB, Magnusson I, Walker CB et al: Efficacy of Perimed antibacterial system on established gingivitis (I). Clinical results, *J Clin Periodontol* 16:630-635, 1989.

30. Rosling B, Hellstrom MK, Ramberg P et al: The use of PVP-iodine as an adjunct to non-surgical treatment of chronic periodontitis, *J Clin Periodontol* 28:1023-1031, 2001.

31. Andrews LW: Commentary: the perils of povidone-iodine use, *Ostomy Wound Manage* 40:68-73, 1994.

32. Fleischer W, Reimer K: Povidone iodine antisepsis. State of the art, *Dermatology* 195(Suppl 2):3-9, 1997.

33. Gjermo P: Chlorhexidine and related compounds, *J Dent Res* 68:1602, 1989.

34. Lobene RR, Lovene S, Soparker PM: The effect of cetylpyridinium chloride mouthrinse on plaque and gingivitis, *J Dent Res* 56:595, 1977.

35. Hanna JJ, Johnson JD, Kuftinec MM: Long term clinical evaluation of toothpaste and oral rinse containing sanguinaria in controlling plaque, gingival inflammation, and sulcular bleeding during orthodontic treatment, *Am J Orthod Dentofacial Orthop* 96:199, 1989.

36. Harper DS, Mueller LJ, Fine J et al: Clinical efficacy of a dentifrice and oral rinse containing sanguinaria extract and zinc chloride during six months of use, *J Periodontol* 61:352, 1990.

37. Kopczyk RA, Abrams H, Brown A et al: Clinical and microbiological effects of a sanguinaria-containing mouthrinse and dentifrice with and without fluoride during 6 months of use, *J Periodontol* 62:617, 1991.

38. Mauriello SM, Bader JD: Six month effects of a sanguinarine dentifrice on plaque and gingivitis, *J Periodontol* 59:238, 1988.

39. Palcanis KG, Sarbin AG, Koertge TE et al: Longitudinal evaluation of the effect of sanguinarine dentifrice on plaque and gingivitis, *Gen Dent* 38:17-19, 1990.

40. Glickman I, Benjamin D: Histologic study of the effect of antiformin, *J Am Dent Assoc* 51:420-424, 1955.

41. Slots J: Selection of antimicrobial agents in periodontal therapy, *J Periodont Res* 37:389-398, 2002.

42. Kalkwarf KL, Tussing GJ, Davis MJ: Histologic evaluation of gingival curettage facilitated by sodium hypochlorite solution, *J Periodontol* 53:63-70, 1982.

43. Forgas LB, Gound S: The effects of antiformin-citric acid chemical curettage on the microbial flora of the periodontal pocket, *J Periodontol* 58:153-158, 1987.

44. Sarbinoff JA, O'Leary TJ, Miller CH: The comparative effectiveness of various agents in detoxifying diseased root surfaces, *J Periodontol* 54:77-80, 1983.

45. Ciancio SG: Agents for the management of plaque and gingivitis, *J Dent Res* 71:1450-1454, 1992.

46. Beiswanger BB, Doyle PM, Jackson RD et al: The clinical effect of dentifrices containing stabilized stannous fluoride on plaque formation and gingivitis—a six-month study with ad libitum brushing, *J Clin Dent* 6:46-53, 1995.

47. Perlich MA, Bacca LA, Bollmer BW et al: The clinical effect of a stabilized stannous fluoride dentifrice on plaque formation, gingivitis, and gingival bleeding: a six month study, *J Clin Dent* 6:54-58, 1995.

48. Mazza J, Newman M, Sims T: Clinical and antimicrobial effect of stannous fluoride on periodontitis, *J Clin Periodontol* 8:203-212, 1981.

49. Krust KS, Drisko CL, Gross K et al: The effects of subgingival irrigation with chlorhexidine and stannous fluoride. A preliminary investigation, *J Dent Hyg* 65:289-295, 1991.

50. DeSalva SJ, Kong BM, Lin YJ: Triclosan: a safety profile, *Am J Dent* 2:185-196, 1989.

51. Cubells AB, Dalmau LB, Petrone ME et al: The effect of a triclosan/copolymer/fluoride dentifrice on plaque formation and gingivitis: a six-month study, *J Clin Dent* 2:63-69, 1991.

52. American Academy of Periodontology: The role of controlled drug delivery for periodontitis, *J Periodontol* 71:125-140, 2000.

53. Drisko CH: Nonsurgical periodontal therapy, *Periodontology 2000* 25:77-88, 2001.

54. Killoy WJ: The clinical significance of local chemotherapies, *J Clin Periodontol* 29:22-29, 2002.

55. Newman MG: Improved clinical decision making using the evidence-based approach, *Ann Periodontol* 1:i-ix, 1996.

56. Goodson JM, Haffajee A, Socransky SS: Periodontal therapy by local delivery of tetracycline, *J Clin Periodontol* 6:83-92, 1979.

57. Henke CJ, Villa KF, Aichelmann-Reidy ME et al: An economic evaluation of a chlorhexidine chip for treating chronic periodontitis: the CHIP (chlorhexidine in periodontitis) study, *J Am Dent Assoc* 132:1557-1569, 2001.

58. Killoy WJ, Polson AM: Controlled local delivery of antimicrobials in the treatment of periodontitis, *Dent Clin North Am* 42:263, 1998.

59. Tonetti M, Cugini M, Goodson J: Zero-order delivery with periodontal placement of tetracycline-loaded ethylene vinyl acetate fibers, *J Periodont Res* 26:440-451, 1990.

60. Goodson JM, Cugini MA, Kent RL et al: Multi-center evaluation of tetracycline fiber therapy. I. Experimental design, methods, and baseline data, *J Periodont Res* 26:361, 1991.

61. Goodson JM, Cugini MA, Kent RL et al: Multi-center evaluation of tetracycline fiber therapy: II. Clinical response, *J Periodont Res* 36:371, 1991.

62. Newman JC, Kornman KS, Doherty FM: A 6-month multi-center evaluation of adjunctive tetracycline fiber therapy used in conjunction with scaling and root planing in maintenance patients: clinical results, *J Periodontol* 65:685, 1994.

63. Drisko C, Cobb C, Killoy R et al: Evaluation of periodontal treatments using controlled-release tetracycline fibers. Clinical response, *J Periodontol* 66:692-699, 1995.

64. Soskolne WA, Chajek T, Flashner M et al: An in vivo study of the chlorhexidine release profile of the PerioChip in the gingival crevicular fluid, plasma and urine, *J Clin Periodontol* 25:1017-1021, 1998.

65. Jeffcoat M, Bray KS, Ciancio SG et al: Adjunctive use of a sub-gingival controlled release chlorhexidine chip reduces probing depth and improved attachment level compared with

scaling and root planing alone, *J Periodontol* 69:989-997, 1998.

66. Soskolne WA, Heasman PA, Stabholz A et al: Sustained local delivery of chlorhexidine in the treatment of periodontitis: a multicenter study, *J Periodontol* 68:32-38, 1997.

67. Jeffcoat M, Palcanis K, Weatherford TW et al: Use of biodegradable chlorhexidine chip in the treatment of adult periodontitis: clinical and radiographic findings, *J Periodontol* 71:256-262, 2000.

68. Polson AM, Southard GL, Dunn RL et al: Periodontal pocket treatment in beagle dogs using subgingival doxycycline from a biodegradable system: I. Initial clinical responses, *J Periodontol* 67:1176, 1996.

69. Garrett S, Johnson L, Drisko CH et al: Two multi-center clinical studies evaluating locally delivered doxycycline hyclate, placebo control, oral hygiene, and scaling and root planing in the treatment of periodontitis, *J Periodontol* 70:490-503, 1999.

70. Wennstrom JL, Newman HN, MacNeil SR et al: Utilization of locally delivered doxycycline in non-surgical treatment of chronic periodontitis. A comparative multi-center trial of 2 treatment approaches, *J Clin Periodontol* 28:753-761, 2001.

71. Williams RC, Paquette DW, Offenbacher S et al: Treatment of periodontitis by local administration of minocycline microspheres: a controlled trial, *J Periodontol* 72:1535-1544, 2001.

72. Ainamo J, Lie T, Ellingsen BH et al: Clinical responses to subgingival application of a metronidazole 25% gel compared to the effects of subgingival scaling in adult periodontitis, *J Clin Periodontol* 19:723-729, 1992.

73. Pedrazzoli B, Killian M, Karring T: Comparative clinical and microbiological effects of topical subgingival application of metronidazole 25% dental gel and scaling in the treatment of adult periodontitis, *J Clin Periodontol* 19:715, 1992.

74. Radvar M, Pourtaghi N, Kinane DF: Comparison of 3 periodontal local antibiotic therapies in persistent periodontal pockets, *J Periodontol* 67:860-865, 1996.

75. Kinane DF, Radvar M: A six-month comparison of three periodontal local antimicrobial therapies in persistent periodontal pockets, *J Periodontol* 70:1-7, 1999.

76. van Steenberghe D, Bercy P, Kohl J et al: Subgingival minocycline hydrochloride ointment in moderate to severe chronic adult periodontitis: a randomized, double-blind, vehicle-controlled, multicenter study, *J Periodontol* 64:637-644, 1993.

77. van Steenberghe D, Rosling B, Soder PO et al: A 15 month evaluation of the effects of repeated subgingival minocycline in chronic adult periodontitis, *J Periodontol* 70:657-667, 1999.

78. Hanes PJ, Purvis JP: Local anti-infective therapy: Pharmacologic agents. A systematic review. *Ann Periodontol* 8:79-98, 2003.

17 Systemic Chemotherapeutic Agents

Denis F. Kinane

The term *periodontitis* covers a range of disease manifestations ranging from extensive and severe periodontitis affecting prepubertal children and young adults (aggressive periodontitis) to the more common form of periodontitis affecting older adults (chronic periodontitis). (See Chapter 2.) The variety of periodontitis disorders is relevant in that a different therapeutic approach must be considered for each condition.

In the general category of systemic chemotherapeutic agents, antimicrobials constitute the majority of agents. However, host response modifiers such as antiinflammatory drugs (e.g., nonsteroidal antiinflammatory drugs [NSAIDs]) also should be considered, along with protease inhibitors such as chemically modified tetracyclines (e.g., low dose doxycycline preparations [Periostat: CollaGenex Pharmaceuticals Inc.; Newtown, PA]) that have been administered systemically for the treatment of periodontitis. It is also important to define some of the terms used for periodontal therapies. In particular, the term *antiinfective* therapy needs to be considered, because this is clearly a term that includes both the mechanical debridement and the chemotherapeutic management of patients. Although mechanical root cleaning, or mechanical debridement, has been undertaken for hundreds of years in the treatment of periodontitis,[1] the use of chemotherapeutic agents is a recent initiative.

The biofilm nature of dental plaque is another important consideration in the discussion of chemotherapeutic agents (see Chapter 6). In the 1990s we witnessed an exponential increase in the field of biofilms and began to fully appreciate the significance of this phenomenon. Biofilms are microbial masses, which develop into complex structures that possess nutrient channels and unique environmental conditions, promoting the growth and interactions of markedly different bacterial species as a sole community. These living masses of microorganisms are extremely resistant to attack by antiseptics or antimicrobial agents. It is estimated that at least 500 times the concentration of an antimicrobial is needed to kill the bacteria within a biofilm, and thus the antimicrobial dosages and antiinfective strategies developed for bacteria in planktonic phases are not effective for the biofilm microbiota.[2,3]

Periodontal disease has presented a significant problem for human populations throughout history; for example, it has been reported to have afflicted the Egyptian civilization. In terms of therapy, periodontal treatment has been featured in medicine and surgical textbooks for more than 1000 years. The Moor, Abu-al-Qasim, in his treatise on surgery "Al-Tasrif," discussed "scraping of the teeth" in his chapter on dentistry.[1] Long before its microbial, mineral, and biochemical complexity was appreciated, the chapter by Abu-al-Qasim discussed calculus and indeed the benefits of its removal using scraping instruments. The

difficulties of root planing were also apparent as he stated that these instruments were to be used on more than one occasion if necessary, until no calculus remains, and the "dirty colour of the teeth disappears."[1]

Even today, the mechanical removal of dental plaque and calculus from tooth root surfaces is considered the standard treatment for chronic periodontitis. Despite advances in medical sciences that would be inconceivable to those early dentists, treatment of periodontal diseases has changed very little, in principle, over the years. A large body of evidence now exists to demonstrate the efficacy of nonsurgical periodontal therapy (as reviewed by Cobb),[4] and despite debate relating to the merits of manual versus ultrasonic instrumentation or the degree of root surface smoothness/hardness to be achieved, scaling and root planing (SRP) remains the "gold standard" treatment for periodontitis against which other treatments are compared. Indeed, the standards of periodontal care and associated treatment philosophies are relatively homogeneous as evidenced by the consensus agreements reached at various European and World Workshops in Periodontology. Moreover, the clinical improvements that can be expected to occur after SRP are remarkably consistent across studies.

Thus it is currently accepted that antiinfective therapy, including mechanical and chemotherapeutic approaches, is the cornerstone of periodontal treatment.[5] Therefore, the scope of this chapter is to discuss the antimicrobial and antiinflammatory agents, protease inhibitors, and related drugs recently introduced to supplement the conventional periodontal therapy. It is worth mentioning that conventional periodontal therapy includes both surgical and nonsurgical techniques, the thorough examination and diagnosis of the condition, the initial and corrective therapies, and the maintenance of the patient. A salient feature of this chapter is the appreciation that any antimicrobial or chemotherapeutic application will be adjunctive to some form of mechanical debridement, and this relates to the fact that we are treating a biofilm-related infection that requires mechanical disruption.[6,7]

It is clear from the previous discussion that two main forms of chemotherapeutic agents are being considered: (1) the antimicrobials that will directly reduce the microbial burden; and (2) the antiinflammatory agents or protease inhibitors that will reduce the level of inflammation. With respect to antimicrobials, one must consider initially why these might be necessary. Clearly, the literature indicates that subgingival root planing, in many cases, is unable to eradicate all periodontal pathogens.[8,9] Explanations for this include the unfavorable anatomy of the root surface or the dimensions of the periodontal pockets making surgical and nonsurgical therapy difficult. Plaque and calculus could be difficult to remove in their entirety, in many cases continuing to exert an influence after mechanical instrumentation has been completed. Adriaens and colleagues[10] have also discussed that microbes may enter dentinal tubules, thus evading removal and the host response. It has been suggested that microbes are capable of invading the periodontal tissues.[11] One additional complication is the possibility of intraoral translocation of bacteria from one site to another that might allow periodontal pathogens to recolonize areas from which they have been removed.[12]

Thus although periodontal treatment through the ages has focused on reduction of bacterial infection by mechanical removal of infectious agents (i.e., SRP), recent clinical research has suggested that adjunctive antimicrobial or host modulators can help in the treatment of periodontal diseases. Adjunctive therapies including systemic antimicrobials and host response modulators can be combined with traditional periodontal therapies to reduce the bacterial burden (e.g., SRP), and also with risk factor modification therapies (e.g., smoking cessation) to constitute a comprehensive treatment strategy for periodontitis.

SYSTEMIC ANTIBIOTICS

As discussed previously, systemic antibiotics or antimicrobials should always be used as an adjunct to mechanical debridement, rather than as a stand-alone treatment (monotherapy), because the clinician is treating a biofilm-related infection. The antibiotics used in periodontics will be considered in some detail. In addition, whether antibiotic sensitivity testing is desirable during periodontal therapy needs to be considered. It could be particularly useful in cases in which specific organisms are not being eliminated by the antimicrobial used. However, sensitivity testing is infrequently used in periodontics because the organisms involved are relatively similar gram-negative anaerobic bacilli and spirochetes to a large extent.[13,14] An antimicrobial that is effective against *Porphyromonas gingivalis* is also usually effective against *Actinobacillus actinomycetemcomitans* and vice versa (as reviewed by Slots and Ting[15]). In addition, disrupting one crucial microorganism within a complex microflora could be effective in removing, disrupting, or killing the others. Systemic antimicrobial usage, as with any pharmacologic intervention, has disadvantages related to drug interactions, adverse effects, and allergies, and particularly for antibiotics, creation of resistant strains, and disruption of commensal flora.

Antibiotics are defined as naturally occurring or synthetic organic substances that can, in low concentrations, kill selective microorganisms. Systemic antibiotics are considered to enter the periodontal tissues and the periodontal pocket through transudation from the bloodstream. The antibiotics within the periodontal connective tissue then cross the crevicular and junctional epithelia into the crevicular region around the tooth, and thus find a way into the gingival crevicular fluid, which is associated with subgingival plaque. As repeatedly stated, the antimicrobial concentration in the gingival crevicular fluid will be inadequate without the mechanical disruption of the microbial biofilm adherent to the tooth, that is, subgingival plaque and calculus. In addition to its effect within the periodontal crevice or pocket, systemic antibiotic therapy might also suppress periodontal pathogens in other parts of the mouth including the tongue and mucosal surfaces. This additional effect on the oral environment is considered beneficial because it may delay subgingival recolonization of pathogens.[16]

The systemic administration of antibiotics includes the negative feature of disrupting commensal or "helpful" organisms in the oral environment and other parts of the body, potentially altering the host-commensal microbiota balance. A particularly good example is the disruption of microorganisms within the gastrointestinal tract by many antibiotics, which can lead to diarrhea and related problems. Tetracycline is notable in its effects in this area, but all other antimicrobials are capable of disrupting the gastrointestinal microflora to varying extents. In the past, antibiotics have been chosen more on the basis of traditional usage rather than on specific indication provided by either antibiotic sensitivity and isolation of specific pathogens, or randomized controlled trials indicating the efficacy of particular antibiotics in particular areas. In addition, the effect of the route of administration and the duration of use of the antibiotics have not been specifically investigated for periodontal therapy. An ideal situation would be that the subgingival flora involved in periodontal lesions would be sampled, the range of microorganisms involved detected, and their resistance to the antimicrobial evaluated before providing systemic antibiotics. As in many branches of dentistry and medicine, this is rarely done given not only the immediate need for antimicrobials in acute situations, but also the expense of doing microbiologic analysis and subsequent antibiotic sensitivity testing. Even if culture and sensitivity were performed for the microbiota from the periodontal pockets, its relevance is still somewhat unclear. The relative importance of organisms other than the periodontopathogens *P. gingivalis*, *Prevotella intermedia*, *A. actinomycetemcomitans*, *Tannerella forsythensis* (*Bacteroides forsythus*), *Fusobacterium nucleatum*, and *Treponema denticola* has not yet been clarified. Clinical and microbiologic research continues to identify more organisms that may contribute to the pathogenesis of periodontal diseases, but casts doubt on the pathogenic capabilities of some species. However, it should be reiterated that periodontal diseases are predominantly gram-negative anaerobic infections involving gram-negative anaerobic bacilli and spirochetes. It is thus likely that antimicrobials that can deal effectively with gram-negative anaerobic organisms will be of benefit in the treatment of periodontal disease.

As can be seen from Table 17-1, the common periodontal antibiotics have significant serum levels after single dosage and maintain this serum level for, in many cases, several hours to almost a day. Adverse effects typically include: (1) those related to the disruption of the gastrointestinal flora such as diarrhea, (2) dermatologic effects related to hypersensitivity as with penicillin rashes, or (3) the photosensitivity caused by tetracycline, which is known to adversely affect the skin's ability to cope with sunlight. Metronidazole has significant effects on liver cytochromes as does its chemically similar drug, Antabuse, which is prescribed to alcoholics to make them feel ill if they use alcohol. Metronidazole is commonly reported to cause nausea and vomiting, and these side effects may be related to its similar liver effects to Antabuse.

It is important to consider the adverse reactions to drugs in relation to the age of patients and other specific systemic conditions. As a general rule it is always wise to avoid any drug therapy, particularly systemic therapy, during pregnancy. Recently, however, the topic has become more complex after studies reporting the potential effect of periodontitis in pregnant women and on their risk for having preterm babies with low birth weight.[17] (See Chapter 32.) Given these data and the emerging data[18] that indicate periodontal therapy is effective in reducing the incidence of preterm low birth weight, some clinicians consider using antibiotics in conjunction with mechanical therapy. Metronidazole, however, should not be used without prior consultation with the patient's physician, because it has the potential to be teratogenic. Penicillins, however, may be safe. Tetracyclines such as doxycycline are contraindicated because they can discolor teeth during the calcification process before birth (Table 17-2). Consultation with the patient's obstetrician should be considered before prescribing any antibiotics.

In children it is crucial to consider the weight and the development of the child, adjusting the dosage of antibiotics accordingly to avoid excessive concentrations in serum. Similar to pregnancy, tetracyclines are contraindicated in children because of their deposition on calcifying

Table 17-1 Pharmacologic Properties of Typical Periodontal Antibiotics

Antibiotic	Absorption from Gastrointestinal Tract (%)	Peak Serum Level After Single Dose (μg/ml)	Serum Half-life (hr)
Penicillin (Amoxicillin)	75	8	1
Tetracycline (Doxycycline)	93	4	18
Metronidazole	90	25	10
Erythromycin	30	2	3
Clindamycin	90	5	2

Adapted from Slots J, Ting M: Systemic antibiotics in the treatment of periodontal disease, Periodontol 2000 28:106-176, 2002.

Table 17-2 Administration, Side Effects, and Contraindications

Drug	Dosage	Features	Pregnancy*
Penicillin or Amoxicillin	250 to 500 mg 3 or 4 times daily (depending on type of penicillin)	Diarrhea, rashes, allergies	Generally safe
Doxycycline	200 mg the first day, then 100 mg once daily (or 50 mg twice daily)	Dental discoloration, photosensitivity, diarrhea, Take 1 hour before food	Avoid
Metronidazole	250 mg 3 times daily, 500 mg twice daily, 200 mg 3 times daily	Nausea/vomiting, care with alcohol (nausea)	Consult physician before prescribing
Erythromycin	250 mg twice daily, 500 mg 3 times daily	Diarrhea	Avoid estolate form
Clindamycin	300 mg 3 times daily	Diarrhea	Generally safe

Consultation with the patient's obstetrician should be considered before prescribing any antibiotics.

enamel, causing tooth discoloration. Furthermore, it has been suggested that tetracyclines can cause depressed skeletal growth.

Care should also be taken with the elderly patient because their altered liver function and other metabolic processes may change the pharmacokinetics of antibiotics and create difficulty in predicting adverse effects. The risks for hypersensitivity reactions might also be increased in the elderly. Penicillin, which can produce allergies or in rare cases anaphylaxis, is a good example. Clearly, the older the patient the larger the possibility of a previous exposure to penicillin, thus the frequency and risk for anaphylaxis are increased. Other drugs used in periodontal therapy include clindamycin and erythromycin. Their most common adverse effects are the disruption of the gastrointestinal flora, causing diarrhea, and episodes of ulcerative colitis sometimes associated with clindamycin. Erythromycin is now rarely used.

If the clinician elects to use a systemic antibiotic as an adjunct to mechanical debridement, key considerations for choosing a particular drug include: (1) route of administration, (2) frequency of administration, (3) dosage to be given, (4) degree of absorption from the gastrointestinal tract, (5) degree and duration of drug concentration in the serum and at the site of infection, and (6) metabolism and excretion of the drug.[19]

Antibiotic Drug Interactions

In general, any drug that is carried in the systemic circulation can displace other drugs from the carrier plasma proteins. For example, the combination of barbiturates and hydantoins can reduce the plasma proteins available for carrying drugs such as metronidazole and tetracycline. Care should be taken in patients taking digoxin and warfarin, because metronidazole and erythromycin can increase the warfarin anticoagulant effect, and tetracyclines can increase the serum levels of digoxin. Metronidazole, as stated earlier, has effects on the liver and interacts with liver cytochromes similar to disulfiram (Antabuse), which is given to alcoholics to reduce enjoyment of alcohol. Any drug that affects the permeability and free ions available in the gastrointestinal tract, such as antidiarrheal agents or antacids, can decrease the absorption of drugs such as clindamycin and tetracycline. The list of antibiotic–drug interactions is enormous and is constantly updated. The practitioner is advised to keep up to date with the current information with respect to these interactions through electronic drug databases, because they may have significant clinical implications.

Clinical Effects of Systemic Antibiotic Therapies

Only a brief summary is attempted in this chapter, but Slots and Ting[15] provide an excellent review on the efficacy of antibiotics in a clinical setting during periodontal therapy. The advantages and disadvantages of specific antimicrobials in relation to clinical therapy are discussed in the following sections.

Recommendations for the Use of Antibiotics in Periodontal Therapy

Antibiotics can be administered for therapeutic, prophylactic, or preemptive purposes. Therapeutic antibiotic regimens are those used to treat established clinical infections such as chronic or aggressive periodontitis. Prophylactic therapy in periodontitis would involve giving antimicrobial agents to the entire population of individuals susceptible to periodontitis, which is approximately 30%. (See Chapter 3.) Clearly, this approach is not advisable because of the high risk-to-benefit ratio involved. The cost-effectiveness of such a prophylactic regimen also would not be considered useful. Therefore, selection criteria should be applied when considering prophylactic antibiotic use in periodontal therapy. In this respect, the prevention of infective endocarditis is a crucial consideration for the dental practitioner. The use of antibiotics during periodontal therapy could aid in the prevention of problematic bacteremias in patients susceptible to infective endocarditis. Moreover, it is increasingly appreciated that periodontally generated bacteremias may be one of the mechanisms in the putative association between oral and systemic diseases. (See Chapter 32.) How this association may affect the use of antimicrobial and antibiotic therapy during the treatment of periodontal diseases remains to be seen.

Selection of antibiotics for periodontal therapy is largely empirical but can, in certain situations, be based on laboratory microbiologic testing. Empirical antibiotic therapy is commonly used when treating acute necrotizing ulcerative gingivitis, which is characteristically associated with gram-negative anaerobic bacilli and treponemes forming pathogenic fusospirochetal complexes. Metronidazole is very effective in this therapy and is currently the regimen of choice.

In treating less acute forms of periodontitis, antibiotic sensitivity and resistance testing on microorganisms within the periodontal lesions may be performed initially before prescribing antibiotics. In many cases, microbiologic testing is unavailable. In these situations, the current view is that combinations of antimicrobials may have positive clinical effects. A recommendation has been made by Slots and Ting,[15] among others, that 250 to 500 mg metronidazole and amoxicillin could be given three times a day for 8 days and would be appropriate in at least 70% of the advanced periodontitis cases.

Another valuable combination of antimicrobials in periodontal therapy is metronidazole and ciprofloxacin, 500 mg of each drug given twice daily for 8 days.[15] This combination is effective against some enteric gram-negative rods not affected by the metronidazole–amoxicillin regimen. Combination antibiotic therapy can also be used for the treatment of localized forms of aggressive periodontitis. The antibiotics recommended for this condition were often tetracycline-based given the understanding that *A. actinomycetemcomitans* was not eradicated by drugs other than tetracyclines. Van Winkelhoff and colleagues,[20] however, suggest that metronidazole plus amoxicillin can be effectively used for the eradication of *A. actinomycetemcomitans*.

Single agent antimicrobial therapy in current periodontics includes metronidazole (500 mg three times daily for 8 days), clindamycin (300 mg three times daily for 8 days), doxycycline (100 mg once daily for 7 to 14 days), and ciprofloxacin (500 mg twice daily for 8 days). However, the use of antibiotic combinations as adjuncts to nonsurgical and surgical therapy is also common.

Clinical Protocol for Periodontal Antimicrobial Therapy

It is interesting to consider the use of antimicrobials in the initial course of periodontal therapy. Antibiotics are commonly administered for a period between 5 and 14 days, depending on the regimen used. In contrast, routine nonsurgical periodontal therapy is normally composed of between two and four appointments at one or two weekly intervals, whereby mechanical debridement of each quadrant or half-mouth is performed. (See Chapter 14.) It is considered ideal to have antibiotics within the serum and available to the periodontal tissues both during therapy and healing. Thus it would probably be most effective to provide the antimicrobials during and after the periodontal therapy. This would entail either continuing antimicrobial therapy for a period greater than 7 to 14 days or attempting to do the majority of the initial mechanical debridement within an 7- to 14-day period. Quirynen and others[21] suggest a protocol of nonsurgical periodontal treatment in appointments spaced 24 hours apart for initial therapy, combined with extensive antimicrobial mouthwash usage. In addition, they have provided full-mouth periodontal therapy within 24 hours without using chlorhexidine, a protocol that had similar efficacy in terms of clinical improvement.[21] Other researchers suggest that full-mouth root planing over 24 hours and quadrant root planing (done over 4 weeks) have similar clinical efficacy.[22] There may be cases in which the clinician would elect to do full-mouth root planing in a single appointment or over two appointments just a day or two apart, so that the majority of periodontal intervention could be achieved early within the 7 to 14 days of antibiotic therapy. Evidence for use of adjunctive antibiotics in combination with nonsurgical or surgical therapy does not clearly delineate the superiority of any one regimen over another.

Use of adjunctive antimicrobial therapy during maintenance care is limited to acute abscesses arising from sites that exhibit recurrence of periodontal disease. As in all cases, the lesions should be treated locally before the adjunctive antimicrobial therapy being used.

Antibiotic Characteristics

Penicillin

Penicillin (benzyl penicillin, penicillin G) is a beta lactam bactericidal compound that acts through inhibition of bacterial cell wall synthesis. Without an adequate cell wall the microorganisms are physiologically incapable of survival. Penicillin has a marked effect on prokaryotic cells with a limited effect on eukaryotic cells, and it is one of the least toxic of all antibiotics. The problem with penicillins, however, is the high rate of hypersensitivity to the drug. It has been shown that 15% of adults have allergic potential to penicillins. Moreover, with its widespread usage, many organisms have developed resistance to penicillin through the production of beta-lactamases, which destroy the beta-lactam ring of penicillin, rendering it inactive.

Augmentin is a proprietary combination of the penicillin derivative amoxicillin and clavulanic acid. Clavulanic acid is an inhibitor of beta-lactamase and thus overcomes the bacterial resistance to amoxicillin. Thus amoxicillin–clavulanic acid combinations are promising in the antibiotic augmentation of mechanical periodontal therapy. However, the combination of amoxicillin–clavulanic acid is significantly more expensive than other penicillins.

Tetracyclines

Tetracyclines traditionally have been the most commonly used antibiotics in periodontitis. Tetracyclines are bacteriostatic broad-spectrum agents that inhibit protein synthesis by blocking the translation of mRNA. They also have the potential to inhibit protein synthesis in eukaryotic cells but to an extremely small extent in comparison to the effect on prokaryotes. The most common tetracycline used in periodontics is doxycycline, followed by minocycline, both semisynthetic types of tetracyclines. Doxycycline and minocycline have the advantage of being completely absorbed through the intestine, and thus are less inhibitory to the indigenous gastrointestinal flora. Their chemical composition entails that they are less readily deposited in calcified tissue, which has long been the problem with tetracyclines. Past literature supports tetracycline use in juvenile periodontitis or, as it is now termed, *localized aggressive periodontitis*. There are also reports that tetracyclines are more concentrated in gingival crevicular fluid than in serum, providing greater concentrations of the drug at the local site of periodontal infection. Probably the most significant feature of tetracyclines, however, is that they have the ability to inhibit tissue collagenases and other matrix metalloproteinases. Golub and colleagues[23] suggest that this collagenase inhibitory activity is probably an aid in the periodontal healing processes after therapy. An increase in resistance to the general tetracyclines constitutes the major problem of these antibiotics, because they have been extensively used over the years and included in the preparation of many foodstuffs and veterinary products, which are administered routinely to animals to improve the meat yield. Doxycycline, however, is currently less problematic with respect to evidence of resistance within the microbiota.

Clindamycin and Erythromycin

Clindamycin is a derivative of lincomycin, whose mode of action is the blocking of protein production by binding to the 50S bacterial ribosome subunit, inhibiting RNA translation into protein. Clindamycin has been shown to be effective against a wide range of bacteria that may be involved in periodontitis, and it is a suitable choice for individuals allergic to penicillin.

Erythromycin is a macrolide antibiotic that inhibits protein synthesis in both gram-positive and gram-negative bacteria. It also binds to the 50S ribosome site and is commonly used as a substitute for penicillin, being preferred because of its reduced risk for causing hypersensitivity reactions. Unfortunately, many strains of A. actinomycetemcomitans, Eikenella corrodens, Bacteroides, and Fusobacterium are highly resistant to this antibiotic. Therefore its use as an adjunct in the control of periodontal microorganisms is not recommended.

Metronidazole

Metronidazole is a nitroimidazole specifically active against anaerobic organisms, particularly spirochetes. Metronidazole is highly effective in the treatment of acute necrotizing ulcerative gingivitis because this disease is closely linked to spirochetal infection. It has also been used extensively in the treatment of chronic periodontitis for which it is particularly suited given its high activity against gram-negative anaerobic organisms and spirochetes, with a very low incidence of resistance. Resistance to metronidazole is evident, however, in facultative microorganisms. A general rule for considering metronidazole efficacy is that the more anaerobic the organisms are, the more effective this antibiotic will be. A recent report has shown, for example, that isolates of A. actinomycetemcomitans (a microaerophilic organism, rather than an anaerobe) recovered from individuals with gingivitis and periodontitis were resistant to metronidazole, but susceptible to fluoro-quinolones (ciprofloxacin and moxifloxacin), ampicillin/sulbactam and doxycycline.[24] Table 17-3 shows the minimal inhibitory concentrations of the strains of A. actinomycetemcomitans tested to these antibiotics. Metronidazole has been typically combined

TABLE 17-3	Range of MIC, MIC_{50}, and MIC_{90} of 45 Strains of Actinobacillus actinomycetemcomitans to 5 Antibiotics		
DRUG	RANGE (μg/mL)	MIC_{50} (μg/mL)	MIC_{90} (μg/mL)
Penicillin/ sulbactam	0.19 to 2	0.38	0.75
Doxycycline	0.125 to 1	0.5	1
Metronidazole	1.5 to ≥296	6	≥296
Ciprofloxacin	≤0.002 to 0.006	0.003	0.006
Moxifloxacin	0.006 to 0.032	0.023	0.032

MIC, Minimal inhibitory concentrations; MIC_{50}, MIC inhibiting 50% of strains; MIC_{90}, MIC inhibiting 90% of strains.
Adapted from Muller HP, Holderreith S, Burkhardt U, et al: In vitro antimicrobial susceptibility of oral strains of Actinobacillus actinomycetemcomitans to seven antibiotics, J Clin Periodontol 29:736-742, 2002.

by clinicians with amoxicillin or penicillin to increase its spectrum, a combination that has been shown to provide highly effective results.

HOST MODULATORS

Protease Inhibitors

Subantimicrobial dose doxycycline (SDD; 20 mg doxycycline twice daily over 6 to 9 months) has been proposed as an adjunctive treatment for periodontitis.[25] A recognized feature of doxycycline is its ability to down-regulate the activity of matrix metalloproteinases, which are active in tissue breakdown during periodontitis. Our current understanding of periodontal pathogenesis suggests that matrix metalloproteinases play a major role in inflammation, tissue remodeling, and the destruction of collagen and bone within the periodontium, leading to clinical signs of periodontitis such as attachment loss, bone loss, and tooth mobility. There are now multicenter clinical studies to support the hypothesis that down-regulation of matrix metalloproteinases by SDD confers measurable benefits to patients with periodontitis.

Caton and colleagues[26] reported on a 190-patient, placebo-controlled trial in which all patients received SRP; half of these subjects also received adjunctive SDD (20 mg doxycycline twice daily). Patients were examined every 3 months over a 9-month period, and for those receiving SDD an improvement in attachment gain of 18% was noted (in patients with 4 to 6 mm pockets at baseline). The differences for SDD over SRP alone were greater in pockets of 7 mm or more, for attachment gain (33%) and pocket depth reduction (40%). Thus the literature suggests that SDD, when prescribed as an adjunct to SRP, results in statistically significant gains in attachment levels and reduction in probing depth when compared with SRP alone. Although the adjunctive use of SDD in addition to mechanical therapy may provide statistically significant improvement in attachment gain when compared with mechanical therapy alone, many have questioned the clinical significance of the differences, which average less than 0.5 mm.[25] One concern that arises with any antimicrobial usage is the emergence of resistant microbial strains, but research implies that SDD is not antibacterial at this dosage (20 mg), and it does not lead to the development of resistant strains or the acquisition of multiantibiotic resistance.[27] The drug is well tolerated by the body, and in clinical trials it is noted that the incidence of unwanted effects is similar to that of the placebo. Walker and coworkers[28] concluded that SDD and placebo did not produce effects on vaginal or intestinal flora over 9 months of usage. SDD is designed to be given over many months and may, therefore, suffer from compliance problems similar to other long-term medications used to treat chronic systemic conditions.

Nonsteroidal Antiinflammatory Drugs

Nonsteroidal antiinflammatories are drugs generally used in dentistry for the treatment of pain. However, as these drugs inhibit antiinflammatory processes related to the cyclooxygenase pathway, such as prostaglandin, thromboxane, and prostacyclin production, they also have the potential to be beneficial as adjuncts in periodontal therapy. It is recognized that prostaglandin E_2 and other arachidonic acid metabolites are important proinflammatory mediators in bone resorption and the various manifestations of periodontal disease.

NSAIDs are certainly of use after surgical periodontal procedures in the reduction of postoperative pain and inflammation. Ibuprofen, for example, has been shown to successfully inhibit prostaglandin E_2 production in the periodontal tissues after surgery, contributing to the healing process.[29] Ibuprofen as an adjunct for SRP, however, has not been demonstrated to be effective. Ng and Bissada,[30] for example, showed that ibuprofen (800 mg/d) administered as an adjunctive treatment to SRP did not improve the results on probing depth and clinical attachment levels when compared with SRP alone. Other drugs such as meclofenamate sodium (Meclomen) have been shown to produce positive results in patients with aggressive periodontitis. The use of systemically administered acetylsalicylic acid (aspirin; 500 mg daily for 6 weeks after mechanical debridement) has also been reported to be an effective adjunct in periodontal therapy.[31]

An important factor that must influence the decision on whether to use NSAIDs on a long-term basis is the gastrointestinal complications that may arise. Some cases may result in considerable ulceration of the gastric mucosa. Newer NSAIDs that selectively inhibit cyclooxygenase (cox-2 inhibitors) are much better tolerated by the gastric mucosa and may one day prove beneficial in modulating the host response in periodontitis.

CONCLUSION

A comprehensive periodontal treatment strategy should aim not only at the reduction of the bacterial burden by mechanical root debridement, but should also consider adjunctive antimicrobial therapy as part of the antiinfective strategy for certain patient populations. Clearly, mechanical therapy alone provides an excellent clinical response in most patients with chronic periodontitis. For these patients, adjunctive systemic agents are not generally indicated. In other patients, especially those with aggressive forms of periodontitis and those who do not respond to mechanical therapy alone, adjunctive agents may be indicated and should be considered as a viable therapeutic intervention.[32] In addition, host-response modulation using protease and inflammatory inhibitors may in the future become widely accepted as an adjunct to periodontal therapy. Furthermore, periodontal risk factor modification such as smoking cessation and simpler measures such as oral hygiene advice and motivation will continue to be crucial in the comprehensive treatment of periodontitis.

REFERENCES

1. Ring ME: *Dentistry: an illustrated history*, St. Louis: 1985, CV Mosby.
2. Anwar H, Strap J, Costerton J: Establishment of aging biofilms: possible mechanism of bacterial resistance to anti-microbial therapy, *Antimicrob Agents Chemother* 36:1347-1351, 1992.
3. Thrower Y, Pinney RJ, Wilson M: Susceptibilities of *Actinobacillus actinomycetemcomitans* biofilms to oral antiseptics, *J Med Microbiol* 46:425-429, 1997.
4. Cobb CM: Clinical significance of non-surgical periodontal therapy: an evidence-based perspective of scaling and root planing, *J Clin Periodontol* 29(Suppl 2):6-16, 2002.
5. Slots J: The search for effective, safe and affordable periodontal therapy, *Periodontol 2000* 28:9-11, 2002.
6. Gilbert P, Das J, Foley I: Biofilm susceptibility to antimicrobials, *Adv Dent Res* 11:160-167, 1997.
7. Socransky SS, Haffajee AD: Dental biofilms: difficult therapeutic targets, *Periodontol 2000* 28:12-55, 2002.
8. Stambaugh R, Dragoo M, Smith DM, Carasali L: The limits of subgingival scaling, *Int J Periodontics Restorative Dent* 1:30-41, 1981.

9. Dragoo MR: A clinical evaluation of hand and ultrasonic instruments on subgingival debridement. I. With unmodified and modified ultrasonic inserts, *Int J Periodontics Restorative Dent* 12:311-323, 1992.

10. Adriaens PA, De Boever JA, Loesche WJ: Bacterial invasion in root cementum and radicular dentin of periodontally diseased teeth in humans. A reservoir of periodontopathic bacteria, *J Periodontol* 59:222-230, 1988.

11. Lamont RJ, Yilmaz Ö: In or out: the invasiveness of oral bacteria, *Periodontol 2000* 30:61-69, 2002.

12. Quirynen M, De Soete M, Dierickx K, van Steenberghe D: The intra-oral translocation of periodontopathogens jeopardises the outcome of periodontal therapy. A review of the literature, *J Clin Periodontol* 28:499-507, 2001.

13. Moore WEC, Moore LH: The bacteria of periodontal diseases, *Periodontol 2000* 5:66-77, 1994.

14. Ximénez-Fyvie LA, Haffajee AD, Socransky SS: Microbial composition of supra- and sub-gingival plaque in subjects with adult periodontitis, *J Clin Periodontol* 27:722-732, 2000.

15. Slots J, Ting M: Systemic antibiotics in the treatment of periodontal disease, *Periodontol 2000* 28:106-176, 2002.

16. Muller HP, Heinecke A, Borneff M, et al: Microbial ecology of Actinobacillus actinomycetemcomitans, Eikenella corrodens and Capnocytophaga spp. in adult periodontitis, *J Periodont Res* 32:530-542, 1997.

17. Offenbacher S, Katz V, Fertik G, et al: Periodontal infection as a possible risk factor for preterm low birth weight, *J Periodontol* 67:1123-1137, 1996.

18. López NJ, Smith PC, Gutierrez J: Periodontal therapy may reduce the risk of preterm low birth weight in women with periodontal disease: a randomized controlled trial, *J Periodontol* 73:911-924, 2002.

19. van Winkelhoff AJ, Winkel EG, Vandenbroucke-Grauls CM: On the dosage of antibiotics in clinical trials, *J Clin Periodontol* 26:764-766, 1999.

20. van Winkelhoff AJ, Rodenburg JP, Goene RJ, et al: Metronidazole plus amoxycillin in the treatment of Actinobacillus actinomycetemcomitans associated periodontitis, *J Clin Periodontol* 16:128-131, 1989.

21. Quirynen M, Mongardini C, De Soete M, et al: The role of chlorhexidine in the one-stage full-mouth disinfection treatment of patients with advanced adult periodontitis, *J Clin Periodontol* 27:578-589, 2000.

22. Apatzidou DA, Kinane DF: Quadrant root planing versus same-day full-mouth root planing. I. Clinical findings, *J Clin Periodontol* 2003 (in press).

23. Golub LM, Ramamurthy N, McNamara TF, et al: Tetracyclines inhibit tissue collagenase activity. A new mechanism in the treatment of periodontal disease, *J Periodont Res* 19:651-655, 1984.

24. Muller HP, Holderrieth S, Burkhardt U, Hoffler U: In vitro antimicrobial susceptibility of oral strains of *Actinobacillus actinomycetemcomitans* to seven antibiotics, *J Clin Periodontol* 29:736-742, 2002.

25. Greenstein G, Lamster I: Efficacy of subantimicrobial dosing with doxycycline. Point/Counterpoint, *J Am Dent Assoc* 132:457-466, 2001.

26. Caton JG, Ciancio SG, Blieden TM, et al: Treatment with subantimicrobial dose doxycycline improves the efficacy of scaling and root planing in patients with adult periodontitis, *J Periodontol* 71:521-532, 2000.

27. Thomas J, Walker C, Bradshaw M: Long-term use of subantimicrobial dose doxycycline does not lead to changes in antimicrobial susceptibility, *J Periodontol* 71:1472-1483, 2000.

28. Walker C, Nango S, Lennon J, et al: Effect of subantimicrobial dose doxycycline (SDD) on intestinal and vaginal flora, *J Dent Res* 79:608, 2000.

29. O'Brien TP, Roszkowski MT, Wolff LF, et al: Effect of a non-steroidal anti-inflammatory drug on tissue levels of immunoreactive prostaglandin E2, immunoreactive leukotriene, and pain after periodontal surgery, *J Periodontol* 67:1307-1316, 1996.

30. Ng VW, Bissada NF: Clinical evaluation of systemic doxycycline and ibuprofen administration as an adjunctive treatment for adult periodontitis, *J Periodontol* 69:772-776, 1998.

31. Flemmig TF, Rumetsch M, Klaiber B: Efficacy of systemically administered acetylsalicylic acid plus scaling on periodontal health and elastase-alpha 1-proteinase inhibitor in gingival crevicular fluid, *J Clin Periodontol* 23:153-159, 1996.

32. Haffajee AD, Socransky SS, Gunsolley JC: Systemic anti-infective periodontal therapy. A systematic review. *Ann Periodontol* 8:115-181, 2003.

18

Contemporary Dental Hygiene Care

Jill Rethman, Connie L. Drisko, and Margaret Hill

DENTAL HYGIENE PROCESS OF CARE

Assessment, diagnosis, planning, implementation, and evaluation comprise the dental hygiene process of care. Mueller-Joseph and Petersen[1] describe the dental hygiene process of care as a cyclic continuum that could also branch into alternative treatments on the basis of the patient's response to therapy. In periodontics, the dental hygienist plays a pivotal role in the assessment and diagnosis of periodontal status, planning of care, implementation of a care plan, and ongoing evaluation of the care plan.

This chapter presents an overview of the dental hygienist's role in periodontal therapy in light of the dental hygiene process of care. Assessment of disease, dental hygiene diagnosis, treatment planning dental hygiene and periodontal care, implementation of the care plan, and evaluation of periodontal therapy are addressed related to the primary functions of the dental hygienist in periodontal care.

ETIOLOGY

Intuitively, understanding the etiologic factors of periodontal diseases seems critical to devising an effective therapy for each patient. Over the years, major efforts to better understand etiologic factors have yielded some progress.

Through the mid-1970s, the nonspecific plaque hypothesis held sway. The basis of this theory was periodontal practitioners' historic observation that therapies that limited plaque and calculus accumulation seemed to be more effective compared with other approaches. In the late 1970s and 1980s, it became clearer that certain patterns of bacterial colonization tended to appear in patients and at sites where destruction of the periodontium had occurred. Therefore, the amount of plaque was probably not as important as the quality of plaque (the specific plaque hypothesis).

Unfortunately, as researchers focused on specific bacteria, it was discovered that deep periodontal pockets might contain hundreds of different species. Further evidence suggested that each person's immunologic response to bacterial attack is not the same and that this response may even vary in the same patient over time. Despite these complications, painstaking research in recent years has implicated a number of bacterial species in the progression of periodontal destruction in humans. Unfortunately, the presence of these putative pathogens does not always mean that subsequent destruction will occur at a given site, and their absence does not guarantee that subsequent destruction will not occur (see Chapter 4).

Where does this knowledge gap in etiologic factors leave us in terms of therapy? Despite the obsolescence of the nonspecific plaque hypothesis, the interim goals of periodontal therapy in the adult patient—that is, therapeutic measures designed to assure improved and more frequent plaque removal by both patient and therapist—have not changed significantly since the 1970s and earlier. What *has* changed is increased recognition that a number of patients may be nonresponsive or only partially responsive to a traditional approach to therapy. Such patients may need to participate in more extensive and sometimes expensive etiologic assessments with subsequent treatment geared toward the results of those tests. Reassessments and retreatments may have to be repeated during these patients' lifetimes. Notably, therapies that may seem to be effective at one time in a patient's life may not work at another time because the patient may have a different periodontal disease or his or her immunoinflammatory response may have changed.

The state-of-the-art approach to therapeutics outlined in the preceding paragraph can place quality periodontal therapy at odds with some business management aspects of dental practice, because a logical end-point exists for most dental endeavors. Most restorative materials last for many years. Quality endodontic therapy is usually successful throughout a patient's lifetime. This is seldom true for thoughtfully conducted periodontal therapy (short of edentulism or death).

In periodontics, such an across-the-board expectation is not realistic. It may be difficult for both practitioner and patient alike to accept the inherent unpredictability of state-of-the art approaches to periodontal diseases. Yet, absent such understanding, many patients and therapists are destined for disappointment because of unrealistic expectations. Indeed, one essay suggested that the mere use of the term "periodontal disease" tends to mislead practitioners, dental vendors, and patients.[2] The author proposed that the term "periodontal syndrome" is more accurate and less misleading in terms of the need to interpret and fit new developments in periodontics into responsible treatment plans for the periodontal diseases. He maintained that precise terminology is key to the development and growth of an accurate dentistry-wide mindset about periodontal maladies and their solutions. Although the term "periodontal syndrome" has not gained wide acceptance, the universal use of the term "periodontal diseases" (plural) or "periodontitis" is more accurate than the singular term "periodontal disease."

The preservation and restoration of a healthy, aesthetic, and functional dentition and oral cavity are the primary goals of all dental therapeutic endeavors. Periodontics can play a part in each portion of this spectrum, but the early stages of the periodontal diseases are easy for both patient and therapist to overlook. Periodontal diseases are typically characterized by asymptomatic clinical signs such as bleeding on probing and loss of clinical attachment. That patients often are unaware of any problems can complicate explanations regarding therapy. Occasionally, the first problems may be discovered as a result of patient complaints about tooth looseness or sensitivity. In either set of circumstances, patients must be educated to understand that unchecked periodontal diseases may eventually lead to tooth loss and that, in occasional cases, tooth loss may occur despite state-of-the-art therapy. Furthermore, unchecked periodontal diseases may contribute to systemic health problems (Fig. 18-1; see also Chapter 31). Together with therapeutic roles, the dental hygienist acts as an educator and patient advocate in periodontal care. These roles are critical to ensuring health and treating disease at an early stage.

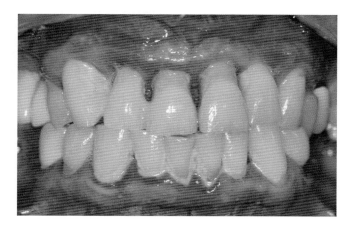

A

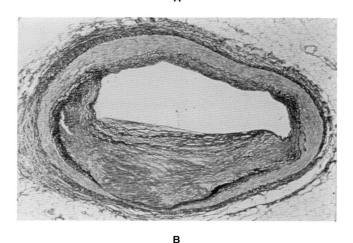

B

Figure 18-1. A, Severe periodontitis in a 70-year-old woman with a history of coronary artery disease. **B,** Histologic section of a coronary artery with a significant arteriosclerotic plaque. The specimen was secured at the time of autopsy.

As was reviewed previously, destruction of the periodontal attachment apparatus may be caused by specific bacteria or the interaction of a number of different bacterial species. The patient (or host) must be susceptible for this tissue breakdown to occur. Repeated comprehensive clinical assessments are critical for successful treatment in all patients with periodontitis. Therefore, traditional assessment methods should be part of all periodic examinations. The intervals between periodontal maintenance examinations should be customized for each patient. The data gleaned at each of these examinations should always be part of a written record. In terms of cost versus benefit, additional etiologic assessments are probably best suited for sites that remain problematic despite quality professional care and self-care.

ASSESSMENT OF DISEASE

Screening Examinations

Assessment is the initial step in the dental hygiene process of care. Two methods of assessment can be used when evaluating the periodontal condition. The first method is a screening technique to determine if a more comprehensive evaluation (the second method) is needed. Various types of screening examination techniques have been used. Screening examinations are used as a means of triage—separating those patients who require more detailed periodontal examination from those patients who do not. One example of such a screening tool that many dental practices in the United States have used is the Periodontal Screening and Recording (PSR).*

Periodontal Screening and Recording

As the name suggests, PSR is a *screening* tool for assessing periodontal conditions. It provides early detection of disease, thus promoting early (and hopefully more successful) treatment. A similar system has been used in Europe for a number of years. The Community Periodontal Index of Treatment Needs (CPITN), sponsored by the World Health Organization and the Federation Dentaire Internationale, was developed in the early 1980s. The CPITN has been used extensively to help clinicians decide if further diagnostic information is required about an individual patient. PSR is an adaptation of the CPITN. PSR simplifies record-keeping and satisfies dental-legal requirements by providing a straightforward method for documenting repeated evaluations. PSR also is a useful tool for educating patients about periodontal diseases and

---

* Periodontal Screening and Recording (PSR) is a registered trademark and service mark of the American Dental Association.

may help motivate them to energetically pursue proper home care procedures.

When should a periodontal screening examination be performed?

Periodontal screening should be performed at every oral examination. Although periodontal screening is designed primarily for use with patients 18 years of age and older, valuable information may be obtained about some younger patients. It is important to remember that periodontal screening does not replace a complete periodontal examination, but it does indicate to the professional when a partial- or full-mouth comprehensive examination is needed. Patients undergoing periodontal maintenance after active periodontal treatment will require periodic comprehensive periodontal examinations. Although screening examinations such as the PSR may be more appropriately used in a general dental office, periodontists and their hygienists may also use such examinations where appropriate. Such use will increase familiarity with the screening system and enhance communication with general practitioners when discussing patient treatment options.

Routine use of periodontal screening examinations allows the general practitioner to use his or her clinical expertise to determine the best treatment methods for a patient. This might involve referral to a periodontist or treatment by the generalist. Periodontal screening gives the examining dentist the option to confer with the periodontist at any time, thus promoting the partnership concept of patient treatment. Where state law allows, the dentist might delegate screening duties to a dental hygienist, thereby involving the hygienist as a cotherapist.

Because the PSR has been used widely in the past and currently remains in use in many dental practices, it is helpful to describe it in detail. Periodontal screening involves two concepts that differ from the traditional comprehensive periodontal examination. First, the mouth is divided into sextants. For each sextant (with one or more teeth or implants), **only the highest score is recorded**. An "X" is recorded when a sextant is edentulous. Second, the use of a special probe is recommended. The probe has a spherical end to limit penetration into the tissues. A color-coded area extends from 3.5 to 5.5 mm on the shank of the probe. A traditional periodontal probe also can be used, but the color-coded design facilitates documentation.

During screening, the tip of the probe is inserted in the gingival crevice around each tooth or implant. The probe is inserted gently until resistance is felt, and the depth of insertion is read according to how much of the colored band remains visible. Notably, pocket depths are not being measured, and only the colored band on the probe is monitored. The total extent of the crevice should be explored by "walking" the probe around each tooth or implant.

A standard coding system has been designed that reflects the amount of the colored band remaining visible (Box 18-1). Codes range from 0 through 4, and the **highest number** for each sextant is recorded on the patient's chart.

According to PSR literature, the therapeutic management of patients, on the basis of their sextant scores, is determined by the examining dentist. The practitioner must decide if an individual patient is best treated by the general dentist or should be referred to a periodontist. Management for Codes 0 through 2 may be relatively simple and routine such as prophylaxis, or scaling in the presence of gingival inflammation, and improved self-care. The correction of defective margins and overhangs may greatly improve the gingival condition. Codes 3 and 4 will likely require more aggressive treatment. Any possible risks, as well as probable outcome, should be discussed with the patient together with treatment recommendations. All communication should be well documented in the patient's chart, with the signatures of both doctor and patient.

PSR is a straightforward, initial step toward periodontal disease detection. The American Dental Association and the American Academy of Periodontology recommend the use of PSR to improve the likelihood of early detection of periodontal maladies. Routine use of PSR provides benefits to both patients and clinicians. For the patient, periodontal screening can become an important link in the process of educating them about the necessity of preventive periodontal care, or effective methods of treatment, or both. For the clinician, PSR is convenient and quick. The widespread use of periodontal screening may facilitate early detection and treatment of periodontal diseases, thereby helping more patients retain their teeth for their lifetimes. It may also help protect practitioners medicolegally.

Comprehensive Periodontal Assessment

A comprehensive periodontal assessment entails more detailed examination. This section is organized into traditional methods, which should be performed on all periodontal patients at each evaluation, and additional, more specific (and expensive) methods, which might best be used for patients who show limited responses to meticulous plaque control (both supragingival and subgingival) performed by the therapist and patient working as a team.

Traditional assessment methods

Traditional methods of comprehensive periodontal examination include measurements of pocket depth and

Box 18-1	**Screening Codes**

Code 0

For a Code 0 score, the colored area of the probe remains completely visible at the deepest site of the sextant (i.e., no probing depth greater than 3.5 mm). This indicates that no probing depths in that sextant are greater than 3.5 mm in depth. No bleeding on probing is detected, and calculus or defective margins are not present.

Code 1

With a Code 1 score, the colored area of the probe also is completely visible at the deepest site in the sextant. However, some bleeding occurs during gentle probing. As with Code 0, no defective margins or calculus are present.

Code 2

A Code 2 score also is indicated when the colored area of the probe is completely visible in the deepest site of the sextant. The difference between Code 2 and Code 1, however, is that a Code 2 is recorded when supragingival or subgingival calculus, or defective margins, or both are detected. Code 2 is *not* related to gingival bleeding.

Code 3

For Code 3, the colored area of the probe remains only partly visible. This indicates that the deepest probing depth of that sextant is between 3.5 and 5.5 mm. A comprehensive periodontal examination and charting of the affected sextant is needed to determine a proper treatment plan. If two or more sextants are scored as Code 3, a comprehensive full-mouth examination and charting is required.

Code 4

Code 4 is recorded when the colored area of the probe completely disappears, indicating a probing depth greater than 5.5 mm. As soon as a Code 4 is discovered for any tooth in a sextant, that sextant is scored accordingly and the next sextant is examined. A Code 4 in any sextant necessitates a full-mouth periodontal examination and charting.

Code ✱

Code ✱ is used to indicate clinical abnormalities. These could include furcation invasion, tooth mobility, mucogingival problems, or gingival recession of 3.5 mm or greater. Specific notation of the abnormality should be made in the patient's record. If Code ✱ exists in the presence of Code 3 or 4, a comprehensive full-mouth periodontal examination and charting is necessary.

clinical attachment level, bleeding on probing, suppuration, radiographs, mobility, and occlusal abnormalities (see Chapter 8). The following sections provide brief descriptions of each method.

Probing depth. This is a linear measurement made from the most coronal extent of the gingival margin to the base of the sulcus and is usually recorded at six sites (i.e., mid-facial, mesial-facial, mesial-lingual, mid-lingual, distolingual, and distofacial) around the perimeter of each tooth. Gentle probing using a periodontal probe is recommended. The most commonly used brands of periodontal probes are round and are 0.4 mm in diameter at their tips. Inflamed gingiva permits a periodontal probe to penetrate through the epithelial attachment into connective tissue. Therefore, probing of inflamed gingiva will almost always overstate the "true" pocket depth by at least 1 mm. This can be misleading and can suggest to inexperienced professionals that minimal therapeutic interventions (e.g., a single prophylaxis and improved self-care) are successfully arresting the progression of peri-

odontal destruction. The reality may be quite different. Therefore, the most useful baseline probing depths (and attachment loss measurements) are those made after initial control of inflammation and during reevaluation appointments at sites where supragingival plaque is reasonably well controlled by daily self-care. It also is important to remember that the six sites chosen for recording of sulcus depths are specified only so that the therapist can generate a written record of examination results. Correct probing is actually conducted all the way around each tooth, not just at the six aforementioned sites. Therefore, the six recorded depths are to some extent extrapolations of data obtained from sites such as mid-mesial or mid-distal aspects, where destruction of the periodontium is most likely to occur, but where it is usually difficult to obtain accurate probing depths in a consistent manner. Because of the high measurement variability at interproximal sites, it is generally accepted that an increase of 2 or more mm of attachment loss over time indicates that a true loss of periodontal support apparatus ("disease activity") has occurred in the interval between measurements. Conversely, at mid-facial or midlingual sites, a smaller change may be suggestive of disease activity.

Clinical attachment level. The clinical attachment level measurement is taken from a fixed reference point (usually the cementoenamel junction) to the base of the sulcus. The probing depth plus the amount of recession equals the amount of attachment loss. The "gold standard" for measurement of past periodontal disease activity is loss of clinical attachment level.[3] Prospective studies have shown that clinical attachment level measurements are the most valid method of assessing treatment outcomes.[4] Accurate baseline measurements are the foundation for effective longitudinal monitoring of attachment loss.

Bleeding on probing. Bleeding on *gentle* probing is an easily obtained clinical sign of inflammation. Some authors have suggested that bleeding on probing may "predict" sites at greater risk for subsequent periodontal breakdown; however, only 30% of sites with repeated bleeding on probing at sequential examinations have attachment loss.[5,6] Therefore, bleeding on probing should be used more as a sign directed toward resolution of inflammation, rather than as a predictor of future events.

Furcation involvement. The area of root separation on multirooted teeth (furcation or furca) can experience interradicular bone loss, which creates a niche for plaque biofilm. Because these areas are difficult to access by the patient and clinician, they can contribute to further breakdown.

Suppuration. Suppuration is sometimes observed accompanying severe inflammation at sites with advanced periodontal destruction and deep probing depths. Its predictive value for subsequent disease activity is low, and in patients who are otherwise healthy, it probably has no more meaning than does bleeding on probing at the same site[6]—that is, suppuration is a clinical indicator of existing inflammation.

Radiographs. Radiographs may depict past periodontal destruction, but they are poor predictors of further breakdown.[7] It has been shown that attachment loss typically precedes bone loss on radiographs by months. However, radiographs provide an important view of changes that have occurred (see Chapter 9). Vertical bitewings generally provide better visualization of bone loss than horizontal bitewings. Subtraction radiography (involving computerized comparisons of geometrically registered radiographs made at different times) is a highly sensitive indicator of subtle changes in bone, which may be related to destruction or repair.[8]

Mobility. Healthy teeth will move a few hundredths of a millimeter in response to normal loading. Greater movement may be caused by either excess loading (termed "primary mobility"), normal loading accompanying diminished periodontal support (termed "secondary mobility"), or both. Either type of mobility may be an important consideration in a tooth's prognosis. Retrospective, private, practice-based studies suggest that high degrees of mobility may facilitate increased periodontal destruction and retard the healing of a treated periodontal lesion.[9,10] Occlusal adjustments, splinting, or both may be indicated in some cases of tooth mobility (see Chapter 29).

Additional assessment methods

Additional assessment methods include microbiologic, immunologic, genetic, and gingival crevicular fluid (GCF) assays. In addition, other means may be necessary to assess the presence or location of subgingival plaque and calculus.

Microbiologic methods. Because periodontal diseases are bacterial infections, microbiologic methods of assessment may help to determine possible etiologic agents and methods of treatment. Although these methods are not used routinely because of cost considerations and limited knowledge about the therapeutic ramifications of their results, they could be useful in determining appropriate antibiotic therapy, in monitoring response to treatment in children and refractory adult periodontal patients, or both. These methods include microscopy, DNA probes, and culturing.

Microscopy. Darkfield and phase-contrast microscopy are probably of minimal value in disease assessment because many of the suspected periodontal pathogens are nonmotile and difficult to identify. Microscopy may have some value as a motivational tool for individual patients.

DNA probes. DNA probes test for specific organisms that may be present in the gingival sulcus. A sterile paper point is inserted into the sulcus to collect the material to be analyzed. The material is sent to a reference laboratory for analysis. DNA probes currently analyze for a limited number of pathogens and do not determine the antibiotic sensitivity of a specific bacterium.

Culturing. Culturing is technique sensitive and costly, but it can be used to detect specific organisms and may be used to help determine their antibiotic sensitivities (Fig. 18-2). Bacterial samples are obtained in the dental office and sent to a reference laboratory for analysis. Organisms are grown in culture media conducive to their survival. Culturing is performed at several laboratories affiliated with major universities.

Genetic assays. One genetic test for susceptibility to periodontitis currently exists. It tests for polymorphisms in the interleukin-1 (IL-1) gene cluster (Fig. 18-3; see also Chapter 3). Approximately 30% of white

```
================================================================================================
LABORATORY ANALYSIS REPORT FOR SPECIMEN NUMBER 00-03046                    DATE  01/03/2001
================================================================================================
```

CULTURE	% Microflora	% INHIBITION		
		Doxycycline-HCL 4 micrograms/ml	Amoxicillin 8 micrograms/ml	Metronidazole 16 micrograms/ml
A. actinomycetemcomitans	0.121	0	100	100
Porphyromonas gingivalis	0.000			
Prevotella intermedia	0.931	85	94	100
Beta-hemolytic streptococci	0.000			
Campylobacter (Wolinella) sp.	0.552	100	100	100
Capnocytophaga species	0.000			
Fusobacterium species	0.000			
Peptostreptoccocus micros	0.000			
Enteric gram negative rods	0.000			
Yeast	0.000			
Enterococcus species	0.000			
Prevotella melaninogenica	0.000			
Non-pigmented Prevotella sp.	0.000			
Staphylococcus aureus	0.000			
Staphylococcus species	0.000			

MORPHOTYPE				
Spirochetes				
Motile rods				
Nonmotile rods				
Cocci				
Other				

```
================================================================================================
ANALYSIS OF SAMPLE RESULTS
Level of A. actinomycetemcomitans exceeds established threshold levels.
================================================================================================
```

Figure 18-2. The oral microbiology testing analysis report identifies the percentage of the specific organisms present, the percent inhibition of the three most common antibiotics, and an analysis of the sample results.

REPORT: PST® GENETIC TEST FOR SUSCEPTIBILITY TO PERIODONTAL DISEASE

Indication for testing: chronic periodontitis.

RESULT: PST-NEGATIVE
This individual's composite genotype is:　　IL-1A:　1,1　　IL-1B:　1,2

INTERPRETATION
This individual does not have the PST-positive genotype and therefore is not at increased risk for periodontal disease by overproduction of IL-1 in the presence of bacteria.

The PST composite genotype is based on the combination of the results for the IL-1A and IL-1B genes. Any combination that includes the presence of a '2' in **both** IL-1A and IL-1B is defined as 'PST-positive' and predisposes an individual to periodontal disease.

This individual's result does not rule out all risk for periodontal disease.

RECOMMENDATIONS
For PST-negative patients with periodontal disease who are non-smokers, supportive periodontal therapy and treatment is indicated.

For PST-negative patients with periodontal disease who are smokers, aggressive treatment and a smoking cessation program are indicated.

The PST test assesses one of several risk factors that should be included in an overall evaluation of risk for periodontal disease. Specific bacteria are associated with the initiation of the disease, and additional risk factors including genetic susceptibility, smoking, diabetes, and oral hygiene have an amplifying effect on disease progression.

Genetic counseling and explanation of test results is available at no charge for clinicians and/or patients.

Figure 18-3. An example of a genetic test for susceptibility to periodontal disease.

Continued

TEST METHODOLOGY

Patient DNA is analyzed for the IL-1A +4845 and the IL-1B +3954 gene polymorphisms by PCR amplification of these specific gene regions followed by digestion with restriction enzyme Fnu4H1 (for IL-1A) or Taq I (for IL-1B). Fragments are separated by polyacrylamide gel electrophoresis. Sensitivity and specificity for detecting each of these mutations is >99.9%. This test evaluates only for the above polymorphisms in IL-1A and IL-1B and cannot detect genetic abnormalities elsewhere in the genome.

An individual can have the following genotypes at each IL-1 gene:
IL-1A: 1,1 or 1,2 or 2,1 or 2,2   IL-1B: 1,1 or 1,2 or 2,1, or 2,2

INFORMATION ABOUT THE IL-1A and IL-1B POLYMORPHISMS

Periodontal disease affects over 30% of the adult population, with severe disease reported in 7-13% of adults. Periodontal disease may be prevented by the early identification of patients with increased susceptibility for rapid disease progression.

A PST-positive genotype impacts periodontal disease in several ways. Individuals who are PST-positive have 1) an increased inflammatory response in the presence of bacteria, 2) increased overall bacterial counts and specific bacterial types associated with active periodontal disease, 3) increased risk for developing severe periodontal disease, and 4) increased risk for tooth loss.

Interleukin-1 (IL-1) is a cytokine known to be involved in the inflammatory component of periodontal disease. PST-positive individuals have a more vigorous inflammatory response to bacteria through the production of up to four times more IL-1 than produced by PST-negative individuals. The presence of the PST-positive genotype, as determined by the PST test, identifies individuals who are at an increased risk to develop periodontal disease. PST-positive individuals are at a 3-7-fold increased risk for severe periodontal disease. The combination of a PST-positive result and smoking leads to an even greater likelihood for severe periodontal disease.

REFERENCES

1. McGuire, MK et al (1999). Prognosis versus actual outcome. IV. The effectiveness of clinical parameters and IL-1 genotype in accurately predicting prognoses and tooth survival. J Periodontal 70:49-56.
2. Kornman, KS et al (1997). The interleukin-1 genotype as a severity factor in adult periodontal disease. J Clin Periodontol 24:72-77.
3. McDevitt, MJ et al (2000). Interleukin-1 genetic association with periodontitis in clinical practice. J Periodontol 71:156-163.
4. Reference List: Risk Assessment and the role of genetics in periodontal disease (1999). Interleukin Genetics, Inc. Available upon request.

PST® is a registered service mark of Interleukin Genetics, Inc.
PST® genotyping is performed under a license from Interleukin Genetics, Inc.

Figure 18-3. cont'd.

individuals are positive for a polymorphism of the IL-1 gene cluster.[11] In some populations, the presence of this polymorphism is low. Only 2.3% of individuals with Chinese ancestry are genotype-positive.[12] Therefore, the test is of little value as a susceptibility test in certain patient populations. Indeed, its usefulness in white individuals is questionable in light of relatively high false-positive and false-negative results.[13]

Gingival crevicular fluid assays. GCF has been the focus of biochemical assessments for disease activity. The flow rate and composition of GCF have been related to periodontal status.

Flow rate. A reduction in GCF flow has been noted after resolution of gingivitis. However, GCF measurements are not an improvement from probing and visual assessment for gingivitis. The value of GCF rates in deep pockets is currently unclear.

Enzymes (collagenase and elastase). Collagenase and elastase enzymes have been shown to increase with increasing disease activity, but the clinical value of these tests remains unclear because of cost factors and because monitoring on a less than daily basis may not be therapeutically meaningful.

Other enzymes. Enzymes such as aspartate aminotransferase, lactate dehydrogenase, and β-glucuronidase are indicators of neutrophil degranulation or cell death. GCF levels of these enzymes have been correlated with evidence of tissue destruction, attachment loss, bone loss, and loss of teeth, but their clinical value remains unclear for the same reasons as stated earlier.

Recent technologic advances aid in the detection of plaque and calculus on subgingival surfaces. The DVD2 Perioscopy System (DentalView, Inc., Irvine, Calif.) is a periodontal endoscope that projects root surface images onto a computer monitor. Images are magnified 24 to 48 times, thus improving visualization. The DetecTar Probe (Ultradent, Salt Lake City, Utah) emits a low infra-red light that identifies calculus in the presence of blood, saliva, or suppuration. When calculus is detected, a light at the juncture of the probe and handle lights up and the unit emits a sound. The probe is the same diameter as a conventional periodontal probe, with graduated markings to measure pocket depth.

DENTAL HYGIENE DIAGNOSIS

After performing a periodontal assessment, the next step is to formulate a dental hygiene diagnosis using current diagnostic parameters[14] (see Chapter 2). To keep a proper perspective of these various states of disease, a definition and clarification of health, gingivitis, and periodontitis are detailed in this section[15] (Table 18-1).

Health is the condition of a patient in which there is function without evidence of disease or abnormality. When discussing the periodontal structures, health could include the following:

1. Sites that are disease-free with no attachment loss or recession
2. Sites that have been successfully treated for periodontal destruction and have attachment loss and recession from previous episodes of disease activity

The probing depth of a healthy sulcus can range from 1 to 4 mm.[16] Bleeding on probing and suppuration are absent. A patient in a state of health requires no periodontal treatment, but is periodically monitored to ensure the healthy state is maintained.

Gingivitis is inflammation of the gingiva, clinically characterized by changes in color, gingival form, position, surface appearance, and presence of bleeding and/or exudate.

Periodontitis is an inflammation of the supporting tissues of the teeth, usually a progressively destructive change leading to loss of bone and periodontal ligament in which inflammation from the gingiva extends into the adjacent bone and ligament.

Case Types

Although patients can be classified by the terms *health*, *gingivitis*, and *periodontitis*, case types are used to describe the stage of destruction or disease progression. These case types have been developed by the American Academy of Periodontology and are used to more fully communicate the condition of the patient, especially for insurance purposes.[17] Types I through IV, as described by the American Academy of Periodontology, are detailed in the following sections.

Case type I: Gingival disease.

Gingivitis presents no clinical attachment loss. Bone loss is not evident when radiographs of the periodontal structures are viewed.

Case type II: Early periodontitis.

Gingival inflammation progresses into the deeper periodontal structures and alveolar bone crest, with slight bone loss. There also usually is a slight loss of connective tissue attachment and alveolar bone (Fig. 18-4).

Case type III: Moderate periodontitis.

This is a more advanced stage of periodontitis than type II, with increased destruction of the periodontal structures and noticeable loss of bone support, possibly accompanied by an increase in tooth mobility. There may be furcation involvement in multirooted teeth.

TABLE 18-1 Periodontal Conditions

TYPE	AGE	MEDICAL HISTORY	DENTAL HISTORY	FINDINGS	MICROBES
Health	Any	Probably good health	Good self-care and professional care	No BOP, attachment loss, or bone loss	Few putative periodontal pathogens
Plaque-induced gingivitis	Any	May be good; possible endocrine system, blood or medication modifiers	Inadequate plaque control	BOP, no attachment or bone loss	No specific flora; generalized increase in plaque biofilm
Nonplaque-induced gingivitis	Any	May be good; possible bacterial, viral, fungal, genetic, systemic, or trauma modifiers	Good or bad self-care and professional care	BOP, no attachment or bone loss	Causative agents vary (e.g., *Neisseria gonorrhea*, *Treponema palladium*, streptococci, candida spp., herpes viruses, and others)
Chronic periodontitis	Any, but most common in adults	May be good; possible systemic (diabetes, HIV), smoking, or stress modifiers	Variable self-care and professional care	Inflammation with progressive attachment and bone loss	Usually gram-negative; *Porphyromonas gingivalis*, *Prevotella intermedia*, *Prevotella nigrescens*, *Tannerella forsythensis*, *Treponema denticola*, *Peptostreptococcus micros*, *Campylobacter rectus*, and others
Aggressive periodontitis	Any; localized (usually circumpubertal onset) or generalized (usually younger than 30 years)	Usually healthy; familial tendency	Variable self-care and professional care	Rapid attachment loss and bone destruction	Gram-negative, *Actinobacillus, actinomycetemcomitans P. gingivalis*; spirochetes, others
Periodontitis as a manifestation of systemic disease	Any	Hematologic or genetic disorders	Variable self-care and professional care	General or local bone loss	Same as above; also reduction in polymorphonuclear leukocytes
Necrotizing periodontal diseases (NUG and NUP)	Any	Increased psychological or physical demand, decreased nutrient intake; HIV; smoking	Possible inadequate self-care and/or professional care, variable deposits	NUG: "punched-out" papillae, bleeding, pain, fetid breath; NUP: gingival, periodontal ligament, and alveolar bone necrosis	Treponema spp., *Selenomonas, Fusobacterium nucleatum, P. intermedia, P. gingivalis*

From Annals of periodontology, Vol 4, No 1: 1999 International Workshop for a Classification of Periodontal Diseases and Conditions, Chicago, 1999, American Academy of Periodontology. *BOP*, bleeding on probing; *HIV*, human immunodeficiency virus; *NUG*, necrotizing ulcerative gingivitis; *NUP*, necrotizing ulcerative periodontitis.

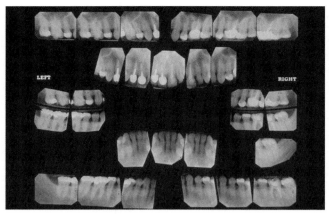

Figure 18-4. Type II early periodontitis in a 50-year-old man.

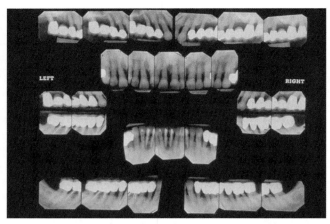

Figure 18-5. Type IV advanced periodontitis in a 55-year-old woman.

Case type IV: Advanced periodontitis.

Periodontitis progresses further in type IV, with major loss of alveolar bone support usually accompanied by increased tooth mobility. Furcation involvement in multirooted teeth is likely (Fig. 18-5).

Formulating the Diagnosis

The dental hygiene diagnosis is defined as "a formal statement of the dental hygienist's decision regarding the actual or potential problems of a patient that are amenable to treatment through the dental hygiene process of care."[18] It is important to recognize that "the purpose of the dental hygiene diagnosis is to keep the planning of care focused on problems or conditions that are amenable to dental hygiene interventions."[1] It is *not* a paraphrasing of a dental diagnosis, and includes only actions that can be rendered by a dental hygienist to improve a condition. Therefore, it should not interfere with state practice acts regarding the legal aspects of professional dental hygiene care.

The dental hygiene diagnostic statements related to periodontal conditions may include the following:

- "Generalized gingival infection related to high levels of plaque biofilm." (This condition could be improved with periodontal debridement performed by a dental hygienist.)
- "Potential for periodontal breakdown related to plaque biofilm and calculus accumulation on distal aspects of third molars." (This condition could be improved with periodontal debridement performed by a dental hygienist; see Fig. 18-6.)
- "Chronic periodontitis related to smoking." (This condition could be improved through tobacco cessation counseling performed by the dental hygienist.)

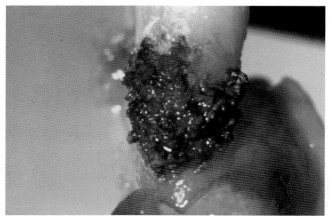

A

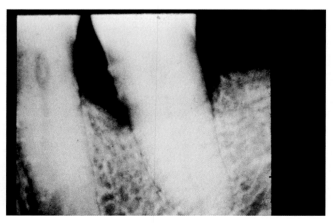

B

Figure 18-6. A, Plaque biofilm and calculus accumulation on a tooth surface. The gingival tissue has been retracted from the teeth. Note the inflamed tissue lining the pocket. **B,** The periapical x-ray reveals a significant accumulation of calculus associated with vertical bone loss on the mesial and distal root surfaces.

- "Root surface decay related to improper oral hygiene." (This condition could be improved through oral hygiene instructions performed by the dental hygienist.)
- "Nonplaque-induced gingival disease (allergic reaction) related to the use of sodium laurel sulfate–containing dentifrice." (This condition could be improved through use of alternative dentifrices recommended by the dental hygienist.)
- "Plaque-induced gingival disease (pregnancy-associated gingivitis) related to accumulation of plaque biofilm and hormonal changes." (This condition could be improved with specific oral hygiene instructions performed by the dental hygienist.)

Considered in concert with the dental diagnosis performed by the dentist, the dental hygiene diagnosis allows the dental hygienist to focus on the specific needs of the patient. The dental and dental hygiene diagnoses complement each other and promote optimum care (Table 18-1).

TREATMENT: PLANNING DENTAL HYGIENE AND PERIODONTAL CARE

The outcome of the assessment and diagnosis procedures will determine the treatment guidelines needed for each patient. It is important to keep in mind that each patient is an individual with a malady that may be largely unique. This suggests that each individual may respond uniquely to the therapy provided. Previously, "periodontal disease" was used as an all-inclusive term to describe periodontal attachment loss. All patients with "periodontal disease" tended to be treated similarly, regardless of susceptibility factors (medically compromised vs. uncompromised), self-care factors (motivated vs. unmotivated), and age factors (early age onset vs. older age onset). This type of treatment frustrated many practitioners and patients. A simplistic "cookbook" approach to treating periodontitis is not possible. Therefore, the results of continued reassessment of responses to therapy should be used to plan and adjust continuing care. Nevertheless, certain general guidelines are useful for managing periodontal patients in the general practice. The PSR coding can be used to suggest directions for treatment.

This section develops guidelines for treating typical chronic periodontitis patients after the scoring used in the PSR examination described earlier in this chapter. These are *suggested* courses of therapy and do not cover all possible situations faced by practitioners. The ultimate decision and responsibility for how to treat a given patient rests with the doctor–hygienist team.

Periodontal Screening and Recording Code 0: Health

Using the PSR probe, the colored area of the probe remains completely visible in the deepest crevice in the sextant. Using a traditional probe, pocket depths measure less than 3.5 mm. No calculus or defective margins are detected. Gingival tissues are healthy with no bleeding after gentle probing.

First appointment: 45 minutes to 1 hour
- Initial (new patients) or periodic examination (patients of record)—both consist of a medical and dental history update (including blood pressure monitoring), head and neck examination, and oral cancer screening
- Complete radiograph series, including vertical bitewings (new patients) or radiographs, as needed (patients of record)
- Adult prophylaxis
- Oral hygiene instruction
- Suitable maintenance interval established (3, 6, or more than 6 months)

The healthy patient is probably "dentally aware" and will likely be open to discussing new advancements and techniques in dentistry. This patient will likely recognize and respond favorably to enhancements in dental therapeutics. The oral hygiene instruction time might be used to discuss new oral hygiene products and their applications. Although further periodontal treatment is unnecessary at this time, the professional must not exhibit a complacent attitude. The patient must realize that future examinations may reveal disease even though his or her current status is healthy.

Periodontal Screening and Recording Code 1: Gingivitis (American Academy of Periodontology Case Type I)

Using the PSR probe, the colored area of the probe remains completely visible in the deepest sulcus in the sextant. Using a traditional probe, pocket depths measure less than 3.5 mm. No calculus or defective margins are detected. There is bleeding after gentle probing.

First appointment: 1 hour
- Initial (new patients) or periodic examination (patients of record)—both consist of a medical and dental history update (including blood pressure monitoring), head and neck examination, and oral cancer screening
- Complete radiograph series, including vertical bitewings (new patients) or indicated radiographs (patients of record)
- Chart sites that bleed on gentle probing
- Stain for plaque and relate stained areas to bleeding sites as part of oral hygiene instruction
- Periodontal scaling
- Nutritional counseling for the control of dental disease

Second appointment: 45 minutes (scheduled 7 to 10 days after first appointment)
- Monitor blood pressure
- Chart sites that bleed on gentle probing

- Stain for plaque and relate stained areas to bleeding sites as part of oral hygiene instruction
- Adult prophylaxis or periodontal scaling, if indicated
- Nutritional counseling for the control of dental disease, if needed
- Suitable maintenance interval established (3 to 6 months) or a third appointment is scheduled for 7 to 10 days later

This patient must be made aware of the problem areas in his or her mouth. Bleeding is a sign of inflammation. All bleeding points should be noted and pointed out to the patient and recorded in the chart. Areas of plaque accumulation also should be entered. Usually these areas will coincide with sites having gingivitis. This relation should be pointed out to the patient. If the patient is made to understand that the disease process is in an early stage and proper professional and self-care will probably reverse the disease, treatment is much more likely to succeed. Involve the patient as a "cotherapist."

Periodontal Screening and Recording Code 2: Gingivitis (American Academy of Periodontology Case Type I)

Using the PSR probe, the colored area of the probe remains completely visible in the deepest probing depth of the sextant. Using a traditional probe, pocket depths measure less than 3.5 mm. Supragingival or subgingival calculus, or defective margins, or both are detected.

First appointment: 1 hour
- Same as PSR Code 1

Second appointment: 45 minutes (scheduled for 7 to 10 days after first appointment)
- Same as PSR Code 1

The PSR Code 2 patient presents with the same conditions as PSR Code 1; however, there are physical irritants present (calculus, defective restorative margins, or both) contributing to the gingival inflammation. Patient involvement with therapy is the key to successful treatment, as discussed with the Code 1 patient. In addition, the removal of all physical irritants is essential. Sites with plaque should be recorded in the record. Sites that bleed on probing also should be recorded.

Periodontal Screening and Recording Code 3: Early or Moderate Periodontitis (American Academy of Periodontology Case Type II or III)

When using the PSR probe, the colored area of the probe remains partly visible in the deepest probing depth in the sextant (Fig. 18-7). Using a traditional probe, pocket depths measure between 3.3 and 5.5 mm.

First appointment: 1 hour
- Initial (new patients) or periodic examination (patients of record)—both consist of a medical and dental history update (including blood pressure monitor-

ing), head and neck examination, and oral cancer screening
- Comprehensive periodontal examination in affected area; sites that bleed on probing also should be recorded
- Complete radiograph series, including vertical bitewings (new patients) or indicated radiographs (patients of record)
- Stain for plaque and relate stained areas to bleeding sites as part of oral hygiene instruction
- Periodontal scaling and root planing, per quadrant
- Nutritional counseling for the control of dental disease
- Application of desensitizing medicaments, if needed

Second, third, and fourth appointments: 45 to 60 minutes (scheduled for 7 to 10 days after previous appointment)
- Monitor blood pressure
- Chart sites that bleed on gentle probing
- Stain for plaque and relate stained areas to bleeding sites as part of oral hygiene instruction
- Periodontal scaling and root planing, per quadrant
- Application of subgingival medicaments, if indicated
- Nutritional counseling for the control of dental disease
- Application of desensitizing medicaments, if needed

Fifth appointment: 30 to 45 minutes (scheduled 4 to 6 weeks after final scaling/root planning appointment)
- Monitor blood pressure
- Comprehensive periodontal examination in affected areas; record sites that bleed on probing
- Chart sites that bleed on gentle probing
- Stain for plaque and relate stained areas to any bleeding sites as part of oral hygiene instruction
- Periodontal maintenance procedures (scaling and root planing, polishing)
- Application of subgingival medicaments, if indicated
- Nutritional counseling for the control of dental disease
- Application of desensitizing medicaments, if needed
- At this time the patient may be put on a suitable recall/reevaluation interval 2 to 4 months later if disease appears arrested (i.e., no bleeding on probing from deep pockets at sites which patient is maintaining plaque free) and there is no other reason to refer to specialist

Maintenance appointments: repeat plan for fifth appointment described earlier. If deeper pockets are still bleeding on probing, it is probably best to refer this patient for possible surgical therapy.

Depending on depth of pockets and extent of bone loss, the PSR Code 3 patient has either early or moderate periodontitis. If Code 3 is detected in only one sextant, a comprehensive periodontal examination including probing depths, mobility, gingival recession, mucogingival problems, and furcation involvements should be performed *in that sextant*. Bacteriologic studies for determination of putative pathogens may be indicated at

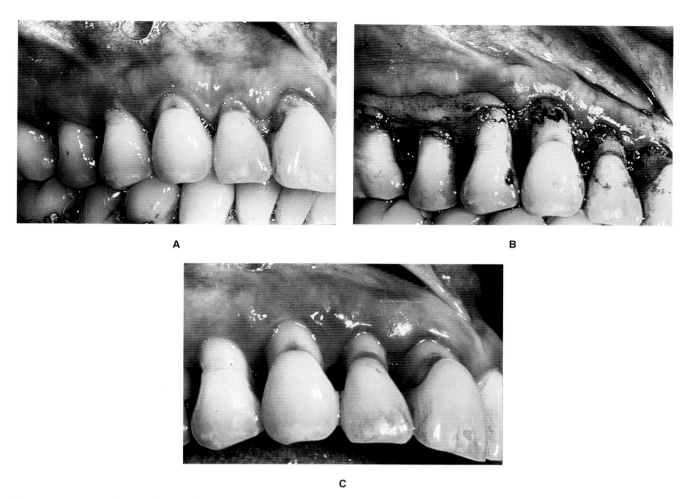

Figure 18-7. A, PSR code 3—early to moderate periodontitis. It is possible to see the dark areas of calculus under the gingival tissue. **B,** Open-flap root planing and scaling were done in order to gain access and thoroughly remove the calculus and plaque on the root surface. **C,** 6 months after root planing and scaling, the patient is maintaining good oral hygiene techniques and the tissue has remained healthy. No other procedures are necessary. The patient is placed into a maintenance recall system.

sites that are kept plaque free by the patient but are still bleeding on gentle probing. If a Code 3 is detected in two or more sextants, the comprehensive periodontal examination is indicated for *the entire mouth*. In this situation, the suggested guidelines for PSR Code 4 may be more appropriate (see later). It is always wise to make note in the record of the sites where the patient's home care fails to remove plaque. It also is important to always record which sites bleed when probed.

Periodontal Screening and Recording Code 4: Advanced Periodontitis (American Academy of Periodontology Case Type IV)

Using a traditional probe, pocket depths measure greater than 5.5 mm (Fig. 18-8).
First appointment: 1 hour

- Initial (new patients) or periodic examination (patients of record)—both consist of a medical and dental history update (including blood pressure monitoring), head and neck examination, and oral cancer screening
- Comprehensive periodontal examination of entire mouth; sites that bleed on probing also should be recorded
- Complete radiograph series, including vertical bitewings (new patients) or indicated radiographs (patients of record)
- Stain for plaque and relate stained areas to bleeding sites as part of oral hygiene instruction
- Nutritional counseling for the control of dental disease
- Application of desensitizing medicaments, if needed

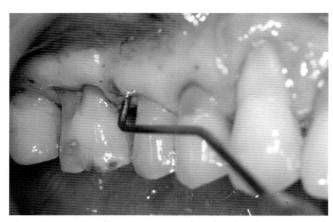

Figure 18-8. PSR code 4: Using a periodontal probe, the pocket depth measures 8 mm on the distal aspect of the maxillary right 2nd bicuspid.

Second appointment: 45 to 60 minutes (scheduled for as soon as possible after initial visit)
- Monitor blood pressure
- Chart sites that bleed on gentle probing
- Stain for plaque and relate stained areas to bleeding sites as part of oral hygiene instruction
- Periodontal scaling and root planing, per quadrant
- Nutritional counseling for the control of dental disease
- Application of desensitizing medicaments, if needed

Third, fourth, and fifth appointments: 45 to 60 minutes (scheduled for every 7 to 10 days)
- Monitor blood pressure
- Chart sites that bleed on gentle probing
- Stain for plaque and relate stained areas to bleeding sites as part of oral hygiene instruction
- Periodontal scaling and root planing, per quadrant
- Application of subgingival medicaments, if indicated
- Nutritional counseling for the control of dental disease
- Application of desensitizing medicaments, if needed

Sixth appointment: 45 minutes (scheduled 4 to 6 weeks after final scaling and root planing appointment)
- Monitor blood pressure
- Comprehensive periodontal examination of entire mouth; record sites that bleed on probing
- Stain for plaque and relate stained areas to bleeding sites as part of oral hygiene instruction
- Periodontal maintenance treatment (scaling and root planing, polishing)
- Application of subgingival medicaments, if indicated
- Nutritional counseling for the control of dental disease
- Application of desensitizing medicaments, if needed
- Referral to a specialist if *any* problems persist—this is likely in these patients

- At this time, patient may be put on a suitable recall/reevaluation interval 2 to 4 months later if disease appears arrested (i.e., no bleeding on probing from deep pockets at sites that *patient* is maintaining plaque-free) *and* there is no other reason to refer to specialist (persistent inflamed pockets, continued attainment loss, and others)

Continuous monitoring of self-care and bleeding on probing is essential in PSR Code 3 and 4 patients. Because of the severity of the condition of the PSR Code 4 patient, more aggressive and more complex treatment often will be necessary. It is important to keep meticulous records so that changes—either beneficial or deleterious—can be noted and addressed promptly. The need to repeatedly stain for plaque cannot be stressed enough—that is, if the patient cannot keep supragingival areas plaque-free at sites that bleed on probing, it complicates decisions about whether the underlying pathology is caused by destructive dynamics deep in the pocket or a mere superficial response to the continuous presence of supragingival plaque.

Conversely, if a patient keeps a site plaque-free (supragingivally) and it continues to exhibit bleeding on probing, it is a reasonable conclusion that an infective process continues deep in the pocket at that site. This clinical presentation suggests more aggressive therapy is probably needed because additional destruction may occur if the infective process is not stopped. Frequently, such sites also will exhibit deep probing depths. Surgical procedures, systemic antimicrobial therapeutic approaches, or both become the next level of intervention. Periodontal surgical procedures are typically designed to produce an anatomy that permits better self-care and professional care at affected sites. Even if these procedures are fully successful at achieving the desired changes in anatomy, a need for maintenance therapy will likely exist for the balance of the patient's life.

PSR Code 4 patients often will be referred to a periodontist. Nevertheless, initial therapy, including a comprehensive full-mouth periodontal examination, often can be performed in the general dentist's office. Other procedures, as outlined earlier, can benefit the entire patient-generalist-periodontist team by better preparing the patient for treatment options that may be presented. If surgery becomes the recommended course of treatment, the chances for success are greater at sites that the patient has been trained and motivated to keep plaque-free at home. The general dentist's team can prepare the patient with thorough oral hygiene instructions geared to point out and mitigate (on a site-by-site and repeated basis) sites that continue to bleed on probing. The generalist, periodontist, and involved hygienists should appear to the patient as a team specially organized to provide each patient the best treatment possible.

Periodontal Screening and Recording Code *: Clinical Abnormalities

Code * is used *with* Codes 0 through 4 when a clinical irregularity is observed, including the following:

- Furcation invasion
- Tooth mobility
- Mucogingival problems
- Recession extending to the colored area of the probe (3.5 mm or greater)

In cases of Codes 0, 1, and 2, the irregularity is specifically described on the patient's record and the appropriate treatment is administered for that abnormality or the patient is referred to a practitioner who can perform the appropriate therapy. With a Code 3 patient, a comprehensive periodontal examination of the asterisked sextant is necessary. A Code 4 patient should undergo a full-mouth comprehensive periodontal examination.

Full-Mouth Disinfection Therapy

Full-mouth disinfection therapy consists of four quadrants of root planing completed within 24 hours, with adjunctive chlorhexidine therapies to include rinsing, subgingival irrigation, and tongue brushing. The rationale for full-mouth disinfection therapy is to reduce bacterial niches in the oral cavity at the time of debridement to reduce the possibility of reinfection and enable better healing. In concept, full-mouth disinfection therapy could reduce the number of appointments and enable more efficient use of appointment time. However, the small sample size of studies that promote full-mouth disinfection therapy, together with noncorroborating data, indicate that further research is needed.[19] The practical implementation of full-mouth disinfection therapy may be difficult for many dental offices, because patients may have to be scheduled for more than one appointment in a 24-hour period.

Referral to a Specialist

The decision to refer to a periodontist is an important one and should be based on a number of considerations. The best interest of the patient always should be the first priority. Whenever satisfactory results are not obtained, the patient should be encouraged to seek treatment by a specialist. Most patients in the general dental practice will present with case type I (gingivitis), case type II (early periodontitis), or case type III (moderate periodontitis). A smaller number will be considered case type IV (severe periodontitis). The dental professional must determine, on a case-by-case basis, whether his or her ability and knowledge are sufficient to properly provide the needed care. If the general dentist or hygienist has the skill to deliver the required standard of care (the same standard as required of the specialist), any periodontal disease may be treated. Otherwise, a referral must be made for the

well-being of the patient and for medicolegal reasons. According to the American Dental Association's "General Guidelines for Referring Dental Patients to Specialists and Other Settings of Care,"[20] referral for specialty care is indicated for the following circumstances:

- Treatment is beyond the limits of the primary care dentist's skills or knowledge
- There is a need for consultation or expert opinion
- The referral increases the overall quality of care for the patient

Good communication between the referring dentist and the specialist is of utmost importance for successful treatment. Dentists initiating the referral should provide the following information to the specialist[20]:

- The name and address of the patient
- The appointment time and date
- The reason for referral
- Medical and dental information, such as medical consultations and specific problems, previous contributory dental history, models, and radiographs
- Projected treatment needs beyond the referral
- The urgency of the situation
- Any information already provided to the patient

The following steps can facilitate communication from the specialist to the primary care dentist:

- An initial report indicating the preliminary diagnosis by the specialist and anticipated treatment
- A progress report if treatment is extended over a considerable period
- A final report that includes information that might alter future courses of therapy; maintenance suggestions plus any other treatment recommendations
- The provision of copies or duplicates of appropriate preoperative or postoperative radiographs
- The return of any original radiographs or forms provided by the referring dentist

Both practitioners must determine who will be responsible for periodontal maintenance once the so-called active stage of treatment is completed. It is important for everyone (clinicians *and* patients) to understand that periodontal diseases usually require meticulous re-care (including periodontal maintenance and even other definitive periodontal procedures at times) for either the rest of the patient's life or until involved teeth are extracted. It may be advantageous to alternate routine maintenance appointments between the general dentist and the periodontist. This returns the patient to the referring dentist's practice while keeping the periodontist involved with the long-term periodontal maintenance care.

Immediately refer to the periodontist any patients exhibiting signs of aggressive periodontitis or periodontitis associated with systemic disease. These types of periodontitis have been associated with rapid destruction of the periodontium. Unresponsive cases and patients showing signs of periimplantitis also require the intervention of a specialist. Teenagers and children with periodontal diseases (other than reversible forms of gingivitis) also should be referred.

IMPLEMENTATION OF PROFESSIONAL CARE

It should be clear from the previous sections that periodontal diseases vary from patient to patient and even in a single patient from site to site or time to time. This variability contributes to the complexity of treatment. Assessment, diagnosis, and planning guidelines have been established; therefore, a description of the next step in the dental hygiene process of care—implementation—is in order. This section focuses first on professionally administered dental hygiene therapies followed by a review of recommended self-care techniques. Both mechanical and antimicrobial therapies are discussed.

Professionally Administered Therapies (Mechanical)

Mechanical therapies include those types of treatment administered by manual implementation, such as scaling and root planing and periodontal surgery (see Chapter 14). Thorough scaling and root planing remains a critical component of therapeutic strategies designed to arrest disease progression. Scaling is defined as the removal of plaque, calculus, and stain from the crown and root surfaces, whereas root planing specifies the removal of cementum or surface dentin that is rough and/or impregnated with calculus, toxins, or microorganisms.[21] As any therapist can attest, thorough root planing is one of the most difficult procedures in dentistry. The primary goal of scaling and root planing is to remove pathogenic microflora and toxins while rendering the root surface more hospitable to new attachment, resulting in gain of clinical attachment level. Previously, the objective of root planing was extensive removal of cementum. It was believed that bacterial endotoxins penetrated the root surface, thus making it necessary to remove as much of the affected cementum as possible. It has since been determined that achieving a glossy smooth surface is unnecessary.[22] Endotoxin does not penetrate root surfaces as deeply as previously thought, and excessive removal of cementum is thought to promote dentinal hypersensitivity.

Types of scaling and root planing instruments

Instruments for scaling and root planing procedures are either hand-activated or power-driven. Hand-activated instruments are available in various designs to effectively reach and treat all areas of the tooth (see Chapter 14) (Table 18-2).

Curettes have the most applications of all the hand-activated instruments. In addition, some curettes are designed to treat specific areas of certain teeth. Curettes have been introduced with longer shanks and smaller working ends to permit improved access to deeper pockets and areas such as furcations. Power-driven instruments, once used primarily as adjuncts to hand-activated instruments, now have a more expanded role. Large-diameter tips are effective in removing gross deposits of calculus and stain, whereas modified, slim inserts are used in deeper periodontal pockets. With power-driven instruments, patient comfort is enhanced and operator fatigue is reduced, because the use of heavy pressured strokes is unnecessary. Some research shows that power-driven instruments are superior to hand-activated instruments in debridement of Class 1 and 2 furcations.[23,24] Furthermore, advances in ultrasonic tips enable clinicians to use them in circumstances where they were once considered detrimental (e.g., specially designed

TABLE 18-2 Scaling and Root Planing Instruments		
INSTRUMENT	PURPOSE	AREA OF USE
Curette	Fine scaling and root planing	Supragingival or subgingival—most tooth surfaces
Sickle	Fine scaling and remove moderate deposits	Supragingival or shallow pockets—buccal, lingual, or interproximal surfaces
Hoe	Gross debridement—remove large deposits of calculus	Supragingival—mandibular lingual surfaces
File	Gross debridement—prepare heavy masses of calculus for curette use	Supragingival—buccal and lingual surfaces
Chisel	Gross debridement—remove large deposits of calculus	Supragingival—lingual surfaces of mandibular teeth

implant tips). Most dental professionals agree that a combination of both hand-activated and power-driven instruments is best for the majority of circumstances.

Power-driven instruments are often termed "ultrasonics." In reality, they may be sonic, ultrasonic, or piezo-electric instruments. Sonic scalers are air-driven. The frequency at which the tip vibrates is less than other types of power-driven scalers; hence, they may be less comfortable to the patient. Ultrasonic scalers are the most widely used type of power-driven instruments. These operate by magnetorestrictive power. (See Chapter 14 for a detailed review of instrumentation for scaling and root planing.)

Surgical versus nonsurgical therapy

As with scaling and root planing, periodontal surgery will likely always have a place in the treatment of periodontitis. Although some studies have concluded that scaling and root planing can be as effective as surgical procedures,[25] several factors should be considered when determining surgical versus nonsurgical treatment for a patient:

1. The goal of therapy. Some goals (e.g., periodontal regeneration) can only be attained using a surgical approach.
2. The skill of the professional and her or his ability to successfully treat a patient non-surgically
3. The depth of the pockets being treated
4. Anatomical difficulties associated with the area being treated
5. The patient's medical history
6. The patient's response to treatment that has already been provided

In the early 1980s it was suggested that the critical determinant in periodontal therapy is not the technique (surgical or nonsurgical) that is used for the elimination of the subgingival infection, but the quality of the debridement of the root surface.[26] This holds true today. Although deep probing depths are not the only criteria for surgery, the success rate in debriding root surfaces is greatly diminished in pockets with probing depths greater than 5 mm. If the infection persists after nonsurgical care, then surgery may be necessary.

Professionally Administered Therapies (Antimicrobial)

Antimicrobial therapy consists of treatments to control the microorganisms that cause disease activity. This therapy can be administered systemically by prescribing antibiotics or locally through controlled-release devices and subgingival irrigation, or both. Although mechanical methods are used primarily to eliminate plaque biofilm and calculus that predispose to disease progression, the use of antimicrobials as adjuncts to help eliminate specific pathogens may be indicated in some cases.

Rationale for antimicrobial therapy

The basic etiologic agent in periodontitis is bacteria. Elimination and suppression of pathogenic organisms will likely halt disease progression. Mechanical therapies are the foundation of all treatment regimens. However, there are some limitations to mechanical procedures. Although bacteria do not deeply penetrate root surfaces, studies have shown that certain bacteria may invade the gingival tissues.[27] This is significant because a bacterial niche for reinfection of the pocket may remain after scaling and root planing and surgical procedures. It also has been proposed that reinfection can occur from other pocket areas in the mouth. In addition, removal of all subgingival calculus and plaque is usually impossible. The anatomic structures of the root surface present physical barriers (furcations, concavities, and others) that make total debridement unattainable, either through "closed" or "open" instrumentation.[28] The following factors limit the effectiveness of scaling and root planing:

1. Anatomy of roots
2. Depth of pockets
3. Position of teeth
4. Inadequate instruments for diagnosis
5. Inadequate instruments for treatment
6. Area of mouth being treated
7. Size of mouth
8. Elasticity of cheeks
9. Range of opening
10. Dexterity of operator

Additional studies have investigated the limitations of scaling and root planing procedures with hand-activated and power-driven instruments.[24] As dental professionals, we hope to provide the best possible therapy for our patients. It is clear that mechanical treatments alone may not be sufficient to control periodontal infections, even when surgical access is obtained. Therefore, the adjunctive use of antimicrobials may help supplement the scaling and root planing and surgical procedures administered.

Systemic antimicrobial therapy: Antibiotics

Systemic antibiotics may be used to treat aggressive forms of periodontitis or those that don't respond to therapy. Other types of periodontal diseases, however, are best treated using basic mechanical procedures and localized delivery of antimicrobials. Systemic antibiotics do not seem to provide long-term improvement for patients with chronic periodontitis.[29] Possible advantages and disadvantages of systemic antibiotics are listed in Table 18-3. (See Chapter 17 for a detailed discussion of systemic antibiotic therapies.)

TABLE 18-3   Systemic Antibiotics: Possible Advantages and Disadvantages

POSSIBLE ADVANTAGE	POSSIBLE DISADVANTAGE
Can readily reach microorganisms	Patient dependent (compliance)
Can completely eradicate many pathogens from pockets	Patient sensitivity (allergies)
Can completely eradicate many pathogens from whole mouth	Superinfections (e.g., vaginitis)
Time efficient	Development of resistant strains
	Drug-specific side effects (gastrointestinal symptoms, dizziness, irritability, insomnia, unpleasant taste, photosensitivity, and others)

Local antimicrobial therapy: Controlled-release devices and subgingival irrigation

"Controlled-release" refers to delivering active chemicals to a specified target at a rate and duration designed to accomplish the intended effect. Advantages to using controlled-release delivery are:

1. High concentration of drugs delivered directly to the site of infection
2. Constant rate of delivery
3. Frequency of application is low
4. Success is not patient dependent

Antimicrobials used in controlled release vehicles include chlorhexidine, tetracycline, doxycycline, minocycline, and others (see Chapter 16). Biodegradable materials dissolve over a specific period together with the drug. As with other types of antimicrobial therapy, controlled-release systems do not replace existing treatment methods but may be used as adjuncts. They might be incorporated into the scaling and root planing phase of treatment. Controlled-release antimicrobials may also be useful in treatment of nonresponding sites, failing implants, and periodontal abscesses. Ideally, the medications should have sufficient concentrations to obtain the desired results (controlling infection, reducing probing depths, and reducing bleeding) without deleterious side effects.

Professional subgingival irrigation is the in-office lavage provided by the dental professional, delivering a medicament directly to the site of infection. Although rinsing will introduce agents into the oral cavity, medicament delivery through irrigation therapy affords targeted delivery of antimicrobials. Rinsing can be an effective method of supragingival bacterial control, but is not effective subgingivally. Professional irrigation therapy uses specialized systems with cannula tips that can readily reach the base of the pocket. The earliest devices used for in-office subgingival irrigation therapy were hand syringes and modified home irrigation units. Hand syringes are simple to use, but they are not ideal irriga-

tion devices because of the inability to control the amount of pressure at which the solution is injected into the pocket. It has been shown that syringes will deliver agents at pressures up to 500 mm Hg.[30] This amount of pressure could cause harm to the tissues and possibly promote abscesses. A safe level would be approximately 60 mm Hg (around 20 psi). Syringes deliver medicaments in a steady stream. An investigation comparing pulsating jet irrigators to hand syringes demonstrated that irrigation of periodontal pockets was more effective with a pulsating jet device than with a syringe.[31] Currently, hand-held syringes, powered irrigation devices, and/or ultrasonic scaling units can be used for professional in-office irrigation. A single episode of in-office irrigation has limited or no beneficial effects.[32] Repeated irrigations over time may be beneficial for some patients.[33]

Professional subgingival irrigation is a safe procedure. Although subgingival irrigation has been shown not to induce bacteremia any more than brushing and flossing,[34] the patient's physician should always be consulted when a high-risk situation is suspected (e.g., patient at risk for bacterial endocarditis). Some of the more common agents used for subgingival irrigation, their level of activity, and possible side effects are listed in Table 18-4.

Although no agent has American Dental Association (ADA) approval as an irrigant, some are approved for reduction of plaque and gingivitis when used as a rinse (chlorhexidine and essential oils products). Other agents that have been used for subgingival irrigation are povidone iodine, metronidazole, cetylpyridinium chloride, chloramine-t, and chlorine dioxide. Currently, there is no "perfect" irrigant. All agents have adverse effects; however, these effects are usually more apparent when rinsing as opposed to irrigating with the product.

It is important to realize that professional subgingival irrigation, together with other types of antimicrobial therapy, is an adjunct to the mechanical procedures necessary to treat a specific patient. The organized structure

TABLE 18-4	Subgingival Irrigants	
AGENT	**ACTIVITY**	**SIDE EFFECTS**
Chlorhexidine	Bactericidal—high substantivity*	Stains teeth, desquamation of tissue, taste alteration, increase in supragingival calculus, discoloration of composite restorations
Tetracycline	Bacteriostatic—high substantivity	No known negative effects
Fluorides	Bacteriostatic—moderate substantivity	Metallic taste, stains teeth (SnF)
Oxygenating agents	Bacteriostatic—low substantivity	Desquamation of tissue (high concentrations)
Zinc chloride	Bacteriostatic—low substantivity	Bad taste
Essential oils	Bacteriostatic—low substantivity	Burning sensation, bitter taste, high alcohol content (Listerine)
Sanguinarine	Bacteriostatic—low substantivity	Burning sensation

* Substantivity refers to the agent's ability to remain effective over a prolonged period. Substantivity for the listed agents has been examined when agents are used as a rinse. Substantivity after subgingival irrigation has not been well documented for any of the agents listed.

of plaque biofilm requires mechanical disruption to achieve a positive outcome. There is little evidence that adjunctive professional subgingival irrigation provides significant benefit over mechanical therapy alone.

IMPLEMENTATION OF SELF-CARE (PATIENT-APPLIED THERAPY)

Patient-applied therapies are composed of mechanical and antimicrobial approaches. Mechanical methods include toothbrushing, flossing and other interdental cleaning aids, and irrigation. Antimicrobials can be delivered through toothbrushes, rinses, and irrigation devices. (See Chapter 13 for a detailed review of patient-applied oral physiotherapy approaches.)

Mechanical Approaches

Toothbrushing

Toothbrushing is the most widely used method of home plaque removal. It has been repeatedly demonstrated to reduce plaque on the buccal and lingual surfaces of the teeth. To a limited extent, toothbrushing also can reach the interproximal surfaces. Brushing is considered a supragingival method of plaque control, because the bristles of a toothbrush will reach only a maximum of 1 to 2 mm subgingivally. Brushes are available in both manual and powered forms. Studies have shown powered brushes to be quite efficacious. A systematic review of the literature comparing manual to power toothbrushing concluded that "powered toothbrushing is at least as effective as manual brushing and there is no evidence that it will cause any more injuries to the gums than manual brushing".[35] The toothbrushing method recommended to a patient depends on his

or her individual periodontal status and ability. Unless a technique is easy to perform for the patient, it will not be used and therefore has no value in controlling plaque.

Floss

Dental floss is the most widely recommended interdental cleaning aid. It is most effective when used regularly and properly by patients with minimal pocket depths and where interdental spaces are filled with interdental papillae. Floss or tape, waxed or unwaxed types demonstrate equal effectiveness in cleaning proximal surfaces.[36] For patients with open gingival embrasures and those who have difficulty using correct flossing technique, another method of interproximal cleaning may be indicated.

Interdental Cleaning Aids

Other cleaning aids that could substitute for floss in various situations are toothpicks, interdental stimulators (wooden, plastic and rubber-tipped), and interdental brushes in various shapes and sizes. Cotton yarn, strips of gauze, and pipe cleaners also have been used for interdental cleaning. All of these methods are best used in areas with large interproximal spaces, open embrasures, exposed furcations, or around pontics in a fixed partial denture. They also may be of benefit with patients who lack the manual dexterity to floss properly.

Irrigation

Irrigation, both supragingival and subgingival, can be considered a mechanical method of plaque removal when water is used as an irrigant. It has been suggested that the flushing action alone, without the use of various medicaments, has an effect on plaque bacteria. An early study in 1973 assessed the impact of pulsating water on plaque bacteria.[37] It was demonstrated that although plaque is not entirely removed by jet-pulsed irrigation, the bacteria contained in the plaque are adversely affected. Bacterial cell walls remained intact, but the cell contents were evacuated or damaged. The properties of plaque as a biofilm reinforce this concept. Irrigation with water can be an adjunctive aid for individuals who have poor oral hygiene or gingivitis. It may also be of benefit to patients who have orthodontic bands, crown and bridge work, and implants. In addition, irrigation may enhance the oral hygiene of patients who have difficulty flossing or using other interdental aids. Small, portable irrigation systems are available to enhance patient concordance.

Antimicrobial Approaches

Patients can apply antimicrobials through delivery vehicles such as toothbrushes, rinses, and irrigation. Because antimicrobial therapy can be an important aspect of periodontal treatment, it is important that the agent reach the site of the bacterial infection. Toothbrushing and rinsing do not significantly penetrate subgingivally. Irrigation, particularly with specially designed subgingival tips, can effectively deliver therapeutic solutions deeper into periodontal pockets.[38]

Toothbrushes, Floss, and Interdental Aids

Brushes are commonly used to deliver dentifrices containing various chemotherapeutic agents such as triclosan and fluorides. A manual brush reaches, on average, less than 1 mm subgingivally.[39] One powered toothbrush, Sonicare (Philips Oral Healthcare, Snoqualmie, Wash.), has demonstrated fluid dynamic action 3 mm beyond the bristle tips *in vitro* (Fig. 18-9).[40] Similarly, floss and other interdental aids can be used as delivery vehicles for antimicrobial agents. For example, a patient can be

instructed to floss before expectorating a fluoride product, or an interdental brush can be dipped into an antimicrobial and then inserted interproximally.

Mouthrinses

Rinsing is simple and quick for the patient to perform. However, like toothbrushing, rinsing does not allow an agent to reach the base of deep periodontal pockets. Some mouthrinses have been accepted by the ADA for use in the treatment of gingivitis (chlorhexidine and essential oils products). The over-the-counter antiseptic mouthrinse, Listerine (Pfizer, Inc., Morris Plains, NJ.) has been demonstrated to be as effective as flossing in the reduction of inflammation at interproximal sites.[41,42] Currently, no mouthrinses are approved by the ADA for treating periodontitis.

Irrigation

Various antimicrobials have been investigated in powered oral irrigation studies. The beneficial properties of chlorhexidine, essential oils, and stannous fluoride have been enhanced when delivered daily through jet-pulsed irrigation by the patient.[38] When a specially-designed subgingival tip is used, solutions can be delivered to the depth of the pocket. In addition, it appears that irrigation therapy presents no particular safety hazard to systemically healthy patients. If irrigation therapy is to be used with patients who require antibiotic premedication (e.g., patient at risk for bacterial endocarditis), it is recommended that the patient's physician be consulted. Because patient-applied irrigation can be performed often, it can play an important role in the treatment of gingivitis and the maintenance of periodontal patients. Irrigation therapy with antimicrobials is one way the doctor–hygienist team can enlist the patient as a cotherapist in treating periodontal problems.

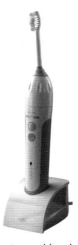

Figure 18-9. Sonicare electric toothbrush. (*Courtesy Philips Oral Healthcare, Snoqualmie, Wash.*)

EVALUATION OF PERIODONTAL THERAPY

Ongoing evaluation is an integral part of periodontal therapy. Evaluation involves feedback on the efficacy of professional treatment and patient self-care and is typically performed during periodontal maintenance. In a sense, the response to periodontal therapy is an important diagnostic tool. Evaluation of professional treatment indicates if additional interventions or referral is necessary. Adjustments in patient self-care regimens may also be warranted.

Successful periodontal therapy is dependent on patient participation in treatment. If the patient does not cooperate in performing necessary oral hygiene procedures, all professionally administered therapies most likely will fail. The patient must be enlisted as a "cotherapist" and must be made aware of the importance of his or her participation.

Gaining patient cooperation is sometimes difficult. Each patient has specific interests or "hot buttons" that will motivate him or her to respond to home care recommendations. Many patients will respond to more than one of these concerns, which could include the following:

1. The longing to achieve aesthetic success
2. The hope of preventing further monetary loss
3. The desire to prevent future pain
4. The need to please the dental professional
5. The will to accomplish a goal

The most effective motivating techniques involve the patient as an equal partner in providing treatment. The patient should never be made to feel inferior. He or she should feel like a responsible participant, recognizing the limited role the dental professional plays in ensuring long-term success and health. Some patients may respond favorably to negativity (e.g., "You will lose all your teeth if you don't . . .") for a short-term period; however, positive reinforcement usually provides better long-term success. The dental professional should outline for the patient in a realistic manner the problem the patient faces, how to best treat the problem, and the chances for success.

The motivational process requires that the clinician and patient work together toward a common goal. Traditionally, clinicians have used the term *compliance* to describe patient cooperation with appropriate treatment recommendations. In reality, compliance is defined as "a yielding, as to a request, wish, desire, demand or proposal; a disposition to yield to others."[43] This definition connotes obedience or submission on the patient's part, not cooperation. The term *concordance* is frequently used in the medical literature when discussing medication use by patients. Concordance implies an open and honest discussion between clinician and patient and requires that they both reach a mutual understanding on the nature of an illness and its appropriate treatment.[44] Concordance suggests that the clinician and patient find areas of health belief that are shared and build on them, rather than the clinician imposing her or his views on the patient (i.e., compliance). Such an approach is appropriate when evaluating periodontal care. It demands a team effort— that is, ongoing communication and guidance (not demands) from the clinician, together with cooperation by the patient. Concordance gives the patient ownership of the periodontal condition and allows him or her to remain a part of the decision-making process.[45]

The patient should always be viewed as an individual. Each patient may respond uniquely to the therapy provided, including self-care procedures. No one method for plaque removal is ideal for all patients during all phases of treatment. In addition, it may even be necessary to modify plaque control methods according to various sites present in the same patient. The dental professional must determine the best techniques and devices for each patient. Adequate instruction and frequent monitoring are essential. The frustration the clinician experiences when a particular method is unsuccessful is probably also felt by the patient. Fruitful self-care often is the result of continuous reevaluation and adaptation, coupled with constant assistance and encouragement. Instructions and techniques should be kept as simple as possible. The number of techniques recommended to the patient at one time should be reasonable. The dental professional often forgets how "second nature" these routines may be for her or him, whereas the patient may be learning them for the first time. The average patient will need several appointments for instructions in plaque removal, and additional techniques will add to this time. The clinician must listen to the patient's problems in using certain methods, adapt the methods to the patient's abilities, and provide guidance at each evaluation.

Acknowledgment

The author would like to thank Mike Rethman, DDS, MS, for his assistance in preparing and reviewing this chapter.

REFERENCES

1. Mueller-Joseph L, Petersen M: The dental hygiene process of care. In Mueller-Joseph L, Petersen M, editors: *Dental hygiene process: Diagnosis and care planning*, Albany, NY, 1995, Delmar Publishers.
2. Rethman M: Periodontal terminology, *J Periodontol* 64:583, 1993 (editorial).
3. Caton J: Periodontal diagnosis and diagnostic aids. In *Proceedings of the World Workshop in Clinical Periodontics*, Chicago, 1989, The American Academy of Periodontology.
4. Armitage G: Manual periodontal probing in supportive periodontal treatment, *Periodontol 2000* 12:33-39, 1996.
5. Haffajee A, Socransky S, Goodson M: Clinical parameters as predictors of destructive periodontal disease activity, *J Clin Periodontol* 12:257, 1983.
6. Badersten A, Nilveus R, Egelberg J: Effect of non-surgical periodontal therapy, VII. Bleeding, suppuration and probing depth in sites with probing attachment loss, *J Clin Periodontol* 12:432, 1985.
7. Lang N, Hill R: Radiographs in periodontics, *J Clin Periodontol* 4:16, 1977.
8. Jeffcoat M, Reddy M: A comparison of probing and radiographic methods for detection of periodontal disease progression, *Curr Opin Dent* 1:45-51, 1991.
9. Nunn ME, Harrel SK: The effect of occlusal discrepancies on periodontitis. I. Relationship of initial occlusal discrepancies to initial clinical parameters, *J Periodontol* 72:485-494, 2001.
10. Harrell SK, Nunn M: The effect of occlusal discrepancies on periodontitis. II. Relationship of occlusal treatment to the

progression of periodontal disease, *J Periodont* 72:495-505, 2001.

11. Kornman K, Crane A, Wang H et al: The interleukin-1 genotype as a severity factor in adult periodontal disease, *J Clin Periodontol* 24:72-77, 1997.

12. Armitage G, Wu Y, Wang H et al: Low prevalence of a periodontitis-associated interleukin-1 composite genotype in individuals of Chinese heritage, *J Periodontol* 71:164-171, 2000.

13. Greenstein G, Hart T: A critical assessment of interleukin-1 (IL-1) genotyping when used in a genetic susceptibility test for severe chronic periodontitis, *J Periodontol* 73:231-247, 2002.

14. *Annals of periodontology, Vol 4, No 1: 1999 International Workshop for a Classification of Periodontal Diseases and Conditions*, Chicago, 1999, American Academy of Periodontology.

15. *Glossary of periodontal terms*, ed 4, Chicago, 2001, American Academy of Periodontology.

16. Haffajee A, Socransky S, Goodson J: Clinical parameters as predictors of destructive periodontal disease activity, *J Clin Periodontol* 10:257-265, 1983.

17. American Academy of Periodontology: Position paper: diagnosis of periodontal diseases, *J Periodontol* 74:1237-1247, 2003.

18. Darby M: Theory development and basic research in dental hygiene: review of the literature and recommendations (1989-90 ADHA Council on Research). Norfolk, Va, School of Dental Hygiene, Old Dominion University.

19. Greenstein G: Full-mouth therapy versus individual quadrant root planning: a critical commentary, *J Periodontol* 73:797-812, 2002.

20. *General guidelines for referring dental patients to specialists and other settings of care*, Chicago, 1992, American Dental Association.

21. Greenstein G: Periodontal response to mechanical nonsurgical therapy: a review, *J Periodontol* 63:118-130, 1992.

22. Nyman S, Westfelt E, Sarhed G et al: The role of 'diseased' root cementum in healing following treatment of periodontal disease, *J Clin Periodontol* 15:64, 1988.

23. Leon L, Vogel R: A comparison of the effectiveness of hand scaling and ultrasonic debridement in furcations as evaluated by differential dark-field microscopy, *J Periodontol* 58:86-94, 1986.

24. Drisko CL, Cochran DL, Blieden T et al: Position paper: sonic and ultrasonic scalers in periodontics, *J Periodontol* 71:1792-1801, 2000.

25. Ramfjord S, Caffesse S, Morrison E: Four modalities of periodontal treatment compared over five years, *J Clin Periodontol* 14:445-452, 1987.

26. Lindhe J, Westfelt E, Nyman S et al: Long-term effects of surgical/nonsurgical treatment of periodontal disease, *J Clin Periodontol* 11:448-458, 1984.

27. Renvert S, Wikstrom G, Dahlen G et al: On the inability of root debridement and periodontal surgery to eliminate Actinobacillus actinomycetemcomitans from periodontal pockets, *J Clin Periodontol* 17:351-355, 1990.

28. Kepic T, O'Leary T, Kafrawy A: Total calculus removal: an attainable objective?, *J Periodontol* 61:16-20, 1990.

29. Slots J, Rams T: Antibiotics in periodontal therapy: advantages and disadvantages, *J Clin Periodontol* 17:479-493, 1990.

30. Kelly A, Resteghini R: Pressures recorded during periodontal pocket irrigation, *J Periodontol* 56:297-299, 1985.

31. Itic J, Serfaty R: Clinical effectiveness of subgingival irrigation with pulsating jet irrigator vs. syringe, *J Periodontol* 63:174-181, 1992.

32. Jolkovsky D, Waki M, Newman M et al: Clinical and microbiological effects of subgingival and gingival marginal irrigation with chlorhexidine gluconate, *J Periodontol* 61:663-669.

33. Christersson L, Nordeyrd O, Puchalsky C: Topical application of tetracycline-HCL in human periodontitis, *J Clin Periodontol* 20:88-95, 1993.

34. Waki M: Effects of subgingival irrigation on bacteremia following scaling and root planing, *J Periodontol* 61:405, 1990.

35. Heanue M, Deacon S, Deery C et al: Manual versus powered toothbrushing for oral health, *Cochrane Database Syst Rev* (1): CD002281, 2003.

36. Hill H, Levi P, Glickman I: The effects of waxed and unwaxed dental floss on interproximal plaque accumulation and interdental gingival health, *J Periodontol* 53:411-414, 1973.

37. Brady JM, Gray WA, Bhaskar SN: Electron microscopic study of the effect of water jet lavage devices on dental plaque, *J Dent Res* 52:1310-1313, 1973.

38. *Position paper: The role of supra- and subgingival irrigation in the treatment of periodontal diseases*, Chicago, 1995, American Academy of Periodontology.

39. Lang N, Raber K: Use of oral irrigators as vehicles for the application of antimicrobial agents in chemical plaque control, *J Clin Periodontol* 8:177-188, 1981.

40. Stanford C, Srikantha R, Wu C: Efficacy of the Sonicare toothbrush fluid dynamic action on removal of human supragingival plaque, *J Clin Dent* 8:10-14, 1997.

41. Sharma N, Charles C, Qaqish J et al: Comparative effectiveness of an essential oil mouthrinse and dental floss in controlling interproximal gingivitis and plaque, *Am J Dent* 15:351-355, 2002.

42. Bauroth K, Charles C, Mankodi S et al: The efficacy of an essential oil antiseptic mouthrinse vs dental floss in controlling interproximal gingivitis. *J Am Dent Assoc* 134:359-365, 2003.

43. *Webster's unabridged dictionary*, New York, 1999, Random House.

44. Britten N: Communication: the key to improved compliance, *Prescriber* 9(10):27-31, 1998.

45. Rethman J: Concordance: a new way to view compliance, *Focus* 5(2):9, 2001.

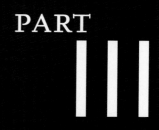

PART
III

SURGICAL
THERAPY

Leonard S. Tibbetts

19 Conscious Sedation

Leonard S. Tibbetts

The goal of conscious sedation is to render the informed and perceptive patient free of anxiety, fear, and apprehension, while being pleasantly relaxed. The objectives of this chapter are to present a review of the various methods of conscious sedation in a logical manner. It is also intended to make dental therapists aware of the current standards of care for the use of in-office enteral, inhalation, or parenteral conscious sedation in the delivery of care, but it is not all-inclusive.

There have been tremendous scientific and clinical advances in the field and scope of periodontics and in the treatment of periodontal diseases over the last half century. As a result of the electronic information explosion that has occurred simultaneously with scientific and clinical progress in periodontics, many computer savvy patients have a heightened awareness of periodontal diseases and the potential consequences of untreated diseases on general health, as well as dental health. Despite the advances in patients' awareness of periodontal diseases and the dental therapists' knowledge base and ability to address and treat the problems resulting from these diseases, much of dentistry remains handicapped in its ability to render or refer such treatment because of the anxiety and fear of pain that patients associate with the delivery of periodontal treatment. In a national health survey, 73% of the respondents indicated that negative dental experiences had changed their attitude about dental care.[1] Pain ranked high as a cause and effect of the change in attitude about not seeking treatment. Fear of pain and pain perception were confirmed as a major barrier to patients seeking dental care in other studies.[2-6] Nearly 80% of the population experience some dental anxiety, with 10% to 15% being highly anxious.[7] Females are inclined to demonstrate greater levels of dental anxiety but similar levels of fear when compared with males.

Minimal to moderate conscious sedation, using either enteral, inhalation, or parenteral conscious sedation, or a combination of these techniques before the delivery of periodontal care, is the ideal way for dentists to control patient anxiety associated with in-office periodontal treatment procedures.[8-10] Treatment of periodontal diseases in a relaxed and stress free environment, however, requires an energized dental practitioner who is willing to use sedation techniques and who feels comfortable doing it.[11] Such individuals must have the educational background of courses, instructions, and experiences deemed necessary to safely and effectively sedate patients. Use of these procedures, with minimal risk to patients, requires that such practitioners have a deep rooted responsibility to be knowledgeable and proficient in taking proper medical and dental histories, to perform thorough dental and physical examinations, and to properly document this information in the patients' records. These practitioners must also be profoundly knowledgeable in drug pharmacology, sedation techniques, airway management, and emergency procedures. Currently, 47 states require specific rules and regulations for the in-office use of conscious sedation.[12] The overall safety and predictability of conscious sedation to effectively control anxiety when administered by thoroughly trained individuals is well documented.[9,10]

The definitions, educational guidelines, and policies presented in this chapter are consistent with the *American Dental Association Policy Statement: The Use of Conscious Sedation, Deep Sedation and General Anesthesia in Dentistry*,[13] the American Dental Association (ADA) documents *Guidelines for the Use of Conscious Sedation, Deep Sedation and General Anesthesia for Dentists*[14] and *Guidelines for Teaching the Comprehensive Control of Anxiety and Pain in Dentistry*,[15] and the Joint Commission on Accreditation of Healthcare Organizations' *Revisions to Anesthesia Care Standards, Comprehensive Accreditation Manual for Ambulatory Care*,[16] which went into effect January 1, 2001. The information is also consistent with the American Academy of Periodontology *Guidelines: In-Office Use of Conscious Sedation in Periodontics*.[17] This chapter focuses on conscious sedation for the adult patient.

TERMINOLOGY

Although a variety of terms have been used in the dental literature to describe various methods of anxiety and pain control, the following definitions are universally used throughout all dentistry disciplines[14,17]:

Analgesia: The diminution or elimination of pain in the conscious patient.

Local anesthesia: The elimination of sensations, especially pain, in one part of the body by the topical application or regional injection of a drug.

Anxiolysis (minimal sedation): A drug-induced, relaxed state of consciousness, during which patients respond to verbal commands. Although cognitive function and coordination may be impaired, ventilatory and cardiovascular functions are unaffected.

Moderate sedation/anesthesia (conscious sedation): A pharmacologic-induced minimally depressed level of consciousness (Stage I of the classic four stages of general anesthesia) during which patients respond purposefully to verbal commands, either alone or accompanied by light tactile stimulation. No interventions are required to maintain a patent airway, and spontaneous ventilation is adequate. Cardiovascular function is usually maintained. In accordance with this definition, the drugs and/or techniques used should carry a margin of safety wide enough to render unintended loss of consciousness unlikely. Furthermore, patients whose only response is reflex withdrawal from repeated painful stimuli would not be considered to be in a state of conscious sedation.

Combined inhalation–enteral conscious sedation (combined conscious sedation): Nitrous oxide/oxygen (N_2O/O_2) when used in combination with appropriate sedation agents may produce anxiolysis (the resolution of restlessness and apprehension achieved through pharmacologic management), conscious sedation, or deep sedation/general anesthesia. Because of the possibility that the combination of N_2O/O_2 and enteral sedation agents may result in mild to moderate conscious sedation, deep sedation, or general anesthesia, it is important for appropriate sedative agents and dosages to be administered when using combined inhalation–enteral sedation to achieve anxiolysis. The enteral route typically exhibits an approximate 30-minute latent period after bolus administration of the drug. Therefore, it is impossible to titrate a patient to a level of sedation that predictably achieves anxiolysis. The dose of an enteral drug should be selected to provide light sedation and then titrated to a level of anxiolysis with the addition of N_2O/O_2 sedation.

Deep sedation/anesthesia: A drug-induced state of depressed consciousness during which patients cannot be easily aroused but respond purposefully after repeated or painful stimulation. Patients may require assistance in maintaining a patent airway, and spontaneous ventilatory function may be inadequate. Cardiovascular function is usually maintained.

Anesthesia: Consists of general anesthesia and spinal or major regional anesthesia; it does not include local anesthesia. General anesthesia is a drug-induced loss of consciousness during which patients can not be aroused, even by painful stimulation. The ability to independently maintain ventilatory function is often impaired. Patients often require assistance in maintaining a patent airway, and positive ventilation may be required because of depressed spontaneous ventilation or drug-induced depression of neuromuscular function. Cardiovascular function may be impaired.

Patient Physical Status

The American Society of Anesthesiologists (ASA) patient classification system is universally accepted as a basis to identify the physical status of candidates for both conscious sedation and general anesthesia. All patients must be dealt with on an individual basis. Patients who are classified as ASA I or II are usually candidates for conscious sedation, whereas patients who are ASA III require special considerations. Patients who are ASA IV are not candidates for in-office conscious sedation. The ASA classifications are listed in Box 19-1.

Box 19-1   American Society of Anesthesiologists Patient Physical Status Classification

ASA I: Normal healthy patient
ASA II: Patient with mild systemic disease
ASA III: Patient with severe systemic disease that limits activity
ASA IV: Patient with an incapacitating disease that is a constant threat to life
ASA V: Moribund patient who is not expected to survive 24 hours with or without the operation
ASA VI: Patients who is declared brain-dead whose organs are being removed for donor purposes
E: Emergency operation of any variety used to modify one of the above classifications (i.e., ASA III-E).

ROUTES OF ADMINISTRATION

It is important that the dentist and office personnel address and be adequately trained in prompt and effective management of sedation complications for all of the sedation administration techniques that are used within an office, as well as have the proper emergency equipment immediately available in the event of a complication. The following sections define terms commonly used to describe the administration routes of drugs and agents used to achieve the various levels of conscious sedation and general anesthesia. General statements regarding the use of the various drug administration routes in achieving conscious sedation in periodontics are included.

Inhalation

Inhalation is a technique of administration in which a gaseous or volatile agent is introduced into the pulmonary tree, and the primary effect is caused by absorption through the pulmonary bed.

Inhalation sedation, with N_2O/O_2 used as the sedation/ anxiolytic agent, is the most commonly used sedation method in dentistry. Jastak[18] states that approximately 50% of dentists practicing in the United States use N_2O/O_2 to achieve light conscious sedation as a supplement to a local anesthetic. N_2O has a rapid onset of action and rate of elimination and clearance.[19,20] These properties make N_2O/O_2 ideal for titration and recovery for light sedation. Titration of N_2O/O_2 requires that no set percentage of N_2O be used. An appointment using N_2O/O_2 sedation should begin and end with the administration of 100% O_2. Titration should start with the administration of 20% N_2O for a full minute, followed by a 10% increase of N_2O per minute until a suitable, ideal level of sedation is reached for each patient. At the completion of the appointment, 100% oxygen should be breathed for at least 5 minutes. Malamed[21] has pointed out that 40% N_2O will produce adequate sedation for most patients receiving it, but also that many patients become uncomfortable, oversedated, and dislike inhalation sedation with 40% N_2O. Approximately 15% of patients receiving N_2O will find it ineffective.

For successful inhalation sedation with N_2O/O_2, it is essential for the dental therapist to psychologically prepare the patient for the experience. The patient should be told, briefly, concisely, and in layman's terms, what to expect in terms of physical subjective symptoms. They should also understand that they will not be "put to sleep," but will be relaxed and calm, with an altered sense of awareness. The properly sedated patient will be fully aware of their surroundings under the influence of N_2O. Before rendering periodontal care under the influence of N_2O inhalation sedation, appropriate preoperative positive suggestions of what the patient will experience will frequently aid the mildly apprehensive patient in overcoming anxiety and an uncooperative attitude about their periodontal care.[22] Ease of use, general patient acceptance, relative safety, and minimal training requirements contribute to its popularity. For several years, N_2O/O_2 inhalation systems purchased in the United States for use in dentistry have had a fail-safe system that will not allow the delivery of less than 25% oxygen to patients. Systems that are capable of delivering less than 25% oxygen to patients must be equipped with an inline oxygen analyzer for patient safety. Although N_2O can be used as a general anesthetic agent, it is effective for conscious sedation in many mildly apprehensive patients. The percentage of N_2O, as delivered by modern dental N_2O inhalation equipment, is not a potent enough agent for patients with moderate to extreme anxiety. The delivery of greater N_2O percentages, however, crosses from light sedation to deep sedation/general anesthesia and presents a high risk potential for therapists not trained to administer deep sedation/general anesthesia.

Enteral

Enteral is any technique of administration in which the agent is absorbed through the oral mucosa or gastrointestinal tract (i.e., oral, rectal, sublingual).

Oral administration of both over-the-counter and prescribed medicines is the most commonly used route of drug administration in the world. Oral sedation has several advantages that make it attractive to many practitioners,[23] including that it is:

1. Convenient
2. Economical
3. Universally accepted by patients
4. Requires no equipment
5. Until recently, it required no special licensure to use.

As a means of managing preoperative stress and stress occurring during periodontal procedures for mildly apprehensive patients, the oral administration of sedative drugs can be used quite effectively.

There are, however, several disadvantages with oral sedation. The primary problem for the therapist is the lack of control over drug action for the following reasons:

1. Reliance on patient compliance
2. A relatively long period of latency from ingestion to effectiveness of the medication (30 to 45 minutes)
3. Long duration of clinical effect (3 to 4 hours)
4. Inability to titrate the effect of the medication
5. Inability to either easily increase or decrease the level of sedation
6. Erratic and/or incomplete drug absorption by the gastrointestinal tract.

The results of oral sedation are often highly variable clinical effects, ranging from minimal or no effectiveness to oversedation. Dosages for oral sedation are empirical: they are generally determined for each patient by body mass, weight, and age.[7] A review of the literature regarding the advantages, disadvantages, and reliability of enteral conscious sedation leads to the conclusion that, with the exception of patients with mild apprehension, there are other sedative drug administration techniques that are more predictably effective and reliable in producing the desired clinical results.[11,24,25]

Rectal sedation is not psychologically acceptable for use in dentistry, with the exception of use in children, and is therefore not often used in periodontal treatment. Currently, the sublingual administration of sedative drugs has little application in periodontics, and if used must be limited to drugs that have a relatively neutral pH, so as not to cause tissue damage by irritation when they are administered. Sublingual sedative drugs are available, but they are primarily used in the field of pediatric dentistry, although Halcion (Upjohn Co.; Kalamazoo, MI) has been recommended for sublingual administration in adults by some authors.

Parenteral

Parenteral is a technique of administration in which the drug bypasses the gastrointestinal tract and is absorbed directly into the cardiovascular system (i.e., intramuscular [IM], intravenous [IV], submucosal, subcutaneous, or intraocular).

Of the parenteral administration techniques of conscious sedation, only IV and IM administrations are routinely used in periodontics. The parenteral administration of drugs has a *decided* advantage over oral administration, because parenteral techniques allow direct entry into the general circulation, rather than having to first pass through the bowel and liver circulation. Drugs administered by IV route have the advantage of more reliable absorption, rapid onset of action (30 seconds to 8 minutes for IV administration and 15 to 20 minutes for IM administration), and faster maximum drug effect.

IM administration of sedation drugs also has as its objective, rapid, maximum attainment of entry into the circulation, with minimal to no complications. IM sedation, however, has several undesirable features, the most significant being the inability to titrate the drug dosage and to rapidly reverse drug action. As in oral sedation, drug dosage is empirical. The physical status and weight of the patient and the experience of the doctor and the staff play an important role in the dosage determination of the sedative agents. With an educated guess regarding the amount of medication that should be administered, three possible results can occur: an ideal level of sedation, an

inadequate or light level of sedation, or oversedation or deep sedation. The duration of action, depending on the drug and the amount administered, can be prolonged.

The greatest patient objection to IM sedation is that an injection is needed, with possible pain or complications of injury from the injection, including hematomas, nerve damage, intravascular injections, tissue irritation, and infection. Proper selection of the injection site is important (Fig. 19-1), with the mid-deltoid area being the most convenient for use in periodontics. The other three locations—the vastus lateralis, the superior outer quadrant of the gluteal area, or the ventrogluteal area—all require some degree of disrobing. If the desired sedation effects are not obtained with the initial injection, or the procedure is prolonged, additional injections may be necessary.

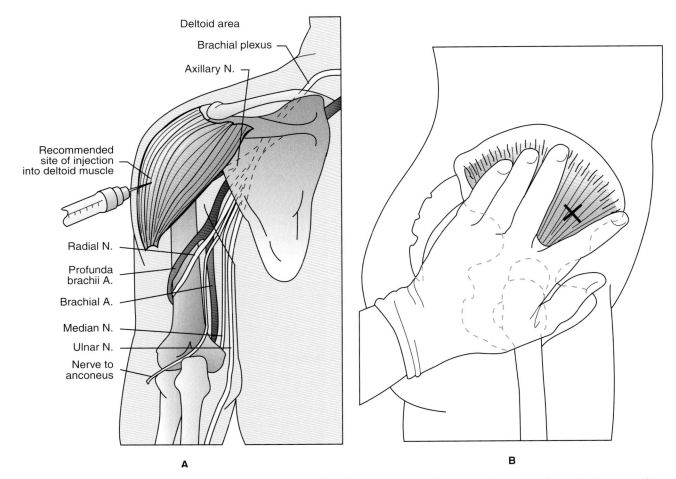

A

B

Figure 19-1. Proper anatomic intramuscular injection sites. **A,** Mid-deltoid area. A rectangle whose upper boundary is formed by the outward extension of the spine of the scapula, the inferior border opposite the armpit, and laterally approximately 1/3 to 2/3 of the way around the upper arm. **B,** Ventrogluteal area. The injection is made between the index finger and the middle finger below the iliac crest (X). The index finger is placed on the superior anterior iliac spine, with the middle finger spread as far apart from the index finger as possible, with the hand pressed onto the hip over the greater trochanter.

Continued

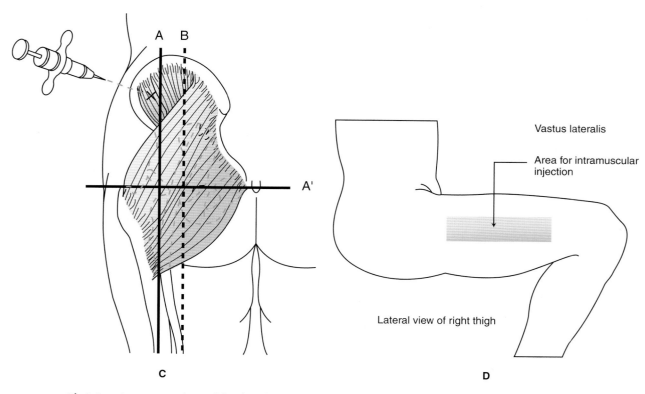

Figure 19-1. cont'd C, Superior outer quadrant of the gluteal area (A and A′), taking care to assure no transgressions into the medial quadrants (B), where the sacral plexus and sciatic nerve are located. **D,** Vastus lateralis area—the anterior and lateral area of the thigh from approximately 4 inches above the knee, to the same dimension below the greater trochanter of the femur. (*From Malamed SF: Sedation: a guide to patient management, ed 4, St. Louis, 2003, Mosby.*)

IV administration of sedative drugs is the route of choice in conscious sedation for several reasons, including the following:

1. Drug administration by the IV route has the most rapid onset of action of all of the sedation techniques. The circulation time for a drug administered in the arm to cross the blood–brain barrier is approximately 1o to 18 seconds.[26]

2. By carefully choosing the sedation medications to be administered intravenously, and by knowing their properties, pharmacology, and particularly their rapid onset of action, the drugs can be titrated to obtain a minimally depressed level of consciousness, with a partial to total amnesia that meets the needs of both the patient and the therapist for successful, anxiety free treatment.

3. The duration of action of intravenously administered drugs is longer than that following inhalation sedation, but generally shorter than oral, rectal, or IM routes.

4. With the maintenance of a patent vein for a continuous IV infusion technique for sedation, additional medication can be given during long procedures without an additional needle stick.

5. Should a medical emergency arise during a continuous IV infusion procedure, emergency drugs can be readily administered.

6. Patient motor activity and the gag reflex are usually diminished significantly with the drugs used in IV sedation.

There are also disadvantages associated with the use of IV sedation, including the following:

1. The necessity of a venipuncture, although the skillfully executed venipuncture tends to be generally well accepted by most patients.

2. Difficulty in finding a suitable vein for the venipuncture can be a problem in obese patients and also in small patients, but proficiency in venipuncture is a learned skill that comes with experience. IV sedation requires cooperation from the patient for the venipuncture; therefore, young apprehensive patients can be a management problem.

3. The possibility of complications at the site of the venipuncture, including phlebitis, hematomas, intraarterial injection of drugs, and other complications.

Transdermal/Transmucosal

Transdermal/transmucosal is a technique of administration in which the drug is administered by patch or iontophoresis (the introduction of a chosen medicament into the tissues by means of an electrical current).

There are currently no sedation techniques using iontophoresis. The use of transmucosal sedation, by spraying water-soluble medications in the nose, has limited general usage, but the technique is used with some tranquilizing medications in pediatric dentistry.

Indications and Advantages

The most frequently stated indication for conscious sedation is the treatment of the apprehensive dental patient. There is a level of awareness in some patients where periodontal procedures can be performed comfortably with no medication other than regional anesthetic. Other patients are essentially unmanageable with just regional anesthetic. The literature points out that levels of awareness[8] may range from one suitable for dentistry without the administration of medication to patients who are unmanageable in a conscious state. The interim levels of awareness are the mildly apprehensive patient, the moderately apprehensive patient, and the severely apprehensive patient. The anticipated level of apprehension that a patient will have when they arrive at the dental office for planned periodontal procedures, based on evaluations made at the initial examination and treatment planning appointments, determines which patients should be consciously sedated, and the type and route of conscious sedation that will produce a level of awareness at which periodontal procedures will be tolerated. Inhalation sedation with N_2O, the weakest agent known for sedation, may satisfactorily manage patients who are mildly apprehensive. Nonetheless, for some mildly apprehensive patients, a combination of enteral–inhalation sedation may offer more effective sedation. Combination enteral–inhalation sedation, however, potentially carries more risks for complications than N_2O alone. For the management of the moderately apprehensive patient, the use of more potent medication(s) with conscious IV sedation is the most effective technique to alleviate the patient's apprehension to the desired level of awareness.

Another commonly cited indication for conscious sedation is to reduce or eliminate the stress that most patients associate with the performance of invasive, tedious, and time-consuming periodontal procedures. Few periodontal surgical procedures are of less than 1 hour in duration, and many are 3 to 4 hours in duration. Patients prefer to have treatment accomplished in a timely manner in as few appointments as possible. They tend to prefer relatively short, atraumatic procedures. Because patients experience an altered sense of awareness with conscious IV sedation, it results in the length of the appointment being perceived as much shorter than it actually is. The partial to total amnesia resulting from the use of some sedative agents also results in patients having relatively pleasant appointment experiences.

With the appropriate conscious sedation technique, the initially uncooperative and apprehensive patient can be rendered calm, less stressed, and cooperative. The application of the proper level of drug-induced conscious sedation results in a reduced level of stress-related, endogenous epinephrine production. Some mentally challenged patients can also be managed by conscious sedation rather than general anesthetic. Conscious sedation likewise tends to dull the psychogenic component of the gag reflex in severe gaggers, often making it possible to work on the posterior aspects of both the maxillary palatal region and the mandibular lingual areas.

Patients who present with compromised medical health (ASA Class II and III patients), in which psychogenic stress is of concern, are further indicated for conscious sedation. With the reduction of psychogenic stress through sedation, stress-induced hypertension is often reduced and controlled, resulting in the patients' vital signs being more stable. Considering that many periodontal patients are 40 years or older, such a reduction of apprehension and stress may prove to be a valuable aid in the prevention of sequelae in undiagnosed cardiovascular patients.[27]

The effective use of conscious sedation ultimately results in safe, conscious patients with intact protective reflexes and the ability to maintain their airway. This results in less stress for the operating dentist and dental assistant, by creating a more cooperative patient, in whom periodontal procedures can be completed during more ideal circumstances, with greater treatment effectiveness and time efficiency.

PSYCHOSOMATIC CONTROL OF APPREHENSION

In many dental practices, the psychosomatic approach to the elimination of anxiety and pain is ignored and neglected. Psychosomatic control of apprehension (iatrosedation) is what can be accomplished without the use of drugs, or as a supplement to drug therapy, when a patient's trust and confidence are gained. Monheim[28] states, "By no other means, can so much be gained with so little effect on the patient." For psychosomatic control of apprehension to be effective, care must be taken with the patient to put them in the proper frame of mind, starting with how the patient is greeted on their initial contact with the office. It continues with all of their subsequent experiences before seeing the dentist, as well as how their treatment concerns are handled. Presenting a warm, caring, personal, and professional approach, with sincerity and honest competence, is an important factor to the patient. Patients should be well informed of office policies, of treatment to be rendered, and what to expect for each appointment in general terms. This may markedly reduce their fears.

Psychologically, no one likes surprises for appointments that they are already concerned about. Appointment times should be prompt true times, to avoid keeping an apprehensive patient waiting, and thereby adding to their apprehensive feeling. In a fearful, apprehensive mental state, a patient's pain threshold is decreased. When nervous and apprehensive, there is a tendency to mentally magnify unpleasant experiences. This often results in the patient's response being out of proportion to the initial painful stimulus. It is therefore extremely important to make a sincere, compelling effort to help the patient have a positive attitude about the setting of their appointment, the therapist, and the anticipated treatment to be rendered during the appointment. Exhibiting a sincere concern for the patient's welfare while under your care tends to help alleviate fear and apprehension. This is particularly helpful in the management of children.[29]

Furthermore, it is important to spare the patient the trauma of any unpleasant sights and sounds, including such things as dental syringes, surgical instruments, soiled gauzes, handpiece sounds, and negative nonverbal communication. The literature reports alleviating anxiety on a long-term basis with behavioral techniques including some of those described earlier.[30] Friedman[31] went into much greater detail, and coined the term *iatrosedation*, which he defined as the act of making a person calm through the doctor's behavior, attitude, and communication stance.

PHARMACOLOGY OF RECOMMENDED DRUGS

Because conscious sedation techniques used in periodontics include oral (enteral) sedation, IM and IV (parenteral sedation) sedation, N_2O/O_2 (inhalation sedation) sedation and combined inhalation/oral (enteral) sedation, the dentist must first choose the technique(s) that has the greatest application for the successful treatment of patients in the environment in which they work, and must be educationally and professionally competent in those techniques.

The use of a wide array of drugs for the various types of conscious sedation is contraindicated, because each drug in the conscious sedation armamentarium should be included only if the practitioner has a detailed working knowledge of the medication and is intimately familiar with the pharmacologic actions, indications, contraindi-

cations, precautions, and drug interactions. Keeping the number of medications in one's armamentarium to a minimum, therefore, is logical and practical from the standpoint of patient safety. The major categories of drugs needed for sedation can be placed into four groups: (1) antianxiety and sedatives–hypnotic drugs, (2) narcotics and narcotic-like analgesics, (3) benzodiazepine antagonist, and (4) narcotic antagonists.

The following discussion is an overview of these drug classes. It is not intended to be a comprehensive review of these drugs. The clinician must have a thorough working knowledge of each drug that is chosen for administration. This requires study of available information from a variety of reference sources.

Antianxiety and Sedatives–Hypnotics

The categories and subcategories of antianxiety and sedative–hypnotics drugs described in the following sections have been used broadly in conscious sedation for periodontal patients.

Benzodiazepines

Benzodiazepines are among the most popular classes of drugs in use today for the safe treatment of anxiety states.[23] Benzodiazepines have extensive clinical applications in medicine and dentistry for anesthesia and sedation procedures, as muscle relaxants, and for sleep disorders. Benzodiazepines potentiate the action of gamma-aminobutyrate (GABA), an inhibitory neurotransmitter, resulting in increased neuronal inhibition and central nervous system (CNS) depression, especially in the limbic system and reticular formation.[32-34] Although all benzodiazepines are relatively effective, their courses of action are variable among patients. They are contraindicated when a patient has hypersensitivity to other benzodiazepines, psychosis, acute narrow-angle glaucoma, pregnancy, shock, acute alcohol intoxication, existing CNS depression, and uncontrolled pain.

Drugs that can affect benzodiazepines include cimetidine, oral contraceptives, disulfiram, fluoxetine, isoniazid, ketoconazole, metoprolol, valproic acid, alcohol, barbiturates, narcotics, antacids, probenecid, ranitidine, rifampin, scopolamine, and theophyllines. Digoxin, levodopa, neuromuscular blocking agents, and phenytoin may be affected by the benzodiazepines.

There is positive evidence of risks (U.S. Food and Drug Administration Pregnancy Category D) to the fetus when used during pregnancy. Investigational or postmarketing data shows risk to the fetus. Use of benzodiazepines during pregnancy is generally not indicated because of these risks.

When benzodiazepines are administered orally, there are significant differences in their absorption rates. Oxazepam is one of the most slowly absorbed, whereas diazepam and flurazepam are among the most rapidly absorbed. The absorption rates of the benzodiazepines with the IM route are often poor and erratic. Most benzodiazepines are not soluble in water, and therefore are not readily available for IV use. Diazepam and midazolam are the two most commonly used agents for IV conscious sedation. Anterograde amnesia is strongly identified with this drug class, but it varies with the route of administration and the specific medication.

The benzodiazepines that are administered orally are listed first in Table 19-1, followed by those with multiple routes of administration in Table 19-2.

Barbiturates

The short-acting barbiturates are the best-suited barbiturates for use in periodontics. Barbiturates were the first drugs used for effective management of anxiety.[23,27] They were more widely prescribed before the development of benzodiazepines. Pentobarbital sodium (Nembutal: Abbot Laboratories; North Chicago, IL) and secobarbital sodium (Seconal: Eli Lilly Co.; Indianapolis, IN) are well suited for use in oral sedation for periodontal therapy, because they have an onset of action in 20 to 25 minutes and last for 3 to 4 hours, which corresponds to the time needed for many periodontal treatment procedures. They also have a long half-life (20 to 28 hours for Seconal and 21 to 42 hours for Nembutal), during which the patient may experience hangover and irritability. Barbiturates are contraindicated in uncontrolled pain. Currently, barbiturates are primarily used when a patient has a history of a reaction to the benzodiazepines, because they are not as effective or as specific as benzodiazepines in their pharmacologic actions. Barbiturates are CNS depressants. At therapeutic dosages, they reduce both anxiety and mental acuity, and they produce a state of drowsiness (hypnosis). At greater dosage levels, barbiturates depress the medulla, causing dosage-related respiratory depression. Uncontrolled respiratory depression can result in progression to cardiovascular depression, coma, and even death.

Barbiturates do not have the ability to obtund pain in therapeutic dosages for conscious sedation and can cause patients to become hyperexcitable to pain or painful stimuli. Adverse effects of sedative dosages of barbiturates have been reported and include paradoxical excitement, antianalgesic effects, nausea, vomiting, hiccoughing, and excessive postoperative drowsiness.[21-24] Pharmacologically, there is a lower therapeutic margin of safety for barbiturates than for benzodiazepines. The use of barbiturates has declined with the advent of more pharmacologically effective antianxiety agents. Barbiturates have many disadvantages, beginning with dose-related respiratory depression, addiction potential, lack of reversal agent, drug interactions, and a lower margin of safety than benzodiazepines. In the past, barbiturates have been drugs highly associated with suicide attempts. Barbiturates are contraindicated in patients with known hypersensitivity; uncontrolled pain; respiratory disease when obstruction or dyspnea is present; a personal or family history of intermittent, latent, or manifest porphyria; and in patients with severe hepatic dysfunction. They are contraindicated for use during pregnancy or during lactation as a potential risk to the fetus or infant. The potential benefits must outweigh the potential risks to use barbiturates during these circumstances. Barbiturates potentiate all types of CNS depressant medications. Table 19-3 lists the barbiturates most commonly used in conscious sedation in dentistry.

Antihistamines

Two drugs—promethazine (Phenergan) and hydroxyzine (Atarax, Vistaril: Pfizer; New York, NY)—under the classification of antihistamines[23] continue to be used in dentistry primarily for sedation before dental procedures. Orally, these medications are given for relief of symptoms of perennial and seasonal allergies and as an adjunctive therapy to anaphylactic reactions. Promethazine, a phenothiazine derivative, continues to be used in dentistry by the oral, IM, and IV routes of administration for preoperative and postoperative sedation, as an adjunct to analgesics for control of postoperative pain, and for relief of apprehension. Promethazine competitively antagonizes histamine at H1 receptor sites, producing sedation, relief of apprehension, and antiemetic effects. Promethazine is often given in combination with a narcotic, which it potentiates, thereby reducing the narcotic dosage by 25% to 50%.[32-34]

The diphenylmethane compound, hydroxyzine, is minimally effective as an antianxiety drug. The oral and IM administration of hydroxyzine do have sedative, antihistaminic, antispasmodic, and antiemetic actions. It will also reduce the narcotic requirement in preoperative and postoperative sedation. Therapy with hydroxyzine was studied in 76 apprehensive and fearful pediatric dental patients,[35] and when 50 mg was administered 1 hour before scheduled appointments, behavioral difficulties were significantly reduced. Table 19-4 lists the antihistamine names, routes of administration, times of onset, and durations of action.

In oral sedation, a large number of the medications listed earlier have been used in the past. Currently, benzodiazepines are the most widely used sedative drugs in both oral and parenteral conscious sedation, because they combine anxiolysis with varying degrees of amnesia and sedation.[36] They also have the major

TABLE 19-1   Orally Administered Benzodiazepines

GENERIC (TRADE) NAME	USE	USUAL ORAL DOSAGE	ONSET	DURATION	AVAILABLE FORMS
Alprazolam (Xanax)	Oral antianxiety	Adults: 0.5-3 mg taken 1 hr before procedure Children: not recommended	Intermediate with oral administration: 1 hr, with peak levels at 1-2 hr	Half-life: 11.2 hr (range: 6.3-26.9 hr)	Sol: 0.5 mg/5 ml Tab: 0.25 mg, 1 mg, 2 mg
Clorazepate dipotassium (Tranxene, Tranxene SD, Gen-XENE)	Oral antianxiety	30-60 mg taken 1 hr before procedure, with rapid and complete absorption	Fast with oral administration: 0.5 hr, with peak levels at 0.5-4 hr	Half-life: 40-50 hr	Cap: 3.75 mg, 7.5 mg, 15 mg Tab: 3.75 mg, 7.5 mg, 15 mg
Estazolam (ProSom)	Oral sedative, hypnotic	1-2 mg taken 1 hr before procedure	0.5-1 hr, with peak levels at 0.5 to 6 hr	Half-life: 10 to 24 hr	Tab: 1 mg, 2 mg
Flurazepam (Dalmane)	Oral sedative, hypnotic	Healthy: 30 mg taken 1 hr before appointment Elderly/debilitated: 15 mg taken 1 hr before appointment	0.5-1 hr	Half-life: 47-100 hr	Tab: 15 mg, 30 mg
Oxazepam (Serax)	Oral antianxiety sedative, hypnotic	Adults: 10-30 mg taken 1 hr before appointment Children: not recommended	1 hr	Half-life: 10-14 hr	Cap: 10 mg, 15 mg, 30 mg Tab: 15 mg
Temazepam (Restoril)	Oral sedative, hypnotic	Adults: 7.5-30 mg taken 1 hr before appointment Children: Not recommended	30 min, with peak levels in 2-3 hr	Half-life: 10 hr	Cap: 7.5 mg, 15 mg, 30 mg
Triazolam (Halcion)	Oral sedative, hypnotic	Adults: 0.125-0.25 mg taken 1 hr before appointment Children: Not recommended	1.3 hr	Half-life: 2.2 hr	Tab: 0.125 mg, 0.25 mg
Zolpidem (Ambien)	Oral sedative	10 mg taken 1 hr before appointment	1 hr, with peak effect in 1.6 hr	Half-life: 2-3 hr (mean half-life in healthy patients: 2.6 hr)	Tab: 5 mg, 10 mg

advantage of having sp   agents available.
The use of barbiturate\   amines for adult
conscious sedation is gen\   \dicated. A limited
number of oral benzodiaz\   \edications, such as
triazolam, diazepam, clorazep\   , estazolam, oxazepam,
or temazepam are suggested for consideration as one or two oral sedation medications to be included in the clinician's armamentarium.

Methohexital (Brevital) and propofol (Diprivan) are not included in the list of medications above, because they

TABLE 19-2   Multiroute-Administration Benzodiazepines

GENERIC (TRADE) NAME	USE	ADMINISTRATIVE ROUTE/USUAL ADULT DOSAGE	ONSET	DURATION	AVAILABLE FORMS
Diazepam (Valium)	Antianxiety, sedative, skeletal muscle relaxant	Oral: 2-10 mg taken 1 hr before appointment IM: 10 mg administered 10-30 min before treatment IV: 2-20 mg, not to exceed 5 mg/min, average sedative dose 12-15 mg	Oral: 1 hr, with peak effect in 2 hr IM: 20-30 min IV: 30-60 sec	Oral: 1-3 hr IM: 1-3 hr IV: 45 min	Tab: 2 mg, 5 mg, 10 mg Inj: 5 mg/ml
Lorazepam (Ativan)*	Antianxiety, hypnotic	Oral: 2-4 mg taken 1 hr before appointment IM: 10 mg IV: 1-2 mg	Oral: 1 hr IM: 15-20 min, with peak plasma effects in 60-90 min IV: 5 min, with peak onset in 20 min, making titration difficult	Oral: 2-4 hr IM: 6-8 hr IV: 6-8 hr	Tab: 0.5 mg, 1 mg, 2 mg Sol: 2 mg/ml Inj: 2 mg/ml and 4 mg/ml
Midazolam (Versed)	Sedation, amnesia	IM: 0.07-0.08 mg/kg (usually 5 mg total) administered deeply in large muscle mass, approximately 1 hr before appointment IV: with 1 mg/ml dilution, administer 1-2.5 mg over 2 min for maximum effect. Titrate to desired level with small increments at 2 min intervals to total dose of <5 mg, particularly if patient is premedicated with other CNS depressants. Total dose should not exceed 10 mg. **Do not administer as a bolus dose**	IM: 15 min IV: 2-2.5 min without narcotic premedication; 1.5 min with narcotic premedication	30-60 min, with half-life of 1.8-6.4 hr	Inj: 1 mg/ml, 5 mg/ml

Lorazepam is rarely used in outpatient or office dentistry because of the long duration of its effects.

Table 19-3   Barbiturates

Generic (Trade) Name	Use	Administrative Route/Usual Adult Dosage	Onset	Duration	Available Forms
Pentobarbital (Nembutal)	Sedative, hypnotic	Oral: 1oo mg taken 1 hr before appointment IM: 1oo-15o mg administered 3o min before appointment IV: 5o-1oo mg	Oral: 15-3o min IM: 1o-15 min IV: 3o sec	Oral: 3-6 hr, with half-life of 21-42 hr IM: 3-4 hr IV: 3-4 hr	Cap: 5o mg, 1oo mg Supp: 3o mg, 6o mg, 1oo mg, 3oo mg Inj: 5o mg/ml
Secobarbital (Seconal)	Sedative, hypnotic	Oral: 1oo-2oo mg taken 1-2 hours before appointment IM: 1oo-2oo mg administered 3o min before appointment IV: 1oo-15o mg	Oral: 1o-3o min IM: 1o-15 min IV: 3o sec	Oral: 3-4 hr, with half-life of 28 hours IM: 3-4 hr IV: 2-3 hr	Cap: 1oo mg Inj: 5o mg/ml

Table 19-4   Antihistamines

Generic (Trade) Name	Use	Administrative Route/Usual Adult Dosage	Onset	Duration	Available Forms
Promethazine (Phenergan)	Sedative, antiemetic	Oral: 25-5o mg taken 1 hr before appointment IM: 25-5o mg , with deep IM administration 1 hr before procedure IV: 25-5o mg	Oral: 2o min IM: 1o-15 min IV: 3o sec	Oral: 4-6 hr IM: 4-6 hr IV: 2 hr	Tab: 12.5 mg, 25 mg, 5o mg Syrup: 12.5 mg/5 ml, 25 mg/5 ml Supp: 12.5 mg, 25 mg, 5o mg Inj: 25 mg/ml
Hydroxyzine HCl (Atarax, Vistaril)	Antihistamine	Oral: 5o-1oo mg taken 1 hr before appointment IM: 25-1oo mg administered 1 hr before procedure, with deep IM administration only	Oral: 15-3o min, with peak effect in 2 hr, with mean elimination half-life in 3 hr IM: rapid onset (15 min)	Oral: 3-4 hr IM: 3-4 hr	Tab: 1o mg, 25 mg, 5o mg, 1oo mg Syrup: 1o mg/5 ml Oral suspension: 25 mg/5 ml Inj: 25 mg/ml, 5o mg/ml

are not considered conscious sedation agents.[37] The use of chloral hydrate as a sedative–hypnotic, either orally or rectally, is also strongly discouraged by the ADA Consultants on Anesthesia and Anesthetic Agents. Chloral hydrate has a significant record of complications as a sedative–hypnotic.

Benzodiazepine antagonist: flumazenil (Romazicon)

Indications for the use of flumazenil are to reverse the pharmacologic effects of benzodiazepines used in anesthesia and sedation and to manage benzodiazepine overdose. Flumazenil,[38] an imidazobenzodiazepine derivative, is a benzodiazepine receptor antagonist that competitively inhibits the activity at the benzodiazepine recognition site on the GABA/benzodiazepine receptor/chloride ionophore complex. Flumazenil does not reverse the effects of opioids and does not antagonize the CNS effects of drugs affecting GABA-ergic neurons by means other than the benzodiazepine receptor, including alcohol, barbiturates, and general anesthetics.[34]

For the reversal of the effects of benzodiazepine-induced conscious sedation, 0.2 mg flumazenil is administered intravenously over 15 seconds. If the desired level of consciousness is not obtained, the 0.2-mg dosage may be repeated at 1-minute intervals up to four additional times for a maximum dose of 1 mg. Most patients respond to a dosage of 0.6 to 1 mg of medication. In the event of resedation, repeated doses may be given at 0.2 mg/min up to 1 mg every 20 minutes. No more than 3 mg should be given in any 1 hour.

For a suspected benzodiazepine overdose, 0.2 mg flumazenil is administered over 30 seconds initially, followed by 0.5 mg over 30 seconds. This is repeated at 1-minute intervals until the patient responds. The maximum cumulative total adult dosage of flumazenil for a suspected overdose of benzodiazepines is 5 mg.

The onset of benzodiazepine reversal is usually at 1 to 2 minutes after the administration is completed, with 80% response reached within 3 minutes. The peak effect occurs within 6 to 10 minutes, with the duration and degree of reversal related to the plasma concentration of the sedating benzodiazepine, as well as the dose of flumazenil given. Resedation is possible if either a large single or cumulative dose of benzodiazepine has been given in the course of a long procedure. In four trials studying the use of flumazenil in 970 patients, the incidence rate of resedation was 3% to 9% during the 3-hour postsedation recovery period. A total of 78% of the benzodiazepine sedated patients receiving flumazenil responded by becoming completely alert. When flumazenil is used to reverse benzodiazepine overdose, one potential complication is the onset of seizures. This is uncommon if the doses of benzodiazepine were near the normal ranges used for conscious sedation.

Analgesics

There are six drugs used as analgesics in parenteral conscious sedation in periodontics. They fall into two categories: narcotic agonists (opioids) and narcotic agonists/antagonists analgesics.

Narcotic agonists (opioids) are potent analgesics and excellent drugs for the relief of moderate to severe pain, as well as sedatives. Their primary side effects are dose-dependent respiratory depression, histamine release (especially with morphine, causing hypotension and

bronchoconstriction), urinary retention, nausea, vomiting, and constipation.

The most commonly used narcotic agonists are morphine and meperidine (Demerol). Fentanyl (Sublimaze) falls into the category of analgesics for deep sedation/general anesthesia. Meperidine is the least potent, with morphine being approximately 10 times more potent than meperidine, and fentanyl being 100 times more potent than morphine.

General contraindications to narcotic agonists include hypersensitivity or intolerance to the drug; acute bronchial asthma; upper airway obstruction; concomitant use with monoamine oxidase inhibitors or within 14 days of such treatment; and when increased cranial pressure or head injuries are present. Narcotics should be used with caution in patients with chronic obstructive pulmonary disease or with any degree of respiratory depression. Elderly or debilitated patients, or those known to be sensitive to CNS depressants, often require decreased doses of narcotics. Table 19-5 lists the narcotic agonists.

Narcotic agonists/antagonists analgesics have two types: those that are antagonists at the mu receptor and are agonists at other receptors (i.e., pentazocine), and those partial agonists that have limited agonist activity at the mu receptor (i.e., buprenorphine). The narcotic agonist/antagonist analgesics are potent analgesic agents with a lower potential for abuse than pure opioid agonists. The agonist actions of these drugs are the same as those of the prototypical narcotic, morphine, whereas the antagonist actions include prevention of narcotic effects if administered in unison or before the narcotic. There is reversal of the narcotic effect when administered after the narcotic, whereas in patients who are physically dependant on opioids, the antagonist action results in almost immediate withdrawal symptoms. Table 19-6 lists the narcotic agonists/antagonists.

Narcotic antagonists

Narcotic antagonists are a class of drugs used to reverse narcotic-induced respiratory depression, sedation, and hypotension. Competitive inhibition at specific opioid receptor sites is the mechanism of action.

Naloxone (Narcan) is a pure opioid antagonist that is a synthetic congener of oxymorphone with no agonist properties.[32,34] It reverses or prevents the effects of opioids including respiratory depression, sedation, and hypotension. It can also reverse the psychotomimetic and dysphoric effects of agonist/antagonists such as pentaxocaine. It does not produce respiratory depression, psychotomimetic effects, or papillary constriction, and in the absence of opioids or agonistic effects of other opioid antagonists, it exhibits essentially no pharmacologic activity.

TABLE 19-5 Narcotic Agonists

GENERIC (TRADE) NAME	USE	ADMINISTRATIVE ROUTE/USUAL ADULT DOSAGE	ONSET	DURATION	AVAILABLE FORMS
Meperidine (Demerol)	Narcotic analgesic	IV: 25-50 mg/70 kg (154 lb) for healthy adult IM, SC: 1-2 mg/kg (0.5 mg/lb), or 50-70 mg/ 70 kg (154 lb) for healthy adult, 15-30 min before beginning procedure.	IV: 2-7 min, with respiratory depression occurring in approximately 3 min	IV: 30-45 min	Inj: 25 mg/ml, 50 mg/ml, 75 mg/ml
Morphine	Narcotic analgesic	IV: 2.5-15 mg/70 kg (154 lb) for healthy adult IM, SC: 5-20 mg/70 kg (154 lb) for healthy adult	IV: 8-10 min, with respiratory depression occurring as early as 2 minutes	2-3 hr	2 mg/ml, 4 mg/ml, 8 mg/ml, 10 mg/ml, 15 mg/ml
Fentanyl (Sublimaze)*	Narcotic analgesic	IV: 0.001-0.002 mg/kg (0.05-0.1 mg for adults) administered at a maximum of 0.05 mg/min	30 sec, with maximum respiratory depression delayed for 7-15 min	30-60 min	Inj: 100 μg/2 ml (0.05 mg/ml), 250 μg/5 ml, 500 μg/10 ml, 1000 μg/20 ml, 1500 μg/30 ml, 2500 μg/50 ml

*Although fentanyl has been used for conscious sedation, it is probably best used by individuals trained in deep sedation/general anesthesia and endotracheal airway management. Significant respiratory depression may occur and will require immediate management. Fentanyl may cause muscle rigidity (especially of the respiratory muscles) with rapid injection. It may also cause significant cardiovascular depression when administered with benzodiazepines. Fentanyl has biphasic elimination.

Precautions: Abrupt reversal of opioids may result in nausea, vomiting, sweating, tachycardia, or tremors. Use with caution in patients with known opioid dependency. The duration of action of some opioids may outlast that of naloxone, therefore the patient should be kept under prolonged surveillance.

Nalmefene (Revex) is a newer opioid antagonist structurally similar to naloxone (a 6-methylene analogue of naltrexone), which can completely or partially reverse opioid drug effects, including respiratory depression, induced by either natural or synthetic opioids. It can be administered intravenously, intramuscularly, or subcutaneously. When administered intravenously, nalmefene should be titrated to reverse the undesired effects of opioids. Nalmefene has no opioid agonist activity; it produces no respiratory depression, psychotomimetic effects, or pupillary constriction. When administered in the absence of opioid agonists, no pharmacologic activity has been observed.[32,34]

Precautions: Less than 3% of patients experienced adverse reactions, including nausea, vomiting, tachycardia, hypertension, postoperative pain, fever, and dizziness.

Table 19-7 lists the administration information of the two narcotic antagonists.

DETERMINATION OF THE EFFECTS OF DRUG ADMINISTRATION

The effects of drug administration are highly dependent on the concentration of the drug in the blood and in the brain tissue. The differences in enteral and parenteral conscious sedation techniques are associated with variations in the absorption, the first pass effect, distribution, metabolism, and excretion of drugs.

Absorption is the process by which a drug enters the circulation. IV drug administration is the most rapid and direct, because the drug is put into immediate contact with the tissues and cells. Circulation time is the elapsing time between the injection of the medication into the blood and maximum distribution of the drug throughout the body. For most medications, circulation time is about 10 to 18 seconds using the IV route.[26] With oral drug administration, most drugs are absorbed by the small intestine.

It is important to remember the intent and contributions of the drug(s) used for conscious sedation. All anesthesia has two essential elements: sedation/hypnosis and analgesia. Because hypnosis is generally associated

TABLE 19-6	Narcotic Agonists–Antagonists					

GENERIC (TRADE) NAME	USE	ADMINISTRATIVE ROUTE/USUAL ADULT DOSAGE	ONSET	DURATION	AVAILABLE FORMS
Butorphanol (Stadol)	Analgesic	IV: 0.5-2.0 mg; average sedative dose of 0.7-1.5 mg; 3.5-7 times more potent than morphine and 30-49 times more potent than meperidine; antagonist activity is 1/40 that of Naloxone	IV: maximum blood levels in 5 min	3-4 hr	Inj: 1 mg/ml, 2 mg/ml
Nalbuphine (Nubain)	Analgesic	IM, SC, IV: 7-10 mg/ 70 kg (154 lb) for healthy adult; at 10 mg, Nalbuphine exerts the same respiratory effect as equianalgesic doses of morphine, and potentiates CNS depressants, especially barbiturates	IV: 2-3 min	3-6 hr	Inj: 10 mg/ml, 20 mg/ml in 1 ml single-dose ampuls and in 10 ml multiple-dose vials
Pentazocine (Talwin)	Analgesic	IM, IV: 30 mg; doses in excess of 30 mg IV or 60 mg IM are not recommended; recommendation is for a single parenteral dose, and SC recommended only when other administration not possible (because of potential for tissue damage)	IV: 2-3 min	3-4 hr	Inj: 30 mg/ml

with sleep and general anesthesia, it is undesirable when the objective is conscious sedation. Because the drugs commonly used to achieve conscious sedation produce a dose-dependent CNS depression, conscious sedation lies on a continuum from minimal sedation (a relaxed, awakened state) to deep sedation/general anesthesia. Medical anesthesiologists feel that because of the rapidity with which a patient can move from conscious sedation to general anesthesia, and the variations in individual patient responses to the same dose of a sedative or analgesic drug, careful monitoring of the patient's vital signs is an essen-

tial property of clinical management.[36] The sedative component medication used should allow careful titration. The analgesic component, when used, is generally a narcotic administered to enhance sedation and anesthesia in relatively low fixed dosages, because the onset of action is too slow for it to be titratable. Both the sedative and the analgesic should be reversible, with minimal respiratory depression, and with a duration of action that match the time needed for the surgical procedure.

The blood level of the drug is dependent on the rate of addition to and removal from the bloodstream.

TABLE 19-7   Narcotic Antagonists

GENERIC (TRADE) NAME	DOSAGE RANGE	ONSET	DURATION	AVAILABLE FORMS
Naloxone (Narcan)	*For excessive sedation*: increments of 0.1-0.2 mg IV every 2-3 min to desired level of reversal *For overdose*: 0.4-2 mg increments repeated at 2-3 min intervals administered through IM, SC, or IV routes *When used*: should be diluted with sterile IV solution to a concentration of 0.1 mg/ml *In emergency situations*: IV administration is the most rapid means of action onset	2 min	30 min to 2 hr; may need to be readministered if narcotic agent being reversed has longer duration of action than naloxone	Inj: 0.2 mg/ml, 0.4 mg/ml, 1.0 mg/ml
Nalmefene (Revex)	*IV administration*: initial dose of 0.25 μg/kg; incremental doses at 2-5 min intervals, stopping as soon as the desired degree of opioid reversal is obtained *Note*: a cumulative dose in excess of 1.0 μg/kg does not produce additional therapeutic effect *Loss of IV access*: single dose of 1 mg Nalmefene administered IM or SC	IM, SC: 5-15 min; If significant improvement does not occur after 2-3 min of IV administration, the respiratory depression is probably not associated with a narcotic overdose	Duration of Nalmefene is as long as most opioid analgesics. However, depending on the half-life and plasma concentration of the narcotic being reversed the duration of action will vary. Low doses of Nalmefene, and the presence or absence of other drugs affecting the brain or muscles of respiration, may prevent the reversal from lasting more than 30-60 min with persistent opioid effects.	Inj: 1 mg/ml

AMERICAN DENTAL ASSOCIATION EDUCATIONAL REQUIREMENTS AND TECHNIQUES FOR SEDATION

Through a cooperative effort, representatives from all of the areas of dentistry that use sedation met in 1999 and 2000 under sponsorship of the ADA. National educational requirements and guidelines for each level of sedation and anesthesia described earlier were established and agreed on. Because training in conscious sedation is con-

tained in the definition of postdoctoral specialty training in periodontics, this chapter includes the educational requirements and guidelines for the methods of sedation commonly used by board-eligible periodontists.[15]

Enteral or Combined Inhalation–Enteral Conscious Sedation

To administer enteral, or combined inhalation-enteral conscious sedation, or both, it is necessary that the periodontist or practitioner satisfy one of the following ADA criteria:

1. Completed training to the level of competency in enteral and/or combined inhalation–enteral conscious sedation consistent with that prescribed in Part I or Part III of the ADA *Guidelines for Teaching Comprehensive Control of Pain and Anxiety in Dentistry.*
2. Completed an ADA-accredited periodontal postdoctoral training program that affords the comprehensive and appropriate training necessary to administer and manage enteral, or combined conscious sedation, or both.

The following guidelines apply to the administration of enteral, or combined conscious sedation, or both, in the periodontal office:

1. The administration of enteral, or combined conscious sedation, or both, by another duly qualified dentist or physician requires the operating dentist and his/her clinical staff to maintain current expertise in Basic Life Support (BLS).
2. When a certified registered nurse anesthetist is permitted to function under the supervision of a dentist, administration of enteral, or combined conscious sedation, or both, by a certified registered nurse anesthetist requires the operating dentist to have completed training in enteral, or combined conscious sedation, or both, consistent with the requirements described in Part I or Part III of the ADA *Guidelines for Teaching Comprehensive Control of Pain and Anxiety in Dentistry* at the time dental training or postdoctoral training was commenced.
3. A dentist administering enteral, or combined conscious sedation, or both, as well as his/her clinical staff, must maintain current expertise in BLS.

Parenteral Conscious Sedation

To administer parenteral conscious sedation, it is necessary for the dentist to satisfy either one of the following ADA criteria:

1. The completion of a comprehensive training program in parenteral conscious sedation, which satisfies the requirements described in Part I or Part III of the ADA *Guidelines for Teaching Comprehensive Control of Pain and Anxiety in Dentistry* at the time dental training or postdoctoral training was commenced.
2. Completion of an ADA-accredited periodontal postdoctoral training program that has the comprehensive and appropriate training necessary to meet the ADA requirements to administer and manage parenteral conscious sedation.

The following guidelines apply to the administration of in-office parenteral conscious sedation:

1. The administration of parenteral conscious sedation by another duly qualified dentist or physician requires

the operating dentist and his/her clinical staff to maintain current expertise in BLS. Many states also require the periodontist to have current completion of a course dealing with either Advanced Training in Dental Emergencies or Advance Cardiac Life Support (or its appropriate equivalent).
2. When a certified registered nurse anesthetist is permitted to function under the supervision of a dentist, the operating dentist must have completed training in parenteral conscious sedation consistent with the standards described in Part I or Part III of the ADA *Guidelines for Teaching the Comprehensive Control of Anxiety and Pain in Dentistry.*

INTRAVENOUS ROUTE OF ADMINISTRATION VERSUS OTHER ROUTES OF ADMINISTRATION

As previously stated, the administration of inhalation, enteral, or parenteral drugs can result in a range of effects extending from conscious sedation to general anesthesia. The result obtained with the drug(s) is dependent on the drug dosage and rate of administration. When properly used, the safest, most predictable, rapid, direct way to administer drugs for conscious sedation is the IV route. Drugs in aqueous solution can be injected directly into the bloodstream, circumventing absorption problems encountered with other techniques of conscious sedation. IV administration also avoids use of arbitrary standard dosages, slow onset times, and the less predictable results of oral and IM sedation. With IV conscious sedation, the effects of the sedative drugs are titratable because of a short circulation time and rapid onset of action. Maximum drug effect for the sedatives commonly used in periodontics is usually achieved in 1 to 5 minutes, thus the pharmacologic action may be accurately titrated in incremental dosages to achieve individually tailored results for each patient. The full effects of Nembutal are realized in approximately 30 seconds, whereas Valium takes about 1 minute, and midazolam takes approximately 2 minutes. These sedatives and others that rapidly pass through the blood–brain barrier are titratable, whereas analgesics are generally less titratable because of their slower onset of action times. Patient response to an intravenously administered sedative allows a more accurate appraisal of the analgesic dosage, because the two classes of drugs generally exhibit an equal tolerance. By titrating the sedative drug and administering an equal tolerance of narcotic, the "dosage guessing" dangers that are seen with the administration of standard dosages for oral and IM sedation based on patient size and weight are avoidable.

PRESEDATION PREPARATION APPOINTMENT

Medical and Physical Evaluation and Documentation

The standard of care in most states requires dentists to evaluate and document a patient's physical, medical, and emotional status before any periodontal care. Initially, patients fill out health questionnaires, followed by dialogue history with the dentist to assess the forms, to gather pertinent health history information, to determine baseline vital signs, and to do a limited physical examination. This should include an assessment of potential IV sites, skin integrity, and color. By doing so, the doctor will be better able to ascertain the physical and psychological status of the patient and to establish an ASA risk factor classification for the patient. When indicated, a medical consultation can be initiated to further clarify the patient's medical and physical well being. Once the patient's medical and physical status is determined, and indicated medical consultations are completed, appropriate periodontal therapy can be planned and modified as necessary. The goals of the medical, physical, and psychological examination and consultations are to determine whether the potential risks that are present can be alleviated with psychomatic control of apprehension, or if some means of chemical anxiety reduction is indicated to help the patient tolerate the stresses involved in therapy. It is also important to determine if additional monitoring is necessary. Stress control begins at the time of the patient's initial contact with the office.

Written presedation instructions should be given to each patient at the presedation appointment. In the current time of electronic patient records, it is easy to give the patient a personalized, written preoperative instruction sheet regarding sedation and preoperative care (Fig. 19-2). Such information is discussed with the patient to assure that it is understood and noted in the patient records. Ensuring that the patient is well informed and knowledgeable about the sedation and planned therapeutic procedure can enhance doctor–patient rapport and patient confidence. Preoperative instructions given immediately before a procedure are generally poorly comprehended and remembered. Postsedation instructions and discussions should also be given to the patient at the time the procedure is planned, rather than waiting until the day of therapy. This will assure that proper planning and treatment can be rendered.

The patient is informed that their surgery will be performed using a combination of conscious sedation and local anesthetic. They are told to take their usual prescribed medications, unless otherwise instructed, as well as those that have been prescribed in preparation for their surgery. The patient is advised to inform the doctor of any medications they are taking, even over-the-counter

drugs, and not to take any medications without the doctor's knowledge and approval. The patient is told not to have anything to eat for at least 6 to 8 hours before their appointment, with the exception of clear liquids, excluding coffee or tea. They are further instructed to refrain from the consumption of any alcoholic beverages within 24 hours of surgery.

The patient is asked to arrive promptly for their appointment, because late arrivals add to the patient's stress level and may necessitate rescheduling of the appointment. Early arrival often allows the staff to help the patient relax before starting the surgery. For IV sedation, the patient is instructed to wear loose comfortable clothing that can easily be drawn up above the elbow to facilitate the venipuncture. No heavy make-up or false eyelashes should be worn, and at least two fingers on each hand should be devoid of fingernail polish or false fingernails to facilitate proper vital sign monitoring. The patient is asked to refrain from wearing contact lenses the day of their appointment to avoid losing valuable time removing and storing the lenses during their scheduled appointment time.

A written preoperative instruction form and prescriptions for medications, should be dispensed to the patient or their guardian in advance. This will allow the information to be reviewed at their leisure. It is emphasized that a responsible adult must accompany the patient to drive the patient home and provide supervision for the remainder of the day. They are made aware that they will not be able to safely or prudently:

1. Operate machinery or drive a car
2. Undertake financial or business matters
3. Drink alcoholic beverages the day of the sedation.

The patient is given telephone numbers to record, file, and call in the event of an emergency.

Written Informed Consent

Dental regulating boards require, and patients are entitled to, appropriate written informed consent forms detailing the benefits of the various conscious sedation procedures, the drugs to be used, and the general actions of the drugs, the risks, and alternatives to conscious sedation. Such sedation and surgical treatment procedure forms given to patients or their guardians in advance enable the patient, parent, guardian, or other responsible adult of a minor, to have a basis of knowledge on which they can make an informed decision and give their permission for the procedure. An informed consent must be obtained on each patient in accordance with individual state laws, specifically stating the risks related to the sedation procedure. To be legally valid, the consent form must be signed before the procedure by the patient; the parent, the guardian, or the responsible adult in the case of a minor; the doctor;

Pre-operative Guidelines for [FirstName LastName]

INSTRUCTIONS FOR PATIENTS WHO WILL BE RECEIVING I.V. SEDATION

For your comfort, your surgery will be performed utilizing a combination of local anesthetics and intravenously administered conscious sedation. For your safely, it is necessary that you follow the instructions below.

1. Take your usual prescribed medications as well as those which have been prescribed for you in preparation for your surgery. *Do not take any aspirin or aspirin-containing medications for at least three days prior to your surgery date.*

2. Advise us of any medications your are taking, even over-the-counter drugs. Please do not take any medicines without the doctor's knowledge and approval.

3. Please *do not have anything to eat for at least 4 hours prior to your appointment.* It is O.K. to have small amounts of clear liquids, but refrain from coffee or tea.

4. Do not drink any alcoholic beverages the day of your appointment. The evening before, do not have more than 1 or 2 glasses of wine or beer, or more than 1 highball or cocktail.

5. Wear loose, comfortable clothing with *sleeves that can easily be drawn up above your elbow.* Do not wear heavy makeup or false eyelashes, and if you wear nail polish or acrylic artificial nails, please remove the nail polish and artificial nails from at least two fingers on your right hand. If you wear contact lenses, please be prepared to remove and store them when you arrive at our office or wear prescription glasses in place of them the day of your appointment. Do not wear your contact lenses for the remainder of the day of your sedation.

6. Please arrive promptly for your appointment. Late arrival may necessitate rescheduling of your surgery. Allow for the usual heavy traffic in planning your departure from home or work so that you can arrive on time. If you are early, the staff will welcome the opportunity to help you relax before your surgery.

7. You must be accompanied home by an adult who will drive and arrange for responsible supervision for the remainder of the day. We are sorry, but we cannot allow you to take a public conveyance or drive yourself home.

8. If any disturbances or problems should develop after you leave our office, you should call our office (or emergency number if after normal working hours) immediately. Parents or guardians of young patients should observe the child continuously upon returning home and call us immediately if disturbances or problems should develop.

9. Full mental alertness will not return for several hours after your sedation. Therefore, for the remainder of the day you should limit activity requiring full concentration power. You will not be able to safely or prudently: (a) drive an automobile or operate machinery, (b) undertake business or financial matters or (c) drink alcoholic beverages the day of your sedation. Remaining sedentary as well as the use of a small ice pack on your face can significantly enhance your comfort. Heavy physical activity shortly after your surgery can cause complications and pain.

10. Please notify us if you develop a cold, sore throat, cough, stuffy nose or fever or any other illness during the days prior to your surgical appointment. If rescheduling your appointment becomes necessary, we would like to have as much advance notice as possible. Please do not wait until the day before, or the day of your surgery to notify us, thinking that you might get better. Our office commonly starts preparing items for your surgery several days in advance, so the lead time related to possible rescheduling can be important.

If you have any questions after reading these guidelines, please do not hesitate to call us for clarification.

Figure 19-2. Personalized, written preoperative instructions sheet for sedation and preoperative care. (*From TiME for Dentistry, Oakland, 2002, DecisionBase, Inc.*)

and a witness. Figure 19-3 is an example of an electronic IV conscious sedation advised consent form.

DAY OF SEDATION APPOINTMENT

Preoperative Preparation

Before patient arrival, all equipment used in conjunction with the sedation procedure must be evaluated for proper operation, including a determination of the presence of an adequate oxygen supply. Sedation supplies are prepared, labeled, checked, and appropriately placed for minimal patient awareness.

On arrival of the patient for the appointment, the front desk must confirm the return of the signed consent forms

and place them in the patient chart. Office personnel must ensure that a responsible adult is present to take the patient home at the completion of the procedure. Any new or unanswered questions regarding the sedation or the surgical procedures should be answered.

Before the start of any sedative procedure, the patient is asked to visit the restroom to take care of any physical needs. For the patient's comfort, and because the patient is not legally responsible for decisions made under the influence of sedation, it is important to review the treatment plan again immediately before the surgery, with the patient understanding what to expect in terms of vital signs monitoring and treatment procedure. The dentist should review what the patient can expect with the procedure and possible surgical complications secondary to

An explanation of intravenously administered sedation, its purpose and benefits, the procedure and drugs used and the possible complications of its use as well as alternatives to its were discussed with you at your consultation. We obtained your verbal consent to undergo this procedure. Please read this document which restates issues we discussed and provide the appropriate signature on the last page. Please ask for clarification of anything you do not understand.

Consent for the Use of Intravenously Administered Conscious Sedation on [FirstName LastName]

ALTERNATIVE TYPES OF ANESTHESIA: I have been informed that my treatment can be performed with a variety of types of anesthesia: (1) local anesthesia as normally used for minor dental treatment; (2) local anesthesia supplemented with I.V. conscious sedation; and (3) general anesthesia in the hospital or out-patient day care surgical center. I have been made aware that the risks with each type of anesthesia very, with local anesthesia generally considered to have the least risk and general anesthesia having the greatest risk. I have been advised that if I am significantly subject to fear, anxiety or emotional stress related to dental procedures, or if a long or stressful procedure is to be undertaken, or if certain medical or physical conditions exist, this risk sequence can change, and I.V. conscious sedation, properly administered, might be beneficial relative to other anesthetics alternatives. I understand that, based on the doctor's judgment, one or more of the choices for anesthesia may not be desirable in every case.

THE PROCESS OF I.V. CONSCIOUS SEDATION: I have been informed that the objective of I.V. conscious sedation is to lessen the significant and undesirable side effects of long and stressful dental procedures by chemically reducing the fear, apprehension, emotional and physical stresses sometimes present. This is accomplished by the administration of small incremental doses of various medications such that they produce a state of relaxation, reduced perception of pain and a degree if drowsiness, but that I will not be put to sleep as with a general anesthetic. In addition, local anesthetics will be administered in my mouth to numb the areas to be operated so as to control pain. I understand that the drugs to be used may include the following:

☐ Versed (midazolam)　　　　　☐ Valium (diazepam)　　　　　☐ Fentanyl

☐ Demerol (meperidine)　　　　　☐ Morphine　　　　　☐ Other: _____

I also understand that other drugs may be used to alter my reaction to these drugs or to enhance my physical status during the procedure.

POSSIBLE RISKS AND SIDE EFFECTS: I have been informed and understand that occasionally there are complications associated with I.V. conscious sedation including but not limited to: pain, hematoma (bruising due to leakage of blood from the vein), phlebitis (inflammation of the vein), infection, swelling, bleeding, numbness, discoloration, nausea, vomiting, allergic reaction, and in extremely rare instance intra-arterial injection with damage to the part of the body supplied by the artery, brain damage or death.

PATIENT COMPLIANCE: I agree to the following: (1) I will refrain from eating for 4 hours prior to my dental appointment; (2) I will refrain from consuming any alcoholic beverages for 12 hours before and 24 hours following this procedure; (3) I will disclose to the doctor any and all drugs and medications I am currently taking; (4) I have disclosed any abnormalities in my current physical status or past medical history including any history of drug or alcohol abuse or any abnormal reactions to any drugs/medications which I have taken; (5) I will arrange for a responsible adult to drive me home and be with me until the effects of the sedation have worn off; and (6) I will refrain from driving a motor vehicle or operating dangerous machinery for the remainder of the day I received sedation.

PATIENT'S ENDORSEMENT: My endorsement (signature) to this form indicates that I have read and fully understand the terms and words within this document and the explanations referred to or implied, and that after thorough deliberation, I give my consent for the performance of any and all procedures related to I.V. conscious sedation as presented to me during consultation and treatment plan presentation by the doctor or as described in this document.

PATIENT'S ENDORSEMENT: My endorsement (signature) to this form indicates that I have read and fully understand the terms used within this document and the explanations referred to or implied. After thorough consideration, I give my consent for the performance of any and all procedures related to I.V. sedation as presented to me during the consultation and treatment plan presentation by the doctor or as described in this document.

_____	_____	_____
Patient's Signature	Date	Patient's Name (please print)
_____	_____	_____
Signature of Patient's Guardian	Date	Relationship to Patient
_____	_____	
Signature of Witness	Date	

Figure 19-3. Electronically prepared conscious intravenous sedation advised consent form. (*From TiME for Dentistry, Oakland, 2002, DecisionBase, Inc.*)

the procedure. The discussion should be noted in the patient's records before sedation.

Postoperative Instructions

Written postoperative instructions regarding conscious sedation should be included as part of the preoperative instruction sheet. Before being released to a responsible adult, the patient must have stable vital signs, be capable of appropriate responses to questions, be easily aroused when lightly sleeping, demonstrate intact protective reflexes, and be capable of sitting upright unassisted. They must have a responsible adult to accompany them to their postoperative recovery quarters and to offer assistance to the patient as needed. Written postoperative instructions specific to the surgical procedure should also be provided. Specific instructions regarding postoperative discomfort, swelling, bleeding, diet, and medications should be given. Oral hygiene instructions and guidance should also be included.

Medical and Physical Evaluation the Day of the Procedure

The patient's medical history should be reviewed at the time the surgical procedure is scheduled and must be reviewed and updated on the day of the procedure. Any changes since the last appointment should be recorded. Questions should include:

1. Is there any change in your overall health?
2. Have you seen or talked to your physician since your last appointment?
3. Have you started taking any over-the-counter or prescription medications since your last appointment?

A positive response to any of these questions must be pursued to ascertain potential risks and contraindications for the procedure. Current vital signs are obtained, including blood pressure, heart rate, and oxygen saturation. An electrocardiographic tracing may be recorded, if desired. The results are compared with the baseline vital signs that were obtained at a less stressful time.

Treatment Room Preparation

To assist in presenting a relaxed environment for the patient and to gain patient confidence, it is important that the treatment room present a pleasant, efficient atmosphere that is conducive to the sedation and operative process. The monitors are used to divert the patient's attention, as they have been previously introduced to them. The remainder of the room should be well organized, with all of the necessary surgical instruments, equipment, and syringes conveniently arranged for ease of use, but either covered or out of the viewing range of the patient. All syringes should be loaded and ready for use. There should be a minimum of distractions, sounds, and excessive movements that may add to the stress level of the patient.

On entering the treatment room, the patient is seated in the dental chair, taking care to ensure that the patient is seated properly for full support of the spine, neck, and head as *the chair is lowered to a semireclining position to start the sedation.*

Vital Signs Monitoring

Anesthesia providers should closely follow the vital signs monitoring standards established by the ADA[14,17] and several other specialty organizations, such as the American Academy of Periodontology. A trained professional provider is required to continually monitor the patient's heart rate, blood pressure, tissue oxygenation, and ventilation by direct clinical observation. For patients with significant cardiovascular disease (ASA III), continuous electrocardiographic monitoring must also be accomplished.

Continuous patient contact is the best method of monitoring the patient's physical status. Ongoing verbal contact with the patient should be maintained. The patient's color can be visually monitored by continually observing the mucosa and nail bed. Circulation (heart rate and blood pressure) can be monitored manually on a time-orientated basis, but it is common to rely on automatic electronic monitors. The oxygen saturation values require the use of pulse oximetry. Respiratory depression and hypoxemia are the primary clinical events of a sequential chain, which if left untreated will result in morbidity and mortality linked to conscious sedation. Pulse oximetry is the single most valuable monitor that is used in conscious sedation. The inexperienced clinician, without the use of proper monitoring, has a tendency to interpret patient movement associated with hypoxemia as an indication for additional drug administration, which will further complicate the situation. Early recognition of respiratory depression and hypoxemia followed by quickly initiating appropriate treatment is paramount to avoiding significant morbidity and mortality with conscious sedation. Auscultation provides some certainty of ventilation adequacy and the presence of a patent airway when used in combination with pulse oximetry. Part of prudent monitoring also involves regular observation of the head position to assure a patent airway. *A sedated patient should never be left unobserved by trained personnel.*

INTRAVENOUS CONSCIOUS SEDATION

Selection of Venipuncture Site

The technique of venipuncture is not difficult to master, but certain precautions should be taken for a venipuncture to be as painless and safe as possible. The superficial veins of the hand and arm are ideal for venipuncture in IV conscious sedation. There are three common areas to evaluate for a venipuncture (Fig. 19-4):

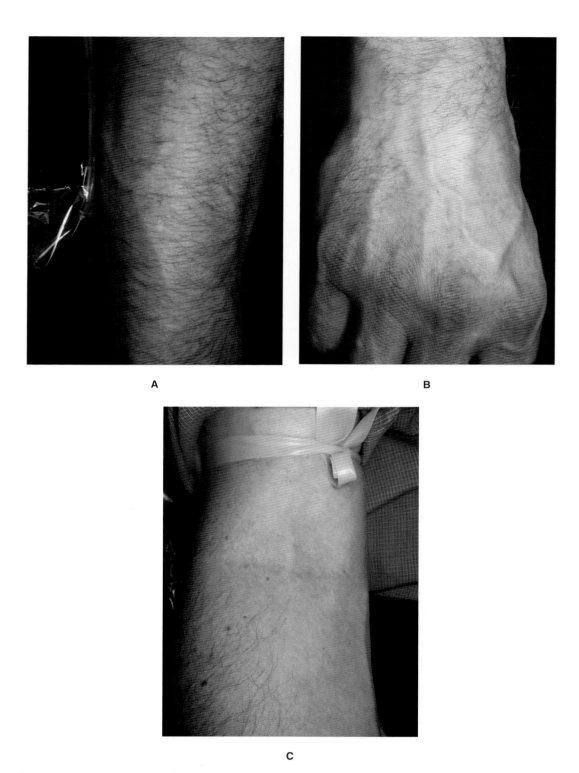

Figure 19-4. Three common areas to evaluate for a venipuncture site. **A,** The dorsal forearm veins (accessory cephalic and median antebrachial veins). **B,** Veins of the dorsal aspect of the hand and wrist (metacarpal and dorsal venous network). **C,** Median basilic and median cephalic veins of the antecubital fossa.

1. The veins in the forearm (accessory cephalic and median antebrachial veins)
2. The veins in the dorsal aspect of the hand (metacarpal and dorsal venous network)
3. The veins in the antecubital fossa (median basilic and median cephalic).

There is a tendency to persistently choose to use the veins in the antecubital fossa for a venipuncture because they are usually large in diameter, thick walled, straight, relatively immobile because of good support by connective tissue, and often easily accessible. Everett and Allen,[39] however, believe that superficial veins on the dorsal aspect of the hand or distal aspect of the forearm have less frequent arterial variations than the antecubital fossa. The order of site selection many practitioners choose for a complication free venipuncture is, therefore, the forearm, the dorsal aspect of the hand, and then the antecubital fossa. A venipuncture site may not be visible until after tourniquet placement for vein engorgement. When possible, superficial vessels should be chosen for the venipuncture, but one must realize that small, thin-walled veins are often poorly supported by connective tissue, roll or collapse easily, and may be fragile and leak blood around the needle penetration. Small veins may not tolerate irritating sedative drugs well, resulting in a greater incidence of phlebitis and thrombophlebitis. Precautions need to be considered, however, when the veins are not superficial, making a venipuncture more challenging. Blind probing with the needle should be avoided when veins are not readily visible. It is important to be extremely aware of the normal anatomic positions of blood vessels and nerves of the three common venipuncture areas, and to choose a site where there is the least chance of an accidental arterial penetration. Deeper positioned veins in the median aspect of the antecubital fossa can lie directly over the brachial artery and median nerve. Aberrant superficially positioned arteries may also be frequently found in the area. *Before tourniquet application and a venipuncture attempt, the selected area needs to be palpated for a pulse, to guard against an intra-arterial puncture* (see Complications section later in chapter).

Because the current standard of care is for maintenance of a continuous infusion of fluid during conscious sedation, a stable vein should be chosen and maintained for the duration of the periodontal procedure. A successful venipuncture in the antecubital fossa, when using a butterfly needle, requires the arm to be immobilized to prevent extravasations during the time that the needle is within the vein. This is a disadvantage, because immobilization can become very uncomfortable during a long conscious sedation procedure. An advantage of a venipuncture in either the dorsal aspect of the hand or the forearm is that they do not require immobilization to maintain a continuous infusion of fluid during an entire surgical procedure. Use of a flexible catheter for a venipuncture in the antecubital area also eliminates the need for arm immobilization.

Components for Continuous Infusion Intravenous Sedation

Historically drugs have been administered both directly and indirectly for conscious IV sedation. The direct method titrated medications by injecting directly into a vein without the benefit of a continuous infusion of one of the standard IV solutions. After the desired effects were obtained, the needle was removed from the vein. The indirect method, however, uses a continuous standard IV fluid infusion into a vein during the entire procedure. Medications are administered into a patent vein with the IV fluid serving as a vehicle. The indirect technique results in decreased venous drug irritation and allows for drug reinforcement during long procedures. The indirect technique is the current standard of care for the administration of drugs for conscious sedation.

For periodontal procedures, the components of an indirect infusion technique include a plastic bag container of IV fluid, an administration set consisting of plastic tubing with an adjustable flow rate, and either a butterfly needle and tubing with a connector or an over-the-needle catheter and tubing with a connector. Plastic containers of 500 ml lactated Ringer's solution, lactated Ringer's solution with 5% dextrose, 5% dextrose in water, or normal saline may be used. The dextrose in some solutions may be valuable to the fasting preoperative patient, who will have low caloric intake after surgery.

The components of the infusion setup should be connected together carefully and aseptically. The administration tubing is cleared of air, before the patient enters the room, by opening the drip control and allowing the fluid to run into a waste receptacle.

With the restricted size of most dental operatories, the IV fluid should be suspended at least 2 to 3 feet above the venipuncture site from a ceiling mount that ideally is not visible to the patient. This will reduce anxiety associated with observation of the infusion flow. A ceiling mount prevents the inconvenience of rolling floor stands or cumbersome pole mounted stands. The position of the mount must be coordinated with other equipment in surgical operatories, so as not to interfere with overhead tract lights, a surgical microscope, or instrument delivery systems.

A prepared tray setup is recommended for all infusion components, the tourniquet, the prepared sedation drug dilutions, sterile alcohol prep-pads, tape and bandages, medications for sedation and systemic complications, and empty syringes (Fig. 19-5).

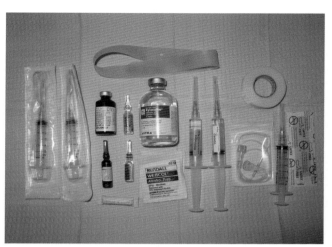

Figure 19-5. Prepared conscious sedation tray set-up with all of the infusion components, the tourniquet, the prepared drug dilutions, sterile alcohol prep pads, tape and bandages, medications for sedation complications, and empty syringes.

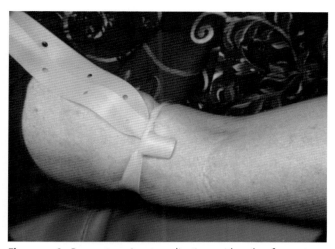

Figure 19-6. Proper tourniquet application, with tails of tourniquet positioned away from the venipuncture site.

Tourniquet Application

Before tourniquet application, the patient is placed in a semi-supine position. This position makes it more difficult for the patient to watch the venipuncture procedure and is an ideal position to minimize the risk for syncope. A Penrose style drain or a 1-inch flat rubber strap is recommended as a tourniquet, or a blood pressure cuff can be used as a tourniquet after blood pressure determination. The tourniquet is applied a short distance proximal to the desired venipuncture site. Applying the tourniquet too tightly will obliterate arterial blood flow distal to the tourniquet placement, with subsequent prevention of venous engorgement. Adequate pressure must be applied with the tourniquet to block venous blood flow, causing venous engorgement, which facilitates easy venipuncture. Application of the tourniquet should be with the tails of the tourniquet medially toward the body midline, or away from the venipuncture site to facilitate tourniquet removal and prevent contamination of the venipuncture site (Fig. 19-6).

Venous Engorgement, Palpation for a Pulse, and Site Preparation

If veins are not prominent in the forearm or dorsal aspect of the hand when the tourniquet is placed a few inches proximal to the desired venipuncture site, placing the arm down by the side of the patient may assist in visualizing them (Fig. 19-7). Application of a warm, moist towel to the desired area may be of value in difficult cases. Light tapping of the site may also assist in better visualization of the veins, as will vigorous site preparation with a radiating circular scrubbing technique of the

skin with a 70% isopropyl alcohol sponge. The alcohol scrub should extend outward in a circular fashion from the center of the venipuncture site for approximately 60 seconds.

Once a venipuncture site is selected, it must be palpated to ascertain that there is no arterial pulse (Fig. 19-8). Then the site is mechanically and chemically cleaned with isopropyl alcohol.[37]

Penetration of a Vein, Tourniquet Release, and Start of Infusion

For a right-handed therapist, the patient's right arm with the engorged veins is grasped with the therapist's left hand just distal to the venipuncture site. The left thumb

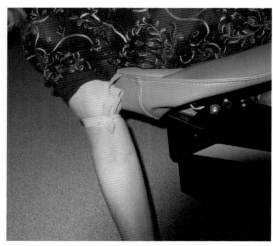

Figure 19-7. Lowering the arm to assist in visualization of veins distal to the tourniquet placement.

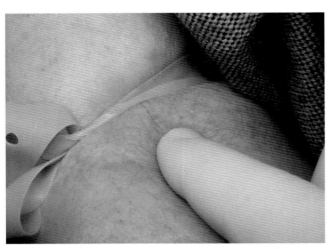

Figure 19-8. Palpating for an arterial pulse at the selected venipuncture site before venipuncture.

is used to extend the skin over the venipuncture site distally to immobilize the vein and facilitate its penetration with either a butterfly needle or an over-the-needle indwelling catheter (Fig. 19-9). With the bevel of the butterfly needle facing up, the winged taps are grasped between the thumb and index finger. A direct approach from the top of the engorged vein is the preferred method, with the needle held at a 30-degree angle to the skin surface. The skin and underlying connective tissue are penetrated to reach to, but not penetrate, the vessel. The angle of the needle is then changed to almost parallel to the skin surface, and the superficial wall of the vein is slowly penetrated, avoiding penetration of the inferior venous wall. The needle is inserted approximately two

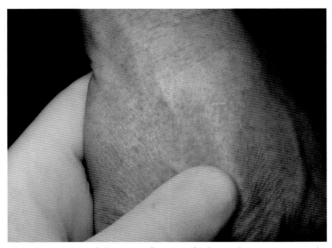

Figure 19-9. Immobilization of vein to facilitate the venipuncture by distal extension of the skin with the left thumb.

thirds of its length for stability. The syringe attached to the butterfly needle is then aspirated to verify that the needle is in a patent vein by drawing blood into the butterfly tubing. For experienced phlebotomists, the butterfly set alone may be used for the venipuncture, with the blood flushing into the tubing indicating a successful venipuncture. If the butterfly needle has been attached to the administration set, the fluid container can be lowered beneath the level of the venipuncture to visualize the back flow of blood into the tubing that occurs with a successful venipuncture.

Use of an indwelling catheter is somewhat more difficult for the novice to place.[36] With the tourniquet in place, the catheter-over-needle device is inserted into the vein with the bevel facing up. Once in the vein, blood will "flash back" into the catheter hub. At this point, the catheter is advanced into the vein as the needle is withdrawn. The major advantage of the indwelling catheter is that there is less likelihood of fluid infiltration than with a butterfly or scalp vein setup, and the arm does not have to be immobilized. Indwelling catheters are slightly more expensive to use. For some patients, subcutaneous administration of a small amount of lidocaine before the venipuncture is helpful to minimize discomfort associated with insertion of the butterfly needle or catheter.

Once the butterfly needle or catheter is in place, the tourniquet is released from the arm by pulling on that portion of the tourniquet tail that was tucked under. The tail is pulled away from the venipuncture site proximally to release it, to prevent displacement of the needle or catheter, and to prevent injection site contamination. On release of the tourniquet and connection of the air-free tubing of the administration set to the scalp needle or catheter, the flow regulator on the fluid administration set is opened to clear blood from the scalp needle or catheter, and to verify a free flow of fluid into the vein. The administration of IV fluid should not be started with the tourniquet in place.

The scalp needle or catheter is then fixed into place by placing two strips of tape parallel to the needle or catheter over the wings of the venipuncture device. A third strip of tape is then placed perpendicular to the wings to form an H-shaped configuration to minimize movement of the needle or catheter, which can be irritating. Alternatively, a variety of tapes are available that are specifically designed to secure the venipuncture site. These tapes usually cover the entire venipuncture site and are clear, allowing visualization of the site. Tubing of the butterfly or scalp needle is often looped and fixed to the arm with tape to secure the administration set (Fig. 19-10). Such fixation prevents tension on the infusion site and the administration set. With the completion of the administration fixation, the infusion is ready for the administration of sedation drugs.

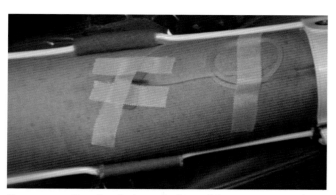

Figure 19-10. Securing the looped tubing of the venipuncture administration device to the arm with tape for venipuncture security.

Preparation of Drugs

A separate, labeled syringe is prepared for each drug that is used in the procedure. The label should delineate the name of the drug it contains and the milligram (mg) dosage present in each milliliter (ml) loaded in the syringe. Single-dose drug ampoules are suggested as a convenience and safety factor, rather than drawing medications out of multidose vials, because it simplifies record keeping for state and federal drug agencies. Because many of the drugs are colorless, it is important to use specific colored labels for each specific drug or to consistently use different, but specific, sized syringes for each drug to avoid accidental administration of a medication.

The concentration of medication per milliliter necessitates that the drug drawn into the administration syringe be diluted so that drug given and the dosage is more convenient to calculate. When a drug (e.g., morphine) comes in a 10-mg/ml ampoule, the drug is aspirated into a color-coordinated 5-ml syringe. It is then diluted with sterile saline or IV fluid to the full 5-ml volume, giving a dilution of 2 mg morphine/ml or 1.0 mg morphine/0.5 ml fluid. By diluting the medication concentrations from 10 mg/ml to 1 mg/0.5 ml, more accurate drug dosages can be administered.

Selection of and Administration of a Drug or Combination of Drugs

IV conscious sedation in the dental office can be managed effectively by using one or more drugs in the following three classes:

1. Benzodiazepines (e.g., midazolam, diazepam)
2. Barbiturates (e.g., pentobarbital)
3. Narcotic analgesics (e.g., morphine, meperidine)

Drugs with a long history of use in conscious sedation are emphasized, although others may be used. Currently, the most common pharmacologic method of controlling anxiety with IV sedation is through the use of one of the benzodiazepines, often in combination with a narcotic analgesic.[23] Benzodiazepines are also commonly used as a sole sedative agent. The benzodiazepines are used to reduce apprehension and fear while providing an amnesia effect. The narcotics provide euphoria and analgesia. In the event of contraindications to the use of benzodiazepines, pentobarbital can be used in combination with meperidine or morphine.

The basic principles and guidelines advocated in managing drugs for conscious IV sedation are well established. They were published by Jorgensen,[38] using pentobarbital and meperidine, and over the years have been modified to include additional medications with the same principles. The drug administration sequence is to:

1. Titrate the benzodiazepine (or the sedative pentobarbital) to establish a baseline.
2. Administer a fixed proportionate dose of the narcotic (morphine or meperidine) relative to the amount of the benzodiazepine or sedative used to achieve the baseline.

The rapid pharmacologic effect of midazolam, diazepam, or pentobarbital allows titration of the drugs in incremental doses to achieve the desired level of sedation, which was referred to as the "baseline" by Jorgensen. The patient experiencing a blurring of vision, symptoms of dizziness, drowsiness, difficulty in enunciating clearly, and an increased blinking of the eyelids can recognize this state of light sedation or mild cortical depression. This recognition is achieved by both close visual observation and by continuing oral communication between the therapist and the patient.

The narcotics, morphine and meperidine, have onset of action in 8 to 10 minutes and 2 to 4 minutes, respectively. Morphine can cause respiratory depression symptoms within 2 minutes, whereas meperidine takes approximately 3 minutes. The durations of action of the two drugs are approximately 30 to 45 minutes for meperidine, and 1.5 to 2 hours for morphine. Because narcotics require relatively long times for onset of action and full pharmacologic effect, they cannot be titrated easily. However, narcotics exhibit equal tolerances relative to diazepam, midazolam, or pentobarbital. Therefore, a predetermined dose of narcotic proportionate to the amount of diazepam, midazolam, or pentobarbital can be given slowly, once baseline sedation has been achieved with the benzodiazepine (or barbiturate). The proportionate dosage range is given in Table 19-8.

The sedatives–narcotics described earlier offer the therapist six combination possibilities for use: (1) midazolam and morphine, (2) midazolam and meperidine, (3) diazepam and morphine, (4) diazepam and meperidine, (5) pentobarbital and morphine, or (6) pentobarbital and meperidine.

Regardless of the drug or combination of drugs that are chosen for administration, the IV infusion set is

TABLE 19-8   IV Sedation Approximate Equivalent Narcotic Dose Relative to Sedative "Baseline" Dose

SEDATIVE AGENT	EXAMPLE DOSE AT WHICH "BASELINE" ACHIEVED	NARCOTIC AGENT	RECOMMENDED APPROXIMATE EQUIVALENT DOSE
Midazolam (Versed)	4 mg 8 mg	Morphine	2.5 mg 5 mg
Diazepam (Valium)	5 mg 10 mg	Morphine	2.5 mg 5 mg
Pentobarbital (Nembutal)*	50 mg 100 mg	Morphine	2.5 mg 5 mg
Midazolam (Versed)	4 mg 8 mg	Meperidine (Demerol)	25 mg 50 mg
Diazepam (Valium)	5 mg 10 mg	Meperidine (Demerol)	25 mg 50 mg
Pentobarbital (Nembutal)*	50 mg 100 mg	Meperidine (Demerol)	25 mg 50 mg

* Pentobarbitol is used if the Benzodiazepines are contraindicated.

opened fully for the drug titration. This allows maximum dilution of the drug as it infuses into the bloodstream, minimizing venous wall irritation complications, such as pain and phlebitis. A minimal amount of the sedative medication is initially administered as a test dose, observing the patient for 1 or 2 minutes for any unusual systemic or local reactions that may occur.

The most obvious local complication is pain at the injection site, indicating fluid seepage into the tissue spaces. Pain in the wrist, hand, or fingers distal to an antecubital fossa or forearm venipuncture site could indicate an intraarterial injection. The sedation medication injection that elicited the pain should be stopped immediately. When an intraarterial injection is suspected, it is important to maintain the venipuncture setup in place, opened fully, to facilitate treatment of the problem. Ten to 20 ml of either 0.5% procaine or lidocaine (with no epinephrine) should be injected into the maintained venipuncture administration cuff, and the patient should be transported to an emergency room for treatment. Anesthesiologists or vascular surgeons are the preferred physicians to direct treatment of this complication. Treatment is to increase the vascular supply to the affected area, by relieving the probable arterial spasm, or thrombosis, or both, and to assess the resulting injury for further treatment.

Although each patient must be managed individually, the following guidelines are offered for administration of sedative agents. For sedation in healthy patients using midazolam, 0.5 mg is administered every 60 seconds until the baseline is reached, on the basis of visual observations and conversation with the patient, the signs previously mentioned, and the vital signs. If diazepam is used, 1 mg is

administered every 30 seconds until the baseline is reached, whereas with pentobarbital, 10 mg is administered every 30 seconds until the desired baseline level is reached.

There are several conditions that can be elicited from the presurgical health evaluation that may indicate a need for a slower drug injection rate or a possible reduced total drug dosage. These conditions may result in unpredictable responses to the medications. In some cases, there may be no increase in the depth of sedation, but there may be an increased time of recovery. Patients younger than 6 years and patients older than 60 years should be closely observed. Patients with cardiovascular disease; impaired respiratory, hepatic, or renal system; endocrine deficiencies; glaucoma; those taking CNS depressants; those with prostatic hypertrophy; and the physically debilitated should also be carefully managed. Such patients can be consciously sedated, but drugs are administered in a more gradual manner, and often in lower doses, to allow a full assessment of the patient's vital signs and physiologic response.

Reinforcement of Sedation

For periodontal procedures in excess of 90 minutes, or for the extremely apprehensive patient, additional sedation medication during the procedure may be required to maintain consistent, stable vital sign responses. Patients taking prescribed medications for systemic health problems may be intentionally undersedated initially to fully assess their response to the sedation medications. Observation of an unsatisfactory level of conscious sedation, judged by patient psychological and physiologic responses to treatment, is the determining factor of when additional medication is required. Both sedative and analgesic drugs can be administered, but although the desired result is euphoria and analgesia, the actual result is a drowsy patient. When the drugs are reinforced, no more than one half of the initial doses are recommended.[27]

Completion of Sedation Procedure

At the completion of the surgical procedure, the patient's stability and alertness is assessed and recorded on the anesthesia record. A stable, healthy patient may be given a single IV dose of a potent nonsteroidal antiinflammatory drug (NSAID), such as ketorolac tromethamine (Syntex Laboratories; Palo Alto, CA), through the wide opened infusion set for the short-term management of moderate to severe postoperative discomfort. The use of a single IV dose of ketorolac at the completion of surgery, followed by the use of enteral NSAIDs after surgery, generally results in the patient having minimal postoperative discomfort. Ketorolac is contraindicated in patients with a history of gastrointestinal bleeding, in patients with renal impairment, and in patients with a high risk for bleeding.

On completion of the surgical procedure and the administration of the postoperative IV medications, vital signs are again checked and recorded before, during, and after the patient is brought to an upright position in slow stages. Patients who have received narcotics and who have been in a semireclined position for an extended time are likely to experience secondary effects, such as postural hypotension, when they are placed in an upright position quickly. Elderly patients are particularly vulnerable to postural hypotension. By slowly altering the patient's postural position, pooling of blood in the peripheral vasculature can be minimized. On returning the patient to an upright position and seeing that the vital signs remain stable, the fluid flow is turned off, which discontinues the infusion. The tape holding the butterfly needle or the IV catheter and plastic tubing is carefully removed, and the venipuncture device is deliberately removed. Firm pressure with sterile cotton gauze is applied to the venipuncture site for several minutes to prevent formation of a hematoma. A bandage strip is then placed over the puncture site.

The responsible adult who is accompanying the patient home is then brought in. The procedure that was performed, the postoperative expectations and limitations, and the postoperative instructions are reviewed with both the patient and the accompanying adult. They are informed that the patient may experience light-headedness with rapid movement. The patient is instructed to slowly turn in the dental chair and extend their legs down to the floor from their elevated, supported position for 30 seconds, after which the patient may slowly stand up, in place, with assistance. If light-headedness is experienced they are cautioned to sit. After standing in place for 30 seconds with no side

effects, the dental assistant accompanies the patient out of the office and to the mode of transportation provided by the responsible adult. The time of patient dismissal, their physical status and alertness, and to whom they were dismissed is documented. The patient and the responsible adult are also asked to immediately call either the office or the emergency number if any problems develop after leaving the office. The parents or guardians of young children should observe the child continuously on returning home and should call immediately if any problems occur.

Complications

Most complications of conscious IV sedation are relatively benign and easily managed, but there are some very significant complications that can result in morbidity and mortality.[21] The discussion herein concerns potential problems that may occur with the use of conscious IV sedation in the practice of periodontics. The complications are broadly grouped in the following sections.

Relatively benign and rapidly correctable venipuncture problems

The most common benign problem, after a successful venipuncture, is for the fluid infusion to be very slow or blocked. The problem may result from any of the following: displacement of the bevel of the infusion needle against the wall of the vein or against a valve when being taped into place; partial or total blockage by extending the needle too far into the vein; and blockage resulting from movement of the limb by the patient. Either of the latter can result in the needle perforating the wall of the vein with subsequent IV fluid infiltration into the tissue. Careful investigation of such problems can usually result in their correction. Use of a catheter instead of a rigid needle reduces the risk for venous wall perforation.

To check for the lumen of the needle being displaced against the vessel wall, the tape used to fix the needle into place is carefully removed to allow a slight elevation of the needle. If elevating the needle improves the flow rate, a folded 2 × 2 gauze square is carefully placed under the wings of the butterfly needle before retaping it into place. Care is taken not to alter the inclination of the scalp needle into the vein. When a catheter has been used, gently pulling distally on the hub may withdraw the catheter away from the vessel wall and improve the flow rate.

If a small, colorless swelling begins to occur in the area of the venipuncture, it usually indicates that the needle has perforated the wall of the vein and the IV fluid is flowing into the interstitial tissue. Such an occurrence is called a *fluid infiltration*. To correct the problem the IV flow rate regulator is closed, firm pressure is applied to the infiltrated area with sterile gauze, and the needle is removed. To prevent a hematoma, steadfast pressure is applied to the area for 5 to 6 minutes.

If a tourniquet is inadvertently left in place after a venipuncture, the infusion fluid will not drip into the vein and blood may rise in the IV tubing. Removing the tourniquet solves the problem.

On noting there is no fluid flow into the vein, the IV infusion bag can be lowered to or slightly beneath the heart level. Blood flow into the tubing indicates a successful venipuncture. Raising the height of the IV bag and getting a fluid flow indicates that the bag was not hung with sufficient elevation to allow fluid infusion. Such a problem may indicate that the dental chair and patient are in an upright position, or that the chair is positioned high enough to affect the infusion rate.

Venospasm

When a vein contracts or appears to collapse or disappear, with a burning sensation, in response to stimulation from a needle in close approximation to, or penetrating the vein, it is a protective reflex called a *venospasm*.[40-42] Needle removal is sometimes unnecessary.[21] By applying moist heat and withdrawing the needle 1 to 2 mm, the vein may dilate. Such dilatation offers an additional opportunity for a venipuncture with a needle that has already punctured the skin.

Phlebitis and thrombophlebitis

Most venous complications of IV sedation are injury or trauma to the vein produced by the needle or drugs administered during the procedure. If the venipuncture site appeared normal during the procedure and at the completion of the procedure and patient release, but approximately 2 days later the venipuncture site becomes sore, puffy, and erythematous, often with an elevated temperature, there is a local venous inflammation called *phlebitis*.[43,44] It can also include a spreading inflammation of the vein and precedes thrombus formation called *thrombophlebitis*.[43,44] Thrombophlebitis usually has a 24- to 48-hour delayed onset, but can develop up to a week after the procedure. The edema, tenderness, and inflammation seen with thrombophlebitis are usually associated with traumatic or chemical irritation of the vein. There is a greater incidence of thrombophlebitis with smaller veins in the hand and forearm than the larger vessels of the antecubital fossa.[45,46] Trauma is usually associated with either the execution of the venipuncture or with improper needle fixation. Chemical irritation is related to the pH of the IV drugs, which can be significantly acidic or basic. The propylene glycol and alcohol solvents in both diazepam and pentobarbital are examples of agents that may irritate small veins with IV administration.

Patients with signs or symptoms of phlebitis or thrombophlebitis must return to the office for an evaluation and documentation of the problem in the patient's chart. The treatment of both phlebitis and thrombophlebitis includes elevation of the limb as much as possible, prescribing aspirin or NSAIDs three to four times per day, moist heat applications to the affected area for 15 to 20 minutes several times per day, and restricted activity of the limb. The postoperative condition needs to be evaluated for improvement after a few days. If improvement is not noted, a physician should be consulted.

Hematoma

A *hematoma* occurs when blood extravasates into the interstitial space around a blood vessel, leading to localized swelling and discoloration. With normal venous elasticity, a seal with no leakage forms around the needle or catheter as it slides into the vein during venipuncture. Hematomas tend to occur either immediately, with the venipuncture attempt, or at the time of the needle removal. The immediate occurrence is generally caused by damage to the vein or loss of vessel elasticity, particularly in the elderly. A hematoma formation after needle removal is usually caused by either inadequate pressure application to the site or adequate pressure application, but for an inadequate time. Pressure to the site is needed for 5 to 6 minutes. Time is the most definitive treatment for resolution of the swelling and discoloration of a hematoma.

Air embolism

Small air bubbles moving down the IV tubing are a bigger psychological problem than a physiologic one. Venous blood will readily absorb infrequent small air bubbles. They can be eliminated from the medication syringes and from the administration tubing before the patient is escorted into the treatment room. The smaller the patient, the more significant air emboli can become; however, Malamed[21] states that a 110-pound adult can tolerate 50 ml of air.

Drug administration complications

Extravascular drug administration. It is important to recognize that the administration of drugs such as midazolam, diazepam, or pentobarbital into the tissues surrounding a vein generally results in a painful, burning sensation at the tip of the needle, delayed absorption of the drug, and consequent tissue damage. To avoid problems, a small test dose (0.1 to 0.2 ml) of medication is initially administered into the IV administration set. If the patient complains of a relatively intense, burning sensation localized to the venipuncture site, it is usually a result of the tip of the needle exiting the vein and drug extravasation occurring, causing some swelling. Treatment of a small amount of drug extravasation involves the removal of the needle and application of pressure for 5 to 6 minutes to stop the bleeding and to disperse the fluid into the surrounding tissue. The skin overlying the swollen tissue may become either ischemic, because of the irritation and resulting blood vessel constriction, or inflamed and erythematous. Extravasation of a larger amount of any of the previously mentioned irritating sedation drugs may require the infiltration of 10 ml 1% procaine or lidocaine in a fan-shaped pattern about the affected site for the local anesthetic properties, to counterbalance the alkaline pH of the sedation drug, as a vasodilator, and as a diluent. In conscious IV sedation, in which the sedative drug(s) are properly titrated, there is minimal probability of a large amount of drug extravasation.

Intraarterial drug administration. The best treatment for intraarterial drug administration is prevention! Arteries exhibit a palpable pulse before tourniquet placement. The anticipated venipuncture site should therefore be palpated for a pulse before the tourniquet is placed. On tourniquet application and vessel engorgement, the placement of the needle in proximity to an artery results in a burning sensation and forceful arteriospasm. An arterial puncture results in intense pain and a burning sensation that radiates from the venipuncture site distally to the hand and fingers. Bright red blood flows into the IV tubing, and tourniquet removal does not result in the blood leaving the IV tubing. With every heart contraction, there is a pulsating fluid flow in the IV tubing. If no medication was injected into the administration set, removal of the needle, followed by a firm, timed pressure application to the puncture site for 10 to 12 minutes will solve the problem.[47]

Injection of one of the sedative agents into an artery, however, will cause major problems from chemical endarteritis resulting in ischemia and thrombosis.[48] Formation of precipitate crystals, resulting from the pH change of the drug in the arterial blood, can result in further occlusion of the vessels distal to the injection site. If not quickly and adequately treated to restore the blood supply to the area, such changes can result in areas of localized gangrene and may lead to amputation of fingers or even total loss of the limb.

Appraisal of the degree of circulation damage can be done by comparing the color and temperature of the affected limb with the unaffected arm, and by parallel evaluations of the radial pulse of both arms. The presence of a regular, but weak pulse is indicative of some blood flow to the hand and fingers, but no pulse indicates an acute problem.

Treatment of such an occurrence is:

1. To leave the intraarterial needle in place to help in the management of the site.
2. To administer 2 to 10 ml 1% procaine into the artery to act as a vasodilator, to decrease the pain, to dilute the sedation medication, and to counterbalance the basic pH of sedation medication.
3. To notify and transport the patient to an emergency room for consultation by an anesthesiologist or a vascular surgeon.

The treating dentist should accompany the patient to the emergency room to advise the consulting physician of the treatment rendered and the drug(s) involved. Careful documentation of the treatment occurrences is of the utmost importance.

Generalized drug-related complications

There are a number of generalized drug-related complications that can be seen with conscious IV sedation. The incidence of nausea and vomiting with this modality is low, but can occur as a result of stress, narcotic administration, hypoxia, and swallowing blood. Oxygen administration often will stem the nausea sensation, but with the use of either midazolam or diazepam in conscious IV sedation, which are antiemetic agents, nausea and vomiting are not significant problems for periodontal procedures. This is another advantage of administering benzodiazepines before narcotic agents: the antiemetic effects of benzodiazepines help prevent nausea often associated with narcotic administration.

The incidence of a localized histamine-related reaction with the use of morphine or meperidine is relatively high. This localized reaction is characterized by itching of the skin at the injection site, and it is associated with the histamine release associated with morphine or meperidine traveling through the vein toward the heart. Clinically, this histamine release results in redness of the tissue about the vein, which will resolve in 5 to 6 minutes, once administration of the narcotic agent is stopped and the IV line is opened to increase fluid flow rate.

Allergies to adhesive tape, used to fix venipuncture needles and administration sets into place, will result in blotchy, erythematous, itchy areas where the tape is placed. With this occurrence, treatment consists of the IV administration of an antihistamine (either 50 mg diphenhydramine or 10 mg chlorpheniramine). The use of hypoallergenic tape in patients known to be sensitive to adhesives is recommended.

Careful questioning of the patient regarding their prior responses and allergies to drugs and medications, tape, and latex is the first line of defense in the prevention of allergies. Prevention or early recognition and management of allergic reactions is also the primary reason for the administration of a small test dose of approximately 0.1 to 0.2 ml sedative and analgesic drugs before further administration. Anaphylaxis usually occurs within 1 to 30 minutes after drug administration.[32,49] On the occurrence of an anaphylactic reaction,[21,32] active treatment must be immediate, as the skin, the respiratory system, and cardiovascular system become involved quickly. On observance of the skin reaction, placement of a tourniquet about the upper arm may slow the general systemic reaction. If the reaction is limited to the limb, antihistamine administration is recommended, but a generalized systemic reaction requires the IV administration of 0.3 to 0.5 mg of 1:1000 dilution of epinephrine, with subsequent administration of antihistamines, administration of oxygen, and airway maintenance. The administration of a corticosteroid will help to prevent a reoccurrence of the reaction. Once stable, the patient should be transported to his or her physician, with a detailed record of the incident, for a thorough evaluation.

Most drugs used in conscious IV sedation are respiratory depressants. Unobserved or undetected respiratory depression leads to respiratory arrest, cardiac arrhythmias, and ultimately cardiac arrest. Most drug-induced respiratory depression is dose related. One of the major advantages of conscious IV sedation is that the chances of respiratory depression are minimized by titrating the sedative medication to the proper level, followed by the slow administration of an equipotent narcotic analgesic. With the prudent observation of ventilatory rate, conversation with the patient, and pulse oximetry to monitor the oxygen saturation level, respiratory depression is easily detected and correctable. With a relaxed sedated patient, the chin position can drop, allowing the tongue to fall into the hypopharynx, causing airway obstruction. If observed, this simple airway obstruction is easily corrected by a simple head tilt and chin lift to open the airway.

In the healthy, alert patient, the respiratory rate is from 12 to 18 breaths per minute, with an oxygen saturation of more than 90%. Benzodiazepines, barbiturates, and narcotics are the drugs used in conscious sedation that are most likely to cause respiratory depression. Barbiturate-induced respiratory depression is characterized by shallow, rapid respiratory attempts, whereas benzodiazepine- and narcotic-induced respiratory depression results in a decreased rate of breathing, to as low as 5 to 6 breaths per minute. There is no antagonist available to reverse barbiturate-induced respiratory depression. This is the main reason barbiturates are rarely used today. On recognizing the problem, barbiturate-induced respiratory depression is treatable only by BLS. This includes maintenance of the airway and assisting or controlling the patient's breathing using a positive pressure oxygen device until the effects subside and the patient can breathe for himself or herself.

Respiratory depression secondary to benzodiazepine administration can be treated with the administration of flumazenil, as described previously. Respiratory depression after the use of a single narcotic, or in combination with a benzodiazepine, can be treated with the administration of a narcotic antagonist. Naloxone or nalmefene are both narcotic antagonists that reverse the effects of opioids, including respiratory depression, sedation, and hypotension. Naloxone should be administered slowly, at a rate of 0.1 mg/min, closely observing for increased respiration. Reversal of respiratory depression usually requires less than 0.4 mg naloxone. Respiratory depression should be reversed with as little naloxone or nalmefene as possible, so as to not reverse the analgesic qualities of the opioid and lead to the onset of the acute surgical pain. Slowly titrating the naloxone reduces the possibility of this action. Because naloxone has a relatively short duration of action (30 minutes), the patient must be observed for possible reoccurrence of respiratory depression. Nalmefene has a duration of action similar to that of the opioids.

INTRAMUSCULAR CONSCIOUS SEDATION

IM sedation for periodontal procedures is only recommended for use when IV routes are not available for drug administration. The IM route of deep muscular drug administration is important to prevent tissue reactions, but can be done when the patient cooperation required for the IV route of drug administration is not available. It is also indicated when submucosal administration is contraindicated by an irritating aqueous solution of a drug, such as midazolam or diazepam. In the event of an emergency, IM drug delivery after a deep IM injection is the most rapid way to achieve a response when the IV route is not available. Because of the greater reliability and faster action that is achieved with IM drug administration, when compared with enteral administration, antiemetic drugs are often given this way. Even though the therapist must rely on an empirical dosage of medication, most injectable agents useful in conscious sedation can be administered by the IM route and are effective within 15 to 40 minutes, with variable effects and duration.

Drug Selection

For light to moderate conscious IM sedation before periodontal therapy, the drug list should be kept to a minimum and should include medications that have a wide margin of safety. The benzodiazepine—midazolam; the antihistamines—hydroxyzine and promethazine; the narcotic agonists—morphine, meperidine, and alphaprodine; and the narcotic agonists/antagonists—pentazocine, butorphanol, and nalbuphine—have onset and duration times that make them amenable to IM conscious sedation. Lorazepam is not often used in dentistry because of the prolonged duration of action. Promethazine is often used in conjunction with narcotics, as a potentiating agent and as an antiemetic. Because of the possibility of complications that can result from combining antianxiety–sedative medications with the narcotics, such combinations are not recommended for

IM conscious sedation, because the medications cannot be titrated.

Site Selection

IM drug administration sites[50] in the dental office most frequently include the mid-deltoid region in the upper third of the arm because of easy accessibility (see Fig. 19-1, *A*). The three other available areas each require some degree of disrobing, but include the upper outer quadrant of the gluteal area (see Fig. 19-1, *C*), the ventrogluteal area (a lateral triangular area between the anterior superior iliac spine, the iliac crest, and the greater trochanter of the femur) (see Fig. 19-1, *B*), and the vastus lateralis area on the anterior aspect of the upper thigh (see Fig. 19-1, *D*). The site chosen for IM drug administration in adults is based on accessibility, the fluid volume to be injected, and patient cooperation. The mid-deltoid region is the most convenient and is able to receive the fluid volume necessary for conscious sedation, but the vastus lateralis and either of the gluteal injection sites can accommodate larger fluid volumes.

Armamentarium

A minimal armamentarium is necessary for IM drug administration, but includes the following:

1. Sterile, disposable 1- to 5-ml syringe with a 20- to 21-gauge 1- to 2-inch needle
2. The desired medication(s)
3. Alcohol sponges
4. Sterile gauze
5. Adhesive bandage

Technique

The following steps are performed for IM injections:

1. An antiseptic sponge is used to clean the injection site (see the IV site preparation) and is allowed to dry before the hypodermic needle penetrates the skin. Penetration of the needle into skin moistened by antiseptic solution can cause irritation by conveying the antiseptic into the underlying tissue.
2. Tense the skin with the free hand, by spreading it between the thumb and index finger (Fig. 19-11, *A*).
3. Holding the 5-ml syringe in a dart grip between the thumb and forefinger (see Fig. 19-11, *B*) of the dominant hand, the needle is inserted approximately three fourths of its length into the skin with a quick thrust almost perpendicular to the skin. The actual insertion depth is dependent on the size of the patient. With a child or young adolescent, the muscle may be reached in 0.5 to 1 inch, whereas an obese patient may require insertion of 2 inches to reach muscle.
4. Aspirate for blood, by pulling back on the plunger of the syringe with the dominant hand, while holding the syringe with the thumb and forefinger of the other hand. The absence of blood, after both aspirating and rotating the needle 90 to 180 degrees in place, means that the lumen of the needle is not in a blood vessel, and can be left in place for the injection.
5. Slowly inject the calculated aqueous drug dosage. The flow should be unobstructed and without force.
6. On completion of the injection of medication, the injection site is pinched with the fingers of the free hand and the needle is withdrawn. After an application of antiseptic, an adhesive bandage is applied to the site. Rapid absorption of the injected drug can be assisted by vigorously massaging the site for a couple of minutes to distribute the drug in the muscle.

Complications

There are several possible complications that can be associated with the IM administration of drugs for sedation, but major complications are generally unusual. Complications associated with IM injections will relate either to the site of the needle penetration, or the area of drug deposition. The therapist can avoid many potential complications by using good judgment and with treatment precautions. Aspiration while circumferentially rotating the needle after its placement in the desired location, but before administration of the aqueous drug solution, protects against IV or intraarterial injections of medication. Should blood be drawn into the syringe while aspirating, the needle is simply withdrawn and another injection site is used after placing pressure on the original injection site for 2 minutes to prevent a hematoma. An air embolism can be prevented by carefully expunging air from the syringe and needle before the injection of the aqueous drug solution. Careful site selection and knowledge of the anatomy of the area chosen for an IM injection minimizes the possibility of resultant nerve damage or paraesthesia. Making sure that sedation medication is deposited deeply into the muscle of the injection site, rather than superficially, decreases the chance of a superficial tissue reaction, such as an abscess, necrosis, and sloughing of the skin at the injection site with subsequent scarring.

The two complications most commonly associated with IM injections are hematomas and periostitis. The hematomas often result when an inadequate amount of pressure is applied to the injection site for too short a time after the needle is removed. When a hematoma occurs, the application of ice to the area for 10-minute intervals for the first 4 hours will help in preventing an increase in its size. The hematoma, as with most traumatic injuries, will resolve over a 10-day period, after going through the normal physiologic discoloration.

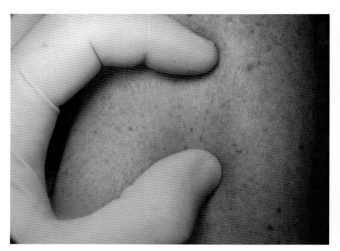
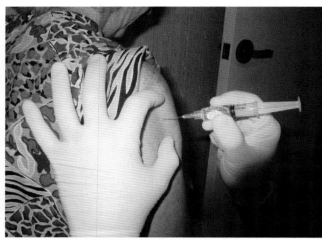

Figure 19-11. Intramuscular injection techniques to assist in carrying out the procedure. **A,** Tensing the skin between the thumb and index finger. **B,** Inserting the needle into the site, holding the syringe in a dart grip between the thumb and forefinger, almost perpendicular to the skin.

Periostitis is usually secondary to hitting the periosteum with the needle. It can be very painful, but can be prevented by using good IM injection technique and judging the size of the patient and their muscle mass correctly.

It is important to document the date, site, time, and drug administered by IM injection in the patient records. Because complications often have a delayed onset, when the patient reports the problem, it is vital to have the patient return to the office to evaluate and document the problem and its treatment. Minor discomfort, resulting from an IM injection, can often be alleviated with NSAIDs, acetaminophen, or aspirin, and time. Such an injury should be periodically checked until it is resolved. If a complication appears to be significant, a medical consultation should be considered. Most complications that do occur are handled in the same manner as the IV sequelae discussed earlier.

Systemic complications can include what begins as respiratory depression, but can quickly progress to circulatory depression. Respiratory depression caused by sedatives and narcotics is clinically evident several minutes before depression of the cardiovascular system. Respiratory depression results in the blood oxygen saturation level being depressed. As it progresses in severity, the oxygen saturation level becomes worse, the patient becomes restless, and their soft tissue coloration changes. Untreated, these symptoms progress to the collapse of the cardiovascular system. Mild narcotic-induced respiratory depression is treated with oxygen through a mask or nasal cannula. Severe respiratory depression is treated with naloxone (Narcan) or nalmefene (Revex), oxygen, assisted ventilation, and positive pressure breathing. The IM dosage administration of naloxone necessary to arouse the patient is equal to the dosage that IV dosage administration requires. Patients with narcotic-induced respiratory depression must be monitored until the effects of the narcotic have subsided, because naloxone often does not have as long a duration of action as the narcotic. It is therefore extremely important to monitor the vital signs until the duration of action of the narcotic is judged to be finished. Secondary naloxone dosing may be required. Nalmefene has a duration of action similar to the opioids and secondary dosing is usually unnecessary.

Respiratory depression secondary to diazepam or midazolam can be treated with flumazenil, as previously discussed. As mentioned earlier, barbiturate-induced respiratory depression is treated with BLS, including positive pressure breathing, assisted ventilation, and supplemental oxygen, until transported to the hospital as quickly as possible for additional treatment and monitoring. Providing respiratory depression is recognized and treated early, the possibility of subsequent circulatory depression is minimized.

PERSONNEL, FACILITIES, AND EQUIPMENT GUIDELINES

During the administration of enteral or combination of inhalation–enteral conscious (combined) sedation, or any type of parenteral conscious sedation, personnel requirements include two people to be present in the room: the dentist, who is appropriately trained in the use of such techniques, and at least one additional person (assistant) trained to monitor appropriate physiologic parameters and to assist in resuscitation measures if necessary. The assistant should have specific assignments, should have current knowledge of the emergency cart inventory, and must be currently competent in BLS. The dentist administering parenteral conscious sedation is required to have current training in BLS, and Advanced Cardiac Life Support or its equivalent is encouraged (ADA Guidelines). Several states require the dentist to be current in either Advanced Cardiac Life Support, its equivalent, or an appropriate, approved advanced emergency course.[51-54] The therapist and all office personnel should participate in periodic reviews of the office emergency protocol.

It is an understood assumption that the dentist who uses any type of enteral sedation, combined conscious sedation, or parenteral conscious sedation will have facilities, personnel, and equipment available to reasonably manage foreseeable emergency situations that a patient may experience associated with the sedation technique used. This is necessary for safe patient care and to satisfy legal requirements. For in-office emergencies, a protocol must be formulated to ensure ready access to a paramedical service or ambulance. It also includes immediate access to pharmacologic antagonists and appropriately sized equipment for establishing a patent airway and providing positive pressure ventilation with oxygen. The positive pressure oxygen ventilation must be capable of administering greater than 90% oxygen at a 5 L/min flow for at least 60 minutes. Before the use of sedation with each patient, it should be determined that there is an adequate oxygen supply available for emergency use. The sedation provider is responsible for the sedation management, the diagnosis of the emergency, and treatment of emergencies associated with the administration of the sedation technique used, until Emergency Medical Services arrive to render emergency management and to transport the patient to an emergency care facility. An automatic defibrillator should be immediately available (on the premises) for the diagnosis and treatment of ventricular fibrillation and fast ventricular tachycardia arrhythmias, particularly when treating ASA type III patients.

When inhalation equipment is used, it must be appropriately calibrated and checked. The equipment must include a fail-safe system that delivers at least 25% oxygen. If a system is used that delivers less than 25% oxygen, an in-line oxygen analyzer must be used. Inhalation equipment must also have an appropriate scavenging system. A positive pressure oxygen system that is suitably sized for the patient being treated must be available, regardless of the type of sedation used.

Equipment appropriate for the technique being used that will monitor the physical status of the patient before, during, and after the procedure must be present. The necessary drugs and equipment to assist in the resuscitation of a nonbreathing, unconscious patient must be immediately available in an emergency cart.

MONITORING AND DOCUMENTATION PROCEDURES

The decision to administer drugs to a patient for conscious sedation necessitates continual monitoring of the heart rate, blood pressure, blood and tissue oxygenation, and ventilation, as well as direct clinical observation of the patient by a trained individual.* Blood pressure and heart rate can be monitored manually, but there are numerous automatic monitors available that automatically record these vital signs at specifically chosen time intervals. Patients with significant cardiovascular disease (ASA Class III) require continuous electrocardiographic monitoring. Some states require electrocardiographic monitoring on all parenteral conscious sedation patients. A pulse oximeter is necessary to continually monitor blood and tissue oxygen saturation.[56] Continuous patient contact through conversation and observation is an excellent method of overseeing the patient's physical status. Such observation includes continually evaluating the color of the skin, mucosa, and blood, as well as frequent observations of chest excursions to satisfy ventilation monitoring requirements. Auscultation of breath sounds with a precordial stethoscope is another ventilation monitoring technique that may be considered. When a sterility barrier is used to drape a patient, a hand or portion of a limb must be left exposed to allow observation of skin color. Once a patient is sedated, the patient should never be left unattended by a trained observer. A patent airway can be assured by frequently checking the patient's head position and by conversing with the patient. For all forms of sedation, it is vital to maintain an appropriate time-oriented anesthesia record, inclusive of the individuals present during sedation.

The vital signs are recorded on a time-oriented anesthesia record at time intervals in accordance with individual state regulations. These usually must include documentation of the heart rate, blood pressure, oxygen saturation, respiratory adequacy, sedation notes, including the route of administration, the site, the type of drugs used, the dosage, and the times of administration. On completion of the treatment procedure, vital signs are recorded. Providing the vital signs are stable and have returned to the preoperative status, the patient is alert and talking, and can sit up unaided, the IV line is disconnected. The patient must be able to stand and walk with minimal assistance to meet discharge criteria, and the patient must be accompanied to their mode of transportation by

---

* References 5, 14, 36, 43, 55, 56.

the assistant after reviewing the postoperative instructions with the adult responsible for transporting the patient home. The time of the patient's discharge, the name of the individual they were discharged to, and the provision of a postoperative instruction sheet are documented.

CONCLUSION

Oral, inhalation, combined oral–inhalation, IM, and IV conscious sedation are adjunctive services that have the potential, by their effective use, to make the practice of periodontics more enjoyable and less stressful for the dentist, the patient, and the staff. These entities also add a patient appreciation factor about treatment that has marketing potential for a practice-building niche. The key to the successful long-term use of conscious sedation is to match the sedation medication(s) and most predictable delivery techniques to the needs of the patient and talents of the practitioner and office staff. Enteral conscious sedation, inhalation conscious sedation, or a combination of the two is useful for alleviating the fear and apprehension of the mildly apprehensive patient undergoing periodontal treatment. IV conscious sedation is the most predictable and safest sedation technique for rendering invasive therapy to the mildly to moderately apprehensive patient. The severely apprehensive patient, as well as mentally challenged patients, can also sometimes be managed with IV conscious sedation. With these challenging patients, good judgment may occasionally dictate assistance with patient management from a dentist–anesthesiologist. Such assistance and shared responsibility can be a wise, time-saving decision, allowing undivided attention by both therapists for the problem at hand. Knowledge, good professional judgment, competency in sedation training techniques that are used, a thorough working familiarity with the conscious sedation guidelines, the proper state sedation permits, and practice marketing to referring dentists makes the rendering of periodontal care to apprehensive patients a realistic probability.

REFERENCES

1. Freidson E, Fedman JJ: The public looks at dental care, *J Am Dent Assoc* 57:325-335, 1958.
2. Klepac RK, Dowling J, Haige G: Characteristics of clients seeking therapy for the reduction of dental avoidance: reactions to pain, *J Behav Ther Exp Psychiatry* 13:293-300, 1982.
3. Woolgrove J, Cumberbatch G: Dental anxiety and regularity of dental attendance, *J Dent Res* 65:209-213, 1986.
4. Kleinknecht RA, Klepac RK, Alexander LD: Origins and characteristics of fear in dentistry, *J Am Dent Assoc* 86:842-848, 1973.
5. Molin C, Seeman K: Disproportionate dental anxiety: clinical and nosological considerations, *Acta Odontol Scand* 28:197-212, 1970.
6. Arntz A, Van Eck M, Heijmans M: Predictions of dental pain: the fear of any expected evil is worse than the evil itself, *Behav Res Ther* 28:29-41, 1956.
7. Mills MP: Periodontal implications: anxiety, *Ann Periodontol* 1:359-389, 1996.
8. Bennett CR: The spectrum of pain control. In *Conscious-sedation in dental practice*, St. Louis, 1974, Mosby.
9. Daniel SR, Fry HR, Savord EG: Intravenous "conscious" sedation in periodontal surgery. A selective review and report of 1,708 cases, *J West Soc Periodontol* 32:133-146, 1984.
10. Ceravolo FJ, Meyers H, Baraff LS, Bennett CR: Full dentition periodontal surgery utilizing intravenous-conscious sedation: a report of 5,200 cases, *J Periodontol* 51:462-464, 1980.
11. Bennett CR: Conscious-sedation versus general anesthesia: the choice is yours, *Compendium* 8:274-279, 1985.
12. American Dental Association, Department of Governmental Affairs: Statutory Requirements for Conscious Sedation Permit, October 11, 2001, The Association.
13. American Dental Association: *American Dental Association Policy Statement: the use of conscious sedation, deep sedation and general anesthesia in dentistry*, Adopted by the American Dental Association's House of Delegates, October 1999.
14. American Dental Association: *American Dental Association Guidelines for the use of conscious sedation, deep sedation and general anesthesia for dentists*, Adopted by the American Dental Association's House of Delegates, October 2000.
15. American Dental Association: *Guidelines for teaching the comprehensive control of anxiety and pain in dentistry*, Adopted by the American Dental Association's House of Delegates, October 2000.
16. The Joint Commission on Accreditation of Healthcare Organizations: *Revisions to anesthesia care standards, comprehensive accreditation manual for ambulatory care*, Effective January 1, 2001.
17. Committee on Research, Science, and Therapy, the American Academy of Periodontology: Guidelines: in-office use of conscious sedation in periodontics, *J Periodontol* 72:968-975, 2001.
18. Jastak JT: Nitrous oxide in dental practice, *Int Anesthesiol Clin* 27:92-97, 1989.
19. Giovannitti JA: Pain control in dentistry: oral premedication and nitrous oxide, *Compendium* 6:647-656, 1985.
20. Berman D, Graber D: Sedation and analgesia, *Emerg Med Clin North Am* 10:691-705, 1992.
21. Malamed SF: *Sedation: a guide to patient management*, ed 4, St. Louis, 2003, Mosby.
22. Thomson KF: The role of suggestion in pain and anxiety control, inhalation sedation-nitrous oxide and oxygen. In Bennett CR, ed: *Conscious-sedation in dental practice*, St. Louis, 1974, Mosby.

23. Byrne BE, Tibbetts LS: Conscious sedation and agents for the control of anxiety. In Ciancio SG, editor: *ADA guide to dental therapeutics*, ed 2, Chicago, 2000, ADA Publishing.

24. Malamed SF: Conscious sedation and general anesthesia techniques and drugs used in dentistry, *Anesth Prog* 33:176-178, 1986.

25. Jastak JT, Paravecchio R: An analysis of 1,331 sedations, using inhalation, intravenous, or other techniques, *J Am Dent Assoc* 91:1242-1249, 1975.

26. Beckman H: The fate of drugs. In *Pharmacology: the nature, action and use of drugs*, ed 2, Philadelphia, 1961, WB Saunders.

27. Loughlin DL, Furman, TH, Scamman FL, Tibbetts LS: Intravenous sedation. In Clark JW, editor: *Clinical dentistry*, Hagerstown, Md, 1979, Harper & Row.

28. Monheim L: *General anesthesia in dental practice*, St. Louis, 1964, CV Mosby.

29. Bennett CR: Pain. In *Conscious-sedation in dental practice*, St. Louis, 1974, Mosby.

30. Klepac RK: Behavioral treatments for adult dental avoidance, *Dent Clin North Am* 32:705-714, 1988.

31. Friedman N: Iatrosedation: the treatment of fear in the dental patient, *J Dent Educ* 47:91-95, 1983.

32. *Drug facts and comparisons: 2003 pocket version*, ed 7, St. Louis, 2002, Facts and Comparisons, pp 509-514.

33. *A to Z drug facts*, ed 3, St. Louis, 2001, Facts and Comparisons.

34. *Physicians' desk reference*, ed 56, Montvale, 2002, Medical Economics.

35. Lang LL: An evaluation of Hydroxyzine (Atarax, Vistaril) in controlling the behavior of child patients, *J Dent Child* 32:253-258, 1965.

36. Sa Rego MM, Watcha MF, White PF: The changing role of monitored anesthesia care in ambulatory setting, *Anesth Analg* 85:1020-1036, 1997.

37. Maki DG, Goldman DA, Rhame FS: Infectious control in intravenous therapy, *Ann Intern Med* 79:867-887, 1973.

38. Jorgensen NB, Hayden J Jr: *Sedation, local and general anesthesia in dentistry*, ed 3, Philadelphia, 1980, Lea and Febiger.

39. Everett GB, Allen GD: Simultaneous evaluation of cardiorespiratory and analgesic effects of intravenous analgesia in combination with local anesthesia, *J Am Dent Assoc* 81:926-931, 1970.

40. Cunningham E, Korbon GA: Venospasm preventing venous access, *Anesthesiology* 59:141-142, 1983.

41. Morgan M, Thrash WJ, Blanton PL, Glazer JW: Incidence and extent of venous sequelae with intravenous diazepam utilizing a standardized conscious technique. Part II: Effects on injection site, *J Periodontol* 54:680-684, 1983.

42. Glazer JW, Blanton PL, Thrash WJ: Incidence and extent of venous sequelae with intravenous diazepam utilizing a standardized conscious sedation technique, *J Periodontol* 53:700-703, 1982.

43. Driscoll EJ, Gelfman SS, Sweet JB et al: Thrombophlebitis after intravenous use of anesthesia and sedation: its incidence and natural history, *J Oral Surg* 37:809-815, 1979.

44. Gelfman SS, Dionne RA, Driscoll EJ: Prospective study of venous complications following intravenous diazepam in dental outpatients, *Anesth Prog* 28:126-128, 1981.

45. Chambiras E, Korbon GA: Sedation in dentistry, intravenous diazepam, *Aust Dent J* 17:17, 1972.

46. Nordell K, Morgensen L, Nyquist O, Orinius E: Thrombophlebitis following intravenous lidocaine infusion, *Acta Med Scand* 192:263-265, 1972.

47. Goldsmith D, Trieger N: Accidental intra-arterial injection: a medical emergency, *Anesth Prog* 22:180-183, 1975.

48. Topazian RG: Accidental intra-arterial injection: a hazard of intravenous medication, *J Am Dent Assoc* 81:410-414, 1970.

49. Mark LC: A lone case of gangrene following intraarterial thiopental 2.5%, *Anesthesiology* 59(2):153, 1983.

50. Holroyd SV, Wynn RL: Adverse drug reactions. In *Clinical pharmacology in dental practice*, St. Louis, 1983, Mosby.

51. Bennett CR: Technical considerations and routes of administration. In *Conscious-sedation in dental practice*, St. Louis, 1974, Mosby.

52. Whitmire HC, Jeske AH, Wilson CF et al, editors: *Enteral conscious sedation & emergency procedures*, Austin, Tx, 2001, Texas Dental Association.

53. Whitmire HC, Redden RJ, Blanton PL et al: *Parenteral conscious sedation & advanced emergency procedures*, Austin, Tx, 2001, Texas Dental Association.

54. Cousins MJ: Monitoring—the anaesthetist's view, *Scand J Gastroenterol Suppl* 25:12-17, 1990.

55. Guidelines for the standard of physiological monitoring of patients during dental anaesthesia or sedation, *SAAD Dig* 7:309-311, 1990.

56. Weaver JM: Intraoperative management during conscious sedation and general anesthesia: patient monitoring and emergency care, *Anesth Prog* 33:181-184, 1986.

57. Council on Scientific Affairs, American Dental Association: The use of pulse oximetry during conscious sedation, *JAMA* 270:1463-1468, 1993.

20

Principles and Practice of Periodontal Surgery*

Howard T. McDonnell and Michael P. Mills

Disclaimer: The views expressed in this chapter are those of the authors and do not reflect the official policy or position of the United States Air Force or the Department of Defense.

The treatment of periodontal diseases encompasses a vast array of nonsurgical and surgical techniques aimed at the elimination of infection and inflammation to establish a healthy periodontium. Nonsurgical therapy often may be sufficient to eliminate the signs and symptoms of mild periodontal diseases. However, cases or sites with moderate to advanced disease often continue to show signs of inflammation after a nonsurgical approach. When periodontal probing depths are sufficiently deep, nonsurgical treatment may be ineffective in establishing health or preventing recurrence of disease. In such cases, gaining surgical access to the various components of the periodontium allows an opportunity for more thorough root debridement and establishment of an oral environment easier to maintain by both the patient and the dental care provider to aid in restoring periodontal health. In addition, surgical treatment provides an opportunity to reconstruct destroyed periodontal tissues and to correct the variety of mucogingival and anatomic anomalies that may present. In essence, periodontal surgery is an irreplaceable therapeutic modality that must be mastered to effectively treat the dental health problems that many patients have. This chapter provides a basic overview of periodontal surgery, emphasizing the principles and practice of good surgical technique.

SURGICAL GOALS, OBJECTIVES, INDICATIONS, AND CONTRAINDICATIONS

The major goals of periodontal surgery are to create an oral environment that is conducive to maintaining the patient's dentition in a healthy, comfortable, and functional esthetic state, and, when feasible, to regenerate and preserve the periodontal attachment. With these goals in mind, four questions should be considered when evaluating the role surgical therapy will have in the overall treatment plan and in determining what type of surgical approach is indicated:

1. Do patient factors (systemic and local) provide a favorable environment for surgery and for postsurgical wound healing?
2. Will surgery be effective and beneficial in correcting the periodontal destruction?
3. What type of defect morphology is present and what are the indications and contraindications that will determine the type of surgical therapy to be used?
4. Which therapeutic approach will best achieve an acceptable and stable periodontal form and meet the needs and desires of the patient?

Patient factors include medical, smoking, and psychological status, patient desires and expected outcomes, oral hygiene effectiveness, and gingival health. Systemic factors should be addressed and modified before and during the commencement of initial therapy. Local factors are addressed during initial therapy to ensure adequate plaque control is obtained and gingival inflammation has been reduced sufficiently to allow atraumatic surgical technique. Usually the answers to the last three questions are finalized after completion of initial therapy, at the time of reevaluation. If, because of the advanced disease state or lack of patient cooperation, surgery will not realistically improve the long-term health and prognosis of the tooth or teeth, then an alternative approach is indicated. With this in mind, the therapeutic choices at the reevaluation stage will be one of the following four options: (1) enter the patient into a maintenance program if a sufficient level of tissue health has been achieved with initial therapy, (2) re-treat persistent diseased sites nonsurgically, (3) enter the patient into a surgical phase of treatment, or (4) enter the patient with disease not amenable to surgery into an intensive program of maintenance and reevaluation.

Table 20-1 lists the indications and contraindications for periodontal surgery. The objectives of surgical therapy are listed in Box 20-1. When treating periodontal disease, the primary indication for surgery is direct access to and visibility of the roots of the teeth and the accompanying osseous deformities that may be present. Thorough debridement of the roots and bony defects is the foundation of all periodontal flap surgery used in treating periodontitis. Multiple studies have demonstrated the increased efficiency and effectiveness of scaling and root planing using a surgical approach.[1-5] Combined with adequate hemostasis, magnification of the surgical field, and use of improved lightening, surgical access will provide excellent visualization of the roots and osseous anatomy, will increase efficiency of root debridement, and will lessen tissue trauma. Access to the osseous defects will allow the surgeon to reestablish physiologic bony architecture through either resective or additive techniques. When the outcome is predictable and if treatment will improve the prognosis of the tooth, additive techniques are usually the preferred treatment because they will result in the gain of attachment and regeneration of destroyed periodontal structures. (See Chapter 21.) When osseous defects are shallow or when factors decrease the predictability of regeneration or new attachment, resective therapy may be the best approach. (See Chapter 23.)

Another proposed benefit of some modes of periodontal surgery, such as the Excisional New Attachment Procedure (ENAP)[6] and the Modified Widman Flap (MWF),[7,8] is the removal of pocket epithelium. The theory of these procedures was the removal of pocket epithelium to allow direct approximation of connective tissue against the root surface, but studies have demonstrated that the use of inverse bevel incisions often resulted in the incomplete removal of pocket epithelium.[9-11] It also has been shown that residual pocket epithelium often degenerates[12] and favorable clinical results may be obtained regardless of whether pocket

TABLE 20-1	Indications and Contraindications for Periodontal Surgery
INDICATIONS	**CONTRAINDICATIONS**
Access to roots and osseous defects	Uncontrolled medical conditions such as:
Resective surgery	• unstable angina
Regeneration of the periodontium	• uncontrolled hypertension
Preprosthetic surgery	• uncontrolled diabetes
• crown lengthening	• myocardial infarction or stroke within 6 months
• gingival augmentation	Poor plaque control
• ridge augmentation	High caries rate
• tori reduction	Unrealistic patient expectations or desires
• tuberosity reduction	
• vestibuloplasty	
Periodontal plastic surgery	
• esthetic anterior crown lengthening	
• soft tissue grafting for root coverage or to obtain a physiologic gingival dimension	
• papilla reconstruction	
Gingival enlargement	
Biopsy	
Implant surgery	
Treatment of periodontal abscesses	
Exploratory surgery	

Box 20-1   Objectives of Periodontal Surgery

Access to roots and alveolar bone
  enhance visibility
  increase scaling and root planing effectiveness
  less tissue trauma
Modification of osseous defects
  establish physiologic architecture of hard tissues through regeneration or resection
  augment alveolar ridge defects
Repair or regeneration of the periodontium
Pocket reduction
  enhance maintenance by patient and therapist
  improve long-term stability
Provide acceptable soft tissue contours
  enhance plaque control and maintenance
  improve esthetics

epithelium is removed.[13,14] Therefore, the removal of pocket epithelium is no longer considered a surgical objective.

Pocket reduction is a desired therapeutic end-point of surgical and nonsurgical therapy. Evidence and clinical practice indicate shallow sulci are easier to maintain by the patient and the dentist[15-18] and may be more stable in the long term.[19,20] In general, surgical therapy provides a more predictable means of pocket reduction.

In concert with pocket reduction is the creation of acceptable soft tissue contours. As previously mentioned, an important periodontal therapy outcome is the creation of an oral environment that is easily maintained. This is reinforced at each recall visit when an evaluation of patient oral hygiene effectiveness and tissue health is accomplished. Easy access for mechanical plaque control devices including interdental aids is important. Soft tissues that consistently impede effective plaque control should be recontoured. In addition, acceptable soft tissue contours in the anterior esthetic region are of primary importance to the patient. Achieving an acceptable level of health, providing gingival symmetry, and maintaining or establishing papillary soft tissue height between anterior teeth is one of the more challenging aspects of periodontal therapy. Esthetics are paramount in the anterior region and must be a critical factor in surgical treatment planning.

SURGICAL PRINCIPLES

Principles of periodontal surgery are similar to general surgical principles applied to other parts of the body. A few notable exceptions challenging dental surgeons are the nonsterile surgical field, the protrusion of teeth from the soft tissues, and the often unfriendly work environment of saliva, the tongue, and the cheeks and lips hindering access and visualization. Box 20-2 outlines the basic principles of periodontal surgery that must be followed if the surgeon and patient are to have a reasonable chance of a predictable healing outcome. These surgical tenets are crucial to wound healing and the final outcome of therapy.

Medical History and Physical Status

According to epidemiologic studies, the overall prevalence and severity of periodontal disease are found to increase as the population ages.[21,22] With aging comes an increased probability that the patient may have at least one significant medical condition that could alter the treatment plan and therapy recommended. To provide safe, effective care, it has become increasingly more important to take an active role in assessing a patient's physical status and ability to tolerate even the less invasive periodontal procedures.

Taking a thorough, comprehensive medical history is a proactive step in identifying potential health problems before they occur suddenly without warning. Eliciting the health history information should include a written questionnaire and dialogue between patient and doctor (see Chapter 36). Relevant aspects of the medical history should include a review of the patient's past and current history with emphasis on a review of the major organ systems; past hospitalization(s) and surgery; current medications, both prescribed and over-the-counter; any known allergies especially to drugs and latex; past and current history of tobacco, alcohol, or substance use or abuse; and

family history of illness. It should be noted that patients generally are poor historians and may unintentionally omit certain elements they deem not significant. In one large study population, 32% of the patients completing comprehensive health histories provided incorrect data or omitted significant information.[23,24] Therefore, the dialogue between patient and doctor becomes even more important to expand on certain parts of the history that require clarification or more specific questioning.

In addition to patient history, a thorough evaluation should include a general assessment of the patient's physical characteristics for abnormalities in gait, body movements, body symmetry, posture, weight, skin, eyes, speech, and ability to think clearly. Other elements of a basic physical examination should focus on the patient's cardiovascular and respiratory functions, which is best accomplished by determining baseline vital signs. This would include blood pressure; rate, rhythm, and quality of the pulse; and rate, depth, and pattern of respirations. Abnormal findings in any of the above assessments should be followed up with more focused evaluation and appropriate medical referral if necessary.

Once a complete patient evaluation has been performed, the patient's physical status may be categorized according to the American Society of Anesthesiologists' (ASA) classification system (see Chapter 19). Currently, this system is used to define not only a patient's physical status but also his or her operative risk. In dentistry, the ASA classification system has been modified to help categorize the physical status of dental patients from the standpoint of risk orientation and dental management.

Whenever there is some question as to the physical status of a patient, the effect that their systemic health may have on dental management, or the effect that dental treatment may have on their systemic condition, a medical consultation is recommended. Generally, a consultation request should be made to the patient's primary physician. However, in cases where the patient does not have a primary physician, the consultation may be sent to a physician of their choosing or by direct referral. It is preferable for the medical consultation to be written (see Chapter 36), but a verbal consultation by phone is acceptable provided the key points of the conversation are recorded in the patient's treatment record. Components of the medical consult should include the following: patient name, age, sex, and race; current systemic condition based on the patient's own history; brief description of current dental condition; brief description of treatment as to duration, proposed drugs, and anesthetic use; expected morbidity and alterations in patient's daily routine; specific questions relative to the patient's ability to safely tolerate the proposed therapy and drugs to be administered; and any suggested alterations in treatment plan.

Box 20-2 **Principles of Periodontal Surgery**

Know your patient and his or her medical status
Develop a thorough and complete treatment plan
Know anatomy of surgical sites
Provide profound anesthesia
Follow aseptic surgical technique
Practice atraumatic tissue management
- sharp, smooth incisions
- careful flap reflection and retraction
- avoid flap tension
Attain hemostasis
Use atraumatic suturing techniques
- smallest needle and suture that can be used in the area
- place sutures in keratinized tissue when possible
- take adequate bites of tissue
- minimum number of sutures to achieve closure
Obliterate dead space between flap and bone
Promote stable wound healing

Diagnosis and Treatment Plan

The surgical phase of periodontal therapy is often only one aspect of the overall plan to establish oral health. Periodontal surgery must be integrated into a well thought out and organized sequence of treatment that is based on previously determined etiologic factors, diagnosis, prognosis, and patient desires and expectations.

Surgical Anatomy

What separates the successful surgeon from all others is his or her knowledge of anatomy and wound healing. The selection of an appropriate surgical technique that can best satisfy the treatment goals and objectives is directly influenced by anatomic relations between bone, soft tissues, and teeth. It is also imperative that the surgeon be familiar with the location of important anatomic structures, especially nerves and blood vessels. Trauma to vital structures may compromise patient safety and comfort and adversely affect proper wound healing.

Anatomic structures

Tables 20-2 and 20-3 list the major anatomic characteristics and features of the mandible and maxilla, respectively. When reviewing these features, it is recommended that the reader refer to an atlas of anatomy or anatomic models to enhance the learning outcome. Anatomic and biologic limitations must be identified prior to initiating treatment. The third column in Tables 20-2 and 20-3 describes some of the considerations that should enter into the surgical plan for a particular anatomic site. These points are meant to assist the surgeon when selecting and planning the most effective procedure to ensure a successful outcome. There can be great variation in the subtleties of anatomy from individual to individual.

Anatomic spaces

Anatomists and surgeons often describe anatomic compartments of the head and neck in terms of anatomic spaces. Table 20-4 lists the major spaces associated with the mandible and maxilla that are of importance to the surgeon. The term *space* refers to the potential for a space to develop, not because one actually exists. Sheets of an areolar type of connective tissue called fascia invest skeletal structures, muscles, viscera, and neurovascular bundles. Fascia either comprises the boundaries of a space or is contained within it. These sheets or layers of fascia are thought of as forming fascial planes. It is along these planes that infection may spread as the fascia is destroyed.

When performing periodontal surgical procedures in the oral cavity, there is always a risk that pathogenic microorganisms could be introduced into the surrounding tissue and anatomic space(s). A healthy immune system is usually capable of eliminating pathogens before they can establish a niche and cause significant infection. The 1%

and 4.4% incidence rates of postoperative infection after periodontal surgery reported by Pack and Haber (1983)[25] and Checchi and colleagues (1992),[26] respectively, seem to support this fact. However, a prudent surgeon should be prepared to identify a problem early and intercede before it develops into a potentially life-threatening scenario. Communication routes between the various anatomic spaces within the head and neck exist by way of fascial planes. Thus, an infection originating in one space may easily spread to an adjacent space and from that space to another and so on. For example, it is possible that an infection originating in the buccal space could spread to the parapharyngeal space and down the neck eventually reaching the thorax and mediastinal space where the heart resides. Therefore, it is critically important for the surgeon to be knowledgeable of the anatomic spaces, their contents, and the possible communication routes.

Blood supply

Maintenance of an adequate blood supply to the tissue is the single most important surgical principle to follow. It is essential for timely and optimal healing of the wound. Having knowledge of the vascular supply to the oral mucosa is a prerequisite for understanding the principles involved in making proper surgical incisions and designing and managing the surgical flap.

The major arterial supply to the oral cavity comes primarily from the lingual, facial, and maxillary arteries, which are branches of the external carotid (Fig. 20-1). Although each of these branches gives off several rami along their course through the head and neck, this review is limited to those arteries that supply the tissue usually involved in periodontal surgical procedures. The first major branch is the lingual artery, which arises between the superior laryngeal artery and facial artery and runs forward beneath the hyoglossus muscle. One of its branches, the sublingual, arises at the anterior border of the hyoglossus muscle and travels between the sublingual gland and genioglossus muscle supplying the sublingual gland, neighboring muscles, mucosa of the floor of the mouth, and the lingual gingival tissue.

Originating just superior to the lingual artery is the facial, which runs forward close to the inferior border of the mandible, lodged in a groove on the posterior surface of the submandibular gland. At the anterior border of the masseter muscle, it curves superiorly over the body of the mandible to travel forward and upward within the cheek to the angle of the mouth. Branches of importance are the submental, inferior coronary, and superior coronary. The submental artery arises as the facial artery emerges from the submandibular gland. It then travels on the mylohyoid muscle below the body of the mandible toward the symphysis where it turns over the chin to divide into deep and superficial branches. Both of these

TABLE 20-2	Surgical Anatomy of the Mandible	
ANATOMIC FEATURES	**CHARACTERISTICS**	**SURGICAL CONSIDERATIONS**
Anterior border of ramus	Anterior border of ramus lies lateral to alveolar process as it extends anteriorly and inferiorly; its anterior extension forms the external oblique ridge; together with the medially located temporal crest it forms the retromolar fossa.	The ramus may be prominent in size and extend more anterior than usual; a flat shelf of bone forms between it and the alveolar process creating a shallow vestibular fornix; surgical flap management can be difficult and access limited; osseous resection to achieve physiologic architecture depends on depth of periodontal defect, thickness of bony shelf, and ability to apically position the surgical flap; keratinized tissue is minimal and must be conserved.
Coronoid process	Anterior/superior extent of ramus; located in infratemporal fossa lateral to pterygoid plate and medial to zygomatic process of maxilla.	A prominent coronoid process may closely approximate the maxillary tuberosity, third molar, and possibly the second molar when opening the jaw; surgical access and flap retraction may be difficult.
Temporal crest (internal oblique ridge)	Located medial and posterior to the anterior border of the ramus; as it approaches distal of last molar, it widens and forms retromolar triangle; together with the laterally located anterior border of ramus it forms the retromolar fossa.	A prominent temporal crest along with the alveolar process may form a broad shelf of bone distal and lingual to the last molar; surgical flap reflection can be difficult and access limited; keratinized tissue is minimal and retromolar mucosa is thick, loose, and difficult to manage; base of the retromolar fossa may be mistaken for an intrabony defect.
External oblique ridge	Formed as a continuation of the anterior border of ramus; may extend as far anteriorly as second premolar.	A prominent or high external oblique ridge may create a shallow vestibular fornix; along with the broad flat alveolar process, it can form a shelf of bone; osseous resection to achieve physiologic architecture depends on depth of periodontal defect, thickness of bony shelf, the and ability to apically position surgical flap; soft tissue grafting procedures may be compromised by a shallow vestibule buccinator and muscle attachment.
Mylohyoid ridge	Attachment for mylohyoid muscle; extends from molar region to premolars on medial (lingual) aspect of mandible.	A prominent or high mylohyoid ridge along with the alveolar process may create a broad bony ledge opposite the molars; horizontal bone loss around molar teeth may accentuate the ledging effect; surgical flap reflection can be difficult, and access for osseous resection or regeneration may be limited without extensive flap reflection and retraction of the tongue.

Continued

	TABLE 20-2 Surgical Anatomy of the Mandible—cont'd		
ANATOMIC FEATURES	**CHARACTERISTICS**	**SURGICAL CONSIDERATIONS**
Mandibular tori	Primarily located on lingual adjacent to premolars.	Mucosal tissue over tori is usually thin and subject to tearing; must exercise care in reflecting flaps and protecting them during tori removal; surgical flap may need to be extended toward midline for better access and tension-free retraction; exostoses may be source of autogenous bone for grafting periodontal intrabony defects.
Genial tubercles	Attachment for the genioglossus (superior tubercle) and genio-hyoid (inferior tubercle) muscles; located at midline near inferior border of mandible.	Usually not a problem except in cases of severe horizontal bone loss or mandibular atrophy as with dental implant placement; flap reflection may be difficult.
Mental protuberance and tubercles	Triangular prominence that comprises the chin bone; mental tubercles are attachment for the mentalis muscles.	A short alveolar process, prominent protuberance and high attachment of the mentalis muscles create a shallow vestibular fornix; may compromise certain soft tissue grafting procedures to cover roots or deepen vestibule; osseous resection may be limited by depth of periodontal defects and ability to apically position the surgical flap.
Mental foramen	Usually located inferior to apices of mandibular premolars yet location may vary.	Neurovascular contents must not be compromised; important to identify location by radiographs and palpation before soft tissue grafting procedures or extensive flap reflection.
Alveolar process	Forms as teeth erupt; continuous with basal bone; cortical bone over the labial or buccal surfaces of the teeth may be thin.	Prominent teeth generally have thin bone and thin mucosa that predispose them to marginal tissue recession; suspect presence of bony dehiscence or fenestration, or both; a short alveolar process is usually associated with a shallow vestibular fornix.

branches supply the muscles and mucosa of the lower lip. The deep branch anastomoses with the mental artery, as does another branch of the facial artery, the inferior labial, which also supplies the muscles and mucosa of the lower lip.

The maxillary artery is the larger of two terminal branches of the external carotid. For descriptive purposes it is divided into three parts on the basis of anatomic location: (1) maxillary, (2) pterygoid, and (3) sphenomaxillary. One branch of great importance is the inferior dental branch, or inferior alveolar artery, which descends

along with the inferior dental nerve to enter the foramen of the mandibular canal. During its course, it gives rise to a dental artery for each root of the molar and premolar teeth. In the region of the first premolar, it divides into the mental and incisive branches, the former emerging from the mental foramen to supply the mucosa of the chin region and the latter continuing forward to supply the incisor teeth. At its origin, the inferior dental artery gives off a lingual arterial branch, which descends with the lingual nerve to supply the lingual mucosa. As it enters the mandibular foramen, the inferior dental artery also gives off a mylohyoid branch, which runs below the mylohyoid muscle sending multiple branches into the muscle.

Branches of the second portion of the maxillary artery are the deep temporal, pterygoid, masseter, and buccal. These arteries travel a short distance to primarily supply muscles of the same name. The first branch arising from the third portion of the maxillary artery is the alveolar or posterior dental artery. It descends onto the tuberosity of the maxilla where it gives off several branches. Some branches enter posterior canals through small foramina to supply the roots of maxillary molars and premolars and

TABLE 20-3	Surgical Anatomy of the Maxilla	
ANATOMIC FEATURES	CHARACTERISTICS	SURGICAL CONSIDERATIONS
Maxillary sinus or antrum	Hollow structure that occupies most of the maxilla; may extend into the alveolarand zygomatic processes, as far anteriorly as the canine and posteriorly as the third molar; may closely approximate the roots of posterior teeth or edentulous ridge; lined by the Schneiderian membrane.	The inferior wall or floor of the sinus may be in close proximity to the base of a periodontal defect limiting osseous resection as a treatment approach; exercise care during defect debridement to avoid perforating into the sinus; pneumatization of the sinus floor in edentulous limit the areas will also extent of alveoplasty to correct adjacent periodontal defects or during preprosthetic surgery.
Zygomatico-alveolar crest	Extends from the tip of the zygomatic process to the alveolar process opposite the first and second molars; forms the posterior border of the malar process (cheek).	A prominent zygomatico-alveolar crest creates a broad shelf ofbone and a shallow vestibular fornix; surgical access will be difficult; osseous surgery and soft tissue grafting procedures may be compromised.
Palate/Palatal vault	Formed by the palatine processes and alveolar processes of the maxilla and the paired palatine bones of the skull; shape of the palatal vault may range from wide and shallow to narrow and high.	A wide and shallow palatal vault is usually associated with a broad bony ledge at the alveolar crest, as well as a wide ledge of palatal mucosa; this anatomy is unfavorable for pocket elimination using osseous resective techniques; in contrast, high and steep vaults are favorable for treating periodontal defects and achieving a physiologic architecture in both bone and palatal mucosa with osseous resective surgery; relative to soft tissue grafts the amount of tissue that can be harvested from the palate is generally less in a shallow vault compared with a high vault.
Greater (anterior) palatine foramen	Located within the palatine bone approximately 2 mm from posterior border of hard palate and 15 mm from midline and superior to the second and third molars; neurovascular bundle courses anteriorly in a groove formed at the juncture of the palatine and alveolar processes.	Care must be taken not to sever or traumatize the neurovascular bundle during surgery; avoid vertical releasing incisions; thinning or harvesting connective tissue grafts to or beyond 7 mm from the alveolar crest in a shallow palate, 12 mm in an average palate, and 17 mm in a high palate may significantly compromise the nerve and vessels.[40]

Continued

TABLE 20-3   Surgical Anatomy of the Maxilla—cont'd

ANATOMIC FEATURES	CHARACTERISTICS	SURGICAL CONSIDERATIONS
Palatal exostoses	Midline palatine torus or palatal exostoses/ledging opposite the second or third molar may be found.	Exostoses in region of second and third molars may hinder surgical access unless adequate flap reflection is obtained; exostoses may be found in close proximity to greater palatine foramen requiring great care in flap reflection, palatal tissue thinning, and osseous contouring; recommend palpation or transmucosal probing through palatal mucosa before dissecting free soft tissue autografts; exostoses may be source of autogenous bone for grafting.
Incisive foramen	Located posterior to the central incisors and deep to the incisive papilla; contains the nasopalatine neurovascular bundle, which supplies the anterior palate from canine to canine.	Care must be taken not to sever or traumatize the neurovascular bundle during surgery; however, its proximity to the teeth often results in some trauma to the nerves and vessels but usually without significant sequelae or morbidity
Alveolar process	Forms as teeth erupt; bone usually thinner over labial/buccal surfaces compared with palatal surfaces.	Prominent teeth generally have thin bone and thin mucosa that predispose them to marginal tissue recession; suspect presence of bony dehiscence or fenestration, or both; a short alveolar process is usually associated with a shallow vestibular fornix. Esthetics of prime concern in anterior region, which may influence choice of therapeutic procedure(s); when surgical access necessary to debride roots and defects, recommend conservative flap design.

the lining of the maxillary sinus, whereas others supply the mucosa, including the gingival tissue on the facial surface. The infraorbital branch is considered a continuation of the trunk of the maxillary artery. It enters the infraorbital canal within the floor of the orbit ascending to supply muscles of the eye and lacrimal gland and descending through anterior dental canals to supply the membrane of the maxillary sinus and the maxillary incisor teeth. It emerges through the infraorbital foramen onto the face to eventually anastomose with branches of the facial artery. Another branch of the maxillary artery important to the periodontal surgeon is the descending palatine artery, which enters the greater palatine canal at the posterior/superior surface of the maxilla. It eventually emerges through the greater (anterior) palatine foramen as the greater palatine artery to travel within a groove formed by the palatine and alveolar processes of the maxilla. In its course it supplies the mucosa and glands of the hard palate and the palatal gingiva of the alveolar process. The terminal branches of the greater palatine artery enter Stenson's foramen to anastomose with the nasopalatine artery. The nasopalatine artery is the internal branch of the sphenopalatine artery, which arises from the maxillary artery before it enters the sphenopalatine foramen. The nasopalatine artery supplies mucous membranes of the nose before it emerges through the incisive foramen to supply the mucosa and gingiva of the anterior palate.

The arterial branches reviewed above give rise to arterioles, which are considered to be the smallest component of the arterial system capable of controlling blood flow to the tissues. The arterioles within the gingiva and alveolar mucosa are supraperiosteal and usually course

TABLE 20-4   Anatomic Spaces Encountered in Periodontal Surgery

ANATOMIC SPACE	BOUNDARIES	CONTENTS
Submental	• Located at base of chin • Boundaries: lateral—anterior belly of digastric muscles; inferior—platysma muscle; superior—mylohyoid muscle	Submental lymph nodes; submental branches of facial artery and vein bilaterally
Submandibular	• Located below mylohyoid muscle • Boundaries: medial—mylohyoid muscle, hyoglossus muscle, and styloglossus muscle; lateral—skin; posterior—stylomandibular ligament inferior—anterior/posterior belly of digastrics; superior—mandible and mylohyoid muscle	Submandibular gland; lingual nerve and vessels; mylohyoid nerve; hypoglossal nerve; facial artery and vein
Sublingual	• Located in submucosal connective tissue of floor of mouth • Boundaries: medial—geniohyoid muscle, genioglossus muscle, and styloglossus muscle; lateral and anterior—lingual aspect of the mandible; inferior—mylohyoid muscle; superior—mucosa of the floor of the mouth	Sublingual gland; Wharton's duct
Buccal	• Lies in the subcutaneous tissue of the cheek between the buccinator muscle and skin • Boundaries: medial—buccinator muscle; lateral—skin; posterior—masseter muscle; anterior—zygomaticus major and depressor anguli oris muscle; superior—zygomatic arch; inferior—mandible	Buccal fat pad; facial artery and vein; parotid duct
Pterygomandibular	• Triangular in shape • Boundaries: medial—medial pterygoid muscle; lateral—ramus of mandible; anterior—pterygomandibular raphe; inferior apex—attachment of the medial pterygoid to the inferior border of the mandible	Inferior alveolar vessels and nerve, and the lingual nerve
Parapharyngeal	• Located at base of skull and delineated by fascial membranes • Boundaries: medial—superior constrictor muscle; lateral—mandible, medial pterygoid muscle, and retromandibular portions of the parotid gland; anterior—pterygomandibular raphe; posterior—apposition of the prevertebral and visceral layers of the deep cervical fascia; superior—petrous portion of temporal bone; inferior—submandibular gland, stylohyoid muscle, posterior belly of the digastric muscle • Separated into two compartments by styloid process • Communicates anteriorly with buccal, sublingual, and pterygomandibular spaces; medially with the retropharyngeal space; and inferiorly with spaces of the neck	Anterior compartment: deep cervical lymph nodes, ascending pharyngeal artery, facial artery; posterior compartment: carotid artery, internal jugular vein, vagus nerve, hypoglossal nerve, cervical sympathetic trunk.

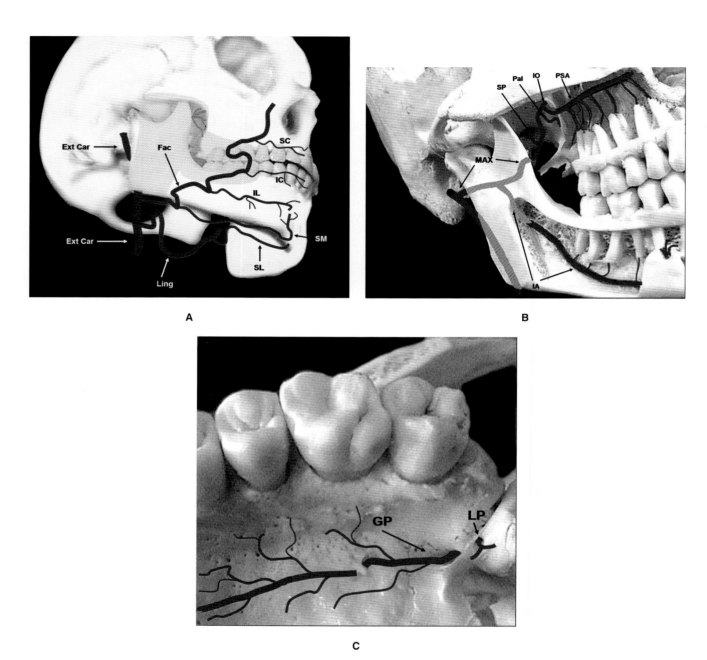

Figure 20-1. Blood supply to oral cavity (schematics of branches off the external carotid). **A,** Lingual and facial arteries. **B,** Maxillary artery and branches. **C,** Greater and lesser palatine arteries. Ext Car, external carotid; Fac, facial; GP, greater palatine artery; IA, inferior alveolar; IC, inferior coronary; IL, inferior labial; IO, infraorbital; Ling, lingual; LP, lesser palatine artery; MAX, maxillary artery; Pal, palatine; PSA, posterior superior alveolar; SC, superior coronary; SL, sublingual; SM, submental; SP, sphenopalatine.

from the posterior to the anterior part of the oral cavity in a horizontal plane parallel to the mucogingival junction (Fig. 20-2). Branches of these arterioles travel in an inferior to superior (apical to coronal) direction to supply the interproximal gingiva and papilla and the gingiva over molar furcations. Capillaries from these blood vessels eventually anastomose with the rich capillary plexus arising from vessels within the periodontal ligament and

alveolar septum (see Chapter 1). Smaller arterioles and capillaries branch from these vertically oriented vessels and travel horizontally to supply tissue over the radicular surfaces of the teeth. This extensive microvascular bed is primarily concerned with the exchange of gases, nutrients, and metabolic waste products with all tissue cells. Capillary exchange takes place with an equally abundant network of postcapillary venules, which drain into veins

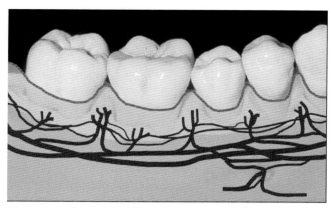

Figure 20-2. Gingival blood supply. Supraperiosteal arterioles course from the posterior to the anterior part of the oral cavity in a horizontal plane parallel to the mucogingival junction. Branches of these arterioles extend vertically (apical to coronal) to supply the interproximal gingiva and papilla and the gingiva over molar furcations.

of increasing size that course in close proximity to the arteries.

An extensive vascular supply is the primary reason that the oral mucosa is able to heal at a rapid rate after being wounded. Proper incision placement, flap design, and atraumatic flap management are critical to the maintenance of this vital blood supply.

Wound healing

The basic events of wound healing are the same regardless of location in the body. The time required for the completion of healing depends on the size and volume of the wound and the availability of adjacent tissue elements to contribute to its repair. The sequence of events can be divided into an inflammatory phase, a proliferative or granulation phase, and a remodeling or maturation phase. A complex array of biological mediators and cellular interactions occur that act in a dynamic but orderly process. For periodontal wounds this involves interaction between the epithelium, connective tissue, and bone, as well as the cells of the periodontal ligament and root cementum.

Three types of surgical wound healing are recognized. All three are related to the degree of wound closure. *Primary intention* healing occurs when the wound margins are directly approximated—that is, primary closure is obtained. This type of healing occurs rapidly compared to other types. Healing by *secondary intention* occurs when the wound margins are not approximated and remain apart; granulation tissue must form to close the gap. In this scenario, the healing phases would be extended in time as new connective tissue and epithelium migrate from the wound edges toward the center. *Tertiary intention* healing is usually associated with a disruption of secondary intention healing as might occur if

the wound is infected. Most periodontal surgical wounds heal by primary and secondary intention.

The inflammatory phase of healing is characterized clinically by the classic signs of redness (erythema), heat, swelling (edema), and discomfort. These signs and symptoms are related to a multitude of events that occur at the cellular and molecular level, which involve the vascular system, immune system, and tissue cells at the site of injury. The redness, heat, and swelling are caused by vasodilation and increased vascular permeability and blood flow, resulting in the buildup of exudate in the extracellular tissue environment. Discomfort is usually mediated by the release of histamine, serotonin, kinins, and the metabolites of arachidonic acid, known as prostaglandins.

Other mediators of inflammation are the cytokines, which are soluble small polypeptides released by cells of the immune system and some tissue cells. Cytokines act at receptor sites on cell membranes to either stimulate or inhibit specific cellular functions. As such, cytokines play an important role in the proliferative and maturation phases of healing. Growth factors comprise another category of signaling proteins, which are produced by several different types of cells. Like cytokines, they mediate their effects through cell membrane receptors. Their effects may be described as being autocrine (act on self), paracrine (act on cells within the local environment), or endocrine (act on distant cells). Growth factors play key roles in cell proliferation, differentiation, and extracellular matrix formation, which are major events associated with the proliferative and maturation phases of healing.

Within hours of wounding, there is an increase in epithelial mitosis in the basal and spinous layers at the wound margin. In 1 to 2 days, epithelium begins to migrate beneath a layer of polymorphonuclear leukocytes called the polyband, which forms under the blood clot. Epithelial cells migrate at a rate of 0.5 to 1.0 mm per day toward the center of the wound. Once epithelium covers the entire wound surface, it takes an additional 28 to 42 days to achieve complete maturation. At approximately 3 to 4 days, fibroblasts begin formation of a new connective tissue matrix. Collagen formation peaks between 7 and 21 days and maturation is complete by 21 to 28 days. Revascularization also begins around 3 to 4 days, with new blood vessels arising from proliferating endothelial cells. Vascular budding and sprouting of new vessels continues for 10 to 15 days.

Injury to bone can occur simply with the reflection of a flap exposing the periosteum or bone proper. Osteoclastic activity to remove necrotic bone begins at around 3 to 4 days and involves either endosteal (undermining resorption) or surface resorption. The resorptive process peaks at around 8 to 10 days but continues along with bone formation between 14 and 21 days. Bone formation predominates between 21 and 28 days and remodeling may take up to 2 years.

Surgical wounds differ from those caused by traumatic events or infection in that the surgeon has the ability to directly influence the course of wound healing by controlling the choice and placement of the incision(s); the design and management of the surgical flap; the extent to which the mucosa and bone are altered; stabilization of the wound; and the postoperative care of the surgical site and patient.

Anesthesia and Pain Control

Control of the physiologic mechanisms of pain is the function of local anesthetics, whereas control over psychological factors that influence the interpretation of stimuli as painful is a function of conscious sedation. (See Chapter 19 for a review of conscious sedation and its indications for the control of anxiety.) Selection of an appropriate local anesthetic for periodontal surgical procedures should be based on pharmacologic and physical properties of the anesthetic agent. These properties determine the effectiveness and duration of action of the anesthetic and potential effects on patient safety.

Local anesthetics traditionally have been classified into two groups: esters and amides.[27] Because of their greater incidence of allergic reactions, the ester-linked local anesthetics are no longer available in dental anesthetic cartridges. Lidocaine, mepivacaine, and bupivacaine are among the most widely used amide-linked local anesthetics; others include prilocaine, tetracaine, propoxycaine, and etidocaine. Potency, onset of action, and duration of action are properties of local anesthetics that are important to the dental practitioner. Potency is defined as the lowest concentration of drug that can block conduction of the sensory impulse. It is most often linked to the lipid solubility of the anesthetic drug; however, its intrinsic vasodilator effect and tissue diffusion properties can also affect potency. Thus, highly lipid-soluble drugs have greater potency than those with low lipid solubility. The lipid solubility coefficient is greatest for etidocaine (141) and bupivacaine (28) and intermediate for lidocaine (2.9) and mepivacaine (1.0).

The onset of action of anesthetic drugs is a function of their ionization constant (pKa) and the tissue pH. Local anesthetics exist in solution as the free base or un-ionized form, a property that makes it possible for them to diffuse across the nerve membrane. Once across the membrane, they dissociate into the ionized form, which initiates the blockade of the nerve. According to the equation pKa − pH = log, a smaller dissociation constant (pKa) for an anesthetic drug at a given pH means that more drug exists in the free base form than a drug with a greater pKa; thus, more drug is available to diffuse across the nerve membrane and the onset of action will be faster.

With a tissue pH of 7.0, mepivacaine (pKa = 7.6) and lidocaine (pKa = 7.7) have a fast onset of action, whereas bupivacaine (pKa = 8.1) is considered intermediate.

Duration of action is linked to the protein-binding capacity of the drug. The greater the binding capacity of the drug, the longer its duration. Protein binding is greatest among the long-acting anesthetics like bupivacaine (94%) and is intermediate for mepivacaine (77%) and lidocaine (64%). Therefore, anesthetics like bupivacaine can provide anesthesia for 4 to 8 hours, which makes it a useful drug for postsurgical pain control. Combining vasoconstrictors such as epinephrine or levonordefrin with the anesthetic agent also can increase the duration of action. Epinephrine is about six times more potent than levonordefrin and is more commonly used. It causes vasoconstriction locally by stimulating α-adrenergic receptors in the vessel wall, thereby reducing blood flow. **Increasing the concentration of epinephrine in the local anesthetic cartridge from 5 (1:200,000) to 20 μg/ml (1:50,000) does not, however, increase the duration of action.**

Another beneficial effect of vasoconstrictors during surgery is tissue hemostasis. Clinically, this is most evident with infiltration techniques where tissue blanching can be observed. Unlike its effects on the duration of action, increasing the concentration of vasoconstrictor in the local anesthetic cartridge from 10 to 20 μg/ml (1:100,000 to 1:50,000) can reduce blood loss in periodontal surgery.[28] After block anesthesia, a small amount of anesthetic agent with vasoconstrictor can be infiltrated into the gingival tissue especially at the gingival margin and papilla. This provides excellent hemostasis and even provides some rigidity to flaccid gingiva. Operator visibility is improved and more accurate, smooth, and sharp incisions can be made.

Depending on the type of periodontal surgical procedure performed and the extent of the surgical field, most procedures may last from 30 minutes to 4 hours. With properly administered anesthesia, a quadrant of surgery may often be performed using as little as two anesthetic cartridges. Situations do arise, however, in which larger volumes of anesthetic agent may be necessary. When four quadrants of surgery are completed in one visit, the maximum dose of local anesthetic may be approached. In these instances, it is more appropriate to calculate the maximum dose allowable on the basis of milligrams per kilograms of body weight rather than number of cartridges. For lidocaine, a maximum safe dose of 4.4 mg per kilogram body weight is advisable, with a maximum dose of 300 mg regardless of whether epinephrine is combined with the anesthetic. This would translate into 8.33 cartridges of lidocaine with 1:100,000 epinephrine. In patients with significant cardiovascular disease and hemodynamic instability, vasoconstrictors may be contraindicated or limited to a maximum dose of 0.04 mg epinephrine, the amount present in two 1.8-ml cartridges with 1:100,000 epinephrine. The use of longer acting anesthetic containing vasoconstrictor must be weighed against the stress created by repeated injections necessary for plain anesthetic to have the same duration of action for a procedure.

The judicious use of local anesthetics is an obtainable goal provided the surgeon is familiar with the distribution of sensory nerves that supply the oral cavity. The primary sensory innervation to the teeth and mucosa are by way of afferent fibers that travel with cranial nerve V, most often referred to as the trigeminal nerve. The cell bodies to the afferent fibers for pain and temperature lie within the trigeminal (gasserian or semilunar) ganglion located in the floor of the middle cranial fossa. The cell bodies to the fibers responsible for proprioception are located within the mesencephalic nucleus of nerve V located within the brainstem. The trigeminal nerve divides into three divisions before leaving the cranial cavity: (1) the first division, or ophthalmic division, (2) the second division, or maxillary division, and (3) the third division, or mandibular division. Branches of the second and third divisions supply all teeth and mucosa of the oral cavity (see Table 20-5 for a list of these branches).

An important aspect of pain control is providing long-lasting anesthesia during the immediate (4 to 6 hours) postoperative healing period. It is often beneficial to take advantage of the long duration of bupivacaine by administering it at the end of the surgical procedure to ensure that the patient remains anesthetized as long as possible after surgery. This allows the patient to return home and take the appropriate postoperative pain medication before anesthesia is lost. Providing profound and lasting anesthesia for the surgical patient is a crucial part of periodontal surgery. Without it, surgical objectives are impossible to obtain, patient and provider stress levels are increased, and the patient's confidence in the surgeon is diminished.

Aseptic Surgical Technique

An unique aspect of periodontal surgery is the environment in which a surgeon must work. It is impossible to sterilize the surgical field. Despite this, it is imperative that the surgical team follow an aseptic surgical technique to ensure the incidence of postoperative infection remains as low as possible in this bacteria laden setting. Surgical caps and surgical masks should be worn. The patient should be draped with sterile towels, including a sterile head wrap to cover the patient's hair and eyes. Sterile surgical glove use

TABLE 20-5	Primary Sensory Distribution to the Oral Cavity		
TRIGEMINAL NERVE	**BRANCHES**	**STRUCTURES INNERVATED**	**TYPE OF ANESTHESIA**
Maxillary division	• Greater palatine nerve	Posterior palatal mucosa	Block at greater palatine foramen
	• Posterior superior alveolar nerve	Posterior teeth; maxillary sinus; maxillary buccal mucosa	Block at posterior superior foramina on maxillary bone
	• Infraorbital nerve	Maxillary sinus; maxillary anterior mucosa	Block at infraorbital foramen
	• Anterior superior alveolar nerve (branch of infraorbital nerve)	Anterior teeth	Infiltrate above apices of teeth
	• Nasopalatine	Anterior palatal mucosa	Block at incisive foramen
Mandibular division	• Inferior alveolar nerve	Mandibular molars and premolars	Block at foramen to the mandibular or inferior alveolar canal
	• Mental nerve	Branch of inferior alveolar nerve; buccal and labial mucosa	Block at mental foramen for premolar and anterior teeth
	• Incisive nerve	Terminal branch of inferior alveolar nerve; mandibular canine and incisors	Block inferior alveolar nerve, or mental nerve
	• Lingual nerve	Lingual mucosa; tongue	Block along with inferior alveolar nerve
	• Buccal nerve	Mandibular buccal mucosa	Infiltrate mucosa over anterior border of mandibular ramus

is the standard of care, and the use of sterile saline or sterile water irrigation, including irrigation through ultrasonic instruments and handpieces, should be a standard of care in surgical treatment rooms. All surgical instruments must be properly sterilized and sterile coverings over light handles are required. A simple technique for covering light handles is to include aluminum foil in surgical kits before sterilization. The sterile foil is then wrapped over the light handles. Although a sterile operating room environment is not required, all efforts must be made to prevent the introduction of nonresident bacteria into the surgical field.

Patient preparation is another important component of aseptic surgical technique. The patient's oral hygiene should be at an acceptable level before surgery. An immediate presurgical rinse with 0.12% chlorhexidine mouthrinse for 30 seconds will provide a significant reduction (ranging from 72% to 97%) in the intraoral bacterial load.[29,30] In addition, a 13-fold reduction in the level of bacteria in aerosol spray has been reported after using chlorhexidine prerinse.[31]

The use of prophylactic antibiotics in healthy immunocompetent patients is not necessary or recommended for most periodontal surgical procedures. Infection rates after routine flap surgery are similar regardless of whether prophylactic antibiotics are used.[26] A notable exception to this philosophy is the empirical use of antibiotics when guided tissue regeneration or implant placement surgery is performed. Although there is no evidence suggesting that patients undergoing these procedures are more prone to postoperative infections, some clinicians will provide a 7- to 14-day course of antibiotics starting the day before or the day of surgery. The stated rationale for use of antibiotics with these two types of surgical procedures is to enhance the predictability of a favorable outcome. Despite the paucity of evidence to support this rationale, empirical use of systemic antibiotics in these cases is accepted by many in the periodontal community.

Although well controlled studies are lacking to support the use of prophylactic antibiotic coverage before invasive procedures, definitive guidelines concerning antibiotic premedication for patients at risk for infectious endocarditis and patients at high risk for infection because of prosthetic joints have been made and should be followed.[32,33] There is less agreement concerning other patients who may be at greater risk for infection—that is, organ transplant recipients; patients with poorly controlled diabetes; patients on long-term, high-dose steroids; asplenic patients; patients with systemic lupus erythematosus; and patients undergoing chemotherapy or hemodialysis. Prophylactic antibiotics may be of benefit for some of these patients, but because there is no universal agreement, consultation with the patient's physician would be prudent.

Atraumatic Surgical Technique: Flap Management

A surgeon must be deft, delicate, and accurate in the management of all tissue within the surgical field. There are several elements in flap management that require planning and atraumatic execution.

Incisions

Surgical access to the various components of the periodontium begins with well thought out incisions. Because there are a variety of gingival, mucosal, and osseous abnormalities that may require treatment, there is no single technique or approach that works well in all cases. Many of these different surgical techniques involve a variety of incision designs. Seven main incision types are commonly used in periodontal surgery (Table 20-6). Incision selection and execution is based on careful planning that takes surgical anatomy, the surgical objective, flap design, and the principles of atraumatic tissue management into consideration. Regardless of the type of incision used, the surgeon must use a sharp cutting instrument with a definitive and smooth movement and minimal drag through tissue. A dull knife will cause unnecessary tissue damage. The scalpel handle should be round and held with a delicate pen grasp, allowing precise, flexible, and accurate movement of the scalpel blade. The knife blade should stay in tissue as much as possible. The more the surgeon lifts the scalpel away from the incision to change its orientation, the greater the chance of having a ragged incision line. Surgical predictability begins with clean, smooth incisions. This will result in faster healing and less patient discomfort.

The external bevel or gingivectomy incision is contained in the gingiva and coronally directed with the surgical objectives of pocket elimination, access to roots, and improved gingival contours (Fig. 20-3). This incision, and the gingivectomy procedure in particular, is indicated to treat gingival enlargement and to perform esthetic crown lengthening when access to the underlying bone is not required. (See Chapter 23.) It is sometimes used in conjunction with flap surgery when it is beneficial to thin the tissues externally before flap reflection. An example would be a case of severe gingival enlargement with lobulated gingiva and highly irregular gingival margins (Fig. 20-4). Recontouring gingiva with an irregular surface morphology is difficult if attempted using an internal thinning technique on the underside of the flap.

Contraindications to the gingivectomy approach include the presence of intrabony defects requiring treatment; a narrow zone of keratinized tissue; probing depths extending apical to the mucogingival junction; unfavorable anatomic considerations, such as a shallow palatal vault or a pronounced external oblique ridge; and when root exposure is contraindicated because of esthetic concerns. Other contraindications include a

TABLE 20-6   Incisions

INCISION	DESCRIPTION	INDICATION	INSTRUMENTATION
External bevel incision (also called gingivectomy incision)	Coronally directed	Gingivectomy: gingival overgrowth, crown lengthening, gingivoplasty	Kirkland knife, Orban knife, scalpel blades #11D, #15 (360-degree knife handle is useful), laser
Internal bevel incision (also called reverse bevel or inverse bevel incision)	Apically directed, placed at the crest of the gingival margin or stepped back from the margin 0.5 to 2.0 mm	Excisional new attachment procedure, modified Widman flap, flap and curettage, crown lengthening, gingival enlargement	Scalpel blades #11, #12 or 12B, #15 or 15c, Beaver blades #67 or #64, Blade breaker
Sulcular incision (also called crevicular incision)	Apically directed, placed in the gingival crevice and directed toward the alveolar crest	When preservation of gingiva is critical, as in esthetic areas or areas of minimal keratinized tissue, guided tissue regeneration (GTR) procedures	Scalpel blades #11, #12 or #12B, #15 or 15c, Beaver blades # 67 or #64, Blade breaker
Releasing incision (also called vertical incision)	Perpendicular to the gingival margin at line angles of teeth	To increase access, to allow apical or coronal positioning of flap	Scalpel blades #11, #15 or 15c, Beaver blades #67 or #64, Blade breaker
Thinning incision	Internal or under-mining incision extending from gingival margin toward the base of the flap to decrease the bulk of connective tissue on the underside of the flap	Palatal flaps, distal wedge procedures, internal bevel gingivectomy, bulky papillae	Scalpel blades #12 or #12B, #15 or 15c, Beaver blades #67 or #64, Blade breaker
Cutback incision	Small incision made at the apical aspect of a releasing incision and directed toward the base of the flap	Pedicle flaps that are laterally positioned	Scalpel blades #11, #15 or 15c, Beaver blades #67 or #64, Blade breaker
Periosteal releasing incision	Incision at the base of the flap severing the underlying periosteum	To release flap tension allowing coronal advancement of the flap	Scalpel blades #15 or 15c, Beaver blades #67 or #64

high caries index or preexisting thermal sensitivity. Although popular in the 1960s and 1970s, the external bevel gingivectomy currently has limited application. The creation of a broad wound that heals through secondary intention increases intraoperative and postoperative bleeding and postoperative discomfort. Simply stated, the classical gingivectomy is not a patient-friendly technique, but it does have advantages in some cases of gingival excess.

The inverse, or reverse, bevel incision is one of the most common types of incisions used in periodontal surgery. As previously mentioned, the initial intent of the reverse bevel incision was to remove pocket epithelium and to provide direct apposition of healthy connective tissue to the root surface. Although this is no longer a surgical objective, the inverse bevel incision is still useful in apically positioning the palatal flap margin by stepping back from the margin and scalloping the flap (Fig. 20-5).

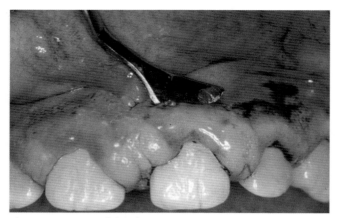

Figure 20-3. External bevel (Gingivectomy) incision. Kirkland knife angled 45 degrees toward the base of the pocket. The gingivectomy incision is started coronal to the mucogingival junction.

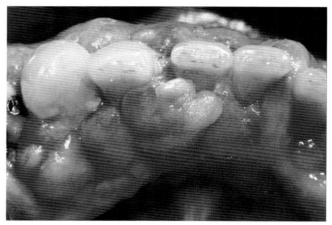

Figure 20-4. Drug-induced gingival enlargement. Irregular gingival contours are more easily treated with an external bevel gingivectomy approach than inverse bevel incisions combined with internal thinning of the flap.

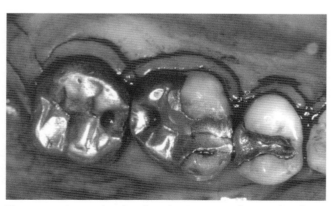

Figure 20-5. Inverse bevel scalloped incision. Initial inverse bevel incisions incorporate a scalloped step-back from the gingival margin. The scallop follows the anatomy of the cervical portion of the tooth and the step-back allows apical positioning of the flap margins.

This incision also may be used on facial surfaces if a broad zone of keratinized tissue is present. The scalpel blade is oriented parallel to the long axis of the teeth and is directed apically toward the alveolar crest or just subcrestal if a greater step-back from the gingival margin is desired and some osseous resection is anticipated (Fig. 20-6). A scalloped incision design is normally incorporated in the flap when an inverse bevel incision is used. The shape of this scallop is dictated by the anatomy of the tooth and underlying root form and the anticipated amount of apical positioning of the flap or flap margin (Fig. 20-7).

A sulcular, or crevicular, incision is selected if preservation of all the existing keratinized tissue is desirable. The scalpel blade is inserted into the gingival crevice, aligned parallel to the long axis of the tooth, and angled

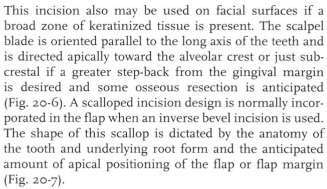

A

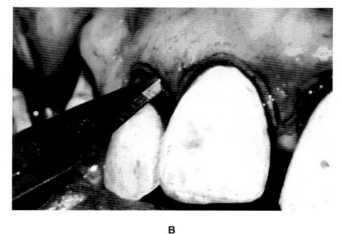

B

Figure 20-6. Inverse bevel incision. **A,** Schematic demonstrating step-back from the gingival margin. The incision is angled toward or just apical to the alveolar crest. **B,** #11 Scalpel blade stepping back from the gingival margin and angling the blade toward the alveolar crest.

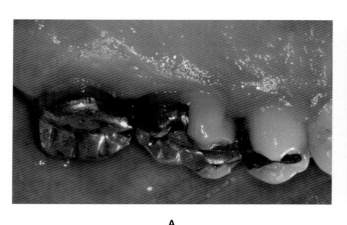 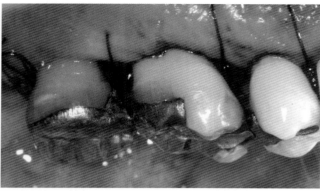

| A | B |

Figure 20-7. Apically positioned flap margin following inverse bevel scalloped incision. **A,** Pretreatment (palatal view) (see Fig. 20-5 for initial incisions). **B,** Apically positioned flap margins—sutured (palatal view).

toward the alveolar crest (Fig. 20-8). Interproximally, the incision is extended into the embrasure space to include as much papillary tissue as possible with the flap.

Vertical releasing incisions are normally perpendicular to the gingival margin and placed at the line angles of the teeth (Fig. 20-9). These incisions increase access to alveolar bone, decrease tension on retracted flaps, allow apical and coronal positioning of flaps, and limit the inclusion of nondiseased sites in the surgical field. Vertical releasing incisions should not be placed in pronounced concavities or over prominent bony ledges or exostoses, and also should not cross over root prominences

or split the interdental papilla unless associated with a double papilla pedicle graft technique used for exposed root surface coverage (Fig. 20-10). As a general rule, when trying to decide on what side of the interproximal space to place the releasing incision, it is best to include the papilla with the flap to enhance the blood supply to the flap and to allow for ease of suturing. An exception to this guideline is in the anterior region where reflection of a papilla may not be warranted because of esthetic concerns.

Thinning incisions reduce the bulk of connective tissue from the underside of the flap and are commonly

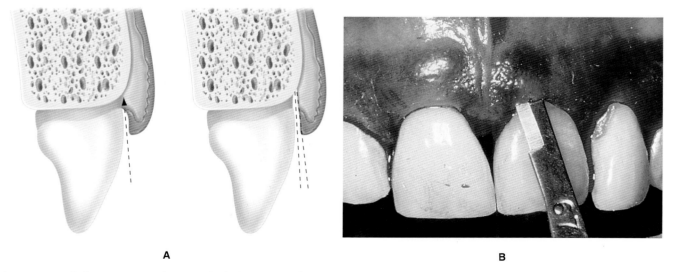

| A | B |

Figure 20-8. Sulcular incision. **A,** Schematic of sulcular incision. The incision is placed within the sulcus and angled toward the alveolar crest. **B,** #67 Scalpel placed in the sulcus and extended to the alveolar crest. The incision is carried into the interdental area where the papilla is either thinned or reflected full thickness.

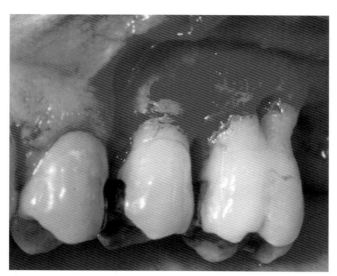

Figure 20-9. Vertical releasing incision. The releasing incision is made at the line angle and the interdental papilla is included in the flap. The vertical release should not cross over the root prominence of the adjacent tooth.

used to reduce the thickness of flaps before reflection (Fig. 20-11). Such incisions are used as part of distal or mesial wedge procedures and also to thin bulky papillae. Thinning incisions are performed either in conjunction with flap reflection (i.e., reflecting the flap as it is thinned) or after completing flap reflection. The novice surgeon may find it less challenging to thin the flap as it is being reflected, because the tissue is less mobile and easier to control. Thinning of bulky tissues, using an

internal approach, allows for better flap adaptation and provides greater patient comfort than thinning tissues with an external bevel incision.

Tuberosity and retromolar pad reduction procedures are used to reduce the bulk of tissue distal to second molars in the maxillary tuberosity and the mandibular retromolar fossa areas.[34] These techniques, of necessity, incorporate internal thinning incisions, with the goal to create primary wound closure and primary intention healing. There are three techniques that are commonly used: the triangular wedge, the linear wedge, and the trap door. (See also Chapter 23.) All three techniques have the advantages over a gingivectomy approach of allowing access to underlying bone, preserving keratinized tissue, and providing for primary closure with more rapid healing and less discomfort. The triangular and linear distal wedge procedures are well suited for reduction of thick tissues characteristic of the maxillary tuberosity.

Triangular wedge incisions are placed creating the apex of the triangle close to the hamular notch and the base of the triangle next to the distal surface of the terminal tooth (Fig. 20-12). These incisions are continuous with the buccal and palatal inverse bevel incisions used in the remainder of the surgical site. The thinning or undermining incisions are accomplished before full reflection of tissue and are extended 2 to 3 mm apical to the crestal aspect of the tuberosity. Flaps can then be fully reflected and the wedge of soft tissue removed from over the tuberosity. If adequate thinning is performed and the wedge is of sufficient length, primary flap closure should be achieved to allow healing by first intention.

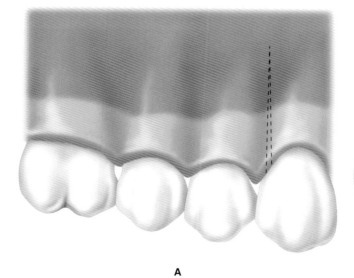

A

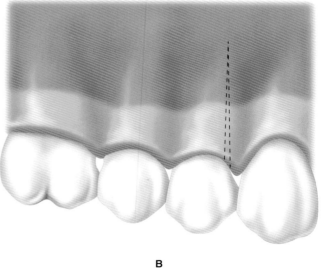

B

Figure 20-10. Correct and incorrect placement of vertical releasing incisions. **A,** Correct vertical releasing incision at the line angle. The papilla is included in the flap. **B,** Correct vertical releasing incision at the line angle. The papilla is not included in the flap.

Continued

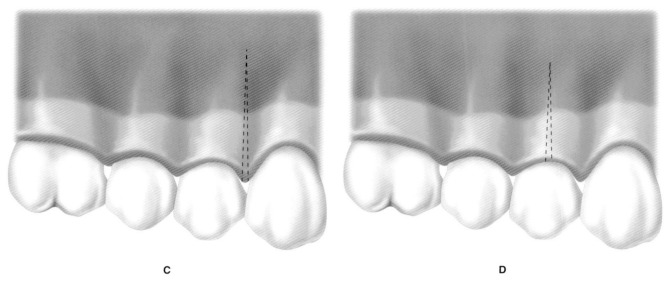

C
D

Figure 20-10. cont'd C, Incorrect vertical releasing incision splitting the papilla. **D,** Incorrect vertical releasing incision over the root prominence.

The linear distal wedge incorporates two parallel incisions over the crest of the tuberosity that extend from the proximal surface of the terminal molar to the hamular notch area. The distance between the two linear incisions is determined by the thickness of the tissues, with wider separation of the incisions in thicker tissue. Vertical releasing incisions placed perpendicular and at the posterior aspect of the linear wedge will allow greater access to the underlying bone (Fig. 20-13). Thinning incisions and removal of the distal wedge are completed in a similar fashion as described for the triangular distal wedge.

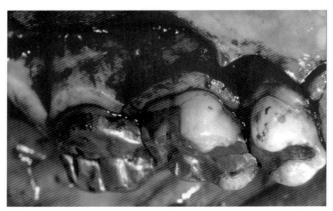

Figure 20-11. Thinning incision—palatal flap. Initial inverse bevel incisions (see Fig. 20-5) are followed by a thinning incision to create a thinned flap that is easily adapted to the teeth at a more apical level. The collar of soft tissue that remains around the teeth (present in this figure) is removed with chisels and curets to allow access to the root surfaces and bone.

Although the triangular or linear distal wedge procedures can be used in the mandibular retromolar pad area if adequate keratinized tissue is present, the trap door technique may be better suited for this area when there is minimal keratinized tissue. The trap door procedure will preserve existing keratinized tissue but still allow internal thinning of tissues and apical positioning of flaps. Various approaches to the trap door procedure may be used depending on the anatomy and tissue type in the mandibular retromolar area. A common technique incorporates a single incision placed from either the distofacial or distolingual line angle of the terminal molar extending posteriorly through keratinized tissue until approximating the ascending aspect of the ramus. At this point, the incision is angled either toward the lingual if initiated from the distofacial line angle or buccally toward the external oblique ridge if started at the distolingual line angle. A rectangular flap (i.e., trap door) is created that is continuous with the buccal mucoperiosteal flap extending anteriorly. This rectangular flap can be thinned as it is reflected and the soft tissue remaining on the crest removed (Fig. 20-14). Although these three retromolar procedures are often described for the management of thick tissues on the distal of terminal molars, they also can be used next to any tooth adjacent to an edentulous space with thick mucosal tissue.

Cutback incisions are small incisions made at the apical aspect of vertical releasing incisions, and they are used in conjunction with pedicle flaps to allow greater movement and less tension when the flaps are moved laterally (Fig. 20-15). Great care must be taken not to extend cutback incisions more than 2 to 3 mm to minimize disruption of the remaining blood supply to the flap.

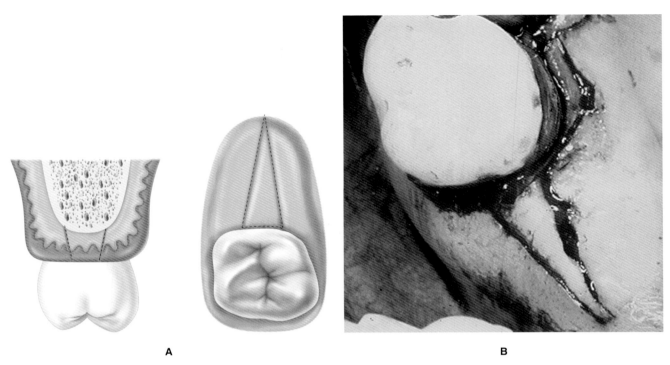

Figure 20-12. Triangular distal wedge. **A,** Schematic demonstrating incisions that diverge as they approach the ridge and converge as they are extended distally. The facial and lingual tissues are thinned before reflection of the flaps. **B,** Initial incisions outlining the triangular wedge. These incisions are best accomplished with an Orban knife or a 12B scalpel.

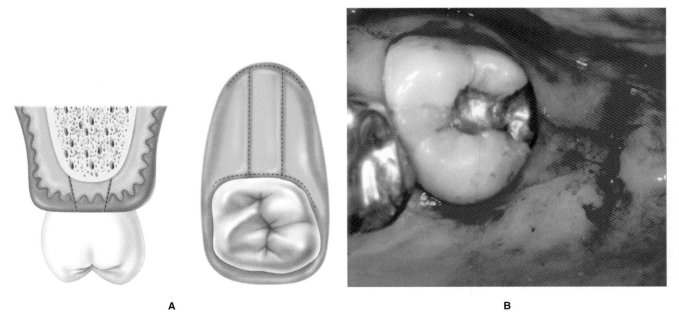

Figure 20-13. Linear distal wedge. **A,** Schematic demonstrating incisions that diverge buccolingually toward the ridge and are parallel as they are extended distally away from the tooth. A releasing "T" incision is placed to allow greater flap reflection and access to the underlying bone. The buccal and palatal tissues are thinned before flap reflection. **B,** The initial parallel incisions may be made with a #12 or 12B scalpel blade or an Orban knife. The "T" incision perpendicular to the linear incisions may be placed with a Kirkland knife. The flaps are thinned with a scalpel as they are reflected. The rectangular soft tissue wedge is removed. The flaps are then approximated and sutured.

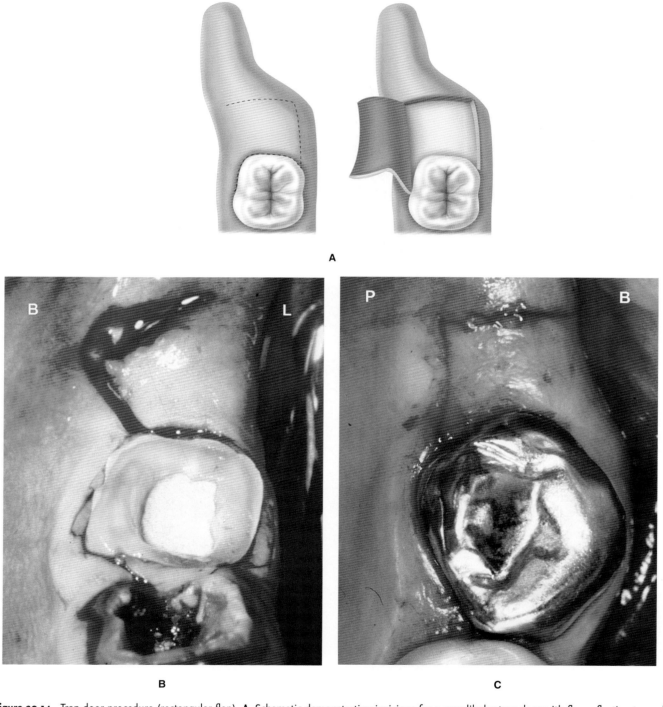

Figure 20-14. Trap door procedure (rectangular flap). **A,** Schematic demonstrating incisions for a mandibular trap door with flap reflection toward the lingual. Incisions should be made over bone and in keratinized tissue. **B,** Mandible: the incision is initiated from the distobuccal line angle and is extended distally and slightly toward the buccal (*B*). A second incision is made toward the lingual (*L*). This approach is beneficial if the underlying osseous defect is located at the distolingual line angle. The flap can be thinned as it is reflected toward the lingual. **C,** Maxilla: The incision is initiated from the distopalatal line angle and carried distally. A second incision is made toward the buccal. This approach may be indicated if the underlying osseous defect is toward the distobuccal aspect of the tooth.

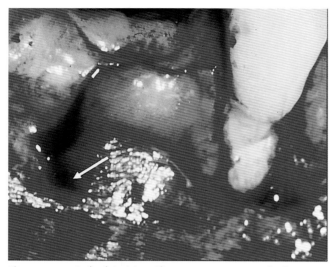

Figure 20-15. Cutback incision. The *arrow* points to a cutback incision placed to increase mobility of a lateral sliding pedicle flap. This partial-thickness flap will be moved mesially (to the right) over the exposed root surface.

Periosteal releasing incisions are used when coronal or lateral advancement of a flap onto the root or crown of the tooth is indicated (Fig. 20-16). This incision, which severs the underlying periosteum at the base of full-thickness flaps, allows tension-free coronal positioning of the flap to cover exposed root surfaces and to provide primary closure over barrier membranes used in guided tissue and guided bone regeneration procedures. Great care must be exercised in making these incisions not to jeopardize the blood supply or detach the flap from its base.

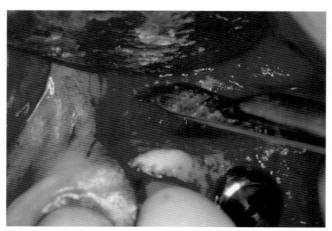

Figure 20-16. Periosteal releasing incision. The periosteum on the underside of the flap is scored with a scalpel blade to increase flap mobility, allowing passive coronal advancement of the flap.

Flap preparation

The surgical flap is defined as the separation of a section of tissue from the surrounding tissues except at its base.[35] A flap that includes epithelium, connective tissue, and periosteum is referred to as a full-thickness or mucoperiosteal flap, and it is the most common type of flap used when access to the bone is indicated for resective or regenerative procedures (Fig. 20-17). When the periosteum is not included in the flap, it is called a partial-thickness or split-thickness flap (Fig. 20-18). This type of flap is used extensively in mucogingival surgery to leave an underlying blood supply where soft tissue grafting is performed to correct deformities in the morphology, position, or amount of gingiva. There are also instances in which part of a flap may be full thickness and the other part may be partial thickness. This combined technique is used in some mucogingival and esthetic crown lengthening procedures.

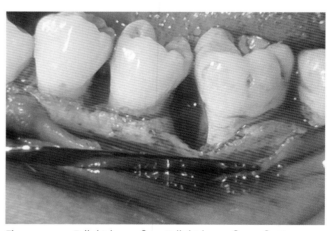

Figure 20-17. Full-thickness flap. Full-thickness flap reflection completely exposing the underlying bone.

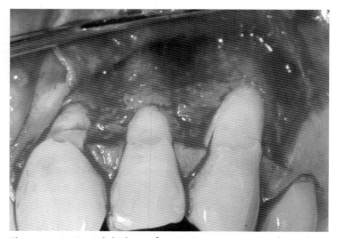

Figure 20-18. Partial-thickness flap. Periosteum is retained over bone before placing a subepithelial connective tissue graft.

Full-thickness flaps are prepared by making an incision through the mucosal layers and the periosteum until the bone is felt. A periosteal elevator is then used to gently separate the periosteum along with the superficial mucosal layers from the bone (Fig. 20-19). The partial-thickness flap is technically more challenging than a full-thickness flap and should not be attempted in areas where the gingiva is thin (≤1 mm). It is also contraindicated in posterior areas of the mandible where the vestibule is shallow and access is difficult. When performing a partial-thickness flap, the use of a new surgical blade, along with soft tissue forceps, is recommended. The tip of the surgical blade is used to split the connective tissue layer into two parts: one, which is left covering the periosteum, and the other, which becomes part of the tissue flap (Fig. 20-20). The tissue forceps aid in the stabilization and retraction of the flap margin as the dissection is carried first laterally, then apically. This approach creates better visibility and reduces tension on the flap. Poor visibility and excessive tension may lead to flap perforation or tearing of the delicate flap. Misadventures such as these will compromise blood supply resulting in flap necrosis and delayed healing.

Flap design

Flap design should be based on the principle of maintaining an optimal blood supply to the tissue. There are generally two basic flap designs: those with and those without vertical releasing incisions. A flap that is released in a linear fashion at the gingival margin but has no vertical releasing incision(s) is called an envelope flap (Fig. 20-21). If two vertical releasing incisions are included in the flap design, it becomes a pedicle flap (Fig. 20-22). If one vertical releasing incision is included in the flap design, some clinicians refer to this as a triangular flap. The teeth, flap, and vertical releasing incision form the sides of the triangle (Fig. 20-23). This flap design should not be confused with the triangular wedge usually associated with the removal of a soft tissue wedge in the tuberosity or retromolar area (Fig. 20-12).

Alterations in gingival circulation resulting from various periodontal flap designs have been studied in human subjects using fluorescein angiography techniques.[36] The major blood supply to a flap was found to exist at its base and travels in an apical to coronal direction. It was also determined that the greater the ratio of flap length to flap base, the greater the vascular compromise at the flap margins. On the basis of this concept, the recommended flap length (height)-to-base ratio should be no greater than 2:1 (Fig. 20-24).

Flap reflection

Once the planned flap design has been established by the initial and thinning incision(s), the following step is the atraumatic elevation of the flap. As previously described, a full-thickness flap is elevated using a sharp periosteal elevator directed beneath the periosteum, and

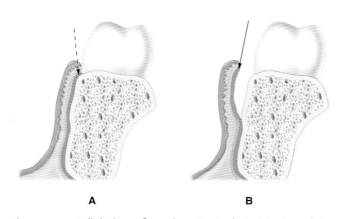

A   **B**

Figure 20-19. Full-thickness flap: schematic. *A*, The incision is made to bone. *B*, The periosteum (*P*) is reflected with the flap.

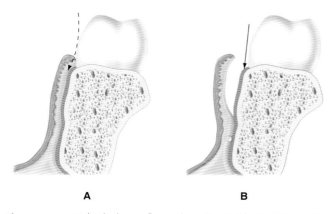

A   **B**

Figure 20-20. Split-thickness flap: schematic. *A*, The incision splits connective tissue. *B*, The periosteum (*P*) is retained over bone.

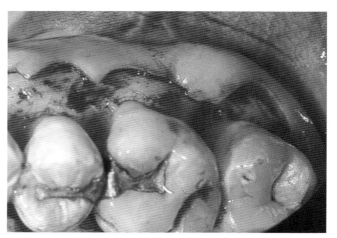

Figure 20-21. Envelope flap. Because no releasing incisions are used, the tissues remains attached to the teeth and alveolar bone anterior and posterior to the freed flap. The longer the flap, the less tension is placed on the envelope flap when it is retracted.

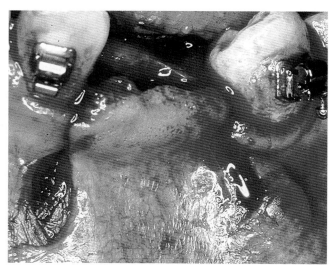

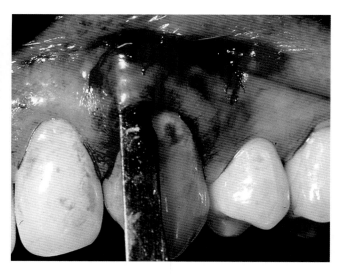

A   B

Figure 20-22. Pedicle flap. **A,** A pedicle flap incorporating two vertical releasing incisions. The blood supply is maintained at the base of the flap. This flap may be moved apically, coronally, or laterally. **B,** A semilunar pedicle flap incorporating a horizontal incision in the sulcus and a second horizontal incision in the vestibule. The blood supply to the flap is maintained laterally. This flap may be moved coronally to cover an exposed root surface.

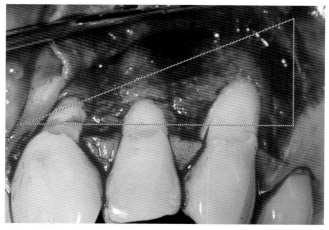

Figure 20-23. Triangular flap. One vertical releasing incision is used to create a triangular-shaped flap. This flap design provides greater access to underlying root and bone with less tension on the flap than the envelope flap.

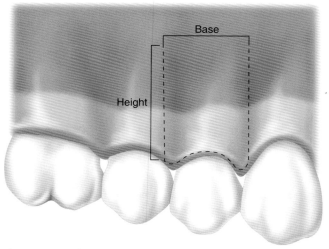

Figure 20-24. Flap height-to-base ratio. To maintain adequate blood supply to the flap, the ratio of flap height-to-flap base should not exceed 2:1.

always kept against the bone. Papillae are reflected first, followed by the marginal gingiva, working across the anterior/posterior extent of the incisions until the flap margin has been freed from the teeth or alveolar crest, or both (Fig. 20-25). This procedure should be accomplished using gentle force. If an abundance of force is required to gain release of the flap, the logical explanation is that the fibrous attachment to the underlying bone has not been completely severed. In such instances, it is

better to retrace the incision(s) with the surgical blade rather than risk tearing the flap. Once the flap margin has been completely released, the periosteal elevator is directed in both a horizontal and vertical plane until adequate access is achieved. It is imperative to follow the morphologic contours of the bone to avoid perforating the flap where the tissue may be thin, particularly when reflecting tissue over bony exostoses or ledges (Fig. 20-26).

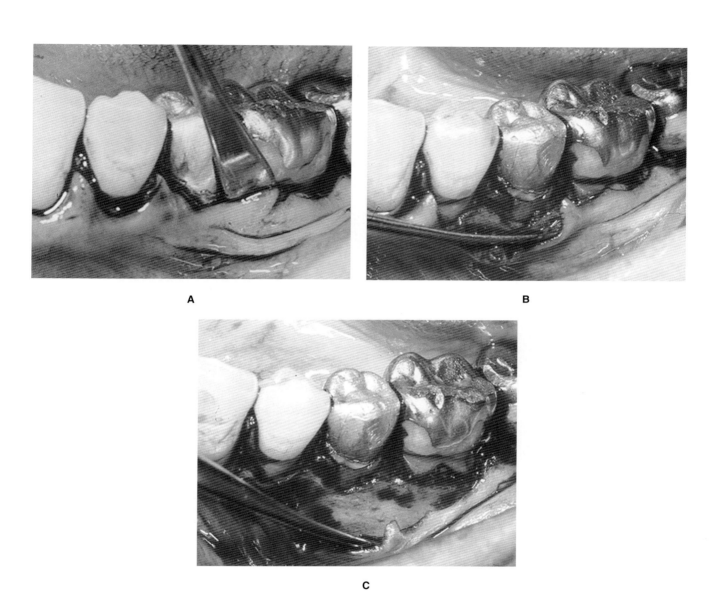

A   **B**

C

Figure 20-25. Flap reflection. **A,** Papillary reflection may be accomplished with a scalpel or with a periosteal or molt elevator. **B,** Marginal tissue reflection is completed with a sharp periosteal elevator or molt elevator. **C,** Flap is reflected apically, then retracted with a Prichard or Minnesota retractor.

In addition to flaps being classified as either full or partial thickness, and as envelope or pedicle, they are also referred to by the anatomic type of mucosa. A flap that includes only gingival tissue is referred to as a gingival flap (Fig. 20-27), whereas if the flap extends beyond the mucogingival junction to include alveolar mucosa, it is a mucogingival flap (see Fig. 20-25). Whether the flap extends to or beyond the mucogingival junction depends on how much access is needed to perform the required procedures. One of the greatest mistakes made by the novice surgeon is a lack of access to the surgical site, caused by inadequate flap reflection. This usually results in greater tissue trauma,

decreased treatment efficiency, and heightened therapist frustration.

Flap retraction

Another element in good flap management that is often given little consideration involves the use of surgical retractors to hold the flap back from the teeth and bone. If the flap has been properly designed and reflected adequately, retraction should be passive without any tension. Force should not be necessary to keep the flap retracted. It is also critically important that the edge of the retractor always be kept on bone (Fig. 20-28). Trapping the flap between the retractor and bone can

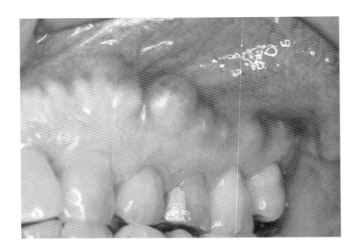

A

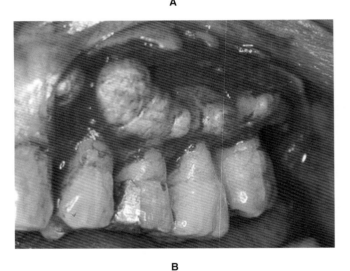

B

Figure 20-26. Reflection over exostoses. **A,** Pretreatment: prominent buccal exostoses provide a challenge to reflect the flap without tearing or perforating the tissue. **B,** Flap reflected without perforation or tearing.

cause tissue ischemia and lead to postoperative flap necrosis. Continuous flap retraction for long periods also is not advised. Such a practice will desiccate the soft tissue and bone causing a delay in wound healing. When the flap is retracted, the surgical assistant should frequently irrigate the surgical field with sterile saline, to keep the tissues moistened, to reduce contamination, and to improve visibility.

Open flap debridement

The prototypical periodontal flap surgery is called open flap debridement or flap curettage.[37] It is against this well established surgical technique that new surgical interventions in clinical trials are often compared. The rationale for this basic surgical approach is the same as all flap surgery:

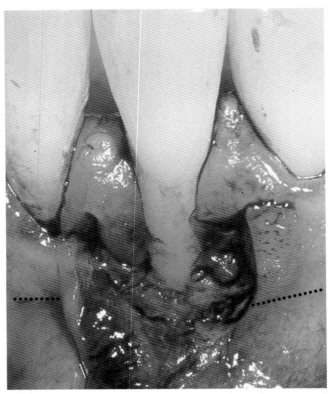

Figure 20-27. Gingival flap. Reflection to but not beyond mucogingival junction (*dotted line*).

to provide access to root surfaces and marginal alveolar bone. Direct visualization of these structures will increase the effectiveness of scaling and root planing and allow debridement of granulomatous tissue from osseous defects. Open flap debridement does not use resective techniques, osseous grafts, or barrier membranes to eliminate osseous defects. Simply stated, roots are planed,

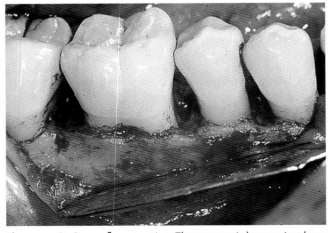

Figure 20-28. Proper flap retraction. The retractor is kept against bone to avoid trauma to the soft tissue.

defects are degranulated, and flaps are closed either at or apical to their original position. Access is initiated with either crevicular or step-back, inverse bevel incisions. Flaps are usually full thickness and reflected beyond the alveolar crest and mucogingival junction to fully expose the alveolar bone and osseous defect. Open flap debridement differs from the MWF procedure in the extent of flap reflection that is performed. Flap reflection with the MWF approach is only 2 to 3 mm beyond the alveolar crest and not beyond the mucogingival junction. Osteoplasty may be performed with either technique if necessary to improve flap adaptation before suturing. Although the MWF procedure dictates a replaced flap, the open flap curettage technique may incorporate replaced, coronally positioned, or apically positioned flaps, as described in the next section.

Flap positioning

Once the planned treatment has been completed, surgical flaps may be repositioned, apically positioned, coronally positioned, or laterally positioned. When possible, the decision as to the final location of the flap margin should be planned before the start of surgery. The final flap location is usually determined by the goal(s) of therapy and the specific periodontal surgical technique performed. A repositioned or replaced flap (Fig. 20-29) is in theory designed to be returned to its original position. It is used most often when surgical access for debridement of the roots is the primary goal, as in flap curettage or the MWF procedure. A repositioned flap also is frequently used in periodontal regeneration procedures where primary closure over a bone graft, with or without a barrier membrane, is of utmost importance. An apically positioned flap is one that is apically displaced from its original position to the level of the alveolar crest or about 1 mm coronal to the crest (Fig. 20-30). This position is chosen when performing "pocket elimination" procedures, which may or may not involve the removal of bone. The coronally positioned flap (Fig. 20-31) is advanced coronal to its original position. This technique is typically used when performing mucogingival surgery where the flap is advanced to cover either an exposed root, a connective tissue graft, or a barrier membrane. To achieve passive positioning of the coronally advanced flap before suturing, the underlying periosteum is released with a sharp scalpel blade (Fig. 20-16). Also used in mucogingival procedures is the laterally positioned flap. This involves the positioning of the flap to an adjacent or contiguous site for the purpose of increasing the width of keratinized tissue or covering of an exposed root (Fig. 20-32).

Hemostasis

Surgical hemostasis is divided into intraoperative and postoperative control of bleeding. Intraoperative hemostasis is essential if visualization of the operative field is to be

obtained. Although bleeding is to be expected when placing incisions and reflecting flaps, prevention of excessive blood loss is initially guarded against by obtaining a thorough preoperative medical history to rule out potential bleeding secondary to systemic disease or medications. In addition, to prevent excessive intraoperative bleeding, the surgeon must develop a sound knowledge of surgical anatomy, achieve adequate tissue health after initial therapy, and implement the principles of atraumatic flap management. Blood loss during periodontal flap surgery is highly variable. In 1977, Baab and colleagues[38] reported blood loss in the range of 16 to 592 ml with a mean of 134 ml. The duration of surgery and the amount of local anesthesia used were correlated with the amount of blood loss. Under normal circumstances, aspiration with a surgical suction should be sufficient to keep the surgical site clear of the limited amount of blood and saliva that appears.

Intraoperative bleeding is usually in the form of oozing from capillaries and small arterioles within the flap, or from nutrient canals and marrow spaces in the bone. If deemed excessive, this type of bleeding is best controlled with pressure using moist gauze for 2 to 5 minutes. Occasionally, a small artery may be the source of bleeding. If direct pressure is ineffective and the vessel can be isolated, vessel ligation using a resorbable suture is the best way to control the arterial bleeding. Another way to control bleeding from a flap is the use of a full-thickness suture at the base of the flap in an attempt to compress the tissues against the vessels. This deep suture technique is also useful when bleeding occurs after the harvest of a free soft tissue autograft from the palate. Placing a suture distal to the donor site will compress the greater palatine artery and provide hemostasis in the area (Fig. 20-33). Bleeding from bone can usually be stopped by burnishing the bone in the area of the bleed with a molt, elevator, or curet. If this is ineffective, bone wax can be compressed into the area of the bleed. Once bleeding is controlled, excess bone wax should be carefully removed to avoid possible delay of normal healing events.

A variety of topical hemostatic agents are available to control surgical bleeding (Table 20-7). Oxidized regenerated cellulose, absorbable collagen, and microfibrillar collagen hemostats act primarily as a lattice to physically promote and stabilize the blood clot through platelet aggregation. These agents usually come in the form of woven fabrics, porous sheets or cubes, or as fibrillar powder. Ferric sulfate acts as an astringent and protein precipitator capable of sealing small blood vessels. Although effective, it may be more irritating to the wound than other hemostatic agents and can possibly cause tattooing of the gingiva. Topical thrombin directly stimulates the formation of fibrin and may be used to control capillary

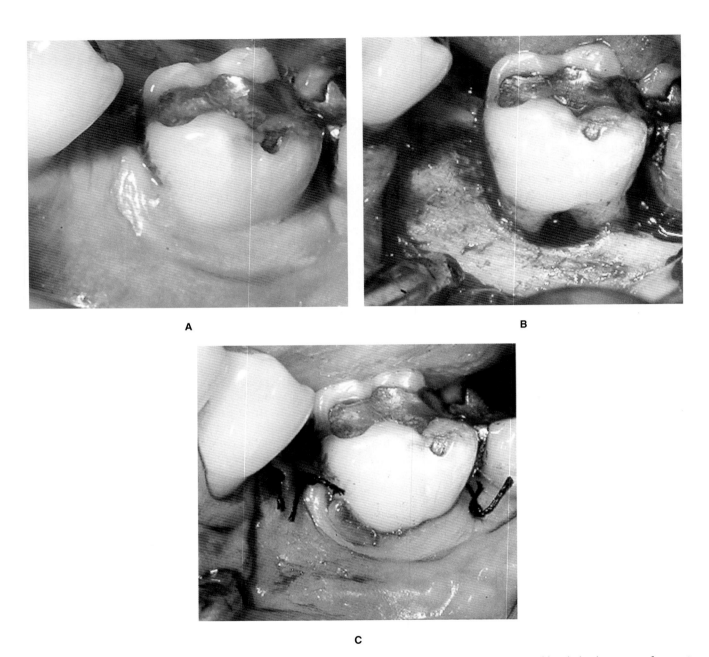

A

B

C

Figure 20-29. Repositioned (replaced) flap. **A,** Pretreatment. **B,** Deep Grade II furcation invasion. Treatment could include placing a graft or periodontal membrane, or both. **C,** Flap replaced to original position and sutured.

oozing. It is bovine derived and is usually applied as a liquid after hydration with sterile water or saline. Topical thrombin also may be used together with an absorbable gelatin sponge or as a dry powder. This hemostatic agent should only be applied topically and never injected into tissues or vessels.

The use of a local anesthetic with vasoconstrictors is a common technique to temporarily control minor intraoperative bleeding. It must be understood, however, that the action of vasoconstrictors is relatively short lived. Postoperative bleeding after the patient returns home may be an unfortunate event if local anesthetic infiltration is used to stop bleeding at the end of surgery. Direct pressure on the flaps for 5 minutes should be the first means to obtain hemostasis at the conclusion of a surgical procedure. If bleeding persists, the use of hemostatic agents other than local anesthetic with a vasoconstrictor is indicated. Under no circumstances should the patient

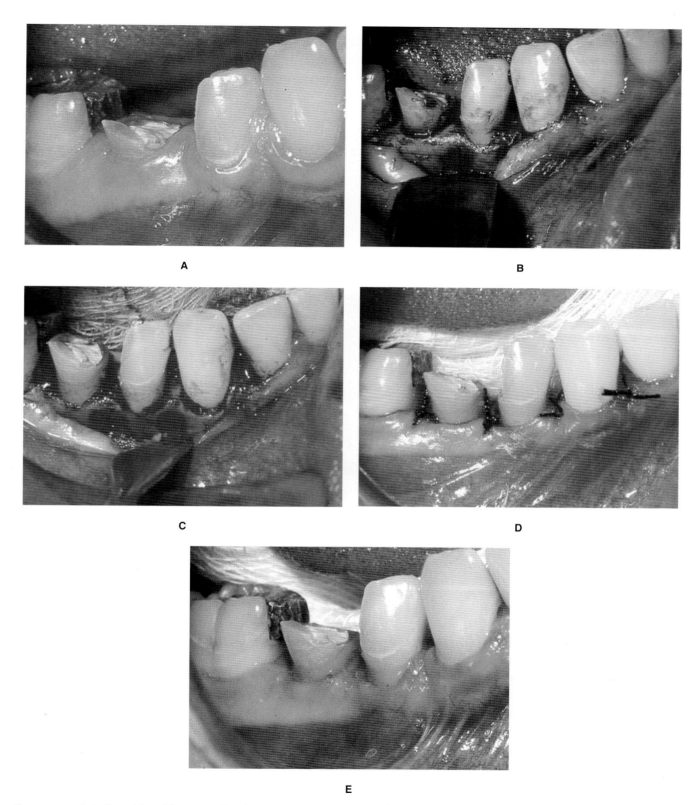

Figure 20-30. Apically positioned flap: crown lengthening. **A,** Pretreatment. **B,** Before osseous resection. **C,** After osseous resection. **D,** Flap apically positioned and sutured. **E,** Three months after treatment.

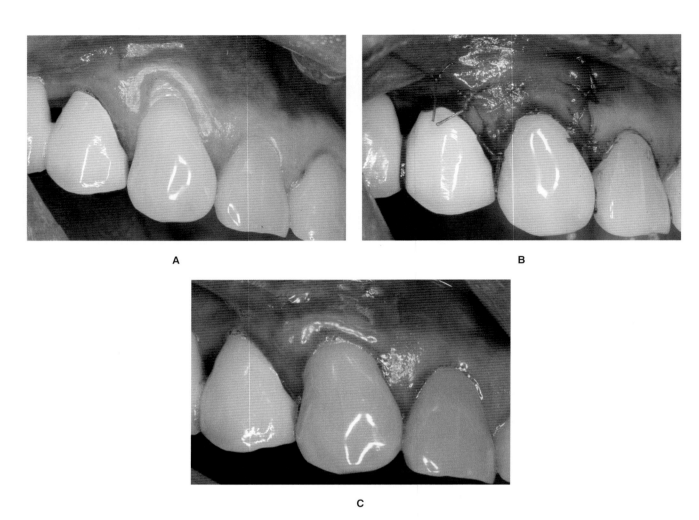

Figure 20-31. Coronally positioned flap. **A,** Pretreatment with gingival recession. **B,** Flap sutured at the level of the cementoenamel junction. **C,** Three months after treatment.

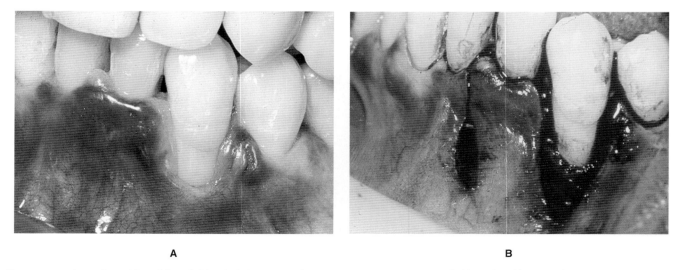

Figure 20-32. Laterally positioned flap. **A,** Marginal tissue recession over canine at pretreatment. **B,** Vertical and horizontal incisions.

Continued

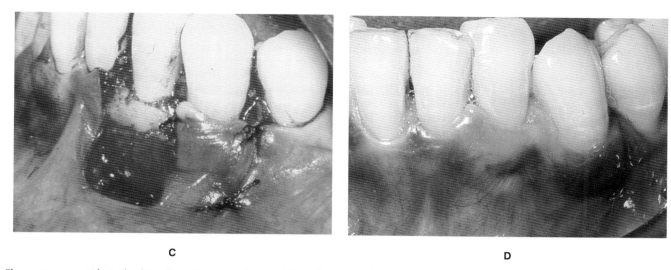

C

D

Figure 20-32. cont'd C, Flap laterally positioned and sutured. **D,** Eighteen months after treatment. Note decreased melanin at donor site.

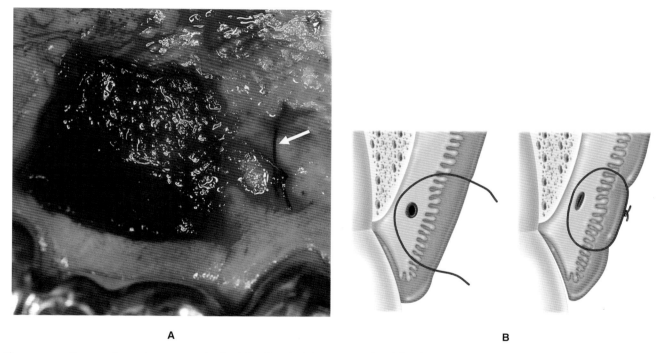

A

B

Figure 20-33. Compression suture to control palatal bleeding. **A,** A deep suture placed distal to the donor site will compress soft tissues against the greater palatine artery to aid in hemostasis after the harvest of a free soft tissue autograft. **B,** Cross-sectional schematic demonstrating compression of soft tissue against the artery causing mechanical constriction of the vessel lumen.

be allowed to leave if significant bleeding is evident. Nausea from ingesting blood, hematoma formation under the flaps with delayed healing, and increased susceptibility to infection are likely sequelae of excessive postoperative bleeding.

Suturing

As important as incision placement and atraumatic flap management are to the outcome of the surgical procedure, flap adaptation and stabilization at the end of the procedure are equally important. After any necessary

TABLE 20-7   Hemostatic Agents

AGENT	BRAND NAMES/DESCRIPTION	USE
Absorbable oxidized regenerated cellulose	SURGICEL (Johnson & Johnson, Somerville, NJ): loosely woven or knitted fabric strips SURGICEL Fibrillar: in form of cotton wisps SURGICEL NU-KNIT: thicker denser woven fabric	Apply dry; acts as scaffold for platelet aggregation and clot stability; quickly loses integrity in blood or saliva; manufacturer claims it is bactericidal; not recommended for implantation in bone defects unless removed before flap closure; should stop bleeding in 2-8 min, absorbed in 7-14 days
Absorbable gelatin sponge	Gelfoam (Pfizer, Cambridge, MA): purified porcine skin (powder or cubes)	Use dry or hydrate with saline; acts as scaffold for platelet aggregation and clot stability
Absorbable collagen	INSTAT (Johnson & Johnson, Somerville, NJ): lyophilized bovine dermal collagen (sponge pad) CollaTape, CollaCote, CollaPlug (Integra LifeScience, Plainsboro, NJ): bovine deep flexor tendon (sheet, thicker sponge, or 1- × 2-cm plug)	Apply dry or hydrated with saline directly to bleeding surface with pressure; acts as scaffold for platelet aggregation and clot stability; maintains integrity in presence of blood; hemostasis achieved in 2-5 min. Excess should be removed.
Absorbable microfibrillar collagen	INSTAT MCH: bovine deep flexor tendon (fibers) Avitene (C.R. Bard, Inc., Murray Hill, NJ): bovine corium collagen (sheet or fibrous powder [flour])	These agents act as a scaffold for platelet aggregation and are applied dry. Microfibrillar form allows application to irregularly shaped bleeding sites. Excess should be removed before closure of flaps.
Topical thrombin	Thrombostat (Pfizer, Cambridge, MA): lyophilized, derived from bovine blood	Use as liquid or powder; may use on an absorbable gelatin or collagen sponge
Ferric sulfate	Monsel's Solution: 20% ferric subsulfate	Astringent and protein precipitate sealing blood vessels; irritating to wound; may delay healing and cause tattooing
Bone wax	Bone Wax (Ethicon) (Johnson & Johnson, Somerville, NJ): semisynthetic beeswax and isopropyl palmitate	Pressed into nutrient canal, acts as mechanical plug; remove excess before flap closure, do not use in areas where bone regeneration is desired.

final recontouring and thinning of gingival tissues, the flaps are placed passively in position. The surgeon must not rely on sutures to pull the flap beyond its passive positioning, as tension is created on the flap. Such tension potentially interferes with blood supply to the gingiva and increases the likelihood of the sutures pulling through the tissues, thereby hindering wound stability. The result may be necrosis of the marginal portion of the flap and delayed healing.

Selection of the type of suture material and needle is dependent on tissue type and thickness, location in the mouth, ease of handling, cost, and the planned time of suture removal. Table 20-8 lists the suture and needle types that are commonly used in periodontal surgery.

TABLE 20-8   **Suture Materials, Needle Designs**

SUTURE MATERIAL	INDICATION	TISSUE REACTION	EASE OF HANDLING	TENSILE STRENGTH
Nonabsorbable				
• Surgical silk	General purpose; used in keratinized tissue	High	Good	Fair
• Expanded polytetra-fluoroethylene (ePTFE; Gore-Tex)	Guided tissue regeneration	Minimal	Fair	Good
Absorbable				
• Surgical gut (plain)	General purpose, gingiva and mucosa	Moderate	Fair	Poor, half-life of 5-6 days
• Surgical gut (chromic)	General purpose; gingiva and mucosa	Moderate	Fair	Poor, half-life of 14 days
• Polyglactin 910 (Coated Vicryl)	General purpose	Minimal	Good	Good, half-life of 2-3 weeks; absorbed in 56-70 days
• Poliglecaprone 25 (Monocryl)	General purpose	Minimal	Good	Fair, absorbed in 91-119 days
Needles				
• P-3	Anterior regions (narrower buccolingual interdental dimension); mucosa; mucogingival procedures			
• FS-2	Posterior regions (wider buccolingual interdental dimension)			
• G-6 (micropoint)	Periodontal plastic surgery			

There is a trend toward the use of smaller suture material and needle diameters. This trend is consistent with the desire to avoid flap trauma and minimize disruption of the remaining blood supply to the flap.

Table 20-9 lists some of the many suturing techniques that are used to secure periodontal flaps. Technique selection is determined primarily by the final flap position, the surgical procedure, and the ease of placement. The interrupted suture is the most common type of suture placed. It works well if both the facial and lingual flaps require similar amounts of tension and heights (Fig. 20-34). Interrupted sutures may be used when flaps are replaced or coronally positioned.

Sling sutures allow positioning of the facial or lingual flap independent of the opposing flap (Fig. 20-35). For example, the sling suture can provide coronal positioning of the facial flap while replacing or apically positioning the lingual flap. Individual sling sutures also work well to secure a laterally positioned pedicle graft around the cervical aspect of the recipient tooth and to secure periodontal barrier membranes around teeth. Continuous or double continuous sling (Fig. 20-36) sutures are used when an entire sex-

tant or quadrant is being sutured. Similar to the single tooth sling suture, these continuous sutures allow opposing flaps to be positioned independently of each other.

External mattress sutures are useful in areas where it is advantageous to keep the bulk of the suture material outside the flap. If interproximal intrabony defects are treated with bone grafts, the external mattress eliminates or minimizes the amount of suture in contact with the graft material. In addition, mattress sutures can better control positioning of the papilla without creating additional tension on the papilla tip. Vertical mattress sutures are better suited for narrower interdental areas (Fig. 20-37), whereas horizontal mattress sutures work well in broader interdental areas (Fig. 20-38). Both of these sutures are frequently incorporated into a double continuous sling suturing technique. Internal mattress sutures are used when it is desirable to have the papilla positioned more upright in the embrasure space (Fig. 20-39). These sutures may be used in anterior regions when esthetics ideally require that the papilla fill the entire interdental area.

Suspensory sutures are best suited to isolated areas where coronal positioning of the flap is required. This type

TABLE 20-9	Suture Techniques
TECHNIQUE	**INDICATIONS**
Interrupted (Fig. 20-34)	Closure of vertical releasing incisions and interproximal areas; replaced and coronally positioned flap closure
Sling (Fig. 20-35)	Allows separate facial or lingual flap positioning in isolated areas
Continuous sling	Single suture to close sextant or quadrant, allows facial and lingual flaps to be closed independently
Double continuous sling (Fig. 20-37)	Apically positioned flap closure, allows facial and lingual flaps to be closed independently
External mattress	Reduces amount of suture under the flap; allows papilla closure over osseous grafts without the suture running through the graft; enhances positioning of the papilla
Vertical (Fig. 20-37)	Narrower interdental spaces
Horizontal (Fig. 20-38)	Wider interdental spaces
Internal mattress (Fig. 20-39)	Anterior interdental areas, knot may be tied on the lingual or palate to improve esthetics; edentulous areas in combination with interrupted sutures to reduce tension on the incision line
Suspensory (Fig. 20-40)	Coronally advanced flaps, useful for root coverage techniques
Anchoring (Fig. 20-41)	Useful in guided tissue regeneration when an adjacent edentulous space is present, achieves primary closure over barrier membranes or bone grafts on the mesial or distal of a tooth
Laurell Loop (Fig. 20-42)	Used in guided tissue regeneration to close over an interproximal barrier membrane

of suture occasionally is used to help stabilize a coronally advanced flap used to treat a recession defect (Fig. 20-40).

The anchoring suture can be used on the distal or mesial of a tooth adjacent to an edentulous space or the retromolar area. This suture is useful when bone grafts or barrier membranes are placed, because it achieves intimate adaptation of the flaps to the mesial or distal surface of the tooth and provides primary closure of the incision (Fig. 20-41).

Another suture that is useful to achieve primary closure over periodontal membranes is the Laurell Loop suture, also known as the vertical sling mattress suture.[39] This suture incorporates an internal mattress type suture that crosses back over the top of the interproximal papilla, through a loop on the lingual, then over the papilla again, and secured on the facial surface (Fig. 20-42). The Laurell Loop suture works well to bring the facial and lingual papillae together when guided tissue regeneration is performed in interproximal sites.

Regardless of the type of suture or technique selected, the following principles of suturing should be followed: (1) use the smallest diameter and least reactive material possible; (2) leave a minimum amount of suture material under the flap; (3) take adequate bites of tissue making sure not to place sutures too close to incision lines or papilla tips; (4) place sutures in keratinized tissue when possible; (5) pass the suture from movable tissue to nonmovable tissue; (6) place suture knots at the side of the incision line, rather than directly over the incision; and (7) remove the sutures carefully and as soon as they stop aiding in wound stability.

Once the flaps are sutured, pressure should be applied to the flaps for 4 or 5 minutes. This will eliminate dead space between the flap, the bone, and the roots. The objective with pressure application is to ensure adequate hemostasis and to prevent hematoma formation and wound separation.

Wound Management

Wound management is a crucial aspect of periodontal surgical therapy. Meticulous surgical technique is not sufficient to prevent delayed or inadequate healing if poor wound management occurs. Postoperative wound stability is paramount for the desired surgical outcome to be achieved. Adequate flap adaptation, obliteration of dead space under the flap, control of postoperative swelling, and carefully explained postoperative instructions are key elements in achieving a stable wound.

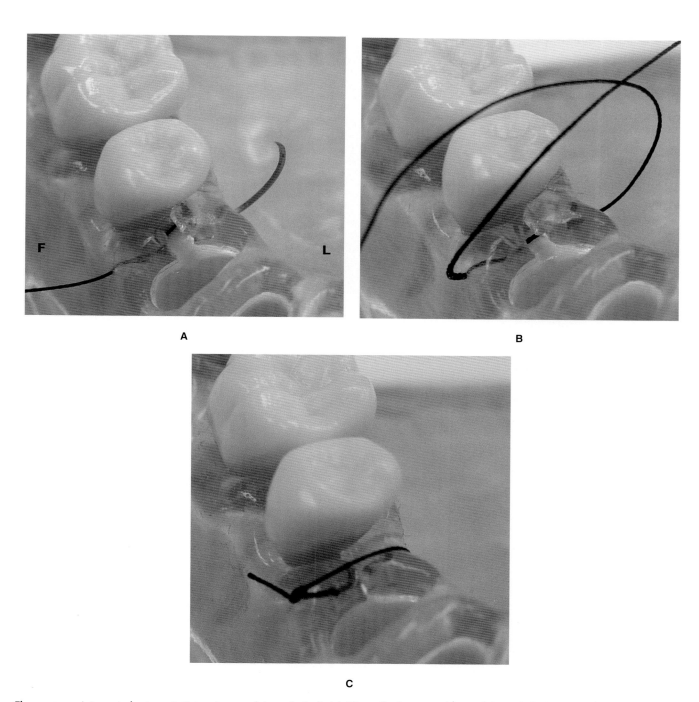

Figure 20-34. Interrupted suture. **A,** Suture is passed through the facial (*F*) papilla from outside-in and through the lingual (*L*) papilla from inside-out. The needle should enter the tissue just coronal to the mucogingival junction. On the palate, the needle should be passed through the tissue several millimeters apical to the base of the papilla. **B,** After passage of the needle through the lingual tissue, the suture is pulled until only 2 or 3 cm of suture material is left outside the facial tissues. **C,** The suture is tied securely without creating excessive tension on the flap.

Periodontal dressings

At periodontal dressing or pack is a protective material applied over a wound created by periodontal surgical procedures. It is most often used to assist in flap adaptation where there are postoperative variations in tissue levels.

Most periodontal dressings currently in use are eugenol-free and are either a two-paste chemical cure material containing zinc oxide, mineral oils, rosin and bacteriostatic, or fungicidal agents (Coe-Pak—GC America, Inc., Alsip, IL; PerioCare—Pulpdent Corp, Watertown, MA), or a visible

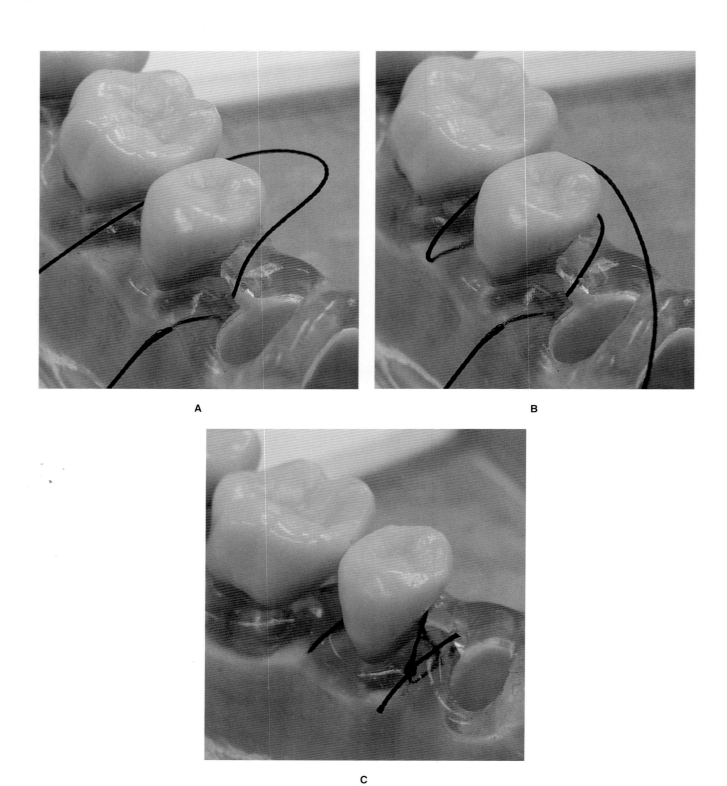

A

B

C

Figure 20-35. Sling suture. **A,** Suture is passed through the facial from outside-in and looped around the lingual of the tooth. The suture does not enter the lingual flap. **B,** The suture is passed through the other facial papilla from the inside-out and looped back around the lingual of the tooth. **C,** The suture is tied securely without creating excess tension on the flap.

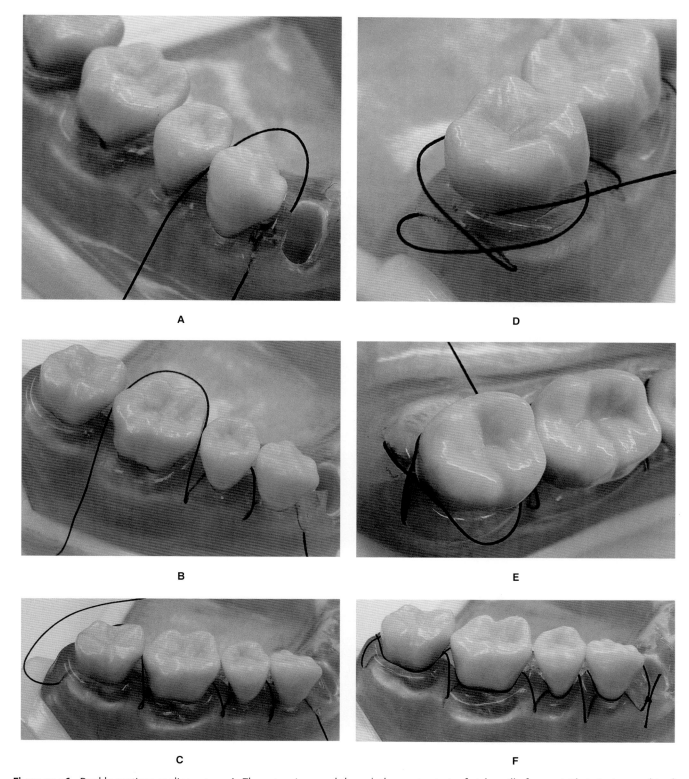

Figure 20-36. Double continuous sling suture. **A,** The suture is passed through the most anterior facial papilla from outside-in just coronal to the mucogingival junction and looped around the lingual of the tooth to engage the next facial papilla. The suture does not enter the lingual flap at this time. **B,** The suture is looped around each successive tooth, penetrating the facial papillae just coronal to the mucogingival junction. **C,** At the distal end of the flap, the suture is passed through the facial tissue and looped back around the lingual of the terminal tooth and through the interdental area mesial to the terminal tooth. The suture is then slung around the facial surface of the terminal tooth toward the distal aspect of the lingual flap. Wrapping the suture around the terminal tooth in this fashion allows the facial flap to be locked in placed and positioned independently of the lingual or palatal flap. **D,** The needle is passed through the most distal aspect of the lingual or palatal flap. The suture is then looped back around the facial surface of the terminal tooth. **E,** The suture is passed through the interdental area to engage the next papilla on the lingual or palatal flap. **F,** The lingual flap is sutured in a similar manner as the facial flap. The suture is tied anteriorly where the suture was initially introduced into the facial tissue.

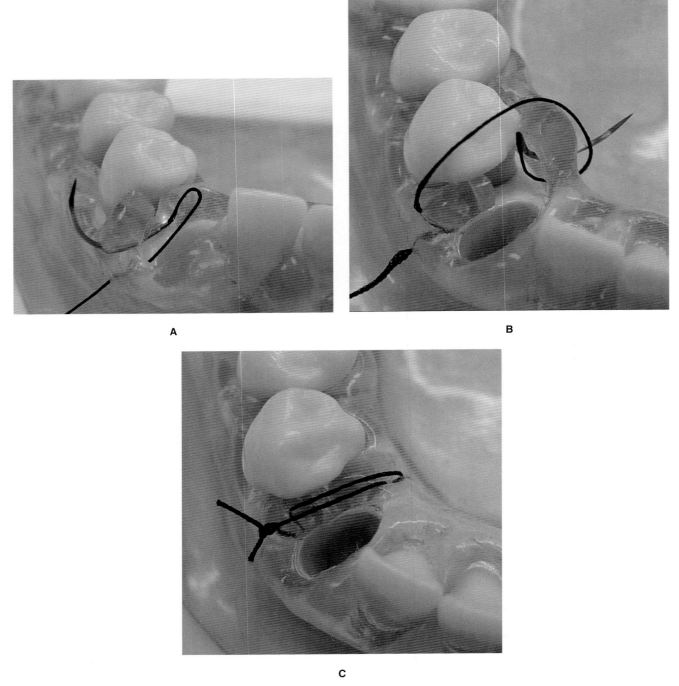

A

B

C

Figure 20-37. External mattress suture (vertical). The external mattress keeps much of the suture material on the outside of the flap. It provides greater stability and positioning of the papilla without placing the suture too close to the tip of the papilla. **A,** Vertical mattress sutures are used in narrower interdental areas when greater control of the papilla tip is required. The suture penetrates the facial papilla just above the mucogingival junction from outside-in. The papilla is stabilized with tissue forceps and the needle is passed from inside-out 2 to 3 mm coronal to the initial suture penetration. **B,** The needle and suture are passed through the lingual (or palatal) papilla in a similar fashion as the facial papilla (from outside-in near the mucogingival junction then inside-out, 2 to 3 mm coronal to the previous suture entry point). **C,** The suture is gently tightened bringing the facial and lingual papilla together. The knot is secured on the facial. Note that the majority of the suture material lies on top of the flaps.

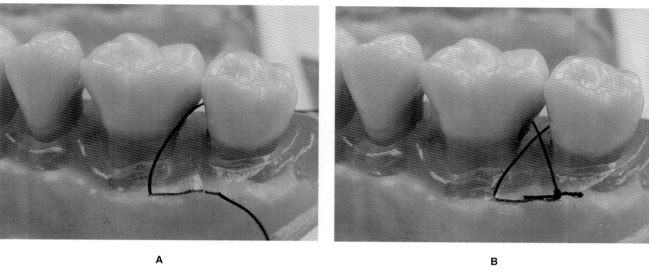

A   B

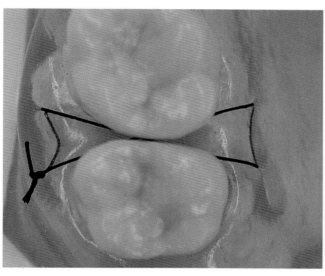

C

Figure 20-38. External mattress suture (horizontal). Horizontal mattress sutures are used in wide embrasure areas to give better control over the papilla tip or in the anterior area to avoid compressing the papilla tips. **A,** The suture penetrates the facial papilla from the outside-in just above the mucogingival junction at the distal aspect of the papilla. The papilla is stabilized with forceps and the needle is passed from the inside-out at a point on the mesial aspect of the papilla along a horizontal plane even with the distal needle puncture. The suture passes through the embrasure space and the suture needle is passed through the lingual tissue in a similar fashion. **B,** The suture crisscrosses over the top of the papilla and is secured on the facial. **C,** Occlusal view of the horizontal external mattress suture.

Continued

light-cured gel, composed of polyether urethane dimethacrylate resin and silanated silica (Barricaid, Dentsply International, Milford, DE) (Fig. 20-43). Cyanoacrylate also has been used as a dressing, especially over free soft tissue autografts. Because cyanoacrylate has not received U.S. Food and Drug Administration approval for this use, it is not discussed in this section. The two-paste dressings are either hand mixed or automixed

with a multiuse cartridge and a single use mixing tip. Both types of dressings rely on a mechanical lock into the embrasure space for retention. When the embrasure spaces are filled with soft tissue, these dressings have a tendency to loosen and displace rather easily. If wound stability is a rationale for dressing placement, their use in these instances may be counter-productive. Barricaid is somewhat more adhesive to the surface of the teeth if applied to

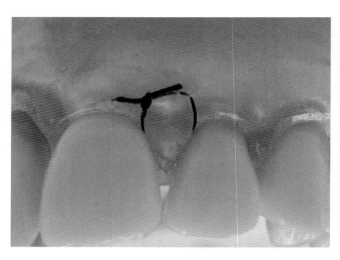

D

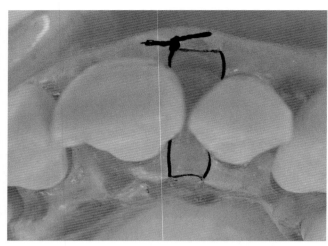

E

Figure 20-38. cont'd D, The horizontal mattress suture may be used in the anterior area placing the suture on either side of the papilla. This will allow the papillary tissue to stay upright filling the embrasure space. **E,** Occlusal view of horizontal mattress suture used in the anterior region.

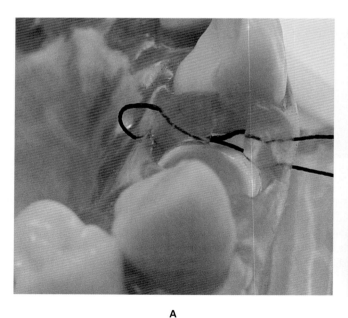

A

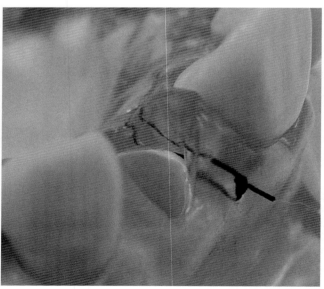

B

Figure 20-39. Internal mattress suture. The internal mattress suture allows both the facial and lingual (or palatal) papillae to stay upright, filling the embrasure space in an esthetic area. **A,** The suture enters the facial tissue just apical to the base of the papilla, runs across the top of the alveolar crest, and penetrates the lingual tissue from the inside-out apical to the base of the lingual papilla. The suture passes back through the lingual papilla from the outside-in, 2 to 3 mm coronal to the previous point of suture penetration, and courses back across the alveolar crest exiting through the facial papilla from the inside-out at a point 2 to 3 mm coronal to the initial facial entry point. **B,** The facial and lingual papillae are positioned together and the suture is tied on the facial. Note that the majority of the suture material lies under the flap in the interdental area.

Continued

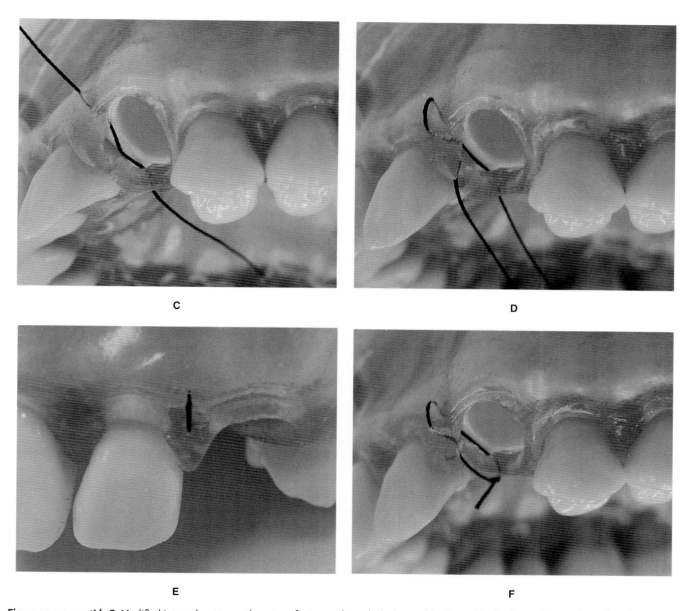

Figure 20-39. cont'd C, Modified internal mattress: the suture first goes through the base of the lingual (palatal) papilla outside-in, then through the base of the facial papilla inside-out, penetrating just coronal to the mucogingival junction. **D,** Modified internal mattress: the suture is then passed through the facial papilla outside-in, 2 to 3 mm coronal to the previously placed suture. At this point the suture does not penetrate the lingual (palatal) papilla again, as it would in a conventional internal mattress. Instead, it is tied to the tail on the lingual aspect. **E,** Modified internal mattress, facial view: suture placement through the facial papilla is a conventional vertical internal mattress. The facial papilla remains upright. **F,** Modified internal mattress: suture placement on the lingual (palatal) is like a conventional interrupted suture. The lingual papilla is positioned apically and the suture is secured on the lingual.

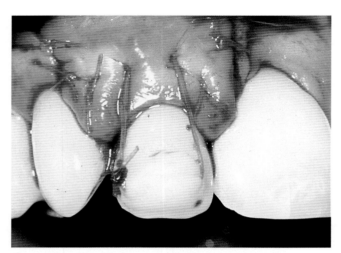

Figure 20-40. Suspensory suture. This technique is used to secure a coronally advanced flap. The suture enters and exits the flap similarly to a horizontal mattress suture and is secured on the coronal aspect of the crown with light cured composite.

dry surfaces. However, these dressings still require a mechanical lock to remain nonmobile during the first 7 to 10 days of healing. An advantage of Barricaid is its translucent gingival coloring making it more suitable for use in esthetic areas than the white or pink paste dressings.

The value of placing periodontal dressings after surgery is controversial. Stated benefits include improved flap adaptation to the underlying bone and root surface, control of immediate postoperative bleeding, wound protection, and immobilization, to help retain osseous graft materials, patient comfort, and temporary splinting of mobile teeth. The effectiveness of periodontal dressings in achieving these proposed benefits is highly variable, and the decision to use or not use dressings appears to be based more on clinical experience and training than on sound evidence-based rationale. Periodontal dressings still have a place in postoperative wound management for many therapists, but the surgeon should focus on good surgical technique and thorough postoperative instructions to provide stable flap adaptation, hemostasis, and patient comfort, rather than relying on surgical dressings to produce the desired outcome.

The decision of when and what type of dressing to use varies greatly from one provider to another. Dressings may be most useful when flaps are apically positioned, in mandibular areas treated with a distal wedge, or after gingivectomy procedures. When flaps are apically positioned, the embrasure spaces are opened, allowing a secure mechanical lock of the dressing. This provides for a stable dressing and prevents the pack from dislodging during the first week of healing. Flaps in the area distal to mandibular second molars are difficult to keep in close approximation to the underlying bone. If a resective approach is used, pocket reduction in these areas could be less than ideal if the tissues

elevate during healing. A periodontal dressing is beneficial to help keep the tissues well adapted to the bone and may improve the predictability for pocket reduction after distal wedge procedures in the mandibular retromolar area.

The use of dressings after gingivectomy procedures is primarily for patient comfort and, to a limited extent, as an aid with hemostasis. The broad wound created by the external bevel incision is notoriously painful. Covering this wound with a dressing can provide some level of comfort, but this varies from patient to patient. If a dressing is placed in the posterior region where esthetics are not a concern, a paste dressing is relatively easy to apply and is often the first choice of dressing. It must be placed while pliable or too much pressure will be exerted on the flap and the blood supply may be jeopardized. In the anterior region, Barricaid provides for a reasonably esthetic dressing.

Postoperative instructions

It is imperative that surgery patients receive thorough verbal and written postoperative instructions before they are released. Patient comfort, wound stability, and plaque control are the three most important considerations during the postoperative phase. Patient comfort and wound stability are provided through a combination of good surgical and suturing techniques and careful postoperative care of the surgical site. In addition, patient discomfort can be controlled with a variety of nonsteroidal or narcotic pain medications, or both. The patient is instructed not to chew or to use mechanical plaque control in the area of surgery until told otherwise. This is usually 10 to 14 days for most flap and gingivectomy procedures, with the exception of guided tissue regeneration and hard or soft tissue grafting surgery. After such procedures, wound stability is important for at least 4 to 6 weeks. To reduce plaque formation during this crucial healing period, a 0.12% chlorhexidine mouthrinse used twice a day is recommended and should be continued until mechanical plaque control is reinstituted in the surgical area. All areas away from the surgical site should be cleansed with normal brushing and interdental plaque control measures.

After surgery, rest and proper nutrition should be stressed to the patient. The diet should be restricted to soft foods and liquids for the first 24 to 48 hours. Chewing should be limited to the side of the mouth opposite the surgical site. Swelling in the area of surgery is to be expected but can be minimized with good surgical technique and intermittent application of an ice pack for the first 8 to 10 hours after surgery. Although smoking is not an absolute contraindication to periodontal surgery, it is a detriment to wound healing and a negative influence on the overall outcome of surgical therapy. (See Chapter 34.) Those surgical patients who have elected to continue smoking must be encouraged to stop the habit during the postoperative healing phase.

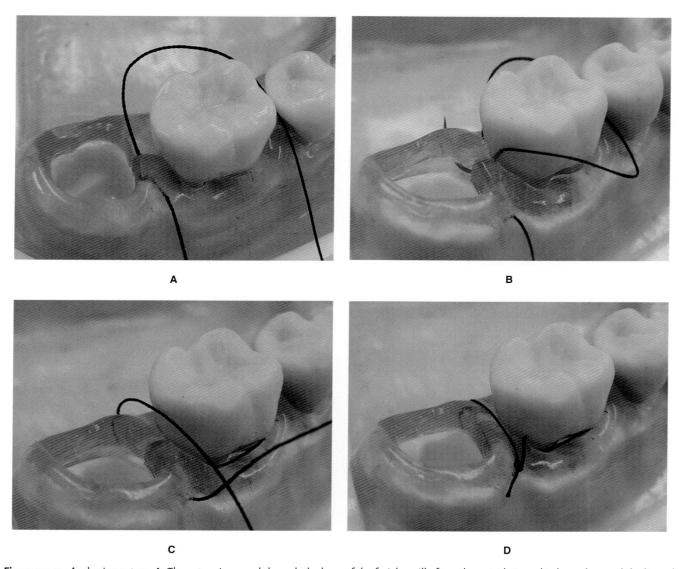

Figure 20-41. Anchoring suture. **A,** The suture is passed through the base of the facial papilla from the outside-in and is looped around the lingual of the tooth, through the interdental space. **B,** The suture loops completely around the adjacent tooth and penetrates the lingual papilla from the inside-out. **C,** The suture crosses over the top of the papilla. As tension is placed on the suture, the papillae are drawn together and toward the proximal surface of the adjacent tooth. This eliminates gaps between the flaps at the proximal tooth surface. **D,** The suture is secured on the facial.

The first postoperative visit is usually 7 to 10 days after surgery. Patient comfort, edema, and tissue healing are assessed. If used, the periodontal dressing is removed and the surgical site is debrided with an antimicrobial solution on a cotton tip applicator. A combination of 0.12% chlorhexidine and 3% peroxide diluted in half with water is useful for mechanical and chemical debridement of the area. If sutures are no longer providing stabilization of the gingival tissues, they are carefully removed at this first postoperative visit. If the sutures are still providing wound stability, they may be left in place and removed at the next postoperative appointment. Additional supragingival plaque removal is accomplished atraumatically with a curet or a rubber cup, or both. If the gingival tissues have been apically positioned at the time of surgery, mechanical plaque control can be instituted 10 to 14 days after surgery. If guided tissue regeneration procedures were performed, the patient

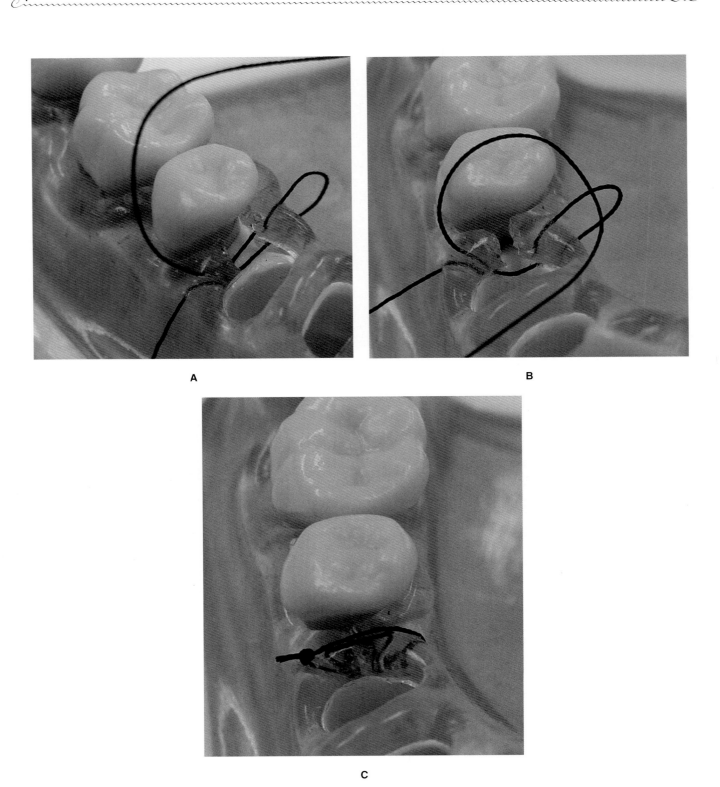

Figure 20-42. Laurell Loop suture. **A,** The suture is passed through the facial and lingual papillae as an internal mattress suture. Instead of being tied on the facial aspect at this point, a loop in the suture is formed on the lingual. **B,** The suture is passed over the top of the papillae toward the lingual, through the lingual loop and back over the top of the papilla toward the facial. **C,** Tension is applied to the suture bringing the flaps and the papillae together and the suture is secured on the facial.

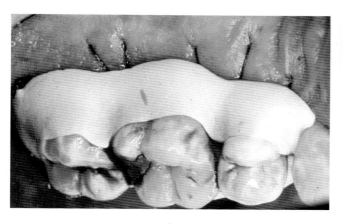

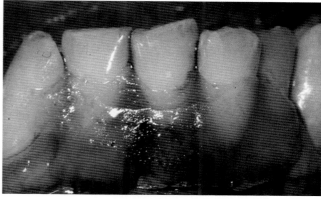

A

B

Figure 20-43. Periodontal dressing. **A,** Coe-Pak (GC America, Inc.; Alsip, IL) dressing is formed into a small roll, looped around the terminal tooth, and gently pressed in place with lateral pressure. Engaging interdental undercuts provides mechanical retention of the dressing. This can easily be accomplished by using a moist cotton tip applicator or curets. **B,** Barricaid (Dentsply International; Milford, DE) dressing is placed as a viscous gel and light cured. It provides a more esthetic dressing for anterior areas.

should continue with chemical plaque control using a 0.12% chlorhexidine rinse until adequate mechanical plaque control can take place in 4 to 6 weeks.

At the second postoperative visit (14 to 21 days after surgery), tissue healing and oral hygiene are assessed. Supragingival prophylaxis is completed as needed. If thermal sensitivity or root caries is a concern, a fluoride gel should be prescribed for daily use. It should be noted that the above procedures are only guidelines. Postoperative care frequently varies from patient to patient based on the type of surgery, wound healing, and the patient's ability to achieve an acceptable level of oral hygiene. The postoperative phase usually lasts 1 to 6 months in most cases. Once wound healing is complete, the patient may enter maintenance therapy.

CONCLUSION

Knowledge of the patient's medical status, surgical anatomy, and basic surgical principles will allow the surgeon to perform safe and effective periodontal surgery. Every surgical procedure must have an end-point in mind before the initiation of treatment. With experience, the mechanics required to reach that surgical end-point are relatively straightforward. The true challenge facing the clinician is determining if the treatment approach selected will predictably achieve the overall therapeutic goals of a healthy, stable, and maintainable dentition over an extended period. With the current emphasis on evidence-based periodontal therapy, scientific knowledge, when available, should become the primary driving force in therapeutic and surgical decision making. Clinical judg-

ment, personal experience, and patient preferences are still valuable entities in this decision-making process, but they must be integrated with sound science to improve the predictability, quality, and efficiency of periodontal care.

Acknowledgments

The authors would like to acknowledge the photographic contributions of many of the former and current teaching staff and residents of the United States Air Force Periodontics Residency Program.

REFERENCES

1. Caffesse RG, Sweeney PL, Smith BA: Scaling and root planing with and without periodontal flap surgery, *J Clin Periodontol* 13:205-210, 1986.
2. Brayer WK, Mellonig JT, Dunlop RM et al: Scaling and root planing effectiveness: the effect of root surface access and operator experience, *J Periodontol* 60:67-72, 1989.
3. Matia JI, Bissada NF, Maybury JE, Ricchetti J: Efficiency of scaling and root planing of the molar furcation area with and without surgical access, *Int J Periodontics Restorative Dent* 6:24-35, 1986.
4. Fleischer HC, Mellonig JT, Brayer WK et al: Scaling and root planing efficacy in multirooted teeth, *J Periodontol* 60:402-409, 1989.
5. Wylam J, Mealey BL, Mills MP et al: Effectiveness of open versus closed scaling and root planing, *J Periodontol* 64: 1023-1028, 1993.
6. Yukna RA, Lawrence JJ: Gingival surgery for soft tissue new attachment, *Dent Clin North Am* 24:705-718, 1980.

7. Ramfjord SP, Nissel RR: The modified Widman flap, *J Periodontol* 45:601-607, 1974.

8. Ramjord SP: Present status of the modified Widman flap procedure, *J Periodontol* 48:558-565, 1977.

9. Bowen W, Bowers G, Berquist J, Organ R: Removal of pocket epithelium in humans utilizing an internally beveled incision, *Int J Periodontics Restorative Dent* 2:9-19, 1981.

10. Fisher M, Bowers G, Berquist J: Effectiveness of reverse bevel incision used in the modified Widman flap procedure in removing pocket epithelium in humans, *Int J Periodontics Restorative Dent* 3:33-43, 1982.

11. Litch JM, O'Leary TJ, Kafrawy AH: Pocket epithelium removal via crestal and subcrestal scalloped internal beveled incisions, *J Periodontol* 55:142-148, 1984.

12. Pippin DJ: Fate of pocket epithelium in an apically positioned flap, *J Clin Periodontol* 17:385-391, 1990.

13. Svoboda P, Reeve C, Sheridan P: Effect of retention of gingival sulcular epithelium on attachment and pocket depth after periodontal surgery, *J Periodontol* 55:563-566, 1984.

14. Smith BA, Echeverri M, Caffesse RG: Mucoperiosteal flaps with and without removal of the pocket epithelium, *J Periodontol* 58:78-85, 1987.

15. Waerhaug J: Healing of the dentoepithelial junction following subgingival plaque control. II. As observed on extracted teeth, *J Periodontol* 49:119-134, 1978.

16. Kho P, Smales FC, Hardie JM: The effect of supragingival plaque control on the subgingival microflora, *J Clin Periodontol* 12:676-686, 1985.

17. Beltrami M, Bickel M, Baehni PC: The effect of supragingival plaque control on the composition of subgingival microflora in human periodontitis, *J Clin Periodontol* 14:161-164, 1987.

18. Katsanoulas T, Reneè I, Attström R: The effect of supragingival plaque control on the composition of the subgingival flora in periodontal pockets, *J Clin Periodontol* 19:760-765, 1992.

19. Badersten A, Nilveus K, Kiger R: Scores of plaque, bleeding, suppuration, and probing depth to predict probing attachment loss: 5 years of observation following nonsurgical periodontal therapy, *J Clin Periodontol* 17:102-107, 1990.

20. Claffey N, Nylund K, Kiger R et al: Diagnostic predictability of scores of plaque, bleeding, suppuration, and probing depth for probing attachment loss: 3.5 years of observation following initial therapy, *J Clin Periodontol* 17:108-114, 1990.

21. Albandar JM, Brunelle JA, Kingman A: Destructive periodontal disease in adults 30 years of age and older in the United States, 1988-1994, *J Periodontol* 70:13-29, 1999.

22. Albander JM: Periodontal diseases in North America, *Periodontol 2000* 29:31-69, 2002.

23. Brady WF, Martinoff JT: Validity of health history data collected from dental patients and patient perception of health status, *J Am Dent Assoc* 101:642-645, 1980.

24. Brady WF, Martinoff JT: Diagnosed past and present systemic disease in dental patients, *Gen Dent* 30:494-499, 1982.

25. Pack PD, Haber J: The incidence of clinical infection after periodontal surgery, *J Periodontol* 54:441-443, 1983.

26. Checchi L, Trombelli L, Nonato M: Postoperative infections and tetracycline prophylaxis in periodontal surgery: a retrospective study, *Quintessence Int* 23:191-195, 1992.

27. Milam SB, Giovannitti JA: Local anesthetics in dental practice, *Dent Clin North Am* 28:493-508, 1984.

28. Buckley JA, Ciancio SG, McMullen JA: Efficacy of epinephrine concentration in local anesthesia during periodontal surgery, *J Periodontol* 55:653-657, 1984.

29. Veksler AE, Kayrouz GA, Newman MG: Reduction of salivary bacteria by preprocedural rinses with chlorhexidine 0.12%, *J Periodontol* 62:649-651, 1991.

30. Buckner RY, Kayrouz GA, Briner W: Reduction of oral microbes by a single chlorhexidine rinse, *Compend Contin Educ Dent* 15:512-520, 1994.

31. Logothetis DD, Martinez-Welles JM: Reducing bacterial aerosol contamination with a chlorhexidine gluconate prerinse, *J Am Dent Assoc* 126:1634-1639, 1995.

32. Dajani AS, Taubert KA, Wilson W, et al: Prevention of bacterial endocarditis. Recommendations by the American Heart Association, *JAMA* 277:1794-1801, 1997.

33. American Dental Association and American Academy of Orthopaedic Surgeons Advisory Statement: Antibiotic prophylaxis for dental patients with total joint replacements, *J Am Dent Assoc* 128:1004-1007, 1997.

34. Robinson RE: The distal wedge operation, *Periodontics* 4:256-264, 1966.

35. *Glossary of periodontal terms*, ed 4, 2001, American Academy of Periodontology, Chicago, IL.

36. Mormann W, Ciancio SG: Blood supply of human gingiva following periodontal surgery. An angiographic study. *J Periodontol* 48:681-692, 1977.

37. Ammons WF, Smith DH: Flap curettage: rationale, technique, and expectations, *Dent Clin North Am* 20:215-226, 1976.

38. Baab DA, Ammons WF, Selipsky H: Blood loss during periodontal flap surgery, *J Periodontol* 48:693-698, 1977.

39. Silverstein LH: *Principles of dental suturing: the complete guide to surgical closure*, Mahwah, Nj, 1999, Montage Media.

40. Reiser GM, Bruno JF, Mahan PE, Larkin LH: The subepithelial connective tissue graft palatal donor site. Anatomic considerations for surgeons, *Int J Periodontics Restorative Dent* 167:131-137, 1996.

21 Periodontal Plastic and Reconstructive Surgery

Mark E. Glover

The goal of periodontal therapy is to establish and maintain the dentition and periodontium in health, comfort, and function with optimal esthetics throughout the lifetime of the patient. This represents a modification in the thought processes of many dentists because the "dentition" now includes both natural teeth and dental implants. Although treatment parameters still include the basics of health, comfort, and function, "esthetics" has recently become an integral portion of the overall goal. Most patients will not accept periodontal treatment without the perception of an acceptable esthetic outcome. The addition of "optimal esthetics" to the goal of periodontal therapy parallels a paradigm shift in all of dentistry. This chapter explores the role of periodontal plastic and reconstructive surgery in the fulfillment of these goals (Fig. 21-1, *A* and *B*).

TERMINOLOGY

Four terms are used to describe this area of periodontics: mucogingival surgery, mucogingival therapy, periodontal plastic surgery, and reconstructive surgery. Each of these terms will be defined, as they developed historically, to clarify the origin and current use of the terms.

The term *mucogingival surgery* was used by Friedman in 1957[1]; he referred to corrective surgery of the alveolar mucosa and the gingiva which included problems with the attached gingiva, shallow vestibule, and the aberrant frenum. Currently, mucogingival surgery is defined as periodontal surgical procedures designed to correct defects in the morphology, position, or amount of gingiva surrounding teeth[2]; neither alveolar bone nor implants are included in this definition.

Mucogingival therapy is defined as the correction of defects in morphology, position, or amount of soft tissue and underlying bone.[3] This is the most comprehensive definition because it includes both nonsurgical and surgical mucogingival therapy of the gingiva, alveolar mucosa, and bone.

In 1988, Miller[4] introduced the term *periodontal plastic surgery* because the term mucogingival surgery did not adequately describe all the periodontal procedures that were being performed under this classification. Such procedures include root coverage, functional crown lengthening, esthetic crown lengthening, ridge preservation (after removal of periodontally involved teeth), ridge augmentation, maintenance of interdental papillae, reconstruction of papillae, esthetic soft tissue surgery around implants, and surgical exposure of teeth for orthodontic purposes. Periodontal plastic surgery is inclusive of surgical procedures to prevent or correct anatomic, developmental, and traumatic or plaque disease-induced defects of the gingiva, alveolar mucosa, or bone. The goal is the creation of form and appearance that is acceptable and pleasing to the patient and the therapist.[3]

The word *plastic* means to mold or shape, therefore *periodontal plastic surgery* literally means to mold or shape the tissues around the teeth or implants to create optimal esthetics. The addition of the word *reconstructive* (meaning to rebuild that which is missing) to the phrase periodontal plastic surgery better describes some of the procedures, such as root coverage, ridge augmentation, and papillae reconstruction, because missing tissues are being reconstructed rather than molding or shaping tissues that are already there. The term *periodontal plastic*

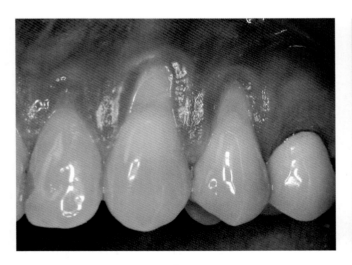
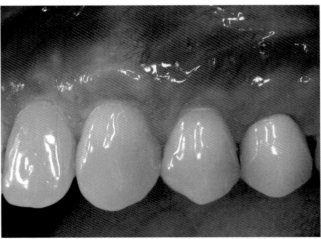

A   B

Figure 21-1. A, Marginal soft tissue recession is recognized by identifying the following: (a) the cementoenamel junction (CEJ), (b) the exposed root surface, and (c) the apically displaced soft tissue margin. **B,** Complete exposed root coverage is achieved by periodontal plastic and reconstructive surgery to establish optimal esthetics; one of the major goals of periodontal therapy was accomplished.

and reconstructive surgery better fits the current definition and goals of periodontal plastic surgery and describes the surgical modalities for both periodontal plastic surgery and mucogingival surgery; therefore, the term periodontal plastic and reconstructive surgery will be used to encompass all the surgical procedures used in this area of contemporary periodontics.

EVIDENCE-BASED APPROACH TO TREATMENT

The identification and interpretation of the signs and symptoms of mucogingival problems will dictate what treatment is performed. A *problem* is anything that will prevent achieving the stated goal of therapy and serves as an indication that treatment is necessary. A *finding* is anything that varies from the perception of normal, and should be documented and monitored. Findings can progress to problems that require treatment when etiologic factors are ignored, whereas they may resolve themselves if the etiologic factors are controlled.

Clinicians are routinely challenged to identify all significant findings, interpret whether a single finding or a combination of findings qualifies as a problem, make a definitive *diagnosis* and then determine which treatment should be used. An *evidence-based approach* to therapy requires a large reliable body of evidence that supports which findings or combination of findings can be identified as a problem, and that the treatment performed successfully alleviated the problem. The long-term success of treatment is determined by how well the etiologic factors of the problem are identified and eliminated. Surgically corrected problems may return again because of an incomplete understanding by the patient or the clinician as to the etiology of the original problem. The clinician must use the current collective knowledge of the literature combined with clinical experience to determine the best treatment for each individual patient, based on the diagnosis for that patient.

NONSURGICAL MUCOGINGIVAL THERAPY

The objectives of nonsurgical mucogingival therapy are to maintain or improve the periodontium and the exposed root surfaces when the findings and diagnosis do not warrant surgical treatment or when contraindications to surgery exist. Documentation of all findings and the identification and control of all etiologic agents is important in preventing a finding from becoming a problem. Careful monitoring of the detailed findings is necessary to determine when change has occurred and if the change in the finding has become a problem. If surgical therapy must be performed, maintenance and monitoring are necessary afterwards to determine the following: the ongoing effectiveness of treatment, the control of

all etiologic agents, and the documentation of other potential problems.

ETIOLOGY OF GINGIVAL RECESSION WITH ROOT EXPOSURE

Marginal soft tissue recession is defined as the displacement of the soft tissue margin apical to the cementoenamel junction (CEJ) with oral exposure of the root surface[3] (Fig. 21-1, *A*). This is a modification of the older but often accurate term *gingival recession*, because marginal soft tissue recession includes recession of either alveolar mucosa or gingiva. The term *exposed root* or *root exposure* is accurate and effective when communicating with patients to explain this diagnosis. Coverage of exposed roots is one of the objectives of periodontal plastic and reconstructive surgery (Fig. 21-1, *B*). The etiologic factors of marginal soft tissue recession can be divided into four major areas: morphology, trauma, inflammatory periodontal disease, and occlusal forces.

Morphology

The morphology or biotype of the periodontium can be described by two extremes: thin and scalloped, or thick and flat.[5] The gingival contour in a thin periodontium mimics the underlying bone, and often there is an exaggerated rise and fall of the marginal gingiva, which is termed *gingival scallop*. It is not unusual for the gingival scallop of the maxillary central incisors of a thin periodontium to be 4 to 6 mm, and the posterior scallop can be 2 to 4 mm (Fig. 21-2, *A* and *B*). A thin periodontium often reveals undulating contours of the prominent roots of the teeth and bone alternating with the interdental bone that is often a depression between the roots of the teeth known as the *interdental sluiceway*.[6] Recession of the papillary and facial gingiva is common because the bone is so thin. This thin bone has a high incidence of dehiscence (an absence of bone over the facial surface of the tooth; Fig. 21-2, *C*) and fenestrations (a window in the bone where the root surface can be seen with some marginal bone intact; Fig. 21-2, *D*). The prevalence of dehiscences and fenestrations may be as high as 20% in the population.[7] When a dehiscence is covered by thin gingiva, a minimal amount of brushing can result in soft tissue recession and exposure of the root. Recession often continues until the soft tissue margin approaches the bone margin where the recession will stop in the absence of inflammation. This phenomenon has been termed *self-limiting recession*.[8]

A thick periodontium is identified by a flat gingival scallop often no more than 3 to 4 mm in the anterior and 1 to 2 mm in the posterior (Fig. 21-3, *A* and *B*). This is a result of thick bone that has a high incidence of exostosis (Fig. 21-3, *C*) and tori. Thick bone supports the marginal

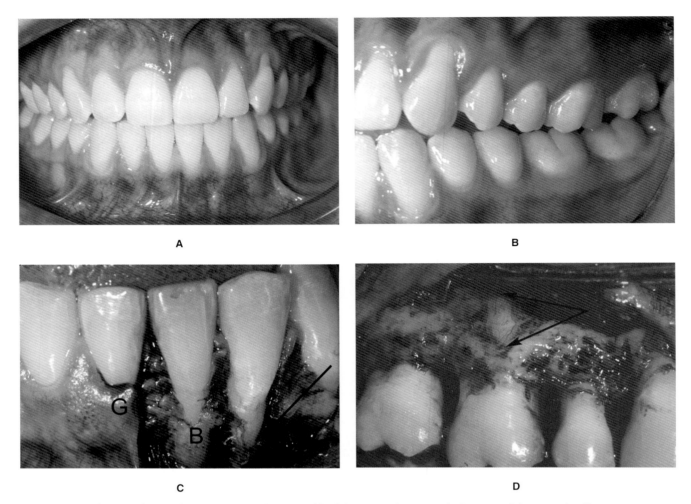

Figure 21-2. A, A thin periodontium has an exaggerated rise and fall of the marginal gingiva, which is termed the *gingival scallop*. Root prominence and the interdental sluiceways between the roots can be seen through the alveolar mucosa and gingiva, giving an undulating effect to the alveolar mucosa. **B,** This lateral posterior view of the same patient with thin periodontium shows generalized posterior gingival scallop of 2 to 4 mm and gingival recession on the maxillary left canine. **C,** The gingiva (G) has been reflected by a full-thickness flap to expose the bone (B) and the roots of two incisors, revealing a bony dehiscence (*arrow*) on the most prominent tooth. **D,** A flap was reflected to reveal a bony fenestration on the mesiobuccal root of the maxillary first molar (*arrows*).

soft tissue and resists the tendency for recession to occur. This lack of recession influences the shape of the gingival margin and creates the minimal rise and fall of the bone and the soft tissue margin. The contours over the roots of the teeth are much less pronounced, and often the roots of the teeth are not prominent because the interdental bone fills out the interdental space revealing minimal undulation between roots (Fig. 21-3, *A* and *B*). If recession does occur in the thick periodontium, there is a much greater chance of stabilizing the gingival recession or even improving it once all of the etiologic factors are controlled.

The eruption patterns of teeth and their eventual tooth position in relation to the buccolingual dimension of the alveolar process have an effect on the position and thickness of the gingiva that will be established around the teeth.[9,10] When a tooth is positioned facially, the bone and soft tissue on the facial of that tooth are thinner and more susceptible to soft tissue recession than the adjacent teeth (Fig. 21-4). The lingual of the same tooth exhibits the exact opposite findings: the lingual bone and gingiva are thicker and located more coronal. There is also a high correlation between root prominence and gingival recession.[8]

In children, the gingival dimensions will increase because of growth in the alveolar process and changed position of the teeth. In a 3-year study with children, 71% of isolated gingival recessions from 0.5 to 3.0 mm were eliminated after improved oral hygiene.[11] Surgical treatment of soft tissue recession in the developing dentition

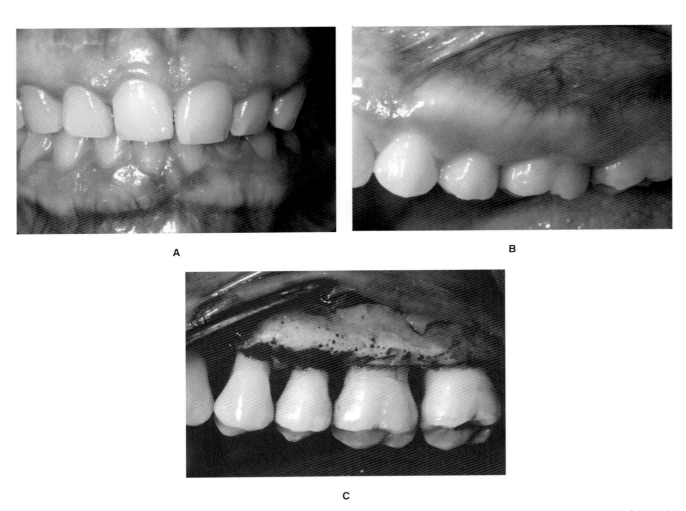

Figure 21-3. **A,** Anterior view of a thick periodontium reveals a flat scallop of 2 to 3 mm and thick gingival contours that are a result of the underlying thick bone. **B,** Posterior view of a thick periodontium showing a flat scallop of 1 to 2 mm and thick gingival contours. **C,** A mucogingival flap has been reflected in the same area as **B** to reveal the underlying flat bony contour with no bony scallop and thick bony margins.

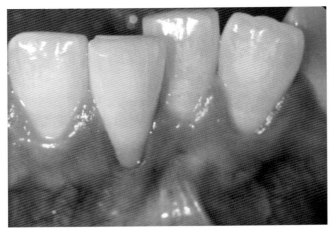

Figure 21-4. A prominent lower central incisor (#25) shows gingival recession, whereas the contralateral central incisor (#24) is lingually positioned with the gingiva more incisal showing that tooth position influences the position of the gingival margin.

may not be necessary in all cases, but careful observation is necessary because 29% of those isolated recessions did not improve. These cases would be the ones that would benefit from gingival augmentation. The changes must be identified on an individual basis, and ongoing documentation is mandatory to identify any changes.

Orthodontic movement itself can change the position of teeth and dramatically alter the marginal and the papillary tissue. If orthodontic movement occurs within the alveolus, then recession rarely is a problem. However, if orthodontic movement creates a dehiscence by moving the teeth off of basal bone, then gingival recession often results.[12] Common areas for this to occur are the lower incisors and the mesiobuccal root of first molars, especially in premolar extraction cases (Fig. 21-5, *A* through *C*), but it can occur in any location. Clinical and scientific studies have shown that the volume (thickness) of soft tissue may be a factor in predicting whether gingival

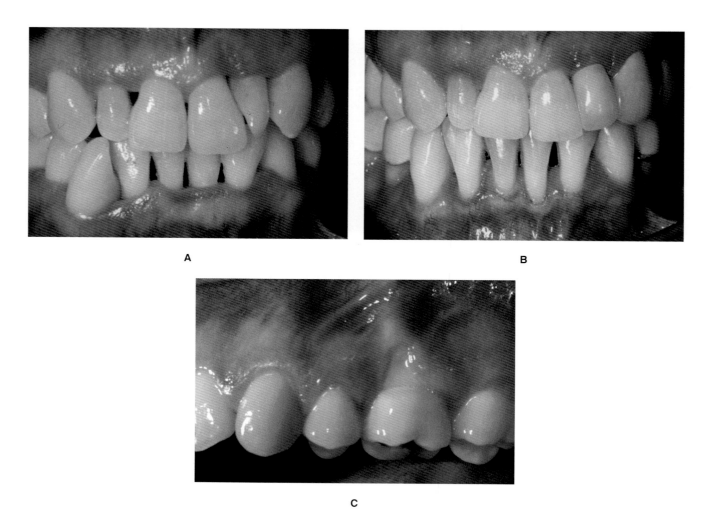

Figure 21-5. A, Before orthodontic treatment. Note the level of gingival margins on the lower incisors. **B,** After orthodontic treatment. The lower incisors have been moved facially, which made the roots of the teeth more prominent and resulted in significant gingival recession. **C,** This premolar extraction case has resulted in moving the first molar into the premolar position, creating a prominent mesiobuccal root and subsequent soft tissue recession.

recession will occur during or after orthodontic therapy.[13,14] Therefore, gingival augmentation is often indicated in the thin periodontium to increase the volume of tissue and reduce the propensity for gingival recession to occur before or during orthodontic therapy.

Trauma

Trauma of the marginal soft tissue can cause an inflammatory response that is capable of destroying gingiva, alveolar mucosa, and bone, resulting in soft tissue recession. Self-inflicted trauma from any oral habit is the most common cause of recession. Toothbrushing practices can inflict microabrasions to the soft tissue, which over time can result in recession (Fig. 21-6). Good plaque control is sometimes directly related to increased soft tissue recession.[15] Patients often feel that scrubbing with a hard brush will result in cleaner teeth, but they are discouraged to find out that aggressive brushing habits create more problems than they prevent. This type of brushing often results in dramatic recession of the facial soft tissue but limited recession on the lingual surfaces. Premolars and canines are most prone to recession because they are stroked twice with each stroke of the brush, whereas molars are often only stroked once; in some instances, patterns of recession can indicate the hand used (Fig. 21-7). The causes of recession must be identified, and then corrected before surgical treatment is instituted to prevent further recession after surgery. Soft tissue recession is often stabilized by good nonsurgical therapy, therefore only a small percentage of teeth with soft tissue recession will require surgical intervention because of progressive recession. The primary concern is to know when soft

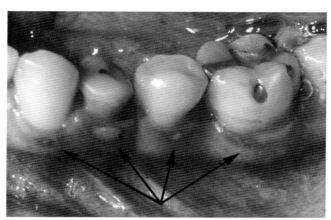

Figure 21-6. The gingival microabrasions at teeth #19, #20, and #21 were caused by toothbrushing. If such abrasions continue on a daily basis, they can create enough trauma to cause gingival recession.

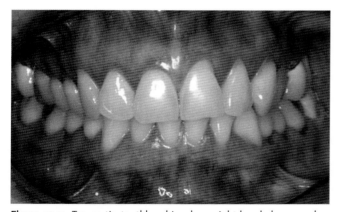

Figure 21-7. Traumatic toothbrushing by a right-handed person has created more recession on the left side (#9, #10, #11) when compared with the right side (#6, #7, #8).

tissue recession is increasing, which teeth are involved, and how much recession has occurred. Excellent, precise documentation and diagnosis is the key to successful determination of teeth that require surgical treatment.

Flossing habits can also create trauma, which leads to loss of attachment and soft tissue recession, and eventually bone loss. The most common mistake is "popping the floss" between teeth and pushing hard into the gingiva, which can cause flossing clefts (Fig. 21-8, *A* and *B*). Patients with no history of periodontal disease and shallow probing depths are usually very health conscious. They are correctly brushing and flossing two or three times a day, and are often faced with significant facial, lingual, and papillary soft tissue recession. These patients are inadvertently using floss to cut the gingival attachment apparatus once or twice a day over many years, resulting in this pattern of recession. The papillary soft tissue and interdental bone in the anterior regions of the mouth are especially vulnerable to damage by flossing because of the accentuated scallop. Watching patients floss will give insight to why the papillary recession may be occurring in the appearance of periodontal health.

Foreign object doodling is another self-inflicted cause of gingival recession. Habits of placing an object on the gingival margin such as the blunt end of a pen, pencil, or fingernail, and rubbing the tooth can traumatize the gingiva and result in gingival recession. Tobacco products made to go between the "cheek and gums" can result in soft tissue recession, as well as periodontitis and oral cancer. Traumatic injuries from sporting and automobile accidents can result in soft tissue recession. All of these self-inflicted injuries can be indications for gingival augmentation if the previously stated criteria are met.

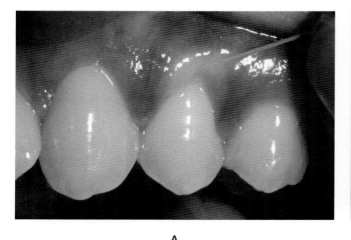

A

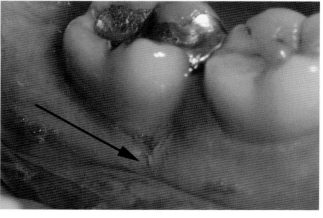

B

Figure 21-8. **A,** Flossing clefts are created by pushing the floss apically well beyond the gingival margin, severing the attachment apparatus and cutting the gingiva. **B,** Flossing clefts are usually seen on the mesial line angles of teeth rather than the distal line angles because of incorrect technique.

Dental procedures themselves can result in trauma and soft tissue recession. Procedures causing direct trauma to the soft tissue such as tooth preparation, rubber dam placement, and gingival retraction can result in gingival recession.[16] Full-coverage preparation of the interproximal region of anterior teeth in the thin periodontium that flattens out the natural scallop results in not only papillary recession, but also facial recession.[17] When restorative procedures violate the biologic width, recession can also occur.[18] Placement of orthodontic bands subgingivally in adults can also lead to gingival recession.

Nonsurgical periodontal procedures such as scaling and root planing to control inflammation can result in recession, because of shrinkage of swollen soft tissue. Surgical treatments that are designed to reduce pockets by apically positioning flaps, such as osseous resective surgery, will result in gingival recession. Any surgical endodontic, periodontal, or oral surgery procedure that requires flap reflection can result in soft tissue recession if the bone margin is more than 2 or 3 mm from the CEJ and the soft tissue is traumatized resulting in marginal flap necrosis.

Inflammatory Periodontal Disease

Inflammatory periodontal disease can cause recession on any surface of any tooth, but it is usually found in the areas of plaque and calculus retention. Recession resulting from inflammatory periodontal disease is much more obvious in cases with a thin and scalloped periodontium where resorption of bone will result in soft tissue recession. The loss of interdental bone and papilla height are visually evident in the esthetic zone, whereas papillary loss between posterior teeth results in lateral food impaction.

Occlusal Forces

Occlusal forces have been related to recession in many periodontal articles with little or no substantiation. However, Solnit and Stambaugh[19] showed resolution of recession by only adjusting the occlusion. Although this does not prove that traumatic occlusion caused the recession, the elimination of the traumatic occlusion did reverse the process and is a noteworthy finding. Conceptually, it is possible for a mobile tooth to resorb a thin cortical plate just like orthodontic movement could create a dehiscence. The presence of a dehiscence and the lack of bone support for the soft tissue margin would be a predisposing factor for recession to occur.

Inconsistent soft tissue margins appear like soft tissue recession, but root exposure has not occurred. The apical movement of the gingival margin is a natural part of the passive eruption of teeth. This can be accelerated on individual teeth for a variety of reasons; the result is inconsistent soft tissue margins in children or adults without root exposure in nonrestored natural teeth. This is not a problem of root exposure, but it may be a problem of tooth position, aberrant frenum, or a decrease in keratinized and attached gingiva. In some cases, especially in the developing dentition, this can look like soft tissue recession, but no CEJ or root surface is exposed; there is no indication for surgical intervention if gingival inflammation can be controlled by proper plaque control (Fig. 21-9). Most cases of this type will not need surgical treatment; therefore, nonsurgical treatment such as plaque control instruction, orthodontics to align teeth, or simply waiting for the maturing of the patient with passive eruption of teeth and concomitant increase in keratinized and attached gingiva, should result in more even gingival margins by the apical movement of the soft tissue margin on the adjacent teeth. Monitoring is important in the mixed dentition to assure improvement in marginal soft tissue contours.

ETIOLOGY OF CERVICAL TOOTH DEFECTS

Cervical tooth defects, also called noncarious cervical lesions, occur in the region of the CEJ and are caused by cervical abrasion, cervical erosion, or occlusal stress (abfraction). They are classified here according to the type of lost tooth structure: cervical enamel defects (loss of enamel), cervical root defects (loss of cementum and dentin), or cervical tooth defects (loss of enamel, cementum, and dentin). Instead of classifying cervical defects based on one of the three etiologic factors, which currently is common, the classification is based on the type of lost tooth structure, because the clinical differentiation among these three entities is still unclear and is usually a combination of more than one etiologic factor.

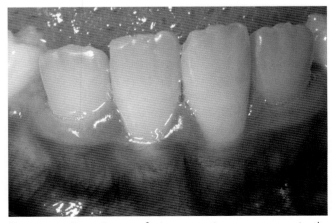

Figure 21-9. Inconsistent soft tissue margins are common in the mixed dentition and are often interpreted as recession; however, no root exposure has actually occurred.

Cervical abrasion is the result of mechanical abrasion in the cervical region of a tooth and is most often caused by excessive use of toothpaste applied with a toothbrush. This is commonly called toothbrush abrasion, but a better term would be *toothpaste abrasion* because an in vitro study has shown that even a hard toothbrush without toothpaste had almost no abrasive effect on acrylic, whereas a soft toothbrush with toothpaste had a dramatic abrasive effect.[20] This is not to negate the traumatic effect of a hard or medium toothbrush on the marginal soft tissues, but rather to point out that cervical tooth loss is caused primarily by the toothpaste with "just" a soft toothbrush. This knowledge is vital to clinicians trying to help patients stop progressive cervical abrasion. The toothbrushing technique is also important because the first area the toothbrush and toothpaste touch will have the greatest concentration of toothpaste, and potentially the most cervical abrasion will occur in this area—usually the maxillary left premolars and canines in right-handed patients (Fig. 21-10, *A* and *B*). However, every patient has his or her own habits, which is why observation of the brushing technique is so important in making a diagnosis and determining the etiology. The facial surfaces are given more attention than the lingual surfaces, and the areas that patients brush for the longest time are also those areas with the greatest propensity for cervical abrasion. It would seem prudent to use a dentifrice with no abrasives or no dentifrice on the toothbrush, when brushing at the gingival margins, in patients that are prone to cervical abrasion. The clinical appearance of cervical abrasion ranges from a wide defect to a slender notch, with varying depths that can affect all teeth (Fig. 21-10, *C*).

Cervical erosion is defined as the irreversible loss of tooth structure by chemical processes not involving bacterial action. The demineralization of the tooth surface can also make it more susceptible to damage by toothbrushing with toothpaste. Enamel is thinnest at the CEJ; therefore, this area is markedly affected by this demineralization process. Loss of the enamel results in a cervical enamel defect that reverses the normal scalloped line of the CEJ and leaves a flat or reversed scallop line (Fig. 21-11, *A*). This is combined with a loss of root structure resulting in a flat, wide, round cervical tooth defect (Fig. 21-11, *B*). This dissolution of mineralized tooth structure occurs on contact with acids that are introduced into the oral cavity from either intrinsic sources, such as gastroesophageal disease or vomiting, or extrinsic sources, such as acidic beverages or citrus fruits.[21] The most common extrinsic dietary sources that have a high acidity (low pH 2.0 to 4.0) are fruits, fruit juices, wine, carbonated drinks, and sports drinks.[22] Chewable vitamin C tablets or hydrochloric acid tablets have been reported to cause dental erosion.[23,24] Factors such as frequency and method of intake will influence the erosive effects. The popular habit of swishing with carbonated beverages is a method of intake that will affect all the facial and cervical surfaces of the teeth, whereas drinking with a straw will decrease exposure of acidity to the teeth. Eating or drinking these dietary sources of acidity immediately followed by tooth brushing will increase the abrasive effect of toothbrushing with toothpaste. Regular toothbrushing with a fluoride gel immediately after intake of these dietary sources of acidity will help remineralization of the root surfaces.

An intrinsic cause of increased oral acidity is from gastroesophageal reflux disease, which is a common condition, estimated to affect 7% of the adult population on a daily basis and 36% at least once a month.[25] Gastroesophageal reflux disease can also be "silent," with the patient unaware of his or her condition until dental changes elicit assessment for the condition.[26] This condition usually will affect the lower lingual and sometimes the palatal molar surfaces of enamel, and it is an important finding to help diagnose the root problem of dental erosion. The second cause of intrinsic acidity is from vomiting, which has long been recognized as causing erosion of the teeth in patients with eating disorders such as anorexia nervosa or bulimia.[27] Dental erosion caused by vomiting typically affects the palatal surfaces of the maxillary anterior and premolar teeth. Both of these conditions primarily affect the lingual and palatal surfaces of anterior teeth, but often patients will complain more about cervical erosion that they are able to see. Therefore, the etiology must be determined to control future cervical erosion.

When acid enters the mouth, *salivary flow rate increases*, the pH increases, and the buffer capacity of saliva also increases, so that within minutes the acid is neutralized and the pH returns to normal. Dental erosion has been associated with decreased salivary flow rates[28] caused by aging, medications, and diseases (such as Sjögren's syndrome), or head and neck radiation treatment. It is well accepted that salivary pellicle protects the teeth from erosion and the lack of salivary pellicle allows for easier demineralization of the tooth surface. One study singles out the presence of serous saliva and salivary pellicle as being one possible reason for a lower prevalence of cervical root defects occurring on the lingual (2%) versus the facial (28%) surfaces of teeth. The facial of maxillary incisors is the most common site for the cervical tooth defects (36%), and the reason was related to the decreased distribution of saliva on these teeth.[29] Therefore, decreased salivary function is an important factor in the etiology of cervical erosion.

Abfraction is the loss of tooth structure at the cervical areas of teeth caused by tensile and compressive forces

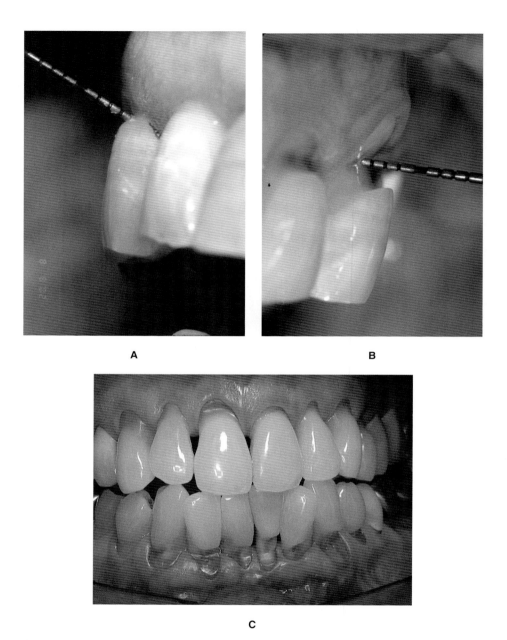

Figure 21-10. **A,** Cervical abrasion of the right maxillary canine in a right-handed patient showing a cervical defect that is 1.0 mm in depth. **B,** Cervical abrasion of the left maxillary canine in the same patient as in Figure 21-10, *A,* showing a cervical defect that is 3.0 mm in depth. The patient began his brushing technique on the left side. The root defect on the left canine is 2 mm deeper than the right canine because of the increased amount of toothpaste and time focused on brushing these teeth. Both teeth have an equal amount of incisal wear, which is evidence of bruxism. **C,** Cervical abrasion of multiple teeth extending into the pulpal region of several mandibular teeth.

during tooth flexure as a result of excessive occlusal forces, which weaken the tooth at the CEJ. The clinical appearance is reported to be a deep, narrow, V-shaped notch that commonly affects the facial surface of single teeth (Fig. 21-12). In 1991, Grippo[30] first originated the term *abfraction* to describe the stresses that biomechan-ical loading forces exert on the teeth causing the enamel[31] and dentin to chip or break away. The hypothesis was not supported with evidence until 1999 when an in vitro abfraction defect was produced in a premolar tooth in a 10% aqueous solution of sulfuric acid and then refer-enced in a brief report.[32] This single case study did use

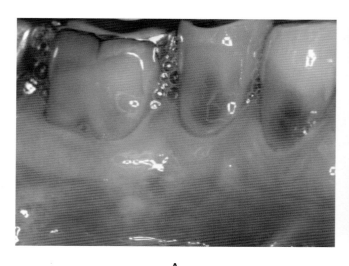
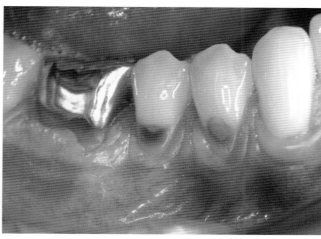

A   B

Figure 21-11. A, Cervical erosion by chemical demineralization of the enamel and dentin, creating a cervical enamel defect and cervical root defect with a resulting reverse scallop of the cementoenamel junction. **B,** Cervical erosion of the enamel and dentin creating a flat, wide, round cervical defect.

acid along with stress to produce the abfraction defect. Other studies have not proven that all wedge- or notch-shaped cervical lesions are caused by occlusion and have attributed some of these defects to toothbrushing habits. One study did relate occlusal wear to 15% of the wedge-shaped defects.[33] This abfraction phenomenon has not been fully researched and cannot be discounted; however, to say it is the only cause of notch-type defects is erroneous. Occlusal stresses on teeth can flex teeth, causing fracture of the thin enamel at the CEJ; however, if stresses

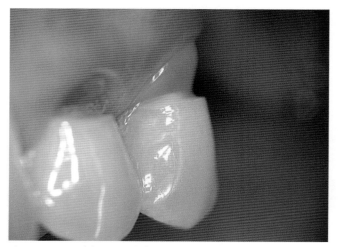

Figure 21-12. Abfraction defects appear as notch-shaped defects created by occlusal forces that weaken the teeth at the cementoenamel junction, resulting in accelerated loss of both enamel and dentin.

on maxillary canines result in abfraction defects on the facial surface, then stress on the lower canine should create abfraction defects on the lingual surface. If occlusal forces were the only cause of the abfraction defects, then teeth would have this type of notch as often subgingivally as supragingivally. Abfraction can rarely be seen on the lingual or subgingival surfaces of teeth. Occlusion does play a role in the flexure of teeth; the greatest force is created not by functional loading, but by parafunctional habits such as clenching and bruxism. These occlusal findings should be controlled when they are found on a tooth that has a cervical notch defect, especially if the defect is to be restored. The occlusal therapy may include both equilibration and bite-guard placement to reduce the functional and parafunctional loading of the teeth in question.

The etiology of cervical root defects is undoubtedly multifactorial. Faster deterioration of the cervical root occurs when multiple factors exist at the same time, and treatment must address all of the known causes to successfully treat the patient. Although there is considerable controversy as to the exact etiology of cervical tooth defects, it can be assumed that they are rare when no root exposure has occurred. It appears that exposure of the root to the oral cavity is usually necessary to create this defect. Conversely, the coverage of exposed roots by periodontal plastic surgery techniques may assist in halting the progressive nature of these defects, especially when complete root coverage is achieved. When the exposed cervical tooth defect is left untreated, it often continues increasing in depth and width over time, even to the point of pulp exposure or tooth fracture (Fig. 21-13). Cervical

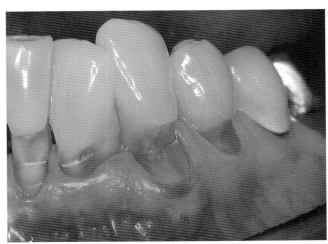

Figure 21-13. Severe loss of cervical tooth structure resulting in pulp exposure of the lower left canine. If steps are not taken to identify and eliminate causative factors, the teeth may be lost.

root defects have been seen in the past as merely a finding and were rarely treated because they were not carious lesions. But, cervical root defects are problems because progressive deepening of the defect can lead to tooth loss. Cervical tooth defects can occur in many shapes and forms, from a simple groove just apical to the CEJ, to a more dished out appearance often involving enamel, to a cleft, notch, or groove with a deep fissure running at an oblique angle. Adhesive restorative solutions to these problems are successful 65% to 100%[34,35] of the time over 1 year, and they can be viewed as a temporary solution, but one worth considering in most cases. As long as the restoration is retained, the loss of root structure is stopped and the cervical defect is eliminated (Fig. 21-14, *A* and *B*). When retention is a problem, full crowns or veneers are the next level of treatment. All of the restorative treatments may result in uneven gingival margins or "long teeth." Root coverage procedures may be preferred rather than restoration in many cases. Often, both root coverage and restorative techniques are needed to reestablish a proper tooth length and to repair the cervical defect when an optimal esthetic outcome is a priority. The etiology of recession must be addressed or the recession will continue after treatment is complete, creating root exposure again. The ideal treatment is to create the proper tooth length and bilateral symmetry by restorative, or root coverage techniques, or both. The increase in incidence and severity of cervical tooth defects is becoming recognized as the most overlooked indication for exposed root coverage surgery. Cervical tooth defects are often a problem in older patients, and they should be carefully evaluated and aggressively treated when seen in a younger patient.

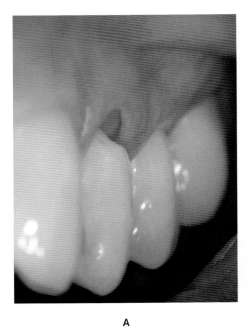

A

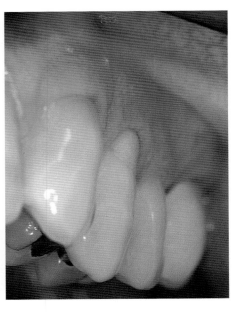

B

Figure 21-14. A, An isolated cervical tooth defect that is 1 mm in depth presents a treatment dilemma. **B,** A Class V restoration was placed to restore the cervical defect and to stop the loss of cervical tooth structure. Long-term retention of this restoration may be a problem if the occlusion has not been properly evaluated and treated to prevent flexion of the tooth.

NONSURGICAL CONTROL OF ETIOLOGIC FACTORS

The control of inflammatory periodontal disease must be the first step in treatment of any periodontal patient. The removal of calculus and plaque from the root surface of the teeth usually can be accomplished without surgery.

Modification of oral hygiene habits must be customized for each patient's needs depending on the findings of the comprehensive examination. Many patients with mucogingival problems are health conscious and concerned about their dental health, as well as esthetics, and a little motivation in this group of people goes a long way toward improving individual oral hygiene habits. Special instructions must be developed for patients with generalized soft tissue recession and cervical root defects without the presence of gingival inflammation from local factors. Patient education regarding the cause of the problem and personalized instruction will help to stabilize or even to reverse the soft tissue recession. Use of an extra soft brush is the best way to reduce soft tissue trauma to the gingiva, along with the proper gentle massage motion rather than a scrubbing motion. When patients realize that brushing is the cause of the problem, the pendulum often swings the other way and the gingival margin is avoided altogether, resulting in increased gingivitis and cervical caries. It is important to stress that there are different brushing techniques and frequencies for each of the following reasons: (1) to remove plaque, (2) to freshen breath, (3) to remove food particles, and (4) to whiten teeth. Many of these patients are brushing the same way three or more times a day, which results in ineffective plaque control and trauma to the gingival margin and root surface. Brushing after every meal is not advised for this group of patients, but if proper brushing is performed to remove plaque once daily, additional brushing can be performed after every meal with focus on the tongue and the chewing surfaces of the teeth to control bad breath. This will result in less trauma to the soft tissue margin and will allow more time for the gingiva to heal between daily brushing episodes. Careful use of interdental cleaners such as floss, toothpicks, or interdental brushes can reduce food retention after each meal, but minimize brushing of the facial and lingual soft tissue margins. Interdental cleaners themselves can cause trauma and should be used gently.

The use of disclosing solution is an important educational tool for the overmotivated patient. It will show how little plaque collects on the facial surfaces of the teeth and will teach the correct end-point of brushing to remove plaque instead of indiscriminate scrubbing of teeth. Once patients realize they are brushing too hard and too often,

they can modify their own schedule to properly remove the visible plaque.

A comprehensive evaluation of intrinsic and extrinsic acidity is needed to determine if modifications in diet or diagnosis of other disease entities such as gastro-esophageal reflux disease, bulimia, or anorexia are appropriate. Abrasive over-the-counter toothpastes are the primary cause of cervical root abrasion and should be avoided in patients with obvious signs of cervical root defects. Careful questioning of how much toothpaste is used and which teeth are brushed first will often coincide with the teeth having the worst cervical root defects. The soft toothbrushes used today hold toothpaste in between the bristles and contribute to abrasion.[20] It is recommended to use a dentifrice with extremely low or no abrasives in these patients. In some instances, the use of no dentifrice at the gingival margins is the best approach. The patient can apply a pea-sized amount of regular dentifrice to their toothbrush and brush the occlusal surfaces of their teeth and their tongue rather than the cervical margins of the teeth. Fluoride gels are also helpful because of the low abrasive content and the potential for root remineralization and increased resistance to cervical erosion.

The patient's flossing technique should be watched carefully because excessive force can traumatize the dentogingival attachment and can lead to a loss of attachment and recession followed by root exposure. This is especially true for highly scalloped periodontiums, where the floss can easily damage the interproximal attachment apparatus (junctional epithelial attachment and the connective tissue attachment), especially in the inflamed condition where there is bleeding when flossing. Papillary recession can occur when first learning how to floss as a result unintentional trauma to the inflamed and compromised gingival attachment apparatus in the thin scalloped periodontium. When the transseptal and circular gingival fibers are damaged, both the papillary and the facial gingival margins can recede as a result. Gentle flossing with a technique that will ensure light apical force, but proper lateral force and floss position, will help to ensure a return of the healthy periodontium without excessive papillary recession.

Orthodontics is one major category of nonsurgical therapy that can improve the status of the periodontium (see Chapter 28). Soft tissue and bone will move with the tooth in the absence of inflammation during orthodontic movement, allowing the therapist control of the gingival margin and bone surrounding that tooth. Many of the indications for periodontal plastic surgery can benefit from orthodontics, and in some cases orthodontics alone can obviate the need for surgical intervention. Orthodontics can make the difference between success and failure with gingival margin discrepancies, inadequate tooth length, papilla preservation and reconstruction, ridge preservation, and a gummy smile.[36] Gingival form and contour in the past have been the primary concern of the periodontist, but currently it is one of the major esthetic concerns under consideration by the practicing orthodontist.[37]

Occlusal traumatism resulting in enamel wear, or the presence of suspected abfraction defects, or both, should trigger questions about parafunctional habits (Fig. 21-12). When bruxism is diagnosed, treatment to reduce occlusal stresses should be initiated, such as a bite-guard. Tooth mobility and fremitus (functional mobility) should also be determined in the initial examination. Excessive occlusal forces should be eliminated by occlusal adjustment, which has been shown to reduce mobility by 28%,[38] and in some cases to reverse gingival recession.[19]

DOCUMENTATION TO MONITOR SOFT TISSUE RECESSION AND CERVICAL ROOT DEFECTS

Documentation for this purpose should include a detailed recording of recession (facial, lingual, and papillary), gingival width (facial and lingual), and six site-probing depths per tooth. The periodontal probe suited for this purpose is divided into 1-mm increments (Fig. 21-15); therefore, documentation of recession can be read in 0.5-mm increments. It is important to be able to recognize small changes, either positive or negative, in the amount of root exposure. Color photography of all gingival and papillary margins in the area of concern is an important tool for documentation, as well as visual communication with the patient (Fig. 21-16, *A*). Patients must be made

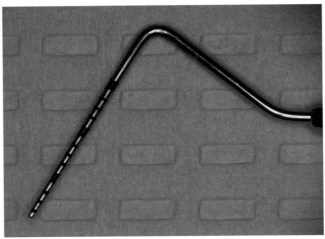

Figure 21-15. University of North Carolina-15 (UNC-15) periodontal probe with 1-mm markings to allow recording measurements of soft tissue recession and cervical defect depths to the nearest 0.5 mm.

aware of the diagnosis so that ownership of the problem is delegated to them, and copies of the photographs can be given to the patient for his or her file. Diagnostic casts of teeth and gingiva can provide the best details of soft tissue recession, root exposure, and extent of cervical root defects that are sometimes hard to visualize on photographs. The impressions must be free of voids at the gingival margins where root defects are present, so that the finished models will accurately duplicate the tooth and soft tissue contours. These models can be given to the patient along with the photographs, so that the patient will have the necessary documentation for future

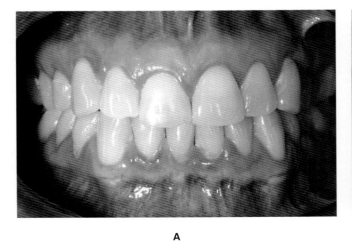

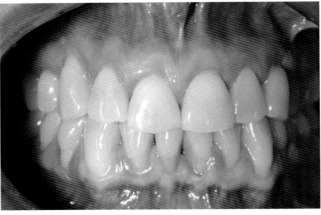

A   B

Figure 21-16. A, Initial documentation photograph of patient with soft tissue recession and gingival inflammation, with no probing depths greater than 3 mm. **B,** Progressive increasing soft tissue recession around several teeth is obvious after less than 1 year.

reference, whether for themselves, for another dentist, or for a periodontist. Radiographs are needed to rule out bone changes when recession occurs. Occlusal evaluation also is necessary to determine the presence of parafunction, fremitus, and mobility.

The intervals of these documented readings vary with each case, but in most instances they are repeated every 3 months until change stops and stability ensues. Then reevaluation appointments for data gathering with photographs and bitewing radiographs can be performed on an appropriate interval from every year to every 3 years, as determined on a case-by-case basis. Maintenance visits should be at the proper interval to maintain periodontal health. Impressions taken on the same schedule as full-mouth radiographs can be compared with the previous impressions.

THERAPEUTIC END-POINTS OF SUCCESS IN PERIODONTAL PLASTIC AND RECONSTRUCTIVE SURGERY

The therapeutic end-points of success or the objectives of periodontal plastic and reconstructive surgery include: gingival augmentation, elimination of the aberrant frenum, exposed root coverage, preservation of ridge morphology after tooth removal, ridge augmentation, esthetic crown lengthening, papilla preservation and reconstruction, and exposure of impacted teeth not likely to erupt. The indications to achieve these therapeutic end-points should be confirmed by the literature, interpreted by the clinician, and then explained to the patient. The elimination of gingival inflammation should be the first step in periodontal therapy. The indications for periodontal plastic surgery that are detailed in the following sections assume that control of inflammation by nonsurgical methods has been completed when indicated. In some instances, gingival inflammation cannot be controlled until surgical procedures have been performed.

INDICATIONS AND CONTRAINDICATIONS FOR GINGIVAL AUGMENTATION

The objectives of gingival augmentation are to increase the width and thickness of gingiva and to establish a proper vestibular depth, to prevent or stop soft tissue recession and facilitate plaque control. The indications for gingival augmentation have changed over the years, primarily as a result of the introduction of new techniques. The current ability to cover exposed roots with soft tissue grafting was not routinely performed before the early 1980's; therefore, the prevention of recession was more important before that time because of the inability to cover exposed roots. Prevention of recession is desirable and remains an important goal of mucogingival

therapy, but it is less often a primary indication for surgical treatment. Prevention of recession is more often accomplished through the methods previously discussed.

The diagnosis of soft tissue recession is not seen as a sole indicator for surgical treatment, because the soft tissue margin can remain stable for years without exposing more root surface.[39,40] However, the amount of soft tissue recession is a finding and should always be documented to determine if the recession is changing. An increase in soft tissue recession and root exposure over time or *progressive soft tissue recession* is an indication for gingival augmentation (Fig. 21-16, *A* and *B*).[3,41] Some authors might argue that the mere presence of root exposure demonstrates that the soft tissue margin has moved; therefore, it should be classified as progressive soft tissue recession. However, the presence of an exposed root surface alone does not predict future soft tissue recession. Other questions that have not been answered are: how much root exposure is acceptable? And does a certain amount of root exposure automatically indicate the need for gingival grafting? It would be impossible to designate a number value for the amount of acceptable root exposure, yet at some point the recession must stop to prevent loss of the tooth; merely because the increased recession was not witnessed does not mean it is not occurring. Therefore, additional findings must be discussed that will help in determining when to recommend gingival augmentation.

Minimal or no attached gingiva was one of the original reasons for performing mucogingival surgery, and the rationale was to return the periodontium to normal form and function. The term *attached gingiva* refers to that portion of the gingiva that is firmly bound down to the bone or tooth. The term *free* or *unattached gingiva* is that portion of the gingiva that forms the unattached soft tissue boundary for the gingival sulcus or pocket. The keratinized gingiva includes both the free gingiva and the attached gingiva. On the basis of observations made in young individuals, it was suggested that a minimum of 2 mm of keratinized gingiva, corresponding to 1 mm of attached gingiva and 1 mm of free gingiva, is adequate to maintain gingival health.[42] This concept continues to be put into practice, but it is not well supported by evidence. One article supporting this practice reports 18% of the sites that were deemed to have inadequate attached gingiva had increased recession and attachment loss over 5 years.[43] The majority of 5- to 10-year studies[44-46] indicate that there is no minimal amount of attached gingiva necessary to maintain a healthy and stable periodontium when traumatic tooth brushing and inflammation are controlled. The absence of keratinized gingiva alone is generally not justification for gingival augmentation,[41,47] and nonsurgical mucogingival therapy is indicated in this group of patients.

When the triad of findings—that is, (1) *gingival inflammation*, (2) *soft tissue recession*, and (3) *no attached gingiva*—are combined, they may be diagnosed as a *mucogingival problem* and an indication for gingival augmentation (Fig. 21-17).[48] Gingival augmentation may also be considered in other situations in which a change in the morphology of the mucogingival complex may facilitate proper plaque control and eliminate gingival inflammation.[47]

When the need for intracrevicular restorations is combined with minimal or no attached gingiva, gingival augmentation is indicated.[49] Greater levels of gingival inflammation are present around teeth with submarginal restorations when a narrow zone (<2 mm) of gingiva is present, compared with teeth having a wide zone of gingiva.[50] Gingival augmentation in this situation is considered a preprosthetic periodontal surgical procedure. Maynard and Wilson[51] stated, "If the clinician plans restorative procedures that will enter the gingival crevice, approximately 5 mm of keratinized tissue, composed of 2 mm of free gingiva and 3 mm of attached gingiva, is necessary to meet restorative objectives." There is little scientific evidence to support this 5 mm minimum; however, experimental studies in dogs have confirmed the need for an adequate amount of attached gingiva before restorative procedures.[52] Other restorative procedures in which continuous mechanical and inflammatory insult may be present in areas of minimal keratinized marginal gingiva, such as with the proximal plate and I-bar design of removable partial dentures and overdentures, are also indications for surgical augmentation procedures.[53]

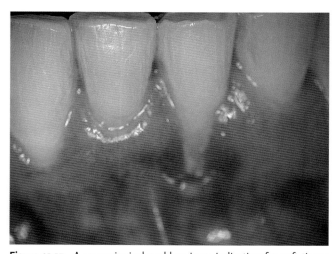

Figure 21-17. A mucogingival problem is an indication for soft tissue grafting when presenting with three findings: gingival inflammation, soft tissue recession, and minimal or no attached gingiva.

The presence of a dehiscence over a root combined with a thin periodontium is an indication for gingival augmentation. The actual presence of a dehiscence is difficult to determine without a surgical flap; therefore, a prominent tooth position or any procedure that is likely to cause a dehiscence in a thin periodontium is an indication for gingival augmentation procedures. Tooth movement, either by orthodontics or by the natural eruption pattern, which will result in moving the tooth out of the alveolar housing and formation of a dehiscence (combined with a thin periodontium), is an indication for gingival augmentation.[9,10,12-14] On the contrary, when teeth with minimal facial gingiva are moved lingually, no augmentation procedures are necessary.[54]

The shallow vestibule was one of the three original mucogingival problems cited by Friedman in the late 1950's that required increasing the apicocoronal dimension of gingiva. The termination of the orofacial muscles into the soft tissues covering the alveolar process forms the vestibular fornix. Shallow vestibular depth can interfere with oral hygiene procedures causing ineffective plaque control (Fig. 21-18, *A*). Bohannan[55] studied ways to deepen the vestibule before the advent of soft tissue grafting and found that the vestibular depth was best maintained when alveolar bone was exposed at the depth of the vestibular incision to achieve a lasting result by producing an "apical scar." This procedure was called the *periosteal separation technique*.[56]

The shallow vestibule is often extended apically by placing a soft tissue graft in conjunction with apical positioning of the mucogingival complex to reposition or resect the adjacent orofacial muscles (Fig. 21-18, *B*). It is rarely necessary to expose alveolar bone to achieve healing by secondary intention and subsequent scarring to bind the vestibule apically, as suggested by Bohannan,[55] rather than placing a soft tissue graft. Even a large vestibuloplasty can be accomplished without exposure of bone because of the current availability of acellular dermal matrix allografts.

Techniques using a split-thickness flap or a periosteal releasing incision to advance a flap can result in a shallow vestibule. Other techniques such as alveolar distraction can also result in a shallow vestibule. These surgically created conditions, as well as naturally occurring shallow vestibules, are indications for increasing the vestibular depth by gingival augmentation procedures.

Dental implants generally have a smaller proportion of attached gingiva and a larger proportion of free gingiva compared with natural teeth. Although natural teeth have a dentogingival attachment apparatus that includes both connective tissue attachment and junctional epithelial attachment, implants have only junctional epithelial attachment[57] (see Chapter 26). Dental

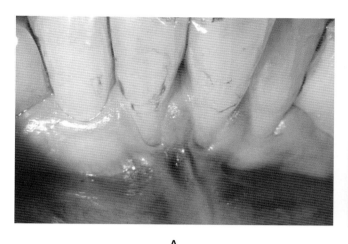

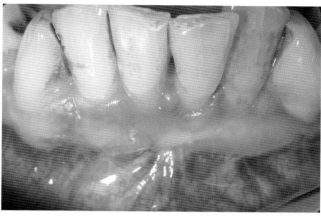

A   **B**

Figure 21-18. **A,** A shallow vestibule may result in ineffective plaque control and gingival inflammation. **B,** A vestibular extension was performed using a free gingival graft to help maintain the vestibular depth.

implants have a high long-term success rate regardless of the type of soft tissue surrounding them.[58,59] The majority of implants in several studies lack the presence of keratinized periimplant mucosa, and in fact have alveolar mucosa surrounding the implants[60,61] (Fig. 21-19). However, the results of one study indicate that the presence of plaque-induced inflammation causes more recession to occur when the periimplant tissue is alveolar mucosa rather than when it is composed of a more collagen-rich masticatory mucosa[62] (Fig. 21-20). Therefore, the presence of keratinized gingiva is desirable, but not clearly necessary for the long-term success of dental implants. A mucogingival problem indicated by soft tissue inflammation, recession, and minimal or no attached gingiva should be present to indicate the gingival augmentation.

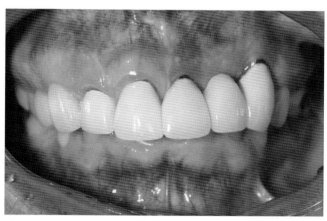

Figure 21-20. These implants have adequate keratinized gingiva and have been stable for more than 5 years but gingival recession has exposed the implant creating an esthetic problem.

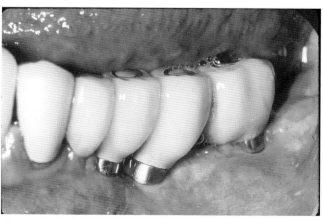

Figure 21-19. These implants have been stable for more than 10 years but they have no keratinized or attached gingiva.

ELIMINATION OF THE ABERRANT FRENUM

The aberrant frenum is a problem that indicates treatment is necessary. The mandibular frenum is evaluated by the amount of attached gingiva coronal to the frenum. When the lip is manually extended, the gingival margin should not move or turn white (blanche). This usually becomes a problem when the free soft tissue margin approaches the frenum as a result of soft tissue recession (Figs. 21-18, *A,* and 21-21, *A*). Originally, this problem was treated by a frenectomy (removal of the frenum) and vestibular deepening. Currently, the mandibular frenectomy is performed as a single procedure in preparation for root coverage procedures where the frenum will create movement of the root coverage graft, thereby resulting in failure to cover the intended root (Fig. 21-21, *C*).

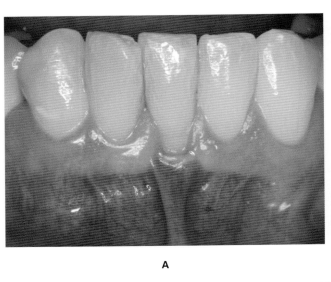

A

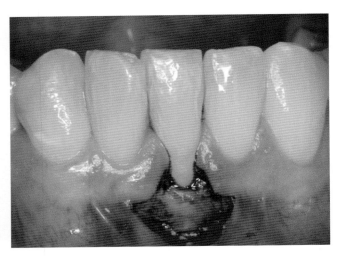

B

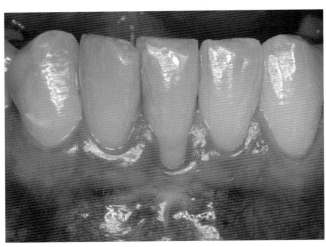

C

Figure 21-21. A, An aberrant frenum will interfere with the proposed root coverage procedures and the marginal gingiva moves slightly when the lip is retracted. **B,** A frenectomy is performed by resection of the frenum and exposure of the root and bone. **C,** The 6-week healing of the frenectomy shows the elimination of the frenum, no movement of the marginal gingiva, and the regeneration of an adequate band of attached gingiva. Root coverage procedures can be performed without interference from the frenum.

A frenectomy is commonly performed in conjunction with a soft tissue graft to increase the amount of attached gingiva and eliminate the aberrant frenum at the same time.

The maxillary frenum is usually evaluated by additional criteria. The frenum can interfere with orthodontic care when a diastema between two central incisors is closed and a frenum inserts directly into the papillary region (Fig. 21-22, A). Surgical correction is delayed until after completion of orthodontic therapy (Fig. 21-22, B). Orthodontic relapse of diastema closure has been shown to be dramatically reduced from an incidence rate of 70% to approximately 7% if a frenectomy is performed after orthodontic therapy is completed.[63] Because a shallow

vestibule is rarely a problem in this area of the mouth, apical positioning of the frenum rather than total elimination of the frenum is often an acceptable goal. A frenotomy (repositioning of the frenum) to a more apical position accomplishes all the objectives without total excision of the frenum. The end result is a normal frenum attachment rather than the total absence of the frenum. If the frenum is large and inserts into the papillary gingiva after surgical removal of most of the keratinized gingiva between the central incisors, loss of the papilla is possible. The placement of a gingival graft to cover this area will improve the ability to prevent papillary recession and to prevent reattachment of the resected frenum.

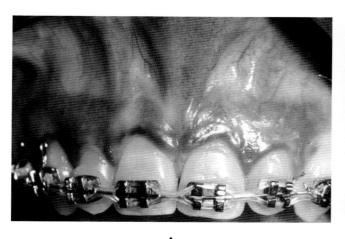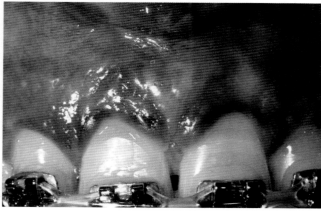

A

B

Figure 21-22. A, A maxillary frenum is shown inserting into the papilla between maxillary central incisors. The midline diastema was recently closed orthodontically. Movement of the lip will slightly move the papillary tissue between # 8 and #9. The patient underwent a maxillary labial frenectomy. **B,** The maxillary frenectomy is healed, but this case has a color discrepancy because of the lack of pigmentation in the regenerated gingiva.

Because this area is in the esthetic zone, donor tissue from the facial surface of the second or third molar region rather than the palate will give a better color match. Pigmented gingiva will lose its pigmentation when grafting; therefore, it does not lend itself to esthetic treatment unless the melanin-containing epithelial cells and the melanocytes are removed by a gingivoplasty resulting in a uniform color match (Fig. 21-23, *A* and *B*).

Esthetic improvements are a primary indication for performing periodontal plastic and reconstructive surgery. Esthetics, or the concept of beauty, is determined by cultural, social, economic, and personal factors. The phrase "beauty is in the eye of the beholder" is very true, and esthetic requirements ultimately are determined by

each patient. The mass media including movies, television, and magazines dictate the philosophy of beauty to patients who see beautiful smiles and then want what they see. Esthetic demands on the dental profession continue to increase as patients become more educated about the available options for improving their smile. It is the responsibility of the dental team to understand optimal esthetics, the indications for treatment, and to be able to effectively communicate with the patient. This is most effective with digital photography and a computer program that provides the patient with a visual concept of the expected results. All of the remaining therapeutic end-points to be discussed are concerned with esthetics, and they are most difficult to evaluate by evidence-based

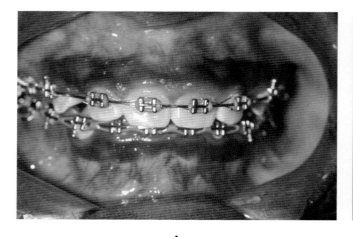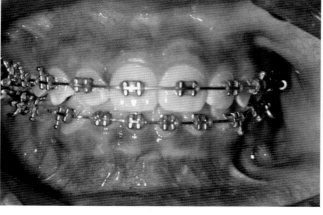

A

B

Figure 21-23. A, Preoperative view of a patient where the pigmentation and short teeth were an esthetic problem for the patient. **B,** Postoperative view shows a dramatic change in the color and contour of the gingiva after gingivectomy and gingivoplasty.

studies because esthetics are subjective. When a specific end-point is attainable, such as root coverage, many articles can be used to determine the degree of root coverage attainable with different procedures, but the esthetic differences among techniques are much more difficult to quantify.

INDICATIONS AND CONTRAINDICATIONS FOR EXPOSED ROOT COVERAGE

The objectives in root coverage procedures are to cover a predictable amount of exposed root surface with attached gingiva resulting in a healthy, shallow sulcus. The rationale is to improve esthetics and/or cover cervical root defects, root caries, or root sensitivity. The amount of root coverage that can be achieved is related to the height of the adjacent interdental bone and papilla. The classification of soft tissue recession defects most commonly used was proposed by Miller (Fig. 21-24)[64]:

Class I: Recession not extending to the mucogingival junction. No loss of interdental bone or soft tissue.

Class II: Recession extending to or beyond the mucogingival junction. No loss of interdental bone or soft tissue.

Class III: Recession extending to or beyond the mucogingival junction. Loss of interdental bone or

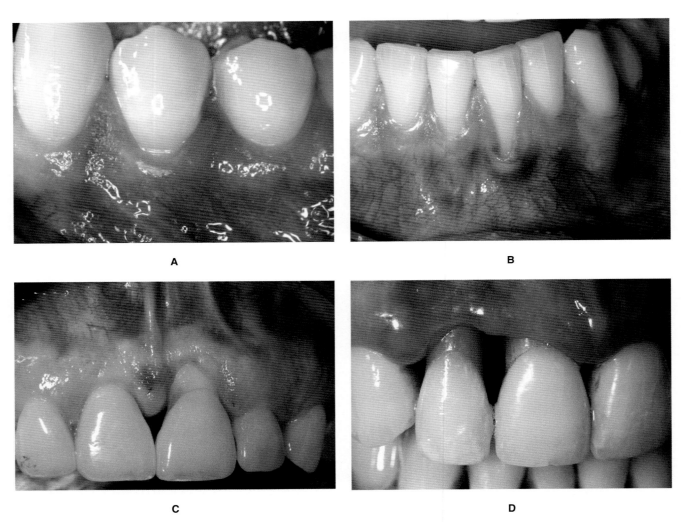

A   B

C   D

Figure 21-24. Marginal soft tissue recession classification. **A,** Class I: Marginal soft tissue recession not extending to the mucogingival junction with no loss of interdental bone or soft tissue. Complete root coverage can be anticipated. **B,** Class II: Marginal soft tissue recession extending to or beyond the mucogingival junction with no loss of interdental bone or soft tissue. Complete root coverage can be anticipated. **C,** Class III: Marginal soft tissue recession extends to or beyond the mucogingival junction with interdental loss of bone or soft tissue, apical to the cementoenamel junction but coronal to the level of soft tissue recession. Partial root coverage can be anticipated. **D,** Class IV: Marginal soft tissue recession extends to or beyond the mucogingival junction with loss of interdental bone or soft tissue apical to the level of the recession defect. No root coverage can be anticipated.

soft tissue is apical to the CEJ, but coronal to the extent of the marginal soft tissue recession.

Class IV: Recession extending to or beyond the mucogingival junction. Loss of interdental bone extends to a level apical to the extent of marginal soft tissue recession.

Notably, in the Miller recession classification, the term *recession* includes both the visible recession and the sulcus or pocket itself. Therefore, if the visible recession or the depth of the sulcus/pocket extends beyond the mucogingival junction, the recession is not a Class I recession defect.

Achieving complete root coverage is possible in Class I and II recession defects (Fig. 21-24, *A* and *B*) primarily because the interdental soft tissue and bone are still intact. Complete root coverage was further clarified to include the following four criteria: (1) the soft tissue margin must be located at the CEJ; (2) there is clinical attachment to the root; (3) the sulcus depth is no more than 2 mm deep; and (4) there is no bleeding on probing.[65] Treatment of Class III recession defects (Fig. 21-24, *C*) will result in partial root coverage because some interdental soft tissue and bone has been lost. Treatment of Class IV recession defects (Fig. 21-24, *D*) will result in no root coverage because of the advanced interdental soft tissue and bone loss. Complete root coverage is more difficult when cervical enamel defects have moved the CEJ farther coronal or incisal (Fig. 21-11, *A* and *B*).

Esthetic improvement is a common indication for exposed root coverage procedures. The decision to cover an exposed root with gingiva or with a restoration is often an esthetic decision based on whether the tooth needs to be shorter or longer. Surgical root coverage procedures can cover up to 100% of the previously exposed root surface; however, not all procedures result in the same esthetic qualities. Many details of the surgical procedures and subsequent healing can make a big difference in the thickness, color, or contour of the healed graft. The esthetic results can be classified as poor, fair, good, and excellent. The excellent result looks identical to the original tissue in thickness, color, and contour.

Cervical root defects are a common biologic indication for root coverage procedures. The shallow root defect (<1 mm; Figs. 21-10, *A*, and 21-11, *B*) is easily treated in Miller Class I and Class II cases to completely cover the root surface. The moderate root defect (1 to 2 mm; Fig. 21-14, *A*) is more difficult to treat because of the extensive amount of root reshaping that must be performed before grafting, but excellent results can be achieved. The presence of deep cervical root defects (>2 mm; Figs. 21-10, *B*, and 21-13) are the most difficult to treat because so much tooth structure is missing, and the remaining tooth is significantly weakened by the cervical root defect.

Root sensitivity is an indication for root coverage procedures if it does not respond to nonsurgical desensitization methods.[66] Root sensitivity often occurs just after the root is exposed and a small amount of root surface is usually visible, as seen in Class I recession defects (Fig. 21-24, *A*). Notably, unless the entire root is completely covered, some sensitivity will likely continue; therefore, complete root coverage is the goal of this procedure. The ability of periodontal plastic surgery to cover these roots will give these patients an improved quality of life.

Root caries that cannot be effectively treated by restorative means can be an indication for root coverage procedures.[67] Smooth surface root caries that are rather shallow can be removed by root planing, but the result will be significant sensitivity and the possibility of more caries because of the exposed root surface. Therefore, a root coverage procedure may be indicated. The depths of root caries that can be successfully treated by root coverage procedures are the same as for cervical root defects.

INDICATIONS AND CONTRAINDICATIONS FOR ALVEOLAR SOCKET AUGMENTATION

In 1981, Ammons[68] stated that the future of ridge augmentation lies in the prevention of the ridge defect at the time of extraction rather than the reconstruction of a resorbed ridge. An intact socket, with the bone present to within 2 to 3 mm of the CEJ of the extracted tooth, represents the best environment for optimal regeneration with or without augmentation (Fig. 21-25). However, even with all four socket walls intact, the buccal, lingual, and interdental bone height will resorb less with the placement of a particulate hard tissue graft at the time of tooth

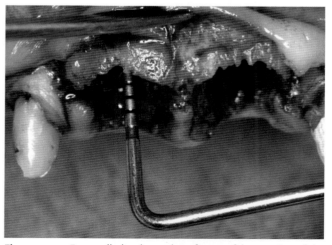

Figure 21-25. Four wall alveolar socket after careful extraction of the central incisors to maintain the thin facial plate of bone, creating an ideal site for maximum potential healing of the alveolar ridge.

extraction when compared with the socket healing without placement of a graft. The thin periodontium will lose much more bone during socket healing than will a thick periodontium.

Alveolar socket defects that will ultimately lead to alveolar ridge defects are indications for surgical ridge preservation after tooth removal, also called *socket wall preservation, socket augmentation,* or *ridge preservation.*[69] Some causes of alveolar socket defects include the following: a surgically created defect to gain access and extract the tooth by removing the buccal wall, a dehiscence defect, a deep periodontal pocket present on one or more sides of the tooth, a split root, previous apical surgery, or advanced periodontitis. When one or more walls of the alveolar socket are missing, the healing potential of the socket is compromised and socket grafting is indicated to preserve the ridge morphology (Fig. 21-26). The need to preserve the maximum height and width of the ridge, as well as the normal soft tissue contour and better papillary height, are indications for socket augmentation.

Immediate placement of a dental implant into the socket will also prevent ridge collapse and is indicated in selected cases (see chapter 26). When an implant is desired, but the socket will not support an immediate implant, socket augmentation to reconstruct a more suitable ridge is indicated. Careful extraction of the tooth and augmentation of a socket can prevent ridge collapse, preserve gingival and papillary tissue, and reduce the number of procedures required to correct the ridge defect after healing.

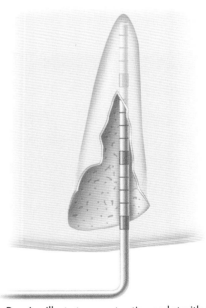

Figure 21-26. Drawing illustrates an extraction socket with a 7- to 8-mm facial dehiscence that will heal with a horizontal and vertical ridge defect.

INDICATIONS AND CONTRAINDICATIONS FOR ALVEOLAR RIDGE AUGMENTATION

Alveolar ridge defects occur when the loss of teeth results in a dimensional loss of bone and soft tissue surrounding the alveolus. The extent of dimensional loss is related to the shape of the underlying bone present at the time of tooth removal. The problem of ridge defects has been primarily esthetic, but with the increased use of dental implants, the needs are evolving into a more functional role. Occasionally, phonetics is a problem and can be managed with the help of ridge augmentation.

Ridge defect classification is based on the visible soft tissue defect and underlying bone defects, which are similar but usually more accentuated when compared with the soft tissue defects. Hard and soft tissue ridge defects can be divided into three classes[70]: Class I, buccolingual loss of tissue with normal apicocoronal ridge height (Figs. 21-27, *A,* and 21-28, *A* and *B*); Class II, apicocoronal loss of tissue with normal buccolingual ridge width (Figs. 21-27, *B* and 21-29); and Class III, combination type with loss of both width and height of the ridge (Figs. 21-27, *C,* and 21-30). Each site can be classified as to the extent of involvement: mild, less than 3 mm; moderate, 3 to 6 mm, and severe, more than 6 mm.[71] A modified system (the HVC System) using the above two classification systems has been proposed.[72] The Class I, II, and III defects are classified as horizontal (H), vertical (V), and combination (C) defects, respectively. Each of the categories is subdivided into small (s, ≤3 mm), medium (m, 4 to 6 mm), and large (l, ≥7 mm) subcategories. Therefore, a defect would be called an H-s for a small horizontal defect or C-m for a medium combination defect. This allows for treatment planning on the basis of the classification of the defect found. A table has been adapted to assist with indications for the different types of ridge augmentation (Table 21-1).

In addition to the soft tissue defect, the underlying bony defect should be evaluated, especially if dental implants are planned. Several classifications have been used for these bone defects as they relate to implant placement.[73,74] Bone sounding to determine the relation of the bone to the soft tissue is extremely useful in evaluating the bony contours. The use of surgical guides, radiographs, tomograms, and computer assisted tomography scans can all be helpful in diagnosing the bone morphology. The relation of the ridge, proposed teeth position, lips, and the smile line must be ascertained. Once the hard and soft tissue morphology of the ridge defect has been evaluated in relation to these factors, a problem list can be generated to determine the best method of surgical treatment to achieve the set goals.

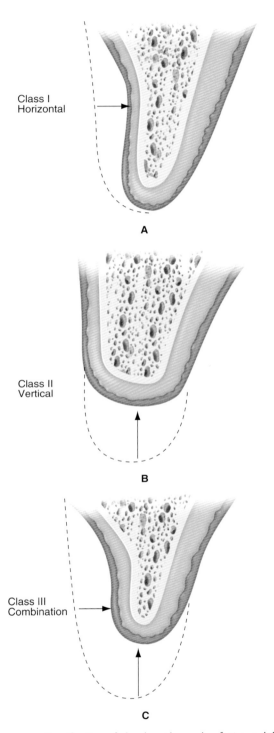

A

B

C

Figure 21-27. Classification of alveolar ridge and soft tissue defects: Mild (small), 3 mm or less; Moderate (medium), 3 to 6 mm; Severe (large), 7 mm or more. **A,** Class I (H-horizontal): has a buccolingual loss of tissue with normal apicocoronal ridge height. **B,** Class II (V-vertical): has an apicocoronal loss of tissue with normal buccolingual ridge width. **C,** Class III (C-combination): has a combination type defect with loss of both width and height.

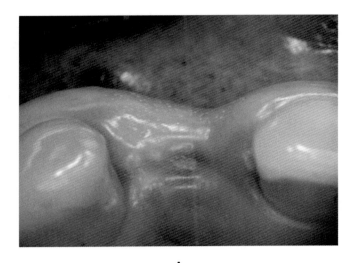

A

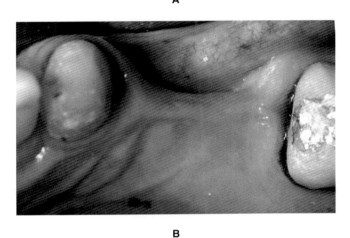

B

Figure 21-28. **A,** Class I: Mild (H-s) ridge defect. **B,** Class I: Moderate (H-m) ridge defect.

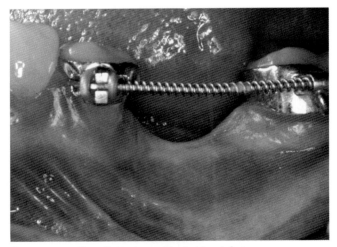

Figure 21-29. Class II: Moderate (V-m) ridge defect.

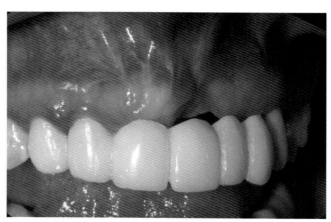

Figure 21-30. Class III: Moderate (C-m) ridge defect.

INDICATIONS AND CONTRAINDICATIONS FOR ESTHETIC CROWN LENGTHENING

Esthetic crown lengthening may be indicated when anterior teeth are shorter than normal, or when *excessive gingival display* or a "gummy smile" (Fig. 21-31) is the problem. The proper treatment can be selected after the diagnosis and etiology is determined, which can be gingival enlargement, altered or delayed passive eruption, short clinical crowns, vertical maxillary excess, or a short upper lip.[75]

Gingival enlargement can be caused solely by gingival inflammation, or it may be complicated by multiple systemic problems such as diabetes, pregnancy, or local irritation from orthodontic appliances (Fig. 21-32). Gingival enlargement caused by medications such as calcium channel blockers, phenytoin, and cyclosporine is also common[76] (Fig. 21-33) (see Chapter 33). Gingival enlarge-

ment caused by hereditary gingival fibromatosis[77] is also a problem occasionally encountered (Fig. 21-34). If the gingival enlargement is still present after elimination of the inflammatory lesion, esthetic crown lengthening may be indicated.

Altered or delayed passive eruption occurs when the dentogingival complex fails to migrate apically and the tooth fails to erupt normally. The width of keratinized gingiva can be quite large. The CEJ is located a significant distance subgingivally; the bone is found at or very close to the level of the CEJ, rather than at its usual position 1 to 2 mm apical to the CEJ[78] (Fig. 21-35, *A* and *B*). This is an indication for surgical crown lengthening.

Short teeth in the esthetic zone may result from attrition caused by bruxism. The teeth usually erupt as the incisal and occlusal wear takes place maintaining the occlusal vertical dimension (Fig. 21-36). This eruption of the teeth increases the width of keratinized gingiva; an excessive gingival display results. In a normal smile, the gingival margins of the maxillary teeth are parallel to, and 0 to 2 mm superior to, the upper lip, with the incisal edges parallel to the lower lip. Esthetic crown lengthening is indicated to establish the proper relation of the gingival margin with the lip and to increase the length of the teeth for improved retention of the crowns. In other cases of incisal attrition where the teeth do not continue to erupt, there is a loss of vertical dimension and the gingival margin is stable and in proper relation with the upper lip. This situation is an indication for restorative treatment to lengthen the teeth and restore the vertical dimension, and it is a contraindication for esthetic crown lengthening. *It is important to determine if the incisal edges of the maxillary anterior teeth are in the correct position, or if the incisal edges need to be restoratively lengthened and the occlusal vertical dimension restored.*

TABLE 21-1	Treatment Options Based on Defect Classification and Type of Donor Tissue	
DEFECT CLASS	**SOFT TISSUE AUGMENTATION**	**HARD TISSUE AUGMENTATION**
Class I mild (H-s)	Pouch procedure	Ridge expansion
Class I moderate (H-m)	Tunnel procedure + CTG	Advanced flap + GBR
Class I severe (H-l)	Advanced flap + CTG	Advanced flap + MBG
Class II mild (V-s)	Advanced flap + CTG	Orthodontic extrusion
Class II moderate (V-m)	Interpositional graft	Advanced flap + GBR/MBG
Class II severe (V-l)	Onlay graft	Distraction osteogenesis
Class III mild (C-s)	Advanced flap + CTG	Advanced flap + GBR
Class III moderate (C-m)	Advanced flap + CTG	Advanced flap + MBG
Class III severe (C-l)	Advanced flap + CTG	Extraoral block bone grafts (tibia, rib, calvaria or hip)

H, Horizontal; s, small; m, medium; l, large; V, vertical; C, combined; CTG, connective tissue graft; GBR, guided bone regeneration; MBG, monocortical block bone graft.

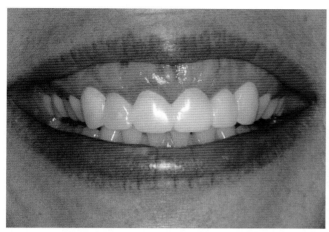

Figure 21-31. A "gummy smile" as a result of excessive gingival display must be closely evaluated to determine the cause.

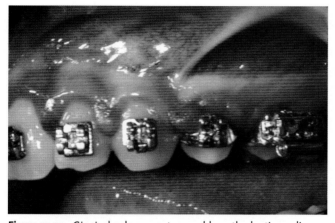

Figure 21-32. Gingival enlargement caused by orthodontic appliances and complicated by pregnancy.

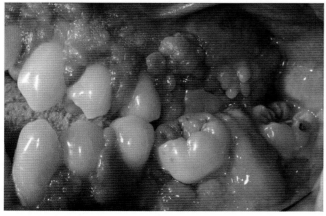

Figure 21-33. Gingival enlargement caused by concurrent administration of a calcium channel blocker, phenytoin, and cyclosporine.

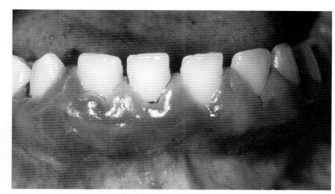

Figure 21-34. Gingival enlargement caused by hereditary gingival fibromatosis.

Vertical maxillary excess results from a skeletal dysplasia such as hyperplastic growth of the maxillary skeletal base. This can be diagnosed by conventional orthodontic and orthognathic surgery criteria. If periodontal surgery is necessary, this should be done before the orthognathic surgery.[79] This gives the oral surgeon a better idea of the relation of the teeth to the upper lip and the amount of impaction necessary. Overintrusion of the maxilla will eliminate visibility of 2 to 4 mm of the incisal edge at rest, resulting in an aging of the patient's appearance. In this type of case, the gummy smile cannot be treated by periodontal plastic surgery alone and achieve a satisfactory result.

A short upper lip is diagnosed when the distance from subnasale to the lower border of the upper lip is less than 20 to 22 mm in young women and 22 to 24 mm in young men[80] (Fig. 21-37). Correction of this problem when indicated usually includes both plastic surgery and orthognathic surgery. The case in Figure 21-37 is not severe enough to warrant either, but the uneven gingival margins do need to be corrected.

Uneven gingival margins can give the appearance of an uneven smile (Fig. 21-37). A beautiful smile is difficult to create unless the gingival framework is bilaterally symmetrical. This framework is created by facial gingival margins and the papillae, which create the gingival scallop around the teeth. Diagnosis of all of these problems can be greatly enhanced by photographs. The causes of the uneven smile become important to the treatment plan. Some causes are unfavorable tooth or implant position, previous crown margins or bridges with missing teeth, periodontal disease, recession, root exposure, or previous trauma resulting in gingival recession. Other problems such as discolored or dark margins around older crowns, implants, or teeth with root canals can result in an unaesthetic smile. Many of the surgical techniques to be discussed can be used to correct these types of symmetry problems.

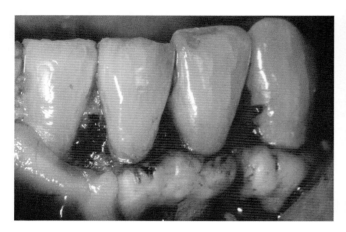
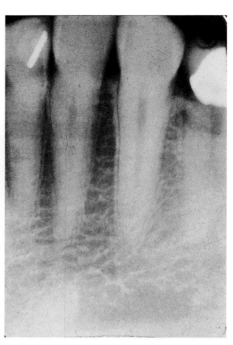

A   B

Figure 21-35. **A,** Altered passive eruption as seen with the bone level at or coronal to the level of the cementoenamel junction and facial exostosis preventing gingival recession. **B,** This radiograph of the previous clinical picture identifies the bone level at the level of the cementoenamel junction.

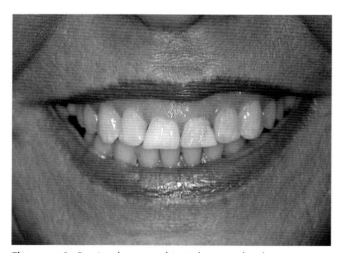

Figure 21-36. Bruxism has caused incisal wear with subsequent eruption of the maxillary incisors, which allowed coronal movement of the gingival margin and resulted in excessive gingival display.

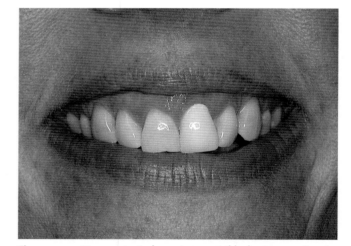

Figure 21-37. Uneven gingival margins are visible due to excessive gingival display, partially because of short upper lip (19 mm); normal upper lip length is 21 to 22 mm.

INDICATIONS AND CONTRAINDICATIONS FOR PAPILLARY RETENTION AND RECONSTRUCTION

The loss of a key papilla in the esthetic zone and the presence of a "black triangle" (Fig. 21-38, *A*) is an indication for evaluation for *papillary reconstruction*. The complete regeneration of lost papillae is unpredictable; therefore, the retention of these papillae is of great importance when an esthetic result is desired from surgical procedures. These procedures include extraction, gingival surgery, or osseous surgery performed in this esthetic region. Tarnow and colleagues[81] have shown that when the distance from the apical extent of the contact point to

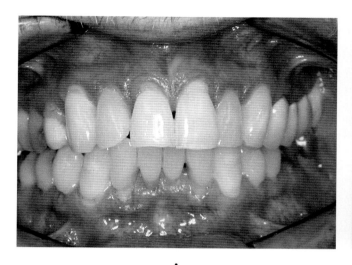

A

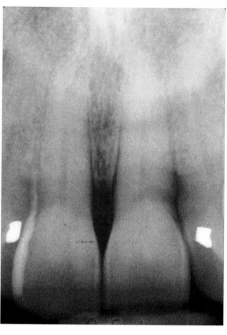

B

Figure 21-38. A, A "black triangle" between the maxillary central incisors is small but is the chief complaint of this patient. Surgical elimination of this space depends on the distance from the contact point to the bone. **B,** The radiograph shows the distance from the bone to the apical extent of the contact point to be 7 mm. The "black triangle" is not likely to diminish in size and a restorative solution would be more advisable rather than surgical intervention.

the bone is 5 mm or less, the papilla should be present or should regenerate to fill the embrasure space after restorative or surgical procedures. When the distance is more than 5 mm, there is a greater chance of papillary recession as the distance increases and open embrasure spaces can be expected. The radiograph in Figure 21-38, *B*, shows that the distance from the contact point to bone is 7 mm. The contact area is positioned relatively close to the incisal edge and is not the ideal length, which is 50% of the central incisor length. Because the regeneration of the papilla is not predictable in this case, a restorative solution should be evaluated to move the contact point 2 mm closer to the bone. This should eliminate the open embrasure and increase the contact area to 50% of the total tooth length.

INDICATIONS AND CONTRAINDICATIONS FOR EXPOSING IMPACTED TEETH FOR ORTHODONTIC REASONS

Impacted teeth not likely to erupt are seen frequently by the orthodontist. Orthodontic movement of teeth can be assisted by surgical exposure of the desired impacted tooth when the tooth will not erupt in a timely manner. After third molars, the most common teeth to be impacted

are the canines. An apically positioned flap will allow adequate gingiva to be developed when the tooth is incorporated into its proper alignment. The bonding of a bracket at the time of surgery will assist in active eruption of the tooth. On occasion, removal of tissue from the occlusal surface will allow for the passive eruption of the tooth. (See Chapter 28 for a more detailed discussion of orthodontic–periodontal relations.)

PERIODONTAL PLASTIC AND RECONSTRUCTIVE SURGERY TECHNIQUES

Periodontal plastic and reconstructive surgery techniques are used when the appropriate indications for treatment are met, as discussed in the previous section, and the rationale for treatment is mutually understood by both the dentist and the patient. Advancements in technology and modifications of techniques are continuously taking place to achieve the best end result for the patient. These techniques will be categorized based on the donor site, the direction of flap movement, and flap design. The major categories are pedicle soft tissue grafts, free soft tissue grafts, guided tissue regeneration, and hard tissue grafts. Combination grafts combine any or all of these techniques.

Pedicle Soft Tissue Grafts

A pedicle graft is a mucogingival flap designed to serve as a soft tissue graft that maintains an intact blood supply from the donor site. Mucogingival flaps can be divided into four major groups based on the direction of the flap movement: rotated flaps, advanced flaps, apically positioned flaps, and replaced flaps.

Rotated flaps

Rotated flaps move laterally while rotating around a pivot point.[82] Many techniques can be placed in this group, and for years these techniques were the only way to predictably cover exposed roots. The first technique was described in 1956 as the "lateral sliding flap"[83] and later as the "laterally positioned flap."[84] This technique uses the donor gingiva from a healthy adjacent tooth to cover the exposed root of a problem tooth. Throughout this chapter, these types of root coverage techniques will be referred to as *laterally positioned flaps*. An isolated area of soft tissue recession with no bone loss on the proximal surface is a good indication for the laterally positioned flap to cover the exposed root (Fig. 21-39, A and B). The adjacent donor tooth should have adequate soft tissue width and thickness, as well as vestibular depth, and there should be adequate bone thickness with no dehiscence. The ideal indication is where the donor site has excessive width and thickness of soft tissue such as in crowded teeth, where the most lingual tooth (donor) will usually have the thickest and most coronally positioned soft tissue and bone. The adjacent tooth is positioned more facial (recipient) and has little or no gingiva with root exposure (Fig. 21-40, A).

The advantage of this technique is that the donor site is adjacent to the recipient site, which produces only one surgical wound, in contrast to techniques that take the donor tissue from another site. This decreases the postoperative pain and bleeding concerns. The pedicle maintains a blood supply through the base of the flap and improves the chances of graft survival and root coverage. The major disadvantage is that recession occurs routinely over the donor site; in some cases, root coverage is accomplished at the donor site only to create recession at the recipient site. The second problem is that the donor tissue is often thin and prone to future recession. It is important to select the case carefully to prevent these problems.

Laterally positioned flap. A clinical example of a laterally positioned flap that has proper indications for treatment is seen in Figure 21-40, A. The first step in this technique is to determine the bone level at the facial of the donor site by sounding to bone after local anesthesia. The distance from the bone to the CEJ should not exceed 1 to 2 mm on the facial unless root exposure of the donor tooth is acceptable. The distance from the CEJ to the bone on the donor lateral incisor in Figure 21-40, B, is 3 mm,

and, as can be seen in Figure 21-40, C, more recession did result. This one disadvantage of the laterally positioned flap can be overcome by leaving a collar of tissue (Fig. 21-39, A). The recipient tooth also should be evaluated to confirm the location of the proximal and facial bone. The recipient root should be smoothed to eliminate all hard and soft tissue deposits and any present root defects. If chemical root treatment is to be performed, it should be done at this point.

The next step is to visualize the incisions and even sketch a design of the procedure before any incisions are made. The parallel incisions will be made at an oblique angle toward the recipient tooth to position the base of the rotation as close to the recipient tooth as possible. The first incision is made beginning at the papilla on the leading edge of the pedicle graft between the donor (D) and recipient (R) teeth at the height of CEJ, continuing parallel to the sulcus of the recipient tooth, and terminating at the opposite side of the recipient tooth at a point apical to the opposite papilla (see Fig. 21-39, A). The incision will end well beyond the mucogingival junction.

The second incision begins at the papilla between the recipient tooth and the tooth on the nondonor (ND) side and extends only 1 to 2 mm horizontally at the proposed height of the graft. The incision then changes direction and extends apically to join the previous first incision well beyond the mucogingival junction. A thin split-thickness dissection to remove the sulcular epithelium of the recipient tooth and the overlying epithelial layer between the first two incisions exposes the recipient bed for the donor flap.

The third incision is made from the line angle of the tooth adjacent (A) to the donor site and parallel to the first incision (Fig. 21-39, A). A fourth incision extends perpendicular to and connects the first and third incisions, ideally leaving 0.5 mm of attached gingiva (sulcus depth + 0.5 mm of keratinized gingiva) over the donor tooth, which usually means 1.5 to 2 mm of keratinized gingiva remains.[85] If there is not enough gingiva to meet these criteria, the entire gingival collar can be moved with the pedicle. The fourth incision can be made in the gingival sulcus, but the donor tooth may end up with recession of 1 to 2 mm depending on the underlying bone levels.

Flap reflection is split-thickness over the papillae and over the facial of the donor tooth if the thickness is adequate (1 mm minimum). Usually a full-thickness flap is necessary over the facial surface of the donor tooth to insure adequate thickness of the donor tissue. Presence of thin donor tissue is a contraindication to this technique because it will not hold up to traumatic brushing, which often is the original cause of recession. Careful attention to the thickness of the donor tissue and the cause of recession will aid in choosing the proper technique. The tissue is now rotated for a trial fit to the donor site. The closer the base of the pedicle is to

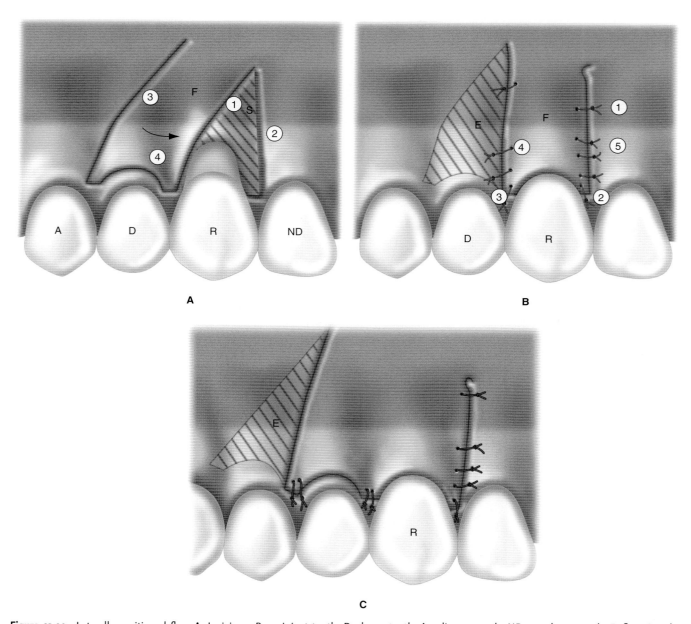

Figure 21-39. Laterally positioned flap. **A,** Incisions: R, recipient tooth; D, donor tooth; A, adjacent tooth; ND, nondonor tooth; F, flap; S, split-thickness dissection; E, exposed bone or periosteum. **B,** Suturing: after rotation of the flap, the sutures are placed in the order seen and the lip is retracted to make sure the graft is immobile. **C,** Multiple teeth: two teeth are easier to stabilize because of the increased size of the flap; therefore, the amount of root coverage is improved.

the recipient tooth, the smaller the arc of rotation is and the less shortening of the flap will be observed. If the base of the flap is over the donor tooth instead of the recipient tooth, the rotation of the flap will cause shortening of the leading edge of the flap, and this will cause inadequate tissue on the leading edge of the flap in the papillary region. If this occurs and a full thickness rather than a partial thickness flap was used, a periosteal releasing incision can be made to allow more mobility

of the flap. Once the flap will lie passively in the desired position, suturing can begin.

The first suture is placed in the mucosa close to the mucogingival line on the leading edge of the flap with a small needle and 5–0 or 6–0 interrupted suture (see Fig. 21-39, B). This will allow for some stability of the flap before suturing the coronal edge of the flap to the nondonor papilla. Suturing of the trailing edge is the same on the opposite papilla between the donor and recipient teeth.

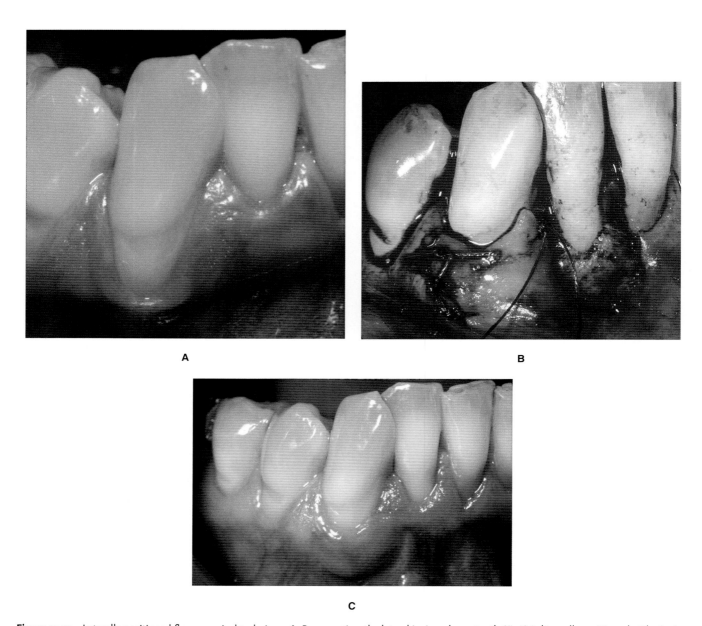

Figure 21-40. Laterally positioned flap—surgical technique. **A,** Preoperative: the lateral incisor donor tooth (#26) is lingually positioned with gingiva at a more coronal level compared with the other incisors, making this an ideal donor tooth because the 1 to 2 mm of recession expected on the donor tooth will create a uniform look among the lower incisors. **B,** Suturing: after rotation and suturing of the flap, the root on #27 is almost entirely covered. The bone level on the donor tooth is as expected. **C,** Postoperative: 3-month healing reveals an increased amount of attached and keratinized gingiva on the canine and a mild increase in recession on the donor tooth. The root coverage was not complete but was average for this technique.

Suturing up the trailing edge can only be performed if periosteum was left intact in this region (i.e., a split-thickness flap was used). If a full-thickness flap was used, no sutures are placed on the trailing edge. Then, additional sutures can be placed to secure the leading edge to the prepared bed. The lip should be moved to make sure the graft is immobile. The graft must be completely stable and immobile. The trailing edge of the pedicle graft is the weakest link because of the lack of stable tissue on which to

suture this edge of the flap. Holding a moistened gauze over the sutured area for 5 minutes will allow a blood clot to form and will assist in stabilizing the area. An area of exposed periosteum or bone (E) will be present over the donor site. This bone will respond with resorption of the crestal bone, regardless of whether the periosteum is present.[86] A small piece of collagen can be placed over the donor site followed by a periodontal dressing, if desired. If periodontal dressing is used, it must be stable. Dressing that moves when the patient talks or chews can severely disrupt the healing process. Light cured periodontal dressings are often the most stable, and they can be secured to the teeth with suture material, if needed.

Postoperative healing occurs quickly; within 1 week the initial healing response will be evident. The success or failure of root coverage is suggested at 1 week but is obvious at 2 weeks. In Figure 21-40, *C*, the healing after 3 months shows there is less root coverage than desired. This likely came from improper stabilization of the graft, whereby slight movement resulted in less than ideal root coverage. There is an improved band of keratinized and attached gingiva, but the amount of root coverage was not complete. The summary data of 10 clinical studies of 216 teeth in 204 patients reveal a 62.5% mean root coverage using laterally positioned flaps or double papilla grafts (Table 21-2).[47]

Multiple teeth. The laterally positioned flap involving multiple teeth (see Fig. 21-39, *C*) is identical to the technique just described but is applied to more than one tooth to increase the size of the flap and provide better blood supply and stabilization to the rotated flap.[87] A combination graft using a *multiple tooth laterally positioned flap over a connective tissue graft* was demonstrated in 1987 by Nelson,[88] achieving better results (91% root coverage) than the use of laterally positioned flaps alone. He also noted that 1 to 3 mm of exposed root was covered 100% of the time, whereas severe recession of 7 to 10 mm was completely covered only 88% of the time. Rotation of larger flaps is much more challenging than small flaps, but the result is better stabilization and improved root coverage.

Free gingival graft. A *laterally positioned flap* can be combined with a *free gingival graft* to cover the exposed periosteum, bone, or exposed root on the donor tooth.[89] This is performed when the donor tooth requires maximum protection to prevent recession because of thin bone or an undiagnosed dehiscence as seen in Figure 21-41, *A*. Normally, this exposed area is very small and the donor area most often used is the gingiva facial to the maxillary second or third molars. Enough gingiva can usually be harvested 0.5 mm apical to the attached gingiva (probing depth + 0.5 mm) on these teeth to cover the donor area (Fig. 21-41, *B*). This donor tissue is gingiva as opposed to palatal mucosa, and the color match is often more favorable after healing than palatal mucosa (Fig. 21-41, *C*). The advantage is no recession on the donor tooth.

Papilla flaps. To prevent recession over the adjacent donor tooth, another modification was made in the rotated flap to achieve root coverage. Papilla flaps were used as the donor source in the "oblique rotated flap,"[90] "rotation flap,"[91] and the "transpositional flap."[92] All of these terms and techniques are occasionally still used and have differences in design, as well as indications and contraindications. The double papilla flap is another design variation of the papilla flap using both papillae mesial and distal to achieve coverage of the exposed root (Fig. 21-42, *A* and *B*).[93] This design is difficult to execute because the wound edges are sutured over an avascular surface, the radicular surface of the previously exposed root. These techniques result in an average root coverage of 63% (see Table 21-2).[47]

Double papilla/connective tissue graft. Improvement in the amount of root coverage finally came when the double

TABLE 21-2	Average Root Coverage Using Different Techniques				
TECHNIQUES	**EXPOSED ROOT COVERAGE, MEAN (%)**	**EXPOSED ROOT COVERAGE, RANGE (%)**	**PRE-TREATMENT RECESSION, MEAN (mm)**	**PATIENTS/ TEETH, n**	**NO. OF STUDIES**
Laterally positioned flap including double papilla	62.5	34-82	3.7	204/216	10
Coronally positioned flap	82.7	70-99	3.7	115/232	5
Guided tissue regeneration + coronally positioned flap	74.1	54-83	5.3	165/177	8
Free soft tissue graft + coronally positioned flap	62.5	36-74	3.3	106/167	8
Thick free soft tissue graft	72.1	11-87	3.4	300/456	15
Combination of various flaps + connective tissue graft	89.3	52-98	3.8	251/349	12
Citric acid root conditioning	78.7	39-98	4.5	266/370	12
Tetracycline root conditioning	98.2	98-99	3.1	92/120	4

Adapted from Wennstrom JL: Mucogingival therapy, Ann Periodontol 1:671-701, 1996.

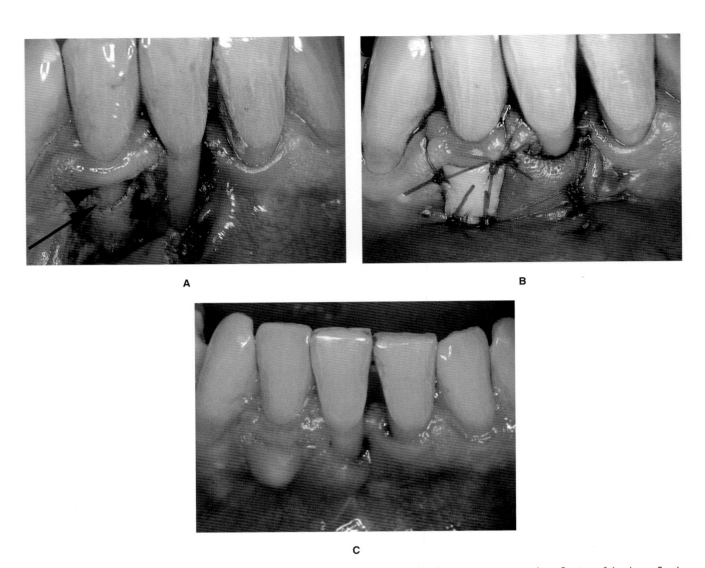

A

B

C

Figure 21-41. Laterally positioned flap combined with free epithelialized graft—surgical technique. **A,** Incisions: the reflection of the donor flap has exposed a dehiscence over the donor tooth (*arrow*), and if not covered the collar of gingiva will not survive over the donor tooth. **B,** Suturing: the donor site for the free epithelialized graft was the facial gingiva of the maxillary second molar. Use of gingiva as the donor tissue, rather than palatal mucosa, may improve color match and tissue contour. The free gingival graft was sutured to cover the dehiscence and to prevent recession on the donor tooth. **C,** Postoperative: the healing shows no recession of the donor tooth with complete coverage of the dehiscence and partial coverage of the Class III recession on the recipient tooth.

papilla technique was combined with a connective tissue graft (Fig. 21-43), achieving 88% to 98% root coverage.[88,94,95] This combination technique is described here. The first incision removes the sulcular epithelium adjacent to the exposed root and extends to the mucogingival junction, which is at the apex of the incision. The second incision is repeated on the opposite side of the exposed root (see Fig. 21-42, *A*). The third incision begins at the level of the desired soft tissue height, usually at the CEJ, and extends horizontally on each side of the tooth stopping no less than 0.5 mm from the gingival margin of the adjacent tooth to avoid creating gingival recession on adjacent teeth. The fourth and fifth incisions are vertical incisions that extend from the termination of the horizontal incisions and extend into the alveolar mucosa. Partial thickness pedicle flaps are reflected to mobilize the papillary pedicles. The pedicle flaps are positioned to ensure they will touch and remain passively in position, and then the two pedicles are sutured together with 5–0 or 6–0 chromic gut suture. The connective tissue is taken from the palate, trimmed to fit the recipient site and is sutured into place with 5–0 or 6–0 chromic gut sutures. The double pedicle

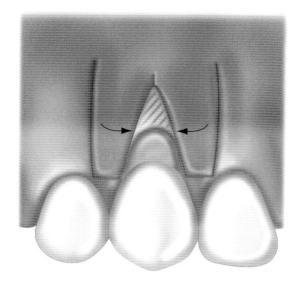

A

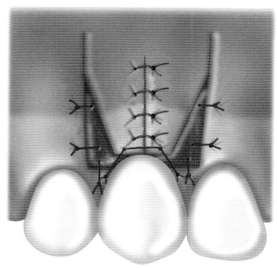

Figure 21-43. Double papilla flap combined with a connective tissue graft (CTG). Diagram shows a connective tissue graft placed under the double papilla flaps. The CTG is sutured to the intact gingiva and mucosa lateral to the root, and the double papilla flap is sutured over the top of the CTG.

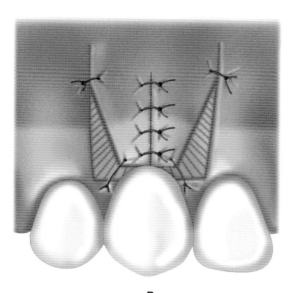

B

Figure 21-42. Double papilla flap. **A,** Incisions: care must be taken to not invade the free gingiva of the adjacent teeth. **B,** Suturing: lateral rotation from each papilla covers the root of the tooth. This technique does not predictably cover root surfaces.

may be necessary. However, it predictably gains 25% to 35% more exposed root coverage than the laterally positioned flap or the double papilla flap alone, which makes this one of the best grafts currently available for single tooth recession problems.[95]

Connective tissue pedicle flap for ridge augmentation. The use of a pedicle connective tissue graft, also called a *split palatal flap* or a *pediculated tissue graft*, for ridge augmentation has been described in several publications.[96-98] This technique has been shown to allow for better soft tissue management in the esthetic zone, because of its ability to maintain a better blood supply to the graft over a larger area, and it may be especially useful in regenerating papillae adjacent to restored teeth or implants. This technique uses a rotated pedicle connective tissue flap from the palate, which can be used to augment the soft tissue ridge in the premolar and incisor region of the maxilla. The base of the pedicle is located in such a position to enable rotating from the deep palate over the recipient site.

Advanced flaps

Advanced flaps move vertically in a coronal direction and do not deviate laterally. These flaps are used to cover exposed root surfaces, and when teeth are not present, this type of flap is used for reconstructive surgery, such as ridge augmentation.[82] The term *coronally positioned flap* is used in this chapter to include techniques used to cover exposed roots with the available gingiva facial to the

is then sutured over the connective tissue graft and is secured with a sling suture. When used properly this technique is very effective in covering exposed roots.

The disadvantages of this technique are: (1) it is primarily used for single tooth root coverage and multiple adjacent teeth are difficult to effectively treat with this technique, and (2) the healing of the keratinized gingiva can be irregular and a gingivoplasty of the irregular tissue exposed root surface (Fig. 21-44, *A* and *B*).[99,100] These techniques have a major drawback because when significant recession occurs, there is rarely enough gingival width or thickness available to coronally position an adequate amount of gingiva and completely cover the exposed root. There is a direct relation between flap thickness and recession reduction when using a coronally positioned flap. Flap thickness that approaches 1.0 mm (>0.8 mm) has a better probability of covering a root surface than a flap thickness of 0.8 mm or less.[101] If the gingiva is too thin, another donor source can be used to increase the thickness of the gingiva.

Coronally positioned flap. The ideal case for a coronally positioned flap has adequate thickness and width of the gingiva on the leading edge of the flap to be advanced. This can be native tissue or it can be the result of a previous procedure used to increase the thickness of tissue to at least 1 mm. The keratinized gingiva has to be wide enough to secure a suture and maintain a stable and secure gingival flap during the healing process. Frenum attachments can limit the amount of coronal positioning and often must be eliminated before a coronally positioned flap can be attempted. There should be adequate quality and height of tissue adjacent to the recipient site to anchor the suture to the desired height.

The advantages of the coronally positioned flap technique are that only one surgical site is involved and an excellent color match occurs if the donor tissue is native tissue. This is the basic technique for many of the future combined techniques; once this technique is mastered it serves as a basis to expand one's expertise. Case selection is important because if the grafted tissue is too thin, only partial root coverage is achieved, and that tissue is prone to future recession. This technique can be difficult to properly stabilize because of the difficulty in suturing, especially with combined techniques.

The basic *coronally positioned flap technique using vertical incisions* is described here in an ideal Class I recession defect with 2 to 3 mm of root exposure and complete root coverage as the desired result (see Fig. 21-44, *A*). The exposed roots should be smoothed to remove any plaque, calculus, or root defects found, and optional root conditioning can be performed at this time. Visualization of the incisions and even sketching the design is a good idea before beginning (Fig. 21-44, *A*). First, measure the amount of root to be covered, which in this case is 2.5 mm. This measurement will be the distance between the coronal and apical horizontal incisions and the height of the recipient bed between the horizontal and vertical incisions. The first two small coronal horizontal incisions are made at the proposed coronal edge of the recipient bed, even with the CEJ, with care not to invade the gingival sulcus of the adjacent tooth. The vertical incisions are extended perpendicular to the first two incisions and well

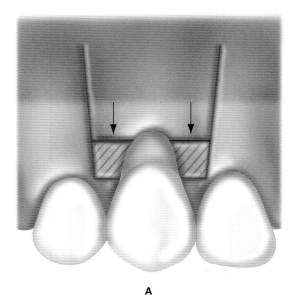

A

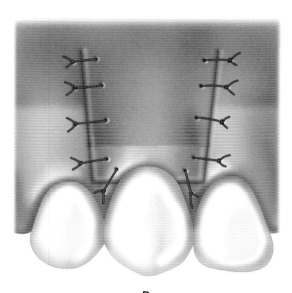

B

Figure 21-44. Coronally positioned flap (with vertical incisions). **A,** The two horizontal incisions are placed the same distance apart as the amount of root to be covered. The vertical incisions can be either parallel or trapezoidal. **B,** The flap is sutured after being adequately advanced and remaining passively in place. Note the coronal displacement of the mucogingival junction.

into the alveolar mucosa. These two incisions may be parallel to one another forming a rectangle, or divergent forming a trapezoid. If the root is prominent, then as the flap is advanced over the root the flap must cover more area because of the root prominence; if the incisions are parallel, the flap will be too short mesial to distal. If there is no root prominence, then the incisions can be more parallel because the mesial to distal distance will not change. The amount of flap divergence is dictated by the amount of root prominence. Figure 21-44 shows a case with slight root prominence, therefore the incisions are slightly divergent. The next horizontal incision is made 2.5 mm apical to the coronal horizontal incisions and it connects the vertical incisions. The surface epithelium is removed from the rectangular area between the vertical and horizontal incisions to yield a connective tissue recipient bed for the graft (Fig. 21-44, A). The thickness of the donor tissue is assessed to determine the type of flap reflection. In some cases, split-thickness dissection is performed in the keratinized tissue, whereas in other cases, a full-thickness flap is used over the radicular surface of the root to maintain a flap thickness of no less than 0.8 mm. The full-thickness portion of the flap is extended to the mucogingival junction where a split-thickness dissection continues from that point apically. The pedicle flap is then advanced in a coronal direction until it comes to rest on the recipient bed for a trial fit. The fit should be a butt joint where the flap is inlayed into or exactly fits into the recipient site with its coronal edge at the CEJ. The donor tissue should stay in place without suturing if the flap reflection was performed well. If the donor tissue does not remain in place, the flap reflection must be extended for adequate release.

Once the tissue lies passively in place, suturing is accomplished with a small reverse cutting needle and 5–0 or 6–0 sutures (see Fig. 21-44, B). Proper suturing should allow adaptation of the donor tissue without any tension on the flap. Pulling the lip out to see if the donor tissue moves is the best way to check for graft stability. If movement is detected, additional sutures may need to be placed. In most cases, periodontal dressing is not used because the flap is stable, but if movement is likely, dressing should be used to stabilize the flap and prevent any movement.

The coronally positioned flap for exposed root coverage may involve a two-stage procedure, because in some cases the native tissue is too thin. The attached gingiva may first be augmented with a free epithelialized graft; then after complete healing a second stage coronally positioned flap is performed to cover the root of the tooth.[99] Currently, an inadvertent two-stage procedure is sometimes used when a connective tissue graft intended to cover the root fails to give the desired amount of root coverage. In this situation, there is usually enough improved thickness and width of the keratinized tissue to successfully cover the exposed root with a secondary coronally positioned flap.

Research shows that the two-stage technique yields a mean exposed root coverage of 62.5% with a range of 36% to 74%, whereas the coronally positioned flap as a one-stage technique with native tissue yields a mean exposed root coverage of 82.7% with a range of 70% to 99% (Table 21-2). This is a confusing result because the thicker coronally positioned two-stage graft gives 20% less root coverage than the coronally positioned flap. One possible explanation is that the two-stage procedure was done only 6 weeks after the initial grafting procedure in these studies. This graft does not have a fully established blood supply and when coronally positioned, the graft does not survive as well as a coronally positioned native graft.

Coronally positioned flap without vertical incisions. The coronally positioned flap without vertical incisions can be performed when multiple teeth are involved with decreasing amounts of recession from the central tooth, which allows for progressive advancement of the flap (Fig. 21-45, A and B). Generally, this technique cannot advance flaps as far as flap advancement with vertical incisions can. This technique requires Class I recession defects with at least 2 mm of attached gingiva with a thickness of 0.8 mm or greater over each tooth in the proposed graft. Root preparation is performed as discussed previously to remove any bacterial or mineralized deposits along with any root defects. The initial horizontal incision is made at the CEJ and extends from the mesial to the distal papilla at each end of the graft. The second incision begins at the termination of the first incision, and this horizontal incision is made apical to the first incision and the radicular level of recession over each tooth. The gingival epithelium is removed over each papilla between the two horizontal incisions leaving a connective tissue bed for the coronally positioned flap. The apical flap is dissected with a split-thickness dissection and is coronally positioned until it passively rests on the prepared bed. One or two sutures are placed at each interdental site to secure the flap into place.

Semilunar flap. The semilunar flap[100] differs in the incision design from the coronally positioned flap, but the direction of movement is the same (Fig. 21-46, A and B). This flap needs a minimum of 2 to 3 mm of keratinized gingiva with adequate thickness to allow for manipulation. The flap can be advanced 1 to 3 mm to cover exposed roots in Class I recession defects (Fig. 21-47, A). The advantages of this technique are that it is a simple technique and often does not require suturing. The disadvantage is that the limit of coronal movement is a maximum of 2 to 3 mm.

After local anesthesia, the bone should be sounded to determine the location of the facial bone. This location will influence the apical extent of the scallop. When the tissue is coronally positioned, it is critical to have tissue cover the root *and the crestal bone* and to avoid having root exposed apical to the semilunar incision. The incision begins at one interdental site, which is slightly coronal to the proposed level of the flap advancement, and continues in a semilunar arc ending at the opposite interdental site (Fig. 21-47, B). The incision begins in gingiva and

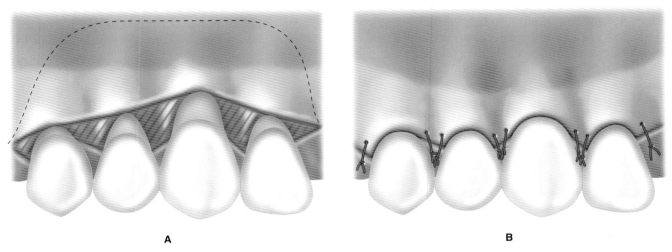

A   **B**

Figure 21-45. Coronally positioned flap (without vertical incisions). **A,** Two horizontal incisions are made the same distance apart as the amount of exposed root, and papillary epithelium is removed to make a recipient bed for the coronally positioned flap. **B,** A split-thickness flap is reflected and coronally positioned with interrupted sutures. Note the coronal displacement of the mucogingival junction.

extends far enough into the mucosa to cover the denuded root, and then courses back into gingiva. The height of the semilunar flap must be greater than the distance from the CEJ to bone, so that the apical border of the flap in its final position rests on bone and not on denuded root. Split-thickness dissection to free the semilunar flap is performed and the tissue is positioned coronally. This dissection is often easier and safer to perform from the apical aspect of the incision toward the gingival margin. The flap is immobilized for 5 minutes with gentle pres-

sure, and then is evaluated for stability; if it is stable, suturing is generally not necessary. If necessary, a small needle and 5–0 or 6–0 sutures can be used to secure the coronally positioned gingiva to the papilla with two interrupted sutures or one suspensory suture (Fig. 21-47, *C*). The final, 3-month healing is seen in Figure 21-47, *D*.

Semilunar flap/free epithelialized soft tissue graft. The major variation of this technique is the combination technique, a semilunar flap and a free epithelialized soft tissue graft (Fig. 21-48, *A* and *B*), where the scalloped

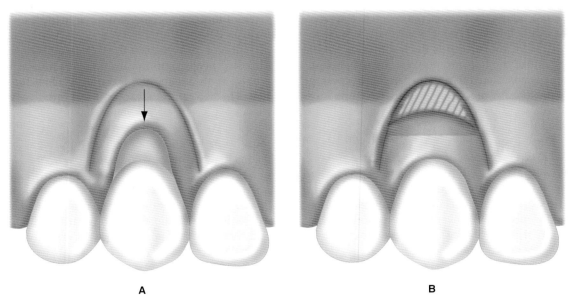

A   **B**

Figure 21-46. Semilunar flap. **A,** Initial incisions are made 2+ mm apical to the mucogingival junction. **B,** Coronal advancement of the semilunar flap and suturing (if needed).

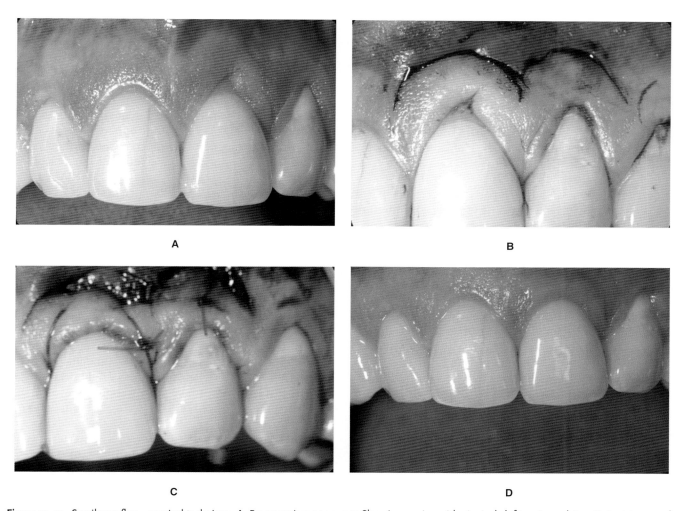

Figure 21-47. Semilunar flap—surgical technique. **A,** Preoperative: 1 to 2 mm Class I recession with gingival clefting #9 and #10. **B,** Incisions made apical to the mucogingival junction. **C,** Coronally positioned semilunar flap sutured with 5–0 sutures. **D,** Three month postoperative view shows complete root coverage.

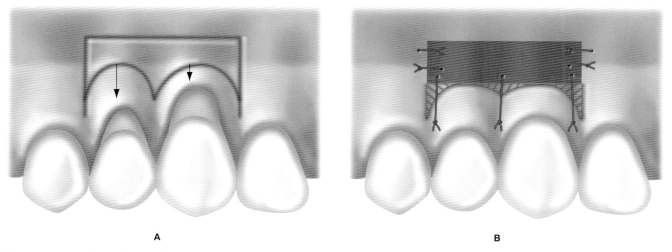

Figure 21-48. Semilunar flap combined with a free epithelialized graft. **A,** Incisions are at the mucogingival junction (no mucosal margins). **B,** Suturing of the coronally positioned gingiva and the supporting free epithelialized graft.

incision is made at the mucogingival junction instead of in the mucosa, as with the previous technique. The semilunar flap combined with a free epithelialized soft tissue graft may be used on one or several teeth. The amount of root surface to be covered is directly related to the width of gingiva to be moved: 1 mm of gingiva can be coronally positioned no more than 1 mm, 2 mm of gingiva can be moved 2 mm, and 3 mm is the maximum root coverage that this technique can accomplish. Then, after coronally positioning the tissue, and suturing if necessary, a free epithelialized soft tissue graft is placed to increase the amount of gingiva and to support the coronally positioned tissue by suturing the graft in place apical to the semilunar flap (Fig. 21-48, B).

Apically positioned flaps

The apically positioned flap moves apically and exposes more of the tooth and sometimes alveolar bone. It was originally designed to increase attached gingiva, deepen the vestibule, and eliminate pocket depth. In addition to the original purposes, this flap technique currently is widely used to maintain keratinized gingiva and to expose more tooth structure. The margin of the flap can be placed in three different positions relative to the marginal bone: (1) 2 to 3 mm apical to the bone, (2) at the level of the bone, or (3) coronal to the margin of the bone but apical to the original gingival margin.

This procedure evolved from vestibular deepening procedures, in particular the denudation procedure,[102] where a flap was reflected, then all of the gingiva was removed with scissors and discarded. The mucosal flap margin contracted and exposed a significant amount of cortical plate. The bone was then left exposed but covered with periodontal dressing and allowed to heal. Gingival fibroblasts proliferated from the periodontal ligament space and reformed the gingiva in approximately 3 months. This procedure produced a long, painful healing time with a deepened vestibule and shallow pockets and has been all but abandoned. In 1954, Nabers[103] suggested the apical positioning of the full-thickness flap to cover the bone, instead of discarding the gingiva and exposing the bone, thereby reducing pain and decreasing the healing time after periodontal surgery. The most common use of this flap is to improve pocket reduction after many different types of periodontal surgery to treat periodontitis.[104,105] In most cases, the bone has been resorbed or surgically reshaped so the flap will be positioned at a more apical position on the tooth exposing more tooth surface.

Crown lengthening. Clinical crown lengthening intentionally seeks to expose more tooth surface by apically positioning the flap with or without osseous surgery. There are two types of crown lengthening: functional and esthetic.

Functional crown lengthening. Functional crown lengthening is used when the clinical crown is too short to retain a crown. The teeth in Figure 21-49 were fractured at the gingival margin, and probing revealed a depth of 2 mm—1 mm of sulcus depth, and 1 mm of junctional epithelial attachment (see Fig. 21-49, A). Sounding depth to bone is 3 mm, which is the total length of the *dentogingival complex* composed of 1 mm connective tissue attachment, 1 mm of junctional epithelium, and 1 mm of sulcus depth. The *biologic width* is the width of the attachment apparatus, which is 1 mm connective tissue attachment and 1 mm junctional epithelial attachment.[106] That will leave only 1 mm of tooth structure for the retention of the crown and the "ferrule effect" for the post and core buildup, which is inadequate.[107] A ferrule is a metal ring or cap used to strengthen the end of a tube. The use of a ferrule as part of the post and core, or a crown, strengthens the tooth and reduces the incidence of recurrent decay and split teeth. This means that when functional crown lengthening is performed there should be a measurement made from the bone to the edge of sound tooth structure. This measurement should be at least 4 mm, which consists of a minimum of 2 mm for the biologic width plus 2 mm for the ferrule effect.[108,109] Reflection of a full-thickness flap reveals that the total tooth length of 3 mm does confirm the sounding measurement (Fig. 21-49, B). Exposure of more tooth surface is necessary to reestablish the biologic width (2+ mm) and leave enough tooth exposed to create adequate retention and the ferrule effect (2+ mm) (Fig. 21-49, C). Therefore, a *minimum* of 4 mm of sound tooth structure, measured from the bone to the coronal edge of sound tooth structure, is needed at the time of surgery. If adequate retention is desired without a post, 5 mm of root should be exposed to give a 3 mm preparation, which is adequate for both retention and the ferrule effect (Fig. 21-49, C). These basic principles of crown lengthening also will apply to esthetic crown lengthening.

Esthetic crown lengthening. Esthetic crown lengthening, is performed when excessive gingival display or the "gummy smile" is a problem, as discussed previously in this chapter (Fig. 21-31). Once the determination has been made that apically positioning the gingiva is the proper course of action, the distance from the CEJ to the bone should be determined. This will help with determining whether osseous surgery will be needed, or if the procedure will involve only the gingiva. The exact amount of lengthening should be determined in consultation with the orthodontist, or general dentist, or both (assuming restorative or orthodontic treatment is needed), and based on the esthetic desires of the patient. The position of the frenum should be evaluated to determine if it would be a complicating factor. If the frenum is a problem, it should be removed using a frenectomy procedure 6 weeks before the flap procedure is performed.

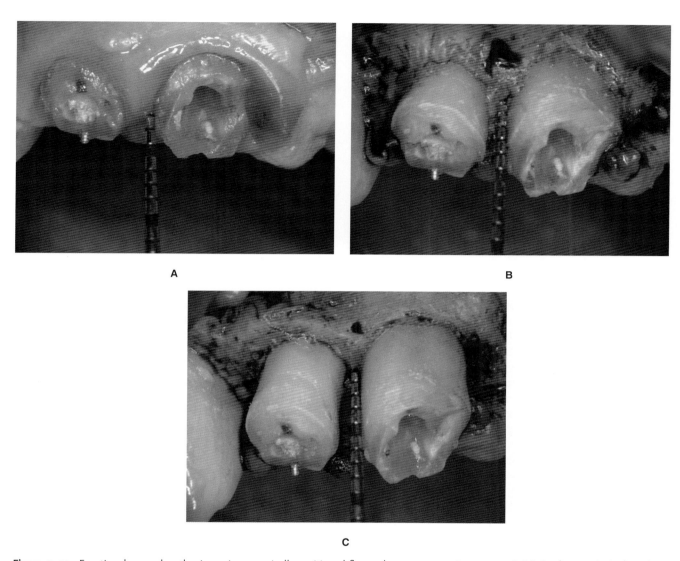

Figure 21-49. Functional crown lengthening using an apically positioned flap and osseous resective surgery. **A,** Minimal supragingival tooth structure was present before surgery; the interproximal probing depth was 2 mm. **B,** Flaps reflected showing the 3 mm of tooth exposed corresponding to the sounding depth and confirming the width of the dentogingival complex (2 mm biologic width or dentogingival attachment, 1 mm sulcus depth). **C,** Osseous surgery exposed 2 mm more of the tooth and gave 5 mm of total tooth length, which will later equal 3 mm of tooth structure for crown preparation. This provides a more than adequate "ferrule effect" for these endodontically treated teeth.

The advantages of the apically positioned flap over the gingivectomy procedure are access to the bone and more rapid healing with less pain. If access to the bone is not necessary, then gingivectomy procedures will give similar results without flap reflection. The apically positioned flap procedure allows access to the bone so that osseous resection can be performed if necessary, as well as precise placement of the gingival margin to ensure a predictable result. The goal is to expose a specific amount of tooth and to maintain a stable gingival margin after the surgical procedure. These procedures are effective in some cases but not in others and the end results seem inconsistent in the

literature.[110,111] In these studies, there was either too much tooth exposed, or in the majority of the cases, too little tooth exposed. Any change in the amount of tooth exposed would be an undesirable occurrence. It is important to understand and recognize the morphology of the case being treated because in the thin periodontium, unwanted bone resorption can lead to increased tooth exposure over the desired amount. Conversely, a finding called *gingival rebound* may occur. There is good evidence that gingival rebound of 0.5 to 1.2 mm at 12 months[112,113] decreases the overall tooth length and reduces the long-term effectiveness of crown lengthening. Ochsenbein and

Ross[5] observed that thick and thin periodontal biotypes behave differently after surgery, and trying to transform a thick periodontium to a thin periodontium is fighting the genetic predisposition of that patient to regenerate the thick periodontium.

Understanding these variations in crown lengthening procedures requires further investigation. In 1961, Gargiulo, Wentz, and Orban[114] reported a wide variation in the dentogingival complex among patients in a study group. Kois[115] clinically evaluated the dimensions of the dentogingival complex by sounding to bone between human maxillary central incisors. He reported that 85% of the population studied had a facial dentogingival complex of 3 mm, whereas the interproximal measurement was approximately 4.5 mm[115]; this distance is close to the 5 mm interproximal measurement seen by Tarnow and colleagues.[81] About 15% of the population still vary from the normal, and Spear[116] reports that variations in biologic width are seen throughout the periodontium within the same patient. Therefore, a baseline reference measurement can be taken for each patient to determine his or her *individual dentogingival complex and biologic width*. This is used to determine how much tooth to expose in the crown lengthening procedure. The reference is taken from an unrestored contralateral tooth if present, or if not, a premolar in the same arch being treated can be used to determine the measurement for that patient. The goal is to properly diagnose the type of periodontium and the width of the total dentogingival complex, which includes the biologic width for that patient. The patient's individually determined biologic width will help to predict the amount of soft tissue rebound after crown lengthening procedures and precisely how much bone to remove at time of surgery for that individual patient. Each patient will return to the baseline width of the normal dentogingival complex for that patient after surgical crown lengthening procedures.

The decision to perform esthetic crown lengthening using a gingivectomy procedure versus an apically positioned flap depends primarily on the distance between the proposed final position of the gingival margin and the underlying bone. If a gingivectomy procedure is used to remove "excess" gingiva, but the new gingival margin position is too close to the underlying bone, the biologic width will be violated and the gingival margin will usually rebound toward its original position. This can result in a "shortening" of the clinical crown over time. If the new gingival margin position is close to the underlying bone, a flap should be reflected and an adequate amount of osteoplasty and ostectomy should be performed to reestablish an adequate biologic width.

The first measurement taken for esthetic crown lengthening is sounding to bone to establish the total dentogingival complex and biologic width for that patient. This measurement is taken on an undisturbed nonrestored tooth, the contralateral tooth if possible. If the contralateral tooth is restored or is not available, another similar tooth should be selected as close to the shape and size of the tooth being treated. The next procedure is to visualize the end result and have a firm idea from consultations with the patient and the dental team of the length, width, and shape of teeth to achieve the desired results. If restorations are planned, the shape of the teeth and the contact points of the crowns will influence the end result. This information must be combined with the biologic width for that patient to determine the proper position of the facial, lingual, and interproximal bone.

Preservation of papillary tissue. The preservation of papillary tissue to prevent "black triangles" from developing interdentally is one of the esthetic goals of treatment. To do this, it is important to determine the distance from the interproximal bone to the contact point. This measurement will determine the probability of regenerating the papilla once surgery has been performed. The papilla will regenerate predictably if the distance from the bone to contact point is 5 mm or less.[81] If the distance is greater than 5 mm, then the papilla will not predictably regenerate and the papilla should be left undisturbed. Many people have an average distance of contact point to bone of 6 mm or even 7 mm without any missing papillary tissue. This measurement is important for those patients and should be carefully evaluated to know how the papilla will respond. If the distance is from 6 to 7 mm, the papillae will not regenerate if the papilla is reflected during surgery; therefore, no flap should be reflected if apical positioning of the papilla is not desired. However, if the distance is 4 to 5 mm, the papilla will fully regenerate filling the embrasure space, but it may take from 3 to 24 months. One mistake is to restoratively close the embrasure space too quickly, before the rebound of the papilla has occurred. If this moves the contact point too close to the bone, there will not be enough space for the papilla, creating gingival swelling and chronic inflammation. Once the initial healing takes place at 6 weeks, the provisional restorations can be placed, if the biologic width that was determined for that patient is not violated and the proper embrasure space of 4 to 5 mm from the bone to the contact point is respected. Placement of final restorations may be delayed several weeks to months to allow tissue maturation. If there is a black triangular space still present interdentally, more time will be required to allow for thickening of the papillary soft tissue and rebound of the papilla. In some cases, the interproximal bone must be reduced for retention of a crown, but, in many cases, the interproximal bone can be left undisturbed. This is preferable when possible because the healing of the facial and lingual soft tissues will occur quickly, compared with the healing of the papilla. If the levels of the interproximal bone must be changed, usually because of inadequate tooth structure, then the contact point between the teeth must be moved toward the bone by decreasing the embrasure space.

To help prevent loss of papillary height and formation of black triangles in the esthetic zone, many clinicians prefer to reflect only a facial or lingual flap at any given surgical appointment. This allows retention of a fixed papilla in each interdental space opposing the reflected flap, improving the stability of the flap after suturing and providing a fixed connective tissue bed for blood supply to the reflected papillary areas. If no restorations are required, esthetic crown lengthening is often restricted to the facial surfaces and may require reflection of only a facial flap.

Excessive gingival display. The first clinical case presents with a right lateral incisor with excessive gingival display (Fig. 21-50, *A*). This tooth had an old crown and 2 mm more gingiva than the contralateral tooth. The facial probing revealed a 3-mm probing depth, and sounding to bone was 5 mm. The other lateral incisor probed 1 mm on the facial and sounded to bone at 3 mm. This means there was enough soft tissue to allow a *gingivectomy* to establish the proper length without involving the bone. A gingivectomy was performed to remove 2 mm of facial gingiva, leaving 3 mm of soft tissue between the new gingival margin position and the bone. The healing at 6 weeks showed the tooth was ready for the new crown (Fig. 21-50, *B*). The final crown 6 weeks later reveals the proper length of the right lateral in comparison to the left lateral (Fig. 21-50, *C*).

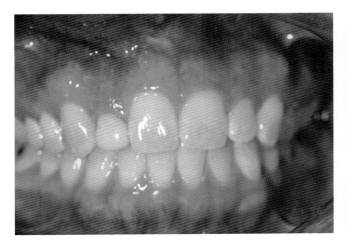

A

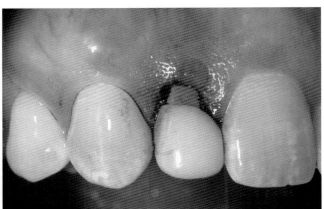

B

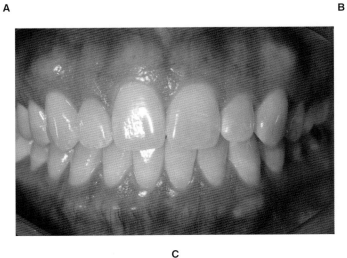

C

Figure 21-50. Esthetic crown lengthening by increasing the gingival scallop (gingivectomy). **A,** Preoperative view of a short lateral incisor (#7) with bilateral asymmetry. **B,** Removal of 2.5 mm of gingiva increases the gingival scallop and leaves a dentogingival complex of 2.5 mm and 2.5 mm of exposed root. Both lateral incisors had equal length after surgery. **C,** Six-week postoperative photograph with new crown #7 and nice bilateral symmetry. (Restorative therapy by Dr. Mark Venincasa.)

Flap reflection and osseous surgery. The next case (Fig. 21-51) will require osseous surgery with flap reflection to achieve the desired result. This patient presents with excessive gingival display of the lateral incisors and canines with a complaint of short teeth and too much gum showing when she smiles (Fig. 21-51, *A*). The extent of the problem was revealed only after sounding to bone under local anesthesia; the facial dentogingival complex on the central incisors measured 3.5 mm, 3.0 mm on the premolars, and 5.5 mm on the laterals and canines. The individual length of the dentogingival complex was taken to be a normal 3.0 mm. The overall length of the central incisors was planned for 10.5 mm (10 mm initial), laterals 9.5 mm (6 mm initial), and canines 10.5 mm (initial 7 mm). This meant that the central incisors could be lengthened 0.5 mm by soft tissue removal, and the canine and laterals would require osseous surgery. The canines and laterals needed to be 3.5 mm longer—2 mm would come from gingivectomy and 1.5 mm from ostectomy (Fig. 21-51, *B*). The point of reference for measurements was a flat metal plate placed in the patient's mouth to establish the occlusal plane and discount for possible variations in the incisal edges of individual teeth. When the proper dentogingival complex is established, uncomplicated healing takes at least 6 weeks (Fig. 21-51, *C*). After final restoration, an ideal result that was pleasing to the patient, restorative dentist, and periodontist was obtained.

The patient in Figure 21-52, *A*, has short teeth as a result of altered passive eruption and will require *osseous*

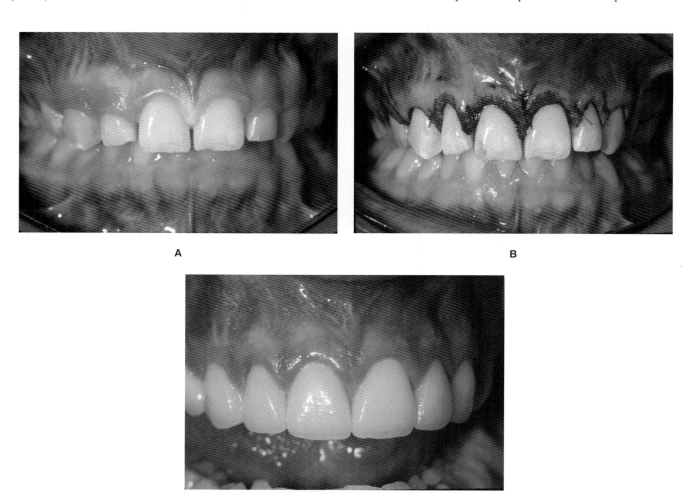

A

B

C

Figure 21-51. Esthetic crown lengthening by gingivectomy and osseous resective surgery. **A,** The patient's chief complaint was short teeth, too much gum showing, and spaces between the front teeth. The individualized dentogingival complex was 3.0 mm. **B,** The teeth were lengthened by a gingivectomy for the central incisors and osseous resective surgery for the lateral incisors and canines to give a total postoperative dentogingival complex of 3.0 mm. **C,** Six-week postoperative photograph shows bilateral symmetry with ideal tooth and papilla length. After placement of porcelain veneers, an ideal esthetic result was achieved. (Restorative therapy by Dr. Dale Robinowitz.)

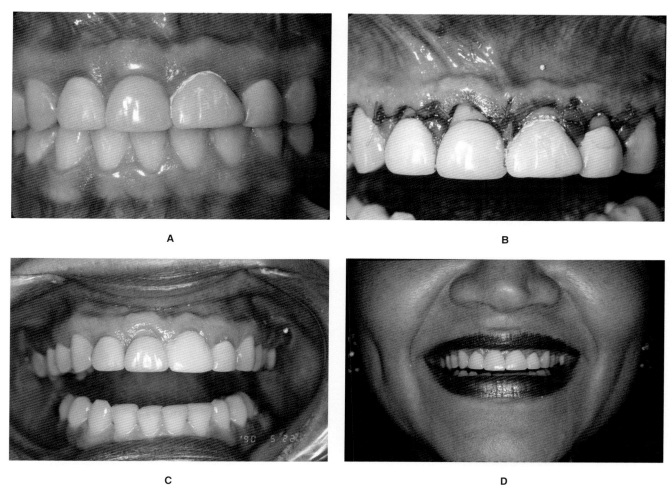

Figure 21-52. Esthetic crown lengthening by osseous resective surgery with papillary retention. **A,** Short, square clinical crowns are seen with the temporary crowns. **B,** Facial gingiva was scalloped to improve the length-to-width ratio. The interproximal tissue was maintained by using a horizontal incision at each papilla to preserve the entire interdental papilla. After osseous resective surgery on the facial surfaces, the flap was sutured at each papilla. **C,** Twelve-week postoperative view showing some marginal rebound compared with the suturing photograph. **D,** The final smile after esthetic crown lengthening and restorative treatment. (Restorative therapy by Dr. Larry Herwig.)

surgery with flap reflection to achieve an acceptable esthetic result. The crowns on the incisors were to be replaced after crown lengthening. The interdental bone and papilla were at an acceptable height, but the facial gingiva and bone needed to be apically positioned to establish bilateral symmetry. The initial incisions are scalloping incisions to increase the tooth length and to establish the new facial gingival margin. Next, horizontal incisions were made at each papilla to preserve the interdental papillae (Fig. 21-52, *B*). This allows for papillary retention and reflection of the flap to expose the facial bone. When osseous recontouring will involve the interproximal bone, a sulcular incision is used and the papillary tissue is included in the reflected flap. When the lingual tissue does not need to be reflected, it is left attached to the

lingual bone and tooth surfaces to maintain the papillary blood supply and prevent interproximal recession. Because the total facial dentogingival dimension was 3.5 mm for the patient in Figure 21-52, osseous surgery was performed to position the bone at the proper position apical to the new location of the gingival margin, thus giving the desired tooth length. Before suturing, optional gingivoplasty of each papilla is performed to allow for an imperceptible incision line. The facial flap is then sutured interdentally, and the apical positioning or lengthening of the teeth comes from the gingival scalloping (Fig. 21-52, *B*). The 12-week healing shows some soft tissue rebound from the suturing slide but the case is ready to be restored (Fig. 21-52, *C*). Because the gingival margin position may shift apically or coronally, even after 12 weeks of healing in some patients, many dentists prefer to place provisional restorations at this time and delay final impressions and crown fabrication for several more months. After restoration, the full smile photograph shows the increased tooth length, intact papillae, proper gingival contours, and relation to each lip (Fig. 21-52, *D*).

Increasing zone of gingiva. One modification of the apically positioned flap technique[117] focuses on increasing the amount of keratinized and attached gingiva while preserving the marginal gingiva, thus avoiding marginal soft tissue recession as with most apically positioned flaps. This technique is indicated in cases in which there is a need for increased keratinized and attached gingiva, and the case must have no bony dehiscence, a minimal sulcus depth, no inflammation, and 0.5 mm or more attached gingiva (Fig. 21-53, *A*). A beveled incision is made in the attached gingiva ending apical to the alveolar crest (Fig. 21-53, *B*). If a dehiscence is discovered, a free

epithelialized soft tissue graft would be placed to cover the dehiscence. The extent of the incision is determined by the area that requires surgery. Two vertical incisions are made to allow for apically positioning the split-thickness flap. The flap is apically positioned the same distance as the desired increase in keratinized tissue width. The flap is secured by sutures, and dry foil may be placed, followed by a periodontal dressing. The dressing is removed in 1 week and chlorhexidine mouthwash is used for 2 weeks. The area usually appears clinically healed in 8 to 12 weeks and the result appears similar to a thin free epithelialized soft tissue graft (Fig. 21-53, *C*). A second stage procedure can be done after 8 to 12 weeks to coronally position the gingiva to cover roots, if needed. There is no increase in pocket depth, but there is on average a 2-mm increase in the amount of attached gingiva. Advantages of this technique are the elimination of the need for donor tissue, the ability to treat multiple teeth, and excellent color match.

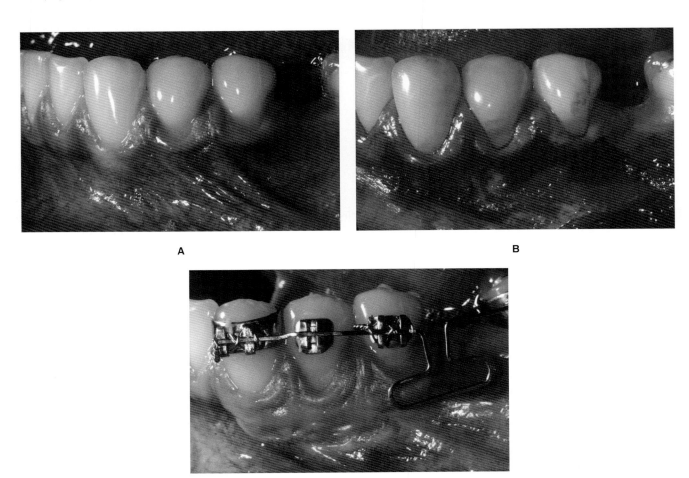

A

B

C

Figure 21-53. Modified apically positioned flap to increase attached gingiva. **A,** Preoperative view of multiple Class I recession defects. **B,** The beveled incision is at the mucogingival junction and the split-thickness flap is apically positioned to expose the periosteum, leaving a collar of gingiva around the teeth. **C,** Ten-week postoperative photograph shows increased attached gingiva that can be coronally positioned if desired.

The disadvantage is the final thickness of gingiva being less than what can be accomplished by other free soft tissue grafting techniques.

Exposure of impacted teeth. The exposure of impacted teeth by the apically positioned flap was first shown to be successful in 75 cases by Vanarsdall and Corn in 1977.[118] With the exception of third molars, the most common maxillary impaction is the canine, followed by the central incisors.[119] The most common mandibular impaction is the second premolar and the second molar.[120] Teeth lose their capacity to erupt after the root apex has closed,[121] therefore surgical intervention is necessary if the tooth is to be brought into occlusion. The most common cause of impacted teeth is an aberrant angulated eruption path.

The most important consideration is to determine whether the tooth is to the facial or to the palatal. Maxillary canines are found labially impacted one third of the time and palatally impacted two thirds of the time. Often the position can be determined by manual palpation, but it may be necessary to use two different dental radiographs such as a periapical film and an occlusal film. In one particularly useful diagnostic technique, one periapical film is taken using standard technique and angulation. A second film is then taken with the X-ray tube head angled 20 to 30 degrees toward the mesial on a horizontal plane. If the impacted tooth is on the labial aspect, the image will "move" toward the distal on the second radiograph. If the impacted tooth is on the lingual/palatal aspect, the image will move toward the mesial. In some difficult cases, a tomographic radiograph may be necessary to locate the position of the tooth.

The major advantage of the apically positioned flap technique for impacted tooth exposure is that it allows formation of an esthetic, adequate band of attached gingiva on the labial surface of these teeth. Other surgical methods of exposing teeth such as gingivectomy that remove all the gingiva leaving only a facial mucosal margin have been shown to significantly reduce the width of buccal keratinized gingiva, increase gingival recession, and increase gingivitis when compared with the apically positioned flap.[122,123] The apically positioned flap technique has some disadvantages when used for very high or laterally displaced impactions where accessory frena can be created in the vertical incision area. Orthodontic relapse has been observed in some patients.[124]

The technique is described here for a maxillary canine (Fig. 21-54, A and B). The apically positioned flap is used when the tip of the impacted canine is apical to the adjacent CEJ. After local anesthesia, an incision is made parallel and far enough away from the mucogingival line to retain 3 to 5 mm of gingiva. Usually this incision is made near the crest of the edentulous ridge. Next, two vertical incisions are made the same width as the edentulous ridge, beginning at the crest of the ridge and extending into the vestibule on either side of the impacted canine as a split-thickness flap is reflected. The desired thickness of the gingival portion of the pedicle flap is at least 1 mm. If two thirds of the tooth is not exposed, some bone must be removed to give adequate access for the bracket. The remaining follicle should be removed through careful curettage.

The split-thickness pedicle flap is then sutured in the apical position to stabilize the gingiva at the desired level to expose one half to two thirds of the crown (Fig. 21-54, C). Periodontal dressing can be used if needed to aid in stabilization of the apically positioned pedicle flap. In 2 to 3 weeks the orthodontist can attach a bracket. The surgeon needs to bond an appliance if the impaction is deeper or if less than one half of the tooth is exposed. A dry field is a problem and sometimes difficult to overcome, but absolutely necessary for successful bonding. The bonded appliance will help with the retention of the periodontal dressing and subsequent stabilization of the pedicle flap. Orthodontic movement can ideally proceed in 1 to 3 weeks (Fig. 21-54, D). The tooth can now be moved into ideal alignment (Fig. 21-54, E).

The position of these impacted teeth varies greatly. The primary problems occur in the deeply impacted cases. In these cases, the bonding of the button or hook is the most difficult and important part of the technique. The application of an absorbable collagen matrix packed around the tooth will help control the bleeding. An etching gel is used to rinse, dry, prime, and bond over the etched surface. The newer generation of light cured orthodontic resin cements aids the speed of setting up the bond, thereby increasing the chances of success.[125]

Replaced flap

The replaced flap is a flap that is reflected and replaced to its original position. The purpose of this flap is for surgical access where the postoperative position of the gingiva is the same as the preoperative appearance. This is the simplest flap of the four types of flaps, but one that must be mastered if periodontal and reconstructive procedures are to be successful. This flap can be used for all types of periodontal flap surgery where esthetics are critical and no recession is desirable, including: guided tissue regeneration, bone grafting, subgingival root surface restorations, and application of enamel matrix protein and other metabolic enhancers of bone and soft tissue regeneration. Other surgical procedures such as closed orthodontic eruption,[126] ridge augmentation surgery,[71] sinus elevation surgery, exploratory periodontal surgery, and endodontic surgery all share the principles of this flap procedure.

Closed orthodontic eruption. Closed orthodontic eruption is a newer technique than the apically positioned flap to expose impacted teeth.[124] The indication for this

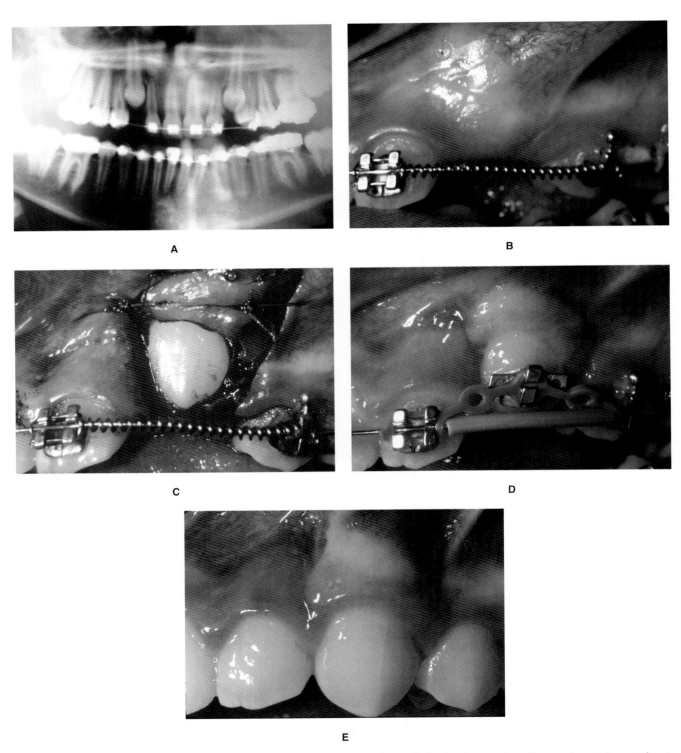

Figure 21-54. Apically positioned flap to expose impacted teeth. **A,** Panoramic radiograph showing impacted maxillary canines. **B,** Impacted canine preoperative clinical view. **C,** A horizontal incision was made at the crest of the ridge, and two vertical incisions were made. The split-thickness flap was apically positioned and sutured to expose the crown of the impacted canine. **D,** Four-week postoperative view shows wide band of facial gingiva. **E,** Six-month postoperative appearance after uncovering and orthodontically erupting the canine.

technique is if the tooth is impacted in the center of the alveolus or high in the vestibule near the nasal spine. Flap access is gained by using a mid-ridge incision with one or two vertical incisions to expose the impacted tooth. If the tooth is covered with bone, the tip of the tooth must be exposed to gain access to the tooth. A bracket or pin is bonded to the tooth and a 0.010-inch ligature wire or gold chain is attached from the bracket to the arch wire. The flap is then replaced and sutured to its original position with only the wire or chain exposed between the flap edges. This technique has been shown to be more esthetically pleasing, causes less tooth exposure, and has less relapse when compared with the apically positioned flap.[126]

This flap technique is often performed on esthetically demanding cases that require exacting control of the postoperative gingival margin position. This often involves a limited area; therefore, vertical incisions are used to assist in flap reflection. The most predictable way to make certain the position of the flap heals properly is to carefully manipulate the tissue, suture, and stabilize the flaps at the proper gingival level. The easiest way to do this is to reflect only the facial or the lingual flap, leaving the other side undisturbed, which ensures that the nonreflected side will maintain its position on the tooth. The reflected flap is sutured to the stable tissue, especially the interdental tissue; consequently, the noncompromised blood supply allows quicker healing with less recession of the reflected flap.

Subgingival restoration placement. The replaced flap technique is sometimes used when subgingival restorations must be placed. Because the flap will be replaced over the restoration, it is ideal to choose restorative materials that are highly compatible with the soft tissues. Dragoo[127] studied three restorative materials, and one material, Geristore (a resin-ionomer restorative material or compomer [Den-Mat Corp., Santa Maria, CA]), had superior handling and healing characteristics. Dragoo was able to show connective tissue fibers functionally aligned and extending into this restorative material. The flap is reflected to allow access to the lesion to be restored. The restoration is placed, smoothed, and finished. The flap is then replaced at its original position.

Tunnel Technique

The tunnel (or envelope) technique gives access to the root and alveolar bone without complete flap reflection; it was developed for use with a connective tissue graft (Fig. 21-55, *A* and *B*)[128] for root coverage procedures[129] and for ridge augmentation procedures. This type of nonconventional pedicle flap maintains a blood supply from two or more sides of the reflected tissue, whereas a conventional pedicle flap maintains an intact blood supply from only one side. This technique uses no conventional incisions; therefore, the blood supply to the papillae is not

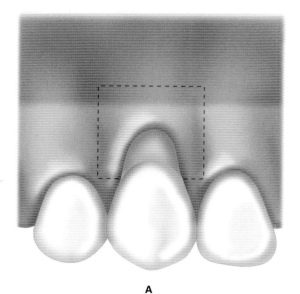

A

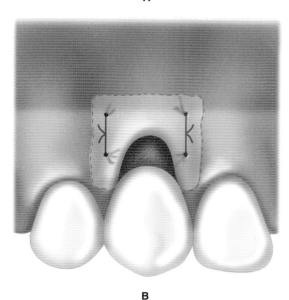

B

Figure 21-55. Single tooth tunnel (envelope technique). **A,** Envelope dissection is outlined. The tunnel or pouch is created through the sulcus and merely undermines the overlying tissue, rather than making superficial incisions. **B,** Autogenous connective tissue graft sutured into envelope.

interrupted. No conventional sutures are needed at each papilla to hold the flap closed. Sutures are only are needed to stabilize the connective tissue graft; therefore, healing is extremely rapid with less papillary healing problems. It is possible to coronally advance, apically position, or replace the soft tissue margin. This technique has promise to be used in the future with endoscopes similar to minimally invasive medical procedures such as endoscopic, arthroscopic, or laparoscopic surgery to reduce trauma and improve healing and esthetics. Because the tunnel technique is rarely used by itself, it is discussed later in this chapter as part of the section that details connective tissue grafts.

Roll technique. The roll technique, a modification of the soft tissue pedicle flap, is used for ridge augmentation and was first described by Abrams in 1980[130] and then revised by Scharf and Tarnow in 1992.[131] It is indicated for small (<3 mm) horizontal maxillary ridge deficiencies. The roll technique involves reflecting a pedicle flap from an edentulous site with the base of the flap toward the facial. The epithelium is removed from the palatal aspect of the flap. An envelope or pouch is made between the base of the pedicle and the bone. The deepithelialized palatal connective tissue pedicle is then rolled into the pouch and sutured to place. This technique is not routinely used because other techniques generally allow for more flexibility and more options with better outcomes.

Free Soft Tissue Grafts

The donor site for this type of soft tissue graft is distant from the recipient site, therefore it maintains none of its own blood supply. The viability of the graft is because of microvascular perfusion from the recipient connective tissue, periosteal, or osseous bed. While Miller[132] is credited with demonstrating the applicability of this technique for root coverage, Bjorn published the first photographic evidence in 1963, and Nabers[133] introduced the term *free gingival graft* in 1966. This technique used tissue removed after performing a gingivectomy, which was the primary surgical procedure for pocket reduction at that time. Instead of discarding the resected gingiva, it was used as the donor tissue. The technique was later modified, and palatal tissue or masticatory mucosa[134] was used as the primary donor source instead of gingiva.

Free epithelialized soft tissue autograft

The free epithelialized soft tissue autograft (Fig. 21-56, A and B) can be subdivided by thickness of the donor tissue (Fig. 21-57): thin (0.5 to 0.8 mm; Fig. 21-58), average (0.9 to 1.4 mm; Fig. 21-59), and thick (1.5 to 2+ mm; Fig. 21-60). The thin epithelialized graft is well suited to increase the amount of attached gingiva and gives the best color match of the three thicknesses (Fig. 21-58). This graft must be placed in intimate contact with an intact blood supply and not over an exposed root to survive; therefore, it is not suited for root coverage. The thin epithelialized graft heals the fastest of the three different graft thicknesses, but shrinks the most after healing (25% to 30%).[135] The palatal wound rarely causes complications because the donor site is so shallow.

The average thickness epithelialized soft tissue graft (0.9 to 1.4 mm) is best suited for all types of grafting except root coverage (Fig. 21-59). This graft is more suited to protect against recession than the thin graft. The appearance is acceptable but not as good as the thin graft. The palatal wound is deeper, which causes more complications

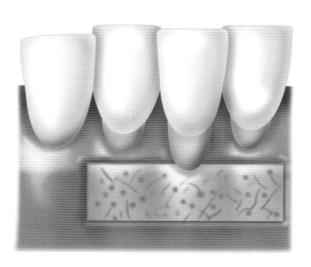

A

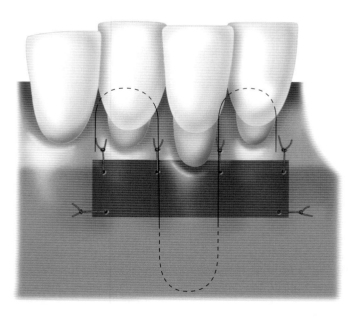

B

Figure 21-56. Thin or average thickness free epithelialized (soft tissue) graft (FEG). **A,** Recipient bed prepared with no attempt at root coverage. **B,** Suturing of FEG showing both interrupted and sling sutures.

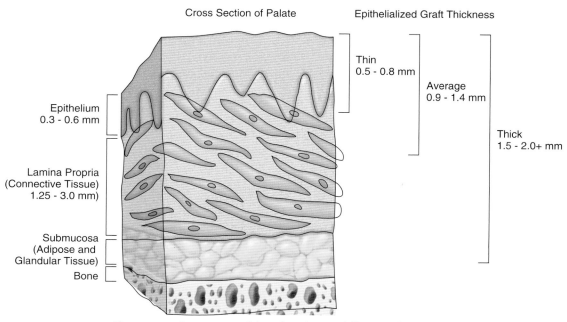

Cross Section of Palate   Epithelialized Graft Thickness

Thin
0.5 - 0.8 mm

Average
0.9 - 1.4 mm

Thick
1.5 - 2.0+ mm

Epithelium
0.3 - 0.6 mm

Lamina Propria
(Connective Tissue)
1.25 - 3.0 mm)

Submucosa
(Adipose and
Glandular Tissue)

Bone

Figure 21-57. Cross section of the palate showing different graft thickness.

such as bleeding, than the thin graft. A palatal stent is recommended to cover the palate and protect the donor site (Fig. 21-61). This stent was made from an impression taken before the surgical appointment, using polymethylmethacrylate powder and liquid with a sprinkle technique. The stent can be made with or without ball clasps, depending on the need for added retention. Other materials can be used, but a properly fabricated palatal stent should be secure so it does not become dislodged when speaking, thereby insuring a stable blood clot. The stent is used for

a pressure application device to stop bleeding and to improve patient comfort.

The technique for a thin or average thickness free epithelialized soft tissue autograft is presented in diagram form in Figure 21-56, *A* and *B*. The case selected has Class III recession and is an indication for treatment because of documented increasing gingival recession after recent orthodontic treatment (Fig. 21-62, *A*). The significant interdental recession precludes complete root coverage, but maintaining a stable and maintainable periodontium is the primary focus of this procedure. The first incision is made at the mucogingival junction and

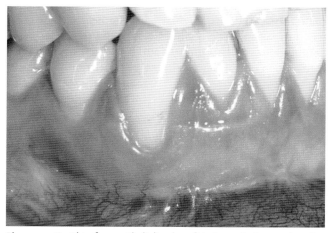

Figure 21-58. Thin free epithelialized graft in lower incisor and canine region—the same thickness and almost the same color as the surrounding gingiva, giving a blended natural look (3 mm increase in attached gingiva on the canine but no coverage of the exposed root, which is typical of thin grafts over wide recession defects).

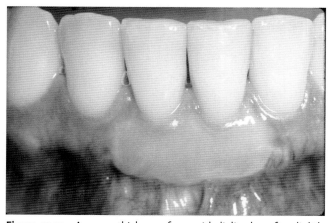

Figure 21-59. Average thickness free epithelialized graft—slightly raised from adjacent native gingiva and color is lighter than native gingiva.

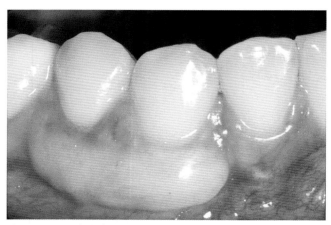

Figure 21-60. Thick free epithelialized graft—significantly raised from adjacent gingiva and the color is much lighter than the native gingiva (3 mm of exposed root was covered on the canine).

defines the length of the recipient site that needs augmentation. The vertical incisions are made in the interproximal sites distal to the terminal teeth to form a right angle with the initial incisions (Fig. 21-62, A). A split-thickness flap is reflected, and then the thin mucosal flap is excised to prepare the recipient bed for the donor tissue. The recipient bed is measured with a periodontal probe and/or a template is cut out of a sterile material such as dry foil or from the sterile foil that is used to enclose most suture materials. This template is then taken to the palate to outline the shape of the donor tissue. The donor tissue is taken at least 2 mm from the palatal gingival margin to prevent recession on these teeth, because recession may occur as a result of the wound edge being too close to the gingival margin. This is often a problem on the palatal root of the maxillary first molar. The template or shape of the donor tissue is

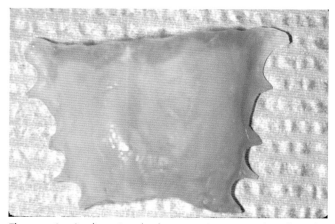

Figure 21-61. Acrylic resin palatal stent used to protect the palate after donor tissue is harvested.

outlined with a scalpel at a right angle to the palate at the desired depth, which can be gauged by the bevel on a #15 scalpel blade (approximately 1 mm). The blade is then turned parallel to the palate and a graft of the desired uniform thickness is removed by sharp dissection from the palate. The prefabricated palatal stent is placed to form a stable blood clot. The donor tissue is transferred to the recipient site to check the fit and modify if needed. Suturing techniques vary widely, but stabilization of the graft is the most important principle. The thin graft requires fewer sutures than the average thickness graft. Stabilization is accomplished by using stable structures adjacent to the surgical site such as interproximal tissue or a sling suture placed around the teeth. The apical muscle group and the periosteum can be used to stabilize the graft using 4-0, 5-0, or 6-0 absorbable sutures (Fig. 21-62, B). Reducing graft mobility and dead spaces will improve the graft success. Because this graft is usually placed over periosteum with a good blood supply, healing will ensue rapidly with a high degree of predictability. After 8 weeks the donor and recipient sites are healed (Fig. 21-62, C).

The thick epithelialized soft tissue autograft can be used for covering exposed roots.[132,136] The thick graft has greater primary (early) contraction than thin or average thickness grafts. This causes collapse of the blood vessels within the graft that may interfere with the revascularization of the graft[137]; however, the secondary (late) contraction will be less during the healing process than with the thin or average thickness grafts. The thick graft should be slightly stretched to reduce primary contraction and keep the capillaries open as much as possible so that a blood supply can be established quickly.[136] Suturing of the graft must completely immobilize the graft to encourage anastomosing of capillaries by maintaining continual intimate contact with its vascular bed. The healed thick graft has the least esthetic qualities of all the grafts because it is much thicker than the surrounding gingiva; therefore, it may look out of place (Fig. 21-60). Currently, it is not often used because of the less than ideal esthetics, and postoperative healing is more uncomfortable than with newer subepithelial techniques.

The thick free epithelialized soft tissue autograft technique is briefly detailed because the principles of the technique of root coverage are important to understand, and this technique is the most difficult to master for predictable root coverage. The initial horizontal incision is made at the level of the desired gingival level, which is usually at the CEJ in a Miller Class I or Class II case (Fig. 21-63, A and B). The incision is extended to the adjacent teeth, but it ends before involving the sulcus of the nongrafted tooth. The next two incisions are vertical incisions made at a right angle to the horizontal incisions. It is important to have prepared a recipient site that extends

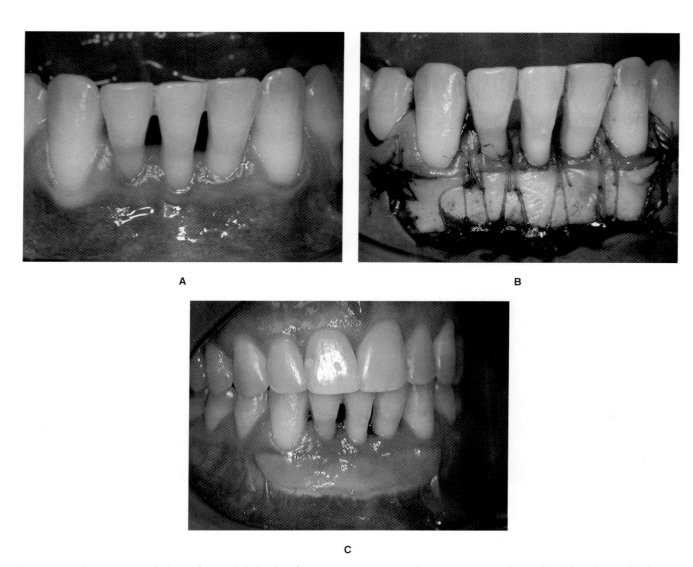

Figure 21-62. Thin or average thickness free epithelialized graft (FEG). **A,** Preoperative Class III recession with interdental bone loss and soft tissue recession. **B,** Suturing of average thickness donor tissue to recipient bed to achieve stability. **C,** Eight-week postoperative healing of average thickness free epithelialized graft.

3 mm past the edge of the denuded root surface. A deep split-thickness dissection is performed to achieve a recipient site that will allow a butt joint to be achieved against all keratinized gingiva. The donor tissue is taken as described before, except that the thickness is 2.0 mm or more; the prefabricated palatal stent as described earlier is placed to encourage blood clot formation (Fig. 21-61). This stent is important for thick grafts because of the potential for postoperative bleeding and pain at the donor site. The stent itself will dramatically reduce pain from the donor site because the open wound is covered, protecting it from the tongue, food, and drink. After the stent is placed, the donor tissue is transferred to the recipient site and suturing must stabilize the graft. The larger the

donor tissue is the easier it is to stabilize, and the more successful it is to cover exposed root surfaces. The small, thick, one tooth graft is the hardest to suture and the least successful graft to cover an exposed root surface. Interrupted sutures are placed at each end of the graft to assure a butt joint and slight stretching of the graft to achieve maximum exposure to a stable blood supply. Then, a sling suture is placed around the affected tooth or teeth to ensure intimate contact of the graft to the interproximal sluiceways, to prevent dead spaces that will delay healing, and to increase the chances of root coverage (Fig. 21-63, *C*). Blood supply is always the most important factor in the survival of any graft procedure; thus the better the circulation the more predictable the

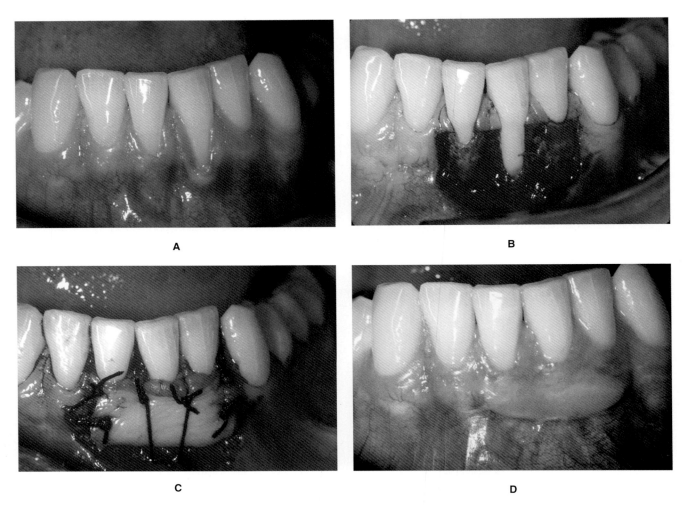

Figure 21-63. Thick free epithelialized graft (FEG)—clinical technique. **A,** Preoperative view of Class II gingival recession #24. **B,** Bed preparation for the thick FEG. **C,** Thick FEG sutured securely to place. **D,** Two-month postoperative view of complete root coverage #24 with the thick FEG.

technique will be. The healing in the case presented in Figure 21-63, *D* resulted in excellent root coverage. The best indications for using the thick graft are: to cover an exposed root, to augment the gingival dimensions (which will increase the resistance to future recession), and to increase the vestibular depth. The literature supports the use of this type of graft to cover root surfaces with an average exposed root coverage of 72.1% (Table 21-2).

The thick graft is more resistant to future recession. Through a process known as *creeping attachment*, there tends to be an increase in root coverage of approximately 1 mm over a 1-year period after graft surgery[138] (Fig. 21-64, *A* and *B*). This creeping attachment has been shown to be stable over a 5-year period.[139] One article shows as much as 7 to 9 mm of exposed roots covered by creeping attachment over a 4-year period, but such dramatic results are rare.[140] Creeping attachment occurs more frequently in cases with a thick graft that replaces the gingival margin. If the margin of native gingiva is retained during graft surgery, creeping attachment is not as pronounced (Fig. 21-63, *C*). This creeping attachment is desirable but rarely occurs with average to thin grafts, and then only when a narrow recession defect (<3 mm in width) is treated. The new creeping attachment tissue that covers the root coronal to the original graft may look different than the grafted tissue and may be more esthetically pleasing than the original graft (Figs. 21-60 and 21-64, *B*). The buccolingual dimension of the graft may also increase in thickness with time, which can be a result of thickening of either soft tissue or the underlying bone,[141] resembling a bony exostosis. This increase in the dimensions of the gingival grafts may continue for several years after the original graft is placed. Creeping attachment has been documented after the placement of free epithelialized soft

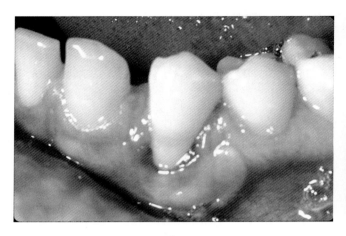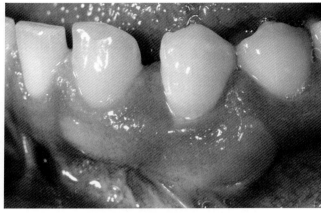

A   B

Figure 21-64. Creeping attachment. **A,** Six weeks after failing to cover the root of a premolar with a thick FEG. Although increased tissue thickness was achieved, root coverage was incomplete. **B,** Creeping attachment has occurred (without additional treatment) to cover the exposed root 16 months later.

tissue grafts,[138-140] subepithelial connective tissue autografts,[142] and allografts.[143]

The decision to perform a soft tissue graft can be accompanied by the knowledge that without surgical intervention the amount of exposed root will usually **stay the same** or *get worse over time*, but after soft tissue grafting the amount of exposed root will usually **stay the same** or *get better over time*.

Soft tissue onlay graft

Ridge augmentation with a thick free epithelialized graft was first published in 1979 by Meltzer[144] to correct an esthetic anterior vertical ridge defect. The soft tissue onlay graft (Fig. 21-65, *A* and *B*) was described by Seibert[70,145] in a series of articles that detailed the technique and its applications. This technique is used primarily to augment vertical ridge defects, but it can be used to augment horizontal or combination defects. When adequate vertical augmentation can be provided, papillary soft tissue augmentation can even be accomplished between the pontics of a fixed partial denture (Fig. 21-65, *C* and *D*).

A soft tissue onlay graft was used to treat the Class III moderate combination ridge defect in Figure 21-66. The defect has 4-mm horizontal and vertical components (Fig. 21-66, *A*). The first step is to remove the epithelium with scalpel, radiosurgery, laser, or rotary diamond burs. Shallow vertical incisions are made into the soft tissue ridge to enhance the bleeding surface and to permit adequate perfusion of the full-thickness graft. One of the best sources of thick epithelialized soft tissue is the maxillary tuberosity. Suturing is important for the stability of this graft (Fig. 21-66, *B* and *C*). Tongue thrusting is one of the biggest causes of failure in any vertical ridge augmentation attempt in the anterior region of the maxilla because the

tongue pushes the graft each time the patient swallows, which interrupts the blood supply by moving the onlay graft. A palatal stent should be made to protect the graft from the tongue during the first 4 to 6 weeks of healing. The stent should be properly relieved to allow for swelling that will occur after augmentation. The major disadvantage with all thick epithelialized grafts is the different appearance of the tissue after healing (Fig. 21-66, *D*). The slight postoperative color variation in Figure 21-66, *D* is not as noticeable as the total lack of tissue that was present before surgery (Fig. 21-66, *A*).

Interpositional-onlay graft

A modification called the interpositional-onlay graft[146] also uses thick epithelialized soft tissue grafts and is indicated for soft tissue augmentation of Class III combination defects (Fig. 21-67, *A*). A split-thickness envelope flap without vertical incisions is reflected (Fig. 21-67, *B*), and a thick wedge of tissue with one epithelialized side (Fig. 21-67, *C*) is placed in the envelope flap. The graft is sutured in place where the epithelialized tissue remains visible (Fig. 21-67, *D*). The advantage of this technique is the increased surface area for improved blood supply and stability during the healing process. The amount of tissue that can be grafted with this technique can increase both vertical and horizontal defects. The disadvantage of this graft is the shape; the wedge can be dislodged if the sutures become compromised early on in the healing process.

Subepithelial connective tissue graft

The connective tissue graft, also called a subepithelial connective tissue graft or a free connective tissue graft, is the second major type of free soft tissue graft. In 1980,

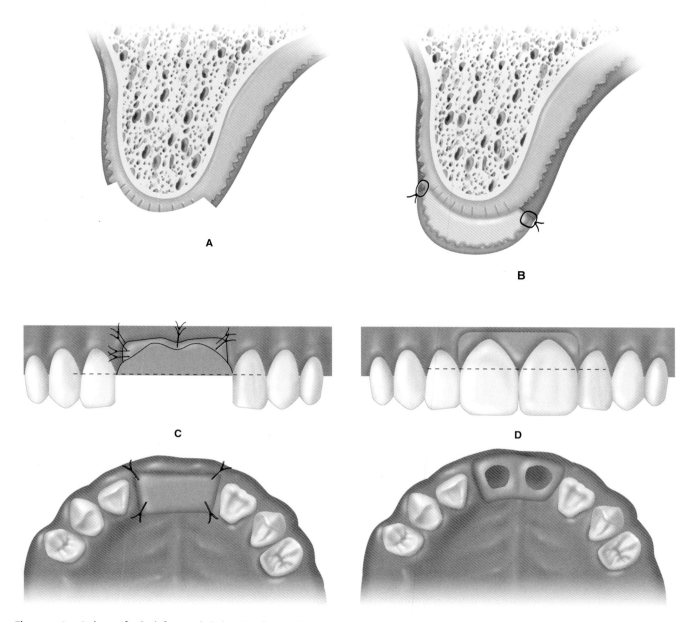

Figure 21-65. Onlay graft (thick free epithelialized graft [FEG] for ridge augmentation). **A,** Class II vertical ridge defect drawing showing removal of epithelium to prepare the recipient bed for the thick free epithelialized graft. **B,** Thick free epithelialized donor tissue sutured to the recipient bed. **C,** Facial and occlusal view of the onlay graft shows the desired height of the graft at the level of the papillae adjacent to the graft. **D,** Ovate pontics for central incisors create the papilla between the central incisors.

Langer and Calagna[147,148] described the subepithelial connective tissue graft for root coverage (Fig. 21-68, *A* and *B*) and ridge augmentation, and this technique currently comprises the bulk of soft tissue grafts used in periodontal plastic surgery. The addition of connective tissue under any pedicle flap yields a mean exposed root coverage of 89.3%, which is the best of all soft tissue grafting tech-

niques used (Table 21-2). It is for this reason that this technique and its many variations are so popular.

The harvesting of donor tissue from the subepithelial connective tissue of the palate requires a complete knowledge of the entire palate. The normal anatomy of the palate consists of masticatory mucosa with a very regular orthokeratinized epithelial layer and a thick, even

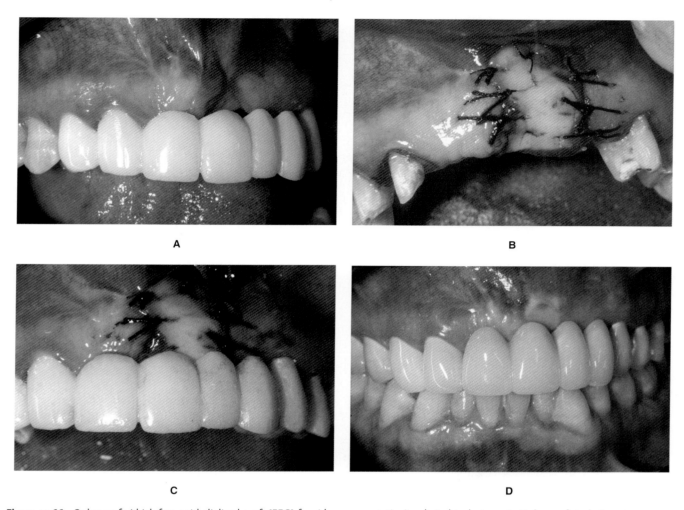

Figure 21-66. Onlay graft (thick free epithelialized graft [FEG] for ridge augmentation)—clinical technique. **A,** Onlay graft technique to correct a Class III combination ridge defect. Preoperative view reveals defect under pontics of provisional fixed partial denture. **B,** Suturing of the thick FEG to immobilize the donor tissue. **C,** Provisional restoration replaced and relieved to allow for swelling. **D,** Final fixed partial denture in place. (Restorative treatment by Dr. Sam Wilbur.)

stratum corneum, compared with gingiva that has an inhomogeneous stratum corneum of varying thickness and an orthokeratinized or parakeratinized surface. Both the epithelium of the hard palate and the gingiva have an average thickness of 0.3 mm[149] and a maximum thickness of 0.6 mm.[150] The lamina propria or connective tissue of the palate extends to a depth of approximately 1.25 to 3.0 mm, and the submucosa extends from there to the bone (Fig. 21-57).

The palatal soft tissue that extends superiorly from the CEJ of the maxillary posterior teeth (for approximately 2 to 3 mm) and the soft tissue near the palatal raphe mediana are composed of very dense lamina propria, which is bound directly to periosteum. The masticatory mucosa between these two sites is the common location of the

donor sites for most connective tissue grafts and is composed of connective tissue and loosely organized glandular and adipose tissue.[151] The pars corporis adiposa contains adipose tissue and resides in the area of the premolars, whereas the pars corporis glandulosum contains glandular tissue and extends posteriorly to the soft palate[152]; the two are roughly separated by the thin mucosa over the palatal root of the first molar.[153]

When the density of connective tissue decreases and becomes loosely organized, the thickness of the donor tissue must increase or it will be too thin to be manipulated and will tear when trying to suture the graft. The best quality connective tissue is found closest to the teeth rather than the midline of the palate; however, taking tissue closer than 2 mm to the teeth puts those teeth at risk for

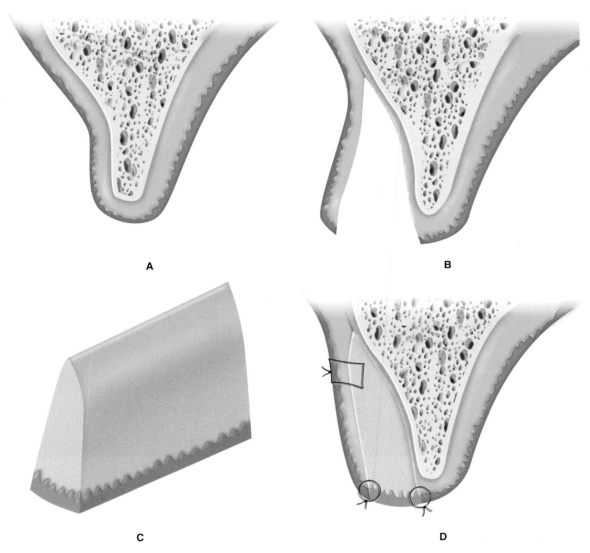

Figure 21-67. Interpositional-onlay graft (thick free epithelialized graft [FEG] for ridge augmentation). **A,** Class III combination ridge defect. **B,** Split-thickness flap reflection is usually a pouch type dissection with no vertical incisions. **C,** A thick wedge of tissue is taken from the maxillary tuberosity or the palate. **D,** The tissue is sutured to place but is easily dislodged if sutures come out prematurely.

postoperative gingival recession. If the donor connective tissue is taken too close to the epithelial layer, the retained flap will not have an adequate blood supply and the palatal flap will slough giving a similar type wound as an epithelialized donor graft wound.

Although there is a distinct anatomic variation between individuals, the thickness of the palate averages slightly more than 3 mm in the area extending from the distopalatal line angle of the canine to the mesial line angle of the palatal root of the first molar, and from the distopalatal line angle of the first molar to the distopalatal line angle of the second molar. The palatal thickness of the third molar averages 4 mm. The thinnest palatal tissue

averages 2 mm over the first molar because of the palatal flaring of this root.[154,155] The second molar can be as thin as the first molar tissue because of a thick alveolar process or exostoses that are often encountered in this palatal region. The palatal root of the first molar requires special attention to prevent postoperative recession, and in thin periodontiums the area should be avoided altogether.

Thin periodontal biotypes vulnerable to gingival recession are often found in the same individuals with generalized thin palatal mucosa that is not suitable for obtaining adequate tissue for connective tissue grafting. In these patients, another periodontal plastic surgery technique may need to be considered. The exact thickness

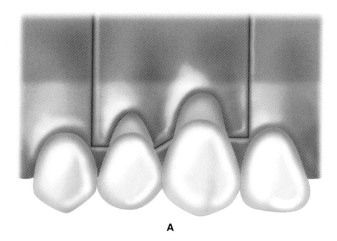

A

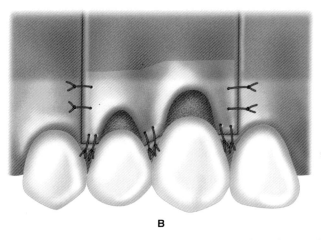

B

Figure 21-68. Partially covered connective tissue graft (with vertical incisions). **A,** Horizontal incision made at the level of the cemento-enamel junction. Vertical incisions can be parallel or trapezoidal. **B,** The connective tissue graft (shown in tan; darker red area demonstrates exposed portion of graft) is placed over the root surface and surrounding bone/periosteum. The flap is then sutured over the connective tissue graft. The overlying flap may be replaced at its original position, as diagrammed, or it may be coronally positioned over the underlying connective tissue graft.

of the palate can be measured after local anesthesia with the anesthetic needle or a periodontal probe, or without anesthesia with the aid of an ultrasonic measuring device that digitally displays the gingival depth to a resolution of 0.1 mm.[153] These aids will help with a treatment plan based on the amount of donor tissue available.

The position of the greater and lesser palatine artery and nerve in the surgical field must be elucidated, and the surgeon must know their location (see Chapter 20 for a detailed discussion of the anatomy of this region). The greater and lesser palatine foramina are located apical to the third molar at the junction of the vertical and horizontal

components of the palate. The greater and lesser palatine vessels and nerves lie in a bony groove, the greater palatine groove, which traverses the palate anteriorly at the junction of the horizontal and vertical palate. It is important to avoid the nerves and vessels located along this neurovascular line. The location of this line varies relative to the CEJ—in shallow palatal vaults the minimal distance is 7 mm, whereas in high vaults the maximum distance is 17 mm. In an average vault there is a distance of 12 mm from the neurovascular line to the CEJ.[151] If the incision is started 2 mm from the soft tissue margin and is ended 2 mm from the neurovascular line, then the maximum width of donor tissue will vary from 3 mm in the shallow vault to 13 mm in the high vault, with an average width of 8 mm in the average vault. The width of connective tissue needed for most grafts is determined by the extent of root exposure and the amount of root coverage anticipated, but 5 to 9 mm is usually an adequate width for donor tissue. This means removing a connective tissue graft from an individual with a shallow palate may result in trauma to the neurovascular structures; thus only 3 to 5 mm of donor tissue can be taken before risking damage to a vessel or nerve. This should be considered and discussed with the patient before deciding on this type of graft because other options may be desired, and the likely sequela of palatal numbness should be thoroughly discussed. When connective tissue is taken for ridge augmentation, the maximum amount of soft tissue is often desired, and the amount of tissue available is relative to the anatomy as described earlier. These limitations in length, width, and thickness are the reasons other sources of donor connective tissues are being evaluated.

Major problems can occur when the above principles are violated. The most common area of violation is when the incision is extended to the lateral incisor or to the horizontal level of the palate; some degree of paresthesia often results. Paresthesia of the anterior palate is more noticeable to the patient because of the phonetic impact that an absence of feeling in this area can have. This paresthesia often dissipates over the next 6 to 12 months because of the regeneration of the damaged nerve fibers, and is rarely permanent.

Suturing is often all that is needed to properly close and stabilize the palatal donor site (Fig. 21-69); however, stents are made for patients who may have bleeding problems (Fig. 21-61). Bleeding can be a major problem when these anatomic barriers are violated; most bleeding can be controlled by ensuring the stent extends past the surgical wound and is inflexible enough to apply sufficient force to stop the bleeding.

The donor connective tissue is divided into the same three thickness categories as the free epithelialized grafts: thin (0.5 to 0.8 mm), average (0.9 to 1.4 mm), and thick (1.5 to 2.0+ mm). The donor tissue can be taken from the palate by two different techniques: *single line incision*

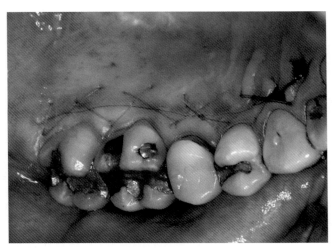

Figure 21-69. A single incision was made to remove the donor tissue without any epithelium on the donor tissue. Suturing of the incision completely closes the wound.

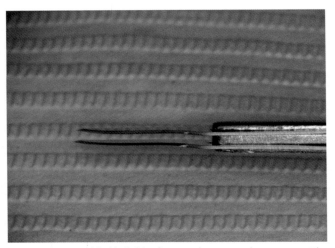

Figure 21-71. Double-bladed knife to easily remove donor tissue. The knife must be handled carefully to avoid injury when placing and removing the blades.

(Fig. 21-69) and *double incision* (Fig. 21-70). The single incision allows for palatal flap reflection and total visualization of the connective tissue donor site before deciding on the desired thickness. The advantage of the single incision is the ability to take larger grafts for ridge augmentation or for root coverage, and to close with primary closure over critical areas such as the palatal root of the first molar without postoperative complications. The double incision is better for smaller grafts of 1 to 3 teeth[156] but requires accurate information about palatal thickness and existing exostoses. When using a double-bladed scalpel handle with a #13 or #15 blade (Fig. 21-71), the harvested tissue is very uniform in thickness. Extreme care must be exercised when loading and unloading this double-bladed instru-

ment to avoid injury. The double incision technique leaves epithelium on the graft tissue (Fig. 21-72, *A*) that can be easily trimmed off if desired (Fig. 21-72, *B*). If connective tissue grafts are completely covered by the flap at the recipient site, all epithelium should be removed from the flap because of the possibility of epithelial cyst formation.[157]

Partially covered connective tissue graft

The clinician has the option of either completely covering the graft with the flap at the recipient site or leaving a portion of the graft uncovered. The partially covered connective tissue graft originally was described by Langer and Langer (Fig. 21-68, *A* and *B*).[158] This technique can be used for Class I, II, or III recession defects. Figure 21-73, *A*, presents a maxillary canine Class II recession defect with 3.5 mm of root exposure and an adjacent lateral incisor pontic with a small Class I horizontal ridge defect. A sulcular incision was made without vertical incisions, which extends from the mesial of the lateral incisor pontic to distal of the second premolar. Vertical incisions were not used, but they could have been used if better visualization was needed. The root of the tooth to be covered was root planed and tetracycline was used to prepare the root surface (Fig. 21-73, *B*). The thick palatal tissue was taken by the double incision technique to augment the ridge of the lateral incisor and to cover the root of the canine. The epithelium was left on the donor tissue and the tissue was sutured to the recipient site by securing the graft with 5–0 chromic gut sutures to each papilla. The flap was then replaced, rather than coronally positioned, and sutured. The flap did not cover the grafted epithelium or connective tissue positioned over the root of the tooth (Fig. 21-73, *C*). The grafted connective tissue was partially covered, and therefore the blood supply was not as good as if the donor

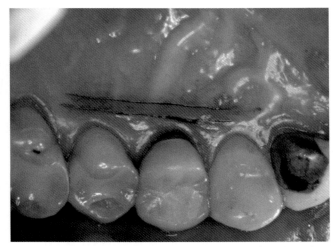

Figure 21-70. Double incision to remove donor tissue from the palate. A narrow band of epithelium is present on the graft.

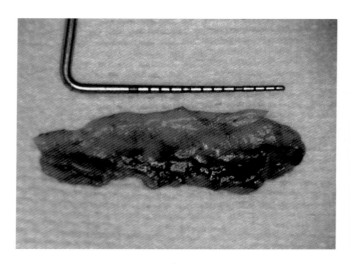
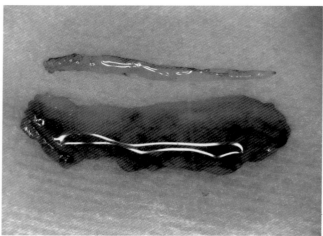

A B

Figure 21-72. A, Epithelium can be seen on this connective tissue graft at the edge nearest the periodontal probe. **B,** The epithelium (average is 0.6 mm in thickness) is removed in this photograph because the graft will be completely submerged under a flap.

tissue was completely covered by a coronally positioned facial flap. The donor tissue must be thick enough to survive over the avascular root of the tooth, and in this case the tissue was a thick graft (1.5 to 2.0 mm thick). The grafted tissue may not look as normal as with the completely covered connective tissue graft; however, the color match can be very close (Fig. 21-73, *D*). Once healing is complete, minor gingivoplasty is sometimes needed to blend the tissue at each papilla. Three years later creeping attachment can be seen covering the margin of the restoration (Fig. 21-73, *E*).

One advantage of this partial graft coverage technique is that the mucogingival junction and the vestibular depth maintain their preoperative dimensions, whereas with a completely covered connective tissue graft, the vestibule becomes more shallow and the mucogingival junction moves incisally because of the coronal positioning of the flap. Another advantage is that when the connective tissue is exposed, it keratinizes and increases the width of keratinized gingiva.[159] This increase in keratinized gingiva makes this technique more desirable in Class II and III recession defect cases because of the ability to increase the keratinized and attached gingiva. The major disadvantage is that thick donor tissue may not always be available, and thinner tissue requires more coverage with the overlying flap.

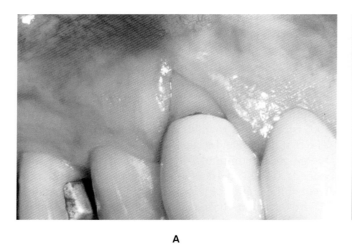
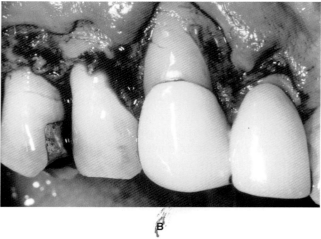

A B

Figure 21-73. Partially covered connective tissue graft (with a replaced flap and no vertical incisions). **A,** Preoperative view of Class II recession #6 and Class I ridge defect (under the lateral incisor pontic). **B,** Flap reflected exposing the broad dehiscence over the canine.

Continued

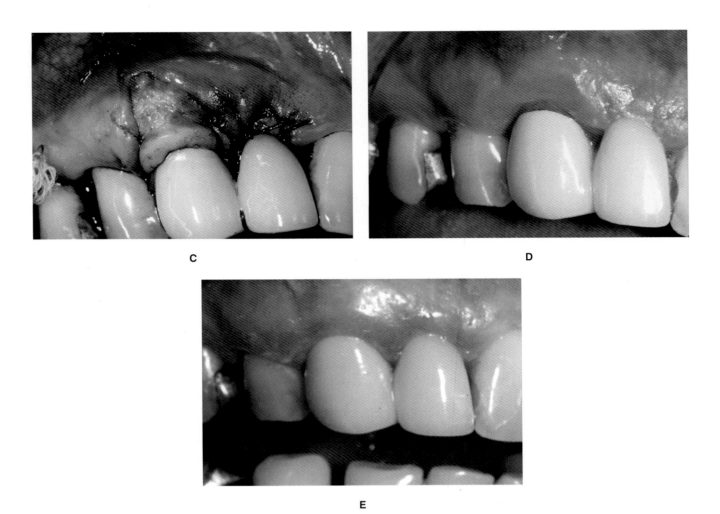

C

D

E

Figure 21-73. cont'd **C,** Suturing of the graft and the replaced flap. The connective tissue of the graft, along with a narrow band of epithelium remains partially exposed. **D,** Postoperative view of healing at 6 weeks shows excellent, but incomplete, root coverage. **E,** Creeping attachment over the next several months has completed coverage of the previously exposed root.

Completely covered connective tissue graft

The completely covered connective tissue graft uses a coronally positioned flap either with vertical incisions (Fig. 21-74, *A* and *B*) or with horizontal incisions (Fig. 21-75, *A* and *B*). The decision to use vertical incisions is the same as with the coronally positioned flap; vertical incisions allow more flap advancement but decreased blood supply and slight scarring of the mucosa. In most cases, the horizontal technique is used initially because vertical incisions can be made if necessary to increase the coronal advancement of the flap. This technique is indicated for Class I recession defects when a thin or average connective tissue graft can be placed under the coronally positioned flap to thicken the soft tissue complex. In Class I defects, a band of keratinized tissue is present at the recipient site before grafting. In more advanced recession defects where little or no keratinized tissue is present before grafting, covering the grafted tissue completely

with a coronally positioned flap often results in complete root coverage, but with the presence of a nonkeratinized mucosal margin at the CEJ.

The clinical case for the completely covered connective tissue graft is shown with horizontal incisions (Fig. 21-75, *A* and *B*) and moderate cervical root defects, with 2 mm of root exposure on mandibular premolars (Fig. 21-76, *A*). The first horizontal incision is made at the desired level of the gingival margin, usually at the level of the CEJ, and it extends to the interdental area adjacent to the terminal teeth of the graft. The second incision should be parallel to the first incision; the same distance apical to the first incision as the amount of desired root coverage. In this case, there is 2 mm of root exposure, therefore the second horizontal incision is made 2 mm apical to and parallel with the first incision (Fig. 21-76, *A*). The incisions converge at the interdental site adjacent to the terminal teeth of the graft, and the soft tissue between the two incisions is

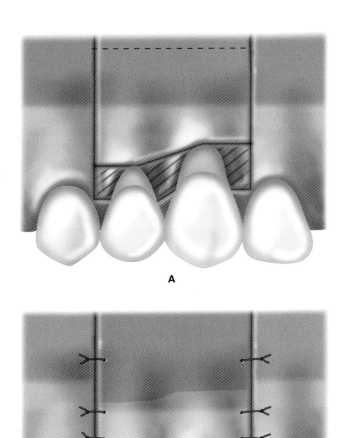

A

B

Figure 21-74. Completely covered connective tissue graft (CTG; with coronally positioned flap and vertical incisions). **A,** Two parallel horizontal incisions are made as far apart as the amount of exposed root. These incisions are then connected with vertical incisions that extend into the mucosa. **B,** The CTG is sutured to place. The split-thickness flap is then coronally positioned over the CTG and sutured to the papillae. The flap may also be sutured to the CTG.

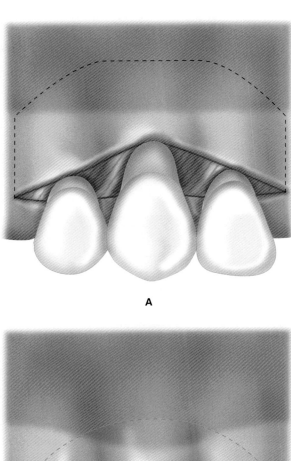

A

B

Figure 21-75. Completely covered connective tissue graft (CTG; with coronally positioned flap and no vertical incisions). **A,** Two horizontal incisions that parallel the cementoenamel junction are as far apart as the exposed roots are made to merge at each end of the incision. Removal of the epithelium between incisions exposes the connective tissue recipient bed (*oblique lines*). The split-thickness dissection continues until the recipient bed has been delineated (*dotted lines*). **B,** The CTG is sutured to place. The coronally positioned flap covers the CTG and is stabilized by one or two interrupted sutures at each interdental site.

removed by a thin split-thickness dissection, leaving the underlying periosteum (Fig. 21-76, *B*). The remaining flap is then reflected by split-thickness dissection to free the flap from the periosteum so the flap can be advanced. The flap must be advanced coronally until the flap edge fits against the most coronal incision. In this case, the flap had to be advanced 2 to 3 mm until the entire root surface was covered. The root defects are then eliminated with rotary instruments and hand instruments to give a smooth root surface. The donor tissue was taken from the palate by

a double incision technique and the epithelium was completely removed (Fig. 21-72, *B*). The palatal wound was sutured and a surgical stent placed. The connective tissue was tried in the recipient site and trimmed until the fit was

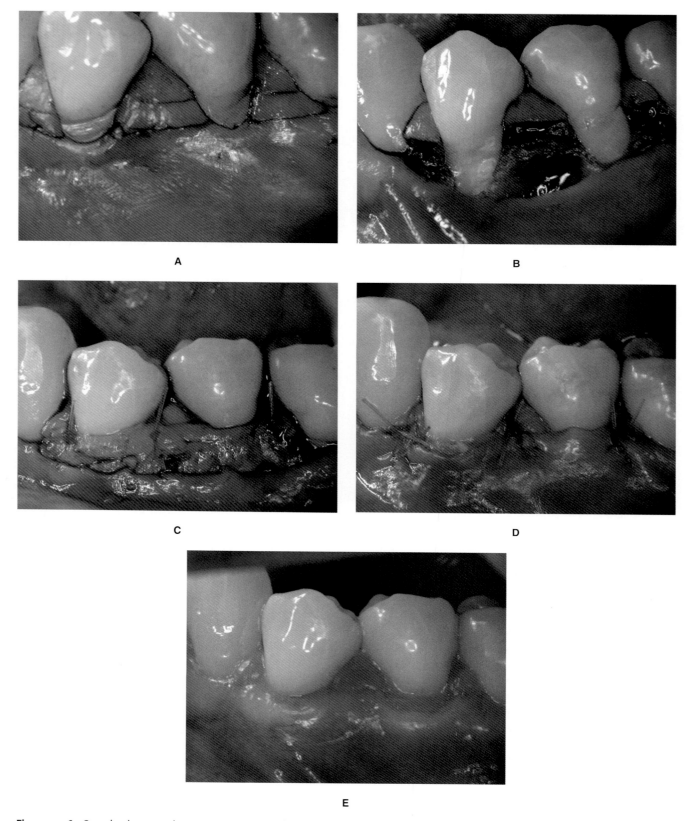

Figure 21-76. Completely covered connective tissue graft (with horizontal incisions)—clinical technique. **A,** Preoperative view of 2-mm root exposure and cervical root defects #20 and #21. Parallel horizontal incisions 2 mm apart converge at end of incisions. No vertical releasing incisions were made. **B,** Split-thickness flap reflection. Papillary gingival epithelium was removed between the two incisions, followed by reduction of cervical defects through root planing. **C,** Connective tissue graft sutured to each papilla. **D,** Coronally positioned flap sutured to each papilla completely covering the connective tissue graft. **E,** Six-week postoperative healing reveals complete root coverage with excellent esthetic results.

ideal; then the tissue was sutured to each interdental papilla with interrupted 5–0 chromic sutures (Fig. 21-76, C). The flap was then coronally positioned to completely cover the connective tissue graft, and the coronally positioned flap was sutured to both the graft and the interdental papillae (Fig. 21-76, D). In many cases the connective tissue graft can be sutured at the same time as the coronally positioned flap. The lack of vertical incisions gives a better blood supply to the flap and more predictable stability to the graft. The 6-week healing shows complete root coverage with a nice color match (Fig. 21-76, E). The papillae are often areas that look irregular, especially if any sutures come out prematurely; however, no significant problems are seen in this case.

The advantages of completely covering a connective tissue graft include better esthetics and the ability to use a thinner graft. A thin graft may not survive over a root surface if it is not completely covered; therefore, a thin connective tissue graft is generally covered completely with a pedicle flap. When a thin connective tissue graft (0.5 to 0.8 mm) is placed under a thin flap (0.5 to 0.8), the total thickness is 1 to 1.6 mm, which closely mimics the thickness of normal gingiva.[160] An average thickness graft is often completely covered by an advanced flap, but it is not mandatory. The goal is to have marginal gingiva that is at least 1 mm in thickness. If small areas of the graft are exposed, they will often survive, especially if the collagen content is high and tissue quality is good.

Acellular dermal matrix allografts

Acellular dermal matrix allografts can be used as an alternative donor source with the completely covered connective tissue graft if autogenous connective tissue cannot be used. An accepted tissue bank should recover the donor allograft tissue. In the United States, the guidelines of the American Association of Tissue Banks and the U.S. Food and Drug Administration should be followed for the donor tissue. The newer methods of processing the allografts have improved the success of acellular dermal allografts procedures.

The current processing technique involves complete removal of the epithelium by uncoupling the bond with the dermis, ensuring no damage to the dermal structure and maintaining the basement membrane. The dermal cells are removed with low molecular weight nondenaturing detergents, whereas the matrix is stabilized through the inhibition of metalloproteinases. The tissue is freeze-dried without damaging components essential for revascularization and repopulation by the recipient's normal cells.[161] This process renders the dermal matrix free from cellular components, but it still contains blood vessel channels, collagen, elastin, and proteoglycans. This allows for a more organized and rapid healing response by using a biologic scaffold for normal tissue remodeling.

The technique used is the same as the complete coverage autogenous connective tissue graft (Fig. 21-75), where the acellular dermal matrix allograft is used instead of the connective tissue autograft (Fig. 21-76, C). The acellular dermal matrix allograft is in the thin to medium range of graft thickness (0.75 to 1.4 mm), and must be totally covered by the advanced flap if root coverage is desired. The major advantages of this technique are the unlimited amount of donor material available and the lack of postoperative complications related to the palatal wound. Because the long-term results are similar to autogenous connective tissue grafting, this option is viable for many people who may desire grafting without the palatal complications.[143] Each patient must be fully informed of the human donor source and the option of using their own tissue, thereby obviating any possible complications related to donor source. When comparing the clinical results of covering exposed roots, autogenous connective tissue grafts and acellular dermal matrix allografts are not statistically different, which means this technique is one of the most successful methods currently available (89%; Table 21-2). However, connective tissue grafts heal an average of 2 to 3 weeks faster, with more keratinized soft tissue than the acellular dermal matrix grafts.[162,163]

Single tooth tunnel technique

The next technique to be discussed is the single tooth tunnel or envelope technique[128] (Fig. 21-55, A and B). This technique uses a connective tissue autograft that is sutured into a tunnel without reflecting a conventional flap. The envelope or tunnel is a nonconventional pedicle flap because it maintains blood supply from the papillary and the mucogingival and mucoperiosteal sides of the tunnel. This gives the best potential of any flap design both in blood supply and in stability of the connective tissue graft.

The single tooth tunnel or envelope technique (sometimes called the *pouch technique*) begins with the root planing of all exposed roots to be grafted. A careful evaluation of the roots will help to determine if this technique can be used. Root defects up to 1 mm in depth can be reshaped with the appropriate armamentarium, consisting of small round diamond burs and curettes to smooth the defect. Root defects deeper than 1 mm present a contraindication to this procedure, and a conventional flap should be reflected to properly access the roots. Proper contouring of the roots regardless of the technique includes enough odontoplasty of the root to give a smooth surface that will accept a graft without any dead spaces created by grooves or notches on the root.

The maxillary premolar to be treated in Figure 21-77, A, has a 3-mm Class I recession defect that was sensitive to cold and was an esthetic problem for the patient. Complete coverage of the root with gingival tissue was the

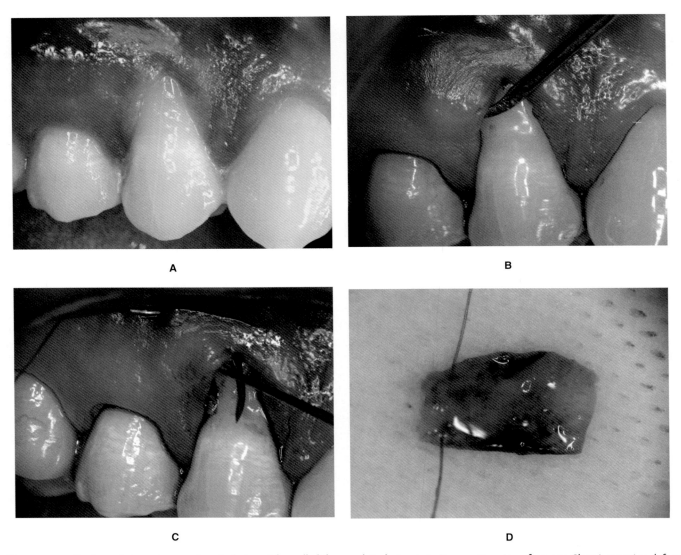

Figure 21-77. Single tooth tunnel or envelope technique (also called the pouch technique). **A,** Preoperative view of a 3-mm Class I recession defect on tooth #5. **B,** A small scalpel blade is used to begin the split-thickness dissection through the sulcus. A very sharp curette may also be used. **C,** The suture is passed from the facial side of the tissue through the gingival sulcus. This needle puncture is made near the apical extent of the pouch and at its farthest distal extent. **D,** The suture is passed through the distal aspect of the connective tissue graft.

Continued

desired result of treatment. After the root was properly smoothed, a split-thickness dissection began to develop the pouch or tunnel. A small scalpel blade or very sharp curette is placed in the sulcus and, with a gentle back and forth pushing motion, a split-thickness "pouch" is developed under the surface of the tissue (Fig. 21-77, *B*). This space was extended coronally to the papilla slightly incisal to the CEJ. The apical extension of the flap results in a split-thickness envelope flap. Because the bone cannot be seen, tactile sensation is the only method of negotiating the space between the periosteum, mucosa, and gingiva. The pouch or tunnel must extend far enough apically and laterally to allow passive placement of the connective tis-

sue graft so that it does not shift out of the pouch with lip, cheek, or tongue movement. This dissection is more difficult and time consuming compared with conventional flap reflection and should be undertaken after many conventional flaps have been reflected and a working knowledge of the anatomy is learned.

Measurements are taken of the recipient site and transferred to the palate. The donor tissue is taken from the palate by either a single or double incision, as previously discussed. The graft is then laid over the teeth to be covered, and the final sizing is performed. The suturing technique is more challenging than other techniques, but fewer sutures are needed and the healing stability and blood

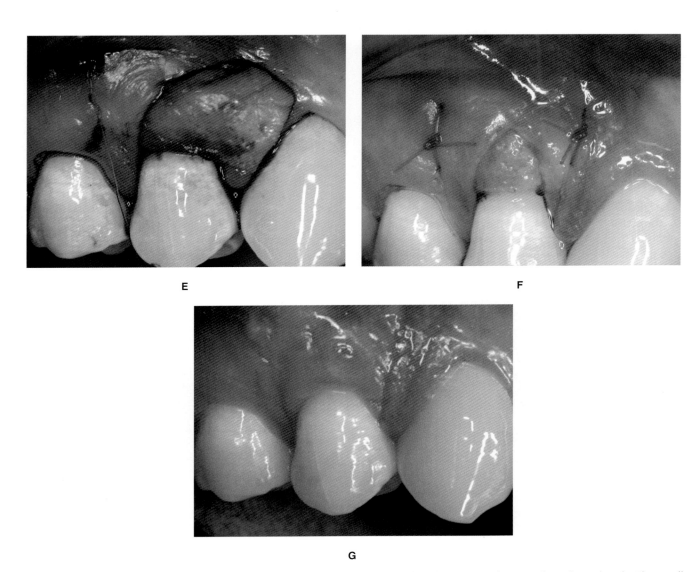

E   F

G

Figure 21-77. cont'd E, The suture needle is then passed back into the gingival pouch and penetrates the tissue from the underside. This needle puncture is placed at the coronal extent of the pouch at a position even with the distal apical suture. The two ends of the suture are pulled distally to introduce the graft into the pouch. An explorer is used to hold the surface tissue of the pouch away from the root surface as the graft is introduced. The suture is tied with a single overhand knot to hold the distal end of the graft in place until the mesial aspect has been introduced into the pouch in a similar manner. **F,** Once the mesial aspect of the graft has been introduced into the pouch, both the mesial and distal sutures are tied securely. The two anchor sutures must not be tied too tight. Stability is primarily created by the envelope. Sutures tied too tight will cause pressure necrosis. **G,** Four-month postoperative result.

supply are superior to other graft techniques because the papillary tissue is not reflected. The suturing technique is designed to pull the donor tissue into the tunnel using sutures; rather than pushing it into the tunnel then trying to suture it. The suture used is 5–0 chromic gut with a 12 to 13 mm reverse cutting 3/8 circle needle. The first needle entry is from the distal edge of the envelope at the most apical position of the two entry points. The needle enters the facial soft tissue of the envelope, directed in a mesial and coronal direction into the tunnel and extending

out of the sulcular opening of that tooth (Fig. 21-77, C). The needle is then inserted through the distoapical corner of the graft (Fig. 21-77, D) from the facial to the lingual, 1 mm from the graft edge. Then the needle is inserted through the distocoronal corner of the graft from the lingual side to the facial side. The donor tissue must be dense enough to allow pulling on the graft with some resistance without pulling the suture out of the donor tissue. The needle is then introduced back into the envelope through its sulcular opening and exits at a point coronal to the previous entry point of the suture and at an equally desired level of the graft at the distal of the tooth. This would be the CEJ in Miller Class I or II cases, as in the example. Both ends of the suture are now on the distal aspect of the last tooth. Both ends are grasped with a needle holder and gently pulled until the tissue is introduced into the space created. Once the graft is pulled into the tunnel completely, one double throw overhand knot is tied to stabilize the graft until the other end of the graft is secured (Fig. 21-77, E). The mesial side of the envelope is opened with an explorer and the suture is passed through the mesioapical location from the facial side of the tissue into the space being held open with the explorer, and the graft is secured with the needle passing through the graft twice just like the distal side. The explorer holds the envelope open again and the needle passes through the space and through the gingiva in a lingual to facial direction at the mesiocoronal exit point at the level of the CEJ. At this point, the donor tissue must be introduced into the envelope using the explorer again to open the space. Once the

graft is in the envelope, the anchor sutures on each end are tied (Fig. 21-77, F).

The advantage of the envelope or tunnel technique is that the sutures play only a minor role in stabilization of the graft, whereas the tissue is the primary stabilizing force. Even if the sutures came out early in the healing process, the graft would remain secure by the interdental papillary tissue; therefore, this technique has a very low failure rate. Because there are no incisions of the papilla, rapid healing ensues because of the stability created by the flap design and suturing techniques, which results in minimal postoperative complications. A disadvantage is that the grafted connective tissue remains partially exposed (Fig. 21-77, F). The exposed connective tissue generally heals to look like the surrounding gingiva and to increase the amount of keratinized gingiva (Fig. 21-77, G).

The tunnel technique[164] treats multiple teeth effectively because of the ability to immobilize long grafts producing exceptional stability, blood supply, and resulting excellent root coverage (Fig. 21-78, A through C). The

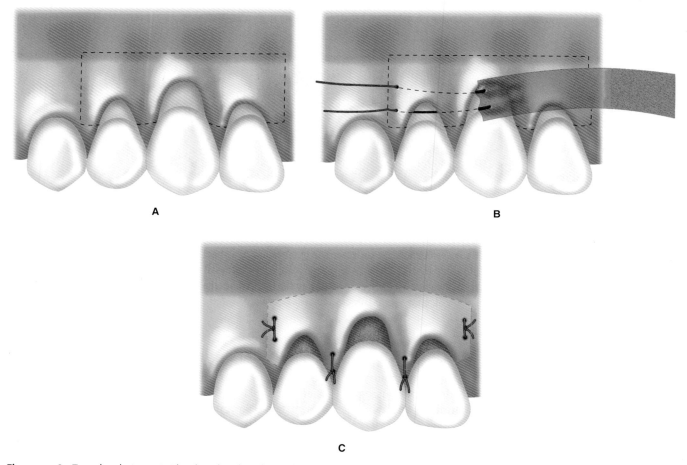

Figure 21-78. Tunnel technique. **A,** The *dotted outline* shows the extent of the split-thickness tunnel dissection. **B,** The suture is used to pull the graft into the tunnel and anchor it at the distal end. **C,** The connective tissue graft is sutured with anchor sutures at the mesial and distal ends and stabilizing sutures at each interdental site.

tunnel is created by soft tissue dissection, as in the envelope or pouch technique described earlier, for every tooth in the proposed tunnel technique. It is imperative that dissection for the tunnel connects all of the individual pouches in the same plane of dissection, and the curette or explorer can be introduced into the tunnel extending from one tooth to the next.

Suturing begins at the interdental site distal to the last tooth in the tunnel at the distoapical point where the needle enters the facial soft tissue of the tunnel and comes out the sulcular opening of that tooth (Fig. 21-78, B). The explorer holds up the next mesial interdental papillary tissue while the needle is passed under this tissue to the next tooth where it is grasped again. This continues until the tooth with the greatest recession is reached. This tooth has the sulcular opening that the graft will be pulled into because it has the largest opening. The donor tissue is then sutured on one end. The suture is then passed back through the tunnel taking care to stay coronal to the previous suture that is in the tunnel. After reaching the last tooth, the needle passes into the tunnel and out of the interdental papilla at the coronal point midway between the interdental tissue at the level of the CEJ. The two ends of the suture are grasped with a needle holder, and pulling on the suture introduces the graft toward the tunnel (Fig. 21-78, B). Care should be exercised at this stage because the graft will often twist and turn. It is important to keep the correct side to the facial, so that when the tissue is positioned there are no twists in the graft. The tissue is guided down the tunnel and over the roots of the recipient teeth with the help of an explorer to open the tunnel so the tissue can be easily pulled to the desired location. Once the tissue reaches the end of the tunnel, a double overhand suture is thrown but no knot is tied. The opposite end of the graft is sutured and positioned to pull into the other end of the tunnel (Fig. 21-78, C) until the donor tissue is properly positioned in the tunnel. The anchor sutures at each end of the graft are then tied to retain the donor tissue in the proper position. One or two interrupted stabilizing sutures are placed at each interproximal site to stabilize the donor tissue at the desired level to attain maximum root coverage (Fig. 21-78, C). Complete coverage is seen the majority of the time, with a mean root coverage of 91% to 92%.[164]

Ridge augmentation

Ridge augmentation using connective tissue grafts was first described by Langer and Calagna in 1980[147] with a completely covered connective tissue graft (Fig. 21-79). This is the primary graft currently used in soft tissue ridge augmentation. The diagram in Figure 21-79, A, shows a Class I ridge defect. If the overlying facial tissue is thick, a split-thickness flap is dissected leaving a connective tissue bed. If the gingiva is thin, a full-thickness flap is reflected

with a deep periosteal releasing incision (Fig. 21-79, B) making the base of the flap a split-thickness flap with mobility to advance the flap (Fig. 21-79, C). The connective tissue donor tissue is taken from the palate, and it should be thicker than is needed if possible. The donor tissue is secured with 6–0 absorbable sutures until it is immobile. It is easier to secure the donor tissue if a split-thickness flap is reflected because the connective tissue bed allows better stabilization. If a full-thickness flap is used, the donor tissue must be sutured to the wound edges and with horizontal stabilizing sutures through the facial flap when necessary (Fig. 21-79, D).

Soft tissue pouch procedure

The soft tissue pouch procedure[165] using an envelope technique was described to augment horizontal defects by making a small incision in the crest of the ridge to create a pouch for a connective tissue graft from the maxillary tuberosity. An improved technique used a split-thickness flap from the palate, which was reflected to the facial to give better visualization and eliminated problems related to opening of the pouch and loss of the graft.[166] This flap was a replaced flap and not an advanced flap, and some of the palatal periosteum was left exposed because of the inability to close the flap after inserting the grafted tissue; therefore, the palatal healing was by secondary intention.

Tunnel technique

A tunnel technique has been described to augment the ridge under an existing pontic by a vertical incision made adjacent to the deficient ridge and a connective tissue graft placed into the tunnel to augment the depression.[167] This technique is similar to that described in Figure 21-78, A through C, except that the tunnel is prepared over an edentulous space rather than over root surfaces. A distal vertical incision is made distal to the ridge deficiency and a split-thickness tunnel is dissected with a small scalpel blade until the mesial end of the ridge deficiency has been reached. A connective tissue graft is then pulled into the pouch using the same suture technique as Figure 21-78, B. This technique is particularly useful in trying to augment a deficient ridge when a fixed partial denture is already in place. Because coronal access to create a tunnel or envelope through a horizontal incision is limited by the presence of the fixed partial denture pontics, creation of a tunnel through a vertical incision may be preferred.

Modified onlay-interpositional graft

Another modification of the onlay-interpositional graft[146] incorporates connective tissue "sides" to the thick epithelialized free graft. This is placed between the facial and lingual split-thickness flaps (Fig. 21-80, A and B) where the epithelialized portion of the connective tissue flap

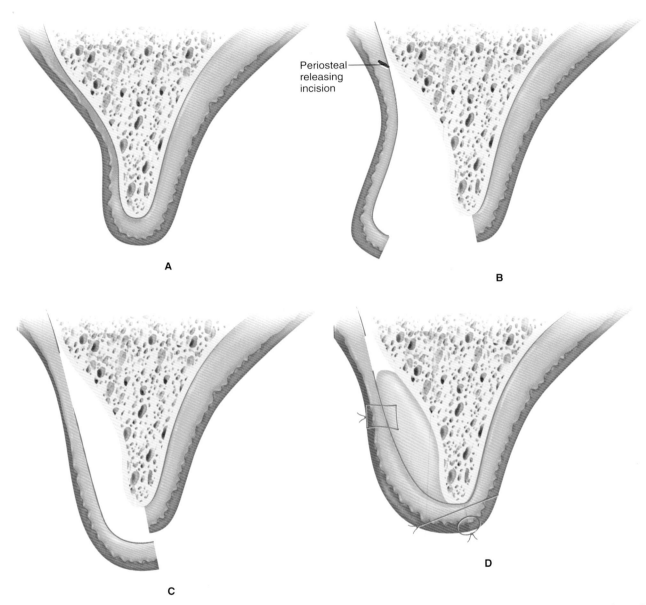

Figure 21-79. Ridge augmentation with a connective tissue graft. **A,** Preoperative view of ridge with a Class I horizontal defect. **B,** The flap reflection was full thickness because of the thin mucosa. A periosteal releasing incision must be made near the base of the flap. **C,** The periosteal-releasing incision allows coronal advancement of the flap because it was full thickness to this point. **D,** The connective tissue graft is sutured to the flap edges with horizontal mattress sutures through the flap to stabilize the graft.

remains exposed to help with vertical augmentation, whereas the connective tissue "sides" are placed under the facial and palatal flaps (Fig. 21-80, *B*). The donor tissue can be prepared by taking a full-thickness palatal graft and removing the epithelium on the sides, or by using a distal wedge with parallel incisions. This type of soft tissue graft may also be used in a socket preservation procedure, where it is placed over the alveolar socket hard tissue graft to prevent the bone graft from coming out of the socket.

In Figure 21-81, *A*, the facial plate of bone was totally absent after tooth extraction, resulting in a ridge that would have had a significant facial depression on healing. The defect was so large that a soft tissue graft alone would not have been thick enough, therefore a hard tissue graft was also used (Fig. 21-81, *B*). The soft tissue graft with a section of epithelium remaining was removed from the palate (Fig. 21-81, *C*). Facial and palatal anchor sutures were placed to secure the graft apically from both the facial and the palatal

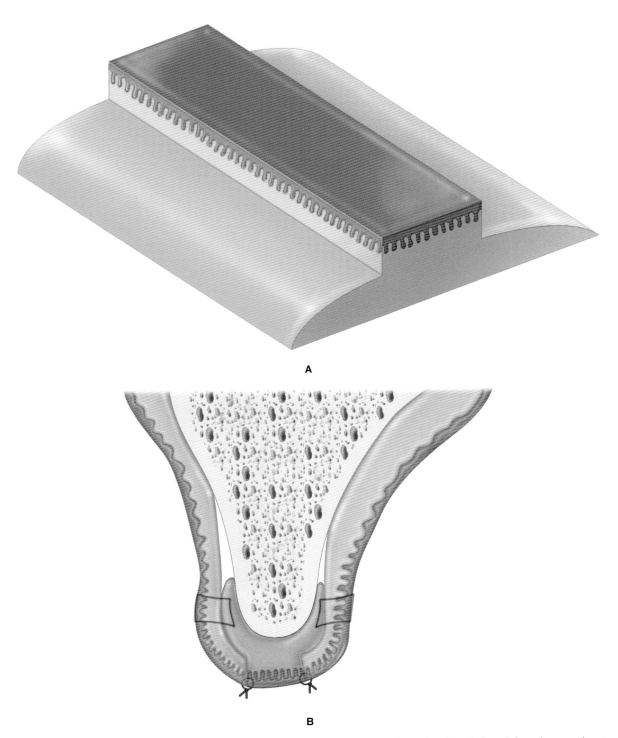

Figure 21-80. Onlay-interpositional completely covered connective tissue graft. **A,** Diagram of a graft with epithelium left on the central region of the graft and deepithelialized connective tissue on the sides. **B,** The cross-sectional view of the graft sutured to the recipient site shows the combination of vertical and horizontal augmentation possible with this technique.

(Fig. 21-81, *D*). The area was overfilled to allow for some shrinkage during healing. Stabilizing sutures were placed at each papilla to completely secure the graft. The 1-year postoperative healing shows the final fixed partial denture in place with normal facial contours (Fig. 21-81, *E*) and no visible evidence of the original bone defect, with both central incisors restored at equal lengths (Fig. 21-81, *F*).

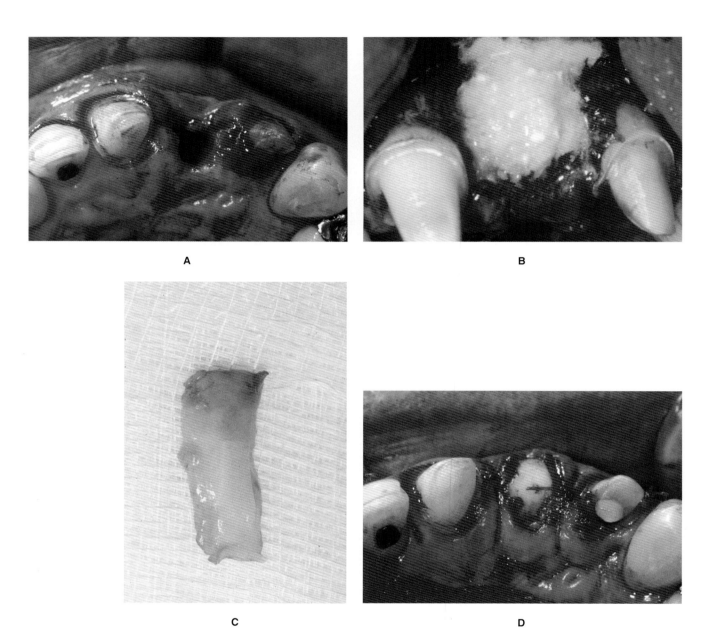

Figure 21-81. Combination onlay-interpositional and a hard tissue graft. **A,** The immediate view after extraction of the central incisor showing a significant loss of the facial plate of bone. **B,** A hard tissue graft (hydroxyapatite) was used to fill the socket defect. **C,** The donor connective tissue is shown. The epithelium remains on the central region of this graft. This epithelialized portion will be placed at the opening in the soft tissue socket, whereas the deepithelialized portions will be placed under the facial and palatal tissues. **D,** The donor tissue was placed over the hard tissue graft and the epithelium was left exposed. Suturing of the graft closes the wound and contains the underlying particulate hard tissue graft.

Continued

Treatment of alveolar ridge defects has improved over the last 20 years as refinements have been made in surgical technique.[168] The limiting factor has always been flap survival over the augmentation material. The autogenous connective tissue ridge augmentation has a distinct advantage over the other methods of augmentation. Because soft tissue is placed under the flaps, problems such as incomplete flap closure, poor healing of the suture line, flap perforations, and flap dehiscences are less significant. Autogenous soft tissue ridge augmentation is a predictable procedure when adequate tissue is available. In large ridge defects, the grafted tissue can be

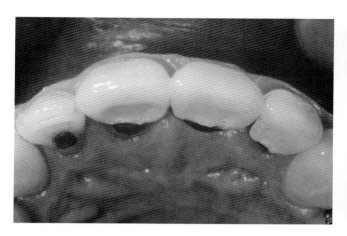

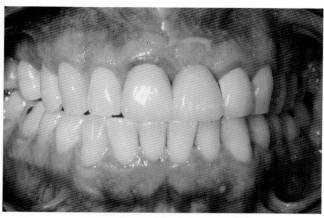

E

F

Figure 21-81. cont'd E, An occlusal view showing the position of the facial tissue, which is very similar to the contralateral tooth. No horizontal ridge deficiency is detected. **F,** The facial view of the finished fixed partial denture 1 year later shows the central incisors are the same length and the esthetic result was good compared with the potential problems that could have occurred without this ridge preservation technique. The pontic at tooth #9 looks like a tooth emerging from the soft tissue. This was possible because the ridge augmentation allowed use of an ovate pontic. Slight inflammation is noted on the facial of tooth #8.

sutured in multiple layers to the periosteum and then covered with an advanced flap.[169]

The greatest disadvantage of the autogenous connective tissue graft is the limited availability of donor tissue. A person who needs 6 mm of ridge augmentation and has thin palatal mucosa will need multiple surgical procedures to complete augmentation of the ridge. It is important to consider the most limiting factor in completing these multiple techniques is not only the thickness of the palate but also the willingness of the patient to undergo several procedures in search of optimal esthetics. The surgeon may need to evaluate other donor sources of both hard and soft tissue when the amount of augmentation exceeds the available tissue. The surgeon's role is to continue searching for the best and least traumatic solutions to difficult problems.

Soft tissue allografts

Soft tissue allografts are also used for ridge augmentation procedures.[170] The amount of augmentation is limited to the thickness of the allograft, but 1 to 2 mm of augmentation is possible and may be performed in conjunction with root coverage procedures. The patients tolerate multiple surgical procedures much better if the palate is not used as the donor source. The technique involves mobilization of an advanced flap to totally cover the underlying soft tissue allograft. Complete passive suturing is needed for success. In Figure 21-82, *A*, an acellular dermal matrix allograft is used both to cover exposed roots and to augment an adjacent edentulous site simultaneously. The acellular dermal matrix allograft was extended over the entire ridge to give additional

thickness of tissue over the implant site (Fig. 21-82, *B* and *C*). The 4-week healing view shows complete coverage of the exposed roots and augmentation of the edentulous site (Fig. 21-82, *D*). The papilla on the mesial of the canine was well preserved. The healing provided this edentulous area with an added 1 to 2 mm of soft tissue thickness and complete root coverage of three teeth without using any palatal donor tissue.

When dental implants are to be placed, the soft tissue must be of adequate thickness to maintain a stable gingival margin over a long period around the implants. Otherwise, exposure of the implant body is likely. Although posterior implants may do well without gingiva, the esthetic zone is not an area where recession over implants is tolerated by patients with a high lip line (Fig. 21-83). The most important focus around implants is to have more soft tissue than is needed. Trying to obtain soft tissue coverage over an exposed implant is much more difficult than obtaining coverage of an exposed root.

Papilla reconstruction

Papilla reconstruction is a major subject of interest for patients receiving soft tissue grafts,[171,172] orthodontic extrusion,[173] and hard tissue grafts.[174] This has been triggered by the increased emphasis on esthetics and the use of dental implants in the esthetic zone. Currently, regeneration of a lost papilla is a difficult process and one that deserves continued improvement in surgical techniques. Predictable regeneration of lost papillae is not possible at this time. However, preventing the loss of papillae is something that is much better understood.

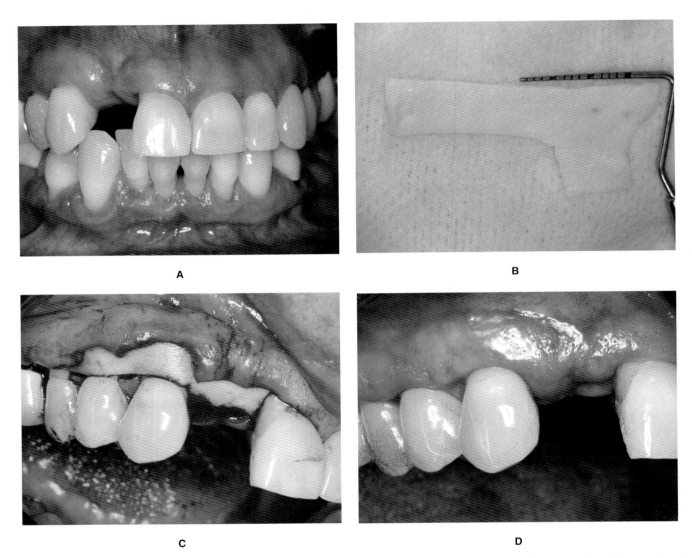

A

B

C

D

Figure 21-82. Acellular dermal matrix allograft for ridge augmentation and root coverage. **A,** Preoperative view shows recession defects on #5 and #6, with a ridge defect at the #7 edentulous site. **B,** An allograft of sufficient size for two premolars, a canine, and an edentulous space was chosen. **C,** Placement of the allograft before the flap was coronally positioned. **D,** Four-week healing shows augmentation of the papilla mesial to the canine and of the tissue over the roots of the premolars.

Focus should be directed toward papilla preservation because of the difficulty encountered in reconstructing this precious soft tissue. Preservation of papillae begins at the time of tooth extraction.[175]

Tooth extraction

A conservative tooth extraction prevents excessive loss of bone and soft tissue and is the best way to preserve soft tissue esthetics. The loss of a single soft tissue papilla after extraction of a tooth is a major concern in the esthetic zone, and papillae are especially vulnerable to reduction or elimination during tooth removal. The goal is to preserve esthetics and the normal gingival contours,

even after the tooth is gone. This includes the papilla tips and the scalloped facial and lingual gingival margins. The thin periodontium has more scallop and papillary height and is more susceptible to recession especially after a tooth extraction. The primary goal is minimal trauma, and if at all possible, removal of the tooth without flap reflection to maintain the soft tissue. This will not only reduce trauma to the gingiva, but also trauma to the bone, resulting in less bone resorption and gingival recession. Tooth extraction without flap reflection focuses on removing root structure rather than bone. Small elevators or periotomes can be used to elevate the root portion; however, if the root cannot be luxated, it must be sectioned

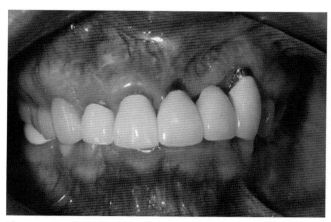

Figure 21-83. A 5-year-old implant supported fixed partial denture is stable and healthy, but is an esthetic failure. The patient regrets having the implants because of the recession resulting from inadequate soft tissue.

without damage to the surrounding bone. The procedure can be time consuming, but maintenance of the facial and lingual plates of bone in the esthetic zone can have a significant esthetic impact.

Retention of papillae

Retention of papillae is best accomplished by the following: (1) the papilla being in good health before the tooth extraction, (2) not reflecting the papilla from the adjacent natural tooth, and (3) supporting the papillae immediately after tooth removal with an immediate implant or by an immediate provisional ovate pontic. If tooth prepara-

tion for a fixed partial denture is performed the day of the extraction, extreme care should be exercised to prevent extending the interproximal preparation too far apically and impinging on the papillary attachment to the root. As soon as the tooth is removed, the papilla will collapse 1 to 2 mm into the space created by the extracted tooth. This is even a greater problem if the papillae must be reflected to surgically remove the tooth. A 5-mm papilla can easily lose 3 to 4 mm of height after a surgical extraction.

When the tooth or teeth to be extracted are to be replaced with a fixed partial denture, the ideal sequence of events occurs when the teeth adjacent to the proposed extractions are prepared and temporarily splinted with a full-coverage acrylic resin provisional restoration before the surgical appointment. This allows the dentist to properly prepare the restoration margins while the tooth to be removed is in place and the papillae are at their original height (Fig. 21-84, *A*). The teeth that cannot be repaired in Figure 21-84, *B*, will be removed because of endodontic failures and advanced periodontal disease. After conservative and atraumatic tooth removal, the papilla and soft tissue are undisturbed (Fig. 21-84, *C*). The sockets were filled with a porous bovine xenograft (Fig. 21-84, *D*). An impression was taken immediately after the extractions and a model was sent to the prosthodontist along with the provisional fixed partial denture. Figure 21-84, *A*, is a photograph of the original provisional restoration before tooth extraction. This same provisional placed on the model of the extraction sites (Fig. 21-84, *E*) demonstrates about 1 mm of soft tissue collapse over the extraction sites. If no bone graft was placed, this recession undoubtedly would have become much worse, making the teeth

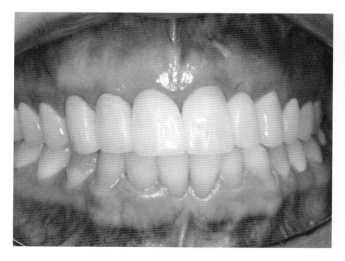

A

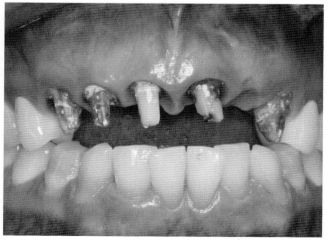

B

Figure 21-84. Conservative extraction and socket augmentation with papilla preservation. **A,** A six-unit provisional fixed partial denture was prepared before tooth extractions. **B,** The incisors (#7, #8, #9) were endodontically and periodontally involved. Tooth #10 was already missing.

Continued

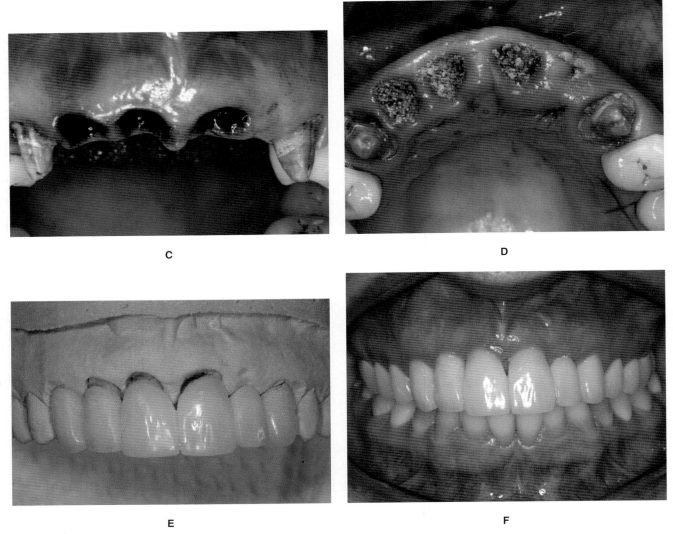

Figure 21-84. cont'd C, The atraumatic extractions left the papilla undisturbed. **D,** The sockets were filled with a bovine xenograft. **E,** The original provisional restoration was placed on a model. The model shows 1 mm of tissue collapse that occurred immediately after tooth extraction. The model was used to fabricate the ovate pontics indirectly, rather than at the surgical site. **F,** Seven-week postoperative view shows continual papillary support and soft tissue stability. The soft tissue over the extraction sites will heal with a concave impression made by the convex surface of the ovate pontics. (Restorative treatment by Dr. Greg Seal.)

even longer than they already were. The model was used to reline the provisional restoration and to make ovate pontics on the model, instead of doing so directly at the surgical site. The provisional restoration ovate pontics mimic the shape of the extracted teeth, supporting the papillae and resisting any more soft tissue recession during the postoperative period (Fig. 21-84, *F*). The pontic should extend into the extraction socket to a depth of at least 2.5 mm to prevent further collapse of the soft tissue. After 4 weeks there will be adequate soft tissue under the pontic so the provisional restoration can be removed and the pontics shortened 1 to 1.5 mm to facilitate flossing.[175]

If the socket has bone supporting all sides, no bone graft is necessary; however, if a bony wall of the socket is missing and the distance from the pontic to the bone is more than 1 mm, socket augmentation will be needed. Another case shows the shape of the healed soft tissue 6 months after tooth extraction and socket preservation (Fig. 21-85, *A* and *B*). The provisional restoration in place shows the soft tissue filling the interproximal sites (Fig. 21-85, *C*). Both of these cases are particularly difficult because all four incisors are missing. When multiple teeth are extracted, the papillae are generally lost and the ridge takes on a flatter form. It is advantageous to maintain

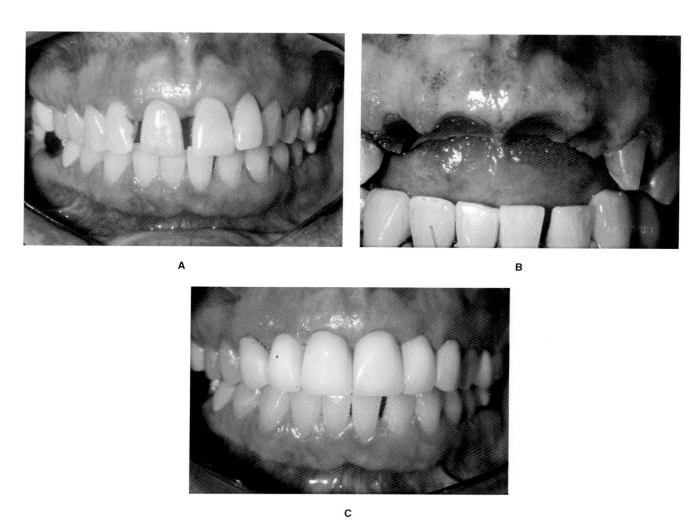

Figure 21-85. Conservative extraction and socket augmentation with papilla preservation. **A,** Preoperative view of advanced periodontitis affecting the maxillary incisors. **B,** Six-month postoperative view of the scalloped papilla. The ovate pontic design was accentuated to increase the amount of papillary support. **C,** One-year postoperative view of the provisional fixed partial denture in place and the papillary tissue present. (Restorative treatment by Dr. Hollon Meadors.)

every other tooth, where possible, because the papillae are easier to maintain adjacent to a natural tooth. Maintaining or creating papillae in an edentulous ridge with more than one pontic space is extremely difficult.[175]

Hard Tissue Grafts

Hard tissue grafts have been used in periodontal plastic surgery primarily to augment deficient ridges.[71] Hard tissue ridge augmentation techniques are designed to treat the defect that is present after healing of extracted teeth. Hard tissue augmentation materials may be autografts, allografts, xenografts, or alloplastic grafts. Which material to use will depend on what type of function is required from the ridge after augmentation. Research and experience favor autogenous grafts for ridge aug-

mentation, with donor sites being from the retromolar area, tuberosity, chin, mandibular ramus, or iliac crest. Allografts are also used and come in different forms: mineralized, demineralized, chip, powder, putty, cortical, or cancellous. Xenografts are usually microporous and can be different particle sizes and either processed chemically or heat-treated.[176] Alloplastic grafts are manufactured out of different materials and are produced in different particle sizes, shapes, and contours. Indeed, the choices are diverse and the research is broad in support of most of these alternatives. (These alternatives are discussed in detail in Chapter 25.) This chapter focuses on how the loss of hard tissue impacts soft tissue esthetics and how the prevention of bone loss and regeneration of hard tissue will preserve esthetics.

Ridge preservation

Ridge preservation, sometimes called *alveolar socket grafting*, is grafting of an immediate extraction socket to prevent collapse of the ridge, which would likely result in an esthetic or functional defect (Fig. 21-26). Bahat[177] initially reported the use of hard tissue grafts in fresh socket defects in 1986. The socket bone graft can also be covered with a soft tissue graft (Fig. 21-81), an absorbable membrane, or a nonabsorbable membrane to promote rapid healing of the bone and prevent loss of the bone graft.

Socket grafting or ridge preservation occurs at the time of tooth removal. Best results can be accomplished when extracted teeth are adjacent to natural teeth so the papilla can be retained; whereas when two adjacent teeth are extracted, the papilla between them is difficult to maintain. When a provisional fixed partial denture has been made before the extraction to replace the lost tooth, the socket graft procedure is immediately simplified because the bone graft is retained by the pontic of the tooth. The procedure for positioning the tooth subgingivally is identical to the above description, except that the pontic rests against a small round piece of collagen that separates the pontic and the underlying bone graft particles, or rests directly on the hard tissue graft. The provisional restoration is then cemented to place. Six weeks later this restoration is removed, and the pontic is shortened if necessary to allow for soft tissue to cover the hard tissue graft. This will help to maintain the position of the facial gingival margin and papillae.

Retention of the hard tissue graft material is improved by using an absorbable membrane (Fig. 21-86). The space for the membrane is created by a tunnel technique to prevent flap reflection. The tunnel is created on both the facial and lingual sides of the tooth. The membrane is cut to the dimension needed and should extend 2 mm past the bony margins of the socket defect, and also should support the papilla if possible. The membrane is inserted into the socket and is positioned between the soft tissue tunnel and the bone. This technique recreates the missing socket walls with membrane material and covers the hard tissue graft material that might otherwise be lost through the socket opening. The membrane can be anchored to the facial and lingual soft tissues with 5–0 or 6–0 sutures (Fig. 21-86), if necessary. The socket, now surrounded with walls consisting of bone and membrane, is filled with bone graft material and allowed to heal. If there is extensive bone loss, a connective tissue graft may be used instead of, or in addition to, the absorbable membrane to better augment the surgical site.

Guided Tissue Regeneration Using Membranes

Guided tissue regeneration using membranes is the last group of techniques mentioned but not completely covered in this chapter, because complete discussions appear in

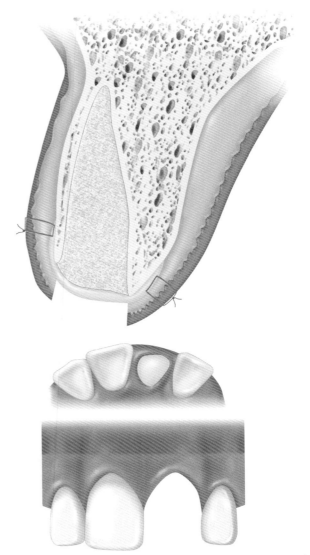

Figure 21-86. Diagram of a ridge preservation technique or socket grafting using a particulate bone graft and an absorbable membrane. The socket is filled with hard tissue grafting material. A split-thickness tunnel is created on the facial and lingual sides of the tooth to allow the membrane to extend beyond all the bony walls of the socket.

Chapter 25. In 1976, Melcher[178] suggested that the cell type that repopulates the root surface after periodontal surgery will determine the type of attachment that forms on the root surface. This redirected the concept of *guided tissue regeneration* in periodontics, in that barrier membranes could be used to promote selective cell population of the root surface, which facilitates periodontal regeneration or the regeneration of the bone, cementum, and the periodontal ligament, while simultaneously excluding the epithelial and gingival cells.[179] The creation of space under the membrane is the primary prerequisite to this regenerative technique.

Root coverage

Root coverage has been attained with guided tissue regeneration when the coronally advanced flap completely covers the membrane and space is created under the membrane for regeneration of not only soft tissue but also bone.[180] In many cases, true regeneration occurs, with formation of new bone, periodontal ligament, and cementum.[181] A mean root coverage of 74% has been obtained using a guided tissue regeneration approach (Table 21-2). When membranes are used for ridge augmentation, the technique has been termed *guided bone regeneration*.[182] This principle was first introduced by Hurley and colleagues[183] in 1959 for the treatment of experimental spinal fusion. Guided bone regeneration techniques are useful in reconstruction of deficient ridges (see Chapter 25). There are two types of membranes used in guided tissue regeneration: *nonabsorbable* and *absorbable membranes* (sometimes called nonresorbable and resorbable, respectively).

Nonabsorbable membranes

Nonabsorbable membranes are usually made of a porous, polytetrafluoroethylene (e-PTFE), or nonporous (high-density) PTFE. When properly used, these membranes will result in the regeneration of bone over alveolar ridges and bone, cementum, and periodontal ligament around teeth. These membranes have been used for both root coverage and ridge augmentation. The porous e-PTFE membranes should stay submerged throughout the healing phase, but the most common complication is exposure of the membrane, which will often lead to infection and failure of the technique. Success occurs when the soft tissue covering the membrane remains intact for a minimum of 30 days and ideally for 6 months or longer as needed for maturing of the newly formed bone. If the membrane can maintain a suitable space under the membrane, no bone grafting materials are needed. Titanium reinforcement helps with shaping of membranes and maintaining space under the membrane. However, bone grafting materials can also be used under the membrane to ensure proper space for bone regeneration. Nonporous high-density PTFE membranes do not have to be covered and can remain exposed to an oral environment until removed at 30 days or later.[184]

Absorbable membranes

Absorbable membranes deteriorate at different rates depending on the type; some resorb in a few days whereas others take months to resorb.[185] The longer the membrane stays intact the longer time the body has to regenerate bone under the membrane. The last bone to mineralize is the bone located directly under the membrane, which is farthest away from the native bone and closest to the soft tissue. When absorbable membranes are exposed to the oral cavity they degrade much faster than they would if contained under a flap. A membrane that takes six months to resorb in tissues can be gone in 30 to 45 days when exposed to the oral cavity. The absorbable membranes have fewer postoperative complications than non-absorbable membranes and do not require a secondary procedure for membrane removal; therefore, absorbable membranes are more widely used. Root coverage has been tried with absorbable membranes, but success rates vary. One report on long term evaluation of an absorbable guided tissue regeneration membrane for root coverage showed a marked decrease in the amount of root coverage over a two year period from 92% to 59%.[186] Some clinicians recommend absorbable membranes for ridge augmentation, but not for root coverage.[187]

Root Preparation

One of the most critical steps in root coverage surgery is proper root preparation before placing the soft tissue graft. The key step is root planing to remove plaque and calculus, and to smooth the root. Some practitioners then use chemicals to condition the root, including citric acid,[132] tetracycline hydrochloride,[188] and ethylenediaminetetraacetic acid. The most common agent is citric acid, which was heavily emphasized in early techniques for root coverage. The biologic rationale for this procedure is to detoxify and demineralize the root surface to encourage a fibrin linkage between the exposed collagen fibers on the root surface and the graft collagen fibers.[189,190] Citric acid has also been shown to remove the smear layer produced when instrumenting the root surface.[191] The use of chemical root conditioning has not been shown to statistically improve the amount of root coverage obtained in controlled clinical trials.[192-194] However, several human block sections support the finding of significant connective tissue attachment and bone regeneration when using citric acid or tetracycline.[141,190,195] Many clinicians continue to use some form of chemical root surface conditioning because of the increased potential for more connective tissue attachment rather than junctional epithelial attachment.

Enamel Matrix Proteins

Enamel matrix proteins are amelogenins that are found during enamel formation, as well as in the initial development of acellular cementum and the associated tooth attachment apparatus. They self-assemble to create a matrix that can mediate the formation of acellular cementum on the root of a developing tooth. Commercially available enamel matrix derivative is derived from developing teeth of porcine origin. The enamel matrix protein is recognized as self when encountered by the human body, and these proteins have been shown to stimulate regeneration of the periodontal ligament, cementum, and bone. This product has primarily been used to treat intrabony periodontal defects but there is general agreement among periodontal surgeons that soft tissue healing is improved with this substance as well. Several studies are in progress to determine if root treatment with enamel matrix derivative will improve clinical root coverage when used in conjunction with soft tissue grafting.

REFERENCES

1. Friedman N: Mucogingival surgery, *Text Dent J* 75: 358-362, 1957.

2. American Academy of Periodontology: *Glossary of Periodontal Terms*, ed 4, Chicago, American Academy of Periodontology, 2001.

3. Genco RJ, Newman MG, editors: Consensus Report—Mucogingival Therapy, *Ann Periodontol*, 1:702-706, 1996.

4. Miller PD Jr: Regenerative and reconstructive periodontal plastic surgery, *Dent Clin North Am* 32:287-306, 1988.

5. Ochsenbein C, Ross S: A reevaluation of osseous surgery, *Dent Clin North Am* 13:87-102, 1969.

6. Johnson RL: Osseous surgery, *Dent Clin North Am* 20(1):35-59, 1976.

7. Elliot JR, Bowers GM: Alveolar dehiscence and fenestration, *Periodontics* 1:245-248, 1963.

8. Gartrell JR, Mathews DP: Gingival recession, *Dent Clin North Am* 20(1):199-213, 1976.

9. Maynard JG, Ochsenbein C: Mucogingival problems, prevalence and therapy in children, *J Periodontol* 46: 543-552, 1975.

10. Andlin-Sobocki A, Bodin L: Dimensional alterations of the gingiva related to changes of facial/lingual tooth position in permanent anterior teeth of children. A two year longitudinal study, *J Clin Periodontol* 20:219-224, 1993.

11. Andlin-Sobocki A, Marcusson A, Persson M: 3-Year observation on gingival recession in mandibular incisors in children, *J Clin Periodontol* 18:155-159, 1991.

12. Coatoam GW, Behrents RG, Bissada NF: The width of keratinized gingiva during orthodontic treatment: its significance and impact of periodontal status, *J Periodontol* 52:307-313, 1981.

13. Wennstrom JL, Lindhe J, Sinclair F, Thilander B: Some periodontal tissue reactions to orthodontic tooth movement in monkeys, *J Clin Periodontol* 14:121-129, 1987.

14. Foushee DG, Moriarty JD, Simpson DM: Effects of mandibular orthognathic treatment on mucogingival tissue, *J Periodontol* 56:727-733, 1985.

15. O'Leary TJ, Drake RB, Jividen GF, Allen MF: The incidence of recession in young males: relationship to gingival and plaque scores, *Periodontics* 6:109-111, 1968.

16. Donaldson D: The etiology of gingival recession associated with temporary crowns, *J Periodontol* 45:468-471, 1974.

17. Weisgold AS: Contours of the full crown restorations, *Alpha Omegan* 70:77-89, 1977.

18. Ingber JS, Rose LF, Coslet JG: The "biologic width"—a concept in periodontics and restorative dentistry, *Alpha Omegan* 70:62-65, 1977.

19. Solnit A, Stambaugh R: Treatment of gingival clefts by occlusal therapy, *Int J Periodontics Restorative Dent* 3:38-55, 1983.

20. Dyer D, Addy M, Newcombe RG: Studies in vitro of abrasion by different manual toothbrush heads and a standard toothpaste, *J Clin Periodontol* 27:99-103, 2000.

21. Gandara BK, Truelove EL: Diagnosis and management of dental erosion, *J Contemp Dent Pract* 1:16-23,1999.

22. Clark DC, Woo G, Silver JG et al: The influence of frequent ingestion of acids in the diet on treatment for dentin sensitivity, *J Can Dent Assoc* 56:1101-1103, 1990.

23. Giunta JL: Dental erosion resulting from chewable vitamin C tablets, *J Am Dent Assoc* 107:253-256, 1983.

24. Maron FS: Enamel erosion resulting from hydrochloric acid tablets, *J Am Dent Assoc* 127:781-784, 1996.

25. Nebel OT, Fornes MF, Castell DO: Symptomatic gastroesophageal reflux: incidence and precipitating factors, *Am J Dig Dis* 21:953-956, 1976.

26. Bartlett DW, Evans DF, Anggiansah A et al: A study of the association between gastro-esophageal reflux and palatal dental erosion, *Br Dent J* 181:125-131, 1996.

27. Milosevic A: Eating disorders and the dentist, *Br Dent J* 186:109-113, 1999.

28. Jarvinen VK, Rytomaa II, Heinonen OP: Risk factors in dental erosion, *J Dent Res* 70:942-947, 1991.

29. Young WG, Khan F: Sites of dental erosion are saliva-dependent, *J Oral Rehabil* 29:35-43, 2002.

30. Grippo JO: Abfractions: a new classification of hard tissue lesions of teeth, *J Esthet Dent* 3:14-19, 1991.

31. Rees JS: The effect of variation in occlusal loading on the development of abfraction lesions: a finite element study, *J Oral Rehabil* 29:188-193, 2002.

32. Whitehead SA, Wilson NH, Watts DC: Development of noncarious cervical notch lesions in vitro, *J Esthet Dent* 11:332-337, 1999.

33. Piotrowski BT, Gillette WB, Hancock EB: Examining the prevalence and characteristics of abfraction-like cervical lesions in a population of U.S. veterans, *J Am Dent Assoc* 132:1694-1701, 2001.

34. Brackett WW, Covey DA, St Germain HA JR: One-year clinical performance of a self-etching adhesive in class V resin composites cured by two methods, *Oper Dent* 27(3):218-222, 2002.

35. Brackett WW, Browning WD, Ross JA et al: 1-year clinical evaluation of Compoglass and Fuji II LC in cervical erosion/abfraction lesions, *Am J Dent* 12(3):119-122, 1999.

36. Kokich VG: Esthetics: the orthodontic-periodontic restorative connection, *Semin Orthod* 2:21-30, 1996.

37. Keim RG: Aesthetics in clinical orthodontic-periodontic interactions, *Periodontol 2000* 27:59-71, 2001.

38. Vollmer WH, Ratietschak KH: Influence of occlusal adjustment by grinding on gingivitis and mobility of traumatized teeth, *J Clin Periodontol* 2:113, 1975.

39. Schoo WH, van der Velden U: Marginal soft tissue recessions with and without attached gingiva. A five year longitudinal study, *J Periodont Res* 20(3):209-211, 1985.

40. Kisch J, Badersten A, Egelberg J: Longitudinal observation of "unattached," mobile gingival areas, *J Clin Periodontol* 13:131-134, 1986.

41. Wagenberg BD, Kennedy JE, Hall WB et al: Proceeding of the world workshop in clinical periodontics. In Nevins M, Becker W, Kornman K, editors: *Consensus report discussion section VII-16-20*, Chicago, 1989, American Academy of Periodontology.

42. Lang NP, Loe H: The relationship between the width of keratinized gingiva and gingival health, *J Periodontol* 43:623-627, 1972.

43. Wilson RD: Marginal tissue recession in general dental practice: a preliminary study, *Int J Periodontics Restorative Dent* 3:41, 1983.

44. Freedman AL, Salkin LM, Stein MD, Green K: A 10-year longitudinal study of untreated mucogingival defects, *J Periodontol* 63:71-72, 1992.

45. Wennstrom JL: Lack of association between width of attached gingiva and development of gingival recessions. A 5-year longitudinal study, *J Clin Periodontol* 14:181-184, 1987.

46. Kennedy JE, Bird WC, Palcanis KG, Dorfman HS: A longitudinal evaluation of varying widths of attached gingiva, *J Clin Periodontol* 12:667-675, 1985.

47. Wennstrom JL: Mucogingival therapy, *Ann Periodontol* 1:671-701, 1996.

48. Camargo PM, Melnick PR, Kenney EG: The use of free gingival grafts for aesthetic purposes, *Periodontol 2000* 27:72-96, 2001.

49. Nevins M: Attached gingiva-mucogingival therapy and restorative dentistry, *Int J Periodontics Restorative Dent* 6(4):9-27, 1986.

50. Stetler KJ, Bissada NF: Significance of the width of keratinized gingiva on the periodontal status of teeth with submarginal restorations, *J Periodontol* 58:696-700, 1987.

51. Maynard JC, Wilson RD: Physiologic dimensions of the periodontium significant to the restorative dentist, *J Periodontol* 50:170-174, 1979.

52. Ericsson I, Lindhe J: Recession in sites with inadequate width of the keratinized gingiva. An experimental study in the dog, *J Clin Periodontol* 11:95-103, 1984.

53. Hall WB: Gingival augmentation/mucogingival surgery, Proceedings of the World Workshop in Clinical Periodontics, Chicago, IL, American Acadamy of Periodontics, July 23-27, 1989, VII-1-VII-20.

54. Dorfman HS: Mucogingival changes resulting from mandibular incisor tooth movement, *Am J Orthod* 74: 286-297, 1978.

55. Bohannan HM: Studies in the alteration of vestibular depth. III. Vestibular incision, *J Periodontol* 34:209-215, 1963.

56. Corn H: Periosteal separation—its clinical significance, *J Periodontol* 33:1-40, 1962.

57. Berglundh T, Lindhe J, Ericsson I et al: The soft tissue barrier at implants and teeth, *Clin Oral Implant Res* 2: 81-90, 1991.

58. Chayto DV, Zarb GA, Schmitt A, Lewis DW: The longitudinal effectiveness of osseointegrated dental implants. The Toronto study: bone level changes, *Int J Periodontics Restorative Dent* 11:113-125, 1991.

59. Lekholm U, van Steenberghe D, Herrmann I et al: Osseointegrated implants in the treatment of partially edentulous jaws. A prospective 5-year multicenter study, *Int J Oral Maxillofac Implants* 9:627-635, 1994.

60. Lekholm U, Adell R, Lindhe J et al: Marginal tissue reactions at osseointegrated titanium fixtures. A cross-sectional retrospective study, *Int J Oral Maxillofac Surg* 15:53-63, 1986.

61. Apse P, Zarb GA, Schmitt A, Lewis DW: The longitudinal effectiveness of osseointegrated dental implants. The Toronto study: Peri-implant mucosal response, *Int J Periodontics Restorative Dent* 11:95-111, 1991.

62. Warrer K, Buser D, Lang NP, Karring T: Plaque-induced peri-implantitis in the presence or absence of keratinized mucosa, *Clin Oral Implant Res* 6:131-138, 1995.

63. Edwards JG: The diastema, the frenum, the frenectomy: a clinical study, *Am J Orthod* 71:489-508, 1977.

64. Miller PD Jr: A classification of marginal tissue recession, *Int J Periodontics Restorative Dent* 2:8-13, 1985.

65. Miller PD Jr: Root coverage with the free gingival graft. Factors associated with incomplete coverage, *J Periodontol* 58:674-681, 1987.

66. Jacobsen PL, Bruce G: Clinical dentin hypersensitivity-understanding the causes and prescribing a treatment, *J Contemp Dent Pract* 15:2(1):1-12, 2001.

67. Goldstein M, Nasatzky E, Goultschin J, Boyan BD, Schwartz Z: Coverage of previously carious roots is as predictable a procedure as coverage of intact roots, *J Periodontol* 73:1419-1426, 2002.

68. Ammons W: Presentation to the Saul Schluger Study Club, Anaheim, Calif, 1981.

69. Bahat O, Deeb C, Golden T, Homarnyckyj O: Preservation of ridges utilizing hydroxyapatite, *Int J Periodontics Restorative Dent* 6:35-41, 1987.

70. Seibert JS: Reconstruction of deformed, partially edentulous ridges, using full thickness onlay grafts. Part I. Technique and wound healing, *Compend Contin Educ Dent* 4:437, 1983.

71. Allen EP, Gainza CS, Farthing GG, Newbold DA: Improved technique for localized ridge augmentation: a report of 21 cases, *J Periodontol* 56:195-199, 1985.

72. Wang H, Shammari K: HVC ridge deficiency classification: a therapeutically oriented classification, *Int J Periodontics Restorative Dent* 22:335-343, 2002.

73. Lekholm U, Zarb G: Patient selection and preparation. In Branemark P-I, editor: *Tissue-integrated prostheses: osseointegration in clinical dentistry*, Chicago, 1985, Quintessence, pp 199-209.

74. Misch CE, Judy KW: Classification of partially edentulous arches for implant dentistry, *Int J Oral Implantol* 4:7-13, 1987.

75. Levine RA, McGuire M: The diagnosis and treatment of the gummy smile, *Compend Contin Educ Dent* 18:757-764, 1997.

76. Meraw SJ, Sheridan PJ: Medically induced gingival hyperplasia, *Mayo Clin Proc* 73:1196-1199, 1998.

77. Bittencourt LP, Campos V, Moliterno LF et al: Hereditary gingival fibromatosis: review of the literature and a case report, *Quintessence Int* 31:415-418, 2000.

78. Coslet JG, Vanarsdall R, Weisgold A: Diagnosis and classification of delayed passive eruption of the dentogingival junction in the adult, *Alpha Omegan* 70:24-28, 1977.

79. Garber DA, Salama MA: The aesthetic smile: diagnosis and treatment, *Periodontol 2000* 11:18-28, 1996.

80. Jorgensen MG, Nowzari H: Aesthetic crown lengthening, *Periodontol 2000* 27:47-58, 2001.

81. Tarnow DP, Magner AW, Fletcher P: The effect of the distance from the contact point to the crest of bone on the presence or absence of the interproximal dental papilla, *J Periodontol* 63:995-996, 1992.

82. Bahat O, Handelsman M: Periodontal reconstructive flaps—classification and surgical considerations, *Int J Periodontics Restorative Dent* 11:481-487, 1991.

83. Grupe HE, Warren RF: Repair of gingival defects by a sliding flap operation, *J Periodontol* 27:92-95, 1956.

84. Staffileno H: Management of gingival recession and root exposure problems associated with periodontal disease, *Dent Clin North Am* 8:111-120, 1964.

85. Grupe J: Modified technique for the sliding flap operation, *J Periodontol* 37:491-495, 1966.

86. Wilderman MN: Repair of the mucogingival surgery with retained periosteum and inclusion of bone surgery procedure, *J Periodontol* 34:487, 1963.

87. Goldman HM, Shuman A, Isenberg G: *An atlas of the surgical management of periodontal disease*, Chicago, 1982, Quintessence.

88. Nelson SW: The subpedicle connective tissue graft, a bilaminar reconstructive procedure for the coverage of denuded root surfaces, *J Periodontol* 58:95-102, 1987.

89. Irwin RK: Combined use of a gingival graft and rotated pedicle procedures: case reports, *J Periodontol* 48:38, 1977.

90. Pennel BM, Higgison JD, Towner TD et al: Oblique rotated flap, *J Periodontol* 36:305-309, 1965.

91. Patur B: The rotation flap for covering denuded root surfaces. A closed wound technique, *J Periodontol* 48:41-44, 1977.

92. Bahat O, Handelsman M, Gordon J: The transpositional flap in mucogingival surgery, *Int J Periodontics Restorative Dent* 10:473-482, 1990.

93. Cohen D, Ross S: The double papillae flap in periodontal therapy, *J Periodontol* 39:65-70, 1968.

94. Harris RJ: The connective tissue and partial thickness double pedicle graft: a predictable method of obtaining root coverage, *J Periodontol* 63:477-486, 1992.

95. Harris R: Root coverage with connective tissue grafts: an evaluation of short- and long-term results, *J Periodontol* 73:1054-1059, 2002.

96. Nemcovsky CE, Serfaty V: Alveolar ridge preservation following extraction of maxillary anterior teeth. Report on 23 consecutive cases, *J Periodontol* 67:390-395, 1996.

97. Nemcovsky CE, Artzi Z: Split palatal flap. I. A surgical approach for primary soft tissue healing in ridge augmentation procedures: technique and clinical results, *Int J Periodontics Restorative Dent* 19:175-181, 1999.

98. Mathews DP: The pediculated connective tissue graft: a technique for improving unaesthetic implant restorations. *Pract Proced Aesthet Dent* 14:719-724, 2002.

99. Maynard JG: Coronal positioning of a previously placed autogenous gingival graft, *J Periodontol* 48:151, 1977.

100. Tarnow DP: Semilunar coronally positioned flap, *J Clin Periodontol* 13:182-185, 1986.

101. Baldi C, Pini-Prato G, Pagliare U et al: Coronally positioned flap procedure for root coverage. Is flap thickness a relevant predictor to achieve root coverage? *J Periodontol* 70:1077-1084, 1999.

102. Goldman HM, Schluger S, Fox L: *Periodontol therapy*, St. Louis, 1956, CV Mosby.

103. Nabers CL: Repositioning the attached gingiva, *J Periodontol* 25:38-39, 1954.

104. Townsend-Olsen C, Ammons W, van Belle G: A longitudinal study comparing apically repositioned flaps, with and without osseous surgery, *Int J Periodontics Restorative Dent* 4:11-34, 1985.

105. Machtei E, Ben-Yehouda A: The effect of post-surgical flap placement on probing depth and attachment level: a 2-year longitudinal study, *J Periodontol* 65:855, 1994.

106. Ingber JS, Rose LF, Coslet JG: The biologic width-a concept in periodontics and restorative dentistry, *Alpha Omegan* 10:62-65, 1977.

107. Sorenson JA, Engelman MJ: Ferrule design and fracture resistance of endodontically treated teeth, *J Prothet Dent* 63:529-536, 1990.

108. Gegauff AG: Effect of crown lengthening and ferrule placement on static load failure of cemented cast

post-cores and crowns, *J Prosthet Dent* 84(2):169-179, 2000.

109. Libman WJ, Nicholls JL: Load fatigue of teeth restored with cast posts and cores and complete crowns, *Int J Prosthodont* 8(2):155-161, 1995.

110. Herrero F, Scott J, Maropis P, Yukna R: Clinical comparison of desired versus actual amount of surgical crown lengthening, *J Periodontol* 66:568-571, 1995.

111. Bragger U, Lauchenauer D, Lang NP: Surgical lengthening of the clinical crown, *J Clin Periodontol* 19(1):58-63, 1992.

112. Pontoriero R, Carnevale J: Surgical crown lengthening: a 12 month clinical wound healing study, *J Periodontol* 72(7):841-848, 2001.

113. van der Velden U: Regeneration of the interdental soft tissues following denudation procedures, *J Clin Periodontol* 9:455-459, 1982.

114. Gargiulo A, Wentz F, Orban B: Dimensions and relations of the dentogingival junction in humans, *J Periodontol* 32:261-267, 1961.

115. Kois J: Altering gingival levels: the restorative connection, Part I: Biologic variables, *J Esthet Dent* 6:3-9, 1994.

116. Spear F: Interdisciplinary management of anterior esthetic dilemmas: an opportunity for personal fulfillment and practice enhancement. Presentation to the American Academy of Periodontology Annual Session in San Antonio, Tx, September 28, 1999.

117. Carnio J, Miller P: Increasing the amount of attached gingiva using a modified apically repositioned flap, *J Periodontol* 70:1110-1117, 1999.

118. Vanarsdall R, Corn H: Soft tissue management of labially positioned unerupted teeth, *Am J Orthod* 72:53-64, 1977.

119. Bass T: Observation on the misplaced upper canine tooth, *Dent Pract Dent Rec* 18:25-33, 1967.

120. Grover P, Lorton L: The incidence of unerupted permanent teeth and related clinical cases, *Oral Surg* 59:420-424, 1985.

121. Witsenberg B, Boering G: Eruption of impacted permanent upper incisors after removal of supernumerary teeth, *Int J Oral Surg* 10:423-431, 1981.

122. Tegsjo U, Valerius-Olsson H, Andersson L: Periodontal conditions following surgical exposure of unerupted maxillary canines—a long term follow-up study of two surgical techniques, *Swed Dent J* 8(6):257-263, 1984.

123. Won-Lee T, Wong F: Maintaining an ideal tooth-gingiva relationship when exposing and aligning an impacted tooth, *Br J Orthod* 12:189-192, 1985.

124. Kokich V, Mathews D: Surgical and orthodontic management of impacted teeth, *Dent Clin North Am* 37:181-204, 1993.

125. Caminiti M, Sandor G, Giambattistini C, Tompson B: Outcomes of the surgical exposure, bonding and eruption of 82 impacted maxillary canines, *J Can Dent Assoc* 64: 572-574, 576-579, 1998.

126. Vermette M, Kokich V: Uncovering labially impacted teeth: apically positioned flap and closed-eruption techniques, *Angle Orthod* 65:23-34, 1995.

127. Dragoo MR: Resin-ionomer and hybrid-ionomer cements: part II, human clinical and histologic wound healing responses in specific periodontal lesions, *Int J Periodontics Restorative Dent* 17(1):75-87, 1997.

128. Raetzke P: Covering localized areas of root exposure employing the "envelope" technique, *J Periodontol* 58: 397-402, 1985.

129. Allen AL: Use of the supraperiosteal envelope in soft tissue grafting for root coverage. I. Rationale and technique, *Int J Periodontics Restorative Dent* 3:217-227, 1994.

130. Abrams L: Augmentation of deformed residual edentulous ridge for fixed prosthesis, *Compend Contin Educ Gen* 1:205, 1980.

131. Scharf DR, Tarnow DP: Modified roll technique for localized alveolar ridge augmentation, *Int J Periodontics Restorative Dent* 12:415-425, 1992.

132. Miller PD Jr: Root coverage using a free soft tissue autograft following citric acid application, *Int J Periodontics Restorative Dent* 2:65-70, 1982.

133. Nabers JM: Free gingival grafts, *Periodontics* 4:243, 1966.

134. Pennel B, Tabor J, King K et al: Free masticatory mucosa graft, *J Periodontol* 40:162-166.

135. Sullivan H, Atkins J: Free autogenous gingival grafts. III. Utilization of grafts in the treatment of gingival recession, *Periodontics* 6:152-160, 1968.

136. Holbrook T, Ochsenbein C: Complete coverage of the denuded root surface with a one-stage gingival graft, *Int J Periodontics Restorative Dent* 3:8-27, 1983.

137. Sullivan H, Atkins J: Free autogenous gingival grafts. I. Principles of successful grafting, *Periodontics* 6:121-129, 1968.

138. Matter J, Cimasoni G: Creeping attachment after free gingival grafts, *J Periodontol* 47:574-579, 1976.

139. Matter J: Creeping attachment of free gingival grafts: a five-year follow up study, *J Periodontol* 51:681-685, 1980.

140. Pollack R: Bilateral creeping attachment using free mucosal grafts. A case report with 4-year follow-up, *J Periodontol* 55:670-672, 1984.

141. Pasquinelli K: The histology of new attachment utilizing a thick autogenous soft tissue graft in an area of deep recession: a case report, *Int J Periodontics Restorative Dent* 15:248-257, 1995.

142. Harris RJ: Creeping attachment associated with the connective tissue with partial-thickness double pedicle graft, *J Periodontol* 68:890-899, 1997.

143. Harris RJ: Acellular dermal matrix used for root coverage: 18-month follow-up observation, *Int J Periodontics Restorative Dent* 22:156-163, 2002.

144. Meltzer JA: Edentulous area tissue graft correction of an esthetic defect: a case report, *J Periodontol* 50:320, 1979.

145. Seibert JS: Reconstruction of deformed, partially edentulous ridges, using full-thickness onlay grafts. Part II. Technique and wound healing, *Compend Contin Educ Gen* 4:549, 1983.

146. Seibert JS, Louis JV: Soft tissue ridge augmentation utilizing a combination onlay—interpositional graft procedure: a case report, *Int J Periodontics Restorative Dent* 16:311-321, 1996.

147. Langer B, Calagna L: The subepithelial connective tissue graft, *J Prosthet Dent* 44:363, 1980.

148. Langer B, Calagna L: The subepithelial connective tissue graft. A new approach to the enhancement of anterior cosmetics, *Int J Periodontics Restorative Dent* 2:22-33, 1982.

149. Schroeder H: *Differentiation of human oral stratified epithelia*, Basel, Switzerland, 1981, Karger AG.

150. Soehren SE, Allen AL, Cutright DE et al: Clinical and histologic studies of donor tissues utilized for free grafts of masticatory mucosa, *J Periodontol* 44:727-741, 1973.

151. Reiser G, Bruno J, Mahan P, Larkin L: The subepithelial connective tissue graft palatal donor site: anatomic considerations for surgeons, *Int J Periodontics Restorative Dent* 16:131-137, 1996.

152. Schroeder H: *Oral structural biology*, New York, 1991, Thieme, pp 350-370.

153. Muller H, Eger T: Masticatory mucosa and periodontal phenotype: a review, *Int J Periodontics Restorative Dent* 22:172-183, 2002.

154. Kydd W, Daly C, Wheeler J: The thickness measurement of masticatory mucosa in vivo, *Int Dent J* 21:430-441, 1971.

155. Studer S, Allen E, Rees T, Kouba A: The thickness of masticatory mucosa in the human hard palate and tuberosity as potential donor sites for ridge augmentation procedures, *J Periodontol* 68:145-151, 1997.

156. Harris RJ: A comparison of two techniques for obtaining a connective tissue graft from the palate, *Int J Periodontics Restorative Dent* 17:260-271, 1997.

157. Harris RJ: Formation of a cyst-like area after a connective tissue graft for root coverage, *J Periodontol* 73:340-345, 2002.

158. Langer B, Langer L: Subepithelial connective tissue graft technique for root coverage, *J Periodontol* 56:715-720, 1985.

159. Cordiolo G, Mortarino C, Chierico A et al: Comparison of 2 techniques of subepithelial connective tissue grafts in the treatment of gingival recessions, *J Periodontol* 72:1470-1476, 2001.

160. Goaslind G, Roberston P, Mahan C et al: Thickness of facial gingiva, *J Periodontol* 48:768-771, 1977.

161. Lifecell Medical Information Center: Patented process for AlloDerm® processing. Available on-line at: www.lifecell.com/healthcare/products/alloderm/patented.cfm, accessed Oct. 10, 2002.

162. Tal H, Moses O, Zohar R et al: Root coverage of advanced gingival recession: A comparative study between acellular dermal matrix allograft and subepithelial connective tissue grafts, *J Periodontol* 73:1404-1411, 2002.

163. Paolantonio M, Dolci M, Esposito P et al: Subpedicle acellular dermal matrix graft and autogenous connective tissue graft in the treatment of gingival recessions: a comparative 1-year clinical study, *J Periodontol* 73:1299-1307, 2002.

164. Zabalequi I, Sicilia A, Cambra J et al: Treatment of multiple adjacent gingival recessions with the tunnel subepithelial connective tissue graft: a clinical report, *Int J Periodontics Restorative Dent* 19:199-206, 1999.

165. Garber DA, Rosenberg ES: The edentulous ridge in fixed prosthodontics. *Compend Contin Educ Gen* 2:212, 1981.

166. Kaldahl WB, Tussing GJ, Wentz RM, Walker JA: Achieving an esthetic appearance with a fixed prosthesis by submucosal grafts. *J Am Dent Assoc* 104:449, 1982.

167. Miller PD Jr: Ridge augmentation under existing fixed prosthesis, *J Periodontol* 57:742-745, 1986.

168. Bahat O, Kaplin LM: Pantographic lip expansion and bone grafting for ridge augmentation, *Int J Periodontics Restorative Dent* 9:345-353, 1989.

169. Maurer S, Leone CW: Use of a serially layered, double connective tissue graft approach to enhance maxillary anterior esthetics, *Int J Periodontics Restorative Dent* 21:497-503, 2001.

170. Fowler EB, Breault LG: Ridge augmentation with a folded acellular dermal matrix allograft: a case report, *J Contemp Dent Pract* 15:2(3):31-40, 2001.

171. Blatz MB, Hurzeler MB, Strub JR: Reconstruction of the lost interproximal papilla—presentation of surgical and nonsurgical approaches, *Int J Periodontics Restorative Dent* 19:395-406, 1999.

172. Nemcovsky CE: Interproximal papilla augmentation procedure: a novel surgical approach and clinical evaluation of 10 consecutive procedures, *Int J Periodontics Restorative Dent* 553-559, 2001.

173. Francischone CE, Costa CG, Francischone AC et al: Controlled orthodontic extrusion to create gingival papilla: a case report, *Quintessence Int* 33:561-565, 2002.

174. Azzi R, Takei HH, Etienne D, Carranza FA: Root coverage and papilla reconstruction using autogenous osseous and connective tissue grafts, *Int J Periodontics Restorative Dent* 21:141-147, 2001.

175. Spear FM: Maintenance of the interdental papilla following anterior tooth removal, *Pract Periodont Aesthet Dent* 11(1):21-28, 1999.

176. Artzi A, Nemcovsky CE, Tal H: Efficacy of porous bovine bone mineral in various types of osseous deficiencies: clinical observations and literature review, *Int J Periodontics Restorative Dent* 21:395-405, 2001.

177. Bahat O, Deeb C, Golden T, Komarnyckyi O: Preservation of ridges utilizing hydroxyapatite, *Int J Periodontics Restorative Dent* 7:35-41, 1987.

178. Melcher AH: On the repair potential of periodontal tissues, *J Periodontol* 47:256-260, 1976.

179. Gottlow J, Nyman S, Lindhe J et al: New attachment formation in the human periodontium by guided tissue regeneration. Case reports, *J Clin Periodontol* 13:604-616, 1986.

180. Pini Prato G, Tinti C, Vincenzi G et al: Guided tissue regeneration in the treatment of human facial recession. A 12-case report, *J Periodontol* 63:554-560, 1992.

181. Garrett S: Periodontal regeneration around natural teeth, *Ann Periodontol* 1:621-666, 1996.

182. Buser D, Dahlin C, Schenk RK: *Guided bone regeneration in implant dentistry*, Chicago, 1994, Quintessence.

183. Hurley AL, Stinchfield FE, Bassett DAL, Lyon WH: The role of soft tissues in osteogenesis. *J Bone Joint Surg* 41A:1243, 1959.

184. Bartee BK: The use of high-density polytetrafluoroethylene membrane to treat osseous defects: clinical reports, *Implant Dentistry* 4:21-26, 1995.

185. Bunyaratavej P, Wang HL: Collagen membranes: a review, *J Periodontol* 72:215-220, 2001.

186. Harris R: GTR for root coverage: a long-term follow-up, *Int J Periodontics Restorative Dent* 22:55-61, 2002.

187. Amarante ES, Leknes KN, Skavland J, Lie T: Coronally positioned flap procedures with or without a bioabsorbable membrane in the treatment of human gingival recession, *J Periodontol* 71:989-998, 2000.

188. Terranova VP, Franzetti LC, Hic S: A biochemical approach to periodontal regeneration: tetracycline treatment of dentin promotes fibroblast adhesion and growth, *J Periodont Res* 21:330-337, 1986.

189. Registar A, Burdick F: Accelerated reattachment with cementogenesis to dentin, demineralized in situ. II. Defect repair, *J Periodontol* 47:497-505, 1976.

190. Cole RT, Crigger M, Bogle G et al: Connective tissue regeneration to periodontally diseased teeth. A histological study, *J Periodont Res* 15:1-9, 1980.

191. Polson A, Frederick G, Ladenhelm S, Hanes P: The production of a root surface smear layer by instrumentation and its removal by citric acid, *J Periodontol* 55:443-446, 1985.

192. Bertrand P, Dunlap R: Coverage of deep, wide gingival clefts with free gingival autografts: root planing with and without citric acid demineralization, *Int J Periodontics Restorative Dent* 8:65-77, 1988.

193. Laney J, Saunders V, Garnick J: A comparison of two techniques for attaining root coverage, *J Periodontol* 63:19-23, 1992.

194. Bouchard P, Etienne D, Ouhayoun J-P, Nilveus R: Subepithelial connective tissue grafts in the treatment of gingival recessions. A comparative study of 2 procedures, *J Periodontol* 65:929-936, 1994.

195. Common J, McFall W: The effect of citric acid on attachment of laterally positioned flaps, *J Periodontol* 54:9-18, 1983.

22 Principles of Periodontal Plastic Microsurgery

Dennis A. Shanelec

PERIODONTAL PLASTIC SURGERY

Plastic surgery is a clinical discipline in which surgical techniques are used to reconstruct bodily structures that are defective or damaged through injury or disease.[1] It relies on mobilization of soft tissue flaps for advancement or retraction in combination with the addition or removal of tissue beneath the flap. Such techniques are capable of molding tissues to restore a lost part or to improve appearance. The adoption of plastic surgical principles to gingival tissues comprises the field of periodontal plastic surgery. Microsurgery is surgery performed under the microscope.[2,3] The influence of microsurgery has changed the surgical disciplines of medicine and will influence periodontal plastic surgery.

CLINICAL PHILOSOPHY OF MICROSURGERY

Microsurgery is a surgical philosophy that embraces three distinct values.[4] The first value is the improvement of motor skills to enhance surgical ability. This is evident in decisive hand movements accomplished with increased precision and reduced tremor. Microsurgical training involves a detailed analysis of those factors that can have positive or negative effects on physiologic tremor.

PHYSIOLOGIC TREMOR AND POSTURE HAND GRIP

Physiologic tremor is an unwanted movement of the hand. It is a naturally occurring phenomenon associated with tension generated by postural antigravity muscles.[5] To limit tremor, specific working posture and handgrip are necessary. Because postural muscles are a cause of tremor, a seated posture that is symmetrical, upright, and balanced is necessary. Support of the forearm and ulnar surface is also important.[6]

INTERNAL PRECISION GRIP OF THE HAND

The internal precision grip is sometimes called the pen grip[7,8] (Fig. 22-1; Box 22-1). When penmanship was a normal part of the education curriculum, skill using this grip was commonplace. Currently, it is relearned with some difficulty, because it supplants poor ergonomic habits previously learned in childhood or even dental school.

With this grip, the external muscles of the hand, its flexors and extensors, are relaxed to resist fatigue. The stage is set for rotating the hand using its intrinsic muscles: those of the thenar and hypothenar eminence (the muscles at the base of the thumb and the base of the little finger, respectively), the interossei, and the lumbricals (small muscles in the palm of the hand). Rotary

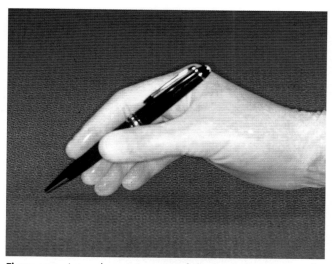

Figure 22-1. Internal precision grip of the hand showing use of a pen grasp.

Box 22-1	Features of the Internal Precision Grip[8]

- It is a chuck grip with the thumb, index, and middle finger.
- The instrument rests at the apex of the first web space.
- The instrument rests on the pads of the fingers.
- The thumb is straight.
- The metacarpal-phalangeal joint is flexed approximately 90 degrees.
- The interphalangeal joints are straight.

movement is the most accurate motion of which the hand is capable.[9,10] Without the proper handgrip, accurate movements and good microsurgical results are not likely.

MICROSURGICAL INSTRUMENTS

The second basic value of microsurgery is the application of microsurgical instruments to reduce tissue trauma. Microsurgical instruments are much smaller, often by tenfold (Fig. 22-2). This creates a smaller surgical field with less injury and bleeding. Microsurgical instruments have subtle design features to accomplish their ends. Their handles have a round cross-sectional diameter to enhance rotary movements using the precision grip (Fig. 22-3). They are frequently made of titanium to reduce weight, prevent magnetization, and provide reliable manipulation of needles, sutures, and tissues. They are manufactured under magnification to high tolerances and resist deformation from repetitive use and sterilization cycles.

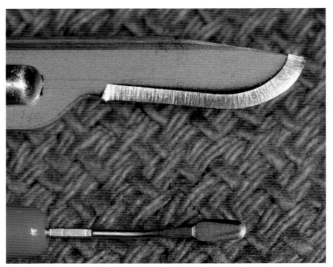

Figure 22-2. Relative size of microsurgical scalpel blade and standard 15C scalpel blade.

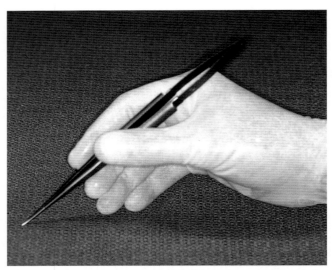

Figure 22-3. A titanium microneedle holder with a round handle fits the precision grip, providing excellent ergonomics.

WOUND APPOSITION AND PRIMARY WOUND CLOSURE

The third basic value of microsurgery is an emphasis on passive wound closure with exact primary apposition of the wound edge. This eliminates gaps and dead spaces, circumventing the need for new tissue formation. An extensive and often painful inflammatory and proliferative phase of wound healing can then be avoided. The ideal microsurgical closure is an invisible incision with little tissue damage and no bleeding, which is closed with small sutures placed precisely under minimal tension (Fig. 22-4, *A* through *E*).

GEOMETRY OF SUTURING

Suturing techniques in microsurgery are quite different from those in traditional surgery. Because the microscope enhances the surgeon's ability to view inaccuracies in

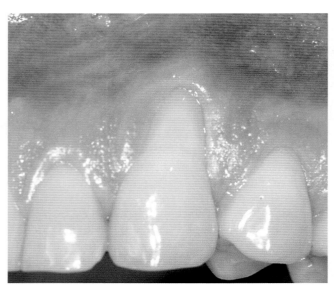

A

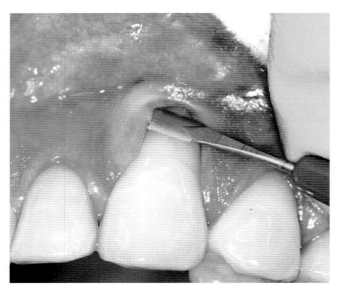

B

Figure 22-4. A, Wide deep recession on maxillary canine, before treatment. **B,** Microsurgical scalpel makes a microsurgical incision in the sulcus.

Continued

Box 22-2	Geometry of Microsurgical Suturing

The following points exemplify the geometry of microsurgical suturing:

Needle angle of entry and exit: Slightly less than 90 degrees
Bite size: 1.5 times the tissue thickness
Symmetry: Equal bite sizes on both sides of the wound
Direction of needle passage: Perpendicular to the wound

ESTHETICS IN PERIODONTICS

In many areas of dentistry, esthetics has become more important in recent years. As separate procedures, or before restorative treatment, esthetic periodontics is an integral part of periodontal practice.[14,15] Esthetics is the basis of periodontal plastic surgery, which has similarities in techniques and objectives to medical plastic surgery. The small scale of this work and the intricate detail required is why surgical microscopy is helpful in

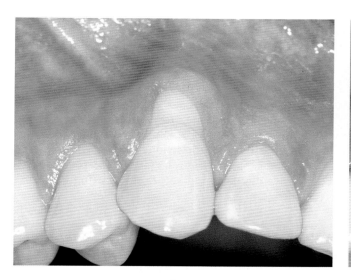

A

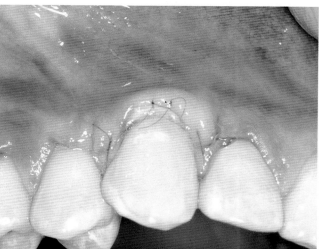

B

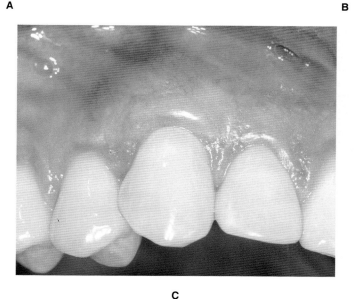

C

Figure 22-6. A, Wide deep recession over a maxillary canine, before treatment. **B,** The connective tissue is sutured into the submucosal space created through the sulcus. No releasing incisions are created. Purse string sutures are placed on the mesial and distal, and interrupted circumferential sutures are used to create apposition between the connective tissue graft and the overlying mucosal flap. This is important to prevent micromovement of the graft against the flap and root surface. A 7-0 monofilament absorbable suture is used. **C,** At 2 weeks, healing shows lack of scarring and inflammation. Again note the increased zone of keratinized tissue.

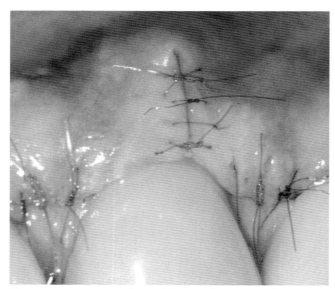

Figure 22-7. Microsurgical wound closure. The interrupted sutures are evenly placed, and the direction of suture passage is perpendicular to the wound edge. The wound is closed passively and no microgaps are present.

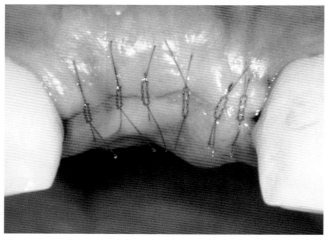

Figure 22-8. A surgeon's knots tied properly is a stable knot. Only two throws are required and the knot lies flat against the tissue. This is a great advantage in the oral cavity where the tongue is a potential source of micromovement of the wound edges. A 7-0 monofilament suture is used.

periodontal plastic surgery. The most dramatic application of periodontal microsurgery is in free transfer of gingival tissues for root coverage. Careful dissection and suturing of adjacent gingival tissue can often remedy small areas of recession without use of major flaps[16] (Fig. 22-9, A through C). When this is impractical,

transfer of distant tissue from the palate or other donor source can be accomplished.

TISSUE TRANSFER FOR ROOT COVERAGE

Grafting is a surgical procedure in which tissue is totally severed from the body and transferred to a new location.[17] Successful grafting depends on the body's ability to restore circulation to the transferred tissue.[18] A recipient bed well supplied with blood vessels is necessary for this to occur.[19] Grafting over avascular root surfaces presents a unique challenge. Autologous grafts (e.g., full-thickness gingival grafts and subepithelial grafts) use tissue borrowed from one area and then transferred to another area within the same individual.[20] Homologous grafts (e.g., freeze-dried human dermal allografts) use tissue from different individuals of the same species. Heterologous grafts (e.g., bovine collagen membranes) use tissue from individuals of different species. Because they revascularize rapidly, autologous grafts from the same individual provide the most predictable means of gingival grafting for root coverage. (Extensive discussion of soft tissue grafting is found in Chapter 21.)

GINGIVAL GRAFTING FOR ROOT COVERAGE

Periodontal plastic microsurgery to cover denuded roots can be routine and predictable using a variety of techniques.[20-23] Functional deficits can be restored, with the grafted autologous gingival tissue attached to underlying bone and root and displaying a normal keratinized epithelial phenotype.[24] The esthetic deficits are corrected by positioning gingival tissue at the cementoenamel junction or a level appropriate to the surrounding teeth to achieve harmonious gingival margin positions. Color match and esthetic appearance of these grafts are often indistinguishable from surrounding gingival tissue[25,26] (Fig. 22-10, A and B).

FULL-THICKNESS GINGIVAL GRAFTS

Full-thickness gingival grafts involve transfer of the entire thickness of the gingiva and a portion of the underlying submucosa. They are better suited for small gingival defects because their donor site cannot be primarily closed.[27] Full-thickness gingival grafts require a large recipient bed for survival. Because it takes time for lateral blood vessels to grow into the graft, the amount of tissue that may be transferred is somewhat limited.[28] Until vascular ingrowth occurs, the graft over the root must survive by plasmatic diffusion from an adjacent recipient bed.[29] Full-thickness gingival grafts produce

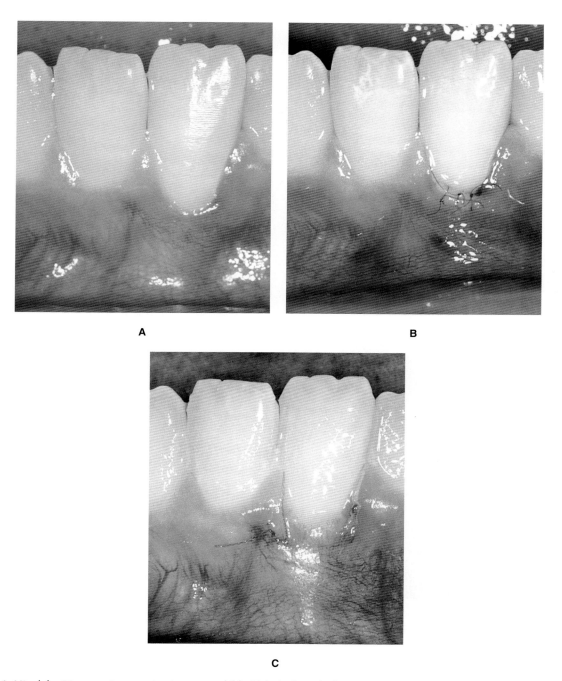

Figure 22-9. A, Mixed dentition eruptive recession in a young child with lack of attached gingiva. **B,** An incision was made through the sulcus with circumferential interrupted sutures to secure the connective tissue graft below the mucosal envelope. Note the minimal level of trauma. A 7-0 monofilament suture is used. **C,** At 1 week, healing shows the thickness of gingival tissue created and its differentiation into keratinized epithelium.

less natural appearing results and are often followed by stricture and shrinkage of the graft. Full-thickness gingival grafts can generally restore narrow recession defects; but for wide recession, subepithelial gingival grafts are often preferred (Fig. 22-11, *A* through *C*). The esthetic result for subepithelial grafts is generally superior to that seen with full-thickness gingival grafts.[30] In esthetic regions of the mouth, this factor may dictate the type of procedure chosen by the clinician. Subepithelial grafts often demonstrate a better color match with the surrounding native tissue than do full-thickness gingival grafts.

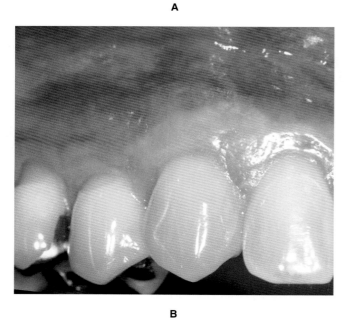

A

B

Figure 22-10. A, Wide shallow recession on maxillary canine, before treatment. **B,** Excellent postoperative color match with increased zone of keratinized tissue accomplished through the subepithelial grafting technique using microsurgery.

SUBEPITHELIAL GINGIVAL GRAFTS

The submucosa is the connective tissue layer beneath the palatal gingival epithelium. It is thick and vascular, making up the bulk of the anatomy in this area. It can quite effectively be grafted beneath flaps when the overlying epithelial layer is removed.[31] Subepithelial grafts may be large, because the donor bed is readily sutured and heals well. Subepithelial grafts revascularize more readily than full-thickness grafts because they receive

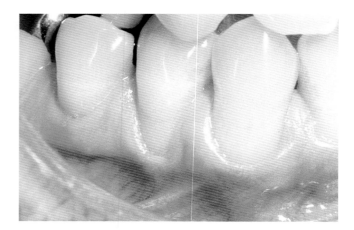

A

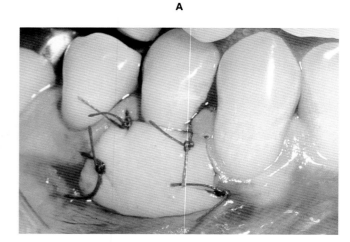

B

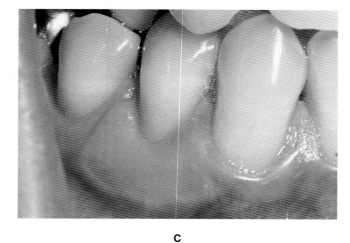

C

Figure 22-11. A, Deep recession over a mandibular premolar with shallow vestibule before treatment. **B,** Full-thickness graft gingival graft. Notice the butt joint and perpendicular apposition at the wound edges. Suture is 5-0 braided filament. **C,** Full-thickness graft postoperative view at 6 weeks shows a definite demarcation between the graft and surrounding mucosa.

initial nourishment from both the underlying recipient bed and the overlying gingival flap.[32] Since the introduction of subepithelial gingival grafts, large blocks of tissue are available for reconstruction of extensive gingival defects.[33] Large areas of gingival recession often call on surgical ingenuity.[34] When microsurgical principles are combined with an understanding of microanatomy, the surgeon frequently becomes the architect of a unique surgical method.[35,36] This innovative spirit has yielded many new procedures that are currently used in periodontal plastic surgery[37,38] (Fig. 22-12, *A* through *E*).

SURGICAL DESIGN

For uncomplicated healing to occur, careful surgical design must be used. Planning incisions with respect to size, location, and direction has enormous impact on outcome. Equally important is the way tissues are handled and positioned beneath the surface.[39] Surgeons must consider the geometry needed to accomplish a desired result and must be cognizant of the effect surgical design has on repair. Gingival tissue frequently must be mobilized to accomplish both primary surgical closure and correction of the esthetic tissue deficit. To mobilize

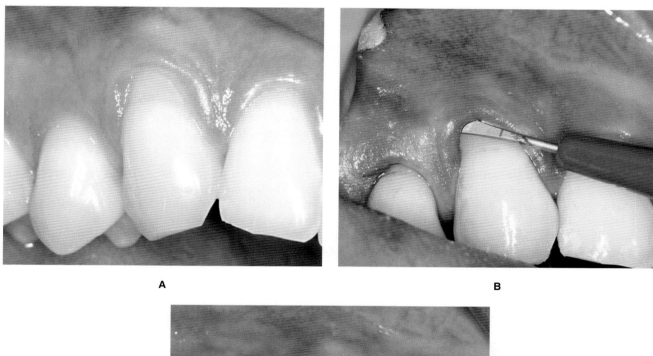

A   B

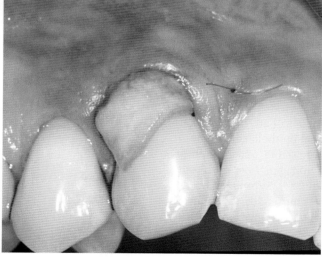

C

Figure 22-12.   A, Wide shallow recession over a maxillary canine, before treatment. **B,** Microsurgical scalpel makes a microsurgical incision in the sulcus. **C,** A 7-0 monofilament suture on the mesial creates a purse string effect to pull the connective tissue graft into the envelope created by the microsurgical scalpel.

Continued

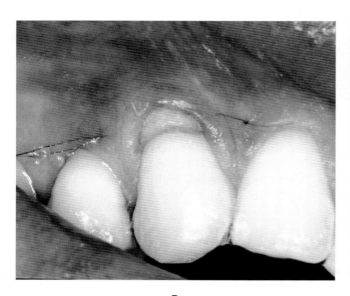

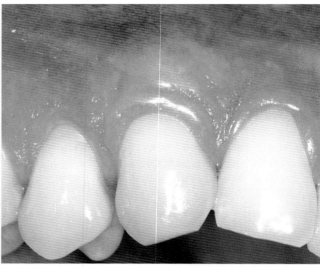

D   E

Figure 22-12. cont'd D, A second purse string suture pulls the graft under the tissue on the distal. No vertical releasing incisions are made. **E,** At 2 weeks, healing of the graft shows complete root coverage with an excellent color match. Normal anatomy of the gingival groove has been established. This reflects the reestablishment of normal supracrestal fiber anatomy.

gingival tissue, it must be separated from a tough, well vascularized tissue known as *periosteum*.[40] It is separated except for a "pedicle" through which circulation is maintained. In some cases, this pedicle will be a broad expanse of tissue without vertical releasing incisions, whereas in other cases, it may be a tiny bridge of tissue containing a few crucial blood vessels. These elevated areas of gingival tissue are referred to as *flaps*. The surgical microscope has made possible refined dissection, suturing, and surgical design of gingival flaps (Fig. 22-13, *A* through *C*).

ROOT PREPARATION

The method of biologic attachment of the gingival tissue to the root surface is of primary importance in periodontics. Most desirable is a ligamentous attachment with new cementum and Sharpey's fibers.[41-43] Some studies have shown the most common means of attachment after flap surgery to be a long junctional epithelial attachment to the root surface.[44] Another possible attachment is through parallel orientation of collagen fibers without actual insertion in the root surface.[45] Several methods of root preparation have been recommended to enhance the possibility of ligamentous attachment to the root surface.[46] Some methods are based on empirical observation and others on histologic evidence.

Mechanical Root Preparation

Empirical observation has shown that gingival tissues heal more readily against root surfaces that have been debrided

of calculus and plaque, and which present a smooth surface. For this reason, most clinicians adhere to meticulous mechanical root preparation. Some authors believe healing is enhanced by extensive removal of pathologically exposed cementum[47] (see Fig. 22-13). Some clinicians prefer to reshape buccally prominent roots to bring their contour

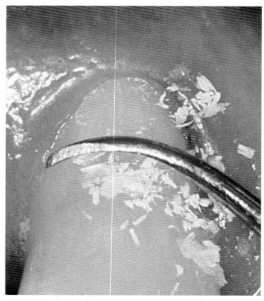

Figure 22-13. Mechanical root preparation under the microscope. Root planing results in small curls of dentin, like wood shavings from a wood plane.

into a more normal profile with the adjacent teeth and to facilitate wound closure.[21] Well accepted principles of surgery require that deep grooves or erosions on the root be contoured to eliminate dead space between the root surface and the graft, thereby preventing hematoma formation under the graft. Hand and ultrasonic instruments, or rotary burs, or both, and rubber cups with pumice may by used to accomplish mechanical root preparation.

Chemical Root Preparation

When the root surface has been scaled and polished, chemical root preparation is sometimes used. Dilute citric acid or ethylenediamine tetraacetic acid (EDTA) is used to chemically decalcify the root surface.[48] Three rationales exist for this approach. First, the smear layer that results after scaling and root planing is removed so that microparticles of debris and salivary mucoids will not delay healing.[49] Second, decalcification also removes endotoxins that may have penetrated the root surface.[50] Third, decalcification exposes collagen fibers to permit collagen "knitting" during initial wound healing.[49] That is, the exposed collagen fibers on the root surface become intertwined with collagen fibers in the grafted soft tissue. Despite the rationale for using chemical root preparation, the preponderance of evidence reveals little difference in final results when root preparation has been used compared with when it has not been used.[51]

Biologic Root Preparation

Biologic root preparation is used by some clinicians before soft tissue grafting. Currently, two biologic root preparation protocols are used. Tetracycline solution may be applied or burnished onto the root surface. In addition to demineralization and exposure of root surface collagen, tetracycline application may promote fibroblast migration to the root surface.[52] Similar to the use of citric acid or EDTA, studies reveal little clinical benefit to tetracycline root preparation. Recently, enamel matrix derivatives have been developed that may enhance healing and new cementum formation. The effects of enamel matrix derivatives on soft tissue grafting procedures is currently unknown.[53]

BENEFIT OF MICROSURGERY FOR PERIODONTAL ESTHETICS

There are many indications for and combinations of periodontal plastic microsurgical techniques. Periodontal plastic surgery is "technique sensitive" and generally thought to be more demanding than other periodontal procedures. For this reason, surgical microscopy appears to be a natural evolution in the area of periodontics[54] (Fig. 22-14). As the benefits of microsurgery in periodontics are realized, its applications will likely be more numerous, as has occurred in medical surgery.

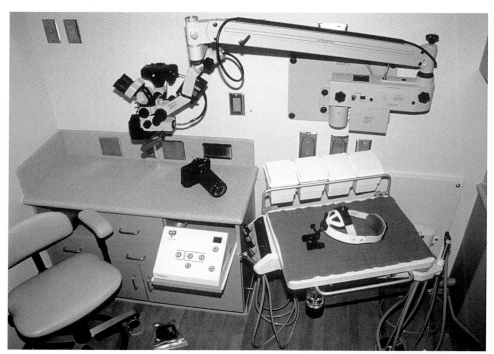

Figure 22-14. The wall-mounted surgical operating microscope is an excellent way to make the microscope accessible. A well positioned microscope in the dental operatory is as effortless to use as a dental light or dental handpiece. It becomes "invisible" after a few weeks of familiarity.

REFERENCES

1. Barsky AJ, Kahn S, Simon BD: *Principles and practice of plastic surgery*, New York, 1964, McGraw-Hill.
2. Daniel RK: Microsurgery: through the looking glass. *N Engl J Med* 300:1251-1258, 1979.
3. Shanelec D: Optical principles of dental loupes. *J Calif Dent Assoc* 20:25, 1992.
4. Acland R: *Practice manual for microvascular surgery*, St. Louis, 1989, Mosby.
5. Serafin D, Georgiade N: *A laboratory manual of microsurgery*, Durham, NC, 1989, Duke University Medical Center.
6. Chang T, Zhu S, Wang Z: *Microsurgery principles, techniques, and applications*, Singapore, 1986, World Scientific Publishing.
7. Barraquer JI: The history of microsurgery in ocular surgery, *J Microsurg* 1:288, 1980.
8. Bunke H, Chater N, Szabo Z: *The manual of microvascular surgery*, San Francisco, 1975, Ralph K. Daves Medical Center.
9. Klopper P et al: *Microsurgery and wound healing*, Amsterdam, 1979, Exerpta Medica, p 280.
10. Sun Lee: *Manual of microsurgery*, Boca Raton, Fla, 1985, CRC Press.
11. Price PB: Shear, stress, and suture, *Ann Surg* 128:408, 1948.
12. Thacker JG, Rodeheaver G, Moore JW, et al: Mechanical performance of surgical sutures, *Am J Surg* 130:374, 1975.
13. Medhorn M, Muller G: Microsurgical exercises: basic techniques anastamosis refertilization transplantation, Stuttgart, 1989, Georg Rhieme.
14. Wennstrom JL: Mucogingival therapy, *Ann Periodontol* 1:671, 1996.
15. Hall WB: Section VII: gingival augmentation/mucogingival surgery. American Academy of Periodontology Proceedings of the World Workshop in Periodontics, Chicago, 1989.
16. Nelson SW: The subpedicle connective tissue graft—a bilaminar reconstructive procedure for the coverage of denuded root surfaces, *J Periodontol* 58:96, 1987.
17. Riediger D, Ehrenfeld M: *Microsurgical tissue transplantation*, Stuttgart, Germany, 1989, Quintessence Co.
18. Janson WA, Ruben MP, Kramer GM, et al: Development of the blood supply to split-thickness free gingival autografts, *J Periodontol* 40:707, 1969.
19. Gordon HP, Sullivan HC, Atkins, JH: Free autogenous gingival grafts. Part II, supplemental findings—histology of the graft site, *Periodontics* 6:130, 1968.
20. Miller PD Jr: A classification of marginal tissue recession, *Int J Periodontics Restorative Dent* 5:9, 1985.
21. Miller PD Jr: Root coverage using a free soft tissue autograft following citric acid application. Part I. Technique, *Int J Periodontics Restorative Dent* 2:65, 1982.
22. Shanelec D: Current trends in soft tissue grafting, *J Calif Dent Assoc* 19:57, 1991.
23. Cohen DW, Ross SE: The double papilla reposition flap in periodontal therapy, *J Periodontol* 39:743, 1968.
24. Karring T, Ostergaard E, Loe H: Conservation of tissue specificity after heterotrophic transplantation of gingiva and alveolar mucosa, *J Periodont Res* 6:282, 1971.
25. Edel A: Clinical evaluation of free connective tissue grafts used to increase the width of keratinized gingiva, *J Clin Periodontol* 1:185, 1974.
26. Miller PD Jr: Root coverage using a free soft tissue autograft following citric acid application. Part III. A successful and predictable procedure in areas of deep wide recession, *Int J Periodontics Restorative Dent* 5:15, 1985.
27. Donn BJ: The free connective tissue autograft: a clinical and histological wound healing study in humans, *J Periodontol* 49:253, 1978.
28. Dorfman HS, Kennedy JE, Bird WC: Longitudinal evaluation of free autogenous gingival grafts, *J Clin Periodontol* 7:316, 1980.
29. Sullivan HC, Atkins JC: Free autogenous gingival grafts. III Utilization of grafts in the treatment of gingival recession, *Periodontics* 6:152, 1968.
30. Shanelec D, Tibbetts L: Recent advances in surgical technology. In Newman MG, Takei HH, Carranza FA, editors: *Carranza's clinical periodontology*, ed 9, Philadelphia, 2002, WB Saunders.
31. Raetzke PB: Covering localized areas of root exposure employing the "envelope" technique, *J Periodontol* 53:397, 1985.
32. Langer B, Calagna L: The subepithelial connective tissue graft, *Int J Periodontics Restorative Dent* 2:22-27, 1982.
33. Shanelec D, Tibbetts L: Periodontal microsurgery, *Curr Opin Periodontol* 3:118-125, 1996.
34. Holbrook T, Ochsenbein C: Coverage of the denuded root with one-stage gingival graft, *Int J Periodontics Restorative Dent* 3:9, 1983.
35. Grupe HE, Warren RF: Repair of gingival defects by sliding flap operation, *J Periodontol* 27:92, 1956.
36. Zabalegui I, Sicua A, Cambra J, et al: Treatment of multiple adjacent gingival recessions with the tunnel subepithelial connective tissue graft. A clinical report, *Int J Periodontics Restorative Dent* 19:199, 1995.
37. Tarnow DP: Semilunar coronally repositioned flap, *J Clin Periodontol* 13:182, 1986.
38. Cohen DW, Ross SE: The double papilla reposition flap in periodontal therapy, *J Periodontol* 39:743, 1968.
39. Oliver RC, Loe H, Karring T: Microscopic evaluation of the healing and revascularization of free gingival grafts, *J Periodontol* 39:84, 1968.
40. Corn H: Periosteal separation—its clinical significance, *J Periodontol* 33:140, 1962.
41. Bowers GM, Schallhorn RG, Mellonig JT: Histological evaluation of new attachment apparatus formation in humans—Part I, *J Periodontol* 60:644, 1989.
42. Bowers GM, Schallhorn RG, Mellonig JT: Histological evaluation of new attachment apparatus formation in humans—Part III, *J Periodontol* 60:683, 1989.
43. Cogen RB, Al-Joburi W, Gantt DG, Denys FR: The effects of various root surface treatments on the attachment

and growth of human gingival fibroblasts: histologic and scanning electron microscopic evaluation, *J Clin Periodontol* 11:531, 1984.

44. Bogle G, Adams D, Crigger M, et al.: New attachment after surgical treatment and citric acid conditioning of roots in naturally occurring periodontal disease in dogs, *J Periodontol Res* 16:130, 1981.

45. Caton J, Nyman S, Zander H: Histometric evaluation of periodontal surgery. II Connective tissue attachment levels after four regenerative procedures, *J Clin Periodontol* 7:224, 1980.

46. Frank RM: Cementogenesis and soft tissue attachment after citric acid treatment in a human, *J Periodontol* 54:389, 1983.

47. Hatfield GC, Bauhammers A: Cytotoxic effects of periodontally involved surfaces of human teeth, *Arch Oral Biol* 16:495, 1971.

48. Liu W, Solt CW: A surgical procedure for the treatment of localized gingival recession in conjunction with root surface citric acid conditioning, *J Periodontol* 51:505, 1980.

49. Polson AM, Frederick GT, Ladenheim S, Hanes PJ: The production of a root surface smear layer by instrumentation and its removal with citric acid, *J Periodontol* 55:443, 1984.

50. Daly CG: Antibacterial effects of citric acid treatment on periodontally diseased root surfaces, *J Clin Periodontol* 9:386, 1982.

51. Mariotti A: Efficacy of chemical root surface modifiers in the treatment of periodontal diseases. A systematic review, *Ann Periodontol* 8:205, 2003.

52. Terranova VP: A biological approach to periodontal regeneration: tetracycline treatment of dentin promotes fibroblast adhesion and growth, *J Periodont Res* 21:330, 1986.

53. Windisch P, Sculean A, Klein F, et al: Comparison of clinical, radiographic, and histometric measurements following treatment with guided tissue regeneration or enamel matrix proteins in human periodontal defects, *J Periodontol* 73:409, 2002.

54. Shanelec D, Tibbetts L: An overview of periodontal microsurgery, *Curr Sci* 2:187, 1994.

23 Resective Periodontal Surgery

Leonard S. Tibbetts and William F. Ammons, Jr.

Gingivitis and periodontitis, as well as certain drugs and systemic conditions, can produce a variety of changes in the clinical appearance, dimension, structure, and function of the gingiva and periodontium. The extent of these changes may range from the usual signs of inflammation, including varying degrees of gingival enlargement, the development of pseudopockets, significant loss of periodontal attachment, and the formation of true periodontal pockets of various depths and configurations (see Chapter 11). As the extent and location of involvement varies, all treatment methods are not applicable to individual periodontal defects, and treatment objectives may vary significantly from one patient to another. The result has been the development of a variety of periodontal treatment regimens.

When periodontal disease is addressed early in its course, the elimination of the etiologic agents and resolution of inflammation through nonsurgical means may be sufficient to resolve and arrest periodontal breakdown. However, if problems persist after the completion of initial nonsurgical therapy, surgical treatment provides a means of altering the oral anatomic environment and enhancing the patient's ability to maintain a sustained, effective daily oral hygiene maintenance program.

In clinical practice, maintenance of a dentition with numerous deep periodontal pockets is difficult when compared with maintenance of a dentition with shallow sulci. Maintenance of deep periodontal pockets requires a highly skilled clinician and a patient willing to attend frequent appointments of longer duration than would be necessary for treatment of shallow sulci. Periodontal resective surgery, which includes both soft tissue procedures and combined soft/hard tissue procedures, was developed and refined to eliminate pockets and to reestablish an architectural form about the teeth that would enable patients, with the periodic help of their dental professionals, to maintain their teeth in an efficient, effective, and economic manner.

The optimal goal of periodontal treatment is the regeneration of the soft and hard tissues lost to inflammatory periodontal diseases.[1] Although bone regeneration is a possibility in specific defects (see Chapter 25), it is not a predictable outcome for all periodontal defects. Therefore, resective therapy remains a major practical component of the treatment of periodontal diseases and the maintenance of functional dentitions. Resective surgical procedures are tools that are necessary for the well trained periodontal therapist to be able to render efficacious, effective treatment of periodontitis with predictable long-term success. These techniques are also required for many procedures that enhance restorative and esthetic treatment in patients without periodontal destruction.

INDICATIONS FOR RESECTIVE PERIODONTAL SURGERY

The indications for resective surgery are: (1) to gain access to an underlying structure; (2) to gain access to achieve more effective removal of calculus and the associated subgingival microbiota; (3) to reduce or to eliminate persistent diseased sites, which often include bony defects resulting from both horizontal and vertical bone loss that are not consistent with the overlying gingival architecture; and (4) to alter the form or dimension of components of the periodontium to enhance and facilitate cosmetic, restorative, and prosthetic procedures.

CONTRAINDICATIONS FOR RESECTIVE PERIODONTAL SURGERY

There are several significant contraindications for resective surgical therapy including the following: (1) ineffective plaque control by the patient; (2) noncompliance with a suggested and accepted treatment plan; (3) shallow probing depths; (4) soft or hard tissue defects amenable to repair or regeneration; (5) severely advanced disease; (6) an anticipated unacceptable cosmetic consequence; and (7) uncontrolled systemic disease. **The clinician must have an accurate diagnosis and a realistic therapeutic end-point formulated for each case, on the basis of the anatomic and clinical information provided in this textbook, before initiating resective surgical therapy. Unrealistic or poorly conceived end-points may result in failure of therapy.**

EXAMINATION AND TREATMENT PLANNING FOR RESECTIVE SURGERY

The potential need for a resective surgical procedure is usually recognized during the performance of a comprehensive periodontal examination (see Chapter 8). Careful probing divulges (1) both normal and abnormal sulcus depths, (2) the presence of furcation involvements, (3) the gingival width, (4) the location of the base of the pocket in relation to the mucogingival junction (the amount of attached versus free gingiva), (5) the anatomy of bony defects (the number of bony walls present), and (6) the location of the base of the pocket to the attachment level on adjacent teeth.[2] Confirmation of the extent and configuration of the suspected bony defects and furcation involvements obtained by normal probing can be achieved by transgingival bone sounding performed under local anesthetic (Fig. 23-1). This clinical information, combined with a complete radiographic survey and a thorough medical and dental history, supports an accurate diagnosis.[3] The results of the diagnosis will assist in establishing the specific treatment needs of the patient.

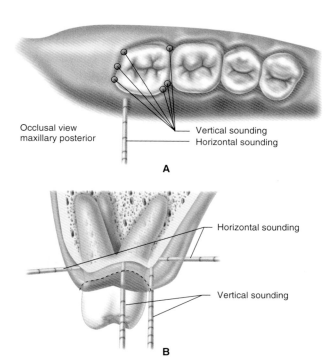

Occlusal view
maxillary posterior

Vertical sounding
Horizontal sounding

A

Horizontal sounding

Vertical sounding

B

Figure 23-1. Transgingival sounding through the soft tissue, using local anesthetic, to delineate the thickness of the soft tissue, the extent and configuration of the alveolar bone, and existing periodontal defects by use of the probe in both a horizontal and vertical manner.

Radiographs of good diagnostic quality are critical to the determination of a need for resective procedures,[3] because they furnish pertinent information regarding root morphology, root trunk length, the presence of angular bone loss, dental decay, pattern and extent of bone loss, and presence of other pathoses that may require attention (see Chapter 9). However, radiographs are not always diagnostically accurate for periodontal disease or for diagnosing the extent of bony defects present on the buccal/facial or palatal/lingual surfaces of either arch. Radiographs cannot show the differentiation between previously treated periodontal diseases and untreated diseases as they serve to help visualize interdental bone levels, but they can act as a means of evidence in evaluating the longitudinal success and stability of hard tissue therapy.

The patient's psychological and physiologic responses to the completion of initial therapy, including oral hygiene instructions, scaling and root planing, occlusal adjustments, and other disease control procedures, are documented and evaluated by reexamining the patient to determine the changes that have occurred. The response to initial therapy can vary significantly, not just from patient to patient, but from one area of the mouth to another. In areas of active inflammation, the soft tissue changes can result in a decrease in swelling and edema and a return to normal sulcus depths and tissue configurations requiring no additional treatment other than periodic maintenance care. This is not as likely to occur in the presence of chronic inflammatory disease. During such conditions, the inflammation may be reduced, but deep periodontal pockets with localized bleeding and suppuration may persist in moderate to advanced periodontitis. Such signs and symptoms are indicative of patient inability to reach these areas and to maintain a satisfactory level of oral hygiene, even with good oral hygiene compliance. Patients with good supragingival plaque control who have residual probing depths of 5 mm or more may be candidates for resective periodontal surgery. Conversely, patients with poor oral hygiene compliance should not be considered good candidates for successful long-term results with resective periodontal surgery, because one of the major causative etiologic factors has not been successfully modified.

TYPES OF RESECTIVE PERIODONTAL SURGERY FOR POCKET REDUCTION

A variety of resective surgical procedures and techniques have been developed to manage the pockets that result from inflammatory periodontal disease. These procedures are listed in Box 23-1 and have been divided into procedures that are applied primarily to the soft tissues and those which involve the resection of both soft tissues and bone. Their application and results are discussed in the following sections.

Box 23-1   Types of Resective Procedures

Soft Tissue Resective Surgery
- Gingivectomy
  - Standard external bevel gingivectomy
  - Internal bevel gingivectomy
- Ledge and wedge technique procedures
- Electrosurgery, laser surgery, chemical gingivectomy
- Open flap curettage (Modified Widman Procedure)

Combined Soft/Hard Tissue Resective Surgery
- Flap access and osseous resection
  - Osteoplasty
  - Ostectomy
- Flap access and osseous resection combined with regenerative therapy

SOFT TISSUE RESECTIVE SURGERY

Indications/Contraindications for Gingivectomy

Gingivectomy and gingivoplasty are terms used to describe the surgical excision of the gingiva performed to treat the pathologic effects of gingivitis, periodontitis, and other conditions that result in alterations in normal gingival form.[4,5] Gingivectomy is generally considered to be the oldest surgical procedure developed to treat the effects of periodontal diseases.[6] By definition, the term *gingivectomy* implies that this procedure is limited to being performed within the confines of the gingiva. The objective of gingivectomy is the elimination of soft tissue periodontal pockets,[7] thereby facilitating the patient's ability to maintain periodontal health.[5] Although gingivectomy was once a commonly performed surgical procedure, it has currently been largely supplanted by a variety of other surgical procedures. Gingivectomy may still be indicated in selected cases.

Gingivoplasty is a term initiated by Goldman.[8] It refers to the plastic reshaping of the gingiva to produce a surface form and topography that simulates those features believed to be characteristic of gingival health. This form has been termed a *physiologic form*, which implies not only a particular shape and structure, but a relation to the function of these tissues. The characteristics of a physiologic form are a free gingival margin with a thin, knife edge–like form that is well adapted to the tooth and tucked under the height of contour of the crown. The interdental papilla should also be thin and well adapted to blend into the interdental groove. A patient displaying the characteristics of a physiologic form is shown in Figure 23-2. Although gingivectomy and gingivoplasty can be performed as separate surgical procedures,[9] most commonly they are performed simultaneously,[8] and subsequent to the completion of nonsurgical procedures designed to resolve the inflammatory signs of active breakdown. The resolution of inflammation that results from oral hygiene procedures and scaling and root planing not only facilitates the performance of gingivectomy/ gingivoplasty and other surgical procedures,[10] it may minimize or even eliminate the need for the surgical intervention.[7]

As the gingivectomy/gingivoplasty procedure is performed within the gingiva, it is therefore limited to areas where (a) bony resorption has resulted in pockets of a generally uniform horizontal form, (b) the apical base of the pockets are located coronal to the mucogingival junction, and (c) sufficient gingiva is present to allow the procedure to be performed without the production of a non-keratinized mucosal margin.

Indications for gingivectomy/gingivoplasty

Gingivectomy/gingivoplasty can be used effectively in the following ways:

1. To eliminate gingival pockets (suprabony pockets), which persist after completion of oral hygiene instruction, scaling and root planing, and other disease control measures
2. To eliminate soft tissue craters resulting from disease or subsequent to other surgical procedures
3. To create an esthetic gingival form in cases of delayed passive eruption
4. To reduce gingival enlargements resulting from medications or genetic factors
5. To create clinical crown length for restorative or endodontic purposes when ostectomy is not required

A typical patient with gingival enlargement, in whom a gingivectomy could be used, is shown in Figure 23-3.

Contraindications to the performance of gingivectomy

1. Acutely inflamed gingiva
2. Inadequate oral hygiene by the patient
3. Pocket depth that is apical to the mucogingival junction; inadequate keratinized gingiva

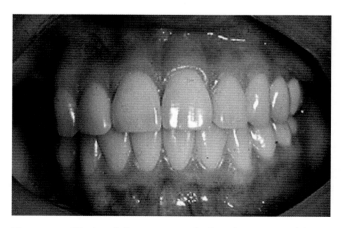

Figure 23-2. Display of characteristics of "physiologic" gingival form.

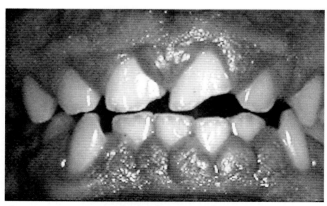

Figure 23-3. Gingival enlargement with pseudopockets, which is appropriate for treatment with gingivectomy/gingivoplasty.

4. Presence of interdental osseous craters and infrabony defects
5. Presence of large osseous ledges and exostoses
6. Inadequate depth of the vestibule
7. An increased caries rate that jeopardizes maintenance of the dentition
8. When removal of the soft tissue would constitute an unacceptable cosmetic compromise

External Bevel Gingivectomy

The performance of gingivectomy/gingivoplasty involves a number of sequential steps. These include the following: (1) anesthesia, which may include either enteral or parenteral conscious sedation, as well as the administration of local anesthetic agents; (2) surgical instrumentation; (3) application of surgical dressings; and (4) postoperative care during the healing period.

Anesthesia

The majority of gingivectomy procedures are performed using nerve block and infiltration of local anesthetic agents. In addition to nerve blocks, many clinicians will routinely infiltrate each interdental papillary area, both buccally and lingually, using a local anesthetic with a vasoconstrictive agent. These infiltrations serve to provide extra turgor to the tissues, facilitating incisions; to produce a transient local ischemia; and to reduce bleeding during the excision of the gingiva. Local anesthesia may be combined with the use of other anesthetic agents such as oral sedatives, nitrous oxide analgesia, or intravenous conscious sedation (see Chapters 19 and 20).

Surgical Instrumentation: External Bevel Gingivectomy

A typical instrument tray for the performance of gingivectomy/gingivoplasty would contain the instruments listed in Box 23-2.

Once adequate local anesthesia has been obtained, the thorough and efficient performance of the gingivectomy procedure requires the precise identification of the depth (base) of the pockets on all surfaces of all teeth within the surgical field. The identification of the base of the pocket is usually accomplished by placement of a series of bleeding points that correspond to the apical extent of pocket. These bleeding points can be made by use of the periodontal probe (Fig. 23-4, A and B) or by use of a mechanical device such as the Crane-Kaplan or Goldman-Fox pocket marker. When a periodontal probe is used, the base of the pocket is measured and that depth is then transferred to the external surfaces of the gingiva. Perforating the gingiva with the periodontal probe then makes bleeding points perpendicular to the base of the pocket. Generally, three points are made per tooth (midradicular area and mesial/distal line angles) on each of the facial/buccal or lingual/palatal surfaces. These bleeding points

Box 23-2	**Gingivectomy/Gingivoplasty Instruments**

- Local anesthetic syringes, needles and anesthetic solution
- Goldman-Fox periodontal scissors
- Hemostat
- Fox gingivoplasty diamond burs
- Cotton surgical sponges
- Periodontal mirror
- Cotton pliers
- Periodontal probe
- Crane-Kaplan periodontal pocket markers
- Kirkland 17 broad bladed GV knife
- Orban sharp bladed GV knife
- Columbia 4R/4L or 2R/2L curettes
- Goldman-Fox tissue nippers
- Minnesota surgical retractor
- Surgical aspirator tip

serve to guide the surgeon during placement of the initial incisions.

After the establishment of the bleeding points, a coronally directed external bevel incision is made, using an appropriate surgical knife. The placement of these incisions to remove the soft tissue pockets is shown in Figure 23-5. The incision is generally begun distal to the first tooth in the surgical area and extended anteriorly, using the bleeding points as guides, to include the last tooth with pocket depth. The incision should begin at the mesial line angle of the tooth adjacent to the first pocket so as to cross the entire papilla and proceed smoothly to end at the mesial line angle of the tooth immediately adjacent to the terminal tooth to be treated. To accommodate an appropriate bevel, the incision on the external gingival surface must of necessity be placed apical to the base of the periodontal pockets, but coronal to the mucogingival junction, and then it must be angled coronally to strike the teeth at the base of the periodontal pocket. Therefore, the incision is begun slightly apical to the "dotted line" created by the bleeding points. The gingivectomy incision should never be started apical to the mucogingival junction, because the incision will eliminate the entire zone of gingiva, as well as the periodontal pockets, and will result in a postsurgical margin consisting entirely of alveolar mucosa.[11,12]

An external bevel incision of about 45 degrees is considered optimal. However, the angulation of the bevel that can be placed is influenced by the (a) width of the band of gingiva, (b) the thickness of the gingiva, (c) the position of the base of the pocket in relation to the crest of the adjacent alveolar bone, (d) the thickness of the crest of the alveolar bone, and (e) the relation of the mucogingival junction to the external bony crest (Fig. 23-6, A and B).

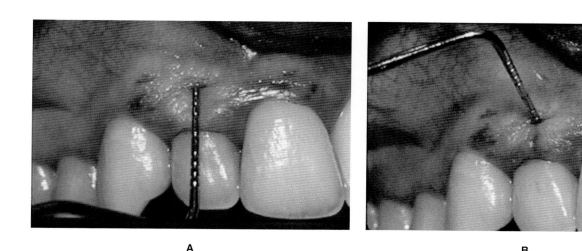

Figure 23-4. Use of periodontal probe to mark pocket depth. **A,** After probing to the base within the pocket, the probe is removed from the pocket and the probing depth is transferred to the external gingival surface. **B,** Puncture marks are made in the external surface of the gingiva corresponding to the position of the pocket base. A specialized instrument such as the Crane-Kaplan or Goldman-Fox pocket marker can also be used. (*From Schluger S, Yuodelis R, Page RC, Johnson RH:* Periodontal diseases, *ed 2, Philadelphia, 1990, Lea & Febiger. Courtesy Dr. Robert Lamb, San Mateo, Calif.*)

The width and characteristics of the gingival band may vary significantly from one tooth to another in the surgical field.[13,14] The greater the thickness of the alveolar process and gingiva the more difficult it is to establish a long beveled incision apical to the bleeding points.

The primary incision is usually made with a broad bladed or round bladed gingivectomy knife such as the Buck #3/4, Goldman-Fox #7/8, or Kirkland #15 K/16 K (Fig. 23-5, *A* and *B*). The rounded contour of the broad bladed gingivectomy knife allows the blade to incise smoothly through the tissue without being arrested by irregularities in the bone or tooth surfaces. The contra-angle design of the typical gingivectomy knifes makes them particularly suitable for this purpose. The only negative factors associated with their use are the need to re-sharpen and re-sterilize the knives after each use. A number of disposable, sterile surgical blades, such as the Bard Parker 15 or 10A, designed to fit a surgical handle are also available and can be used during the performance of gingivectomy.

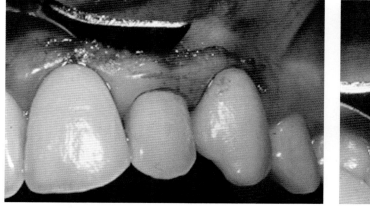
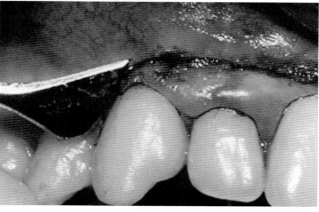

Figure 23-5. Incisions to eliminate pocket depths. **A,** Using a broad-bladed periodontal knife such as a Kirkland 17 gingivectomy knife, the incision is begun at the distal of the surgical area. **B,** The incision is continued to the distal of the most terminal contralateral tooth in the surgical area.

Continued

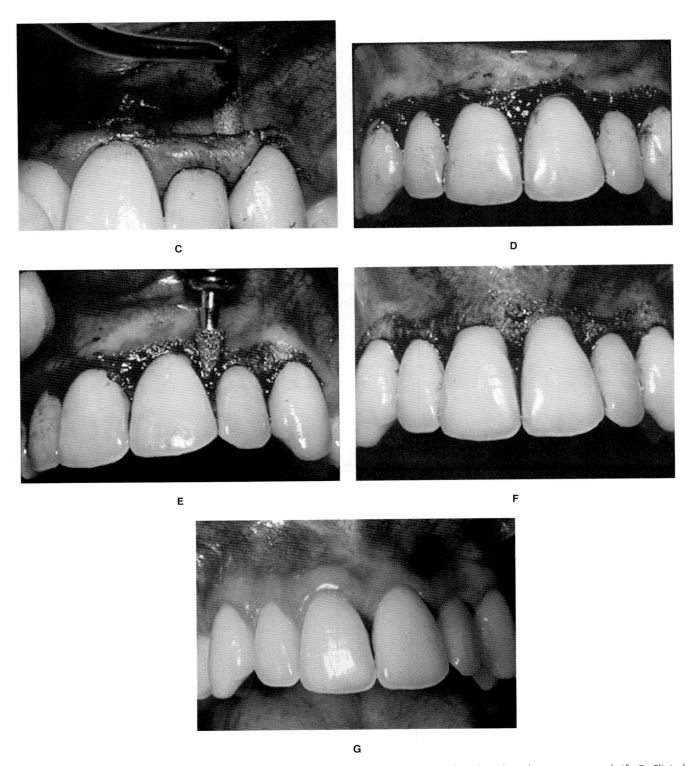

C

D

E

F

G

Figure 23-5. cont'd C, The interproximal areas are severed with a sharp-pointed periodontal knife such as the Orban gingivectomy knife. **D,** Clinical view of facial tissues after removal of the soft tissue pocket depth. Any tissue tags may be removed with sharp curettes, a gingivectomy knife, scissors, or an instrument such as Goldman-Fox tissue nippers. **E,** Use of a tapered Fox diamond bur to perform gingivoplasty. **F,** Facial soft tissue contours after completion of gingivoplasty. **G,** Post-surgical healed appearance of gingival tissues following gingivectomy and gingivoplasty. Observe the physiologic contours. (*From Schluger S, Yuodelis R, Page RC, Johnson RH:* Periodontal diseases, *ed 2, Philadelphia, 1990, Lea & Febiger. Courtesy of Dr. Robert Lamb of San Mateo, Calif.*)

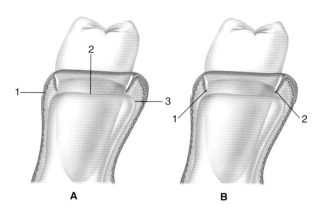

Figure 23-6. Factors affecting the angle of incision. **A,** (1) The width of the band of gingiva; (2) the depth and configuration of the pocket; (3) the presence of ledges of bone. **B,** (1) A 45-degree beveled incision to the base of the pocket is ideal. However, in an area with little gingiva, this incision may result in the total elimination of gingival tissue, resulting in a mucosal margin. (2) The presence of a bony ledge may prevent placement of an incision to base of the soft tissue pocket.

After completion of the primary incisions on the facial/buccal and palatal/lingual surfaces, the interdental incisions are made with a tapered, narrowed bladed knife such as Goldman-Fox #8 or #11 DE, Towner #19/20, Orban 1/2, or Buck 5/6 (Fig. 23-5, *C*). These narrow knives are commonly triangular or spear-shaped, and the shank is offset to allow them to be directed into the interproximal area. These knives are used to sever the interproximal portion of the soft tissue pockets with the same interproximal slope (angle) that was used in the primary incision. When properly performed, the primary facial and secondary interproximal incisions completely release that portion of the gingiva comprising the soft tissue pocket. This allows the excised tissue to be dislodged and removed from around the teeth. Appropriate instruments for removal of the soft tissue include the PR 1-2 Prichard curette, a mosquito hemostat, K-29 chisel, a periosteal elevator, or other types of universal curettes (Columbia 2R/2L; 4R/4L; 13/14). Sharp, decisive initial and secondary incisions not only provide a surface that is smooth and free of tags, but they make removal of the tissue faster and easier.

After removal of the excised tissues, the surgical site is carefully inspected for any residual debris and probed to ensure that residual pocket depth does not remain. Tissue tags can be removed with sharp curettes, tissue nippers, or surgical scissors. The exposed root surfaces are examined and instrumented to insure removal of all calculus. After debridement, the margins of the gingiva and the adjacent mucosa may be refined by gingivoplasty, if needed.

Gingivoplasty

The purpose of gingivoplasty is to reshape the remaining gingiva to a so-called physiologic form. Gingivoplasty can be performed using a number of different instruments. Appropriately shaped coarse diamond stones may be used[15] (Fig. 23-5, *E*). These stones, designed for use in high speed and conventional speed dental handpieces, must be used with copious irrigation and high volume aspiration during abrasion of the wound surface to prevent the generation of heat. An additional problem of rotary abrasion for gingivoplasty is the production of a significant amount of aerosol contaminated by the patients' blood and tissue fragments. Other instruments used for gingivoplasty include tissue nipper and surgical scissors. The edge of the round-bladed gingivectomy knife may also be used in a scraping motion along the tissue surface and margins.

Ledge and Wedge and Internal Bevel Gingivectomy Techniques

In 1965, Ochsenbein[16] proposed the use of the ledge and wedge gingivectomy technique as a means of eliminating the guesswork involved with placement of the primary incisions, thereby ensuring pocket elimination. This technique is generally believed to require less experience and clinical sophistication and yet affords a means of eliminating the pocket and producing an acceptable postoperative form.[17]

Two variations of the ledge and wedge technique can be used (Figs. 23-7 and 23-8). The first technique being with a primary incision that is placed perpendicular (90 degrees) to the tissue surface to connect the bleeding points that were initially created by marking the pocket depth (Fig. 23-7, *B*). The incision can be made with a broad-bladed gingivectomy knife or a disposable blade such as a Bard Parker 10A or 15 beginning at the distobuccal and distolingual surfaces of the most distally involved tooth. The incisions should contact the tooth surfaces and extend interproximally as far as the teeth permit. The purpose of these incisions is to eliminate that portion of the gingiva that encompasses the periodontal pockets. The result is elimination of the soft tissue pockets, but with the production of a horizontal soft tissue ledge.

The secondary incisions are coronally directed (Fig. 23-7, *C*) and produce an **external** bevel, the length of which is dependent on the thickness of the remaining gingiva and the width of the buccal and lingual radicular bone. The objective of the secondary incisions is the creation of an appropriate external gingival contour, a so-called physiologic form. The same principles and instruments as previously mentioned should be used in excising and removing the tissue, in the removal of any tissue tags, and in refining the external

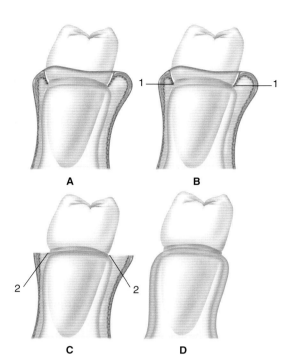

Figure 23-7. Ledge and wedge gingivectomy technique 1. **A,** Preoperative diagram showing gingival enlargement. **B,** The initial facial and lingual incisions (1) are made perpendicular to the gingiva to strike the base of the soft tissue pockets. **C,** Secondary incisions (2) are made on the facial and lingual at a 45-degree *external* bevel to remove the remaining soft tissue ledges. **D,** Postoperative result.

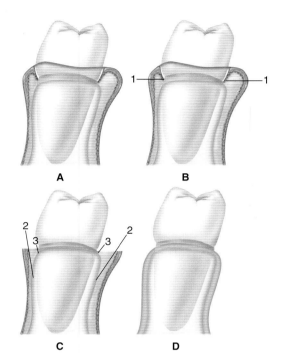

Figure 23-8. Ledge and wedge gingivectomy technique 2. **A,** Preoperative diagram showing gingival enlargement. **B,** The initial facial and lingual incisions (1) are made perpendicular to the gingiva to strike the base of the soft tissue pockets. **C,** The secondary *internal* bevel incisions (2) are made parallel to the external gingival surface, retaining a connective tissue base sufficient to retain the blood supply, to thin the tissue mass. The gingiva is scored with the third incision (3) at the bony crest to allow the removal of the connective tissue wedge. The soft tissue flap is then sutured to cover the bone. **D,** Postoperative result.

contours of the tissues to obtain a result as shown in Figure 23-7, *D*.

In the second ledge and wedge technique, the primary incisions are performed in a similar manner, directed perpendicular to the external gingival surface at the level of the pocket base (Fig. 23-8, *B*). The secondary incision, however, is directed parallel to the external tissue surface to form an **inverse** bevel (also called an internal bevel) incision (Fig. 23-8, *C*). This internal bevel gingivectomy technique is particularly useful in cases of gingival enlargement, where thick tissues are present. The internal bevel gingivectomy technique does not leave a large external bevel and therefore is associated with less postoperative pain and bleeding. This technique also allows the reflection of a conventional flap, if access is required to the underlying bone.

In clinical situations in which gingival enlargement has resulted in pocket formation (both pseudopockets and true pockets) and also in an increased mass of the gingiva apically to the base of the pockets, use of an external bevel incision would result in an extensive wound.[18] In such conditions, an external bevel incision of sufficient length not only to eliminate the periodontal pockets but to reduce the tissue bulk as well would result in an extensive wound (Fig. 23-9, *A* and *B*).

The internal bevel gingivectomy may begin with either a ledge incision (Fig. 23-8, *B*) or with a scalloped internal bevel incision placed several millimeters apical to the gingival margin and following a scalloped contour associated with a normal gingival margin. Either technique results in the production of a mucoperiosteal flap, which can then be positioned and sutured to cover the alveolar bone (Fig. 23-9, *C* through *E*). The internal bevel gingivectomy procedure is not a true gingivectomy, because it is not confined to the gingiva. It is more appropriately described as a partial-thickness flap procedure (see Chapter 20).

Electrosurgery, Lasers, and Chemical Gingivectomy

In the past there has been considerable interest in other modes of instrumentation for gingivectomy. These have included the use of electrosurgery,[19] various chemical agents,[20] and more recently the use of lasers.[21,22]

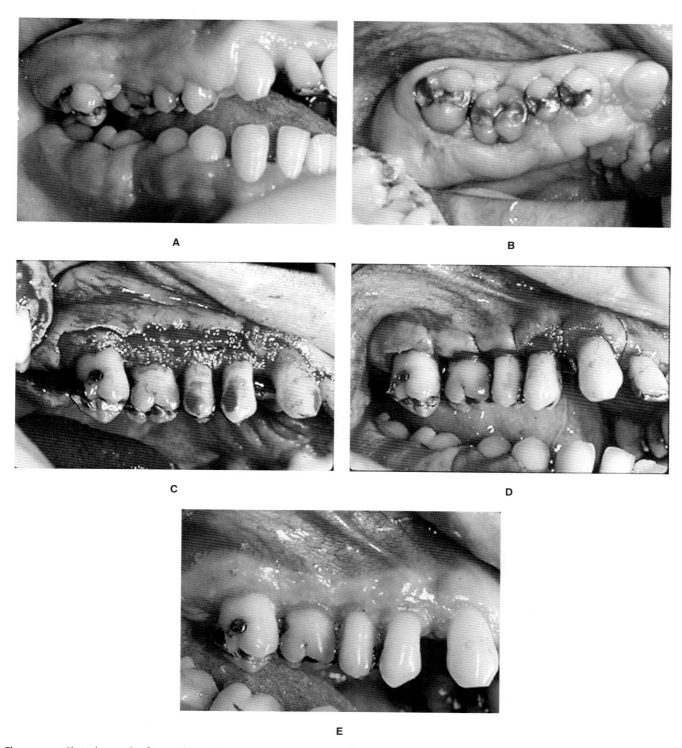

A

B

C

D

E

Figure 23-9. Clinical example of internal bevel gingivectomy. **A,** Preoperative facial gingival contours demonstrating gingival enlargement. **B,** Occlusal view demonstrating gingival enlargement. External bevel gingivectomy would result in a large wound. **C,** Following incisions to reduce and remove the large bulk of excess tissue, a flap may be elevated. **D,** Continuous sling sutures used to close the flap. No significant external wound is present. **E,** Facial view 8 weeks after surgery. Note the dramatic reduction in tissue mass. (*Courtesy Dr. Stanley Sapkos, Seattle, Wash.*)

With electrosurgery a high frequency electric current (fully rectified) is used to cut and coagulate soft tissue. Electrodes, which are available in a number of shapes, are applied in a brushing motion to remove incremental portions of the soft tissue lesion. Its use was promoted because of an ability to cauterize and to sterilize as soft tissue was removed, which resulted in an essentially bloodless field. In addition, the design of the electrodes allows their use in areas where the application of conventional gingivectomy knives is difficult or impossible. Disadvantages of electrosurgery include possible heat damage, increased time required for instrumentation compared with conventional surgery, and unpleasant odor created during cutting. Also, electrosurgery cannot be used in patients with noncompatible or poorly shielded cardiac pacemakers. Although proponents of electrosurgical gingivectomy may disagree,[23,24] the prevailing evidence is that electrosurgical gingivectomy may result in delayed wound healing,[25] loss of periodontal support,[26,27] and cemental burns if the electrodes contact alveolar bone or the tooth root.[25,28] Therefore, electrosurgery is best limited to superficial soft tissue procedures where the potential adverse effects of contacting bone or tooth root can be avoided.

Chemical agents such as potassium hydroxide and paraformaldehyde have also been advocated as a means of removing soft tissue periodontal pockets.[20] So-called chemical gingivectomy, however, is not currently recommended. The depth and form of the action of chemical agents on the gingival tissues is difficult to control; therefore, reshaping of the tissues cannot be accurately accomplished and healthy tissues may be adversely affected. In addition, some studies suggest that wound healing may be retarded with chemical gingivectomy.[29]

A number of types of dental lasers have been suggested for use during periodontal therapy including gingivectomy/gingivoplasty. Most reports in the dental literature have addressed the use of CO_2,[28,30-32] Nd:Yag,[32] and diode[33] lasers. These lasers have different characteristics, which are related to their wavelengths, power, and design. Although these instruments have been applied to both soft and hard tissues, and a substantial number of research publications have been presented, current evaluation suggests that they have some of the same general limitations as electrosurgery.[34] With proper shielding of the root surfaces to prevent damage, they can be used for some cases of gingivectomy and gingivoplasty. However, they are less useful for most cases.[35]

Periodontal Dressings

The gingivectomy/gingivoplasty procedure can result in the creation of a substantial surgical wound that is devoid of epithelium and with connective tissues exposed. These wounds are not only a potential source of postoperative discomfort and bleeding, but they are subject to additional trauma. Therefore, patients treated by gingivectomy/gingivoplasty should be provided with the protection of a surgical dressing (Fig. 23-10, *A* and *B*). There are a number of commercial products available that may be applied to cover the wound surface.[36,37]

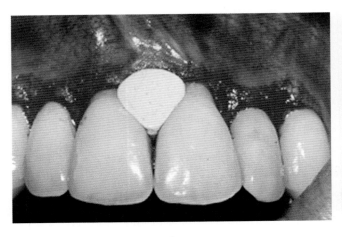
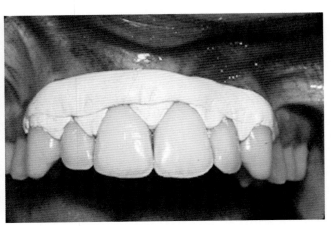

A   **B**

Figure 23-10. Application of periodontal dressing after the gingivectomy procedure. **A,** Wedges of dressing are placed interproximately on both the buccal and palatal surfaces. **B,** A roll of dressing is positioned over the interproximal wedges of dressing. The roll of dressing is then blended to cover the surgical site. (*From Schluger S, Yuodelis R, Page RC, Johnson RH: Periodontal diseases, ed 2, Philadelphia, 1990, Lea & Febiger. Courtesy Dr. Robert Lamb, San Mateo, Calif.*)

Early periodontal dressings, such as that developed by Ward in 1923, relied on an interaction between zinc oxide and eugenol to produce a cement-like material to protect the surgical wound[38,39] and for antibacterial effects.[40] Other materials such as tannic acid, zinc acetate, and asbestos fibers were also commonly added to such dressings to alter their properties. Surgical dressings containing these materials have generally been eliminated from use because of the potential for adverse effects.[41,42]

Periodontal dressings using metallic oxide and fatty acids have largely replaced the zinc oxide eugenol types of dressings. These dressings are packaged in two tubes. When equal lengths of each are mixed together, they interact and thicken to produce a material of rubbery-like consistency; Coe-Pak (GC America, Inc.; Alsip, IL) and Periocare (Pulpapent Corp.; Watertown, MA) are examples of such products. Other noneugenol packs have contained cyanoacrylates[43] and methacrylic gels. Clear, translucent light cured dressings, such as Barricaid VLC periodontal surgical dressing (Dentsply Caulk Co.; Milford, DE), are available and are preferred by some clinicians in esthetic regions of the mouth. Some authors have advocated the addition of antibiotics to surgical dressings, to improve comfort and reduce odor and bad taste that can result during healing.[44] However, such agents may produce hypersensitivity or promote resistant strains of microorganisms.

These dressings usually require replacement every 5 to 7 days for approximately 2 to 3 weeks. After this period, healing has usually progressed to the point that the surgical site may be left uncovered. During this period, patients should perform their normal oral hygiene procedures in areas of the mouth not involved in the surgical procedure. Oral hygiene procedures can be supplemented with oral saline rinses or with antibacterial mouthwashes such as 0.12% chlorhexidine digluconate.[45] After the dressing is removed, the surgical site can be cleansed with judicious use of a soft, multitufted toothbrush. The surgical site needs to be kept free of plaque and oral debris for an optimal surgical result.

Wound Healing After Gingivectomy

The response of the tissues during wound healing after gingivectomy have been well described at both the clinical and histologic levels.[46-48] When correctly performed, gingivectomy results in the surgical elimination of the pocket, but the patient is left with a surface wound that exposes periodontal ligament and gingival connective tissues that cover the adjacent alveolar bone. The wound surface is devoid of its epithelial covering.

The initial healing events after the procedure are directed toward establishing hemostasis and the production of a fibrin clot to cover the wound surface. This initial lag phase is followed by cellular proliferation of epithelium at the wound margins as demonstrated by increased DNA synthesis (12 to 24 hours)[47] and a proliferation of vascular tissues, which peaks at 3 to 4 days after surgery.[48] These events are necessary to replace the missing epithelium and to restore tissue continuity. After about 35 to 48 hours, the epithelial cells resulting from the cellular replication begin to migrate across the cut connective tissue surface under the fibrin clot to cover the wound. These cells migrate at a rate of approximately 0.5 mm per day until the wound surface is covered. Depending on the extent of the wound surface, it may take 1 to 2 weeks to complete surface epithelialization.[49] The source of these migrating epithelial cells is from the wound margin and the residual epithelial cells that were not totally eliminated by the external bevel incision. The epithelial growth proceeds until it contains the root surface and a new junctional epithelial attachment is established. The subsequent proliferation of connective tissues adjacent to the root results in the formation of a new gingival sulcus. By approximately 14 days the tissues assume a normal clinical form, although some hypervascularity (redness) may persist. Remodeling of the tissues, as evidenced by changes in form and color, may continue for a period of approximately 3 months.[50]

Oral Hygiene

An optimal therapeutic result is dependent not only on thorough diagnosis, careful case planning, and technical surgical excellence, but on appropriate postsurgical care by both the therapist and the patient.

The extent of discomfort after periodontal surgery varies widely from patient to patient and may limit postoperative oral hygiene efforts by the patient. Surgical dressings and oral medications may suffice to manage the patient's discomfort; however, other steps need to be taken to ensure optimal wound healing. Patients should continue their usual oral hygiene regimen in the areas of their mouth not affected by the surgery. This regimen should be supplemented with antibacterial rinses such as chlorhexidine. Surgical dressings should be changed at appropriate periods, usually every 5 to 7 days, as needed. Inadequate oral hygiene can lead to the formation of excessive granulation tissue that can compromise the surgical result. After a period of 2 weeks, most patients no longer require periodontal dressings and may reinstitute plaque control measures in the surgical site using ultrasoft dental brushes. Brushing should be supplemented by oral rinses to suppress bacterial plaque. The exposure of dentinal surfaces, in the presence of dental plaque formation, can result in dentinal hypersensitivity. This hypersensitivity, however, usually responds rapidly to effective plaque removal combined with topical applications of fluoride gels or fluoride rinses.

Therapeutic Result of Gingivectomy/ Gingivoplasty

There have been many reports of the use of gingivectomy, but few longitudinal studies that would meet the criteria of evidence-based research.[51] Surgical studies indicate that when the tissues are excised to the base of the pocket, the junctional epithelium is completely removed. Instrumentation usually results in an average of 0.5 mm severance of connective tissue during the root planing portion of gingivectomy. Root planing during a gingivectomy usually results in a down-growth of the new epithelium during sulcus formation. Surgery therefore results in a loss of attachment, but also tends to produce more shallow gingival sulci if the pretreatment pocket depths are greater than 3 mm.[52]

In a large group of patients who received gingivectomy and were managed for up to 7 years, gingival health and sulcus depth of up to 2 mm were restored, except when there was incomplete removal of plaque and calculus, inadequate curettage, overhanging restorations, food impaction, or poor physiotherapy by the patient.[11] Relapse was greatest in patients with poor oral hygiene. Donnenfeld and Glickman[46] show that periodontal pockets could be eliminated after gingivectomy without significant changes in the location of the base of the gingival sulcus, that is, without loss of attachment. However, there was a reduction in the width of the attached gingiva, as might be expected from this excisional procedure.

Although there are little published long-term data documenting the results of treatment using gingivectomy and gingivoplasty, clinical experience indicates that gingivectomy remains an acceptable surgical treatment for patients who meet the limited selection criteria. This procedure is used less often now than 20 years ago primarily because of the evolution of various flap techniques that allow access to underlying periodontal structures and the presence of less postoperative discomfort associated with these procedures when compared with gingivectomy. It should always be remembered that regardless of the adequacy of the surgical procedure, without good oral hygiene by the patient and routine maintenance, pocket reduction will not be achieved or maintained.

FLAP PROCEDURES

Once a significant amount of attachment is lost, or osseous deformities of complex morphology develop, gingivectomy/gingivoplasty is not a surgical treatment option, because its application would leave the patient with residual bony deformities and would present mucogingival problems by eliminating the buccal or lingual gingival tissues, or both. Patients with such problems become candidates for periodontal flap surgery. Flap surgery provides a means of gaining access to the alveolar ridge, the root structure of the teeth, and adjacent bony periodontal pockets for instrumentation. The access and visibility with flap surgery improves the efficiency and efficacy of debridement and allows the retention of a sufficient zone of gingiva for function. The reduction of the tissue mass through internal thinning and subsequent repositioning of the flap, combined with the subsequent resolution of inflammation, can result in a reduction in pocket depth.[53-55] An additional benefit to flap surgery is that proper closure does not result in extensive deepithelialized wound surfaces, therefore postsurgical discomfort is usually reduced.

Indications for Periodontal Flap Surgery

The use of flap surgery is indicated in the following situations:

1. When there is a need to gain access to any structure not clearly visible in the oral cavity, for example, subgingival caries, root resorption, impacted teeth, a root tip, cyst or other area of pathosis
2. To provide access for visibility and instrumentation of deep periodontal pockets, areas of furcation involvement, or other areas of complex anatomy not readily instrumented through the sulcus
3. To eliminate or reduce the depth of periodontal pockets in areas of minimal gingival width, where excision of the pocket would result in the formation of a mucosal margin
4. To provide access for grafting, ridge augmentation, guided tissue regeneration, and guided bone regeneration procedures

Flap Design and Elevation

The first step in a flap operation is incision and elevation of the flap. A properly designed flap will provide access and visibility to the operative site, allow debridement with a minimum of associated trauma, and preserve the blood supply so that rapid healing occurs. The design and placement of incisions allowing the reflection and elevation of surgical flaps is described in detail in Chapter 20.

Although a variety of flap designs may be used during periodontal flap surgery, most flap debridement procedures are performed using sulcular or submarginal inverse bevel scalloped incisions, to allow the reflection of a full-thickness mucoperiosteal flap. The incisions are begun sufficiently distal to the terminal tooth in the planned surgical field to provide access using an appropriate blade, such as the Bard-Parker (BD Medical [Becton, Dickinson, and Company]; Franklin Lakes, NJ) 15 or 15C. If pocket depth is associated with an enlarged tuberosity or retromolar pad, one of the specific techniques described later in this chapter may be used to reduce the tuberosity or retromolar pad area. When a terminal tooth is not involved, the incision is begun on a tooth adjacent to the area of concern, in an area of normal gingiva. On the buccal aspect, a sulcular or submarginal inverse bevel incision is directed from the gingival crest and angled toward the bony crest to strike the coronal aspect of the alveolar bone. The incision is directed anteriorly, following the scalloped, labial configuration of the teeth until the incision is terminated at the distal line angle of the tooth immediately anterior to the most anterior involved tooth in the surgical field. The periosteum overlying the bone must be incised cleanly to allow flap reflection. As the buccal flap can be readily repositioned, the majority of the buccal gingiva can be preserved. The buccal incision can also be placed largely in the sulcus without adversely affecting the postoperative pocket depth.[56] However, the placement of an incision in the sulcus may make it more difficult to cleanly elevate the flap. An example of the use of sulcular and submarginal incisions to allow access for debridement in a mandibular posterior sextant is seen in Figure 23-11, *A* through *F*.

The process of elevating a palatal flap is different from that of a buccal flap. Because of the structure of the palatal mucosa, it is not possible to apically position the palatal flap. The palatal flap, therefore, must be incised precisely so that any soft tissue pocket depth will be eliminated and the flap will cover the bony margin when it is sutured. When the palatal tissue is thick and the bulk of the flap is to be reduced, the flap, of necessity, will have to be thinned. Palatal flaps, therefore, are commonly partial-thickness dissections. A properly dissected flap should have a flaccid nature and should not have a thickened base that is resistant to flap coaptation. An example of flap surgery, requiring the elevation of a partial-thickness palatal flap to reduce pocket depth associated with advanced attachment loss, is shown in Figure 23-12, *A* through *E*.

Debridement and Scaling and Root Planing

After the flap is reflected and thinned, the tenacious tissue remaining around the necks of the teeth and on the alveolar process, including the pocket wall and any excess soft tissue, must be removed. Placing the scalpel blade into the sulcus and extending it to bone at the most anterior aspect of the flap, the blade is extended distally around the necks of the teeth in contact with the bone to cleanly incise this tissue at its base. An Ochsenbein #2 or a K-29 chisel is then placed into the sulcus between the retained but loosened tissue and the most anteriorly involved tooth. By maintaining contact between the end of the chisel and the bone and using a slight twisting action on the chisel, the retained tissue can be further loosened, elevated, and reflected. As the tissue is reflected off of the underlying bone, a 5-inch curved hemostat is

used to grasp the tissue and assist in its removal. Once the collar of tissue has been removed, the roots of the teeth are curetted to remove any calculus or debris. A variety of techniques may then be used to treat the bony defects, including various resective and regenerative approaches. The debrided surgical site is then thoroughly rinsed, and the flaps are reapproximated and sutured in place using appropriate interrupted or continuous sutures (see Chapter 20).

Modified Widman Flap Procedure

In 1974, Ramfjord and Nissle introduced a variation on the flap operation that they termed *the modified Widman Flap*.[56] They reported that variations of the Widman flap procedure had been used for more than 30 years and described the currently used modification of the procedure. This modified Widman Flap procedure was incorporated into a longitudinal surgical study comparing the results of a number of treatment procedures on attachment level and pocket depth,[57,58] and results using the procedure have subsequently been reported.[59-62]

Features of the modified Widman Flap were (a) an intracrevicular or marginal buccal incision, (b) exaggerated palatal scallops to ensure interproximal flap adaptation, (c) minimal flap reflection, (d) retention of any residual connective tissue attachment coronal to the bone,[63,64] and (e) close interproximal flap adaptation to maximize healing.

The objective of the modified Widman Flap was not eradication of pocket walls, but rather to obtain a "maximum healing in areas of previous periodontal pockets with minimum loss of periodontal tissues during and after the surgery."[56] The advantages of the procedure were stipulated to be an intimate postoperative adaptation of healthy collagenous tissues to all tooth surfaces, reattachment with formation of new cementum from the apical aspects of the lesion, optimal coverage of root surfaces, conservation of bone, and greater potential for bone regeneration.[56]

A significant number of studies using this procedure have been published and the results have been analyzed. When appropriately performed, the long-term results obtained appear to be similar to that obtained with other surgical debridement procedures[54,55] in that there is a gain in clinical attachment level and a reduction in probing depth that appears to be maintained long-term when combined with professional maintenance.[58,61,62,65,66] Wound healing studies indicate that the procedure results in the production of a long junctional epithelial attachment that is located at or near the point of root instrumentation, and that if bone fill occurs on the walls of vertical defects, it is generally not accompanied by new attachment.[59,60]

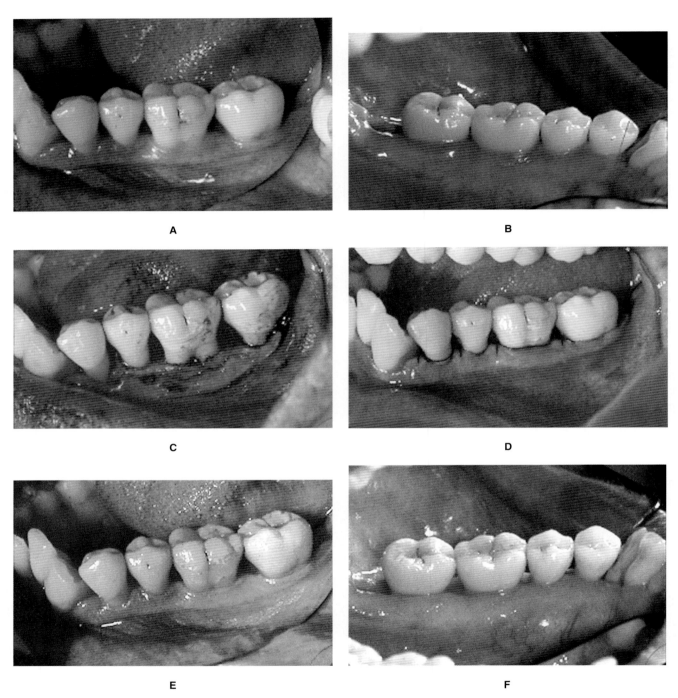

Figure 23-11. Use of sulcular and crestal incisions for flap reflection and debridement. **A,** Buccal preoperative view. Note the minimal band of gingiva on the buccal of the second molar. Sulcular incisions will allow the flap to be reflected, while preserving the band of gingiva. **B,** Lingual preoperative view. The band of gingiva is wide on this surface and the soft tissue is more coronally positioned. Submarginal inverse bevel incisions will be used to elevate the flap. **C,** Buccal view after flap reflection. Note the Class II bifurcation defect on the mandibular first molar. Flap reflection and debridement provides access for root instrumentation and treatment of the interdental bony defects (in this case, through osseous resection). **D,** The flaps are closed with continuous sling sutures. **E,** Three-week buccal postsurgical view, noting the residual soft tissue cratering after surgery. These soft tissue deformities will resolve in subsequent weeks as the interdental tissues reform. **F,** Three-week lingual postsurgical view. (*From Schluger S, Yuodelis R, Page RC, Johnson RH:* Periodontal diseases, *ed 2, Philadelphia, 1990, Lea & Febiger. Courtesy Dr. Dennis H. Smith and Dr. W.F. Ammons, Seattle, Wash.*)

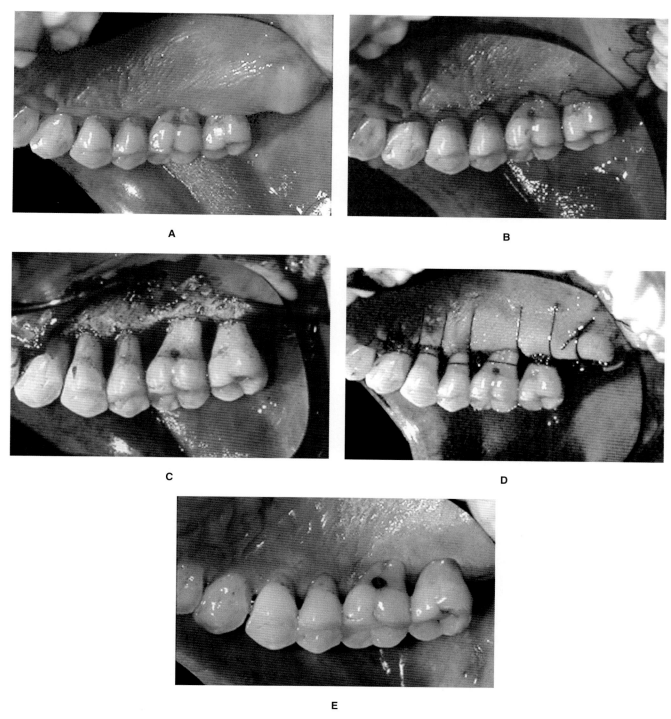

Figure 23-12. Use of a partial thickness palatal flap during flap debridement. **A,** Palatal preoperative view. Note the marginal tissue position in the presence of advanced attachment loss and pocket depth. **B,** Outline of palatal incisions, with partial thickness flap dissection used to allow thinning of the palatal flap and to allow a more apical postsurgical position of the soft tissue margin. **C,** Osseous defects from the palatal view after debridement. The flap operation provides access for multiple treatment options directed at managing the bony defects. **D,** Palatal flap closed with continuous mattress sling sutures. Note the more apical position of the palatal flap margin when compared with the preoperative view. **E,** Palatal 8-year postoperative view. (*From Schluger S, Yuodelis R, Page RC, Johnson RH:* Periodontal diseases, *ed 2, Philadelphia, 1990, Lea & Febiger. Courtesy Dr. Dennis H. Smith and Dr. W.F. Ammons, Seattle, Wash.*)

TUBEROSITY REDUCTIONS

The size and position of the maxillary tuberosity and mandibular retromolar pad in relation to the clinical crown of the terminal molar varies greatly. Probing depths in excess of normal often occur distal to the terminal tooth as a result of the adjacent tissue covering a portion of the crown. The presence of impacted third molars, or the soft tissue result of previous surgical removal of the third molars, frequently contributes to the severity of probing depths found distal to the maxillary second molars. The existence of such problems is an indication for surgical soft tissue reduction. A number of surgical techniques have been developed to provide a means of management of the tuberosity and retromolar areas during the performance of resective periodontal surgery.[67-72]

A relatively normal bone pattern around the terminal tooth would seem to indicate that an external bevel gingivectomy would be the simplest method to reduce either an enlarged tuberosity or retromolar pad. However, the use of gingivectomy leaves a broad external wound and may result in a stormy and prolonged postoperative healing period compared with an internal bevel flap reduction approach with primary closure. The presence of bony aberrations, such as exostoses, bony ledges, or interproximal defects, either individually, or in combination with pocket depth, is a contraindication to the use of the gingivectomy, because the pocket depth will reoccur if the bony deformities are not eliminated. For a less traumatic and more effective surgical management of tuberosity and retromolar pocket depths, there are a number of alternatives to a gingivectomy (see Chapter 20).

Tuberosity reduction procedures are commonly combined with buccal and palatal flap reflection, to gain access to the teeth and underlying bone for both debridement and osseous surgery procedures. The three most common approaches are the triangular wedge (inverse bevel distal wedge or "Mohawk" procedure), the inverse bevel linear wedge technique, and the pedicle flap procedure (trapdoor procedure).

Inverse Bevel Triangular Distal Wedge (Mohawk) Procedure

The inverse bevel distal wedge technique is usually integrated with buccal and palatal inverse access incisions and flap reflection.[67,70,72] The probe is used to sound through the mucogingival complex to bone, both horizontally and vertically, to map the thickness of the overlying tissue and the underlying bone configuration (see Fig. 23-1).

The location of the initial incision is dependent on the magnitude and thickness of the gingiva present, the presence and severity of the bone defects, and the therapist's estimation of where the final tissue position will be (Fig. 23-13). An initial palatal "tracing" incision, approximately 1 mm in depth, is placed from the most mesial involvement, distally to the hamular notch with either a #12B Bard-Parker double-edged scalpel blade or a custom broken carbon steel blade in a blade breaker, to create a moderately scalloped bleeding line. A push stroke is used, because the push stroke provides the greatest effectiveness and control. At the distopalatal aspect of the terminal tooth, the scalloped incision is accentuated, and then it is extended distally along the crest of the tuberosity with a straight-line incision to the hamular notch. The initial buccal incision, also approximately 1 mm in depth, is then outlined with a #15C Bard-Parker scalpel blade or a custom blade breaker blade. The buccal incision is started at the hamular notch, with a straight-line incision initiated from the ending point of the palatal incision, with a pull stroke toward the distobuccal line angle of the terminal tooth. The exact location of the incision is dependent on the tissue thickness and desired reduction of tuberosity tissue. Thicker tissue requires greater separation of the two incisions. The tuberosity incision outline is then extended anteriorly along the buccal aspect of the teeth with a moderate scallop, until the most mesially involved tooth has been included in the incision. A distal triangular wedge is thus outlined with the initial incisions, with the base of the triangle at the distal surface of the terminal tooth, and the apex formed by converging buccal and palatal straight-line incisions that meet in the mucosa of the hamular notch.

Once the "tracing" incisions are completed, the palatal and buccal incisions are extended apically in lamina propria to the level of the bone, using a #15C Bard-Parker blade to establish flaps of uniform thickness. Reduced sized Kirkland gingivectomy knives are preferred by some to thin the tissue and extend the incisions to bone, but the sharpest surgical blade possible allows for a more precise and clean incision. Once all incisions have been extended to bone, the distal wedge tissue and the collar of marginal soft tissue can be removed (Fig. 23-14). An Ochsenbein chisel is placed in contact with the bone between the collar of tissue and the tooth surface, and gently twisted to free the wedge and marginal collar from the underlying bone. Initially, this soft tissue tends to be removed in fragments by the novice surgeon, but with experience, the excess tissue can be removed in one continuous band resembling a Mohawk haircut in the tuberosity region, hence the name Mohawk procedure.

After thorough soft tissue debridement, the roots of the teeth can be curetted and smoothed, and the anatomic defects definitively surveyed. Resective osseous surgery can then be used in mild to moderate periodontitis to

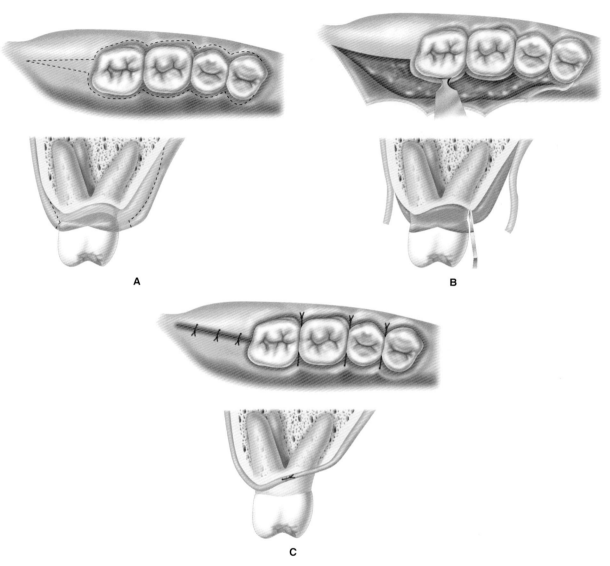

A

B

C

Figure 23-13. Inverse bevel triangular distal wedge (Mohawk) tuberosity procedure. **A,** Occlusal illustration depicting a maxillary posterior segment with a large tuberosity, illustrating a thick periodontal biotype. Cross-sectional illustration of the distal surface of the second molar. Note the shallow bony crater and the magnitude and thickness of the gingiva. The *dotted line* indicates the outline of the initial tracing incisions, which extend from the most mesial involvement distally to the hamular notch. This incision is made approximately 1-mm deep into the tissue to establish a bleeding line for further dissection before flap reflection. The initial tracing incision is extended apically to bone, thinning the flap as it is made. **B,** Once these incisions have been extended to bone, the tuberosity tissue and collar of marginal tissue can be removed with the aid of a twisting action with the Ochsenbein #2 chisel inserted between the teeth and the tissue. The *darker red* tissue in the cross-sectioned view represents the tissue to be removed during soft tissue debridement. **C,** After removal of this soft tissue, osseous resective surgery is completed, and the distal bony defect is eliminated. The thinned flaps and tuberosity region are closed primarily and sutured. Note the reduction in the tissue mass on the distal aspect of the second molar.

establish a suitable physiologic bony contour. Once a satisfactory architecture is achieved, the moderately scalloped flaps are approximated for trial closure to visualize whether further sculpting with a scalpel blade is necessary for proper flap positioning. Ideally, healing by primary closure means the scalloped flaps should cover the alveolar bone and a large portion of the exposed interproximal areas, as well as approximately 1 mm of root surface. The flaps may be secured using a variety of suturing techniques (see Chapter 20).

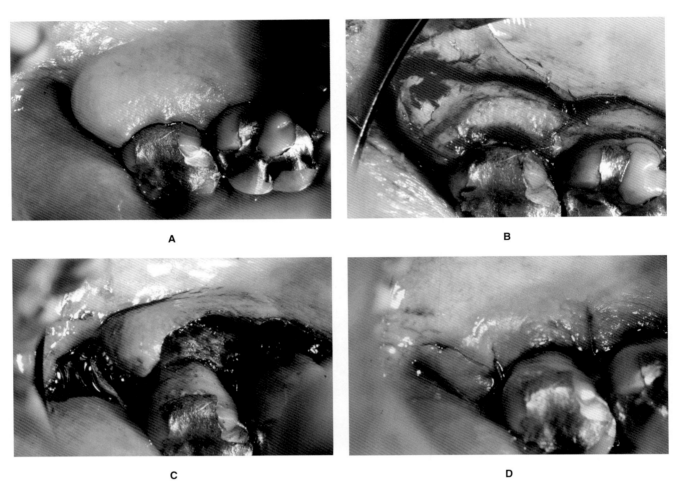

Figure 23-14. Clinical example of an inverse bevel triangular distal wedge (Mohawk) procedure. **A,** Preoperative palatal view of the enlarged tuberosity region with excessive probing depth and need for clinical crown lengthening for restorative purposes. After local anesthesia, the pocket on the distal aspect should be sounded to bone, and the probe should be placed through the soft tissue of the tuberosity to bone to determine the thickness of the tissue. **B,** The initial scalloped incision is made around the teeth and extended into the tuberosity region in a triangular shape. The incisions are then extended apically to bone, creating an evenly thinned flap. This palatal view shows the flap being retracted to reveal the underlying mass of soft tissue in the tuberosity and the collar of marginal tissue around the teeth. An Ochsenbein chisel is placed between the teeth and this marginal collar and twisted while being guided apically to removed the collar from the underlying bone. **C,** The collar of tissue and the distal wedge have been removed, revealing excellent access to the roots and underlying bone. **D,** The flaps are positioned to gain primary closure and sutured. Note the reduction in soft tissue height in the tuberosity region and along the palatal aspect of the second molar. The restorative dentist has excellent access for tooth preparation.

Inverse Bevel Linear Distal Wedge Procedure

The inverse bevel linear wedge procedure is similar to the triangular distal wedge procedure from a technique standpoint, except that after determining the soft tissue thickness of the tuberosity region or the edentulous area and the bony topography, parallel initial linear incisions are made from the distal of the terminal tooth to the distal of the keratinized tissue in the hamular notch area (Fig. 23-15). These tracing incisions act as guidelines for the apical dissection of the buccal and palatal flaps. The distal incision, which is made perpendicular to the linear incisions, joins the two linear incisions and extends to the mucogingival junction buccally and into palatal mucosa to the point where the palatal flap will be thinned. The distal incision must not be extended so far palatally as to risk incision of the greater palatine artery (see Chapter 20).

The parallel linear incisions are blended into the scalloped incisions at the distal of the terminal tooth and are extended anteriorly for buccal and palatal

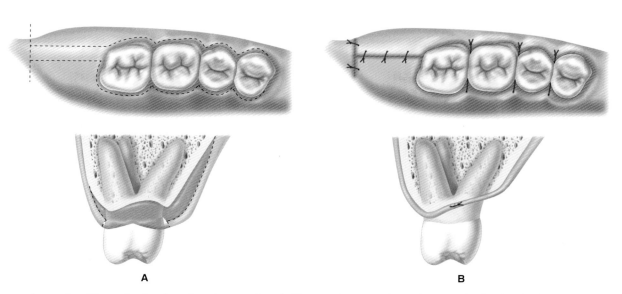

Figure 23-15. Inverse bevel linear distal wedge tuberosity procedure. **A,** The procedure is similar to the triangular distal wedge, but the distal incision is made perpendicular to the parallel linear incisions, extending past the mucogingival junction buccally to end in mucosa. Palatally the distal incision is extended as far as the palatal tissue will be thinned. The tissue that will be removed is darkened in the cross-sectional illustration. **B,** The thinned flaps and tuberosity region are closed primarily and sutured. Note the reduction in the tissue mass on the distal aspect of the second molar.

access. The resected tissues are removed using the same instruments and principles previously described for a distal wedge procedure. This technique offers the same advantages as the triangular distal wedge procedure but is of greater use in edentulous areas between existing teeth. It is particularly useful when the tuberosity has a short anterior-posterior dimension. In these cases, the triangular distal wedge procedure can be difficult to perform.

Tuberosity Pedicle Flap (Trapdoor) Procedure

The "trapdoor procedure" was designed to manage the maxillary tuberosity region in the presence of pocket depths.[70] For the inexperienced clinician, the procedure has the same potential complications of a gingivectomy, as well as the probability of leaving bone exposed when poorly planned and performed. It does provide excellent access to bone deformities and complete coverage of the tuberosity when properly executed and sutured (Fig. 23-16).

The initial incision is an inverse beveled straight-line palatal incision extending from the distopalatal line angle of the terminal molar to the end of the masticatory mucosa at the distal of the tuberosity. A vertical incision is then begun starting from the straight-line palatal incision at the distopalatal aspect of the terminal molar and moving buccally, through the distal periodontal pocket region and into the buccal gingiva and mucosa immediately adjacent to the distobuccal line angle of the terminal tooth. A second vertical incision is then made at the

terminus of the tuberosity that extends toward the buccal, at a right angle to the palatal incision. The incision extends into the buccal alveolar mucosa. By undermining and thinning the tuberosity pedicle flap tissue through split-thickness dissection from the palatal to the buccal, the pedicle flap is elevated and reflected buccally. This exposes a dense pad of connective tissue that remains over the tuberosity region. Internal bevel incisions are then extended from the distal of the terminal tooth anteriorly, on both the buccal and palatal surfaces of the teeth, to reflect mucogingival flaps and expose the residual connective tissue remaining from the buccal and palatal flaps. The connective tissue pad of the tuberosity and the residual connective tissue remaining from reflection of the flaps is then removed, using instrumentation described earlier, to achieve access. After completion of the planned procedure, trial flap closure, and necessary tissue trimming to prevent soft tissue overlap, the area is closed with suture after primary flap adaptation is achieved.

MANDIBULAR RETROMOLAR PAD REDUCTION

Soft and hard tissue anatomic differences between the maxilla and mandible require modifications in soft tissue access when tissues distal to the terminal mandibular molar are to be resected. The soft tissue immediately distal to the terminal molar consists of a small retromolar papilla, composed of gingiva, situated in varying proximity to the base of the anterior border of the ramus.

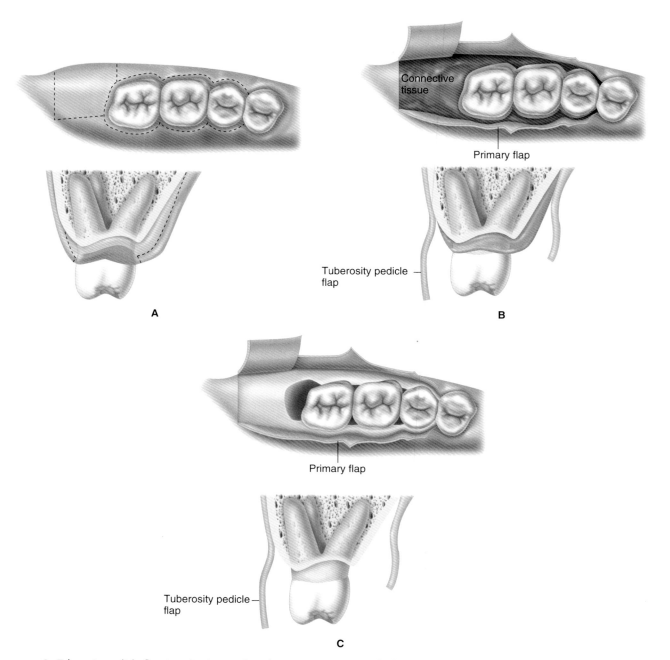

Figure 23-16. Tuberosity pedicle flap (trapdoor) procedure diagrams. **A,** Diagram of tuberosity pedicle flap incisions. A straight incision is made from the distopalatal line angle of the terminal molar to the most posterior extent of the tuberosity. Two incisions are then made perpendicular to the initial incision. The first courses buccally through the distal pocket region and into the buccal gingiva and mucosa. The second extends from the most distal aspect of the straight-line incision out into the buccal mucosa. **B,** Thinned and reflected tuberosity "trapdoor." Note that the bulk of the tuberosity tissue remains attached to bone, as does the collar of tissue along the buccal and palatal aspects of the teeth. This tissue will be removed from the underlying bone to allow access to bony defects. **C,** The tuberosity tissue and collar of marginal tissue are removed to reveal the underlying bony anatomy. After root debridement and osseous treatment, the flaps are closed primarily and sutured.

Distally, the retromolar papilla extends into mucosa, which contains an aggregation of retromolar glands. The result is a prominence covered by loosely attached mucosa that forms the base of the cheek. Together, the firm, pale papilla and the retromolar glandular prominence are often mistakenly called the retromolar pad. The anatomic retromolar pad, in reality, is the soft, dark red glandular prominence.[73]

Retromolar Inverse Bevel Triangular Distal Wedge Procedure

Management of tissues posterior to the mandibular terminal molars is done by means similar to maxillary tuberosity procedures. However, the clinician must be aware of anatomic structures unique to the mandibular retromolar region (see Chapter 20). In particular, there is often an anatomic concavity on the lingual aspect in this region, created by the lateral flare of the ascending ramus and posterior mandible. **Incisions must be placed over bone,** and the clinician must avoid placing scalpel blades too far to the lingual. The lingual nerve often courses close to the tissue surface and may be damaged by incisions placed too far to the lingual.

An inverse bevel triangular distal wedge can be used for the reduction of the retromolar area[68] (Fig. 23-17). The base of the triangle is at the distal of the terminal molar. Rather than coursing straight posteriorly, as is often done in the maxillary tuberosity, the apex of the mandibular wedge is angled toward the buccal, following the course of the ascending ramus. Moderate scalloping incisions are place around both distal line angles of the tooth, intersecting with the straight-line incisions coming from the apex of the wedge. From these incisions, the tissue can be thinned laterally and apically to bone to create flaccid, passive flaps. The wedge of dissected tissue is then removed in a similar fashion to that described in the tuberosity region.

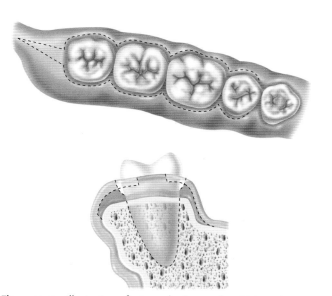

Figure 23-17. Illustration of retromolar inverse bevel triangular retromolar wedge procedure. Occlusal view shows a heavy mylohyoid ridge and lingual tori, with a thick periodontal biotype. Initial incisions extend from the base of the triangle, at the distal aspect of the terminal molar, posteriorly to the apex, which is skewed somewhat toward the buccal to maintain contact with the underlying bone.

Retromolar Inverse Bevel Linear Wedge Procedure

The inverse bevel linear wedge procedure can also be used (Fig. 23-18), initiating the parallel incisions far enough distally to adequately reduce the retromolar pad and to gain visual and instrumentation access to the underlying bone. The lingual incision must be kept in contact with bone and must not be placed so far lingually as to risk trauma to the lingual nerve. **The distal perpendicular incision carries great risk to the lingual anatomic region.** For this reason, most clinicians prefer either the triangular or trapdoor approaches to the mandibular retromolar procedure.

Retromolar Modified Pedicle Flap Procedure (With Braden Modifications)

In 1969, Braden[67] suggested a modification to the retromolar surgical approach that simplifies the procedure and is especially useful in areas where the retromolar pad is fibrous in nature. In the Braden modifications, the retromolar tissue remains a component of either the buccal or the lingual flap. In the first approach (Fig. 23-19, *A*), the buccal scalloped incision that is made around the teeth is carried around the distal aspect of the terminal molar to the distolingual line angle. The lingual scalloped incision extends from the distolingual line angle posteriorly to the retromolar pad. This incision courses parallel to the underlying disto-oblique ridge of the mandible, maintaining contact with the underlying bone. The extent of the incision posteriorly determines the degree of flap release achievable during the surgery. The buccal flap is then undermined and thinned distal to the terminal molar as it is reflected. The thinning incision is carried to bone on the buccal aspect, and the tissue that remains attached to bone is then removed. When the thinned flap is replaced and sutured, the removal of this underlying bulk of soft tissue results in apical positioning of the flap.

The second Braden modification (Fig. 23-19, *B*) is similar to the first technique, but it is the buccal incision that

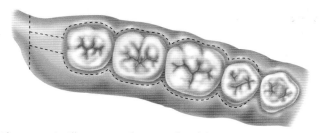

Figure 23-18. Illustration of inverse bevel linear retromolar wedge procedure. Incision outlines almost mirror the inverse bevel linear wedge tuberosity technique, but care must be exercised because of the anatomic location of the lingual nerve.

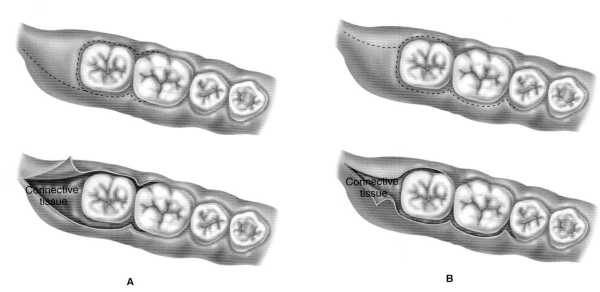

A   B

Figure 23-19. Braden buccal and lingual modifications of the retromolar flap procedures. **A,** Braden buccal retromolar flap reflection modification. Initial facial scalloped inverse bevel incision is carried around the distal aspect of the tooth to the distolingual line angle, where it meets the scalloped lingual incision. A secondary incision then extends from the distolingual line angle distally, but parallel and slightly buccal to the lingual border of the retromolar triangle, to the distal of the retromolar pad. The retromolar flap is thinned from the distal of the retromolar pad to the distal of the terminal tooth as it is reflected buccally. **B,** Braden lingual retromolar flap reflection modification. Initial lingual scalloped inverse bevel extends around the distal aspect of the tooth to the distobuccal line angle, where it meets the buccal scalloped incision. A secondary buccal incision extends from the distobuccal line angle of the terminal tooth, parallel to the disto-oblique ridge, to the distal of the retromolar pad. The retromolar flap is thinned by dissecting and undermining toward the lingual to bone, removing the excessive tissue and creating access to the lingual retromolar area.

is carried posteriorly, rather than the lingual incision. The lingual scalloped incision that is made around the teeth is carried around the distal aspect of the terminal molar to the distobuccal line angle. The buccal scalloped incision extends from the distobuccal line angle posteriorly to the retromolar pad. The lingual flap is then carefully undermined and thinned as it is reflected. The thinning incision is carried to bone and the tissue that remains attached to bone is removed. When the flap is replaced and sutured, the removal of this underlying bulk of soft tissue results in the apical positioning of the flap.

RESULTS OF FLAP DEBRIDEMENT SURGERY

Flap debridement surgery provides improved access for instrumentation over the closed scaling and root planing approach and results in more thorough removal of plaque, calculus, and debris.[53,74] When flaps are positioned to cover the alveolar bone, healing is rapid and generally uneventful.[54,56,75] Pocket depth is reduced by the resolution of residual inflammation, reduction in the bulk of the tissues, apical placement of the tissues, and reattachment of the flaps. Probing depth is reduced, and there is commonly some gain in probing attachment level, which may be maintained in patients who participate in a regular

recall program.[58,62] However, in the absence of three wall bony defects, new attachment is minimal, and the usual result is the formation of a long junctional epithelial attachment.[59,60]

PERIODONTAL OSSEOUS RESECTIVE SURGERY

History indicates that thought leaders in periodontics have been practical in their approaches to the treatment of periodontitis. They have tried to apply their knowledge of the anatomy of the periodontium and the etiology of periodontal disease to achieve the goal of maintaining the patient's dentition. As that knowledge evolves, therapeutic approaches have also evolved. For many years the "gold standard" in the treatment of periodontal "pockets" was scaling and root planing with hand instruments. Indeed chronic periodontitis has been successfully treated with nonsurgical debridement by skilled therapists.[76] Other therapists advocated surgical treatment because of the limitations of the closed approach.[69] Still others advocated surgical treatment because of mechanical concepts[77] or the belief that the alveolar bone in pockets was infected.[78] Schluger, considered the "father of osseous resective surgery," advocated osseous resective treatment of periodontitis, rather than scaling and root planing or the gingivectomy, as the most effective use of the limited available dental manpower.[69] He pointed out it was more economic and time efficient to treat 5- to 7-mm pocket depths with resective osseous surgery and to maintain the postsurgical shallow sulci than to try to maintain deep periodontal pockets with regular, periodic root planing and curettage.

Rationale for Osseous Resection

The primary objective of resective osseous surgery is the elimination of periodontal pockets and the creation of shallow gingival sulci that can be readily maintained by the patient and dental professionals. Gingiva has an architectural pattern that it follows with or without the support of underlying alveolar bone. After periodontal surgery, gingiva tends to "level" out and revert to a form similar to its original architecture. If the underlying bony architecture is not consistent with the architectural pattern of the gingiva, pocket depths reoccur. Thus the primary goal of the surgical eradication of periodontal pockets is accomplished by ensuring that the underlying bone form mimics the normal bony architecture at a somewhat more apical level on the tooth root, or that the final bony architecture is modeled after the form the therapist anticipates the gingiva will attain after surgery.

Such surgery requires both ostectomy and osteoplasty.[79] Osteoplasty, although reducing the volume of bone, does not involve the removal of any bony attachment from the tooth—that is, osteoplasty does not remove alveolar bone proper. Osteoplasty is a common component of a variety of surgical techniques. Conversely, ostectomy involves the removal of bone that is attached to the tooth. Because ostectomy results in the immediate loss of some attachment, the use of ostectomy has been more controversial. However, ostectomy, even with some resulting attachment loss, is necessary if certain types of bony defects are to be eradicated and pocket depth is to be reduced.[69] Properly done, ostectomy and osteoplasty result in soft tissue contours that reflect the under-lying bone form. When this occurs the soft tissue and the bone are said to be consistent with each other. Osseous resective surgery aimed at achieving such architecture is best performed in patients with early to moderate periodontitis.

FACTORS INFLUENCING THE PERFORMANCE OF OSSEOUS RESECTION

The performance of resective surgery to eliminate significant osseous defects requires a knowledge of and an appreciation for not only normal soft and hard tissue anatomy, but what the morphology of the osseous architecture will be after the elimination of the bony defects. The surgeon must be able to conceptualize before surgery how the desired osseous anatomy will appear after surgery and what biologic and anatomic limitations exist. An optimal result also requires a subtle understanding of the differences between flap design for access and debridement and flap design that will be required in order for the flap to be intimately adapted to the osseous platform that will result after either resection of the osseous deformities or the placement of materials to induce new attachment or regeneration (see Chapter 25).

Influence of Root Form and Root Trunk

Knowledge of root forms gives tremendous insight into the normal form and depth of each alveolus and acts as a basis for the diagnosis and treatment of anomalies in the periodontium. Root trunk length is an important anatomic factor in the diagnosis and treatment planning for posterior multirooted teeth. By definition, the root trunk extends from the cementoenamel junction (CEJ) to the furcation.[80] Gargiulo, Wentz, and Orban[81] found the distance from the CEJ to the marginal bone in health to be 1.5 to 2 mm, depending on the site and the tooth involved. Ochsenbein[80] classified the molar root trunks into maxillary and mandibular categories with different dimensions for the teeth in the two arches (Table 23-1).

TABLE 23-1	Classification and Dimensions of Molar Root Trunks	
ARCH	**CLASSIFICATION**	**DIMENSION (FROM CEJ TO BUCCAL FURCATION ENTRANCE)**
Maxillary	Short root trunk	3 mm
	Medium root trunk	4 mm
	Long root trunk	5 mm or more
Mandibular	Short root trunk	2 mm
	Medium root trunk	3 mm
	Long root trunk	4 mm or more

CEJ, *Cementoenamel junction.*

Because the distance from the CEJ to the buccal marginal bone has been found to be 1.5 to 2 mm,[81] the type of molar root trunk determines the amount of bone coronal to the furcation entrance in health. A short root trunk may have only 1 mm of crestal bone coronal to the furcation entrance in health. This information is of paramount importance to the dentist in treating interdental defects with osseous resective surgery.

Influence of Tooth Inclinations

Anatomic patterns and tooth inclinations seen in relation to the maxilla and the mandible have a significant effect on normal periodontal architecture and on the types and locations of bony defects encountered. The degree of axial root inclination in both a mesiodistal and buccolingual direction is varied for each tooth and class of teeth when measured from a vertical line perpendicular to the occlusal table of each arch. Maxillary teeth show the least amount of variation in root inclination.[82] Mandibular canines and incisors have the greatest deviation in root inclination, whereas the premolars and molars exhibit the most stable axial inclination. Axial tooth inclinations are significant because of their effects on alveoli and root form. Krause and colleagues[83] developed a table of axial inclinations (Table 23-2) and illustrations (Fig. 23-20) that are important in visualizing the influence of tooth inclinations on the thickness of the facial and lingual or palatal plates.

The maxillary and mandibular central incisor roots range from an almost perpendicular mesiodistal alignment to a slight mesial inclination. The root of the maxillary canine has a distal inclination of approximately 17 degrees, whereas the posterior teeth have root inclinations to the distal that range from 5 to 10 degrees. The mandibular canines and first premolars both have roots that range from being almost perpendicular to a slight distal inclination of approximately 6 degrees. There is an increased distal tilting of the root surfaces of the posterior teeth and a corresponding mesial inclination of the clinical crowns. The mesial root of the second molar is inclined distally approximately 14 degrees, whereas the palatal roots of the maxillary first and second molars have a distal inclination of 10 and 8 degrees, respectively. Because of their highly variable form, position, and eruption pattern, the third molars in either arch were not considered.

The maxillary central incisors, on a faciolingual axis, have the greatest degree of root inclination, with the roots being inclined lingually approximately 29 degrees. The palatal inclination of the canine root is approximately 16 degrees, whereas the premolars are generally aligned with their axial centers almost perpendicular to the occlusal plane. The axial inclination of the maxillary molars seldom exceeds 15 degrees, and except for the distobuccal root of the first molar, all roots tend to extend palatally. The buccal roots of the molars are not normally palatally inclined as much as the palatal roots.

The mandibular incisors have a lingual tilt to the root apex, as is the case for the canine and first premolar. The remaining posterior teeth have a facial root inclination ranging from 9 degrees on the second premolar to

TABLE 23-2	Subjective Clinical Average Axial Tooth Inclinations	
	ANGLE OF MESIODISTAL INCLINATION OF THE ROOT TO THE DISTAL OF THE TOOTH CENTRAL AXIS WITH A VERTICAL LINE (IN DEGREES)	ANGLE OF BUCCOLINGUAL INCLINATION OF THE TOOTH CENTRAL AXIS WITH A VERTICAL LINE (IN DEGREES)
Maxillary		
Canine	17	16*
First premolar	9	5*
Second premolar	5	6*
First molar	10	8*
Second molar	8	10*
Mandibular		
Canine	6	12*
First premolar	6	9*
Second premolar	9	9†
First molar	10	20†
Second molar	14	20†

*Root apex inclined lingually.
†Root apex inclined labially.
From Krause BS, Jordan RE, Abrams L: Dental anatomy and occlusion, Baltimore, Md., 1969, Williams and Wilkins, pp 223-231.

20 degrees on the first and second molars. Although the only published study states that the mandibular molars have a 20-degree axial inclination to the lingual, the authors,[82] after studying numerous dry mandibles, believe that the lingual inclination of the molars is often greater than 20 degrees.

The axial center of a tooth is clinically significant, because it relates directly to the height of the radicular

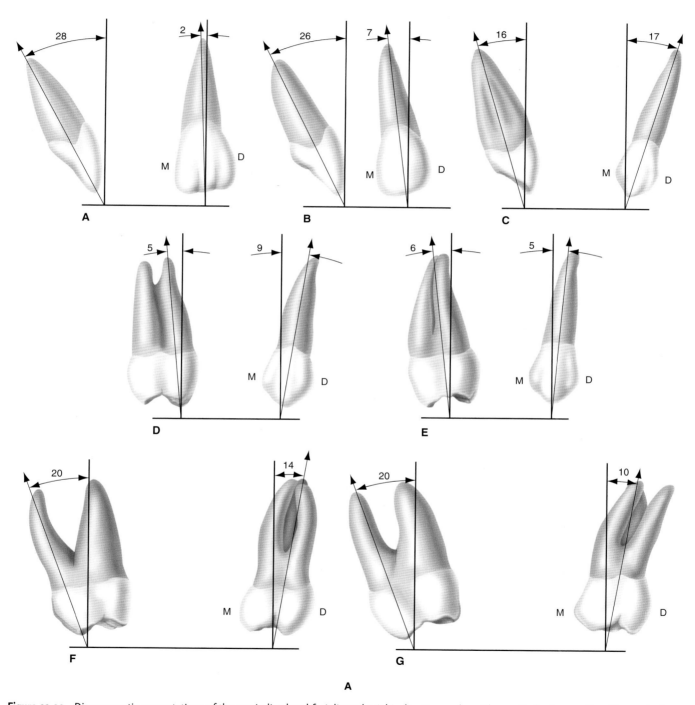

Figure 23-20. Diagrammatic presentations of the mesiodistal and faciolingual axial inclination angles with a vertical reference line. The tooth sizes are *not* proportional. **A,** Maxillary teeth (*A-G*): *A,* central incisor; *B,* lateral incisor; *C,* canine; *D,* first premolar; *E,* second premolar; *F,* first molar; *G,* second molar.

Continued

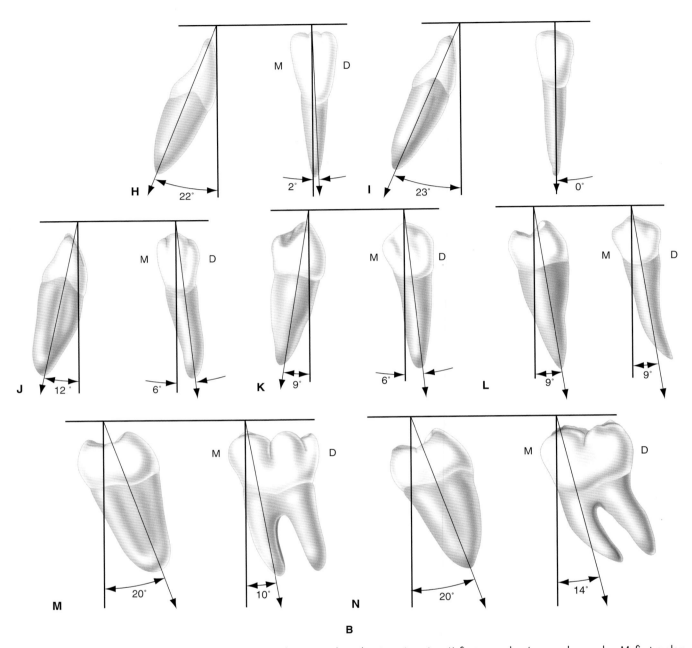

Figure 23-20. cont'd B, Mandibular teeth (*H-N*): *H,* central incisor; *I,* lateral incisor; *J,* canine; *K,* first premolar; *L,* second premolar; *M,* first molar; *N,* second molar.

alveolar bone and the natural sloping of the interproximal alveolar bone. The axial center of a maxillary central incisor results in the facial height of crown contour being positioned more apically and the lingual height of crown contour being elevated incisally.

The positioning of the axial center of a mandibular molar results in the lingual height of crown contour being positioned apically and the facial height of crown contour being heightened occlusally. *The enamel on the lingual surfaces of the mandibular molars and second premolars consequently tends to extend further apically than that on the buccal surfaces, resulting in a natural sloping of the interproximal alveolar bone from an occlusally higher buccal plate to a more apically positioned lingual plate.*

Ritchey and Orban[84] pointed out that the configurations of the crest of the interdental alveolar septae are defined by the relative positions of the adjacent CEJs in health. The alveolar crest ordinarily parallels the CEJ of the teeth throughout the mouth. The interproximal areas of the molar regions are predominately flattened, whereas the anterior teeth mesial to the second premolar are unusually convex or pyramidal in shape.[85] The tooth forms present determine the width of the interproximal alveolar bone. Bell-shaped or convex mesial and distal tooth surfaces normally present with wide interdental septae, whereas narrow septae exist when proximal tooth surfaces are relatively flat.

The facial housing of the alveolar bone frequently is thin from the midline distally through the premolar areas. The blood supply to these areas is also different: a circulatory bed or network supplies the radicular bone surfaces, rather than a central complex of nutrient vessels characteristic of interdental bone. Bone resorption follows the pathway of inflammation, but the pathway is different for radicular bone versus interdental bone.[69,86,87] Where the marginal bone is thin, inflammation can result in a bony dehiscence, which is thought to result in gingival recession.[88,89] When the alveolar bone has a thick biotype, inflammation will result in a circumferential type defect with an intrabony component.

Location and Type of Bony Defects

As stated earlier in this chapter, the normal anatomic configuration of alveolar bone and overlying soft tissues are harmonious, but with variations in the thickness and degree of scalloping of the tissues about the teeth. In periodontal diseases, however, ubiquitous resorptive bony lesions create significant variations

from normal morphologic features of the bone and the bone height.

Bone loss is often referred to as localized or generalized and as either horizontal or vertical in nature. Horizontal bone loss tends to be the more common pattern of bone loss.[80] The interdental and interradicular areas generally show similar degrees of resorption. Loss of midradicluar bone (facial, or lingual, or both) often depends on the thickness of bone, with thin areas more likely to dehisce. When there is sufficient volume of bone surrounding the root(s) of teeth, resorptive bone patterns may take a vertical or funnel form, resulting in formation of intrabony defects.

Bone resorption caused by inflammatory periodontal disease alters the configuration of the alveolar bone around the dentition and can result in an infinite variety of bony defects. Goldman and Cohen[90] classified bony defects based on the number of bony walls that they presented (Fig. 23-21). The presence of bony walls provides potential for in-growth of bone-producing cells.

The most common bony lesion described and encountered in periodontal disease is the interdental crater.[91-93] Interdental osseous craters are concavities in the crest of the alveolar septa centered under the contact point of adjacent teeth. Facial and lingual walls are present, but the mesial and distal "walls" of the defect are composed of the root surfaces of the adjacent teeth. An early to moderate interdental crater is a saucer-shaped concavity in the alveolar septum. Early to moderate interproximal craters often do not cause a loss in papillary height. Manson and

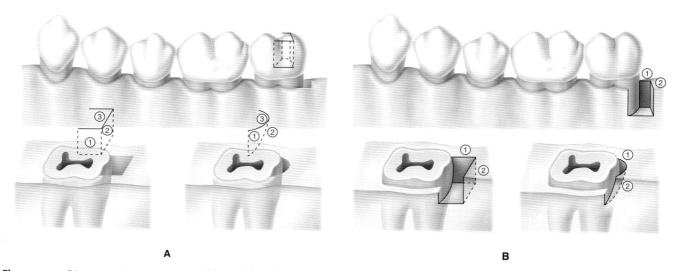

A   **B**

Figure 23-21. Diagrammatic presentations of bony defects based on the number of walls that the defects present. **A,** Three-wall bony defect at the distal of a mandibular second molar in diagrammatic box form and as it might actually appear intraorally. The facial, lingual, and distal bony walls are present. The fourth "wall" of the defect is formed by the avascular root surface. **B,** Two-wall bony defect represented diagrammatically in box form, and then as a two-wall defect might actually appear. The lingual and distal bony walls are present, but the facial wall is not.

Continued

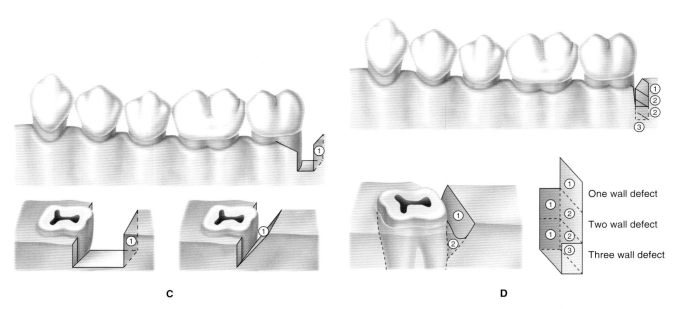

C   **D**

Figure 23-21. cont'd C, One-wall bony defect. Only the distal bony wall remains. **D,** Diagrammatic representation of a combined one-wall, two-wall, three-wall bony defect. Bony defects can take on a number of combinations in reference to the number of walls and the width of the defects that are present. Such factors may have a significant bearing on the predictability to be expected with regenerative procedures.

Nicholson[91] report that the interdental crater was found to represent one third (35.2%) of all maxillary defects and about two thirds (62%) of all mandibular defects recorded. The prevalence of crater defects is greater in the posterior than in the anterior regions of the mouth. Ochsenbein[80] divided bony craters into three basic types: shallow, medium, and deep (Box 23-3).

Alveolar Margin Alterations

The next most commonly encountered type of bony defects was an alteration to the alveolar margin.[94] Such alterations were present in the form of thickened bony ledges and exostoses (Figs. 23-22 and 23-23), resorption of radicular bone causing facial or lingual alveolar defects such as dehiscences or fenestrations (Fig. 23-24), and presence of "reverse architecture" (Fig. 23-25). Comparatively, thickened margins were found much more

frequently in the maxilla than in the mandible.[92] Marginal defects were most frequently found in the maxillary posterior segments, but the pattern of resorption was found to be random. Reverse architecture, also called inconsistent bony margins, results when the interproximal crest is more apical than the buccal or palatal/lingual radicular bone height, producing a reverse pattern in comparison to the normal scalloped alveolar process.

Furcation Involvements

The invasion of the trifurcations and bifurcations of multirooted teeth is termed a furcation involvement.[95] The probability of furcation involvements is dependent on the degree of bone loss and the length of the root trunk of the teeth in question. Furcation involvements are classified according to the amount of bone loss (see Chapter 24). The prevalence of furcation involvements increases with age. There is disagreement as to whether mandibular first molars or maxillary molars have the greatest prevalence of furcation involvement.[94] Bone loss in the furcation of maxillary first premolars is least prevalent.[96]

Vertical (Angular) Defects

Vertical bony defects are intrabony lesions classified by the numbers of osseous walls that are present in the slanting or oblique direction beside a tooth. There may be one, two, or three walled defects, or combination osseous defects.[90] The base of a vertical defect is located apical to

Box 23-3	**Classification of Maxillary and Mandibular Osseous Craters, and Depth (Dimension from Crest of Facial/Lingual Bone to Crater Base)**

Crater Type	Dimension
Shallow crater	1-2 mm
Medium crater	3-4 mm
Deep crater	5 mm or more

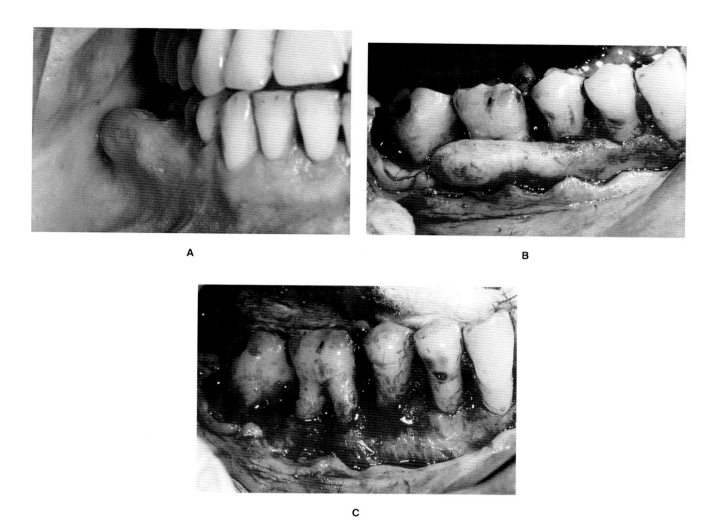

Figure 23-22. Alveolar margin aberrations. **A,** Buccal exostosis viewed from the anterior region of the second premolar and molar areas. **B,** After reflection of a buccal flap, the magnitude of the aberration can be seen. **C,** Buccal view after both ostectomy/osteoplasty. The thickness of the exostosis precluded visualization of the furcation area radiographically. However, bone sounding before incisions revealed a Class II furcation involvement.

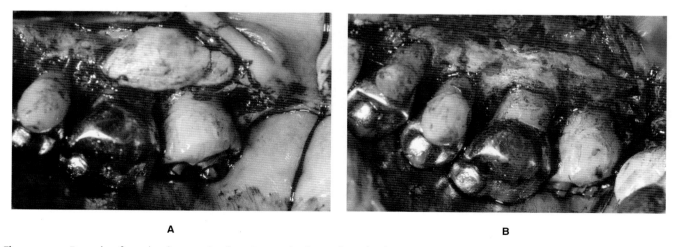

Figure 23-23. Example of an alveolar margin alteration in the form of a palatal exostosis. **A,** View of palatal exostosis after flap reflection and debridement. Note the thickness of the bony aberration and the effects the aberration may have on normal physiologic contours. **B,** View of area after osteoplasty and ostectomy. Most of the recontouring that was performed was osteoplasty, and little alveolar bone proper was removed.

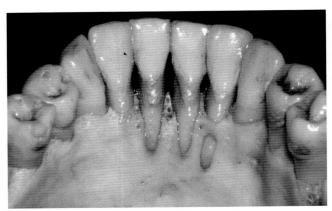

Figure 23-24. Resorption of radicular bone causing bony dehiscences and fenestration on the lingual aspect of mandibular incisors (dry skull specimen).

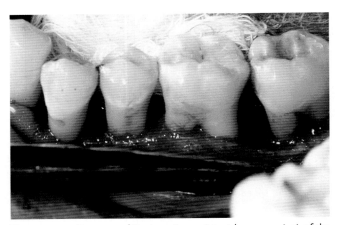

Figure 23-25. Reverse architecture (inconsistent bony margins) of the lower posterior region, where the bone margins in the midradicular areas are positioned further occlusally than the interproximal bone height. This can be noted especially between the two molars.

the surrounding bone (Fig. 23-21). The occlusal aspect of a vertical defect often exhibits fewer walls of bone than the apical portion, meaning a vertical defect may be a combination one-, two- and three-wall bony defect. A vertical defect may occur interproximally, or on the buccal and palatal/lingual radicular surface of a tooth. A one-wall defect is also called a hemiseptum.

Interproximal vertical defects can often be detected radiographically, whereas radicular surface vertical defects are not readily visible.[92,97,98] The presence of three-wall vertical defects is seen most frequently on the mesial surfaces of maxillary and mandibular molars. With age, vertical defects increase, but a large percentage of individuals with interdental vertical defects have only a single defect.[93,96,97]

TECHNIQUE OF OSSEOUS RESECTION

The successful performance of periodontal osseous resective surgery requires the application of the entire spectrum of the therapist's diagnostic and surgical knowledge and skills. The sequence of steps involved in the performance of resective osseous surgery are listed in Box 23-4.

Gaining Access for Osseous Resection

Presurgical examination and periodontal probing provides information regarding the position, depth, and configuration of the periodontal pockets, as well as the anatomic parameters of the overlying soft tissues.[99] This information is essential for planning surgical access. Position of the initial incisions can have a profound effect on the success or failure of the procedure. Access and instrumentation must be carefully planned so as not to have a detrimental effect on the final result. Inadequate access to a surgical site can result in a torn flap as a result of the retraction pressure while attempting to visualize and instrument the area (see Chapter 20).

Debridement and Assessment of Defects to be Corrected

After establishing adequate flap thickness with the initial and thinning incisions, the buccal and palatal/lingual flaps are reflected for surgical access. The remaining connective tissue is removed from the bony surfaces to fully visualize the underlying defects. Any remaining

---

Box 23-4   Principle Sequence of Osseous Resective Surgery

1. Assess nature and location of the bony defects and aberrations using a periodontal probe and diagnostic quality radiographs
2. Formulate a treatment plan regarding how to handle the bony aberrations and the incisions for access
3. Primary, secondary incisions for flap thinning; reflection and removal of soft tissue
4. Visual and tactile confirmation of location and nature of bony defects and aberrations
5. Scaling and root planing
6. Reduction of thick buccal and palatal/lingual bone (osteoplasty)
7. Elimination of the interproximal bony defects
8. Refinement of the bony contours with hand instruments and finishing burs
9. Complete odontoplasty where necessary
10. Final assessment of osteoectomy/osteoplasty and the recontoured bony morphology
11. Apically position the reflected flaps in a position harmonious with the recontoured bone for primary healing, and close with sutures.

tissue tags are removed using a combination of ultrasonic and hand instrumentation, giving a clear view of the marginal bone and bony defects that are present. The root surfaces are thoroughly instrumented to remove plaque and calculus.

Elimination of Osseous Defects

After confirming the presence and configuration of the osseous defects, the bony deformities are systematically eliminated by initially using osteoplasty and then ostectomy. It should be the surgeon's goal to eradicate the defects, but to accomplish this by the removal of the least amount of attachment possible (ostectomy). The ability to accomplish such a result is dependent on the extent of attachment loss that has occurred and the intrinsic anatomic variables of the patient's dentition. Observations of the problems encountered when resective osseous surgery is performed without full consideration and understanding of the anatomic factors of the dentition resulted in the development of two primary approaches to performing posterior resective osseous surgery to minimize any adverse effects. These two approaches are the palatal approach for the posterior maxillary interproximal craters[100,101] and the lingual approach for similar defects in the mandibular arch.[102]

PALATAL APPROACH TO OSSEOUS RESECTIVE SURGERY

Historically, the surgical management of early to moderate periodontitis of the maxillary anterior and bicuspid region has met with a much greater degree of success than that of the molar region. Accessibility is partially responsible, but careful study and consideration of the anatomic factors associated with the posterior maxilla and mandible explains more fully the lesser degree of successful therapy, especially when the presurgical morphology of the molar teeth and surrounding bone is taken into account. Taking these anatomic factors into consideration, Ochsenbein and Bohannan[100,101] described the palatal approach to osseous surgery to refine and complement the treatment of interdental craters in the maxillary molar region. The architectural factors recognized as favoring a palatal approach to osseous surgery are listed in Box 23-5. An example of the correction of periodontal osseous defects using the palatal approach to correction is shown in Figure 23-26.

LINGUAL APPROACH TO OSSEOUS RESECTIVE SURGERY

In 1976, Tibbetts and colleagues[102] reported on the importance of performing resective osseous surgery in the posterior mandible primarily from a lingual approach

Box 23-5   Architectural Factors Favoring a Maxillary Palatal Approach

- Avoidance of buccal furcations, which are located further occlusally than the mesiopalatal and distopalatal furcations
- Buccal root proximity in molar areas (narrow buccal embrasure spaces)
- Wider embrasures palatally, therefore wider spaces, because the molars are considered single rooted from the palate
- Poor posterior access for proper instrumentation from a buccal approach
- Thin buccal radicular bone; dehiscences and fenestrations from central incisor through first molar (bone is thicker over the second and third molars)
- Greater palatal bone thickness around the arch from second premolar to second premolar, but thinner over the palatal aspect of the molars
- Shallow buccal vestibular depth, or a narrow width of gingiva, or both
- Palatal tissue is all keratinized

to achieve successful long-term treatment results. By doing so, iatrogenic periodontal problems can be avoided on the buccal surfaces of the mandibular posterior teeth. An example of the correction of periodontal osseous defects using the lingual approach is demonstrated in Figure 23-27.

Although the palatal and lingual approaches to osseous surgery are not panaceas, the premise of the procedures is to create acceptable and maintainable periodontal architectural forms, by using anatomic relationships unique to the topography of the regions. The use of these techniques prevents some of the intrinsic problems primarily encountered with buccal approaches, such as exposure of buccal furcations and the presence of shallow vestibular depth with a narrow width of gingiva over the facial radicular surfaces of the teeth. Thin, compact bone is often present over the radicular surfaces of the molars. Wound healing studies show significant permanent bone resorption with surgical compact bone exposure.[89]

Resective osseous surgery from a palatal or lingual approach does not prevent the necessity of surgical intervention from the buccal aspect, because almost all cases require some buccal contouring, but the bulk of the crater reduction is done palatally or lingually to preserve the height and integrity of the buccal bone, particularly where the root trunk is short and the buccal furcation, which is positioned further occlusally than the mesiopalatal and distopalatal, or lingual furcations may be compromised.

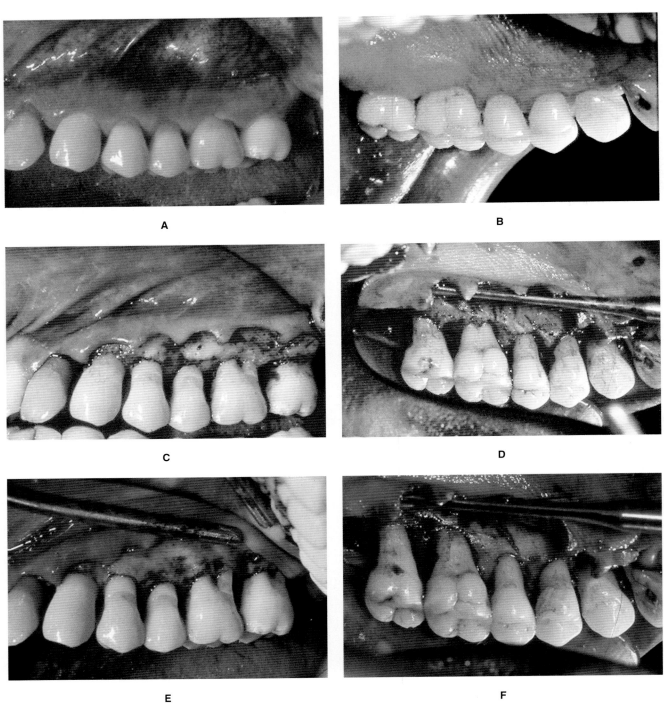

Figure 23-26. Correction of periodontal osseous defects using a palatal approach to surgical correction. **A,** Buccal preoperative view from maxillary lateral incisor distally. **B,** Palatal preoperative view from maxillary lateral incisor through second molar. **C,** Buccal view after flap reflection and debridement, showing Class I furcation involvement and interdental cratering from the premolars distally. **D,** Palatal view after flap reflection and debridement, showing defects from the canine distally, with the most severe defect interproximal to the molars. **E,** Buccal postosseous resective surgery. Minimal ostectomy was performed, with the majority being in the molar region. The height of interproximal bone from the facial aspect is unchanged, except between the molars where slight reduction at the distobuccal line angle of the first molar can be seen. Extensive osteoplasty was performed to thin the bony ledging, before the ostectomy procedure. **F,** Palatal postosseous resective surgery, showing the results of ramping the defects toward the palate.

Continued

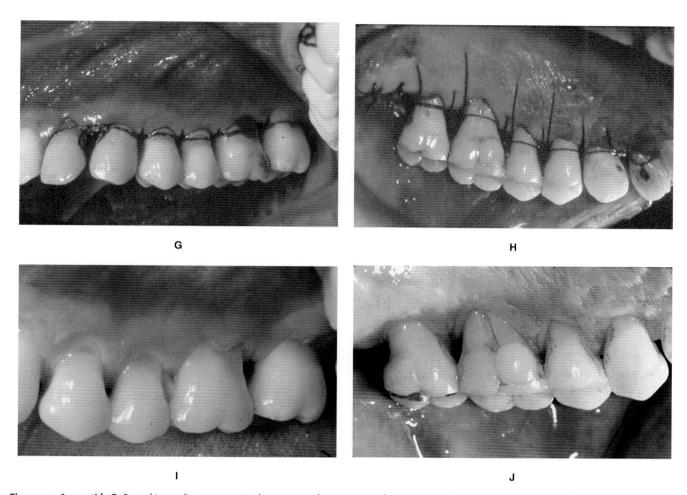

Figure 23-26. cont'd **G,** Buccal immediate postsurgical suturing with continuous sling sutures. Note the apical positioning of the flap. **H,** Palatal use of continuous vertical sling mattress sutures to drape the tissue at the desired level and to position the interdental papillae correctly. **I,** Five-year postoperative buccal view, with probing depths within normal limits. **J,** Five-year postoperative palatal view, with probing depths within normal limits.

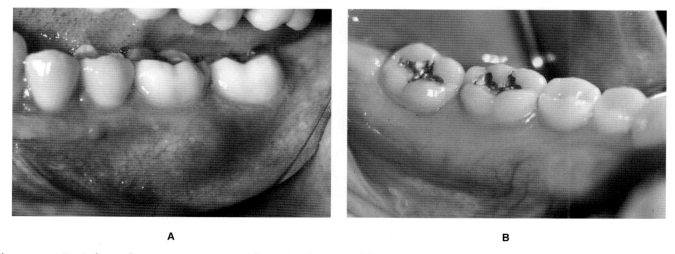

Figure 23-27. Surgical case demonstrating correction of periodontal osseous defects using lingual approach to resective surgery. **A,** Presurgical buccal view of mandibular posterior segment, with a buccal exostosis and a relatively thick periodontal biotype. **B,** Lingual presurgical view of mandibular posterior segment, with a thick biotype, a lingual torus, and interproximal probing depths of 5 to 6 mm.

Continued

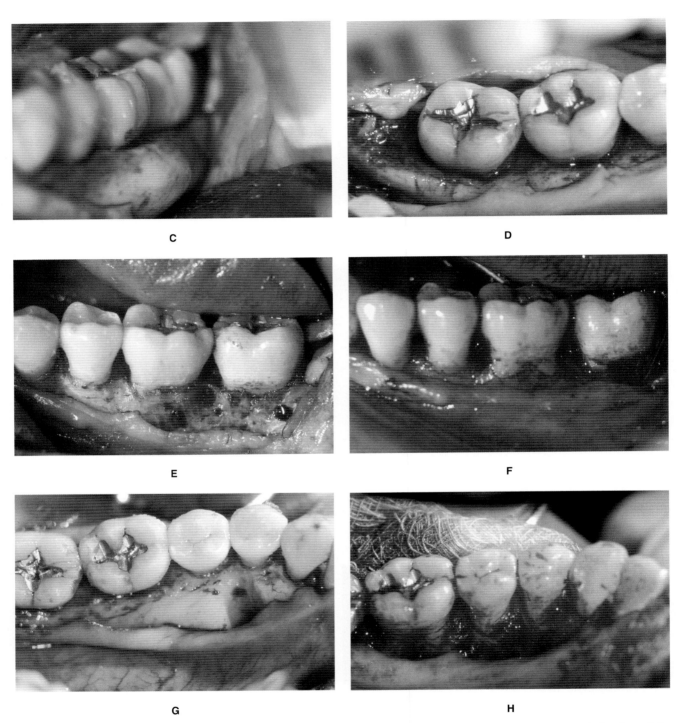

Figure 23-27. cont'd C, Direct anterior–buccal view of teeth and bone after flap reflection and soft tissue debridement. Note shallow bony defects on buccal tooth surfaces and thickness of buccal bone. **D,** Lingual-occlusal view of retromolar area, enabling visualization of thick bony ledge extending to distal of retromolar area, and shallow crater in molar region. **E,** Buccal view after osteoplasty. No ostectomy has been performed. The interdental crater between the molars can be seen. **F,** Buccal view after ostectomy. A positive architecture is formed, with interproximal bone height being located more coronally than midfacial bone height. **G,** Beginning of lingual osteoplasty, with groove in premolar area illustrating thickness of alveolar bone. **H,** Lingual view after osteoplasty/ostectomy in premolar–molar region.

Continued

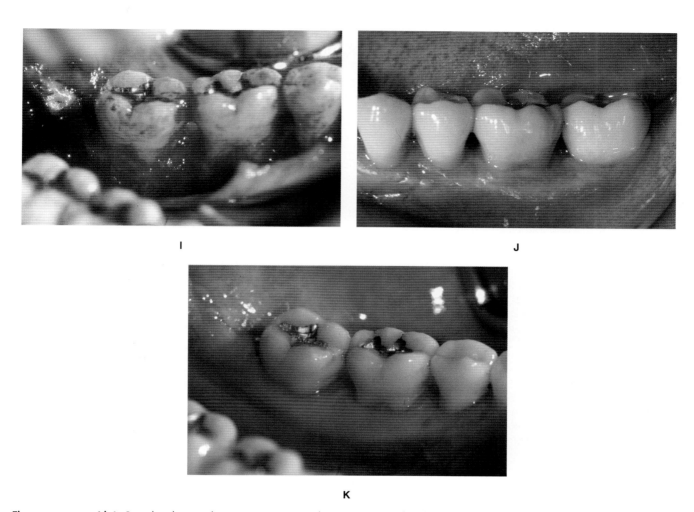

Figure 23-27. cont'd I, Completed osteoplasty/ostectomy in molar region. Note the elimination of the large lingual shelf in the retromolar region. The flaps are the apically positioned and secured with suture. **J,** Buccal postoperative view at 8 weeks. **K,** Lingual postoperative view at 8 weeks.

TECHNIQUE AND INSTRUMENTATION FOR OSSEOUS RESECTION (MODELS)

The sequence for resective osseous surgery presented in Box 23-4 is performed on a model typical of a mandibular segment, with architectural factors favoring a lingual approach, as enumerated in Box 23-6. Ochsenbein developed the anatomic model used in the photographic sequence illustrating the procedures performed by the authors.

The surgeon must carefully examine the area(s) of concern from several different angles and views to formulate a three-dimensional picture of the architectural anatomy that is present. Observation of the buccal surface from a 90-degree angle to the mandible shows no bony variations from normal (Fig. 23-28, *A*), whereas the same area viewed at a 45-degree angle reveals a shallow crater between the two premolars and the thickened marginal bone combined with an early Class II furcation involvement of the first molar (Fig. 23-28, *B*). A lingual surface inspection from a 90-degree angle reveals the presence of a torus lingual to the premolars, simulated root caries at the mesiolingual line angle of the second molar, and a prominent mylohyoid ridge (Fig. 23-28, *C*). A 45-degree view (Fig. 23-28, *D*) and an anterior–occlusal view (Fig. 23-28, *E*) greatly supplement the visualization of the bone thickness and bony architecture present about the teeth. Seeing the anatomy of the shallow crater and the torus with the teeth removed (Fig. 23-29, *A*) allows a much clearer conceptual picture of the crater anatomy and the effect that the torus has on the crater, as does a cross-sectional view of the interproximal area distal to the first premolar (Fig. 23-29, *B*). With the three-dimensional picture, achieved by thoroughly viewing the surgical site, the therapist can ascertain whether the treatment planned before clinical flap reflection and debridement needs modification or can be rendered as planned.

<table>
<tr><td>Box 23-6</td><td>Anatomic Factors Favoring a Mandibular Lingual Approach</td></tr>
</table>

- Prominent external oblique ridge on buccal aspect extends obliquely from beneath the mental foramen to the anterior border of the ramus, often resulting in shallow buccal vestibule.
- Posterior teeth have lingual crown inclination; facial root inclination ranges from 9 degrees on the second premolar to 20 degrees on the molars.
- Enamel on the lingual surfaces of the mandibular molars and the second premolar extends further apically than on the buccal surfaces.
- Natural sloping of the interproximal bone from an occlusally higher buccal plate to a more apically positioned lingual plate.
- Because of lingual axial inclination of the crowns of posterior teeth, the base of the interdental crater is positioned lingually.
- Lingual bony plate is thicker.
- Thin buccal radicular bone over the premolars and mesial root of the first molar.
- Avoidance of buccal furcation, which is located further occlusally than the lingual furcations.

After thorough examination, it is obvious that there are five variations from normal anatomy on the technique model, including:

1. A shallow interdental crater between #28 and #29
2. A lingual torus in the #28-#29 area
3. Thickened radicular bone on the labial of #30, with a Class I buccal furcation involvement
4. A physiologic violation of the attachment apparatus at the mesiolingual line angle of #31 caused by root caries
5. A prominent mylohyoid ridge

With the confirmed diagnosis of the five deviations from normal, the therapist should first mentally determine what the ideal treatment is for each individual deviation. The shallow crater can be readily treated by resective surgery to reduce the deepened pocket depth and facilitate more effective oral hygiene efforts. The torus requires treatment because it is an integral part of the lingual crater wall between the premolars. The furcation involvement of #30 requires treatment. Both resective therapy and regeneration are potential treatment modalities for this furcation. Regeneration might be the ideal theoretic treatment, but the furcation is shallow and may respond more predictably to a resective approach.

Treatment options for the violation of the physiologic dimension of the attachment apparatus by caries on the mesiolingual of #31 include surgical crown lengthening, extraction, extraction and ridge preservation surgery followed by implant placement after the socket heals, or

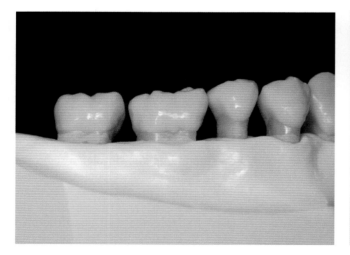

A

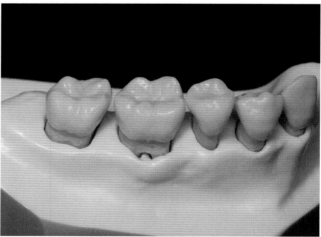

B

Figure 23-28. Examination of technique model from several different angles allows therapist to formulate three-dimensional mental picture of architectural anatomy. **A,** Buccal view from 90-degree angle to mandible shows flat anatomy, with no visible bony variations from normal. **B,** Buccal view from 45-degree angle reveals shallow interdental crater between premolars and thickened marginal bone combined with early Class II furcation involvement of first molar.

Continued

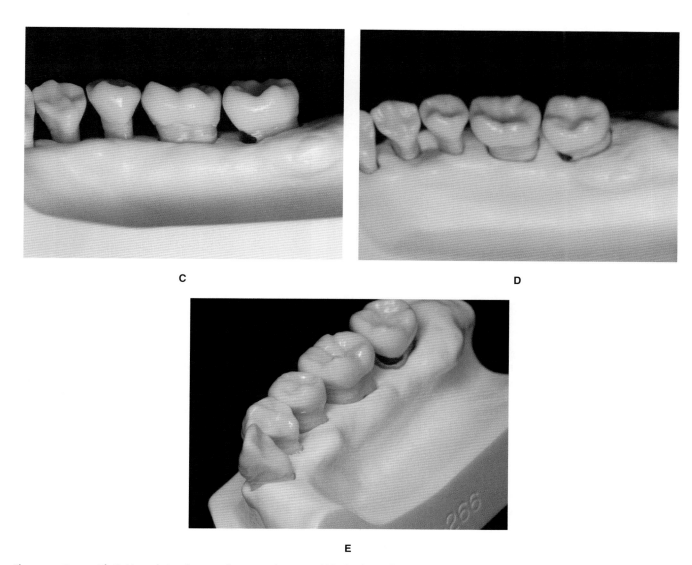

C

D

E

Figure 23-28. cont'd C, Lingual view from 90-degree angle to mandible displays a flat marginal anatomy, a thickened mylohyoid ridge from straight lingual of second molar, a torus in premolar region, and caries violating physiologic dimension at mesiolingual of second molar. **D,** Shallow interdental crater between the two premolars, lingual torus, physiologic dimension violation, and prominent mylohyoid ridge is visible from a 45-degree lingual view. Root caries on the mesiolingual aspect of the second molar can be appreciated. **E,** Anterior–lingual–occlusal view gives much better concept of lingual bony anatomy and thickness, as well as the physiologic dimension violation at the mesial of the second molar. Note the presence of the torus in the premolar area and the thick mylohyoid ridge at the second molar.

immediate extraction and placement of an implant to replace the tooth. Crown lengthening is a viable option if there is a medium to long root trunk with no furcation involvement, and root form and root length are adequate. If the bone reduction necessary for a crown lengthening procedure theoretically jeopardizes the possibility of future implant placement in the event of tooth loss, other treatment options should be discussed with the patient and considered. Because the bone level around the second molar is relatively normal, and the tooth has a medium root trunk with mildly diverging roots, surgical crown

lengthening for the tooth is a viable treatment option. The prominent mylohyoid ridge only requires treatment because it interferes with proper flap positioning. Like the lingual torus adjacent to the premolars, the prominent mylohyoid ridge would otherwise require no treatment if it was asymptomatic.

When the five aberrations from normal are present simultaneously, treatment options should be blended into a combined treatment plan that addresses all of the deviations concurrently. With the exception of the buccal bony aberration on the first molar, the labial

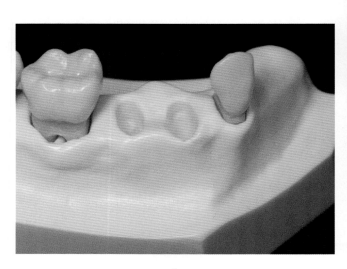

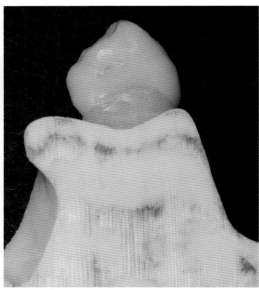

A   B

Figure 23-29. Visualization of the interproximal crater between the premolars. **A,** With the two premolar teeth removed from the model, the crater, with its prominent buccal and lingual wall, is more visible. Note that the lingual wall corresponds to the position of the torus. Treatment of the crater requires torus reduction. Interproximal bone anatomy is within normal limits at distal of canine and mesial of molar. Labial radicular bone thickness is also within normal limits. **B,** Proximal cross-section distal to first premolar shows much thicker bone lingually, with the crater being positioned to the lingual of the contact area. Less supporting bone will be sacrificed by lingual ramping of the defect than would occur if the crater was ramped to the facial.

architecture is within acceptable limits. The prudent therapist will limit labial treatment to the first molar and the immediately adjacent proximal areas, extending no further than blending the anatomy to the midline of the adjacent teeth. The labial resective osseous contouring initially involves osteoplasty, followed by ostectomy. The crater between the premolars should be ramped lingually, with no labial bony recontouring. Lingual ramping will necessitate both osteoplasty, to thin the marginal bone, and ostectomy, to reduce supporting alveolar bone, and will create a normal architectural form at a more apical level. Because the interdental crater is to be ramped lingually, the lingual torus should be reduced by osteoplasty before the ostectomy aspect of treatment is initiated.

Lingual osteoplasty is initiated at the mesial of the torus, using a #8 or #10 surgical length bur in an apical–occlusal direction, with a light feather brush stroke (Fig. 23-30, A). The apical–occlusal brush stroke in an actual clinical case, with a Prichard retractor at the apical extent of the retracted flap, will prevent flap laceration as often seen when an occlusal–apical stroke of the surgical bur is used. On starting the osteoplasty procedure, the area must be continually irrigated and aspirated, which allows the work in progress to be visualized and evaluated to

determine the degree to which further osteoplasty is necessary. By periodically stopping and evaluating the progress of the surgeon's efforts, modifications necessary to achieve the desired results can be seen, so as not to overreduce or underreduce the torus.

The osteoplasty will be extended distally to thin the lingual marginal bone and the mylohyoid ridge as it extends obliquely from the apex of the first premolar to the distal of the retromolar triangle, meaning that the prominent mylohyoid ridge at the lingual and distal of the second molar will be reduced by osteoplasty (Fig. 23-30, B). The osteoplasty does nothing to reduce the shallow interproximal crater between the two premolars, but adequate osteoplasty will make ostectomy easier when it is started because the thin bone is easier to remove from the root (Fig. 23-30, C). Osteoplasty of the prominent mylohyoid ridge in the second molar area requires good flap access. Inadequate access to the retromolar area contributes significantly to only being able to complete partial reduction of the prominent mylohyoid ridge.

The clinical crown lengthening of #31 will initially involve osteoplasty of both #30 and #31, followed by ostectomy. To easily perform ostectomy, the thick lingual bone in this area must be recontoured by osteoplasty. Inexperienced resective surgeons are often hesitant at flap

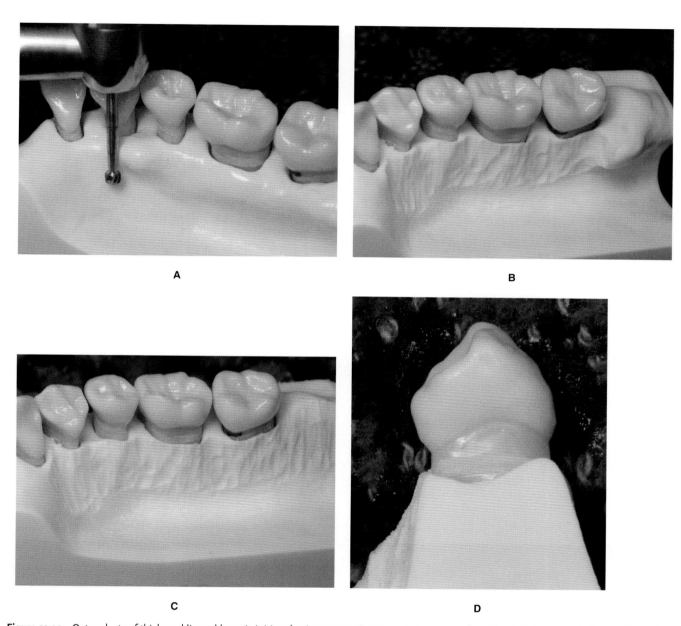

A

B

C

D

Figure 23-30. Osteoplasty of thickened lingual bone is initiated using an anterior-to-posterior approach until satisfactory completion. **A,** Osteoplasty is performed using a light feather brush stroke in an apical–occlusal direction, starting at the most mesial involvement and progressing distally. **B,** On completion of torus reduction, osteoplasty progresses distally, continuing to use rotary instrument in a light apical–occlusal stroke. Excellent flap access is required, especially in the posterior lingual area. Without adequate access, a thick and sharp portion of mylohyoid ridge is often left by a novice surgeon. The flap must be protected from the rotating bur by placement of a retractor between the tissue and the bur. **C,** Adequate lingual osteoplasty reduces the thickened mylohyoid ridge to the distal of the retromolar area and makes ostectomy an easier task, because there is less supporting bone thickness to remove. **D,** Distal of first premolar interproximal cross-section demonstrating result of osteoplasty. The bone contour is thinner in this region (compare to Fig. 23-29, **B**), but no ostectomy has yet been performed.

reflection in the retromolar region, which often results in incomplete exposure and reduction of the enlarged mylohyoid ridge. Partial reduction results in the creation of a sharp bony spicule. The postoperative result of such sharp bony aberrations during osteoplasty is flap perfora-

tion during healing. Such perforations can also be caused by catching the lingual flap with a rotary instrument in a high-speed handpiece. These perforations are difficult to suture and often present a stormy postoperative course. **The undersurface of the lingual flap should be protected**

from the rotating bur by proper placement of a flap retractor between the flap and the bur.

The buccal osteoplasty over the first molar is started with a #8 surgical length round bur. This too should be done in an apical–occlusal direction (Fig. 23-31, *A*). Thinning of the buccal bone on #30 will be extended to include the buccal of the second molar, and to the midline of the second premolar, to blend the osteoplasty contouring into the adjacent anatomy (Fig. 23-31, *B*). No osteoplasty or ostectomy is necessary on the buccal of the canine or two premolars.

The elimination of the shallow interproximal crater between the premolars will be accomplished by ramping the defect to the lingual (Fig. 23-32). Reduction of the lingual wall of the crater leaves bone on the lingual radicular surfaces and the distolingual line angle of #28 and the mesiolingual line angle of #29 positioned at a further occlusal level than the lingual proximal bone level. This is commonly referred to as *reverse architecture*. The reverse architecture in these areas is reduced using the end-cutting bur to blend the marginal bone at the line angles and on the radicular surfaces smoothly into the proximal bone, with no irregularities or thin spines to create a base from which the gingiva will establish itself. Alternative instrumentation can be either the Ochsenbein #1 chisel or the Wedelstaedt chisel, with the assistance of the Tibbetts back-action chisels. The object is to create a scalloped architecture similar to the preoperative scalloped gingival form. In cases of more advanced periodontal destruction, reverse architecture may not be completely eliminated, to prevent excessive removal of bone on adja-cent root surfaces. This compromise may result in some residual pocket depths after healing.

The clinical crown lengthening of #31 requires ostectomy on both #30 and #31 (Fig. 23-33, *A* and *C*). The amount of ostectomy is determined by the position of the apical margin of the eventual restoration. It is desirable to attain a distance of approximately 4 mm between the restoration margin and the most coronal bony margin. Beginning at the lingual proximal surfaces of both #30 and #31, the end-cutting bur is used to remove supporting bone around the affected line angles of both teeth and to scallop the bone over the distolingual root surface of #30 and the mesiolingual root surface of #31. Exposure of the lingual furcation entrances should be avoided. No supporting bone is removed from the buccal surface, but a lingually inclined ramping slope is created to provide adequate root surface exposure for restorative purposes (Fig. 23-33, *B*).

Final Assessment of the Surgical Area

Once the resective osseous recontouring is completed, the bony architecture is closely evaluated, from the same series of views used before surgery, to determine whether further ostectomy/osteoplasty in needed to achieve the desired results. The flaps are positioned and closed on a trial basis, contoured if necessary to an appropriate level, and the surgical area palpated again to determine the need for further recontouring. On obtaining the desired results, the area is sutured closed. Good presurgical planning frequently results in minimal soft tissue changes being necessary.

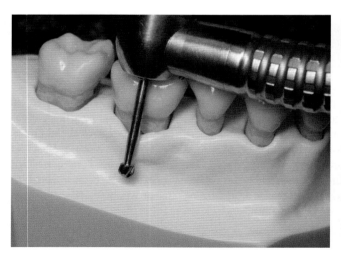

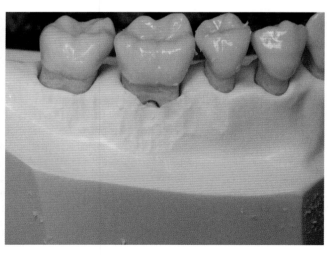

A

B

Figure 23-31. Buccal osteoplasty is limited to the first molar and approximately one half of a tooth in both a mesial and distal direction. **A,** Osteoplasty is initiated over first molar, continuing with use of rotary instrumentation in an apical–occlusal direction with periodic evaluation of necessity of further osteoplasty. **B,** View of completed buccal osteoplasty from midradicular surface of second premolar to interradicular surface between second molar roots.

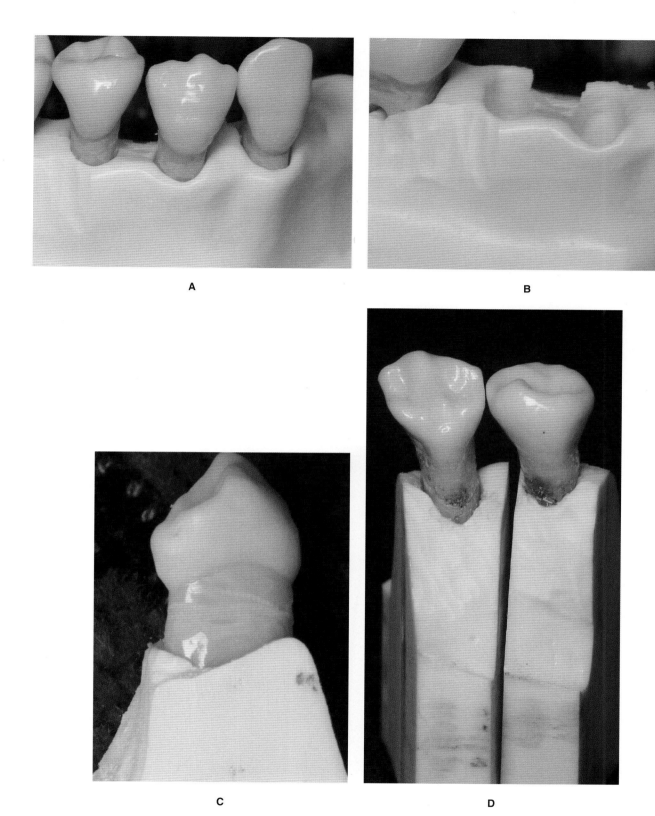

Figure 23-32. Shallow interdental crater between premolars is ramped lingually, with ostectomy only necessary on the distal and lingual surfaces of first premolar, and mesial and lingual surfaces of second premolar. **A,** Buccal view of effects on lingual ramping of crater between premolars. No buccal support was sacrificed. **B,** With premolars removed, a clearer concept is gained of the effect of only ramping interdental crater to lingual, with no ostectomy. Reverse architecture is present, with the interproximal bone adjacent to the canine and the first molar at a more apical level than the midlingual bone on the premolars. The peaks of bone must be removed, and the bone scalloped along the lingual surface of the premolars. **C,** Cross-sectional view of distal of first premolar, showing effect of ramping interproximal defect to lingual. The peak of bone on the distolingual line angle, often referred to as a *widow's peak*, must be removed through ostectomy. **D,** Lingual block section of both premolars after completion of osteoplasty/ostectomy. Shaded root surface areas represent supporting bone lost in resective surgical procedure to establish a scalloped physiologic architectural form.

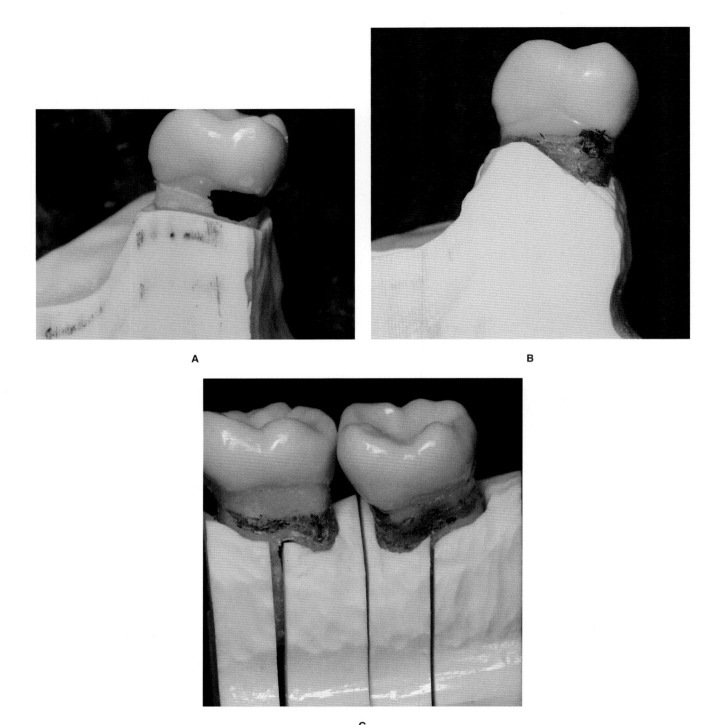

A

B

C

Figure 23-33. Crown lengthening for restorative purposes requires exposure of adequate root surface beyond decayed tooth margin for restoration margin placement and physiologic attachment apparatus (approximately 4 mm). **A,** Mesial interproximal cross section of second molar with mesiolingual decay after osteoplasty on both buccal and lingual surfaces. **B,** Mesial interproximal cross-section post-resective view of second molar, illustrating amount of interproximal bone and lingual radicular bone sacrificed in restorative crown lengthening procedure. **C,** Lingual view of the bony physiologic architecture after completion of restorative crown lengthening procedure. Shaded root surfaces represent loss of supporting bone with procedure. Note there is no furcation involvement, because this molar has moderate root trunk length and the lingual furcation entrance is positioned further apically than the buccal furcation entrance.

WOUND HEALING AFTER OSSEOUS SURGERY

The wound healing of the soft tissue component of the osseous resective surgical procedure is the same as that described for flap debridement in the previous section of this chapter (see also Chapter 20). Wound healing events will vary depending on a number of variables: management of soft tissues during incision, flap thinning, flap elevation, and flap closure; the extent of attachment loss; the configuration of the osseous defects; and the amount of trauma to which the periodontium is exposed during the surgical procedure.

Osteoplasty and osteoectomy produces an additional amount of surgical trauma. Osteoplasty reduces the volume of the bony periodontium; however, it does not immediately reduce the height of attachment of the periodontium. The trauma associated with the surgery, however, subsequently leads to some bony resorption, and thus the loss of attachment. Patients subjected to frequent reflection and debridement alone, without osteoplasty, displayed a mean loss in alveolar bone height of 0.2 mm 6 months after surgery.[54,103] Remodeling after osteoplasty is similar to that which occurs after debridement alone,[104] except that grinding during ostectomy/osteoplasty contributes to greater bone loss. Osteoplasty in seven patients using full-thickness flaps showed a mean loss of crestal bone height of 0.62 mm, with the patients having the thinnest radicular bone consistently demonstrating the most bone loss,[105] which is comparable to that reported in other studies.[75,104,106]

Osteoectomy results in an immediate loss of bony attachment, as well as some additional attachment loss during remodeling. The resection of the walls of interdental bony defects results in a reduction in height of the alveolus and a loss of connective tissue attachment on affected and adjacent teeth. The procedure results in the elimination of the angular bony defects and reduction in the height of the interdental soft tissue.[107] If patients are appropriately selected (early to moderate periodontitis, with one-wall, two-wall, or combination defects) and skillfully treated, the extent of ostectomy is a mean of about 0.6 mm circumferentially around the affected tooth.[54,108] The greatest extent of resection occurs at the line angles and on the facial or lingual surfaces, or both. Proponents of osseous resection believe that this loss of attachment is justified to eliminate the periodontal pockets and facilitate long-term maintenance of the patient.[108-110]

Exposure of the interdental bony crest usually does not permanently alter the attachment level significantly. Although some resorption of the crest may occur during the immediate postoperative period, by 6 months the interdental crest appears to reform, and the extent of interdental loss, as determined by direct sounding to bone crest, is commonly not measurable by routine clinical means.[54] If the facial and lingual bony periodontium is relatively thick and the trauma is minimized by good surgical technique, a similar result occurs. However, if the facial/lingual plates of bone over the radicular surfaces are thin, affected by bony dehiscences or fenestrations, or subjected to significant trauma from heat generated during surgical instrumentation, a substantial degree of bony resorption may occur. In general, osseous resection of thick bone results in less overall loss of bone height than similar procedures done in areas of thin bone.

The bony architecture produced during resective osseous surgery is quite stable if the patient is well maintained free of significant inflammation. According to Matheson, "alveolar bone is capable of maintaining surgically produced contour and soft tissue is reflective of that contour." Matheson also states that osseous resection "appears to be more effective in maintaining surgical contour than interdental osteoplasty alone."[107]

CLINICAL CROWN LENGTHENING: RESECTIVE SURGERY AS A PERIODONTAL–RESTORATIVE INTERFACE

Presurgical Considerations

Esthetic dentistry has become a buzzword for the patient and the dentist. Referrals are often made for a crown lengthening procedure with the request that esthetics not be compromised. There are, however, two different types of surgical crown lengthening, and both are basic surgical concepts based on biologic principles that delineate how clinical crown lengthening can be accomplished. These principles and concepts are based on anatomic relations including those of the dentogingival junction, tooth morphotypes, gingival contours, root trunk anatomy, and width/thickness of gingival tissues. The literature states that from 3 to 5.5 mm of tooth must be exposed in crown lengthening, measuring from the alveolar crest occlusally to the most apical margin of the restoration.[111-115] Such principles and concepts are sometimes not appreciated when the requests for surgical crown lengthening are made by the restorative dentist. One definite misconception is that crown lengthening is a single tooth procedure, which is clearly untrue. Attempting surgical crown lengthening on a single tooth results in inconsistent gingival margins that are difficult to maintain.[112] Such procedures do not take periodontal tissue behavior and anatomy into consideration. By extending the procedure to include, at least minimally, the teeth mesial and distal to the problem area, adequate crown lengthening can be achieved, as well as an anatomic form that is maintainable in an otherwise healthy periodontium.

Surgical crown lengthening is therefore a procedure needing discussion with both the restorative dentist and the patient, but particularly in the following situations:

1. It may compromise esthetics
2. There will be compromised periodontal support after surgery
3. There is a high smile line and the affected teeth are visible
4. There is moderate periodontal disease with horizontal bone loss
5. There is furcation involvement

During these circumstances, selective extraction should sometimes be considered as a possible alternative in conjunction with a ridge preservation procedure, followed by tooth replacement with either an implant-retained restoration or a fixed partial denture.

Indications for Surgical Crown Lengthening

Rosenberg and colleagues[113] listed the following indications for surgical crown lengthening:

1. Tooth decay at or below the gingival margin
2. Tooth fracture below the gingival margin, with adequate remaining periodontal support and attachment
3. Teeth with excessive occlusal or incisal wear
4. Teeth with insufficient interocclusal space for necessary restorative procedures
5. Delayed passive eruption (where the gingival margin is coronal to the CEJ) for esthetic or restorative purposes

An Alternative to Surgical Crown Lengthening: Orthodontic Forced Eruption

An alternative to surgical crown lengthening of a single tooth is orthodontic crown lengthening by forced eruption. Such a procedure offers a method of treating a nonrestorable tooth by extruding it orthodontically for the placement of a dowel core, on which a crown will be placed. It requires extrusion to expose at least 1 to 2 mm of solid tooth structure for the fabrication of the dowel core, and it also requires adequate supporting root length for the procedure to be successful. The crown that is placed on the tooth must encircle the tooth structure (ferrule effect) apical to the core to prevent fracture by the dowel.[112]

Surgical Crown Lengthening for Restorative Purposes

Crown lengthening for restorative purposes is begun after the administration of the necessary sedation and local anesthetic, as indicated. Inverse bevel submarginal incisions are made in the presence of a moderate to thick biotype, preserving as much labial gingiva as possible (Fig. 23-34). Presurgically there should be a band of gingiva at least 3 mm in width to allow a final postsurgical gingival width of at least 2 mm. In the presence of a thin biotype, initial sulcular incisions should be used, with gentle tissue handling, to maintain all of the keratinized tissue. On flap reflection, the granulation tissue is removed. An evaluation of the clinical crown coronal to the alveolar crest is made to determine how much clinical crown exposure is necessary or whether simple apical positioning of the flaps will create adequate clinical crown length (Fig. 23-34, C and D). The preoperative gingival form should act as a pattern for any bone reshaping that is necessary, particularly in reference to the difference between the labial and lingual/palatal radicular bone height and the interproximal crestal shape and height. If there is 3 mm or less of clinical crown from the alveolar crest, crown lengthening will be necessary to create 4 to 5.5 mm of clinical crown length. When contouring is necessary, osteoplasty with a #8 surgical length round bur is completed initially to thin the buccal and palatal/lingual plates, so that the bone removal necessary for crown lengthening by ostectomy will be easier to accomplish. The ostectomy is performed with the surgical length end-cutting bur or hand chisels until the appropriate amount of bone is removed circumferentially (Fig. 23-34, E). When the end-cutting bur is held parallel to the long axis of the tooth, the root surface is not scarred and most of the interproximal can be reached. Hand instruments can be used to finish any difficult to reach areas. Once the desired crown lengthening and bone form is achieved, the adjacent proximal teeth must also be lengthened and blended into a form that flows smoothly and slowly from proximal areas distal and mesial to the involved teeth to the apical position of the crown-lengthened tooth. The flaps are then positioned for trial apically positioned flap closure. Any necessary soft tissue modifications are made and the flaps are repositioned and sutured closed (Fig. 23-34, F and G). A periodontal dressing may be used to maintain flap stability, if needed. Within 6 to 8 weeks, the area should be ready for the restorative procedure (Fig. 23-34, H and I).

Crown Lengthening for Esthetics

When a patient has delayed passive eruption, or short clinical crowns, in the esthetic zone (Fig. 23-35, A), the objective is to give the patient normal clinical crown lengths without affecting or destroying the papillary form that fills the interproximal space (Fig. 23-35, B). Such loss of interdental papilla height will create "dark triangles" between the teeth. This situation requires a different surgical crown lengthening procedure.

Initially it must be determined how much the clinical crown should be lengthened, by establishing where the CEJ is located on the labial surface of the teeth, and if any ostectomy is necessary. Bone sounding under local

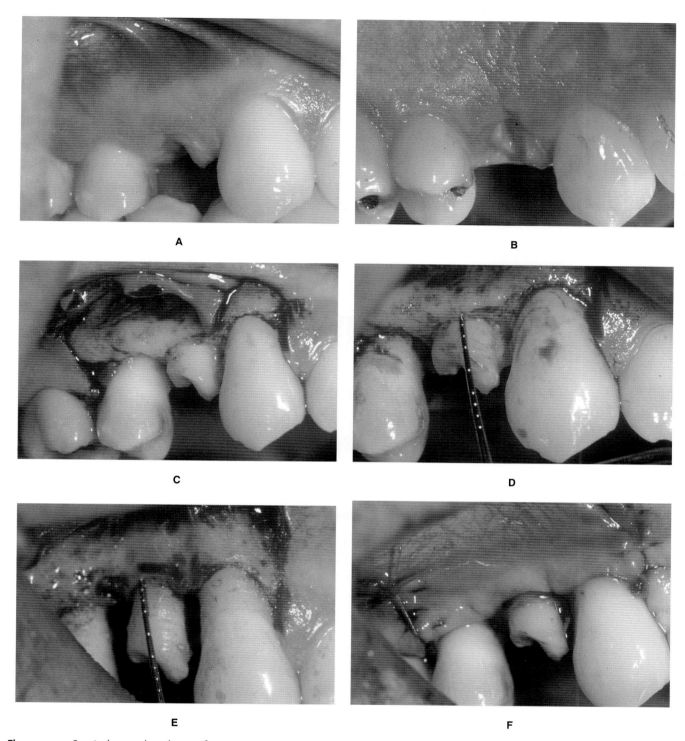

Figure 23-34. Surgical crown lengthening for restorative purpose cannot be performed successfully on a single tooth, but must include at least three teeth to facilitate blending resultant architectural features into a maintainable form. **A,** Buccal preoperative view of fractured first premolar clinical crown with inadequate tooth surfaces for restorative purposes. **B,** Lingual view of tooth fractured subgingivally. Probing depths are minimal. **C,** Flap reflection with vertical incisions for postsurgical apical flap positioning. Note relatively normal bone form and anatomy. **D,** Measuring root surface exposed coronal to bone height. **E,** Completion of osteoplasty and ostectomy, blending from more occlusally positioned proximal bone at mesial of canine and distal of second premolar, to more apically positioned bone levels at the mesial and distal of fracture tooth. The distance from the fracture line to the bony crest measures 5 mm. **F,** Buccal suturing of flap in an apical position. Suture positioning prevents apical flap displacement past desired position. Application of surgical dressing, if needed, prevents occlusal flap displacement.

Continued

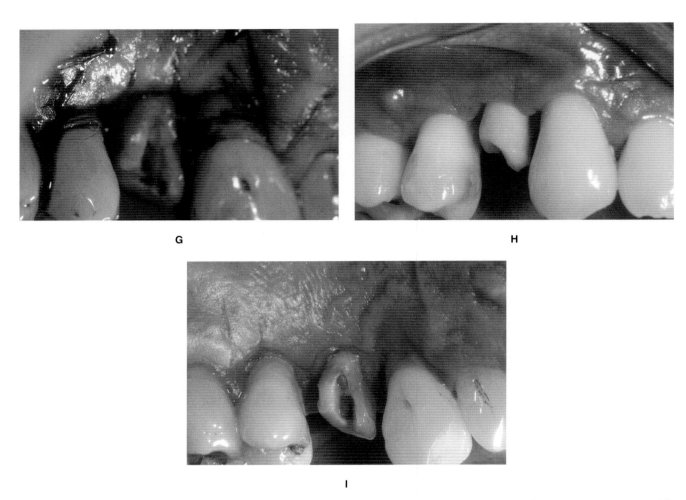

G

H

I

Figure 23-34. cont'd G, Palatal flap suturing, using interrupted sutures for vertical incisions, and a continuous sling suture to prevent apical flap positioning beyond desired level. **H,** Buccal postoperative view at 6 weeks. **I,** Lingual postoperative view at 6 weeks.

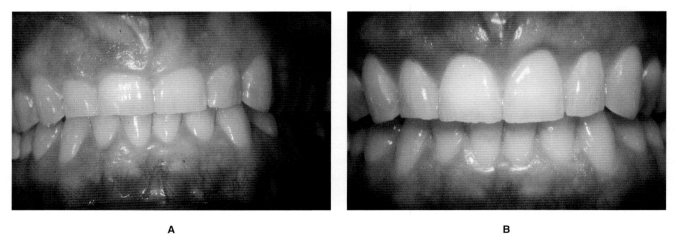

A

B

Figure 23-35. Short clinical crowns of concern to the patient can often be treated with esthetic crown lengthening, resulting in normal clinical crown lengths and no loss of interdental papillae. **A,** Preoperative short clinical crowns of concern to the patient and family. **B,** Postesthetic crown lengthening at 6-month postoperative visit.

anesthesia can identify the CEJ and its position relative to the bony crest. If the bony margin is 2 to 3 mm apical to the CEJ, osseous resection may not be required. If the bony margin is less than 2 mm apical to the CEJ, osseous resection will most likely be indicated. Ostectomy must be performed in such a manner that the bony crest follows the contour of the CEJ, which in the anterior region of the mouth has a much more scalloped form than in the posterior region. The flaps must be intimately adapted to the underlying bone and to one another in the interproximal region. Atraumatic suturing with small diameter suture will help minimize trauma to the papillary tissues and prevent recession in this area (see Chapter 21).

Resective Osseous Therapy in Treatment

The current American Academy of Periodontology Practice Profile Survey lists osseous surgery as the most commonly used form of periodontal surgery.[116] Despite this, osseous resective surgery is not a technique that is easily learned, because optimal performance of the procedure requires an in-depth knowledge of periodontal and dental anatomy and the proper application of basic surgical principles. Furthermore, the anatomic factors important to osseous resective surgery are not always taken into consideration when performing the procedure. It is a procedure best applied to early or moderate attachment loss. Osseous resective therapy is not applicable to the treatment of a single tooth in a contiguous arch because of the physiologic and anatomic behavior patterns of the periodontium. Taking the various anatomic factors reviewed earlier in this chapter into consideration, a minimum of three or more teeth and/or anatomic spaces are necessary for inclusion in osseous resective surgery to create a satisfactory architectural form that will be maintained.

If success after periodontal surgery is related to the degree of plaque control that is established and thereafter maintained, it appears to be a rational decision to apply the surgical procedure that will produce a periodontium that is most easily maintained by the patient and dental therapists. When appropriately applied, resective surgery provides a predictable means of eliminating or reducing the depth of periodontal pockets, establishing physiologic dimensions for restorative crown lengthening procedures, creating esthetic crown lengths, and providing an oral environment that is readily maintained by the patient and dental auxiliaries.

REFERENCES

1. Garrett S: Periodontal regeneration around natural teeth, *Ann Periodontol* 1:626-670, 1996.
2. Tibbetts LS: Use of diagnostic probes for detection of periodontal disease, *J Am Dent Assoc* 78:549, 1969.
3. Prichard JF: The role of the roentgenogram in the diagnosis and prognosis of periodontal disease, *Oral Surg* 14:182, 1961.
4. Goldman HM: Gingivectomy indications, contraindications and method, *Am J Orthod* 32:323, 1946.
5. Ramfjord S: Gingivectomy—its place in periodontal therapy, *J Periodontol* 23:30, 1952.
6. Zentler A: Suppurative gingivitis with alveolar involvement. A new surgical procedure, *JAMA* 71:1530, 1918.
7. Goldman HM: Gingivectomy, *Oral Surg* 4:1136, 1951.
8. Goldman HM: The development of physiologic gingival contours by gingivoplasty, *Oral Surg* 3:879, 1950.
9. Glickman I: The gingivectomy technique. In *Clinical periodontology*, ed 4, Philadelphia, 1972, WB Saunders.
10. Gottsegen R: Should the teeth be scaled prior to surgery? *J Periodontol* 32:301, 1961.
11. Glickman I: The results obtained with an unembellished gingivectomy technic in a clinical study in humans, *J Periodontol* 27:247, 1956.
12. Wennstrom J: Regeneration of gingiva following surgical excision. A clinical study, *J Clin Periodontol* 10:287, 1983.
13. Ainamo J, Loe H: Anatomical characteristics of gingiva—a clinical and microscopic study of the free and attached gingiva, *J Periodontol* 37:5, 1966.
14. Bowers GM: A study of the width of attached gingiva, *J Periodontol* 34:201, 1963.
15. Fox L: Rotating abrasives in the management of periodontal soft and hard tissues, *Oral Surg Oral Med Oral Path* 8:1134, 1955.
16. Ochsenbein C: Ledge and Wedge Technique. Formal Presentation, American Academy of Periodontology, Las Vegas, Nev., 1965.
17. Schluger S, Yuodelis RA, Page RC, Johnson RH: Principles of periodontal surgery. In *Periodontal disease*, ed 2, Philadelphia, 1990, Lea & Febiger.
18. Schluger S, Yuodelis RA, Page RC, Johnson RH: Resective surgery. In *Periodontal disease*, ed 2, Philadelphia, 1990, Lea & Febiger.
19. Oringer MJ: Electrosurgery for definitive conservative modern periodontal therapy, *Dent Clin North Am* 13:53, 1969.
20. Loe H: Chemical gingivectomy. Effect of potassium hydroxide on periodontal tissues, *Acta Odontol Scand* 19:517, 1961.
21. Pick RM, Pecaro BC, Silberman CJ: The laser gingivectomy: the use of CO_2 laser for the removal of phenytoin hyperplasia, *J Periodontol* 56:492, 1985.
22. Catone GA: Lasers in periodontal surgery. In Catone GA, Aling CC, editors, *Laser applications in oral and maxillofacial surgery*, Philadelphia, 1997, WB Saunders, pp 181-196.
23. Eisenmann D, Malone WF, Kusek J: Electron microscopic evaluation of electrosurgery, *Oral Surg Oral Med Oral Path* 29:660, 1970.

24. Malone WF, Eisenmann D, Kusch J: Interceptive periodontics with electrosurgery, *J Prosthet Dent* 22:555, 1969.

25. Pope JW, Gargiulo AW, Staffileno H, Levy S: Effects of electrosurgery on wound healing in dogs, *Periodontics* 6:30, 1968.

26. Nixon KC, Adkins KF, Keys DW: Histologic evaluation of effects produced in alveolar bone following gingival incision with an electrosurgical scalpel, *J Periodontol* 46:40, 1975.

27. Glickman I, Imber IR: Comparison of gingival resection with electrosurgery and periodontal knives—a biometric and histologic study, *J Periodontol* 41:142, 1970.

28. Wilhemsen NR, Ramfjord SP, Blankenship JR: Effects of electrosurgery on the gingival attachment in Rhesus monkeys, *J Periodontol* 47:160, 1976.

29. Tonna E, Stahl SS: A polarized light microscopic study of rat periodontal ligament following surgical and chemical gingival trauma, *Helv Odontol Acta* 11:90, 1967.

30. Fisher SE, Frame JW, Browne RM, Tranter RMD: A comparative histological study of wound healing following CO_2 laser and conventional surgical excision of the buccal mucosa, *Arch Oral Biol* 28:287, 1983.

31. Pogrel MA, Yen CK, Hansen LS: A comparison of carbon dioxide laser, liquid nitrogen cryosurgery and scalpel wounds in healing, *Oral Surg Oral Med Oral Pathol* 69:269, 1990.

32. McDavid VG, Cobb CM, Rapley JW et al: Laser irradiation of bone. III. Long-term healing following treatment by CO_2 and Nd:YAG laser, *J Periodontol* 72:174, 2001.

33. Moritz A, Schoop U, Goharkhayi K, Sperr W: Treatment of periodontal pockets with a diode laser, *Lasers Surg Med* 22:302, 1998.

34. Loumanen M: A comparative study of healing of laser and scalpel incision wounds in the rat oral mucosa, *Scand J Dent Res* 95:65, 1987.

35. American Academy of Periodontology: Lasers in periodontics, *J Periodontol* 73:1231, 2002.

36. Sachs HA, Farnoush A, Checchi L, Joseph CE: Current status of periodontal dressings, *J Periodontol* 55:689, 1984.

37. Watts TAP, Combe EC: Periodontal dressing materials, *J Clin Periodontol* 6:3, 1979.

38. Ward AW: The surgical eradication of pyorrhea, *J Am Dent Assoc* 15:2146, 1928.

39. Ward AW: Postoperative care in the surgical treatment of pyorrhea, *J Am Dent Assoc* 16:635, 1929.

40. Haugen E, Gjermo P, Orstavik D: Some antibacterial properties of periodontal dressings, *J Clin Periodontol* 4:62, 1977.

41. Haugen E, Mjor IA: Bone tissue reactions to periodontal dressings, *J Periodont Res* 14:76, 1979.

42. Koch G, Magnusson B, Nyquist G: Contact allergy to medicaments and materials used in dentistry. IV. Sensitizing effect of eugenol/rosin in surgical dressing, *Odontol Revy* 24:109, 1973.

43. Levin MP, Cutright DE, Bhaskar SN: Cyanoacrylate as a periodontal dressing, *J Oral Med* 30:40, 1975.

44. Baer PN, Sumner CF, Scigliano J: Studies on a hydrogenated fat-zinc bacitracin periodontal dressing, *Oral Surg* 13:494, 1960.

45. Sanz M, Newman MG, Anderson L et al: Clinical enhancement of post-periodontal surgical therapy by a 0.12 per cent chlorhexidine gluconate mouthrinse, *J Periodontol* 60:570, 1989.

46. Donnenfeld OW, Glickman I: A biometric study of the effects of gingivectomy, *J Periodontol* 37:447, 1966.

47. Engler W, Ramfjord S, Hiniker JJ: Healing following simple gingivectomy. A tritiated thymidine radioautographic study. I. Epithelialization, *J Periodontol* 37:298, 1966.

48. Ramfjord SP, Engler WD, Hiniker JJ: A radioautographic study of healing following simple gingivectomy. II. The connective tissue, *J Periodontol* 37:179, 1966.

49. Stahl SS, Slavkin HC, Yamada L, Levine S: Speculations about gingival repair, *J Periodontol* 43:395, 1972.

50. Afshar-Mohajer K, Stahl SS: The remodeling of human gingival tissues following gingivectomy, *J Periodontol* 48:136, 1977.

51. Palcanis KG: Surgical pocket therapy, *Ann Periodontol* 1:589-617, 1996.

52. Waite IM: A comparison between conventional gingivectomy and a non-surgical regime in the treatment of periodontitis, *J Clin Periodontol* 3:173, 1976.

53. Ammons WF, Smith DH: Flap curettage: rationale, technique, and expectations, *Dent Clin North Am* 20(1):215, 1976.

54. Smith DH, Ammons WF, Van Belle G: A longitudinal study of periodontal status comparing osseous recontouring with flap curettage. 1. Results after six months, *J Periodontol* 51:367, 1980.

55. Townsend-Olsen C, Ammons WF, Van Belle C: A longitudinal study comparing apically repositioned flaps, with and without osseous surgery, *Int J Periodontics Restorative Dent* 5(4):11, 1985.

56. Ramfjord SP, Nissle RR: The modified Widman flap, *J Periodontol* 45:601, 1974.

57. Ramfjord SP, Knowles JW, Nissle RR et al: Longitudinal study of periodontal therapy, *J Periodontol* 44:66, 1973.

58. Ramfjord SP, Knowles JW, Nissle RR et al: Results following three modalities of periodontal therapy, *J Periodontol* 46:522, 1975.

59. Caton J, Nyman S: Histometric evaluation of periodontal surgery. I. The Modified Widman flap procedure, *J Clin Periodontol* 7:212, 1980.

60. Caton J, Nyman S: Histometric evaluation of periodontal surgery. II. Connective tissue attachment level after four regenerative procedures, *J Clin Periodontol* 7:224, 1980.

61. Kaldahl WB, Kalkwarf KL, Patil KD et al: Evaluation of four modalities of periodontal therapy. Mean probing

depth, probing attachment level and recession changes, *J Periodontol* 59:783, 1988.

62. Kaldahl WB, Kalkwarf KL, Patil KD et al: Long term evaluation of periodontal therapy. I. Response to 4 therapeutic modalities, *J Periodontol* 67:103, 1996.

63. Levine HL: Periodontal flap surgery with gingival fiber retention, *J Periodontol* 43:91, 1972.

64. Levine HL, Stahl SS: Repair following periodontal flap surgery with the retention of gingival fibers, *J Periodontol* 43:99, 1972.

65. Caton J, Zander HA: The attachment between tooth and gingival tissues after periodic root planing and soft tissue curettage, *J Periodontol* 50:462, 1979.

66. Ramfjord SP, Knowles JW, Nissle RR et al: Results following three modalities of periodontal therapy, *J Periodontol* 46:522, 1975.

67. Braden BE: Deep distal pockets adjacent to terminal teeth, *Dent Clin North Am* 13(1):161, 1969.

68. Robinson RE: The distal wedge operation, *Periodontics* 4(5):256, 1966.

69. Schluger S, Yuodelis RA, Page RC, Johnson RH: Resective periodontal surgery in pocket elimination. In *Periodontal disease*, ed 2, Philadelphia, 1990, Lea & Febiger, pp 501-526.

70. Tibbetts LS, Loughlin DM: Management of problems in the posterior maxilla and mandible. In Clark JW, editor: *Clinical dentistry 3*, Hagerstown, Md., Lippincott, 1985, D-9:1-25.

71. Kramer GM, Schwartz MS: A technique to obtain primary healing in pocket elimination adjacent to edentulous areas, *Periodontics* 2:252, 1964.

72. Tibbetts LS, Shanelec D: Periodontal microsurgery, *Dent Clin North Am* 42(2):339-359, 1998.

73. Sichel H, Dubrul EL: *Oral anatomy*, ed 5, St. Louis, 1970, CV Mosby, p 487.

74. Wylam JM, Mealey BL, Mills MP et al: The clinical effectiveness of open versus closed scaling and root planing on multi-rooted teeth, *J Periodontol* 64:1023, 1993.

75. Kohler CA, Ramfjord SP: Healing of gingival mucoperiosteal flaps, *Oral Surg Oral Med Oral Path* 13:89, 1960.

76. Hirshfeld I, Wasserman B: A long-term survey of tooth loss in 600 treated periodontal patients, *J Periodontol* 49:225, 1978.

77. Black GV: *Special dental pathology*, Chicago, 1911, Medico-Dental Publishing.

78. Stern IB, Everett FC, Robicsek K: S. Robicsek—a pioneer in the surgical treatment of periodontal disease, *J Periodontol* 36:265, 1965.

79. Friedman N: Periodontal osseous surgery: osteoplasty and osteoectomy, *J Periodontol* 26:257, 1955.

80. Ochsenbein C: A primer for osseous surgery, *Int J Periodontics Restorative Dent* 6(1):9, 1986.

81. Gargiulo AW, Wentz FM, Orban B: Dimensions of the dentinogingival junction in humans, *J Periodontol* 32:261, 1961.

82. Dempster WI, Adams WJ, Duddles RA: Arrangement in the jaws of the roots of teeth, *J Am Dent Assoc* 67:7, 1963.

83. Krause SK, Jordan RE, Abrams L: The dentition: it's alignment and articulation. In *Dental anatomy and occlusion*, Baltimore, Md, 1969, Williams and Wilkins, pp 226-228.

84. Ritchey B, Orban B: The crest of the interdental alveolar septa, *J Periodontol* 24:75, 1953.

85. O'Connor WT, Biggs NL: Interproximal bone contours, *J Periodontol* 35:326, 1964.

86. Kronfeld R: Condition of alveolar bone underlying periodontal pockets, *J Periodontol* 6:22, 1935.

87. Waerhaug J: The infrabony pocket and its relationship to trauma from occlusion and subgingival plaque, *J Periodontol* 50:355, 1979.

88. Stahl SS, Canter M, Zwig E: Fenestrations of the labial alveolar plate in human skulls, *Periodontics* 1:99, 1963.

89. Wilderman MN, Pennel BM, King K, Barron JM: Histogenesis of repair following osseous surgery, *J Periodontol* 41:551, 1967.

90. Goldman HM, Cohen DW: The infrabony pocket: classification and treatment, *J Periodontol* 29:272, 1958.

91. Manson JD, Nicholson K: The distribution of bone defects in chronic periodontitis, *J Periodontol* 54:88-92, 1974.

92. Manson JD: Bone morphology and bone loss in periodontal disease, *J Clin Periodontol* 3:14, 1976.

93. Neilson JI, Glavind L, Karring T: Interproximal periodontal intrabony defects: prevalence, location and etiological factors, *J Clin Periodontol* 7:187, 1980.

94. Tal H: Relationship between interproximal distance of roots and the prevalence of intrabony defects, *J Periodontol* 55:604, 1984.

95. Larato DC: Some anatomical factors related to furcation involvement, *J Periodontol* 46:608, 1975.

96. Papapanou PN, Tonetti MS: Diagnosis and epidemiology of periodontal osseous lesions, *Periodontol 2000* 22:8, 2000.

97. Papapanou PN, Wennstrom JL, Grondahl L: Periodontal status in relation to age and tooth type. A cross-sectional radiographic study, *J Clin Periodontol* 15:469, 1988.

98. Woulters FR, Salonen LE, Hellden LB et al: Prevalence of interproximal periodontal infrabony defects in an adult population in Sweden. A radiographic study, *J Clin Periodontol* 16:144, 1989.

99. Easley J: Methods of determining alveolar osseous form, *J Periodontol* 38:112, 1967.

100. Ochsenbein C, Bohannan HM: The palatal approach to osseous surgery I. Rationale, *J Periodontol* 34:60, 1963.

101. Ochsenbein C, Bohannan HM: The palatal approach to osseous surgery II. Clinical application, *J Periodontol* 35:54, 1964.

102. Tibbetts L, Ochsenbein C, Loughlin D: Rationale for the lingual approach to mandibular osseous surgery, *Dent Clin North Am* 20:61, 1976.

103. Wilderman MN, Wentz FM, Orban BJ: Histogenesis of repair after mucogingival surgery, *J Periodontol* 31:283, 1960.

104. Donnenfeld OW, Hoag PM, Weissman DP: A clinical study on the effects of osteoplasty, *J Periodontol* 41:131, 1970.

105. Wood DL, Hoag PM, Donnenfeld OW, Rosenfeld LD: Alveolar crest reduction following full and partial thickness flaps, *J Periodontol* 43:141, 1972.

106. Tavtigian R: The height of the facial radicular alveolar crest following apically positioned flap operations, *J Periodontol* 41:412, 1970.

107. Matheson DG: An evaluation of healing following periodontal osseous surgery in monkeys, *Int J Periodontics Restorative Dent* 8(5):9, 1988.

108. Selipsky HS: Osseous surgery. How much need we compromise? *Dent Clin North Am* 20(1):79, 1976.

109. Caton J, Nyman S: Histometric evaluation of periodontal surgery. III. The effect of bone resection on the connective tissue attachment level, *J Periodontol* 52:405, 1981.

110. Schluger S: Osseous resection: a basic principle in periodontal surgery, *Oral Surg Oral Med Oral Path* 2:316, 1949.

111. Maynard Jr JG, Wilson RDK: Physiologic dimensions of the periodontium significant to the restorative dentist, *J Periodontol* 50:170, 1979.

112. Becker W, Ochsenbein C, Becker BE: Crown lengthening: the periodontal-restorative connection, *Compend Contin Educ Dent* 19:239, 1998.

113. Rosenberg ES, Garber DA, Evian CI: Tooth lengthening procedures, *Compend Contin Educ Dent* 1:161, 1980.

114. Ingber JS, Rose LF, Coslet JG: The biologic width: A concept in periodontics and restorative dentistry, *Alpha Omegan* 10:62, 1977.

115. Wagenberg BD, Eskow RN, Langer B: Exposing adequate tooth structure for restorative dentistry, *Int J Periodontics Restorative Dent* 9:323-331, 1989.

116. The American Academy of Periodontology: 2000 Practice Profile Survey: characteristics and trends in private periodontal practice, 2001, p 132.

24

Treatment of Molar Furcations

William F. Ammons, Jr.

Loss of attachment in the furcation area has long been considered an adverse event in the prognosis of multi-rooted teeth. The furcation is an area of complex anatomy and its involvement complicates treatment planning and the performance of therapeutic procedures, and directly affects the ability of both the patient and therapist to successfully maintain the dentition after active treatment. A thorough knowledge of the anatomy of the furcation is as essential to successful treatment as a mastery of the various methods of furcation therapy.

ETIOLOGY OF FURCATION INVOLVEMENT

The primary cause of furcation involvement is the progressive loss of attachment that results from inflammatory periodontal disease. In most patients, the response to bacterial plaque, in the absence of therapy, is a progressive and site-specific loss of attachment. Although the rate of response may vary from individual to individual, local anatomic factors that affect the deposition of plaque or hamper its removal can exert a significant impact on the development of attachment loss.[1-3] Local factors such as the defective margins of restorations and cervical enamel projections[4] complicate dental plaque removal, and in the case of the enamel projections, may represent biologic weak links in the attachment that decrease resistance to furcation involvement[5] (see Chapter 7). Variations in root form, dental anatomy, and dental anomalies may also play a role because the extent of attachment loss necessary to produce furcation involvement is related to the local anatomy of the affected tooth.[6,7] Root trunk length is a key factor that affects both the development of furcation involvement and the mode of treatment (Fig. 24-1).

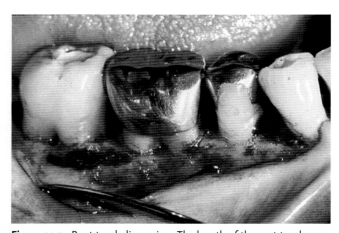

Figure 24-1. Root trunk dimension. The length of the root trunks may be highly variable. In very short root trunks, like these mandibular molars, the attachment level even with health may be near or at the entrance into the furca. The shorter the root trunk, the less attachment that has to be lost before involvement of the furcation.

Dental caries, pulpal disease, iatrogenic dentistry, and factitial injury can also contribute to furcation involvement. Because the prevalence and extent of attachment loss increases with age,[8] the prevalence and severity of furcation problems tend to be related to age.[9,10]

DIAGNOSIS OF FURCATION INVOLVEMENT

For most diseases, the sooner the disease is recognized and a diagnosis is established, the more effective the therapy will be and the better the long-term prognosis. This is true for inflammatory periodontal disease and is particularly relevant to the problem of treating furcation involvement. The earlier the clinician recognizes furcation involvement, the simpler the treatment required to manage the problem will be. Conversely, the greater the extent of attachment loss before furcation involvement is diagnosed, the more complicated the treatment required to manage the problem will be and the poorer the prognosis. The therapist needs to detect furcation problems before a significant amount of attachment is lost.

If an early diagnosis of furcation invasion is to occur, the therapist must be looking for furcation involvement. The entrance to the furcation can be quite small and difficult to identify. In 1979, Bower provided data about the anatomy and the mean width of the entrance into the furcation.[11,12] The entrance varies from 0.5 to 2.0 mm, but 58% of all furcations studied were narrower (≤0.75 mm) than commonly used periodontal curettes.[12] Early detection of furcation invasion, therefore, requires thorough periodontal probing with an instrument of an appropriate dimension. Probing of all potential furcation areas is an integral part of any thorough periodontal examination.[13] Treatment planning for the therapeutic management of furcation problems requires documenting the extent of furcation involvement, the morphology of the tooth and furcation, and the presence and configuration of any bony defects. In addition, the presence of developmental anomalies, the position of the tooth relative to adjacent teeth, and any local factors that may require correction during therapy should be identified and recorded in a systematic manner in the patient's electronic or paper chart using appropriate symbols. (The process of periodontal examination is described in Chapter 8.)

CLASSIFICATION OF FURCATION INVOLVEMENT

The need to document the extent and severity of furcation involvement has led to the development of a number of classification systems or indexes. These systems are usually based on the extent of horizontal and vertical involvement of the furcation and its relation to the adjacent soft and hard tissues. A number of systems have been developed to allow the clinician to classify the extent of furcation involvement. Among these systems are those developed by Glickman (1958),[14] Heins and Canter (1968),[15] Easley and Drennan (1969),[16] Hamp, Nyman, and Lindhe (1975),[17] and Tarnow and Fletcher (1984).[18] Although most systems record the horizontal extent of furcation involvement, the systems developed by Easley and Drennan and Tarnow and Fletcher also provide information about the vertical component of the furcation.

One of the most widely used furcation classification systems was developed by Glickman.[14] In this system, furcation involvement is divided into four categories, primarily on the basis of the horizontal component of destruction:

Grade I: Early furcation involvement just into the fluting of the furcation is present. There is no significant destruction of bone or connective tissue in the furcation proper.

Grade II: Distinct horizontal destruction of the furcation area is present. This lesion has been called a "cul de sac" because destruction may extend to any depth within the furcation, but does not extend all the way through the furcation to its other side. The extent of horizontal probing determines whether the Grade II furcation is shallow or deep. Vertical bone loss may or may not be present.

Grade III: Destruction of bone and connective tissue all the way through the furcation such that an instrument can be passed from its opening to its exit. The furcation defect is not visible to the eye because the gingival tissues cover the furcation entrance.

Grade IV: Destruction of bone and connective tissue all the way through the furcation. Gingival recession has occurred to the point that the entire furcation invasion can be seen on visual examination. A "tunnel" thus exists between the affected roots.

An example of various degrees of furcation involvement using Easley and Drennan's classification system is shown in Figure 24-2.[16] This classification system provides information relative to the vertical component of furcation involvement. Figure 24-2, *A*, is normal, with no significant attachment loss. Figure 24-2, *B*, demonstrates Class I furcation involvement because there is attachment loss that involves the root flutings, but there is no horizontal component to the involvement. In this classification system, Class II and III furcations (Fig. 24-2, *C* and *D*) are separated into subtypes 1 and 2 on the basis of the configuration of the alveolar bone at the entrance to the furcation. Horizontal resorption into the furca is subtype 1, whereas subtype 2 indicates a significant vertical component to the defect. This separation contributes to treatment planning as a vertical component may contribute to the ability to "fill" the deformity.

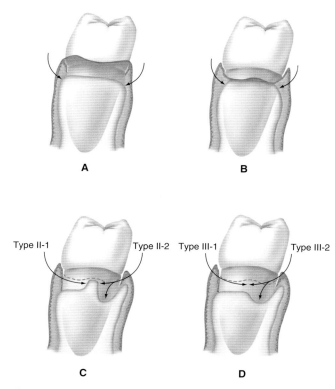

Figure 24-2. Easley and Drennan's classification of furcation involvement. **A,** Normal anatomy. No furcation involvement. **B,** Class I: Incipient involvement in which the fluting coronal to the furcation entrance is affected but there is no definite horizontal component to the furca. **C,** Class II: Type 1—A definite horizontal loss of attachment into the furcation, but the pattern of bone loss is essentially horizontal. There is no definite buccal or lingual ledge of bone. Type 2—There is a buccal or lingual bony ledge and a definite vertical component to the attachment loss. **D,** Class III: A through and through loss of attachment in the furcation. As with Class II furcation defects, the pattern of attachment loss may be horizontal (1) or there may be a vertical component (2) of varying depth.

THERAPEUTIC MANAGEMENT OF EARLY FURCATION INVOLVEMENT

The identification of incipient to early furcation involvement during a periodontal examination may or may not be an indication for treatment of the furcation problem. Although documentation of the furcation is essential for longitudinal monitoring of the site, the mere presence of furcation involvement may not be an indication for treatment. The presence of inflammatory periodontal disease and the etiologic and local factors that are associated with the disease are the keys to a making a treatment decision. Questions to be answered include the following: Does the patient have clinical signs of gingivitis or periodontitis?; Is marginal inflammation present?; Is the sulcus deepened (pocket depth)?; and Does the area bleed on periodontal probing? Second, are plaque, calculus, or an inflammatory exudate present? If so, therapy is indicated. However, the therapy required[14,19] is dependent not only on the presence of disease but on the local dental/periodontal anatomy associated with the disease.

For example, if the inflammation is related to the presence of bacterial plaque and there are no complicating local anatomic factors, the only therapy required may be the removal of the plaque. Although this may be accomplished by the therapist, a more permanent solution requires implementation, by the patient, of an oral hygiene program that will remove the plaque on an ongoing daily basis. If both plaque and calculus are present, scaling and root planing is required to resolve the inflammation. The presence of a local factor, such as an overhanging margin of a restoration or a cervical enamel projection,[4] requires not only the removal of the plaque and calculus but also the removal of the local factor. This may be accomplished by odontoplasty or may require the placement or replacement of a dental restoration.

THERAPY FOR MODERATE TO ADVANCED FURCATION INVOLVEMENT

A significant horizontal component to the furcation defines a Class II furcation. The primary objective of Class II furcation treatment is the production of a local environment that the patient and the dental therapist(s) can maintain free from further attachment loss. The treatment of a Class II furcation may be simple or may become relatively complex. Therapy for Class II furcations varies with the extent of the horizontal and vertical attachment loss, the configuration of any associated bony defect, and the anatomy of the tooth. The most successful long-term result will occur if the furcation can be obliterated.

Significant horizontal or vertical involvement of the furcation can pose a number of local anatomic problems that may complicate therapy. The furcation area of molars is not smooth and regular, but may be highly irregular in form.[6,20] Intermediate bifurcation ridges, which run in a mesial–distal direction at the entrance to the furcation, may result in a significant "domed" area being present.[20] If this domed area is exposed to the oral environment, it becomes a trap for plaque formation that is not readily accessible by the patient or a dental therapist. The efficacy and efficiency of furcation debridement by conventional instrumentation has been investigated. Studies suggest that it may be virtually impossible to effectively remove plaque and calculus from some furcations.[21-23] Such furcations can become continually inflamed and are potential sites for the development of dental caries and further attachment loss. The dome of the furcation is also a common exit site for accessory pulpal canals.[24] Although pulpal infection through accessory pulpal canals is theoretically possible, the current dental literature does not indicate that retrograde infection of the dental pulp from a periodontal pocket is a common source of pulpal pathosis.[25,26]

The variability in the size and configuration of the roots of mandibular and maxillary molars poses additional anatomic problems. For example, the dimension between the roots can vary significantly. The roots of molars may be fused, partially fused, closely approximated, or widely divergent. The dimension between closely approximated roots may be less than the width of curettes and ultrasonic scalers, and thus inaccessible to instrumentation.[12] Not only may the dimension between the roots preclude access for removal of plaque and calculus, but roots that are separated at the root trunk may become fused at their apex, further complicating therapy. In contrast with the distal roots of mandibular molars and the distobuccal roots of maxillary molars, which are generally rounded, the mesial root of mandibular molars and the mesiobuccal root of maxillary molars frequently have a deep vertical groove that extends from the dome of the furcation to near the apex of the root.[27] These grooves further complicate plaque removal and restoration of the root. The mesial root of such molars frequently is sharply curved and commonly has more than one pulp canal, which may complicate root canal treatment.

SURGICAL TREATMENT OF CLASS II FURCATION INVOLVEMENTS

A significant horizontal involvement of one or more furcations of a multirooted tooth, if combined with other local anatomic problems, is a common indication for the use of a surgical treatment approach. The primary indication for surgery is an inability to adequately instrument the furcation by routine scaling and root planing through the gingival sulcus. Persistence of inflammation or exudation after instrumentation, in the presence of good oral hygiene, indicates inadequate debridement and may dictate surgical debridement or the obliteration of the furcation to facilitate successful long-term maintenance. Different procedures with differing therapeutic objectives have been used successfully to treat molars with furcation involvement.

SURGICAL DEBRIDEMENT OF FURCATIONS

The most elementary surgical method used is debridement of the furcation by means of a periodontal flap procedure. Flap design and the process of surgical debridement are described in Chapters 20 and 23. The reflection of a flap provides access and visibility to the furcation. This facilitates the thorough removal of plaque, calculus, and any bacterial contaminants from the root surfaces of the furcation. If the bony resorption is of a horizontal nature without a significant intrabony (vertical) component or heavy ledging, thorough debridement will result in a resolution of inflammation and potentially to a diminishment of pocket depth because of tissue shrinkage or a gain in clinical attachment, or both.

Odontoplasty and Osteoplasty

The addition of odontoplasty or localized osteoplasty, or both, to surgical debridement, provides a means of further altering the physical dimension of the furcation defect in more advanced situations.[28,29] Odontoplasty provides a means of reducing the intermediate bifurcation ridge and the extent of dome over the furcation, thereby reducing the volume of the furcation defect.[28] Osteoplasty does the same for any bony deformity.[29] Reducing the physical dimension of bony ledges and placement of strategic grooving allows the therapist to reduce both the soft and hard tissue component of the furcation. The result is a shallow furcation area, which facilitates the patient's ability to remove plaque during oral hygiene. An example of the management of Class II furcations using a combination of debridement, odontoplasty, and osteoplasty is shown in Figure 24-3.

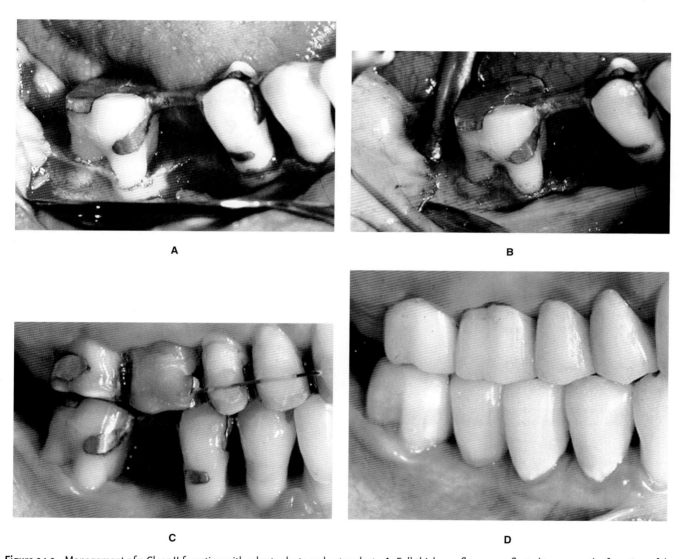

Figure 24-3. Management of a Class II furcation with odontoplasty and osteoplasty. **A,** Full-thickness flaps are reflected to expose the furcation of the mandibular right second molar and adjacent areas. Note the Class II, type 1 involvement. There are also combination one-, two-wall bony defects on the mesial and distal aspects of the molar. **B,** Odontoplasty has been performed to remove a portion of facial aspect of the furcation dome; osteoplasty has been performed to remove the horizontal component of the Class II furcation. In addition, osteoplasty and some ostectomy has been used to eliminate the adjacent bony deformities. **C,** Facial 3-week postoperative view. **D,** An 8-week postoperative view after placement of provisional restorations. Note that the provisional restoration reconstructs the desired fluting between the mesial and distal roots of the second molar, with a flat emergence profile extending coronally from the crown margin.

The efficacy of simply debridement procedures is generally limited to the buccal and lingual furcations of mandibular molars; the buccal furcations of maxillary molars with early to moderate degrees of involvement; and those furcations where aberrations in root/furcation morphology and significant osseous defects are absent. The long-term success of debridement procedures is ultimately dependent on access for plaque removal and the patient's willingness to perform daily oral hygiene procedures.

ROOT RESECTION

The simultaneous involvement of two furcations by deep Class II furcations or the presence of a Class III furcation may be an indication for removal of a root of a molar. Root resection is the process by which one or more roots of a tooth are removed at the level of the furcation while leaving the crown and remaining roots in function.[30] Root resection has been a component of the periodontal surgical armamentarium since the 1800s.[31,32] The indications and contraindications to root resection were well described by Basaraba in 1969[33] and are summarized in Boxes 24-1 and 24-2. The objective of root resection is the obliteration of the furcation as a problem in periodontal maintenance. Root resection, when performed in an appropriate and timely manner, can convert an affected tooth to a tooth free of a furcation defect.

The decision to use root resection during periodontal treatment should be carefully considered, because it commonly commits the patient not only to endodontics, but also frequently to a major restorative dentistry procedure. Root resection can be a costly and time-consuming procedure and often requires the patient to seek interdisciplinary care by a number of therapists. Therefore, the advantages, disadvantages, and treatment alternatives

---

Box 24-1　Indications for Root Resection

1. Severe vertical bone loss on one root of a multirooted tooth not amenable to regeneration/reattachment
2. Furcation invasion not correctable by odontoplasty
3. Proximal furcation invasion in combination with root approximation
4. Furcation invasion that is not maintainable
5. Periodontally involved abutment teeth with a hopeless prognosis associated with one root
6. Vertical or horizontal root fracture
7. Uncorrectable root dehiscence
8. When endodontic therapy is impossible on one root of a multirooted tooth

Modified from Basaraba N: Root amputation and tooth hemisection, Dent Clin North Am 13(1):121, 1969.

Box 24-2　Contraindications to Root Resection

1. Advanced bone loss with an unfavorable crown-to-root ratio
2. Fused roots that cannot be separated
3. If an endodontically inoperable canal would be retained
4. If the remaining root(s) would be inadequate to serve as a prosthetic abutment
5. If indicated splinting cannot be performed
6. When periodontal support after resection is inadequate to withstand normal occlusal forces
7. Inability to create a good postsurgical gingival environment
8. If socioeconomic conditions preclude necessary treatment procedures
9. In the presence of inadequate oral hygiene

Modified from Basaraba N: Root amputation and tooth hemisection, Dent Clin North Am 13(1):121, 1969.

should be thoroughly discussed with the patient before committing the patient to root resection procedures.

Which Root and Why?

The selection of a root to resect requires knowledge of dental anatomy, the anatomy of the alveolar bone in the area, and an appreciation for other dental procedures that may be required to adequately treat the patient. The therapist should remove the root that (a) has the least amount of remaining bony support, (b) will obliterate the furcation and contribute to the elimination of any associated periodontal defect, (c) will facilitate plaque removal by the patient and instrumentation by the dentist or dental hygienist during periodontal maintenance, and (d) is the most difficult for the endodontist or restorative dentist to treat. Another consideration is the ability of the remaining root or roots of the tooth, after resection, to serve as an abutment if a fixed or removable partial denture is planned.

The most common root resection is the removal of the distobuccal root of the maxillary first molar (Fig. 24-4).[34-36] The anatomy and relation of the first and second molars plus the incidence of furcation involvement dictate this particular resection. A two-wall bony pocket is frequently located between the first and second molar. This pocket is commonly associated with root approximation of the distobuccal root of the first molar and the mesiobuccal root of the second molar. The result is inadequate access for plaque removal once these furcations are involved. The clinical result of a distobuccal root resection is shown in Figure 24-5.

Vital versus Nonvital Root Resection

Once the decision is made to use root resection, the patient should be referred for endodontic therapy. Although root resections can be successfully performed

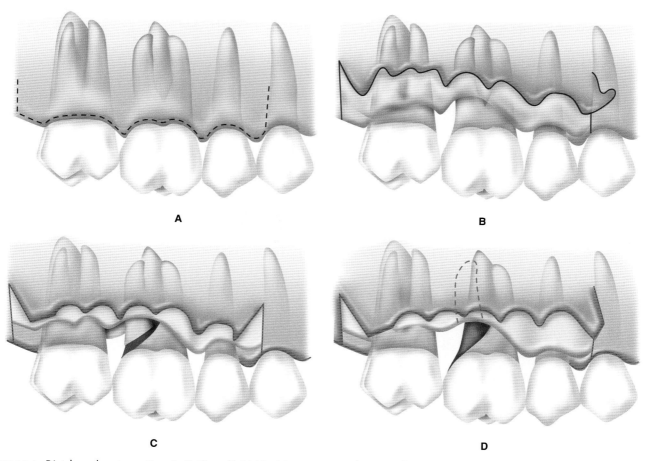

Figure 24-4. Distobuccal root resection. **A,** Outline of initial incisions to expose the surgical area for removal of a distobuccal root from the maxillary right first molar. **B,** Full-thickness flap reflected and area degranulated to expose the furcation and the adjacent bony structures. **C,** Removal of some facial marginal bone over the distal root and the root sectioned to allow elevation and removal. **D,** Final contour of area before flap closure.

on vital teeth,[37,38] it is preferable to have pulp extirpation precede the resection. This facilitates the performance of root canal obturation and allows the endodontist to determine that the canals can be adequately instrumented. The endodontist can remove the radicular pulp from the tooth and seal the orifice of the canal of the root to be resected; therefore, contamination of the pulp chamber by oral fluids does not occur. The completion of endodontics and filling of the pulp chamber before root resection facilitates the surgical removal of the root, because it allows more extensive odontoplasty[28] to be performed. It also reduces the potential contamination of the surgical field by metallic fragments from a restoration. If one is certain which root is to be removed, it is wise to have the endodontic therapy completed on the roots that are to be retained. It is quite distressing to perform a vital root resection and to subsequently discover that the remaining roots cannot be instrumented or to have one of the remaining roots inadvertently split or perforated. Completing endodontic treatment before root resection also minimizes the potential for postoperative pain.[38]

Conversely, it is equally disconcerting to have the endodontic therapy performed and then to discover during surgery that extraction of the tooth is indicated, rather than root resection. The clinician must carefully weigh the certainty of root resection and tooth retention before performing endodontic therapy. If the clinician feels strongly that root resection will be performed, consultation before periodontal surgery with the clinician performing the endodontic treatment allows an assessment of the likelihood of successful root canal therapy.

The only potential contraindication to completing endodontics before root resection may be a possible adverse effect on regeneration of the periodontal attachment. Prichard[39] believed that obturation of the canals should be delayed if a regenerative procedure is to be performed on the affected tooth. However, sectioning vital teeth and submerging the roots, without endodontic treatment, does not adversely affect regeneration attempts as compared with nonsubmerged controls.[40,41] Currently, there are no evidence-based studies that preclude regeneration attempts on devitalized teeth.

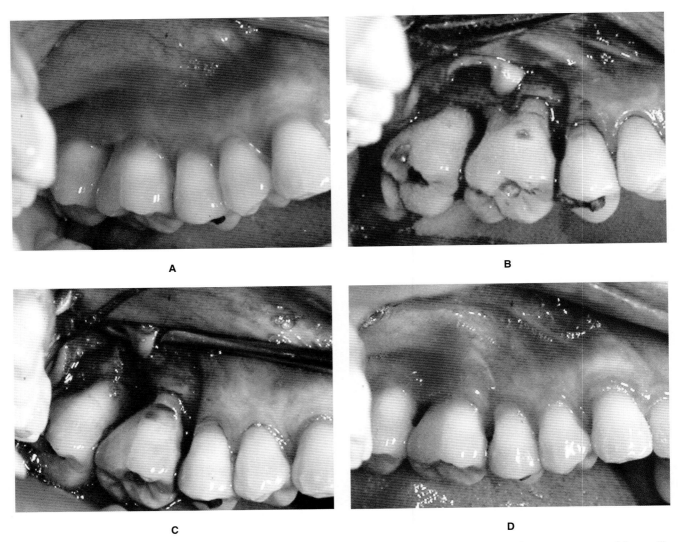

Figure 24-5. Distobuccal root resection to eliminate a distal Class II furcation and root approximation. **A,** Buccal preoperative view of the maxillary right molar area. **B,** Full-thickness flap reflected. Note the interproximal bone loss and the root approximation as the distal root of the first molar flairs toward the mesial of the second molar. The area between the first and second molars has severe bone loss. **C,** Distal root of the first molar resected and removed. Odontoplasty has been performed to reduce the bulge of the crown contour where the resected root resided. **D,** Buccal view 6 months after surgery. Note the dimension for access to the interproximal area for maintenance. (*From Prichard JF: The diagnosis and treatment of periodontal disease in general dental practice, Saunders, Philadelphia, 1979.*)

PERFORMANCE OF ROOT RESECTION

Root resection may be performed as an isolated procedure or as a component of other procedures being performed within the surgical field. After surgical draping of the patient and anesthesia, the surgical field is probed and examined. If resection of the root requires cutting through metallic restorations, it is generally wise to reduce or section through the metal before incision and reflection of the flap. This prevents metallic fragments from becoming embedded in the soft tissues. If an advanced Class II or a Class III furcation is present associated with a short root trunk, the root may occasionally be resected without the elevation of a flap; however, this situation is not common. Insertion of a curved furcation probe, such as the Nabors probe or a pig-trailed explorer into the furcation can serve to guide the plane of the surgical section. The removal of a portion of the crown of the tooth immediately coronal to the root (odontoplasty[28]) and the placement of a long beveled section into the dome of the furca also facilitates the subsequent removal of the root (Fig. 24-6).

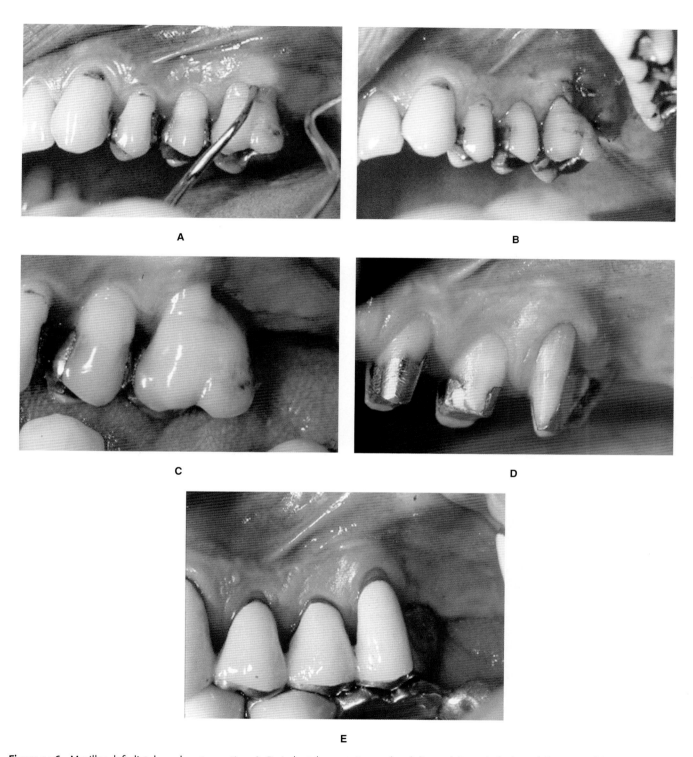

A

B

C

D

E

Figure 24-6. Maxillary left distobuccal root resection. **A,** Periodontal curette inserted and directed through the buccal furcation of the involved maxillary molar toward the distal furcation. There was a Class III furcation involvement that was associated with a short root trunk. **B,** Distobuccal root resected and flap sutured. **C,** A 6-week postoperative view of resection site. Note the shrinkage of the soft tissue that follows the remodeling of the underlying bony periodontium. **D,** Preparations of the root resected molar and bicuspids for fixed restorations. **E,** A 15-year postoperative view of the area of the root resection. The root resected tooth remains in excellent health. (*From Prichard JF: The diagnosis and treatment of periodontal disease in general dental practice, Saunders, Philadelphia, 1979.*)

If a vital root resection is to be performed, flap elevation should precede sectioning of the root. A clinical example from a patient with advanced attachment loss is shown in Figure 24-7. Although fixed splinting was planned, the molar was so severely compromised that the ability to perform a root resection was unclear; therefore, the area was surgically exposed to determine the feasibility of resection before endodontic therapy. After removal of the distobuccal root, odontoplasty was performed to ensure that no "lip" of tooth structure was left in the dome of the furcation. Leaving residual tooth structure in this area provides a niche for plaque retention and is impossible for the patient to clean. After distobuccal root resection, intact bone was found in the remaining mesial furcation, and the remaining periodontal attachment was adequate to support the planned restoration. Subsequent to removal of the root, ostectomy and osteoplasty were required to eliminate the remaining bony deformities and to prepare the edentulous ridge for pontic adaptation. The restoration was made to allow excellent oral hygiene access for the patient and clinician. Although the place of root resection in the periodontal surgical realm during the era of dental implant therapy has been questioned, the long-term results in this case demonstrate the potential for this type of treatment.

Root resection is commonly performed as a portion of the surgical treatment of a larger area of the mouth and may be combined with other resective or regenerative procedures. The design of the flap to gain access requires consideration not only of the root to be resected but planning for any other surgical objectives to be accomplished. In the example shown in Figure 24-8, a distobuccal root resection on the first molar was combined with an apically positioned flap procedure to reduce pocket depth and to facilitate restoration and maintenance. Note the effect that removal of this root has on the contours of the molar restoration and access to the molar embrasure. The extent of the flap elevated must be sufficient to provide access and visibility for instrumentation and to facilitate proper wound closure. Surgical access must allow the optimal performance of procedures, because inadequate access is one of the most common mistakes made during periodontal surgery. It should always be remembered that large flaps heal just as rapidly as small flaps, provide better visibility, facilitate instrumentation, and are less likely to be traumatized during the procedure.

During root resection, once the root is cleanly divided from the remaining roots and crown of the tooth, it can be carefully elevated from its socket. This is accomplished with a suitable instrument such as an elevator or a chisel. Pressure should be carefully applied to the root and care taken not to luxate or damage the remaining roots of the tooth or of an adjacent tooth. Root curvature may pose a problem during elevation. The mesial root of mandibular

molars and the mesiobuccal root of maxillary molars commonly are curved distally. The result is that the root is directed distally into the furcation and against the distal root during elevation. This is particularly true if the interradicular zone of the furcation is narrow and the roots are closely approximated. In such cases, it may be necessary to progressively section and remove the coronal portion of the root as it is elevated until the root can be removed from the socket. Otherwise a significant amount of the facial bone over the root may have to be removed to allow removal of the sectioned root. The removal of bone over the facial may be of little consequence if the interradicular dimension is great and/or the embrasure with the adjacent tooth is wide. However, removal of a large amount of the facial bony plate can result in a significant reduction in the width of the ridge, can compromise pontic adaptation, and may pose a potential cosmetic problem.

After delivery of the root, the area is examined to insure that no root stump remains. Odontoplasty to facilitate plaque removal, and osteoplasty to remove any sharp edges or defects from the bony alveolus may be performed. The area is thoroughly irrigated with sterile saline, and the flap(s) are reapproximated with appropriate sutures. Surgical dressings may or may not be used. Postoperative instructions and care are similar to that following other periodontal surgical procedures.

ROOT RESECTION OR HEMISECTION OF MANDIBULAR MOLARS

Hemisection is the surgical process by which a two rooted tooth, usually a mandibular molar, is converted into a single rooted tooth by the removal of one root and the associated portion of the crown.[42] Hemisection, like root resection, may provide a means of salvaging a mandibular molar that would otherwise have a hopeless prognosis. The economic consequences of hemisection and the advent of other therapeutic methods such as dental implant placement have resulted in a reduction in the frequency of hemisection. It remains, however, a valuable procedure for carefully selected patients. Appropriate examples include: (a) patients who experience vertical root fracture or root perforation during endodontic therapy; (b) patients who have endodontically treated mandibular molars with advanced bone loss on only one root that are serving as terminal abutments of a prosthesis; and (c) patients who have local anatomy that precludes extraction and simple implant placement.

As with root resection, endodontic treatment should precede hemisection whenever possible. After obturation of the canal of the root that is to be retained, the pulp chamber of the tooth should be filled with amalgam, composite resin, or glass ionomer. This seals the root canal space and prevents leakage after hemisection or root resection.

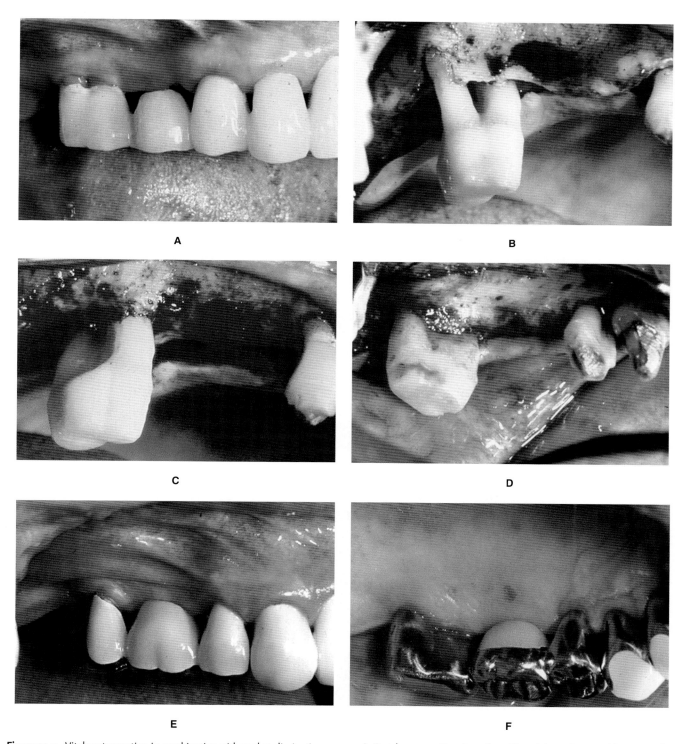

A

B

C

D

E

F

Figure 24-7. Vital root resection in combination with pocket elimination surgery. **A,** Facial preoperative view of maxillary right molar area. The patient has advanced attachment loss and has had provisional splints placed because of hypermobility. **B,** Facial view of the surgical area showing the advanced degree of bone loss on the molar. There is a Class III buccal-to-distal furcation invasion. **C,** A vital root amputation of the distobuccal root has been performed in conjunction with osteoplasty to eliminate the bony defects and to alter the form of the adjacent edentulous ridge area. **D,** Palatal view after vital root resection and osteoplasty. Note that the mesial furcation of the molar is intact. **E,** Facial view of the area 8 years after restoration. **F,** An 8-year postoperative view after restoration. The contours of the restoration allow excellent access for oral hygiene. Note the areas of tooth brush abrasion on the palate.

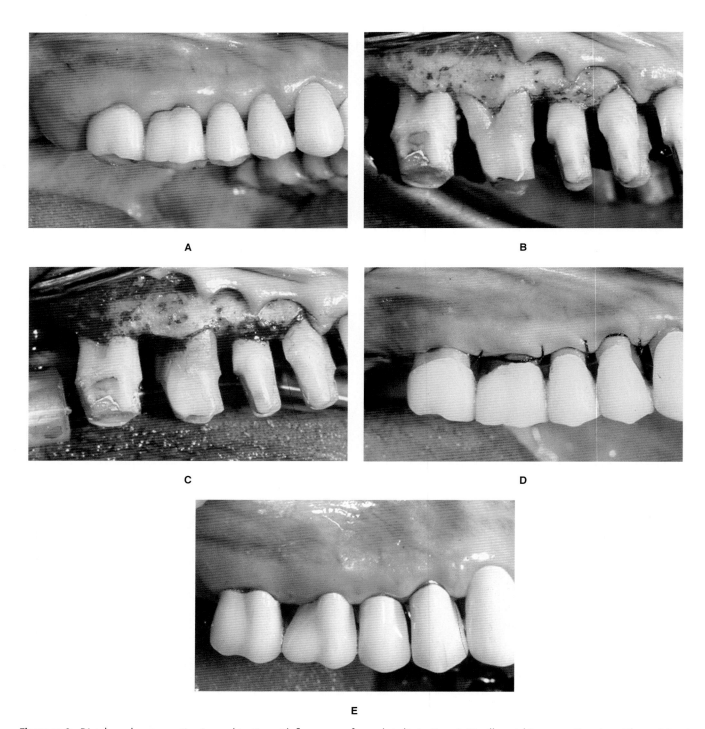

Figure 24-8. Distobuccal root resection in combination with flap surgery for pocket elimination. **A,** Maxillary right preoperative view with provisional restorations in place. **B,** Facial view after full-thickness flap reflection and debridement. Note the root approximation between the distal root of the first molar and the mesial root of the second molar. There is an early Class II buccal furcation involvement of the maxillary second molar and a generalized horizontal pattern of bone loss. **C,** Facial view after resection of the distobuccal root of the first molar and localized osteoplasty to reduce the buccal bony profile. The root proximity problem between the molars has been resolved. **D,** Facial view of apically positioned flap adaptation using continuous sling sutures. **E,** Facial view of the area of root resection 5 years after restoration. Note the effect of root resection on the contours between the first and second molars. There is clear access for an interproximal brush to facilitate oral hygiene.

SURGICAL PERFORMANCE OF HEMISECTION

The performance of a hemisection is shown in Figure 24-9. The patient has a mandibular left second molar with advanced attachment loss and a Class III furcation defect. Previously the molar has had successful endodontic therapy. Full-thickness flaps were reflected and the area debrided to reveal significant osseous deformities associated with this Class III furcation involvement. The amount of attachment remaining on the distal root was sufficient to provide adequate support for the fixed restoration. In such an example, the removal of the severely affected and highly fluted mesial root may result in the maintenance of the tooth and allow construction of a fixed partial denture for additional years of service.

The path of the furcation is explored to guide the hemisection and separation of the root. If necessary a curved explorer or periodontal probe may be passed through the furcation to guide the hemisection of the root (Fig. 24-9, *C*). A high-speed handpiece with a carbide bur or diamond stone of appropriate length is then used to separate the roots. If a crown or other metallic restoration is present, it is wise to section through the metallic portion of the crown before elevation of the flap to prevent contamination of the surgical area with metal particles.

The root to be sacrificed is then removed with an appropriate forcep or elevator. Most patients requiring hemisection have significant bony deformities associated with the furcation involvement. Therefore in addition to removal of the hopeless root, other therapies such as osteoplasty, ostectomy, or regeneration procedures may be required to provide adequate clinical crown length, a biologic width of attachment, or ridge alteration to provide for prosthetic rehabilitation. In this patient, resective

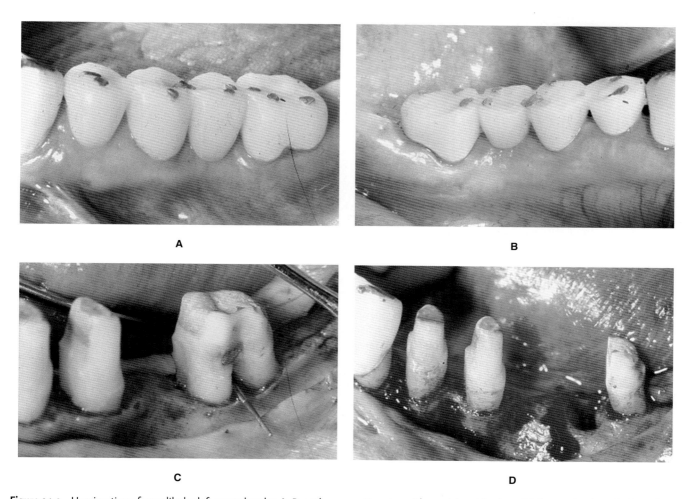

A	**B**
C	**D**

Figure 24-9. Hemisection of mandibular left second molar. **A,** Buccal preoperative view with provisional fixed partial denture in place. **B,** Lingual preoperative view. **C,** Buccal view showing periodontal probe inserted through the Class III furcation to guide the hemisectioning of the molar. **D,** Buccal view after removal of the mesial root and osseous recontouring to eliminate the bony defects.

Continued

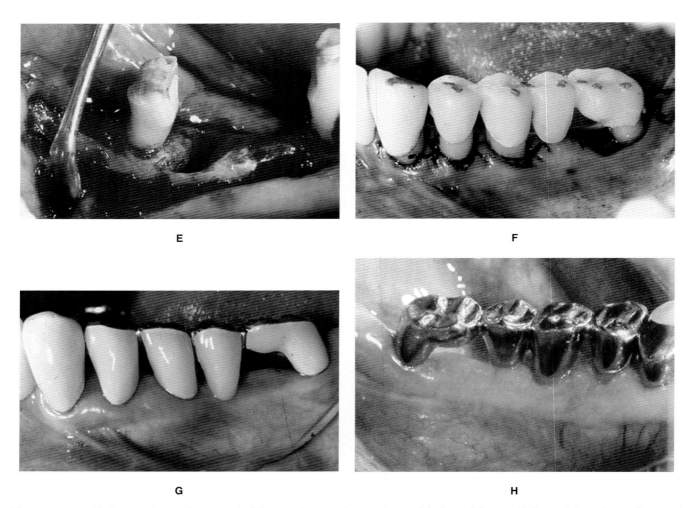

E

F

G

H

Figure 24-9. cont'd **E,** Lingual view after removal of the mesial root and recontouring of the bony defects and ledging. **F,** Buccal view after apical positioning and suturing of flaps and recementation of the provisional restoration. **G,** Buccal view of the hemisected molar 5 years after restoration. Excellent access for oral hygiene has been created in the final restoration. **H,** Lingual view of the hemisected molar 5 years after surgery.

osseous surgery was used to eliminate the osseous defects. The surgical flaps are then closed with appropriate sutures, temporary restorations replaced, surgical dressings applied, and the patient is provided with postoperative instruction and medications.

RESTORATIVE CONSIDERATIONS OF ROOT RESECTION/HEMISECTION

The need to restore the root or roots remaining after resection or hemisection is also a key consideration in the decision to use these therapies. The length of the roots that remain and their external and internal configuration may be major complications if restoration is required. As previously discussed, the flutings and multiple canals present in the mesial root of mandibular molars pose significant restorative challenges, particularly if it is necessary to

place a post to restore the tooth. Deep flutings in these roots complicate preparation of the root and may preclude adequate finishing of the margin during cementation. In addition, such roots may be at risk for vertical root fracture during cementation or subsequently when subjected to heavy occlusal forces.

If a significant portion of the crown of the tooth has been lost from caries or previous dental restorations, the root trunk length and the width of the pulpal floor that remain after resection must be considered. In 1992, Mazjoub and Kon[36] suggested that poor root anatomy may be a contraindication to root resection. In the case of the maxillary first molar, after resection and removal of the distobuccal root, an average of only 2.7 mm of tooth structure remains between the pulp chamber floor and the most coronal aspect of root separation in the remaining furcation dome. In 84% of the teeth studied, the dimension was 2 to 3 mm. If a biologic width of 2.04 mm is to be preserved,[42] then little tooth is present for a restorative finish line. Thus violation of the biologic width during restoration is quite likely. The consequences of such a violation, however, may be overestimated as longitudinal studies do not indicate that subsequent periodontal attachment loss is a common cause of failure of root resected molars.[43-45] However, these dimensions must be considered during treatment planning.

TUNNELING

An alternative to root resection and hemisection that has been used to treat Class II and III furcation involvement in two rooted teeth such as mandibular molars is "tunneling."[17] This is the process of deliberately removing bone from the furcation to produce an open tunnel through the furcation. The result is to produce what Glickman[14] would classify as a Grade IV furcation. The rationale for this is to provide ready access for a variety of home care instruments to be passed through the furca to remove dental plaque. This access would also facilitate instrumentation and the application of topical medicaments such as fluorides or chlorhexidine.

There are a number of potential problems associated with this therapy. Only a few molars have roots sufficiently long or widely divergent to allow tunneling and the establishment of a local anatomy that is readily maintained. Soft tissues tend to rebound and obstruct the furcation and many patients are unwilling or unable to perform the home care procedures necessary to keep the furcation free of plaque. As a result, the development of dental caries in molars with tunnels is common.[17,46]

BONE GRAFTS AND GUIDED TISSUE REGENERATION PROCEDURES

During the last 30 years significant research effort has been devoted to materials and techniques designed to regenerate attachment on teeth affected by periodontitis.[47] A variety of materials and techniques have been proposed and investigated. Among these are bone autografts, allografts and xenografts, and alloplastic materials designed as either bone substitutes or biologic barriers[47] (see Chapter 25). These materials have been applied to the treatment of molar furcations and other periodontal defects.

Radiographic evidence of "bone fill" and repair with a variety of techniques has been published.[39,48-50] Clinical evidence of regeneration and bone fill in the furcation area has also been provided. Histologic evidence documenting regeneration, however, has been less common. Evidence of regeneration using autogenous bone and allograft bone in combination with surgical debridement has been provided by a number of investigators.[40,41,51,52]

Autogenous hip marrow has been used, but the potential morbidity and cost of this procedure has limited its use. Another common periodontal grafting material is osseous coagulum. Osseous coagulum is a mixture of autogenous bone, connective tissue, and blood elements. The use of this material was described by Robinson in 1969.[48] In this procedure, after thorough debridement of the affected area, the patient's own bone collected during osteoplasty and ostectomy is placed into the bony defect and covered by a surgically reflected flap. Clinical and histologic evidence of bone fill or regeneration, or both, with osseous coagulum has been published in both human and animal models.[49,52] However, histologic study of teeth treated with osseous coagulum frequently indicated that although some new attachment occurred, the majority of the radiographic change was caused by bone fill with an interposed long junctional epithelial attachment.[53,54] Although this may be considered a successful clinical result, the long-term stability of the fill with osseous coagulum is unknown.[47]

Since 1988 a large number of investigations have reported on the use of resorbable and nonresorbable barrier membranes to treat molar furcation defects. These membranes are used to isolate the furcation and exclude soft tissue elements so that healing will be accomplished by elements from the periodontal ligament and adjacent alveolar bone.[55] Many so-called guided tissue regeneration (GTR) and guided bone regeneration (GBR) procedures were reported using membranes manufactured of e-PTFE (Teflon). Teflon is a uniquely stable, inert material and e-PTFE membranes in a number of different configurations are available for clinical application. The coronal margin of these membranes is designed to impede epithelial downgrowth into the wound. After an appropriate period of healing, usually at least 6 weeks, the e-PTFE GTR procedure requires a second stage procedure to remove the nonresorbable membrane. The use of a GTR Teflon membrane for treatment of the furcation in a mandibular right second molar is shown in Figure 24-10.

Subsequent to the advent of e-PTFE membranes, a variety of resorbable membranes constructed of collagen, dermis, or synthetic polymers were developed for GTR and GBR purposes. The operative procedure is essentially identical to that of e-PTFE with the exception that a second stage removal of the membrane is not required. Although GTR procedures were originally performed with only a barrier membrane to isolate the furcation, their use has been extended to include combinations of the membranes with grafts of bone, bone substitutes, and various root surface preparations or growth factors, or both.[47] These modifications of the procedure are an indication of the limitations observed with the original technique. The application of combinations of membranes with other materials is potentially costly for the patient and some reports indicate no

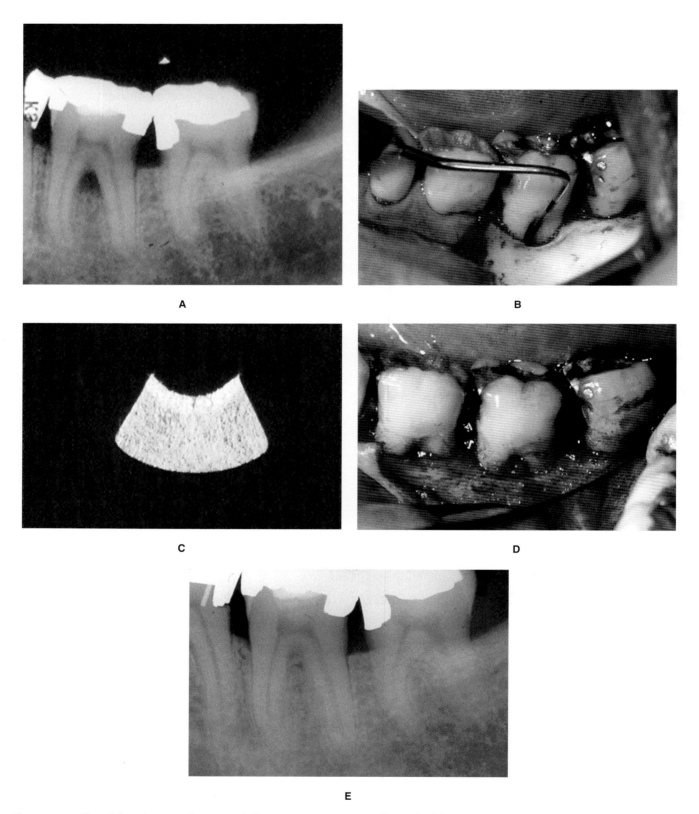

Figure 24-10. Class II furcation treated using guided tissue regeneration. **A,** Radiograph of the mandibular second molar with a furcation defect. **B,** Buccal view of the furcation debrided. **C,** ePTFE (Teflon, W.L. Gore Inc., Flagstaff, AZ) membrane used to cover the furcation. **D,** Buccal view 6 weeks after surgery, at time of membrane removal. The furcation is filled with newly formed granulation tissue. **E,** Radiograph of area 1 year after surgery showing apparent bony fill of the furcation.

significant clinical differences with other less complex procedures, except for Class II furcations.[47] The GTR procedure is technique sensitive and requires more than average clinical skills. It is most successful in the intrabony portion of the defect and is best applied to Class II furcations.[47,56,57] It is least successful in Class III or Glickman Grade IV furcation deformities.[47,58,59] Therefore these procedures are indicated for teeth of critical importance when other treatment approaches are not likely to be successful.

EXTRACTION OF MOLARS WITH FURCATION INVOLVEMENT

One treatment option that must always be considered for molars with advanced attachment loss in the furcation or in the presence of unfavorable tooth anatomy is extraction. Although molars with advanced Class II or Class III furcation involvements may be maintained for significant periods by frequent instrumentation, they should be removed before allowing the development of bony deformities that would require major surgical repair or would preclude routine prosthesis. The ability to replace missing members of the dentition and to restore function by a variety of restorative and prosthetic means makes the potential loss of one or more members of the dentition less threatening now than in the past.

PROGNOSIS OF ROOT RESECTION/HEMISECTION

The long-term results of root resection and hemisection are well described in the periodontal literature.[17,34] The success rate is quite high when resections are preceded by careful diagnosis and the procedures are appropriately performed.[43-45] Likewise the reasons for failure are equally well known.[17,60-63] The primary causes of failure after root resection are root fracture, caries, endodontic complications, cement washout, restorative failures, and periodontal attachment loss (Table 24-1).

Dental caries is one of the major causes of failure after furcation therapy. This is particularly true if access to the furcation is poor or if the patient is unwilling or unable to perform appropriate plaque removal. For this reason patients who are unwilling or unable to perform appropriate plaque removal are not candidates for root resection or hemisection. Indeed, except for isolated instances they likely are not appropriate candidates for periodontal surgical treatment.

In the majority of studies in which the long-term survival of root resections/hemisections were evaluated it would appear that recurrent or ongoing periodontal attachment loss is not the major cause of failure (Table 24-1). Tooth loss from attachment loss after resection ranges from about 3% to 26%, and most periodontal failures occur after 5 to 10 years.[63] Indeed, current literature suggests that failure from recurrent periodontal disease is a relatively low risk and that the survival rate for root amputations is similar to that for osseointegrated dental implants.[43-45,64,65]

PROGNOSIS OF TREATMENT OF MOLAR FURCATIONS

It is evident from study of the periodontal literature that the presence of furcation involvement on a maxillary or mandibular molar does not always lead to loss of that tooth. Indeed, molars with varying degrees of furcation involvement can be effectively treated and preserved in function for periods equal to or superior to that of other teeth with intact furcations. Effective management of furcation defects requires knowledge of the anatomic problems associated with furcation involvement and the application of treatment methods that are consistent with the nature and extent of

TABLE 24-1 **Root Resection and Hemisection Failures**

STUDY	NO. OF TEETH	CAUSE OF FAILURE				TOTAL NO. OF FAILURES	% FAILURE
		CARIES	ENDO	PERIO	OTHER		
Bastin et al 1996	49	2	1	0	1	4	8.2
Bergenholtz 1972	45	0	1	2	0	3	6.7
Buhler 1988	28	1	5	2	1	9	32.1
Carnevale et al 1991	488	9	4	3	15	28	5.7
Carnevale et al 1998	175	3	4	3	2	12	6.9
Erpenstein 1983	34	0	6	1	0	7	20.6
Hamp et al 1975*	7	3*	0	0	0	3*	42.9*
Klavan 1975	34	1	0	0	0	1	2.9
Langer et al 1981	100	3	7	10	18	38	38.0
Fugazzotto 2001	701	7	5	8	4	24	3.4

*Data reported only for tunnel problems.

the involvement. Surgical debridement, oral hygiene procedures, and periodic periodontal maintenance will retain affected members of the dentition for long periods.[66,67] Other therapeutic procedures are available that will restore lost attachment, eliminate periodontal pockets, or eliminate hopelessly affected roots.

This is not to suggest that root resection is indicated for all molars with furcation involvement, but rather that resection is one of the therapies that may be used in the performance of a well designed and performed periodontal treatment plan. The keys to successful treatment of molar furcation involvement are the same as for any other periodontal problem—that is, early diagnosis, thorough treatment planning, good oral hygiene by the patient, careful technical execution of the therapeutic modality, and a well designed and implemented program of periodontal maintenance.

REFERENCES

1. Goodson JM, Tanner ACR, Haffajee AD et al: Patterns of progression and regression of advanced destructive periodontal disease, *J Clin Periodontol* 9:472, 1982.

2. Socransky SS, Haffajee AD, Goodson JM, Lindhe J: New concepts of destructive periodontal disease, *J Clin Periodontol* 11:21, 1984.

3. Hancock EB: Prevention, *Ann Periodontol* 1:225, 1996.

4. Masters DH, Hoskins SW: Projection of cervical enamel into molar furcations, *J Periodontol* 35:49, 1964.

5. Hou GL, Tasai CC: Relationship between periodontal furcation involvement and molar cervical enamel projection, *J Periodontol* 58:715, 1978.

6. Gher ME, Vernino AR: Root morphology-clinical significance in pathogenesis and treatment of periodontal disease, *J Am Dent Assoc* 101:627, 1980.

7. Larato DC: Some anatomical factors related to furcation involvement, *J Periodontol* 46:608, 1975.

8. Papapanou PN: Periodontal diseases: epidemiology, *Ann Periodontol* 1:1, 1996.

9. Tal H: Furcal bony defects in dry mandibles: Part I: biometric study, *J Periodontol* 53:360, 1982.

10. Tal H, Lemmer J: Furcal defects in dry mandibles: Part II. Severity of furcal defects, *J Periodontol* 53:364, 1984.

11. Bower RC: Furcation morphology relative to periodontal treatment. Furcation root surface anatomy, *J Periodontol* 50:366, 1979.

12. Bower RC: Furcation morphology relative to periodontal treatment: furcation entrance architecture, *J Periodontol* 50:23, 1979.

13. Tibbetts LS: Use of diagnostic probes for detection of periodontal disease, *J Am Dent Assoc* 78:549, 1969.

14. Glickman I: The treatment of bifurcation and trifurcation involvement. In *Clinical periodontology*, Philadelphia, 1958, WB Saunders, pp 693-704.

15. Heins PJ, Canter SR: The furca involvement: a classification of bony deformities, *J Periodontol* 6(2):84, 1968.

16. Easley JR, Drennan GA: Morphological classification of the furca, *J Can Dent Assoc* 35:104, 1969.

17. Hamp S-E, Nyman S, Lindhe J: Periodontal treatment of multirooted teeth: results after 5 years, *J Clin Periodontol* 2:126, 1975.

18. Tarnow D, Fletcher P: Classification of the vertical component of furcation involvement, *J Periodontol* 55:283, 1984.

19. Goldman HM: Therapy of the incipient bifurcation involvement, *J Periodontol* 29:112, 1958.

20. Everett F, Jump E, Holder T, Wilson G: The intermediate bifurcational ridge: a study of the morphology of the bifurcation of the lower molar, *J Dent Res* 37:162, 1958.

21. Matia JB, Bissada NF, Maybury JE, Ricchetti P: Efficiency of scaling of the molar furcation area with and without surgical access, *Int J Periodontics Restorative Dent* 6(6):25, 1986.

22. Parashis AO, Anognou-Vareltzides A, Demetrious N: Calculus removal from multirooted teeth with and without surgical access: (1) efficacy on external and furcation surfaces in relation to probing depths. *J Clin Periodontol* 20:63, 1993.

23. Wylam JM, Mealey BL, Mills MP et al: The clinical effectiveness of open versus closed scaling and root planing on multi-rooted teeth, *J Periodontol* 64:1023, 1993.

24. Gutmann JL: Prevalence, location and patency of accessory canals in the furcation region of permanent molars, *J Periodontol* 49:21, 1978.

25. Harrington GW, Steiner DR: Periodontal-endodontic considerations. In Walton RE, Torabinejad M, editors: *Principles and practice of endodontics*, ed 3, Philadelphia, 2002, WB Saunders, pp 466-484.

26. Harrington GW, Steiner DR, Ammons WF Jr: The periodontal-endodontic controversy, *Periodontology 2000* 30:123-130, 2002.

27. Keough B: Root resection, *Int J Periodontics Restorative Dent* 2(1):17, 1982.

28. Lindhe J: Treatment of furcation involved teeth. In *Textbook of clinical periodontology*, ed 2, Philadelphia, 1989, Monksgaard.

29. Friedman N: Periodontal osseous surgery: osteoplasty and osteoectomy, *J Periodontol* 26:257, 1955.

30. *Glossary of periodontal terms*, ed 4, Chicago, 2001, The American Academy of Periodontology.

31. Farrar JN: Radical and heroic treatment of alveolar abscess by amputation of roots of teeth, *Dental Cosmos* 1884;26:79.

32. Black GV: *The American system of dentistry*, In Litch W, editor: Philadelphia, 1886, Lea Brothers, pp 990-992.

33. Basaraba N: Root amputation and tooth hemisection, *Dent Clin North Am* 13(1):121, 1969.

34. Klavan B: Clinical observations following root amputation in maxillary molar teeth, *J Periodontol* 46:1, 1975.

35. Eastman JR, Backmeyer J: A review of the periodontal, endodontic and prosthetic considerations in odontogenous resection procedures, *Int J Periodontics Restorative Dent* 6(2):34, 1986.

36. Majzoub Z, Kon S: Tooth morphology following root resection procedures in maxillary first molars, *J Periodontol* 1992; 63:290.

37. Haskell EW, Stanley HR: A review of vital root resection, *Int J Periodontics Restorative Dent* 2(6):29, 1982.

38. Smukler H, Tagger M: Vital root amputation. A clinical and histological study, *J Periodontol* 47:324, 1976.

39. Prichard J: A technique for treating infrabony pockets based on alveolar process morphology, *Dent Clin North Am* 1:85, 1960.

40. Bowers GM, Chadroff B, Carnevale R et al: Histologic evaluation of a new attachment apparatus formation in humans. Part I, *J Periodontol* 60:664, 1989.

41. Bowers GM, Chadoff B, Carnevale R et al: Histologic evaluation of new human attachment apparatus formation in humans. Part II, *J Periodontol* 60:675, 1989.

42. Gargiulo AW, Wentz FM, Orban B: Dimensions of the dentinogingival junction in humans, *J Periodontol* 32:261, 1961.

43. Carnevale G, DiFebo G, Tonelli MP, et al: A retrospective analysis of the periodontal-prosthodontic treatment of molars with interradicular lesions, *Int J Periodontics Restorative Dent* 11:188, 1991.

44. Carnevale G, Pontoriero R, Di Febo G: Long-term effects of root resective therapy in furcation-involved molars: a 10 year longitudinal study, *J Clin Periodontol* 25:209, 1998.

45. Basten CHJ, Ammons WF, Persson R: Long-term evaluation of root resected molars. A retrospective study, *Int J Periodontics Restorative Dent* 16(3):206, 1996.

46. Hellden LB, Elliot A, Steffensen B, Steffensen JEM: The prognosis of tunnel preparations in treatment of class III furcations. A follow-up study, *J Periodontol* 60:182, 1989.

47. Garrett S: Periodontal regeneration around natural teeth, *Ann Periodontol* 1(1):621, 1996.

48. Robinson RE: Osseous coagulum for bone induction, *J Periodontol* 40:503, 1969.

49. Rivault AF, Toto PD, Levy S, Gargiulo AW: Autogenous bone grafts: osseous coagulum and osseous retrograde procedures in primates, *J Periodontol* 42:787, 1971.

50. Stahl SS, Froum SJ, Kushner J: Healing response of human intraosseous lesions following the use of debridement, grafting and citric acid root treatment: II. Clinical and histologic observations one year post surgery. *J Periodontol* 54:325, 1983.

51. Dragoo MR, Sullivan HC: A clinical and histological evaluation of autogenous iliac bone grafts in humans. Part I. Wound healing 2 to 8 months, *J Periodontol* 44:599, 1973.

52. Coverly L, Toto P, Gargiulo A: Osseous coagulum: a histologic evaluation, *J Periodontol* 46:596, 1975.

53. Froum SJ, Thaler R, Scopp IW, Stahl SS: Osseous autografts. II. Histologic responses to osseous coagulum-bone blend grafts, *J Periodontol* 46:656, 1975.

54. Caton J, Nyman S: Histometric evaluation of periodontal surgery. II. Connective tissue attachment level after four regenerative procedures, *J Clin Periodontol* 7:224, 1980.

55. Becker W, Becker BE, Berg L, et al: New attachment after treatment with root isolation procedures. Report for treated class III and class II furcations and vertical osseous defects, *Int J Periodontics Restorative Dent* 8(3):9, 1988.

56. Leckovic V, Kenney EB, Kovacevic K, Carranza FA Jr: Evaluation of guided tissue regeneration in class II furcation defects. A clinical re-entry study, *J Periodontol* 60:694, 1989.

57. Macheti EE, Shallhorn RG: Successful regeneration of mandibular class II furcation defects: an evidence-based treatment approach, *Int J Periodontics Restorative Dent* 15(2):146, 1995.

58. Demolon IA, Persson GR, Ammons WF, Johnson RH: Effects of antibiotic treatment on clinical conditions with guided tissue regeneration: one year results, *J Periodontol* 65:713, 1994.

59. Garrett S, Gantes B, Zimmerman G, Egelberg J: Treatment of mandibular Class III periodontal furcation defects. Coronally positioned flaps with and without expanded polytetrafluoroethylene membranes, *J Periodontol* 65:592, 1994.

60. Buhler H: Evaluation of root-resected teeth. Results after 10 years, *J Periodontol* 59:805, 1988.

61. Buhler H: Survival rates of hemisected teeth: an attempt to compare them with survival rates of alloplastic implants, *Int J Periodontics Restorative Dent* 14:537, 1994.

62. Erpenstein H: A 3-year study of hemisected molars, *J Clin Periodontol* 10:1, 1983.

63. Langer B, Stein SD, Wagenberg B: An evaluation of root resections. A ten-year study, *J Periodontol* 52:719, 1981.

64. Blomlof L, Jansson L, Applegren R, et al: Prognosis and mortality of root-resected molars, *Int J Periodontics Restorative Dent* 17:190, 1997.

65. Fugazzotto PA: A comparison of the success of root resected molars and molar position implants in function in a private practice: results of up to 15-plus years, *J Periodontol* 72:1113, 2001.

66. Ross I, Thompson RH: A long term study of root retention of maxillary molars with furcation involvement, *J Periodontol* 49:238, 1978.

67. Hirschfeld L, Wasserman B: A long-term survey of tooth loss in 600 treated periodontal patients, *J Periodontol* 49:225, 1978.

25 Periodontal Regeneration and Reconstructive Surgery

Richard T. Kao

One of the initial objectives of periodontal therapy is infection management. Our understanding of the putative pathogenic periodontal microflora has altered our therapeutic approach from one of elimination of microbes to one of controlling pathogenic microorganisms and the immunoinflammatory response. Using treatments such as scaling and root planing, maintenance therapy, and antimicrobial therapy, our goal is to control the pathogenic microflora to prevent further periodontal destruction. Despite successful disease management, however, anatomic changes resulting from past disease activity often occur and must be corrected. Left untreated, these defects can provide a potential harbor for the reestablishment of pathogenic microflora. Thus, to facilitate long-term management of a healthy dentition, the periodontal defects must be eliminated. Therapeutic approaches for correcting these anatomic defects include procedures such as flap debridement/flap curettage, resective procedures, and periodontal regenerative therapy. Of these therapies, periodontal regeneration, or the complete restoration of the structure and function of damaged periodontal tissue, is the ideal goal. Over the last three decades several different techniques have been developed to achieve periodontal regeneration. Each technique has strengths and weaknesses. This chapter summarizes our current understanding of periodontal regeneration and examines how regenerative approaches toward correcting periodontal bony defects have changed over the years.

PERIODONTAL REGENERATION AND REPAIR

When the periodontium is damaged by inflammation or as a result of surgical treatment, the defect heals either through periodontal regeneration or repair.[1] In periodontal *regeneration*, healing occurs through the reconstitution of a new periodontium, which involves the formation of alveolar bone, functionally aligned periodontal ligament (PDL), and new cementum. Alternatively, *repair* is healing by replacement with epithelium or connective tissue, or both, that matures into various nonfunctional types of scar tissue, termed new attachment. Histologically, patterns of repair include long junctional epithelium, new connective tissue adhesion, and/or ankylosis (Fig. 25-1).

On the cellular level, periodontal regeneration is a complex process requiring coordinated proliferation, differentiation, and development of various cell types to form the periodontal attachment apparatus. During tooth development, periodontal stem cells, originating from dental follicle cells, differentiate into cementum, PDL, and alveolar bone. Some stem cells remain in the PDL after tooth development. During periodontal wound healing, these stem cells, as well as those from the perivascular region of the alveolar bone, are stimulated to proliferate; migrate into the defects; and differentiate to form new cemento-

blasts, PDL fibroblasts, and osteoblasts.[2] This process of cell proliferation, differentiation, and maturation must occur in a synchronized fashion to form new alveolar bone, PDL, and cementum in a sequence such that these three individual tissues are integrated to function as a new periodontal supporting apparatus.

A number of periodontal regenerative approaches have been attempted with varying degrees of success, including the following:

- Root conditioning procedures: This strategy focuses on treatment with citric acid, tetracycline, or edetate disodium (EDTA) to demineralize the root surface. The conditioned root surface reportedly enhances the formation of new connective tissue attachment.
- Osteogenic vital bone grafts (autografts): Intraoral bone sites and iliac crests have been used as autogenous bone sources to correct intrabony and furcation defects.
- Osteoinductive nonvital bone grafts (allografts): Demineralized freeze-dried bone allografts (DFDBAs) and freeze-dried bone allografts (FDBAs) have been shown to induce bone formation.
- Osteoconductive materials: These materials include inert materials acting as biologic fillers (alloplastic materials), such as β tricalcium phosphate-hydroxyapatite, calcium ceramics-tricalcium phosphate, biocompatible composite polymers, and bioactive glass polymers; also included are organic materials such as coral and bone xenografts.
- Guided tissue regeneration (GTR): This process involves applying to the surgical wound site an occlusive barrier membrane that will prevent epithelial and connective tissue ingrowth. This enables stem cells from the PDL and perivascular tissue to repopulate the root area and differentiate into a new periodontal supporting apparatus. Occlusive barriers may be used either alone or in combination with a bone graft or alloplastic material.
- Biologic and biomimicry mediators: Purified biologic (enamel matrix derivative) or synthetic biomimicry agents (platelet-derived growth factors and bone morphogenetic proteins [BMPs]) have emerged as potential agents to enhance periodontal regeneration.

In this chapter, these various approaches to periodontal regeneration are reviewed. A comparative analysis of these various techniques is provided in Table 25-1. When analyzing this information, readers should consider the following questions:

1. What are the indicators for success with periodontal regeneration?
2. Are the clinical results superior to other therapeutic approaches (scaling/root planing, flap curettage, osseous resective surgery, and strategic extraction followed by implant placement)?
3. Which clinical approach, alone or in combination, will provide the best result?
4. Are the improved clinical results because of periodontal regeneration or repair?

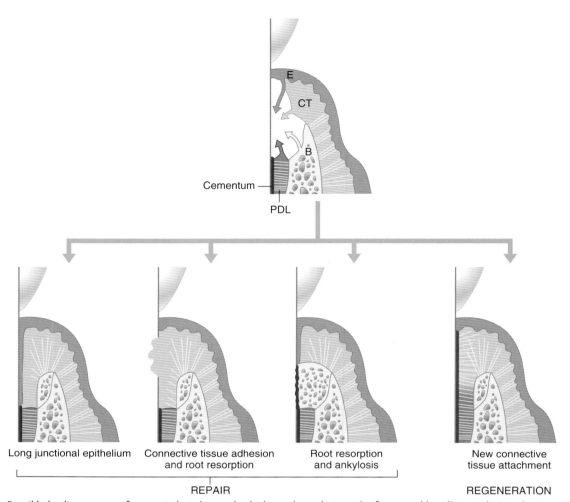

Figure 25-1. Possible healing patterns for a periodontal wound, which are dependent on the four possible cell types that predominate that wound site. The downgrowth of epithelial cells (*E*) results in a long junctional epithelium. The proliferation of connective tissue (*CT*) may result in connective tissue adhesion ± root resorption. With the predominance of bone cells (*B*), there may be root resorption, ankylosis (although this is relatively uncommon in humans when compared with animal models), or both. With the ingress of periodontal ligament (*PDL*) and perivascular cells from the bone, a regenerated periodontium with new cementum develops.

5. How stable are the clinical improvements? Are there 5-, 10-, 20-, or 30-year data to support the value of these techniques?

6. What are the clinical determinants that may influence the success of the periodontal regenerative approach?

7. Is patient compliance important?

8. How does one assimilate the information into a clinical decision tree for patient management?

ASSESSMENT OF PERIODONTAL WOUND HEALING

The periodontal literature is replete with articles discussing various approaches for correcting periodontal defects. In these studies, a number of techniques are used for assessing periodontal wound healing. To properly evaluate each technique, it is important to understand the advantages and weaknesses associated with each.

Clinical assessment usually involves periodontal probing. Probing depth, the measurement from the gingival margin to the base of the sulcus, may vary depending on the amount of pressure applied to the probe and the degree of health versus inflammation present (see Chapter 8). With inflamed tissue the probe may penetrate past the initial connective tissue attachment to the root surface, whereas in periodontal health the probe may fall short of the connective tissue attachment.[3,4] Complicating this method of measurement is the amount of gingival recession that can result from past disease. Given these problems, changes in probing depth are of little value in assessing healing. The measurement that is usually used for clinical assessment is clinical attachment level—the distance from the cementoenamel

TABLE 25-1 Comparative Analysis of Regenerative Approaches

GRAFT MATERIAL	CAL GAIN, mm	DEFECT FILL, % OR mm	HISTOLOGIC ASSESSMENT	COMMENTS
Autologous				
• Extraoral (iliac crest)	3.3-4.2[47] 2.60 mm in o-wall 3.75 mm in 1-wall 4.16 mm in 2-wall	—	33 of 39 defects showed evidence of regeneration[48]	Only evidence of regeneration in o-wall and (2.5 mm) supracrestal regeneration. Only one controlled study with 2.98 mm of bone gain vs. 0.66 mm with debridement.[51]
• Intraoral autologous	2.88-3.44 mm[50-53]	73%[51]	0.7 mm of regeneration[48,55]	No significant difference in one study.[54]
Allograft (vital)				
• Human vital	3.6 mm mean[48,60] 3.6 mm in 1-, 2-, and 3-wall 2.1 mm in o-wall	—	Evidence of regeneration[48]	Potential risk for disease transmission.
Allograft (nonvital)				
• FDBA	2.0 mm mean[61-64,66]	60-68% of 1401 defects had ≥50% fill[61-64]	None available	Only controlled study using paired defects showed no difference between FDBA vs. debridement.[65] No histologic study of healing pattern. The addition of autologous osseous coagulum enhances healing.
Comparative studies				
• FDBA vs. FDBA + autologous graft	—	63-67% had ≥50% fill (FDBA) vs. 78-80% had ≥50% fill (FDBA and autologous)[62]		
Allograft (nonvital)				
• DFDBA vs. debridement	2.3-2.9 vs. 0.3-1.3 mm[72-74]	65% vs. 11%[72-74]	1.21 mm of periodontal regeneration[70,71]	
Comparative studies				
• DFDBA vs. FDBA	1.7 vs. 2.4 mm[75]	59% vs. 66%[75]		
Ceramics				
• HA vs. debridement	1.3-2.8 vs. 0.5-0.9 mm[96-99]	67% vs. 10%[96] 55-60% vs. 31-32% had ≥50% fill[97-99]	No new periodontal attachment, osteogenesis, or cementogenesis.[102]	

Continued

TABLE 25-1   Comparative Analysis of Regenerative Approaches—cont'd

Graft Material	CAL Gain, mm	Defect Fill, % or mm	Histologic Assessment	Comments
• PHA vs. debridement	3.6 mm vs. 1.2 mm[104-106]	24% vs. 9%[105] 58% vs. 22%[106]	Bone formation in the implant pores and periphery. No new attachment. Pocket reduction by long JE.[109-111]	
• TCP	2.3-2.7 mm[112-115]	67%[112]	Fibrous encapsulation followed by rapid resorption. No evidence of new attachment. Healing by long JE.[117]	
Comparative studies				
• PHA vs. FDBA • PHA vs. DFDBA	1.3 vs. 2.2 mm[65] 1.6 vs. 2.1 mm[76] 2.8 vs. 2.1 mm[77]	— 53% vs. 61%[76] —		No significant differences. No significant differences. Suggest PHA is superior to DFDBA.
Biocompatible composite polymer				
• HTR vs. debridement	1.9 vs. 1.0 mm[118] 3.4 vs. 2.7 mm[119]	61% vs. 33%[118]	No regeneration but some evidence of new connective tissue attachment.[121,122]	
Calcium carbonates				
• NCS vs. debridement	2.3 vs. 0.7 mm[126]	67% vs. 26%[126]		NCS is superior to debridement.
Comparative study				
• NCS vs. PHA vs. debridement	—	57.4% vs. 58.1% vs. 22.2%[106]		NCS is comparable to PHA and both are superior to debridement.
Bioactive glass ceramics				
• BGC vs. debridement	3.40 vs. 1.56 mm[132] 2.96 vs. 1.54 mm[134]	— 4.36 vs. 3.15 mm[134]	Bone fill is by osseous infiltration of implant. Healing by long JE.[129,130]	No significant difference in one study.[133]
Comparative study				
• BGC vs. DFDBA	2.27 vs. 1.93 mm[135]	61.8% vs. 62.5%[135]		No significant differences.
Anorganic bovine bone (xenografts)				
• ABB vs. DFDBA • ABB vs. ABB + GTR (histologic case study)	3.5 vs. 2.6 mm[95] —	55.8% vs. 46.8%[95] —	New cementum and bone with ABB being osteoconductive. GTR membrane addition enhanced healing.[95]	No significant differences.

GTR

• ePTFE	2.0-5.3 mm[155-157]	0.5-1.7 mm of new attachment[155-157]	
• Resorbable barrier Polyglactin-910 vs. ePTFE	4.0 vs. 3.5 mm[166,167]	77.5% vs. 70.7%[166,167]	

Comparative studies

• ePTFE + DFDBA + citric acid root conditioning	4.7 mm[153]		Clinical series suggest improved results with DFDBA + citric acid root conditioning.
• ePTFE + DFDBA vs. DFDBA	2.8 vs. 3.2 mm[172,173]	58% vs. 71%[172,173]	Improved results with DFDBA.
• ePTFE vs. ePTFE + HA-collagen graft vs. HA-collagen graft alone	3.70 mm[154] vs. 3.80 mm vs. 2.60 mm	1.50 mm[154] vs. 1.55 mm vs. 0.85 mm	ePTFE membranes ± HA-collagen graft was better than HA-collagen graft alone.
• ePTFE vs. debridement	2.1 mm	0.60 mm	

EMD

• EMD vs. placebo control or debridement	2.2 vs. 1.7 mm[193] 4.26 vs. 2.75 mm[196]	— 74.0% vs. 22.7%[196]	Suggests EMD can stimulate new attachment. Histologic analysis of two cases. Both cases had new cementum and attachment but only one had new bone.[190,191]

Comparative studies

• EMD vs. GTR (evaluated after 24 and 48 months)	3.0 vs. 2.9 mm[199]	—	Both techniques improve CAL and appear to be stable over 4 years.
• EMD + bioactive glass vs. bioactive glass	3.22 vs. 3.07 mm[200]	—	No significant difference.
• EMD + anorganic bovine bone vs. EMD + fibrin glue	2.89 vs. 2.83 mm[202]	—	Improved results over published debridement results, but no difference between treatment modality.

ABB, anorganic bovine bone; BGC, bioactive glass ceramics; CAL, clinical attachment level; DFDBA, demineralized freeze-dried bone allograft; EMD, enamel matrix derivative; ePTFE, expanded polytetrafluoroethylene; FDBA, freeze-dried bone allograft; GTR, guided tissue regeneration; HA, hydroxyapatite; HTR, hard tissue replacement; JE, junctional epithelium; PHA, porous hydroxyapatite; NCS, natural coral skeleton; TCP, tricalcium phosphate.

junction to the base of the pocket. Most studies report changes in clinical attachment level. However, gains in clinical attachment level, although desired, do not necessarily imply that the new attachment is the result of actual regeneration (i.e., new bone, PDL, and cementum). The resolution of tissue inflammation, formation of a long junctional epithelial attachment, connective tissue attachment, and increased bone fill all result in clinical attachment level gain. In some studies, surgical stents have been used to ensure that the placement and angulation of the periodontal probe can be duplicated in subsequent dental visits, resulting in more accurate clinical attachment level measurements.

Bone fill is the only aspect of regeneration/healing that can be accurately assessed clinically. Formerly, bone fill measurements were performed by surgical reentry. This approach, however, is no longer recommended for routine clinical use because it requires an unnecessary second surgical procedure. Studies using nonsurgical means, such as bone probing or "sounding" performed with local anesthesia, have demonstrated accuracy in measuring changes in bone height equal to surgical reentry.[5,6] Although this can give an indication of how much bone has been produced, it is important to note that bone fill does not necessarily equate with regeneration. Bone fill is simply the formation of new bone within the periodontal defect; it does not describe how the tissue relates to the root surface. Histologic analysis has demonstrated that new bone fill may occur, and yet be separated from the root surface by formation of a long junctional epithelium or connective tissue adhesion, indicating periodontal repair.[7-9] In periodontal regeneration, functionally aligned PDL fibers are observed between newly formed bone and the root surface.

Standardized radiographic evaluation of bone regeneration provides qualitative evidence of bone fill, but yields little information in terms of the nature of the attachment and the density of the bone (Fig. 25-2). The amount of mineralization required to cause a detectable change in radiographic pattern makes this method of assessment less reliable than clinical probing techniques or surgical reentry.[10,11] With the advent of subtraction radiography, however, linear analysis has improved the radiographic assessment of bone fill.[12,13] This technique, used in conjunction with computer-assisted densitometric image analysis (CADIA), offers the greatest level of accuracy.[14,15]

Histologic analysis is the only definitive method for determining whether the healing tissue was formed by repair or by regeneration (Fig. 25-3). This method provides an accurate assessment of the various components and their interrelationship in the newly formed periodontal attachment apparatus. In regeneration studies, reference notches are placed at the base of bony defects or at the apical extent of calculus deposits, and periodontal regeneration is considered to have occurred when the newly formed periodontium is coronal to the apical extent of the notches. Unfortunately, this approach cannot be used in human studies because it would be unethical to extract the treated tooth, especially when it responded positively to therapy. On rare circumstances, human histology is available if the tooth is to be extracted in conjunction with orthodontic or restorative therapy.

Several animal model systems can be used to study periodontal healing. Currently, the most widely used model systems include beagle dogs and nonhuman primates.[16] Because it is difficult to find an adequate number of naturally occurring periodontal osseous defects, the defects are either surgically produced or experimentally induced. Although the surgically produced defects may control the nature of the defect, they lack the chronic infectious properties observed with the naturally occurring disease process. The experimentally induced lesions have the chronic infectious properties, but it is difficult to control the type of osseous defects that result. Despite these weaknesses, these animal models permit the clinical and histologic study of the healing process.

The importance of histologic evaluation in confirming periodontal regeneration is exemplified in a classic primate study.[17] At the time of this study, the literature had described positive clinical outcomes from the modified Widman flap procedure, flap procedure with frozen autologous bone transplant, flap procedure with tricalcium phosphate (TCP) graft, and periodontal root planing and soft tissue curettage. When these four therapeutic approaches were examined histologically in the treatment of a monkey experimental periodontitis model system, all therapies resulted mostly in the formation of long junctional epithelium, a characteristic of repair, not regeneration. Although bone regeneration was detected in the intrabony defect, junctional epithelium was present between the newly formed bone and the root surface. These results suggested that apical migration of epithelial cells occurs more rapidly than colonization by other cell types. This study emphasized the importance of histologic confirmation of periodontal regeneration.

As the various approaches toward periodontal regeneration are reviewed, it is important to distinguish the type of defects being corrected and the results described. Improvement in clinical attachment level or bone fill radiopacity associated with the defect does not necessarily mean periodontal regeneration has occurred. The reconstitution of a new periodontium is a histologic determination that is difficult to obtain. Currently, the most widely used methods of evaluating whether a treatment modality can potentially result in periodontal regeneration are to provide histologic evaluation of periodontal regeneration in animal models when human biopsy materials are not available and to provide supportive clinical and radiographic data.

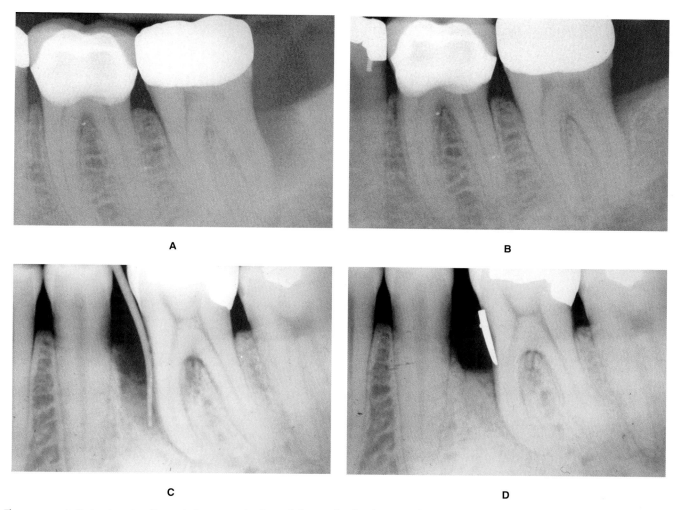

Figure 25-2. A, Pretreatment radiograph demonstrating bony defect on the distal aspect of #18. **B,** Posttreatment radiographic appearance consistent with good bone fill. **C,** Pretreatment radiograph with gutta percha point noting bony defect. **D,** New osseous level with Hirschfield point postregenerative procedure. Although radiographs may indicate the presence of new bone, they may underestimate the amount of bone loss or gain, and they do not define the true nature of the newly formed tissue. (**A** and **B,** Courtesy of Dr. J. Salzman, Larkspur, PA; private practice.)

The healing tissue often will contain areas of periodontal regeneration and areas of repair. Therefore, it is important to remember that, even in the presence of histologic evidence of regeneration, not all of the improvement in clinical attachment level is because of regeneration; some improvement is because of new attachment.

THERAPEUTIC APPROACHES TOWARD PERIODONTAL REGENERATION

Root Conditioning Procedures

One approach toward improving periodontal healing is to clean and to enhance the root surface so that it is biologically compatible. Although scaling and root planing will

remove bacterial endotoxins, early animal experiments indicated that demineralizing the root surface with citric acid at pH 1 for 2 to 3 minutes resulted in new connective tissue attachment and cementogenesis.[18-20] Histologically, the new connective tissue attachment appeared as perpendicularly arranged collagenous fibers, which were continuous with the newly formed cementum. Several studies analyzed the healing sequence of the citric acid–treated root surface. With treatment, the smear layer (a surface layer of protein and debris) was removed and the root surface was demineralized to expose a 2- to 15-μm zone of thick collagenous fibrils anchored to a root surface with opened dentinal tubules.[19,20] After 1 to 3 days, a fibrin linkage was present between the PDL and root surface. By 21 days, the fibrin network appeared to be well attached to the

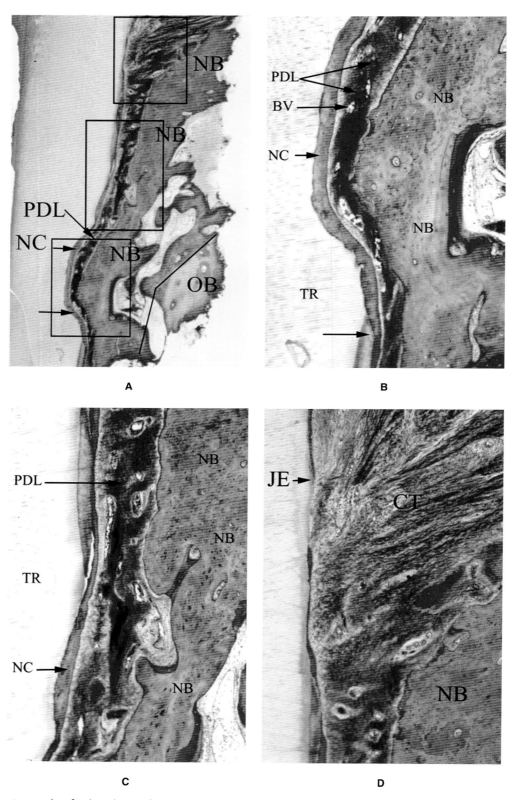

Figure 25-3. Photomicrographs of a clinical case of periodontal regeneration 9 months after the application of recombinant human platelet-derived growth factor. Histologic landmarks as evidence of regeneration include the following: a low magnification view of the regenerated area (**A**); a detailed view of the notched root surface (**B**) and the newly regenerated periodontium coronal to this landmark (**C**); and the coronal aspect of the regenerated periodontium in relation to the junctional epithelium (**D**). BV, blood vessel; CT, connective tissue; JE, junctional epithelium; NB, new bone; NC, new cementum; OB, old bone; PDL, periodontal ligament; TR, root trunk. (Courtesy of Dr. S. Lynch, Biomimetic Pharmaceuticals, Inc.; Franklin TN.)

root surface. This fibrin linkage has been shown to impede the apical migration of epithelium and result in a rapid ingress of cells, which putatively will develop the new connective tissue attachment.[21-24] Interpretations of histologic studies suggest that the formation of new attachment is the result of interdigitation between newly synthesized collagen fibrils and established collagenous fibrils of the cementum or dentin. The histologic findings of citric acid treatment have been confirmed in human studies.[25-29]

The positive attributes of citric acid treatment are supported by two clinical studies.[30,31] In a split-mouth design to evaluate the effect of citric acid treatment after replacement flap surgery, citric acid at pH 1 was applied to the root surface for 3 to 5 minutes. An average clinical attachment level gain of 2.1 mm was observed for the citric acid–treated side as compared with a 1.5 mm gain for the control side. In a similar study evaluating citric acid use with root surfaces associated with intrabony defects, the gain in clinical attachment level was 2.0 mm, whereas the nonacid-treated control had a clinical attachment level gain of only 1.2 mm. Approximately 73% of the acid-treated teeth gained 2 mm or more in clinical attachment level. Contrary to these studies, others have not been able to reproduce histologic evidence of new attachment[32-34] or beneficial clinical results.[35-38]

Root conditioning with tetracycline and EDTA also has been advocated. The suggested benefit is that it may produce a histologic phenomenon similar to citric acid treatment without inducing pulpal or epithelial injuries.[39,40] Histologic information on these agents, however, is limited. There are other indications that may warrant the use of tetracycline. Tetracycline has been shown to bind to dentin with the maximum binding occurring when tetracycline is applied at 50 mg/ml or greater. The bound tetracycline is released and serves as a local antimicrobial delivery vehicle for up to 14 days.[41,42] In addition, tetracycline-treated dental slabs have been shown in cell culture experiments to bind fibronectin, a cell adhesion protein that mediates cell attachment and migration of mesenchymal cells. The presence of fibronectin permits increased cell adhesion and colonization. Conversely, tetracycline reverses the binding of laminin, an epithelial cell attachment protein.[43] These studies suggest that tetracycline treatment preferentially permits the colonization and migration of fibroblasts over epithelial cells.

Two clinical studies have disputed the efficacy of tetracycline root conditioning. In the first study, diseased root surfaces underwent root planing and were treated with tetracycline burnished for 3 minutes, tetracycline burnished with an application of exogenous fibronectin, or no treatment. No new attachment was present in any of the groups. The tetracycline treatment resulted in a statistically significant improvement in clinical attachment level, but the difference was clinically insignificant.[44] When

tetracycline treatment was used in conjunction with GTR, there were no clinical improvements observed when compared with control.[45] A comprehensive, systematic review of all the evidence for root conditioning with citric acid, tetracycline, and EDTA in humans found no statistically or clinically significant benefit to use of any of these agents.[46] Despite the lack of evidence, some practitioners continue to perform root conditioning in certain cases. There appear to be no adverse effects of such treatment.

Bone Grafts and Grafting Materials

The classical approach to periodontal regeneration in the last 30 years has been the use of bone grafts or bone substitutes in repairing periodontal defects (Box 25-1). Grafts are generally classified according to their original source as follows:

Autograft: Tissue transferred from one position to another within the same individual.

Box 25-1   Bone Grafts and Bone Substitutes Used in the Correction of Periodontal Defects

Bone-Derived Material

Vital Bone Graft
- *Autograft*
  - Oral
    - Osseous coagulum
    - Bone blend
    - Bone harvested from extraction site, tuberosity, edentulous ridge
  - Extraoral
    - Iliac crest
- *Allograft*
  - Cryopreserved bone
  - Fresh bone from iliac crest

Nonvital Bone Graft
- *Allografts (human bone)*
  - Freeze-dried bone allograft
  - Demineralized freeze-dried bone allograft
- *Xenograft*
  - Anorganic bovine bone

Nonosseous Material

Organic
- *Dentin*
- *Cementum*
- *Coral*

Anorganic (alloplasts)
- *Calcium sulfate (plaster of Paris)*
- *Calcium phosphate-hydroxyapatite*
- *Calcium ceramics*
- *Bioactive glass polymers*

Allograft: Tissue transferred from one individual to another genetically dissimilar individual of the same species.

Xenograft: Tissue transferred from one species to another species.

Alloplast: A synthetic graft or inert foreign body implanted into tissue.

Early clinical series reported that bone regeneration was enhanced by the use of cancellous bone autografts from the iliac crest. These fresh autografts are *osteogenic*, that is, vital cells present within the grafted material are capable of forming new bone. Although this method proved clinically successful, the necessity of a secondary surgical harvest using an extraoral site (the hip) and surgical complications of ankylosis and root resorption of the treated tooth or teeth made this approach less popular. Therefore, during the last decade, FDBA and DFDBA have become the materials of choice. These materials are widely available and may induce new bone formation. However, studies have questioned the bone inducing properties of bone allografts, suggesting that this potential may vary depending on the bone bank or batch within the bank used, processing procedures, and donor characteristics. Alternatively, a variety of xenograft and alloplastic grafting materials have become available for use in periodontal regeneration and repair. This section reviews the clinical and histologic results after the use of these materials.

Bone grafts and bone substitutes used in regenerative therapy are derived from bone or nonosseous materials. Correction of osseous aspects of the periodontal defect occurs by osteoinduction or osteoconduction. A graft material is *osteoinductive* when it can induce bone formation. This implies that the material is able to recruit undifferentiated mesenchymal cells, be mitogenic for preosteoblasts, and induce differentiation of these cells into bone-forming osteoblastic cells. A material is *osteoconductive* when its structure and chemical composition facilitate new bone formation from existing bone. Osteoconductive materials generally act as scaffolding on which new bone forms. This often results in the amalgamation of the material into the newly formed bone mass.

Osteogenic autogenous bone grafts (autografts)

Iliac bone and marrow autografts have proven to be the most predictable graft materials for bone growth. However, because of the necessity of harvesting from a secondary surgical site and the possible morbidity associated with these procedures, they are no longer popular. In an early study, Schallhorn and colleagues[47] treated 182 osseous defects ranging from 3.3 to 4.2 mm in 52 patients with iliac graft. The resultant mean bone fill was 2.6 mm in "zero wall or no wall" defects, 3.75 mm in one-wall defects, and 4.16 mm in two-wall defects. Approximately 87% of the

Class II furcations had complete fill. Histologically, new bone, cementum, and functionally oriented PDL were observed.[48] Complications associated with the use of fresh iliac bone and marrow included a high rate of root resorption and anklyosis.[49] These complications were later shown to be minimized by either freezing the bone graft in a storage medium or adding autologous intraoral bone to the harvested iliac crest bone graft mixture. To date, iliac bone and marrow have the most osteogenic and regenerative potential, and are one of two graft materials with the reported ability to regenerate periodontium horizontally or with "zero wall" defects, meaning actual crestal apposition of new bone.

Intraoral autogenous bone grafts have been harvested from various intraoral sites including edentulous ridges, the maxillary tuberosity, 8- to 12-week postextraction healing sites, and tori or exostoses. Three clinical case series described the use of intraoral cortical-cancellous grafts, which resulted in bone fill of 2.88 to 3.44 mm in 373 defects.[47,50,51] One controlled study of 37 paired defects demonstrated 2.98 mm of bone gain when autogenous intraoral bone grafts were used, as compared with 0.66 mm for debrided controls that received no grafts.[52] With the exception of furcations and crestal defects, intraoral bone grafts were comparable to iliac grafts. Contrary to these findings, two controlled studies indicated no significant differences in bone gain.[53,54] These conflicting reports may be because of site morphology and donor tissue. Studies have indicated that the degree of success and increased amount of bone fill are related to the increased number of osseous walls associated with the defect. The source of intraoral bone also is important. When bone is predominantly cortical in nature, it has little osteogenic potential. Cancellous bone, which contains hematopoietic marrow, such as red bone marrow from the maxillary tuberosity or from healing bone sockets 8 to 12 weeks after extraction, provides better osteogenic potential. According to two reports,[48,55] when intraoral autogenous bone is used in a composite graft with FDBA, regeneration is enhanced as compared with FDBA alone (78%-80% vs. 63%-67% of defects exhibiting greater than 50% bone fill). Histologically, several studies[48,55] and case reports[56-59] have shown that intraoral autogenous bone is able to form new attachment.

These clinical studies suggest that autografts can effectively enhance bone fill by an average of 3 to 4 mm. Currently, this is considered the "gold standard" for periodontal graft material.

Osteoinductive nonvital bone grafts (allografts)

In a series of animal experiments and clinical case series, Schallhorn and Hiatt[48,60] reported that when allografts of iliac bone and marrow were used, the results were similar to autogenous iliac grafts with mean bone gain of

3.6 mm in one-, two-, and three-walled defects; 2.1 mm vertical increase in "zero wall" defects (crestal apposition in cases with horizontal bone loss patterns); and 3.3 mm bone gain in furcation defects. Notably, this is the only other graft material with reported ability to correct "zero wall" defects. However, despite these encouraging results, the risk for disease transmission from the donor to the graft recipient has eliminated the potential use of frozen allografts in periodontics. Allografts used in periodontics are primarily in two forms: FDBA and DFDBA. These allografts are processed in such a way as to minimize the risk for disease transmission.

In four uncontrolled studies, FDBA has been shown to be effective in correcting osseous defects. These studies involved a total of 1401 defects, and results consistently indicated that 60% to 68% of the defects had 50% or more bone fill on reentry.[61-64] Osseous regeneration was least pronounced in furcation defects.

FDBA used alone and augmented with other graft materials also has been tested and compared with other grafting procedures. Studies using FDBA augmented with autogenous bone found that an additional 11% to 17% of these defects had 50% or more fill when compared with defects treated with FDBA alone.[62,64] A comparison of FDBA with granular porous hydroxyapatite (PHA) indicated that FDBA was superior, with 2.1 mm of bone fill compared with 1.3 mm for granular PHA.[65]

Currently, there is no histologic evidence of periodontal regeneration after FDBA grafting procedures. Although clinical reports of osseous fill are impressive, with approximately 60% of the defects having 50% or more fill and the mean bone fill approximately 2 mm, the only controlled study to date showed no difference between the use of FDBA versus debridement in a small number of paired defects.[66]

Animal studies by Urist and colleagues[67,68] and other studies[69] have shown that demineralization of cortical bone allografts will improve the osteogenic potential by exposing BMPs, an inductive factor known to increase bone formation. Tissue banks have used modifications of this protocol to process DFDBAs. In human histologic studies, Bowers and colleagues[70,71] demonstrated that the mean new attachment formation for 32 defects was 1.21 mm when DFDBA was used, whereas no new attachment was observed in 25 debrided defects that received no grafts. Clinical studies have shown that using DFDBA results in more bone fill as compared with controls in which only debridement is performed (2.3-2.9 mm vs. 0.3-1.3 mm and 65% vs. 11-37% bone fill).[72-74] In clinical comparison studies, DFDBA has been shown to be comparable to FDBA[75] and comparable[76] or inferior to PHA.[77]

Recent studies have focused on three issues: (1) Are DFDBA grafts osteoinductive?; (2) Can the osteoinductive potential of DFDBA be improved?; and (3) What is the long-term outcome of DFDBA-treated sites?

Are demineralized freeze-dried bone allografts osteoinductive? The clinical premise for using DFDBA was based on Urist's studies[67,68] that suggest demineralization of FDBA will make BMP accessible for osteoinduction. Although BMPs are genetically highly conserved, FDBA and DFDBA are immunogenic between species.[78] To eliminate the immunogenicity issue, Becker and colleagues[79] implanted human BMP preparations and DFDBA from four commercial bone banks into muscle pouches of athymic mice, which were genetically immunosuppressed. Histologically, commercial DFDBA induced minimal amounts of new appositional bone (7.5-21.6%). However, Urist's partially purified human BMP preparations resulted in 96% of the field filled with new appositional bone.[80] The discrepancy between Urist's preparation and commercial DFDBA preparations may be because of the modification of the bone-processing protocol used by the bone bank to minimize risk for infection. Furthermore, denaturation of BMPs may occur during large batch processing of commercially available DFDBA.

To address the issue of whether laboratory-prepared DFDBA is different from commercially available DFDBA, Shigeyama and colleagues[81] compared the protein extracts from these DFDBA preparations in terms of their effects on early events of bone formation—for example, cell recruitment, attachment, and proliferation. The laboratory preparation was more mitogenic and resulted in a faster rate of cell proliferation than the extracts from commercial DFDBA. All extracts enhanced cell attachment, whereas no extracts were effective in cell recruitment and chemotaxis. When matrix proteins were analyzed, although both preparations contained BMP-2, -4, and -7, the laboratory-prepared DFDBA had greater concentrations of BMP-2, the primary osteoinductive protein of the BMP family. This study suggests that even though commercially prepared DFDBA may retain proteins that have the capacity to influence cell differentiation and possibly regeneration *in vivo*, many of these proteins are lost during tissue processing.

Schwartz and colleagues[82] subsequently examined 14 batches of commercially available DFDBA from 6 bone banks. The investigators found discrepancies between and even within lots from the same bone banks in terms of particle size, surface morphometry, and pH properties. When implanted into muscle pouches of athymic mice, three of the bone bank samples formed new bone after 1 to 2 months, whereas no bone was formed after the implantation of graft materials from the other bone banks. When different preparation lots from each bone bank were analyzed, there were variations in the rate and the amount of new bone formed. A subsequent study examined 27 lots from the same bone bank, which previously had been shown to manufacture DFDBA that was consistently osteoinductive.[83] Five lots had little or no osteoinductive properties; 12 (40%) were found to be associated with new bone present in 40% or more of the surface areas examined; and only 5 lots (18.5%) produced new bone in more than 50% of the surface areas. This study suggests there is a wide variation in osteoinductive properties of DFDBA from commercial bone banks, and even among lots from the same bone bank.

Because DFDBAs have varying levels of osteoinductive properties, are there technical procedures that can maximize the osteogenic potential? Histologic sections from the controlled study by Reynolds and Bowers[84] were reviewed to study the fate of DFDBA. Approximately 72% of the grafted sites exhibited residual DFDBA particles. When comparing sites containing residual DFDBA versus those without residual DFDBA, greater amounts of new attachment formation (1.72 vs. 0.2 mm), new bone (2.33 vs. 0.23 mm), and cementum (1.74 vs. 0.23 mm) were associated with sites containing some residual DFDBA. Graft containment may thus be an important factor in influencing the regenerative response.

Can the osteoinductive potential of demineralized freeze-dried bone allograft preparation be improved? Findings suggest that preparations of DFDBA differ in their ability to induce new bone formation, and some batches may not induce any activity at all. This has resulted in studies that have attempted to describe methods for monitoring the osteogenic potential of various DFDBA batches, as well as factors that will influence the osteogenic potential of each batch.

Although the implantation of various batches of DFDBA into athymic mice may be an effective way of predicting their osteogenic potential, this system is costly and impractical. Previously, human PDL cells and ROS osteosarcoma cells have been used to predict the osteogenic potential of various batches of DFDBA.[85] The ability to induce new bone formation *in vivo* was highly correlated with cell proliferation and alkaline phosphatase production in these cells. This approach was used by Zhang and coworkers,[86] in which alkaline phosphatase activity *in vitro* was shown to be correlated with calcium uptake into the DFDBA-implanted area *in vivo*. These *in vitro* assays, together with the implantation of DFDBA into athymic mice, have indicated the influence of various factors on the osteogenic potential of a DFDBA preparation. Several tissue banks are providing *in vitro* assay and athymic mice implantation data to demonstrate the osteogenic potential of their products. Although these data are interesting, the more valuable information would be the specific data for each batch distributed. This not only would serve as quality assurance standards, but would eventually validate the usefulness of these assays.

The osteogenic potential of DFDBA appears to be dependent on the extent of demineralization. FDBA, the mineralized precursor to DFDBA, when prepared from various animal sources has been shown to be ineffective in osteoinduction. This was confirmed in a study using human DFDBA, which was effective only after demineralization. Maximum osteoinduction was observed when there was only a 2% or less residual calcium level in the DFDBA material.[87]

The osteogenic potential of DFDBA may also be dependent on the age of the bone donor. Previously, animal experiments have indicated that the osteogenic potential of rat DFDBA is age dependent. Bone harvested from middle aged donor animals had better bone forming potential than bone from younger animals, and bone formation was better in younger recipients than in older ones.[88] This finding was repeated in a study using 27 lots of human DFDBA from the same bone bank in which the age and sex of the donor for each lot was identified and each sample was implanted into athymic mice.[83] The osteogenic potential was not dependent on the sex of the bone donor, but was improved in younger compared with older donors. A study of donor age and sex suggested that DFDBA processed from donor bone of women aged 31 to 40 years and men aged 41 to 50 years possess the greatest osteoinductivity.[87] Thus, the ability to induce new bone formation appears to be age dependent, with DFDBA from older donors having the lowest osteoinductive potential. Osteoinductive potential appears not to be influenced significantly by the sex of the donor.

What is the long-term outcome of demineralized freeze-dried bone allograft–treated sites? Although there are case reports that indicate gains in clinical attachment may be maintained for up to 5 years after implantation of DFDBA in combination with expanded polytetrafluoroethylene (ePTFE) membranes, there have been few assessments of the long-term stability of sites grafted with DFDBA alone.[89] A randomized controlled study compared DFDBA-grafted and debrided sites in eight patients.[90] After 6 months, the mean bone gains for the DFDBA-grafted and the debrided sites were 2.2 and 1.1 mm, respectively. After 3 years, with 3- to 6-month intervals of periodontal maintenance therapy, the mean bone gain changed by only 0.1 mm. These data indicate that alveolar bone gain after DFDBA implantation may be maintained over 3 years.

Xenografts—anorganic bovine bone

Anorganic bovine bone (ABB) is bovine bone that has been chemically treated to remove its organic components, leaving a trabecular and porous architecture similar to human bone. It has been proposed that this bone has no osteoinductive properties, but acts as a scaffold for new bone formation (osteoconduction). Studies in rabbits and dogs have shown it to be effective in correcting experimental bone and intrabony defects.[91,92]

Animal studies provide new insights regarding the healing pattern of ABB. In a comparison of anorganic bone with bioactive glass ceramics (BGC) in a critical-sized defect in rabbits, the anorganic bone-grafted sites were more radiopaque and had more new bone.[93] Whereas five of six anorganic bone grafted sites healed with bony union and restoration of the anatomic contour after 8 weeks, only one out of six BGC sites demonstrated similar findings. In dogs, the regenerative potential of anorganic bone plus collagen in experimental periodontal defects was evaluated at 6, 18, and 36 weeks by contact microradiography and scanning electron microscopy.[94] The anorganic bone plus collagen showed increased bone formation as compared with the flap curettage–treated sites. These two animal studies suggest that anorganic bone may be superior to BGC in experimental nonperiodontal bony defects and that, when augmented with collagen, it may be useful in correcting periodontal defects.

One study compared ABB with DFDBA in intrabony defects.[95] Significant improvement in pocket depth and clinical attachment level were observed for both graft materials after 6 months. A comparison of ABB with DFDBA indicated comparable pocket depth reduction (3.0 vs. 2.0 mm), clinical attachment level gain (3.5 vs. 2.6 mm), and bone fill (55.8% vs. 46.8% bone fill). Thus, there was no difference between the clinical healing responses with the two graft materials.

The use of ABB alone and in conjunction with GTR has been compared histologically.[95] In four anterior defects, two were grafted with ABB and two with ABB in conjunction with a bovine collagen GTR membrane. Clinical and histologic examination revealed that for the ABB^- and ABB^+ GTR-treated sites, the lengths of newly formed cementum were 5.1 to 5.2 mm and 7.0 to 7.6 mm, respectively; the height of new bone was 4.2 to 4.8 mm and 4.5 to 5.3 mm, respectively. Histologically, ABB was incorporated into the new bone, which suggested that healing was osteoconductive. When used in conjunction with a GTR membrane, the new connective tissue attachment extended to the coronal level of the original intrabony defect and an increase in new bone was observed. Thus, ABB may result in gains in clinical attachment that may be accompanied by regeneration when combined with use of an occlusive membrane.

Inert biologic fillers (alloplastic materials)

Alloplastic bone grafts used in periodontics consist of ceramics, such as hydroxyapatite (HA) and TCP, and biocompatible composite polymers. These inert biological fillers represent the first generation of alloplastic bone graft materials. They have been extensively studied and were comprehensively reviewed, showing these materials to be safe and well tolerated. Although effective in procedures such as ridge preservation and ridge augmentation,

these materials have been shown to be of more limited effectiveness in treating osseous defects around teeth.

Ceramics. Ceramics consist primarily of HA $[Ca_{10}(PO_4)_6(OH)_2]$ and β TCP $[Ca_{13}(PO_4)_2]$. HA is a solid calcium phosphate compound that is sintered. The physical and chemical properties of HA affect the rate of resorption and subsequently influence its clinical application. The density (dense or porous) determines the compressive strength of the graft material and the extent of vascular ingrowth. These two characteristics will influence the rate of resorption. Larger crystalline particles are nonresorbable, whereas smaller or amorphous particles are resorbed more rapidly. In general, the larger crystalline HA particles are used for ridge preservation and augmentation, and the small particles are used for periodontal applications. In clinical applications, dense HA has been shown to compare favorably with debridement in reducing probing depth (1.3 to 2.8 mm) and increasing clinical attachment gain.[96-99] A 5-year follow-up study indicated that HA-treated sites, particularly those exhibiting deep pockets (≥6 mm), were stable and less susceptible to subsequent attachment loss when compared with debrided sites.[100-102] Human histologic studies indicate that dense HA does not induce new attachment or bone formation, that pocket reduction is primarily through fibrous encapsulation of the HA particles in the intraosseous defect, and that pocket closure is through long junctional epithelium and connective tissue adhesion.[102,103] PHA has been shown to be effective in reducing probing depth and increasing attachment gain in both intraosseous defects[104-106] and Class II furcation defects.[107,108] Comparison of PHA with other grafting materials has shown PHA to produce similar clinical results to FDBA,[66] DFDBA,[76] and natural coral.[106] Other comparisons indicate that PHA is superior to DFDBA[77] and inferior to dense HA.[105] Three histologic analyses of clinical PHA-grafted defects indicated no new attachment, the presence of long junctional epithelium, and varying extents of bone associated with the PHA particles.[109-111]

β TCP is a calcium phosphate that is mixed with naphthalene at high temperatures. As the composite cools, the naphthalene evaporates, forming a porous calcium phosphate structure. Like HA, the rate of resorption is dependent on the porosity and particle size. Limited research of TCP as a periodontal graft material consists of six small noncontrolled studies with varying positive results of 1.2 to 2.8 mm bone gain and 2.3 to 2.7 mm of clinical attachment level gain.[112-115] Although animal studies indicate TCP is rapidly resorbed and replaced by bone,[116] a histologic study of human periodontal defects indicated that TCP particles are encapsulated by fibrous connective tissue and pocket closure is primarily through long junctional epithelium.[117] Thus, ceramic fillers (HA and TCP) are unlikely to result in true regeneration.

Biocompatible composite polymer. Biocompatible composite polymer (Bioplant HTR [Bioplant Inc.; South Norwalk, CT], or "hard tissue replacement" material) consists of poly-methylmethacrylate-poly-hydroxyl-ethylmethacrylate beads coated by calcium hydroxide. This calcium hydroxide surface forms a calcium carbonate apatite when introduced into the body. HTR has been shown to be superior to debridement alone in correcting intraosseous defects (60.8% vs. 32.2% mean defect fill)[118,119] and Class II furcation defects.[120] Clinical comparison studies have shown HTR to be equally as effective as autogenous bone grafts. Histologically, HTR rarely promotes new attachment.[121,122]

One report found that the improved clinical attachment level after implantation of HTR into furcation defects was stable after 6 years.[123] Thirteen patients with 16 maxillary and 10 mandibular grade II furcation defects were treated with HTR. Reentry after 6 to 12 months indicated an improvement of mean horizontal attachment level of 2.2 to 4.4 mm, and mean vertical attachment gain of 1.2 mm. After 6 years, the mean attachment level was maintained, indicating that implantation of HTR may be beneficial and stable in the treatment of maxillary and mandibular grade II furcations.

Calcium carbonates. Calcium carbonates are processed natural coral skeletons (NCSs) from *Porites* coral, which can serve as resorbable bone graft substitutes. Cell culture and animal studies have indicated the material enhances osteoblastic cell attachment and growth[124] and can be converted to bone in experimental defects.[125] It enhanced healing by resorption and replacement with newly formed bone. NCS itself was not osteoinductive, but rather osteoconductive, acting as a scaffold for formation of new host bone. The first controlled study of NCS in comparison with debridement alone was performed in 20 patients with at least two defects each. In a nonpaired controlled comparison of 40 defects receiving NCS and 39 treated by debridement alone, surgical reentry after 6 months indicated a mean defect fill of 2.3 mm (67%) for the NCS-treated sites and 0.7 mm (25.9%) for those treated with debridement alone.[126] Of the sites examined, 88% of the NCS sites had more than 50% defect fill versus 18% in the control sites. This finding was confirmed by a study in which NCS was compared with PHA or debridement alone.[106] Ten patients with three intrabony defects each were treated and assessed. After 12 months, bone fill of 2.2 mm (57.4% bone fill) for NCS treatment, 2.5 mm (58.1%) for PHA treatment, and 1.1 mm (22.2%) for control were observed. These studies suggest that NCS augmentation is clinically superior to debridement alone and comparable to PHA.

Bioactive glass ceramics. BGC are made of CaO, Na$_2$O, SIO$_2$, and P$_2$O$_5$ in the same proportions as in bone and teeth and are referred to as *45S5 bioactive glass*. This material was initially introduced as an amorphous material (Bioglass; NovaBone Products, Alachua, FL) and has been demonstrated in animal studies to regenerate bone and soft tissue attachment to teeth.[127] The material has subsequently been produced in a particulate form with a 90- to 710-μm diameter (PerioGlas; NovaBone Products, Alachua, FL) and with a 300- to 350-μm (BioGran; 3i, Palm Beach Gardens, FL) diameter. Bioactive glass enhances bone formation by ionic dissolution of the ceramic particles such that a silica gel layer forms over the particles on contact with body fluid. Over this silica gel layer, a calcium phosphate layer forms, which is quickly converted into a hydroxycarbonate apatite layer.[128] This apatite layer has been shown to be identical to bone mineral and to provide the surface for osteoblast cell attachment and bone deposition.[129,130] The continuous ionic exchange results in dissolution of the ceramic particles such that after 1 to 3 years, the particles have been shown to be replaced by bone.[131] Only recently has clinical information been available regarding its use in the correction of periodontal defects.

In a report of a case series where BGC were placed in 17 intrabony osseous defects in 12 patients, the healing was monitored over 6 months.[132] At the end of the study, the mean probing depth was reduced 3.40 mm, and a mean attachment gain of 1.56 mm and a mean radiographic bone fill of 2.60 mm were achieved. These clinical results remained stable over a 24-month period.

In a controlled study comparing the use of BGC to debridement alone, there were significant increases in radiographic density and volume of bone in defects treated with BGC when compared with those treated only with surgical debridement.[133] Probing depth and attachment levels for both groups improved. Comparison between the groups in these parameters indicates that even though there was a greater trend toward improvement with the BGC-treated group, it was not statistically significant.

In another large, controlled, split-mouth design study, BGC was found to be superior to surgical debridement alone, as evidenced by mean probing depth reduction (4.26 vs. 3.44 mm), increased clinical attachment level (2.96 vs. 1.54 mm), and less gingival recession (1.29 vs. 1.87 mm) at 12 months.[134] Surgical reentry indicated greater defect fill with BGC (4.36 vs. 3.15 mm). This study suggests that BGC results in significant improvement in clinical parameters compared with open debridement.

BGC was compared with DFDBA in a paired study of 15 patients.[135] After 6 months, sites treated with BGC were similar to those receiving DFDBA in mean probing depth reduction (3.07 vs. 2.60 mm), mean attachment level gain (2.27 vs. 1.93 mm), and mean bone fill (2.73 vs. 2.80 mm). Surgical reentry indicated BGC resulted in 61.8% bone fill and 73.3% defect resolution, whereas DFDBA achieved 62.5% bone fill and 80.9% defect resolution. No statistical differences in soft and hard tissue improvement were observed between BGC and DFDBA during the 6-month study.

Guided Tissue Regeneration/Guided Bone Regeneration

Our current understanding of periodontal healing is based on a hypothesis by Melcher,[2] who proposed that the cell type that repopulates the exposed root surface at the periodontal repair site will define the nature of the attachment or repair that takes place. If mesenchymal cells from the PDL or perivascular region of the bone proliferate and colonize the root surface, regeneration occurs. Alternatively, if lost tissue is replaced by the surrounding tissue to form a scar, repair occurs. The anatomy of the scar is dependent on the cell types that predominate the defect. The four cell types of concern in the periodontium are gingival epithelial cells, mesenchymal cells from gingival connective tissue, alveolar bone cells, and PDL cells (see Fig. 25-1). If epithelial cells proliferate along the root surface, a long junctional epithelium will result. If gingival connective tissue populates the root surface, a connective tissue attachment will form and root resorption may occur. If bone cells migrate and adhere to the root surface, root resorption and ankylosis occur. Root resorption is much more common in animal models than it is in humans.

Animal models studying GTR have confirmed the importance of PDL cells as progenitor cells for periodontal regeneration.[136,137] Evaluation of cell proliferation kinetics revealed that both the PDL and perivascular cells from the bone proliferate and migrate into the osseous defect to form the early healing tissue.[138] Melcher[139] has amended his original hypothesis to include the contribution of the perivascular cells of the bone in periodontal regeneration—that is, cells from both the PDL and alveolar bone are important in formation of new bone, cementum, and functionally oriented PDL (regeneration). This current theory influences much of our therapeutic approaches toward management of periodontal defects.

A classic nonhuman primate study evaluated histologic healing after four different treatments: a modified Widman flap procedure, a flap procedure with a frozen autologous bone graft, a flap procedure with a TCP graft, and periodontal root planing and soft tissue curettage.[17] All four therapies resulted in repair in the form of long junctional epithelium with limited regeneration restricted to the base of the periodontal defects. These results suggest that the apical migration of epithelial cells occurs more rapidly than the colonization of the reparative surfaces by other cell types.

Early clinical approaches toward epithelial exclusion suggested this approach may enhance regeneration.[140] Denudation procedures were used to excise all interdental soft tissue, granulation tissue, and calculus from three-walled intrabony defects. Surgical dressings were applied to prevent epithelial ingrowth from the surrounding wound margins. Using this approach, two studies[141,142] reported a mean clinical attachment level gain of 2.44 mm and a mean defect fill of 47.5%. Defect improvement resulted from a combination of crestal resorption (mean, 0.48 mm) and defect repair (mean, 2.55 mm). These results are similar to other osseous grafting studies in terms of percent of defect fill.

A series of experiments and clinical studies[143-146] demonstrated that if the apical migration of epithelial cells can be impeded and PDL cells allowed to repopulate the root surface, regeneration will occur. The use of an occlusive membrane barrier to promote the formation of new periodontium is called GTR (guided tissue regeneration).

As early animal studies confirmed Melcher's postulate that the cells that populate the root surface during healing will define the healing tissue, this approach was developed into clinical procedures for human defects. To promote the proliferation of PDL cells, membrane barriers were used to exclude epithelial, bone, and gingival connective tissue cells. Classically, GTR is associated with the use of membranes, either nonresorbable or resorbable (Box 25-2). However, other forms of barriers also have been used.

Nonresorbable membranes

In classic animal and human studies demonstrating the efficacy of GTR, cellulose acetate filters were used. As this technique became more prevalent, the first commercial membrane was produced from ePTFE. This membrane has all the properties necessary for GTR barriers; for example, it (1) is a cellular barrier, (2) is biocompatible, (3) provides space for the healing tissue, (4) permits tissue integration, and (5) is clinically manageable. Much of our current understanding of GTR is based on studies using ePTFE membranes. Although currently used less frequently, ePTFE

Box 25-2   Guided Tissue Regeneration Membranes

Nonbioresorbable membranes

1. Expanded polytetrafluoroethylene (ePTFE)
2. Miscellaneous membranes (Millipore membrane, rubber dam)

Bioresorbable membranes

1. Synthetic polymers
   - Polyurethane
   - Polylactic acid
   - Lactide/glycolide copolymers (e.g., polyglactin-910)
   - Polylactic acid blended with citric acid ester
2. Natural biomaterials (e.g., collagen)
3. Calcium sulfate

membranes are still popular for guided bone regeneration (GBR) and ridge preservation; therefore, it is important to understand the clinical procedures for managing these membranes.

The clinical effectiveness of ePTFE membranes is dependent on technique. Preservation of the keratinized gingiva and a relatively thick overlying surgical flap are critical to avoid perforation of the flap by the membrane during healing. After flaps have been reflected in the surgical area, the defect is degranulated and the root surface scaled and root planed. The ePTFE membrane is trimmed to adapt to tooth configuration, secured by ePTFE sutures, and the flap is repositioned. Notably, although much of the emphasis in the literature is on adapting the membrane to the defect, no membrane can ever be perfectly adapted. Despite the presence of gaps between the membrane and the root surface, these membranes seem to work. After membrane placement, healing is allowed to proceed for 4 to 6 weeks. Barring any membrane exposure, a second surgery is performed to remove the membrane. During this removal, the healing tissue often appears reddish and granulomatous, although more mature bonelike tissue is sometimes noted. After membrane removal, the area should not be probed for 3 to 6 months. Radiographic evidence of bone fill is usually present after 6 months and should continue during the course of 1 year (Fig. 25-4).

Clinical studies have shown that ePTFE membranes used in GTR procedures are more effective than surgical debridement alone in correcting intrabony defects.[147-154] In intrabony and furcation defects, there are gains in clinical attachment level (3 to 6 mm), improved bone levels (2.4 to 4.8 mm), and probing depth reductions (3.5 to 6 mm). Studies have demonstrated that these regenerative results can be maintained during the course of several years.[89,155-157]

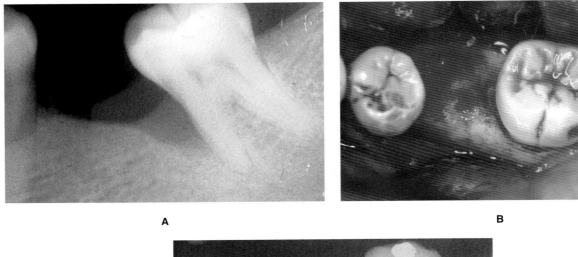

A   B

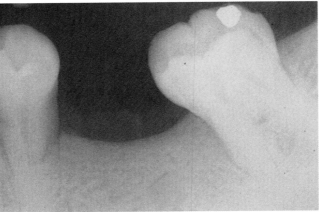

C

Figure 25-4. Radiographs and clinical photograph of a guided tissue regeneration case using a nonresorbable expanded polytetrafluoroethylene (ePTFE) membrane. The mesially inclined molar is associated with a three-walled intraosseous defect (**A**). The defect was filled with demineralized freeze-dried bone allograft, and ePTFE membrane was used (**B**). Membrane became exposed after 8 weeks and was removed 2 weeks later. Radiographic "fill" was approximately 50% after 6 months, and maximum fill was present after 12 months (**C**).

The advent of titanium-reinforced ePTFE membranes allowed for the formation of larger spaces, thus permitting correction of larger defects (Fig. 25-5).[158] These membranes are embedded with strips of titanium that can be bent and shaped to fit the bony defects and prevent collapse of the membrane into the defect. This resulted in significant clinical improvements using titanium-reinforced ePTFE compared with ePTFE.

To determine how regeneration can be enhanced with GTR technique, the prolonged retention of ePTFE membranes was evaluated.[159] After allowing the membrane to be retained for 4 months, surgical reentry after 1 year determined that the mean bone fill of intrabony defects was 95%. This suggests that prolonged retention of a barrier membrane is desirable if no tissue perforation is present. This is consistent with many clinical reports of the improved bone quality associated with GBR in implant site development.

The major problem with using nonresorbable membranes is that the membrane may become exposed to the oral environment during healing. On exposure, the membrane is contaminated and colonized by oral microflora.[160-162] Several studies have shown that contamination of the surgical field can result in decreased formation of new attachment.[16,163,164] If the membrane is exposed, the infection can be temporarily managed with topical application of chlorhexidine. This may minimize the infection and extend the time the membrane can be retained in place. However, any sign of frank infection such as swelling or pus formation suggests the membrane should be removed.

Bioresorbable membranes

For many clinicians, bioresorbable membranes have replaced the routine use of ePTFE membranes in GTR. There are basically three types of bioresorbable membranes: (1) polyglycoside synthetic polymers (i.e., polylactic acid, polylactate/polygalactide copolymers), (2) collagen, and (3) calcium sulfate. Polyglycoside membranes degrade as the result of random nonenzymatic cleavage of the polymer, producing polylactide and polyglycolide, which are converted to lactic acid and pyruvate, respectively, and metabolized by the enzymes of the Krebs cycle. Collagen membranes currently available are of porcine or bovine origin, and consist of either type I collagen or a combination of type I and type III collagen. Collagen membranes are degraded by collagenases and subsequently by gelatinases and peptidase. There has been a resurgence in the use of calcium sulfate as a regeneration material because it can be used as a pavable resorbable barrier when used in combination with bone or bone substitutes. The calcium sulfate is bioresorbed through a giant cell reaction. Several features make these bioresorbable membranes easier to manage clinically: (1) they are more tissue compatible than nonresorbable membranes; (2) the timing for resorption can be regulated by the amount of cross-linkage in the synthetic polymer and collagen membrane or the amount of heat-processed calcium sulfate chips in calcium sulfate barrier; and (3) a second surgical procedure is not required to retrieve the nonresorbable membrane. A disadvantage of many resorbable membranes is a relative lack of rigidity, because resorbable membranes, unlike titanium-reinforced ePTFE membranes, have no embedded support structures.

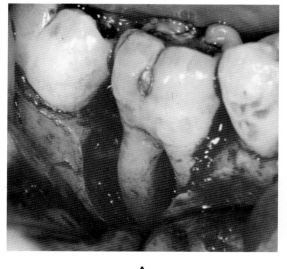
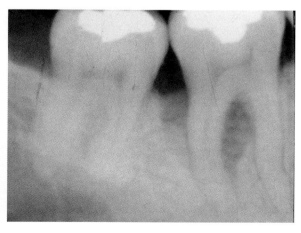

A   **B**

Figure 25-5. Clinical photographs and radiographs of a guided tissue regeneration case using titanium-reinforced expanded polytetrafluoroethylene membrane. The osseous defect was along the distal interproximal area wrapping buccally over the furcation (**A** and **B**). Tooth #30 was vital.

Continued

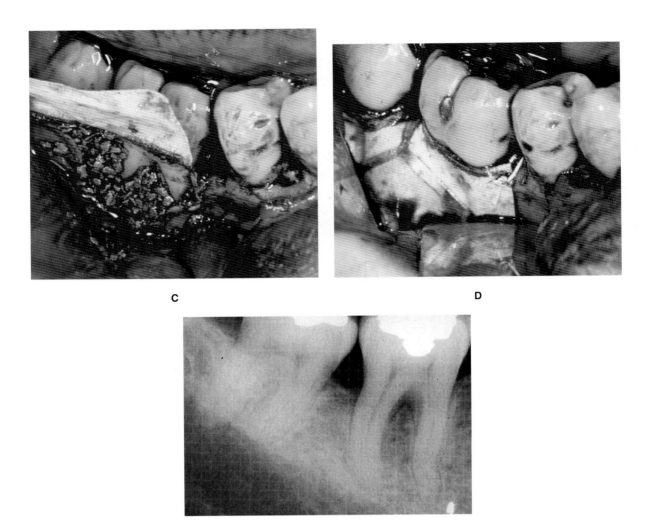

C

D

E

Figure 25-5. cont'd To prevent the membrane from collapsing into the osseus defect and over the root surfaces, demineralized freeze-dried bone allograft was placed in the defect and the titanium-reinforced membrane was molded to provide a larger space for regeneration (**C** and **D**). One year later, the radiographic and clinical signs are consistent with achieving significant bone fill (**E**).

In a 1-year GTR study comparing the use of bioresorbable membranes (polylactate/polygalactate copolymer), ePTFE membranes, or surgical debridement alone, significant gains in clinical attachment level were observed in all three groups.[165] There was no difference in clinical attachment level gain between the two membrane groups, with both of them gaining 2 mm or more. In both membrane groups, 83% of the sites improved 4 mm or more, which was significantly better than the surgical debridement control group. These findings indicate GTR procedures are equally effective using resorbable and nonresorbable membranes. This finding has been confirmed by other investigators.[166-168]

A large multicenter clinical study reported the use of bioresorbable membranes in 203 consecutively treated intrabony defects.[169] After 1 year, investigators found that

clinical attachment level improved by 79%, and 78% of the sites improved by 4 mm or more. An average of 3 mm of bone fill was measured radiographically. Compromised clinical results occurred in cases where membranes became exposed to the oral environment or where patients had poor plaque control.

Use of guided tissue regeneration with bone grafting

Although regeneration may be attempted with various graft materials used alone or with membranes alone, combinations of the two may also be indicated. The use of GTR in conjunction with various regenerative approaches has been attempted with reported success. In a large case series using GTR in combination with root conditioning and DFDBA, significant gains in clinical attachment level were observed in a variety of furcation and intrabony defects.[153] Importantly, the regenerated results were stable over 5 years.[89] Others have reported similar positive clinical results with DFDBA alone.[170] When this combination was used and studied histologically, the amount of newly regenerated attachment varied from 0 to 1.7 mm.[171] In a split-mouth paired control study comparing GTR versus GTR with DFDBA, both groups had improved bone fill, but there were no statistically significant differences between the two groups.[172,173] A similar study was performed comparing GTR alone with GTR plus HA-collagen grafts.[154] Improved results were seen in both groups, with no significant differences between groups. These and other studies suggest that GTR techniques may be somewhat improved with the use of bone grafts or other defect fillers. In a comprehensive, systematic review of human data, use of a bone augmentation material in combination with a membrane was shown to provide clinically superior results compared to use of a membrane alone in the treatment of molar furcation defects.[174] In treating interproximal intrabony defects, the two approaches gave similar results.

The use of GTR with bone grafting has been applied with the use of calcium sulfate. Calcium sulfate has been safely used in periodontics for the last four decades.[175-177] Animal studies indicated that calcium sulfate can create a "sealing" effect that permits orderly bone replacement of the osseous defect. The calcium sulfate resorption time averaged 2 to 4 weeks.[175] Early clinical application to periodontal defects reported favorable results, but it did not demonstrate any capacity for osteoinduction.[178,179] Because the barrier effect was minimal, this technique was abandoned until its revival this past decade. Sottosanti[180] altered the technique to gain adequate time for regeneration by modifying the use of calcium sulfate to include a bone graft. The technique involves two basic components. The first component is composite graft of approximately 80% DFDBA and 20% calcium sulfate, which is placed into the defect. Over this composite graft is a second placement of a calcium sulfate barrier. The advantage of this technique is that the material is highly tissue compatible, it permits the management of large irregularly shaped defects, and gaps in flap coverage do not appear to be significant. Several clinical case reports and series have suggested this as a viable technique,[181-183] but no large clinical, controlled, or comparable studies are available.

Using guided tissue regeneration principles for implant site development (guided bone regeneration)

The principle of selective cell repopulation has been useful in enhancing site development for implant placement. Whereas GTR requires the regeneration of bone, PDL, and cementum to form a new periodontal apparatus, the requirements for implant site development are less complicated in that only bone formation needs to be

enhanced. By using a barrier membrane at an extraction site or a deficient alveolar ridge, bone can be regenerated. At the time of tooth extraction, the socket can be augmented with a graft material and "sealed" with a barrier membrane. In some cases, a membrane may be used without graft material in the socket. This procedure is termed ridge preservation (see also Chapters 21 and 26). Similarly, an alveolar ridge with a volumetric deficiency can be improved with the use of graft material and a barrier. This procedure is termed GBR (guided bone regeneration) and is a commonly used technique for osseous ridge augmentation. Both of these approaches use the barrier concept to selectively permit osteoprogenitor cells to colonize the site such that an increased volume of bone may be formed.

In ridge preservation, the need for a barrier membrane is highly dependent on the nature of the alveolar housing. In a site with thick gingiva and a thick labial alveolar plate, there is minimal postextraction remodeling and the management required is minimal. In these cases, ridge preservation may not be needed after extraction. Alternatively, the thin gingiva case with a thin labial plate is susceptible to remodeling. As the ridge heals, there is a tendency for the ridge to remodel apically and lingually, resulting in a vertical and a horizontal deficiency. To prevent this, ridge preservation procedures can minimize ridge atrophy, especially in the vertical dimension. This is especially important because most ridge augmentation techniques work fairly predictably in correcting horizontal defects, but they are more limited in restoring the vertical dimension. As a preparatory procedure, ridge preservation can minimize the number of subsequent augmentation procedures needed. With this technique, it is critical to extract the tooth atraumatically. The socket is degranulated thoroughly and grafted. Though various graft materials have been advocated, it is important to remember that an implant needs to be placed in this space approximately 3 to 6 months after extraction. The ideal graft material needs to act as a scaffold for new bone formation, and also to be minimal in volume at the time of implant placement. This is important to maximize the amount of bone available for osseointegration. It has been noted that when implants are placed in grafted sites, nonresorbed graft materials are displaced laterally and do not interact with the implant surface. If the newly healed site is predominately filled with residual graft material, the site may not be structurally ideal for osseointegration and site integrity. Consequently, some have advocated that no graft material be placed and only a membrane barrier should be used. In these cases, it is hoped that the socket will fill completely with new host bone.

Several types of membranes, as well as calcium sulfate barriers, have been reported to be effective in "sealing" the socket. When used, ridge preservation minimizes the amount of remodeling. Invariably, there will be some degree of ridge resorption, and the patient should be advised that further treatment such as ridge augmentation may be needed to develop the ideal implant placement site (see Chapter 26).

GBR is one of the many approaches for ridge augmentation. In this technique, the deficient alveolar site is surgically exposed and all soft tissue adherent to bone is removed. Many clinicians have advocated perforating the cortical plates to open the marrow spaces and allow for osteoprogenitor cell migration into the site. Graft materials are used to serve as volumetric scaffolds and a membrane is used to "seal" the area. Membrane requirements that appear important include its ability to be maintained during the course of treatment and its ability to support the increased tissue dimension. Early studies focused on the use of ePTFE because many of the resorbable membranes initially on the market were not intact after a few months. The advent of titanium-reinforced ePTFE membranes also helped with maintaining the space under the membrane required for regeneration. The difficulty with ePTFE membranes is that their stiffness and thickness often resulted in soft tissue perforation. The ensuing infection often compromised the amount of regeneration achieved. More recently, the more tissue-compatible resorbable membranes have been modified to slow their resorption, so the barrier effect can be maintained up to 6 months. Regardless of the type of membrane used, the difficulty with this approach of ridge augmentation is that it is not highly predictable, the volume of bone regeneration attainable is limited, and the ridge can be improved mainly in the horizontal dimension. In situations where extensive augmentation is needed ($\geq$3 mm), other augmentation techniques such as alveolar monocortical grafts or distraction osteogenesis should be considered.

Ridge preservation and GBR are best used at the time of extraction to preserve and possibly improve the alveolar ridge in preparation for implant placement (Fig. 25-6). Importantly, after these procedures, additional augmentative procedures may be necessary. These options and other implant site development approaches are discussed in detail in Chapter 26.

NEW APPROACHES TO PERIODONTAL REGENERATION

Experimental and clinical studies on GTR have validated Melcher's postulate that the germinal cell type that colonizes the periodontal wound healing site will determine the fate of the healing tissue. Although the use of a barrier membrane enhances our ability to regenerate the periodontium, its efficacy is limited to certain periodontal defects. Periodontal regeneration is unpredictable in circumferential, one- or two-wall intraosseous defects, and in Class III and advanced Class II furcation defects. This past decade, research has focused on two main approaches involving the use of biological mediators to selectively enhance cellular repopulation of the periodontal wound. The first approach involves the use of peptide sequences, protein preparations, and growth factors to regenerate tissues through the principle of biomimicry. Biomimetics is the science of constructing or mimicking natural processes or tissues, with the expectation that the regeneration cascade will proceed spontaneously. Enamel matrix derivative (EMD), platelet-rich plasma (PRP) preparation–fibrin glue, and growth factors such as platelet-derived growth factor (PDGF) purportedly function in this fashion. The second approach involves the use of growth differentiation factors to enhance periodontal regeneration. BMPs are differentiation factors that have been studied extensively for periodontal and bone regeneration. Several of these growth factors and derivatives are present in bone and teeth (Table 25-2), and they have been shown to have *in vitro* effects on various types of cells within the periodontium (Table 25-3).

Enamel Matrix Derivative

EMD harvested from developing porcine teeth has been reported to induce periodontal regeneration. The rationale for the mechanism of action is that EMD contains a protein preparation that mimics the matrix proteins that induce cementogenesis. During root development, the Hertwig's epithelial sheath deposits enamel matrix proteins on the newly formed root dentin surface. These proteins stimulate the differentiation of surrounding mesenchymal cells into cementoblasts, which form acellular cementum.[184] Once a new cementum layer is formed, collagen fibers form in the adjacent PDL, attaching into the new cementum.[185,186]

EMD is an acetic acid extracted protein preparation from developing porcine tooth buds that contains a mixture of low molecular weight proteins. The major constituents are amelogenins, which are highly hydrophobic proteins that aggregate and serve as a nidus for crystallization. Other proteins identified include ameloblastin and enamelin. This protein preparation uses propylene glycol alginate (PGA) as a carrier. The EMD-containing PGA remains highly viscous when stored in the cold or at room temperature. Once it is applied to the tissue at a neutral pH and at body temperature, the PGA carrier decreases in viscosity, and the EMD preparation precipitates. EMD is absorbed into the HA and collagen fibers of the root surface, where it induces cementum formation followed by periodontal regeneration.

In vitro studies indicate EMD may influence the cellular activities of the various cell types in the periodontium. When PDL cells are exposed to EMD, the cells exhibit enhanced protein production, cell proliferation, and the ability to promote mineral nodule formation.[187] More recently, cementoblasts treated with EMD and osteoblasts in cell culture increased cell proliferation, altered the gene expression of osteocalcin and osteopontin, and inhibited mineral nodule formation.[188] Understanding how cells

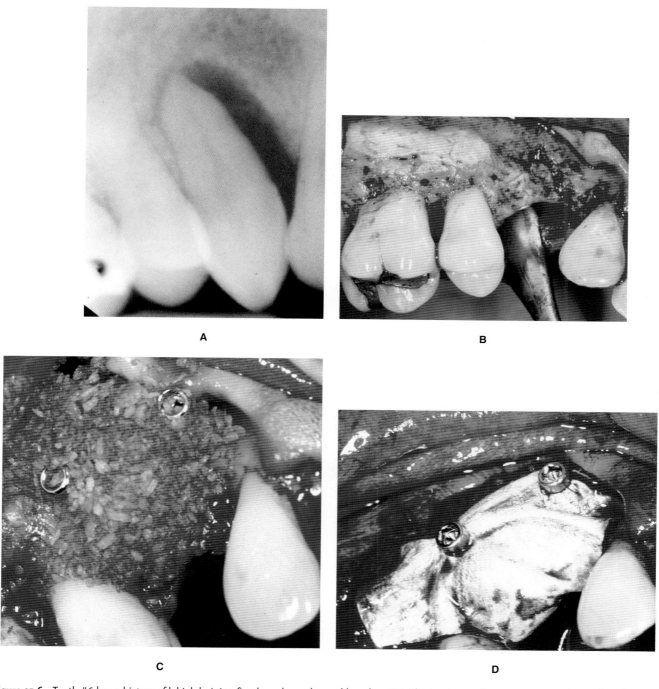

A

B

C

D

Figure 25-6. Tooth #6 has a history of labial draining fistula and was deemed hopeless (**A**). The treatment plan was to extract the tooth and prepare the site for a dental implant by using a combination of socket wall preservation and guided bone regeneration. The tooth was extracted and the socket degranulated (**B**), and the labial defect was managed with tenting pins and demineralized freeze-dried bone allograft (DFDBA) (**C**). The tenting pins and DFDBA provide space for new bone formation. An expanded polytetrafluoroethylene membrane was placed over the augmented area (**D**).

Continued

respond to EMD may elucidate how biomimetic agents work in general. It is only through this understanding that there can be a more predictable clinical therapy.

In an animal study, experimental dehiscence defects were created with bilateral removal of the alveolar bone, PDL, and cementum.[189] Before repositioning the flap, one side was treated with acid-etching and EMD, whereas the control side was acid-etched only. After 8 weeks, histologic examination of the specimens indicated that the EMD-treated side generally showed no gingival recession

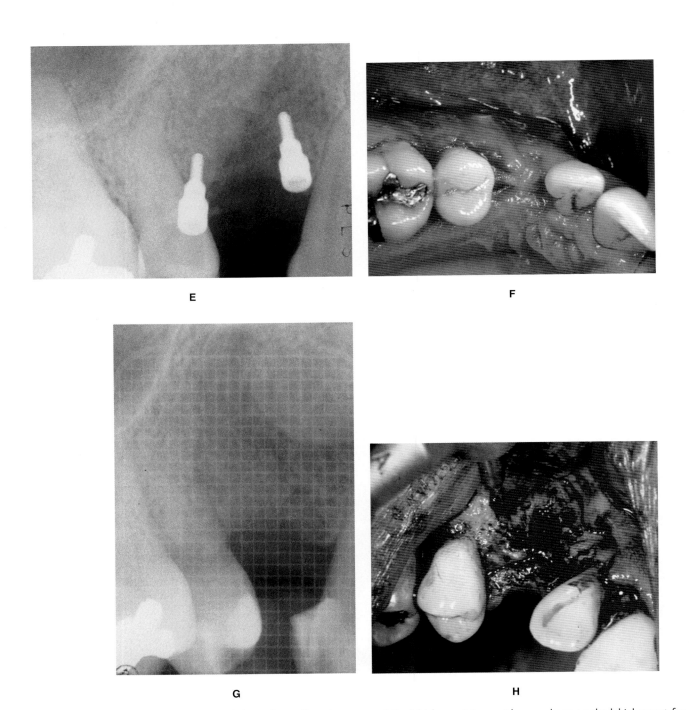

E

F

G

H

Figure 25-6. cont'd This functionally preserved the socket walls and augmented the labial aspect to provide more bone on the labial aspect for implant placement. After 3 months of healing, radiographic evidence of fill was present (**E**). The two tenting pins are clearly visible on the radiograph. These pins will be removed at the next surgery. At 6 months after extraction, the ridge is clinically healed (**F**) and radiographic evidence of increased mineralization was present (**G**). On reentry for implant placement surgery, the site was successfully augmented to allow the implant to be placed in an ideal position (**H**).

or formation of a long junctional epithelium, and 60% to 70% of the surface was covered with regenerated acellular cementum. The control sites displayed gingival recession with only 10% of surfaces regenerated.

The histologic finding of EMD-induced periodontal regeneration has been confirmed in a clinical case report.[190] A mandibular lateral incisor destined for orthodontic extraction was treated with acid-etching and EMD. After

TABLE 25-2   **Growth Factors in Bone Matrix**

GROWTH FACTORS IN BONE MATRIX	SIZE, kD	BONE CONTENT, mg/kg	SOURCE IN BONES (OSTEOBLAST/SERUM)
• TGF-β	35	200	+/+
• BMP-1 to -12	16-30	2-5	+/−
• PDGF AA, AB, BB	36	50	+/+
• IGF-1, -2	7, 6	400	+/+

BMP, *bone morphogenetic protein;* IGF, *insulin-like growth factor;* PDGF, *platelet-derived growth factor;* TGF, *transforming growth factor.*

TABLE 25-3   *In Vitro* **Effects of Growth Factors on Periodontal Ligament Cells and Osteoblasts**

	TGF-β	BMP-2, -3	BMP-7	PDGF	IGF-1,-2
PDL cells					
• Cell proliferation	−	++	++	++	+
• Chemotaxis	o	+	+	++	++
• Collagen synthesis	+	+	+	++	++
• Protein synthesis	+	+	+	+	+
Osteoblasts					
• Cell proliferation	+++	o	+	++	++
• Chemotaxis	+++	+	ND	+++	+
• Collagen synthesis	++	o	+	o	+
• Protein synthesis	+/−	ND	+	o	o
• Alkaline phosphatase synthesis	+/−	++	+++	o	o

(−), *inhibitory effect;* o, *no effect;* (+), *slight effect;* (++), *moderate effect;* (+++), *strong effect;* BMP, *bone morphogenetic protein;* IGF, *insulin-like growth factor;* ND, *not done;* PDGF, *platelet-derived growth factor;* PDL, *periodontal ligament;* TGF, *transforming growth factor.*

4 months, the tooth was extracted and examined histologically. Regenerated cementum covered 73% of the defect and regenerated alveolar bone covered 65%. This histologic finding has been confirmed in another case series.[191,192]

In a multicenter study, 33 patients with at least two intrabony defects were treated in a split-mouth design in which the experimental site was acid-etched and EMD was applied to the denuded root surfaces.[193] At the control site, a placebo was applied. Patients were examined at 8, 16, and 36 months after surgery. Increased bone fill of the osseous defect was observed over time for 25 of the 27 (93%) EMD-treated teeth, but no bone fill was detected in the controls. The mean radiographic bone fill was greater for the EMD-treated defect compared with the control sites (2.7 vs. 0.7 mm). Statistically significant improvements were observed for EMD-treated sites over control sites in mean pocket reduction (3.1 vs. 2.3 mm) and mean attachment level gain (2.2 vs. 1.7 mm). These clinical findings have been supported by several other studies.[194-196]

The biosafety of EMD was tested on 107 patients who were treated with EMD at two separate visits.[197,198] No adverse clinical or immunologic reactions were observed.

None of the serum samples analyzed for total and anti-EMD antibodies indicated deviations from established baseline ranges. After 3 years of clinical use, approximately half the patients were reevaluated and there was no report of adverse reaction. This study suggests that the immunogenic potential of EMD is extremely low when applied in conjunction with periodontal surgery.

There have been four studies comparing the use of EMD alone or in conjunction with other regenerative approaches. When EMD treatment was compared with GTR using bioresorbable membranes, the clinical results were comparable and stable over a 4-year period.[199] No significant difference was found when EMD with BGC was compared with bioactive glass as the sole grafting material.[200] Similar comparable results were found when EMD was used in conjunction with anorganic bone graft material.[201,202]

Growth Factors for Biomimicry

Growth factors are naturally occurring proteins that regulate various aspects of cell growth and development.[203,204] Several growth factors have been identified and characterized. Several of these growth factors are found in the bone matrix (Table 25-2). In wound healing, these growth factors modulate cell proliferation, migration, extracellular matrix formation, and other functions of selected cell types. In addition, some growth factors may also function as cell differentiation factors. In periodontal regeneration, much of the focus has been on PDGF, insulin-like growth factor (IGF), and, more recently, PRP preparation.

Most of the information about growth factors comes from cell culture experiments. Before biotechnology, crude preparations of growth factors were applied to various cells in culture, and their effects on selected target cell types (i.e., fibroblasts, osteoblasts, epithelial cells, and others), cell proliferation and function, extracellular matrix formation, and phenotypic expression were studied (Table 25-3).

PDGF is one of the early growth factors studied for its effect on wound healing because it is a potent mitogenic and chemotactic factor for mesenchymal cells. IGFs are growth factors that are highly homologous with proinsulin. Two of the most well characterized growth factors in this group are IGF-1 and IGF-2, which are somewhat similar, but have different receptors and properties. IGF-1 has been shown to be an effective chemotactic agent and mitogen for osteoblasts and PDL cells. Early cell culture experiments using PDGF and IGF-1 indicated that these two growth factors produced greater mitogenic responses when used together than when used individually. This synergistic effect resulted in distinguishing growth factors as either competence growth factors, which prime the cell to enter the cell proliferation cycle, or as progression growth factors, which are required for cell division. In these classic experiments, PDGF was determined to be a competence factor and IGF-1 to be a progression factor.

Using the information from these cell biology experiments, PDGF and IGF-1 were topically applied to periodontally diseased root surfaces in beagle dogs.[205,206] Substantial amounts of new bone, cementum, and PDL were present after 2 weeks. The results of this study were subsequently confirmed in three other studies using beagles and experimentally induced periodontitis in nonhuman primates.[207-209] A human clinical trial was conducted using recombinant human PDGF/recombinant human IGF-1 (rhPDGF/rhIGF-1).[210] Using a split-mouth design, defects were treated with either a low dose (50 μg/ml) or high dose (150 μg/ml) of rhPDGF/rhIGF-1. After 9 months, high-dose rhPDGF/rhIGF-1 induced 2.08 mm of new bone with 43.2% osseous defect fill, as compared with 0.75-mm vertical bone height and 18.5% bone fill in placebo controls. Low-dose rhPDGF/rhIGF-1 was statistically similar to control.

Simultaneous with the human clinical trial, a primate study examined the regenerative effects of PDGF/IGF in combination or individually.[209] PDGF alone was found to be as effective as the PDGF/IGF combination in producing new attachment after 3 months. No significant effect was found when IGF was used alone. This study suggests that IGF may not be important at the dose level tested. A multicenter clinical trial of rhPDGF is currently being evaluated (Fig. 25-7).

The animal studies and human clinical trials suggest that PDGF may be useful in enhancing periodontal regeneration. Although encouraging, the regenerative response reported in the first clinical trial is not dissimilar to that found with GTR or with the use of bone graft materials. Additional clinical trials are needed to test greater dosages

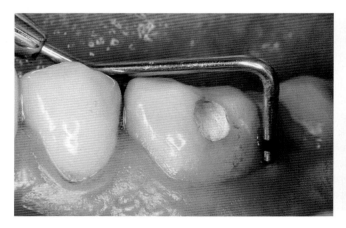

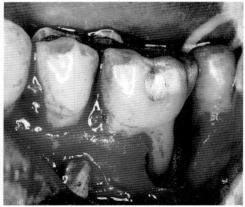

A

B

Figure 25-7. A case from the clinical trial for the use of recombinant human platelet derived growth factor (rhPDGF) for the treatment of periodontal defects. Initial probing depth was 14 mm and the tooth tested vital (**A**). After flap reflection and degranulation, the osseous defect was 9-mm-deep and 4-mm-wide (**B**).

Continued

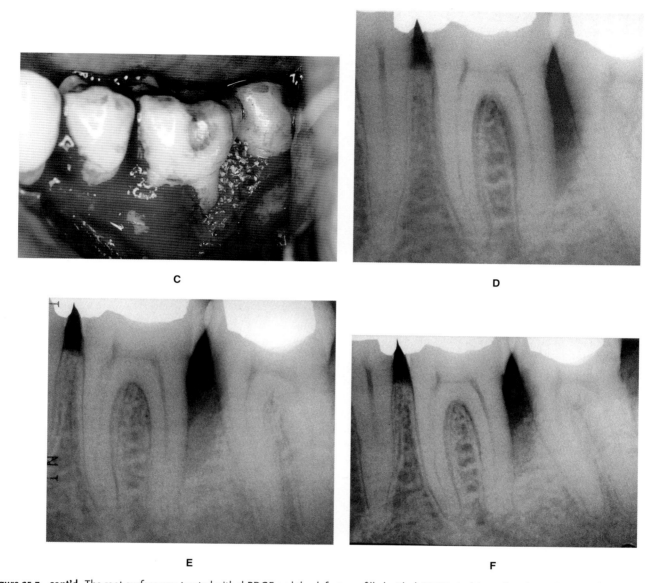

Figure 25-7. cont'd The root surface was treated with rhPDGF and the defect was filled with rhPDGF-tricalcium phosphate (**C**). Note that no guided tissue regeneration (GTR) membrane was used. The radiographs indicate increased radiopacity from the initial surgical radiograph (**D**) to the 3-month (**E**) and 6-month (**F**) postsurgical radiographs. This pattern of radiographic improvement is approximately twice as fast as those observed with GTR cases. Final probing depth was 4 mm, with 4 mm of recession. The gain in clinical attachment level was 6 mm. Histologic evidence of regeneration for a similarly treated case is presented in Figure 25-3.

of PDGF and PDGF in combination with GTR to determine whether regeneration can be enhanced. Lastly, the role of IGF-1 needs to be elucidated, and studies need to be conducted to determine whether the effects of competence and progression growth factors are *in vitro* events only, or a clinical phenomenon as well.

Platelet-Rich Plasma Preparation

The use of PRP preparation as a source of growth factors in bone and periodontal regeneration has been pro-posed.[211] In this approach, autologous blood is drawn and separated into three fractions: platelet-poor plasma (fibrin glue or adhesive), PRP, and red blood cells. Platelets are enriched by 338% in the PRP preparation and concentrations of PDGF and TGF-β in PRP are 41.1 and 45.9 ng/ml, respectively.[212] Monoclonal antibodies have identified the presence of PDGF, IGF, and TGF-β in the cytoplasmic granules of platelets. This preparation also contains a high concentration of fibrinogen. In clinical use, calcium and thrombin are added to the PRP preparation to activate the proteolytic cleavage of fibrinogen into fibrin. Fibrin formation initiates clot formation, which, in turn, initiates wound healing. Although many case reports attribute improved healing results to these growth factors, it is questionable whether the concentrations used are adequate to elicit clinically measurable results. The level of PDGF in PRP is 3000-fold less than that reported to be effective in other studies of PDGF.[210] Alternatively, the accelerated healing may be the result of the presence of a fibrin clot, which stabilizes the early wound healing matrix.

Differentiation Factors: Bone Morphogenetic Proteins

Bone morphogenetic proteins (BMP) are a group of regulatory glycoproteins that are members of the TGF-β superfamily. These molecules primarily stimulate differentiation of mesenchymal stem cells into chondroblasts and osteoblasts. At least seven BMPs have been isolated from bovine and human sources. In the field of periodontal regeneration, much of the research interest has focused on BMP-2 (OP-2), BMP-3 (osteogenin), and BMP-7 (OP1).[213]

The osteoinductive effect of BMPs was characterized by using crude protein preparations derived from decalcified bone. When these crude preparations were placed in muscle or subdermal pouches, an ectopic focal formation of cartilage was present after 12 days, and bone was present after 28 days. The induction of mesenchymal stem cell differentiation to recapitulate endochondral bone formation stimulated clinical interest in using bone preparations (FDBA and DFDBA) as osteogenic graft materials. However, when the actual concentration of BMPs in commercial bone preparations was measured, the amount present was quite low. Approximately 10 kg of bovine bone yields 2 μg of BMP.[82] This has resulted in research efforts to purify, identify, and characterize BMPs so they can be synthetically produced by recombinant DNA technology.

Experiments using crude and recombinant BMPs have provided insight as to their potential use. Crude preparations of BMP-2 and BMP-3 applied in surgically induced furcation defects appeared to stimulate periodontal regeneration.[214] Studies have used recombinant human BMPs (rhBMPs) to determine their potential for correcting horizontal bone loss and intrabony, furcation, and fenestration defects.[215-219] When rhBMP-2 was used in horizontal periodontal bony defects, the gains in bone and cementum were 3.5 and 1.6 mm, respectively, compared with 0.8 and 0.4 mm for controls.[217] Histologic analysis revealed periodontal regeneration with areas of ankylosis. Contrary to these findings, BMP-7 augmentation resulted in a significant increase in periodontal regeneration without any ankylosis.[217] Healing through ankylosis has been a concern; therefore, most of the research using rhBMPs has involved its effect in stimu-

lating new bone formation through GBR before or in conjunction with implant placement, where ankylosis is of no concern.[220-227]

Gene Therapy for Correcting Periodontal Defects

Major limitations associated with the use of growth and differentiation factors include their short biological half-lives. The factors, once applied, are subject to proteolytic breakdown and receptor binding problems and are dependent on the stability of the carrier system. Gene therapy can be used for extended local delivery of these factors. Gene delivery of PDGF was accomplished with the successful transfer of the PDGF gene into the cementoblast and other periodontal cell types.[228] This study demonstrated that gene delivery of PDGF stimulated more cementoblast activity than a single application of recombinant PDGF. In another report, periodontal wounds were transduced effectively by the use of gene transfer.[229] The use of gene delivery offers a new approach to delivering growth factors. The safety and efficacy for using gene therapy for regeneration have yet to be evaluated.

Factors That Influence Therapeutic Success

Factors that adversely affect periodontal regeneration were reviewed at the 1996 World Workshop in Periodontics and 2003 Workshop on Contemporary Science in Clinical Periodontics.[230,231] A number of factors have been implicated or shown to adversely influence periodontal regenerative therapy. These include:

- *Poor plaque control/compliance*: Classical studies of poor plaque control and poor postoperative recall compliance have indicated that much of the therapeutic gain from periodontal surgery will deteriorate over time.[232-236] This response also is observed in GTR regenerated sites.[237-239] Progressive deterioration and a greater incidence of infection with putative periodontal pathogens (*Porphyromonas gingivalis, Prevotella intermedia, and Actinobacillus actinomycetemcomitans*) were more prevalent in patients with poor plaque control and compliance as compared with those with excellent plaque control and maintenance.[240] Furcation repairs also respond similarly, with deterioration for patients with poor plaque control and compliance, and increased stability in patients exhibiting the converse behavior.[241] The difficulty is that patient compliance is hard to maintain.[242-244] Motivating patients to remain highly enthusiastic about oral hygiene and to be compliant with periodontal maintenance is difficult but extremely important (see Chapter 13).
- *Smoking*: Smoking is a major risk factor not only for disease progression, but also for adverse therapeutic outcomes.[245-247] Not only has smoking been implicated as having a detrimental effect on peri-

odontal wound healing after surgical procedures,[248-250] it also has been linked to impaired healing response to GTR procedures in both intrabony defects and furcation repairs.[251]

- *Tooth/Defect factors*: Therapeutic success is influence by the tooth's importance in the prosthetic rehabilitation, its endodontic status, and the defect characteristics.
  - The critical question to be addressed is whether the involved tooth is strategically important in the final restorative plan.[252] If not, the procedure may not be justified because of its technical difficulty and expense, potential postsurgical complications, and the difficulty in obtaining excellent patient oral hygiene and compliance.
  - Once a tooth is deemed essential, it is important to assess its endodontic status. Frequently, chronic endodontic–periodontal defects have the same appearance as an advanced intrabony defect. Treatment of the periodontal component of an endodontic–periodontal defect without first addressing the endodontic component will result in failure.[253,254] The chronicity of the endodontic–periodontal infection may be more important in predicting the outcome of regenerative procedures. Teeth with adequate endodontic therapy appear to respond to regenerative therapy in a way similar to vital teeth without pulpal pathology. Given the expense for endodontic treatment, periodontal regenerative procedures, crown buildup, and the crown strategic extraction and possible replacement with a prosthesis or a dental implant should be considered.
  - Characteristics of the defect, such as the overall defect depth, width, and number of walls, can influence clinical outcome in response to regenerative surgery.[50,52,54,55,255] Studies have consistently shown that an increased depth of the defect is correlated with increased improvement in clinical attachment level and probing depth.[52,55] Therefore, a 7-mm-deep intrabony defect can be expected to demonstrate a greater percent defect fill, greater defect resolution, and greater clinical attachment gain than a 3-mm-deep defect. Conversely, an increased width of the bony defect has been correlated with decreased bone fill and clinical healing response. Defects with more acute angles at the base of the defect (i.e., a steeper vertical inclination of the bony walls) have greater regenerative potential than defects with less acute angles at the base. Lastly, intrabony defects characterized

by three- or three- and two-walled configurations will generally respond more positively to regenerative procedures.[235,236,256,257] Barring early reports on the use of iliac and autologous grafts, current regenerative approaches have not been consistently successful in regenerating one- or zero-walled defects. It is likely that defects with a greater number of bony walls have better regenerative potential because of the increased area for influx of bone-forming cells into the defect.

- *Surgical management*: As with any surgical procedure, flap management and wound stability are important (Fig. 25-8). In the regenerative management of intrabony defects, it is important to ascertain presurgically whether there is sufficient keratinized tissue to allow complete tissue coverage of the defect. Surgical flap design should be such that after sulcular or inverse bevel incisions, buccal and lingual full-thickness flaps are reflected extending to at least one to three teeth mesially and distally to the treated tooth. In the case of a missing proximal tooth, the flap should be extended at least 5 to 10 mm proximal to assure adequate visualization of the defect. Visualization often can be enhanced with the placement of vertical releasing incisions. In addition, these incisions can permit the coronal positioning of the flap. Care should be taken to preserve as much of the keratinized gingiva as possible. In many cases, sulcular incisions are used to maintain the entire zone of keratinized tissue and to ensure complete coverage of any grafts or regenerative membranes that are placed. Interdental tissues should be preserved in their entirety so that flap margins in this region can be coapted to prevent graft or membrane exposure during healing. After flap reflection, it is important to remove all granulation tissues associated with the defect and to thoroughly root plane the surfaces adjacent to the defect. Root defects, such as severe irregularities, cemental pearls, or cementoenamel projections, must be corrected with odontoplasty. After evaluation of the defect, root conditioning may be performed. Regenerative materials may be placed and a GTR membrane applied, if desired. It is important to have good tension-free surgical closure over the defect after suturing and for the wound to remain clinically closed throughout healing. Studies have implicated poor regenerative response because of surgical exposure and infection of membranes used in GTR procedures. These problems were prevalent with nonresorbable membranes; however, current resorbable membranes are more tissue-compatible and it is easier to maintain good tissue coverage over the GTR membrane.

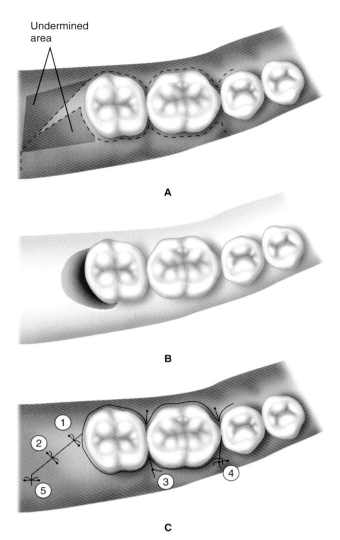

Figure 25-8. Flap management and suturing sequence for periodontal regeneration. Good flap design is essential for visualizing and debriding the osseous defect. In areas of redundant tissues, such as over an edentulous area, the soft tissue may be thinned by undermining. It is essential to achieve tension-free primary closure, which can be accomplished with surgical extension and vertical releasing incisions when needed. Vertical releasing incision should be at least one tooth away from the regeneration site (**A** and **B**). After debridement, the defect is managed and sutured in the sequence as numbered (**C**). The suturing sequence should start at the regeneration site and continue away from the defect area. This ensures good closure over the site of the defect.

CONCLUSION

Over the last three decades, the periodontal literature has been filled with numerous reports related to periodontal regeneration. This therapeutic goal, although ideal, is difficult to achieve. A variety of graft materials and regenerative strategies are currently available; however, they all have limitations. The surgical procedures can be technically demanding, and when successful results are achieved, the maintenance of positive results is highly dependent on patients' oral hygiene habits and compliance with periodontal maintenance. Despite all these difficulties, periodontal regeneration is a clinical possibility that can be offered to patients. The clinician must carefully evaluate the various regenerative and reparative approaches, and then decide which technique may result in the best clinical outcome. With the advent of new regenerative approaches, such as biological modifiers like EMD and growth factors, we must critically evaluate how they may improve our ability to regenerate periodontal defects.

Treatment planning in periodontics also has changed dramatically in the last decade because of the acceptance of dental implants as a viable long-term option for replacing missing teeth. With the increased predictability of implants, the question arises as to when to treat severe periodontal defects with regenerative or other procedures and when to perform strategic extraction in preparation for implant placement. Sometimes the best management of a periodontal defect may be extraction in lieu of periodontal regeneration or when regenerative efforts have been unsuccessful. Extraction would minimize further bone loss and provide the maximum volume of bone at the future implant healing site. This paradigm shift has complicated our views about regeneration. With dental implants as a viable alternative, we may need to redefine periodontal prognosis and consider strategic extraction more often. Heroic regenerative procedures may be contraindicated when extraction and implant placement is considered more predictable and cost effective.

A clinical decision tree is provided to help guide the clinician in deciding the appropriate situations for selecting regenerative procedures over other therapeutic approaches (Fig. 25-9). As with any guidelines, these are intended as a roadmap rather than as a strict set of rules. Clinicians are strongly advised to stay current with changes in the field of regeneration, as well as in other aspects of periodontics and implantology. As periodontics evolves, the clinical decision tree may need to be modified to accommodate for advances in science and technology.

Periodontal regeneration continues to be one of the primary therapeutic approaches toward the management of periodontal defects. Although evidence suggests that current regenerative techniques can lead to periodontal regeneration, the use of GTR and biological modifiers can enhance these results. The crucial challenge for the clinician is to critically assess whether a periodontal defect can be corrected with a regenerative approach or whether it would be better managed with other treatment options.

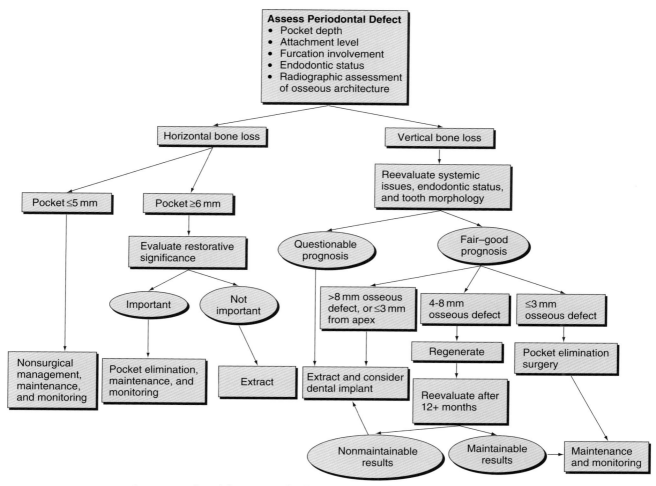

Figure 25-9. Clinical decision tree for the management of advanced periodontal defects.

REFERENCES

1. American Academy of Periodontology: *Glossary of periodontal terms*, ed 4, Chicago, 2001, American Academy of Periodontology.

2. Melcher AH: On repair potential of periodontal tissues, *J Periodontol* 47:256, 1976.

3. Listgarten MA: Periodontal probing: what does it mean?, *J Clin Periodontol* 7:165, 1980.

4. Greenstein G: The significance of pocket depth measurements, *Compend Contin Educ Dent* 5:49, 1984.

5. Greenberg J, Laster L, Listgarten MA: Transgingival probing as a potential estimation of alveolar bone level, *J Periodontol* 47:514, 1976.

6. Ursell MJ: Relationships between alveolar bone levels measured at surgery, estimated by transgingival probing and clinical attachment level measurements, *J Clin Periodontol* 16:81, 1989.

7. Listgarten MA, Rosenberg MM: Histological study of repair following new attachment procedures in human periodontal lesions, *J Periodontol* 50:333, 1979.

8. Moskow BS, Karsh F, Stein SD: Histological assessment of autogenous bone graft. A case report and critical evaluation, *J Periodontol* 50:291, 1979.

9. Nyman S, Lindhe J, Karring et al: New attachment following surgical treatment of human periodontal disease, *J Clin Periodontol* 9:290, 1982.

10. Lang NP, Hill RW: Radiographs in periodontics, *J Clin Periodontol* 4:16, 1976.

11. Theilade J: An evaluation of the reliability of radiographs in the measurement of bone loss in periodontal disease, *J Periodontol* 31:143, 1960.

12. Eickholz P, Hausmann E: Evidence for healing of interproximal intrabony defects after conventional and regenerative therapy: digital radiography and clinical measurements, *J Periodont Res* 33:156, 1998.

13. Jeffcoat MK, Williams RC, Reddy M et al: Flurbiprofen treatment of human periodontitis: effect on alveolar bone height and metabolism, *J Periodont Res* 23:381, 1988.

14. Bragger U, Pasquali, Weber H et al: Computer assisted densitometric image analysis (CADIA) for the assessment

of alveolar bone density changes in furcations, *J Clin Periodontol* 16:46, 1989.

15. Topback GA, Brunsvold MA, Nummikoski PV et al: The accuracy of radiographic methods in assessing the outcome of periodontal regenerative therapy, *J Periodontol* 70:1479, 1999.

16. Page RC: Animal models in reconstructive periodontal therapy, *J Periodontol* 65:1142, 1994.

17. Caton J, Nyman S, Zander H: Histometric evaluation of periodontal surgery: II. Connective tissue attachment levels after four regenerative procedures, *J Clin Periodontal* 7:224, 1980.

18. Register A, Burdick F: Accelerated reattachment with cementogenesis to dentin, demineralized in situ. I. Optimum range, *J Periodontol* 46:646, 1975.

19. Garrett J, Crigger M, Engelberg J: Effects of citric acid on diseased root surfaces, *J Periodont Res* 3:155, 1978.

20. Polson A, Proye M: Effect of root surface alterations on periodontal healing. II Citric acid treatment on the denuded root surface, *J Clin Periodontol* 11:441, 1982.

21. Polson A, Proye M: Fibrin linkage: a precursor for new attachment, *J Periodontol* 54:141, 1984.

22. Woodyard S, Synder A, Henley G, O'Neal R: A histometric evaluation of the effect of citric acid preparation upon healing of coronally positioned flaps in non-human primates, *J Periodontol* 55:203, 1984.

23. Polson A, Hanes P: Cell and fiber attachment to demineralized dentin. A comparison between normal and periodontitis-affected root surfaces, *J Clin Periodontol* 14:357, 1987.

24. Polson A, Ladenheim S, Hanes P: Cell and fiber attachment to demineralized dentin from periodontitis-affected root surfaces, *J Periodontol* 57:235, 1986.

25. Cole R, Crigger M, Bogle G et al: Connective tissue regeneration to periodontally diseased teeth. A histologic study, *J Periodont Res* 15:1, 1980.

26. Albair W, Cobb C, Killoy W: Connective tissue attachment to periodontally diseased roots after citric acid demineralization, *J Periodontol* 53:515, 1982.

27. Common J, McFall W: The effects of topical citric acid application on attachment of laterally positioned flaps, *J Periodontol* 54:9, 1983.

28. Frank R, Fiore-Donno G, Cimasoni G: Cementogenesis and soft tissue attachment after citric acid treatment in a human, *J Periodontol* 54:389, 1983.

29. Lopez N: Connective tissue regeneration to periodontally diseased roots, planed and conditioned with citric acid and implanted into the oral mucosa, *J Periodontol* 55:381, 1984.

30. Cole R, Nilveus R, Ainamo J et al: Pilot clinic studies of the effect of topical citric acid application on healing after replaced periodontal flap surgery, *J Periodont Res* 16:117, 1981.

31. Renvert S, Englberg J: Healing after treatment of periodontal intraosseous defects. II. Effect of citric acid conditioning of the root surface, *J Clin Periodontol* 8:459, 1981.

32. Stahl S, Froum S: Human clinical and histological repair responses following the use of citric acid in periodontal therapy, *J Periodontol* 48:261, 1977.

33. Kashani H, Magner A, Stahl S: The effect of root planing and citric acid applications on flap healing in humans. A histologic evaluation, *J Periodontol* 55:679, 1984.

34. Cogen R, Al-Jaburi W, Gantt D et al: Effect of various root surface treatments on the attachment of human gingival fibroblasts: histologic and scanning electron microscopic evaluation, *J Clin Periodontol* 11:531, 1984.

35. Parodi R, Esper M: Effect of topical application of citric acid in the treatment of furcation involvement in human lower molars, *J Clin Periodontol* 11:644, 1982.

36. Renvert S, Garrett S, Schallhorn R et al: Healing after treatment of periodontal intraosseous defects. III. Effects of osseous grafting and citric acid conditioning, *J Clin Periodontol* 12:441, 1985.

37. Marks S, Mehta N: Lack of effect of citric acid treatment of root surfaces on the formation of new connective tissue attachment, *J Clin Periodontol* 13:109, 1986.

38. Moore J, Ashly F, Waterman C: The effect on healing of the application of citric acid during replaced flap surgery, *J Clin Periodontol* 14:130, 1987.

39. Ryan P, Newcomb G, Seymour J et al: The pulpal response to citric acid in cats, *J Clin Periodontol* 11:633, 1984.

40. Valenza V, D'Angelo M, Farina-Lipari E et al: Effects of citric acid on human gingival epithelium, *J Periodontol* 58:794, 1987.

41. Wikesjo UME, Baker P, Christersson L et al: A biomedical approach to periodontal regeneration: tetracycline treatment conditions dentin surfaces, *J Periodont Res* 21:322, 1986.

42. Demirel K, Baer P, McNamara T: Topical application of doxycycline on periodontally involved root surfaces in vitro: comparative analysis of substantivity on cementum and dentin, *J Periodontol* 62:312, 1991.

43. Terranova V, Franzetti L, Hic S et al: A biochemical approach to periodontal regeneration: tetracycline treatment of dentin promotes fibroblast adhesion and growth, *J Periodont Res* 21:330, 1986.

44. Alger F, Solt C, Vuddhakanol S et al: The histologic evaluation of new attachment in periodontally diseased human roots treated with tetracycline-hydrochloride and fibronectin, *J Periodontol* 61:447, 1990.

45. Parashis A, Mitsis F: Clinical evaluation of the effect of tetracycline root preparation on guided tissue regeneration in the treatment of class II furcation defects, *J Periodontol* 64:133, 1993.

46. Mariotti A: Efficacy of chemical root surface modifiers in the treatment of periodontal disease. A systematic review. *Ann Periodontol* 8:205, 2003.

47. Schallhorn RG, Hiatt WH, Boyce W: Iliac transplants in periodontal therapy, *J Periodontol* 41:566, 1970.

48. Hiatt WH, Schallhorn RG, Aaronian AJ: The induction of new bone and cementum formation: IV. Microscopic

examination of the periodontium following human bone and marrow allograft, autograft and non-graft periodontal regenerative procedures, *J Periodontol* 44:495, 1978.

49. Schallhorn RG: Postoperative problems associated with iliac transplants, *J Periodontol* 43:3, 1972.

50. Hiatt WH, Schallhorn RG: Intraoral transplants of cancellous bone and marrow in periodontal lesions, *J Periodontol* 44:194, 1973.

51. Froum SJ, Thaler R, Scopp IW, Stahl SS: Osseous autografts. I. Clinical responses to bone blend or hip marrow grafts, *J Periodontol* 46:515, 1975.

52. Froum SJ, Ortiz M, Witkin RT et al: Osseous autografts. III. Comparison of osseous coagulum-bone blend implants with open curettage, *J Periodontol* 47:287, 1976.

53. Carraro JJ, Sznajder N, Alonso CA: Intraoral cancellous bone autografts in the treatment of infrabony pockets, *J Clin Periodontol* 3:104, 1976.

54. Renvert S, Shallhorn RG, Egelberg J: Healing after treatment of periodontal intraosseous defects. III. Effect of osseous grafting and citric acid conditioning, *J Clin Periodontol* 12:441, 1985.

55. Dragoo MR, Sullivan HC: A clinical and histological evaluation of autogenous iliac bone grafts in humans. Part I. Wound healing 2 to 8 months, *J Periodontol* 49:599, 1973.

56. Nabers C, Reed O, Hammer J: Gross and histologic evaluation of an autogenous bone graft 57 months postoperatively, *J Periodontol* 43:702, 1972.

57. Hawley CE, Miller J: A histologic examination of a free osseous autograft. Case report, *J Periodontol* 46:289, 1975.

58. Ross SE, Cochen DW: The fate of free osseous tissue autograft: a clinical and histologic case report, *Periodontics* 6:145, 1968.

59. Langer B, Gelb DA, Krutchkoff DJ: Early reentry procedure. Part II. A five year histologic evaluation, *J Periodontol* 52:135, 1981.

60. Schallhon RG, Hiatt WH: Human allografts of iliac cancellous bone and marrow in periodontal osseous defects. II. Clinical observations, *J Periodontol* 43:67, 1972.

61. Mellonig JT, Bowers GM, Bright RW, Lawrence JJ: Clinical evaluation of freeze-dried bone allografts in periodontal osseous defects, *J Periodontol* 47:125, 1976.

62. Sanders JJ, Sepe WW, Bowers GM et al: Clinical evaluation of freeze-dried bone allograft in periodontal osseous defects. Part III. Composite freeze-dried bone allografts with and without autogenous bone grafts, *J Periodontol* 54:1, 1983.

63. Sepe WW, Bowers GM, Lawrence JJ et al: Clinical evaluation of freeze-dried bone allografts in periodontal osseous defects-Part II, *J Periodontol* 49:9, 1978.

64. Mellonig JT: Freeze-dried bone allografts in periodontal reconstructive surgery, *Dent Clin North Am* 35:505, 1991.

65. Barnett JD, Mellonig JT, Gray JL, Towle HT: Comparison of freeze-dried bone allograft and porous hydroxylapatite in human periodontal defects, *J Periodontol* 60:231, 1989.

66. Altiere ET, Reeve CM, Sheridan PJ: Lyophilized bone allografts in periodontal intraosseous defects, *J Periodontol* 50:510, 1979.

67. Urist MR, Sato K, Brownell TI et al: Human bone morphogenetic protein (hBMP), *Proc Soc Exp Biol Med* 173:194, 1983.

68. Urist MR, Strates B: Bone formation in implants of partially and wholly demineralized bone matrix, *Clin Orthop* 71:271, 1970.

69. Harakas N: Demineralized bone-matrix-induced osteogenesis, *Clin Orthop* 188:239, 1984.

70. Bowers GM, Chadroff B, Carnevale R et al: Histologic evaluation of new attachment apparatus formation in humans, Part III, *J Periodontol* 60:683, 1989.

71. Bowers GM, Chadroff B, Carnevale R et al: Histologic evaluation of new attachment apparatus formation in humans. Part II, *J Periodontol* 60:675, 1989.

72. Pearson GE, Rosen S, Deporter DA: Preliminary observations on the usefulness of a decalcified, freeze-dried cancellous bone allograft material in periodontal surgery, *J Periodontol* 52:55, 1981.

73. Mellonig JT, Captain DC: Decalcified freeze-dried bone allograft as an implant material in human periodontal defects, *Int J Periodontics Restorative Dent* 6:41, 1984.

74. Meadows CL, Gher ME, Quintero G, Lafferty TA: A comparison of polylactic acid granules and decalcified freeze-dried bone allograft in human periodontal osseous defects, *J Periodontol* 64:103, 1993.

75. Rummelhart JM, Mellonig JT, Gray JL, Towle HJ: A comparison of freeze-dried bone allograft and demineralized freeze-dried bone allograft in human periodontal osseous defects, *J Periodontol* 60:655, 1989.

76. Bowen JA, Mellonig JT, Gray JL, Towle HT: Comparison of decalcified freeze-dried bone allograft and porous particulate hydroxyapatite in human periodontal defects, *J Periodontol* 60:647, 1989.

77. Oreamuno S, Lekovic V, Kenney EB et al: Comparative clinical study of porous hydroxyapatite and decalcified freeze-dried bone in human periodontal defects, *J Periodontol* 61:399, 1990.

78. Sampath TK, Reddi AH: Homology of bone-inductive proteins from human, monkey, bovine, and rat extracellular matrix, *Proc Nat Acad Sci USA* 80:6591, 1983.

79. Becker W, Urist MR, Tucker LM et al: Human demineralized freeze-fried bone: inadequate induced bone formation in athymic mice, a preliminary report, *J Periodontol* 66:822, 1995.

80. Becker W, Urist MR, Becker BE et al: Clinical and histologic observation of sites implanted with intraoral autologous bone grafts or allografts. 15 human case reports, *J Periodontol* 67:1025, 1996.

81. Shigeyama Y, D'Errico JA, Stone R, Somerman MJ: Commercially prepared allograft material has biological activity in vitro, *J Periodontol* 66:478, 1995.

82. Schwartz Z, Mellonig JT, Carnes DL et al: Ability of commercial demineralized freeze-dried bone allograft to induce new bone formation, *J Periodontol* 67:918, 1996.

83. Schwartz Z, Somers A, Mellonig JT et al: Ability of commercial demineralized freeze-dried bone allograft to induce new bone formation is dependent on donor age but not gender, *J Periodontol* 69:470, 1998.

84. Reynolds MA, Bowers GM: Fate of demineralized freeze-dried bone allografts in human intrabony defects, *J Periodontol* 67:150, 1996.

85. Shteyer A, Kaban L, Kao R: Effect of demineralized bone powder on osteoblast-like cells in culture, *Int J Oral Maxillofac Surg* 19:370, 1990.

86. Zhang M, Powers RM, Wolfinbarger L: A quantitative assessment of osteoinductivity of human demineralized bone matrix, *J Periodontol* 68:1076, 1997.

87. Zhang M, Powers RM, Wolfinbarger L: Effect(s) of the demineralization process on the osteoinductivity of demineralized bone matrix, *J Periodontol* 68:1085, 1997.

88. Jergessen HE, Chua J, Kao R et al: Age effects on bone induction by demineralized bone powder, *Clin Orthop* 268: 253, 1991.

89. McClain PK, Schallhorn RG: Long-term assessment of combined osseous composite grafting, root conditioning, and guided tissue regeneration, *Int J Periodontics Restorative Dent* 13:9, 1993.

90. Flemming TF, Ehmke B, Bolz K et al: Long-term maintenance of alveolar bone gain after implantation of autolyzed, antigen-extracted allogenic bone in periodontal intraosseous defects, *J Periodontol* 69:47, 1998.

91. Thaller SA, Hoyt J, Dart A et al: Reconstruction of calvarial defects with inorganic bovine bone mineral (Bio-Oss) in a rabbit model, *J Craniofac Surg* 4:79, 1993.

92. Thaller SA, Hoyt J, Dart A et al: Repair of experimental calvarial defects with Bio-Oss particles and collagen sponges in a rabbit model, *J Craniofac Surg* 5:242, 1994.

93. Schmitt JM, Buck DC, Joh S-P et al: Comparison of porous bone mineral and biologically active glass in critical-sized defects, *J Periodontol* 68:1043, 1997.

94. Clergeau LP, Danan M, Clergeau-Guerithault S, Brion M: Healing response to anorganic bone implantation in periodontal intrabony defects in dogs. Part I. Bone regeneration—a microradiographic study, *J Periodontol* 67:140, 1996.

95. Camelo M, Nevins ML, Schenk R et al: Clinical, radiographic, and histologic evaluation of human periodontal defects treated with Bio-Oss and Bio-Gide, *Int J Periodontics Restorative Dent* 18:321, 1998.

96. Meffert RM, Thomas JR, Hamilton LM, Brownstein CN: Hydroxylapatite as an alloplastic graft in the treatment of human periodontal osseous defects, *J Periodontol* 56:63, 1985.

97. Yukna RA, Mayer ET, Brite DV: Longitudinal evaluation of durapatite ceramic as an alloplastic implant in periodontal osseous defects after 3 years, *J Periodontol* 55:663, 1984.

98. Yukna RA, Harrison BG, Caudill RF et al: Evaluation of durapatite ceramic as an alloplastic implant in periodontal osseous defects. II. Twelve month reentry results, *J Periodontol* 56:5400, 1985.

99. Yukna RA, Cassingham RJ, Caudill RF et al: Six month evaluation of calcite (hydroxyapatite ceramic) in periodontal osseous defects, *Int J Periodontics Restorative Dent* 3:35, 1986.

100. Yukna RA, Mayer ET, Miller S, Amost S: 5-year evaluation of durapatite ceramic alloplastic implants in periodontal osseous defects, *J Periodontol* 60:544, 1989.

101. Galgut PN, Waite LM, Brookshaw JD, Kingston CP: A 4-year controlled clinical study into the use of a ceramic hydroxylapatite implant material for the treatment of periodontal bone defects, *J Clin Periodontol* 19:570, 1992.

102. Froum SJ, Kusher L, Scopp TW, Stahl SS: Human clinical and histologic responses to durapatite implants in intraoseous lesions, *J Periodontol* 53:719, 1982.

103. Ganeless J, Listgarten MA, Evian CI: Ultrastructure of durapatite-periodontal tissue interface in human intrabony defects, *J Periodontol* 57:133, 1986.

104. Kenney EB, Lekovic V, Han T et al: The use of a porous hydroxyapatite implant in periodontal osseous defects. I. Clinical results after 6 months, *J Periodontol* 58:521, 1985.

105. Krejci CB, Bissads NF, Farah C, Greenweit H: Clinical evaluation of porous and non porous hydroxyapatite in the treatment of human periodontal bony defects, *J Periodontol* 58:521, 1987.

106. Mora F, Ouhayoun JP: Clinical evaluation of natural coral and porous hydroxyapatite implants in periodontal bone lesions: results of a 1-year follow-up, *J Clin Periodontol* 22:877, 1995.

107. Kenney EB, Lekovic V, Elbaz JJ et al: The use of a porous hydroxyapatite implant in periodontal defects II. Treatment of Class II furcation lesions in lower molars, *J Periodontol* 59:67, 1988.

108. Kenney E, Lekovic V, Sa Ferreira et al: Bone formation within porous hydroxyapatite implants in human periodontal defects, *J Periodontol* 57:76, 1986.

109. Carranza FA, Kenney EB, Lekovic V et al: Histologic study of healing of human periodontal defects after placement of porous hydroxyapatite implants, *J Periodontol* 58:682, 1987.

110. Stahl SS, Froum SJ: Histologic and clinical responses to porous hydroxyapatite implants in human periodontal defects, *J Periodontol* 58:689, 1987.

111. Nery EB, Lee KK, Czajkowski S et al: A Veterans Administration cooperative study of biphasic calcium phosphate ceramic in periodontal osseous defects, *J Periodontol* 61:734, 1990.

112. Evans GH, Yukna RA, Sepe WW et al: Effect of various graft materials with tetracycline in localized juvenile periodontitis, *J Periodontol* 60:491, 1989.

113. Strub JR, Gaberthuel TW, Firestone AR: Comparison of tricalcium phosphate and frozen allogenic bone implants in man, *J Periodontol* 50:624, 1979.

114. Snyder AJ, Levin MP, Cutright DE: Alloplastic implants of tricalcium phosphate ceramic in human periodontal osseous defects, *J Periodontol* 55:273, 1984.

115. Baldock WT, Hutchens LH, McFall Jr WT, Simpson SM: An evaluation of tricalcium phosphate implants in human periodontal osseous defects of two patients, *J Periodontol* 56:1, 1985.

116. Barney VC, Levin MP, Adams DF: Bioceramic implants in surgical periodontal defects. A comparison study, *J Periodontol* 57:764, 1986.

117. Froum S, Stahl SS: Human intraosseous healing responses to the placement of tricalcium phosphate ceramic implants II. 13 to 18 months, *J Periodontol* 58:103, 1987.

118. Yukna RA: HTR polymer grafts in human periodontal osseous defects. I. 6 month clinical results, *J Periodontol* 61:633, 1990.

119. Stahmiri S, Singh IJ, Stahl SS: Clinical response to the use of the HTR polymer implant in human intrabony lesions, *Int J Periodontics Restorative Dent* 12:295, 1992.

120. Yukna RA: Clinical evaluation of HTR polymer bone replacement grafts in human mandibular class II molar furcations, *J Periodontol* 65:342, 1994.

121. Plotzle E, Barbose S, Nasjleti CE et al: Histologic and histometric responses to polymeric composite grafts, *J Periodontol* 64:342, 1993.

122. Stahl SS, Froum SJ, Tarnow D: Human clinical and histologic responses to the placement of HTR polymer particles in 11 intrabony lesions, *J Periodontol* 61:269, 1990.

123. Yukna RA, Yukna CN: Six-year clinical evaluation of HTR synthetic bone grafts in human Grade II molar furcations, *J Periodont Res* 32:627, 1997.

124. Sautier JM, Nefussi JR, Forest N: Surface reactive biomaterials in osteoblast cultures: an ultrastructural study, *Biomaterials* 13:400, 1992.

125. Guillemin G, Patat JL, Fournie J, Chetail M: The use of coral as a bone graft substitute, *J Biomed Mater Res* 21:557, 1987.

126. Yukna RA: Clinical evaluation of coralline calcium carbonate as a bone replacement graft material in human periodontal osseous defects, *J Periodontol* 65:177, 1994.

127. Wilson J, Low SB: Bioactive ceramics for periodontal treatment: comparative studies in the Patus monkey, *J Appl Biomater* 3:123, 1992.

128. Ducheyne P, Broen S, Blumenthal N et al: Bioactive glasses, aluminum oxide and titanium. Ion transport phenomena and surface analysis, *Ann NY Acad Sci* 523:257, 1988.

129. Kitsugi T, Nakamura T, Oka M et al: Bone bonding behavior of three heat-treated silica gels implanted in mature rabbit bone, *Calcif Tissue Int* 57:155, 1995.

130. Greenspan DC, Zhong JP, La Torre GP: The evaluation of surface structure of bioactive glasses in vitro. In Wilson J, Hench LL, Greenspan D, editors: *Proceedings of the 8th International Symposium on Ceramics in Medicine; Bioceramics, Vol 8*, London, 1995, Pergamon, 477-482.

131. Hench LL, Andersson OH: Introduction. In Hench LL, Wilson J, editors: *An introduction to bioceramics, Advanced series in ceramics, Vol 1*, Singapore, 1993, World Scientific Publishing.

132. Low SB, King CJ, Krieger J: An evaluation of bioactive ceramic in the treatment of periodontal osseous defects, *Int J Periodontics Restorative Dent* 17:359, 1997.

133. Zamet JS, Darbar UR, Griffiths GS et al: Particulate bioglass as a grafting material in the treatment of periodontal intrabony defects, *J Clin Periodontol* 24:410, 1997.

134. Froum SJ, Weinberg MA, Tarnow D: Comparison of bioactive glass synthetic bone graft particles and open debridement in the treatment of human periodontal defects. A clinical study, *J Periodontol* 69:698, 1998.

135. Lovelace TB, Mellonig JT, Meffert RM et al: Clinical evaluation of bioactive glass in the treatment of periodontal osseous defects in humans, *J Periodontol* 69:1027, 1998.

136. Aukhil I, Simpson DM, Suggs C, Pettersson E: In vivo differentiation of progenitor cells of the periodontal ligament. An experimental study using physical barriers, *J Clin Periodontol* 13:862, 1986.

137. Isidor F, Karring T, Nyman S, Lindhe J: The significance of coronal growth of periodontal ligament tissue for new attachment formation, *J Clin Periodontol* 13:145, 1986.

138. Iglhaut J, Aukhil I, Simpson DM et al: Progenitor cell kinetics during guided tissue regeneration in experimental periodontal wounds, *J Periodont Res* 23:107, 1988.

139. Melcher AH, McCulloch CAG, Cheong T et al: Cells from bone synthesize cementum-like and bone-like tissue in vitro and may migrate into periodontal ligament in vivo, *J Periodont Res* 22:246, 1987.

140. Prichard JP: Present state of the interdental denudation procedure, *J Periodontol* 48:566, 1977.

141. Becker W, Becker BE, Berg L, Samsam C: Clinical and volumetric analysis of three-wall intrabony defects following open flap debridement, *J Periodontol* 57:277, 1986.

142. Becker W, Becker BE, Berg L: Repair of intrabony defects as a result of open debridement procedures. Report of 36 treated cases, *Int J Periodontics Restorative Dent* 6(3):8, 1986.

143. Karring T, Nyman S, Lindhe J: Healing following implantation of periodontitis affected roots into bone tissue, *J Clin Periodontol* 7:96, 1980.

144. Nyman S, Karring T, Lindhe J et al: Healing following implantation of periodontitis affected roots into gingival connective tissue, *J Clin Periodontol* 7:394, 1980.

145. Nyman S, Gottlow J, Karring T, Lindhe J: The regenerative potential of the periodontal ligament: an experimental study in the monkey, *J Clin Periodontol* 9:257, 1982.

146. Nyman S, Lindhe J, Karring T et al: New attachment following surgical treatment of human periodontal disease, *J Clin Periodontol* 9:290, 1982.

147. Gottlow J, Nyman S, Lindhe J et al: New attachment formation in the human periodontium by guided tissue regeneration, *J Clin Periodonol* 13:604, 1986.

148. Becker W, Becker B, Berg L et al: New attachment after treatment with root isolation procedures. Report for treated Class II and Class III furcations and vertical osseous defects, *Int J Periodontics Restorative Dent* 3:9, 1988.

149. Cortellini P, Pini Prato G, Baldi C, Clauser C: Guided tissue regeneration with different materials, *Int J Periodontics Restorative Dent* 10:137, 1990.

150. Cortellini P, Pini Prato G, Tonetti MS: Periodontal regeneration of human infrabony defects. II. Re-entry procedures and bone measures, *J Periodontol* 64:261, 1993.

151. Tonetti M, Pino Prato G, Cortellini P: Periodontal regeneration of human infrabony defects. IV. Determination of healing response, *J Periodontol* 64:934, 1993.

152. Stahl SS, Froum S, Tarnow D: Human histologic responses to guided tissue regenerative techniques in intrabony lesions. Case reports on 9 sites, *J Clin Periodontol* 17:191, 1990.

153. Schallhorn RG, McClain PK: Combined osseous grafting, root conditioning and guided tissue regeneration, *Int J Periodontics Restorative Dent* 4:9, 1988.

154. Kilic AR, Efeoglu E, Yilmaz S: Guided tissue regeneration in conjunction with hydroxyapatite-collagen grafts for intrabony defects. A clinical and radiological evaluation, *J Clin Periodontol* 24:372, 1997.

155. Gottlow J, Nyman S, Karring T: Maintenance of new attachment gained through guided tissue regeneration, *J Clin Periodontol* 19:315, 1992.

156. Weigel C, Brugger U, Hummerle CH et al: Maintenance of new attachment 1 and 4 years following guided tissue regeneration (GTR), *J Clin Periodontol* 22:661, 1995.

157. Cortellini P, Pino Prato GP, Tonetti MS: Long-term stability of clinical attachment following guided tissue regeneration and conventional treatment, *J Clin Periodontol* 23:106, 1996.

158. Cortellini P, Pini Prato G, Tonetti MS: Periodontal regeneration of human intrabony defects with titanium reinforced membranes. A controlled clinical trial, *J Periodontol* 66:797, 1995.

159. Murphy KG: Interproximal tissue maintenance in guided tissue regeneration procedures. Description of surgical technique and 1-year re-entry results, *Int J Periodontics Restorative Dent* 16:463, 1996.

160. Selvig KA, Nilveus RE, Fitzmorris L et al: Scanning electron microscopic observations of cell populations and bacterial contamination of membranes used for guided periodontal tissue regeneration in humans, *J Periodontol* 61:515, 1990.

161. Nowzari H, Slots J: Micro-organisms in polytetrafluoroethylene barrier membranes for guided tissue regeneration, *J Clin Periodontol* 21:203, 1994.

162. Nowzari H, MacDonald ES, Flynn J et al: The dynamics of microbial colonization of barrier membranes for guided tissue regeneration, *J Periodontol* 67:694, 1996.

163. Simion M, Trisi P, Maglione M, Piettelli A: Bacterial penetration in vitro through GTAM membrane with and without topical chlorhexidine application. A light and scanning election microscopic study, *J Clin Periodontol* 22:321, 1995.

164. Mombelli A, Lang NP, Nyman S: Isolation of periodontal species after guided tissue regeneration, *J Periodontol* 64:1171, 1993.

165. Cortellini P, Pino Prato GP, Tonetti MS: Periodontal regeneration of human intrabony defects with bioresorbable membranes. A controlled clinical trial, *J Periodontol* 67:217, 1996.

166. Christgau M, Schmalz G, Reich E, Wenzel A: Clinical and radiographical split-mouth study on resorbable GTR membranes, *J Clin Periodontol* 22:306, 1995.

167. Christgau M, Schmalz G, Wenzel A, Hiller KA: Periodontal regeneration of intrabony defects with resorbable and nonresorbable membranes: 30-month results, *J Clin Periodontol* 24:17, 1997.

168. Weltman R, Trojo PM, Morrison E, Caffesse R: Assessment of guided tissue regeneration procedures in intrabony defects with bioabsorbable and non-reabsorbable barriers, *J Periodontol* 68:582, 1997.

169. Falk H, Laurell L, Ravald N et al: Guided tissue regeneration procedures of 203 consecutively treated intrabony defects using a bioabsorbable matrix barrier. Clinical and radiographic findings, *J Periodontol* 68:571, 1997.

170. Anderegg CR, Martin SJ, Gray JL et al: Clinical evaluation of the use of decalcified freeze-dried bone allograft with guided tissue regeneration in the treatment of molar furcation invasions, *J Periodontol* 62:264, 1991.

171. Stahl SS, Froum SJ: Histologic healing responses in human vertical lesions following the osseous allografts and barrier membranes, *J Clin Periodontol* 18:149, 1991.

172. Guillemin MR, Mellonig JT, Brusvold MA: Healing in periodontal defects treated by decalcified freeze-dried bone allografts in combination with ePTFE membranes. I. Clinical and scanning electron microscope analysis, *J Clin Periodontol* 20:528, 1993.

173. Guillemin MR, Mellonig JT, Brusvold MA et al: Healing in periodontal defects treated by decalcified freeze-dried bone allografts in combination with ePTFE membranes. Assessment by computerized densitometric analysis, *J Clin Periodontol* 20:520, 1993.

174. Murphy KG, Gunsolley JC: Guided tissue regeneration for the treatment of periodontal intrabony and furcation defects. A systematic review. *Ann Periodontol* 8:266, 2003.

175. Bier SJ: Plaster of Paris, an adequate bone substitute to bone for filling periodontal defects, *Clin Dent* 2:1, 1974.

176. Bell WH: Resorption characteristics of bone substitutes, *Oral Surg Oral Med Oral Pathol* 17:650, 1964.

177. Radentz WH, Collings CK: The implantation of plaster of Paris in the alveolar process of the dog, *J Periodontol* 36:357, 1965.

178. Alderman N: Sterile plaster of Paris as an implant in the infrabony environment, *J Periodontol* 40:11, 1969.

179. Shaffer CD, App G: The use of plaster of Paris in treating infrabony periodontal defects in humans, *J Periodontol* 42:685, 1971.

180. Sottosanti JS: Calcium sulfate: a biodegradable and a biocompatible barrier for guided tissue regeneration, *Compend Contin Educ Dent* 13:226, 1992.

181. Anson D: Saving periodontally "hopeless teeth" using calcium sulfate and demineralized freeze-dried bone allograft, *Compend Contin Educ Dent* 19:284, 1998.

182. Anson D: Using calcium sulfate in guided tissue regeneration, *Compend Contin Educ Dent* 21:365, 2000.

183. Bier SJ, Sienensky MC: The versatility of calcium sulfate: resolving periodontal challenges, *Compend Contin Educ Dent* 20:655, 1999.

184. Hammarstrom L: Enamel matrix and cementum development, repair and regeneration, *J Clin Periodontol* 24:658, 1997.

185. Ten Cate RC, Mills C, Solomon G: The development of the periodontium, A transplantation and autoradiographic study, *Anat Rec* 170:365, 1971.

186. Andreasen JO: Interrelation between alveolar bone and periodontal ligament repair after replantation of mature permanent incisors in monkeys, *J Periodont Res* 16:228, 1981.

187. Gestrelius S, Andersson C, Lidstrom D et al: In vitro studies on periodontal ligament cells and enamel matrix derivative, *J Clin Periodontol* 24:685, 1997.

188. Tokiyasu Y, Takata T, Saygin E et al: Enamel factors regulate expression of genes associated with cementoblasts, *J Periodontol* 71:1829, 2000.

189. Hammarstrom L, Heijl L, Gestrelius S: Periodontal regeneration in a buccal dehiscence model in monkeys after application of enamel matrix derivative, *J Clin Periodontol* 24:669, 1997.

190. Heijl L: Periodontal regeneration with enamel matrix derivative in one human experimental defect. A case report, *J Clin Periodontol* 24:693, 1997.

191. Yukna RA, Mellonig JT: Histologic evaluation of periodontal healing in humans following regenerative therapy with enamel matrix derivative, *J Periodontol* 71:752, 2000.

192. Sculean A, Chiantella GF, Windisch P et al: Clinical and histologic evaluation of human intrabony defects treated with an enamel matrix derivative (Emdogain), *Int J Periodontics Restorative Dent* 20:375, 2000.

193. Heijl L, Heden G, Svardstrom G, Ostgren A: Enamel matrix derivative (EMDOGAIN) in the treatment of intrabony periodontal defects, *J Clin Periodontol* 24:705, 1997.

194. Okuda K, Momose M, Miyazaki A et al: Enamel matrix derivative in the treatment of human intrabony osseous defects, *J Periodontol* 71:1821, 2000.

195. Heden G: A case report study of 72 consecutive Emdogain-treated intrabony periodontal defects: clinical and radiographic findings after 1 year, *Int J Periodontics Restorative Dent* 20:127, 2000.

196. Froum SJ, Weinberg MA, Rosenberg E et al: A comparative utilizing open flap debridement with and without enamel matrix derivative in the treatment of periodontal intrabony defects: a 12-month re-entry study. *J Periodontol* 72:25, 2001.

197. Zetterstron O, Andersson C, Eriksson L et al: Clinical safety of enamel matrix derivative (EMDOGAIN) in the treatment of periodontal defects, *J Clin Periodontol* 24:697, 1997.

198. Heard RH, Mellonig JT, Brunsvold MA et al: Clinical evaluation of wound healing following multiple exposures to enamel matrix protein derivative in the treatment of intrabony periodontal defects, *J Periodontol* 71:1715, 2000.

199. Sculean A, Donos N, Blaes A et al: Comparison of enamel matrix proteins and bioabsorbable membranes in the treatment of intrabony periodontal defects. A split-mouth study, *J Periodontol* 70:255, 1999.

200. Sculean A, Barbe G, Chiantella GC et al: Clinical evaluation of an enamel matrix protein derivative combined with a bioactive glass for the treatment of intrabony periodontal defects in humans, *J Periodontol* 73:401, 2002.

201. Scheyer ET, Velasquez-Plata D, Brunsvold MA et al: A clinical comparison of a bovine-derived xenograft used alone and in combination with enamel matrix derivative for the treatment of periodontal osseous defects in humans, *J Periodontol* 73:423, 2002.

202. Lekovic V, Camargo PM, Weinlaender PM et al: A comparison between enamel matrix proteins used alone or in combination with bovine porous bone mineral in the treatment of intrabony defects in humans, *J Periodontol* 71:1110, 2000.

203. Lind M: Growth factors: possible new clinical tools. A review, *Acta Orthop Scand* 67:407, 1996.

204. American Academy of Periodontology: Position Paper: the potential role of growth and differentiation factors in periodontal regeneration, *J Periodontol* 67:545, 1996.

205. Lynch SE, Williams RC, Polson AM et al: A combination of platelet-derived and insulin-like growth factors enhanced periodontal regeneration, *J Clin Periodontol* 16:545, 1989.

206. Lynch SE, Ruiz de Castilla G, Williams RC et al: The effects of short term application of a combination of platelet-derived and insulin-like growth factors on periodontal wound healing, *J Periodontol* 62:458, 1991.

207. Rutherford RB, Ryan ME, Kennedy JE et al: Platelet-derived growth factor and dexamethasone combined with a collagen matrix induce regeneration of the periodontium in monkeys, *J Clin Periodontol* 20:537, 1993.

208. Giannobile WV, Finkelman RD, Lynch SE: Comparison of canine and non-human primate animal models for periodontal regenerative therapy: results following a single administration of PDGF/IGF-I, *J Periodontol* 65:1158, 1994.

209. Giannobile WV, Hernandez RA, Finkelman RD et al: Comparative effects of platelet-derived growth factor-BB and insulin-like growth factor-I, individually and in combination, on periodontal regeneration in Macaca fascicularis, *J Periodont Res* 31:301, 1996.

210. Howell TH, Fiorellini JP, Paquette DW et al: A phase I/II trial to evaluate a combination of recombinant human platelet-derived growth factor-BB and recombinant human insulin-like growth factor-I in patients with periodontal disease, *J Periodontol* 68:1186, 1997.

211. Marx RE, Carlson ER, Eichstaedt RM et al: Platelet-rich plasma: growth factor enhancement for bone grafts, *Oral Surg Oral Med Oral Pathol Oral Radiol Endod* 85:638, 1998.

212. Landesberg R, Roy M, Glickman RS: Quantification of growth factor levels using a simplified method of platelet-rich plasma gel preparation, *J Oral Maxillofac Surg* 58:297, 2000.

213. Massague J: TGF-β signal transduction, *Ann Rev Biochem* 67:753, 1998.

214. Ripamonti U, Heliotis M, van den Heever B et al: Bone morphogenetic proteins induce periodontal regeneration in the baboon (Papio ursinus), *J Periodont Res* 29:439, 1994.

215. Toriumi DM, Kotler HS, Luxenberg DP et al: Mandibular reconstruction with a recombinant bone-inducing factor. Functional, histologic and biochemical evaluation, *Arch Otolaryngol Head Neck Surg* 117:1101, 1991.

216. Ishikawa I, Kinashita A, Oda S et al: Regenerative therapy in periodontal disease. Histological observation after implantation of rhBMP-2 in surgically created periodontal defects in dogs, *Dent Jpn (Tokyo)* 31:141, 1994.

217. Sigurdsson TJ, Lee MB, Kubota K et al: Periodontal repair in dogs: recombinant human bone morphogenetic protein-2 significantly enhances periodontal regeneration, *J Periodontol* 66:131, 1995.

218. Giannobile WV, Ryan S, Shih MS et al: Recombinant human osteogenic protein-1 (OP-1) promotes periodontal wound healing in class III furcation defects, *J Periodontol* 69:129, 1998.

219. King GN, King N, Cruchley AT et al: Recombinant human bone morphogenetic protein-2 promotes wound healing in rat periodontal fenestration defects, *J Dent Res* 76:1460, 1997.

220. Xiang W, Baolin L, Yan J et al: The effect of bone morphogenetic protein on osseointegration of titanium implants, *J Oral Maxillofac Surg* 51:647, 1993.

221. Hanish O, Tatakis DN, Boskovic MM et al: Bone formation and reosseointegration in peri-implantitis defects following surgical implantation of rhBMP-2, *Int J Oral Maxillafac Implants* 12:604, 1997.

222. Cochran DL, Schenk R, Buser D et al: Recombinant human bone morphogenetic protein-2 stimulation of bone formation around endosseous dental implants, *J Periodontol* 70:139, 1999.

223. Boyne PJ, Marx RE, Nevins M et al: A feasibility study evaluating rhBMP-2/absorbable collagen sponge for maxillary sinus floor augmentation, *Int J Periodontics Restorative Dent* 17:11, 1997.

224. Van den Bergh JP, ten Bruggenkate CM, Groeneveld HHJ et al: Recombinant human bone morphogenetic protein-7 in maxillary sinus floor elevation surgery in 3 patients compared to autogenous bone grafts, *J Clin Periodontol* 27:627, 2000.

225. Howell TH, Fiorellini J, Jones A et al: A feasibility study evaluating rhBMP-2/absorbable collagen sponge device for local alveolar ridge preservation or augmentation, *Int J Periodontics Restorative Dent* 17:124, 1997.

226. Cochran DL, Jones AA, Lilly LC et al: Evaluation of recombinant human bone morphogenetic protein-2 in oral applications including the use of endosseous implants: 3-year results of a pilot study in humans, *J Periodontol* 71:1241, 2000.

227. Barboza EP, Durate ME, Geolas L et al: Ridge augmentation following implantation of recombinant human bone morphogenetic protein-2 in the dog, *J Periodontol* 71:488, 2000.

228. Giannobile WV, Lee CS, Tomala MP et al: Platelet-derived growth factor (PDGF) gene delivery for application in periodontal tissue engineering, *J Periodontol* 72:815, 2001.

229. Zhu Z, Lee CS, Tejeda KM et al: Gene transfer and expression of platelet-derived growth factors modulate periodontal cellular activity, *J Dent Res* 80:892, 2001.

230. Garrett S: Periodontal regeneration around natural teeth. *Ann Periodontol* 1:621, 1996.

231. Reynolds MA, Aichelmann-Reddy ME, Branch-Mays, Gunsolley JC: The efficacy of bone replacement grafts in the treatment of periodontal osseous effects: A systematic review. *Ann Periodontol* 8:227-265, 2003.

232. Nyman S, Lindhe J, Rosling B: Periodontal surgery in plaque infected dentitions, *J Clin Periodontol* 4:240, 1977.

233. Rosling B, Nyman S, Lindhe J: The effects of systematic plaque control on bone regeneration in intrabony pockets, *J Clin Periodontol* 3:38, 1976.

234. Lindhe J, Westfelt E, Nyman S et al: Long-term effects of surgical/non-surgical treatment of periodontal disease, *J Clin Periodontol* 11:448, 1984.

235. Ramfjord S, Caffesse R, Morrison E et al: 4 modalities of periodontal treatment compared over 5 years, *J Clin Periodontol* 14:445, 1987.

236. Axelsson P, Lindhe J, Nystrom B: On the prevention of caries and periodontal disease. Results of a 15-year-longitudinal study in adults, *J Clin Periodontol* 18:182, 1991.

237. Cortellini P, Pini Prato G, Tonetti MS: Periodontal regeneration of human intrabony defects. I. Clinical measures, *J Periodontol* 64:254, 1993.

238. Cortellini P, Pini Prato G, Tonetti MS: Periodontal regeneration in human intrabony defects. II. Re-entry procedures and bone measures, *J Periodontol* 64:261, 1993.

239. Cortellini P, Pini Prato G, Tonatti M: Periodontal regeneration of human infrabony defects (v). Effect of oral hygiene on long-term stability, *J Clin Periodontol* 21:606, 1994.

240. Machtei EE, Cho MI, Dunford R et al: Clinical, microbiological, and histological factors which influence the success

of regenerative periodontal therapy, *J Periodontol* 65:154, 1994.

241. Hugoson A, Ravald N, Fornell J et al: Treatment of class II furcation involvement in humans with bioresorbable and non-resorbable guided tissue regeneration barriers. A randomized multi-center study, *J Periodontol* 66:624, 1995.

242. Wilson TF, Glover ME, Schoen J et al: Compliance with maintenance therapy in a private periodontal practice, *J Periodontol* 55:468, 1984.

243. Wilson TG: Compliance: a review of the literature with possible applications to periodontics, *J Periodontol* 58:706, 1987.

244. Mendoza AR, Newcomb GM: Compliance with supportive periodontal therapy, *J Periodontol* 62:731, 1991.

245. Haber J, Wattles J, Crowley M et al: Evidence for cigarette smoking as a major risk factor for periodontitis, *J Periodontol* 64:16, 1993.

246. Grossi SG, Zambon JJ, Ho AW: Assessment of risk for periodontal disease. I. Risk indicators for attachment loss, *J Periodontol* 65:260, 1994.

247. Grossi SG, Genco RJ, Machtei EE: Assessment of risk for periodontal disease. II. Risk indicators for alveolar bone loss, *J Periodontol* 66:23, 1995.

248. Preber H, Bergstrom J: Effect of cigarette smoking on periodontal healing following surgical therapy, *J Clin Periodontol* 17:324, 1990.

249. Ah MKB, Johnson GK, Kaldahl WB et al: The effects of smoking on the response to periodontal therapy, *J Clin Periodontol* 21:91, 1994.

250. Jones JK, Triplett RG: The relationship of cigarette smoking to impaired intraoral wound healing: a review of evidence and implications for patient care, *J Oral Maxillofac Surg* 50:237, 1992.

251. Tonetti MS, Pini Prato G, Cortellini P: Effect of cigarette smoking on periodontal healing following GTR in infrabony defects. A preliminary retrospective study, *J Clin Periodontol* 22:229, 1995.

252. Hall WB: Periodontal reasons to extract a tooth. In Hall WB, editor: *Decision making in periodontology*, St. Louis, 1998, Mosby.

253. Jansson L, Ehnevid H, Lindskog S, Blomlof L: Relationship between periapical and periodontal status. A clinical retrospective study, *J Clin Periodontol* 20:11, 1993.

254. Jansson LE, Ehnevid H, Blomlof L et al: Endodontic pathogens in periodontal disease augmentation, *J Clin Periodontol* 22:598, 1995.

255. Prichard J: A technique for treating infrabony pockets based on alveolar process morphology, *Dent Clin N Am* 1:85, 1960.

256. Selvig KA, Kersten BG, Wikesjo UME: Surgical treatment of intrabony periodontal defects using expanded polytetrafluoroethylene barrier membranes: influence of defect configuration on healing response. *J Periodontol* 64:730, 1993.

257. Klein F, Kim TS, Hassfeld S et al: Radiographic defect depth and width for prognosis and description of periodontal healing of infrabony defects. *J Periodontol* 72:1639, 2001.

26

Dental Implants in the Periodontally Compromised Dentition

Louis F. Rose and Laura Minsk

IMPLANTOLOGY

History

Humans have attempted to replace natural teeth with artificial implants for more than 1500 years.[1] Dental implant treatment did not become a reliable option, however, until 1952 when P. I. Brånemark's studies of bone marrow in the rabbit fibula introduced the concept of osseointegration.[2] The first human patient was treated in 1965, and since then dental implants have become one of the most significant advancements in dentistry. From the original protocol limiting implants to the anterior mandible in fully edentulous patients, the concepts and techniques have evolved to include both the mandible and the maxilla, edentulous and partially edentulous patients, and orthodontic and orthognathic applications. Currently, the use of dental implants is common in clinical practice.

Osseointegration

Osseointegration is defined as a "direct structural and functional connection between ordered, living bone and the surface of a load-carrying implant."[2] It involves the incorporation of nonbiological material within the human skeleton without initiating a rejection phenomenon and allows for permanent penetration of the soft tissues without a chronic inflammatory response. Osseointegration is a dynamic phenomenon made possible by the characteristics of the implant's composition. The most widely used dental implant material is titanium and its alloy. Titanium is nearly always covered by an external oxide layer that prevents direct contact between the host's living tissues and the potentially harmful metallic ions.[2] This surface layer, titanium oxide (TiO_2), is biologically inert, thus permitting the implant to be accepted and gradually surrounded by new bone.

Unlike natural teeth, osseointegrated implants lack a periodontal ligament. Mineralized bone grows in close proximity along the length of the implant surface. At the coronal end, the soft tissues around osseointegrated implants form a tight connective tissue barrier, containing a larger proportion of collagen and a lower proportion of fibroblasts than does tissue adjacent to natural teeth. Because of the lack of cementum for collagen fiber insertion, the fibers around dental implants are oriented parallel to the implant's surface. As with natural teeth, epithelial cells attach to the implant's surface by means of hemidesmosomes and a basal lamina, and a sulcus forms lined by sulcular epithelium that is continuous apically with the junctional epithelium. The term biologic width is used when describing the soft tissue dimensions around implants[3] (Figs. 26-1 and 26-2).

According to the original Brånemark protocol, an implant must be sterile and made of a highly biocompatible material, such as titanium, to be osseointegrated. It must be inserted with an atraumatic surgical technique that avoids overheating the bone during preparation of the recipient site, and the implant must have initial stability. Also, the implant must not be subjected to any functional forces during the initial 4- to 6-month healing period. Well controlled clinical studies demonstrate that when these guidelines are followed, osseointegration occurs with a high degree of predictability.[4-8]

Outcomes of Treatment

The criteria used to evaluate the success of oral implant treatment have changed considerably during the last 35 years. The criteria proposed during the first National Institutes of Health consensus meeting on this subject in 1979 are now considered inadequate according to current standards.[9] At that time, up to 1.0 mm of implant mobility was considered acceptable. In 1986, Albrektsson and colleagues[10] proposed a more stringent set of criteria that is currently used to evaluate the functional success of implant systems:

- Individual unattached implant that is immobile when tested clinically
- Radiograph that does not demonstrate evidence of periimplant radiolucency
- Bone loss that is less than 0.2 mm annually after the implant's first year of service
- Individual implant performance that is characterized by an absence of persistent and/or irreversible signs and symptoms of pain, infections, necropathies, paresthesia, or violation of the mandibular canal
- A success rate of 85% at the end of a 5-year observation period and 80% at the end of a 10-year observation as a minimum criterion for success

Dental implant patients currently demand more than merely functional restorations. Esthetics are also tremendously important. Although patient satisfaction is generally high with osseointegrated restorations, appearance is the most common cause of dissatisfaction.[2] Smith and Zarb[11] added to the criteria for implant success by suggesting that the implant design should not preclude placement of a crown or prosthesis with an appearance that is satisfactory to the patient and dentist. To meet these goals, we must balance the risks involved in achieving a restoration result that is biologically and functionally acceptable, as well as esthetically agreeable.

Indications

One of the first indications for dental implant treatment was to treat complete edentulism. Edentulism can result in anatomic and functional deformities that may prevent the use of removable appliances (Fig. 26-3). In addition to the functional compromises (Box 26-1), edentulism and

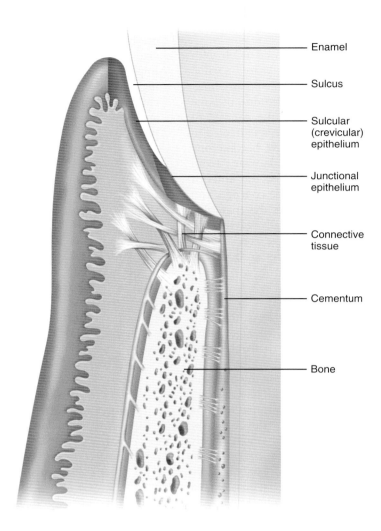

Enamel

Sulcus

Sulcular
(crevicular)
epithelium

Junctional
epithelium

Connective
tissue

Cementum

Bone

Figure 26-1. Biological attachment to a natural tooth. Connective tissue fibers insert into the root apical to the junctional epithelium.

the loss of supporting bone can result in significant esthetic deformities (Box 26-2).

Patients with these anatomic and esthetic compromises, as well as patients who have a hyperactive gag reflex, are frequently unable to wear a removable prosthesis with palatal coverage. These patients may, therefore, benefit from implant-supported or implant-assisted prostheses.

Implant-assisted prostheses

Implant-assisted prostheses are removable, tissue-supported dentures (overdentures) that benefit from the additional retention offered by endosseous dental implants. They are recommended when a limited number of implants can be placed, when hard or soft tissues must be replaced to accommodate the prosthetic device, or when unfavorable ridge morphology may result in poorly positioned implants. In the maxilla, implant-assisted over-dentures may be fabricated without palatal coverage. This is extremely beneficial for patients with a pronounced gag reflex. Because they are easy to remove, implant-assisted prostheses may also be the treatment of choice for patients who are physically or mentally challenged and who are unable to perform proper oral hygiene procedures. For patients with financial constraints, implant-assisted restorations may be more feasible because as few as two implants may be needed for support (Fig. 26-4).

Implant-supported prostheses

Implant-supported prostheses are only anchored by the dental implants and, therefore, require a minimum of

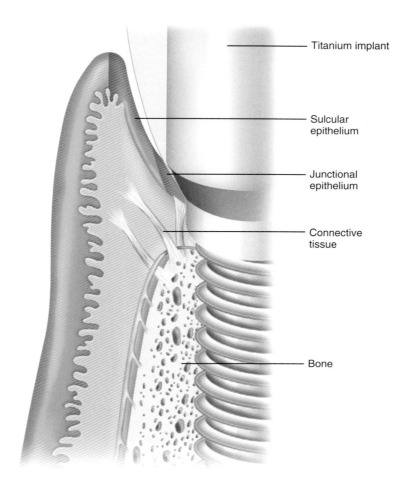

— Titanium implant

— Sulcular epithelium

— Junctional epithelium

— Connective tissue

— Bone

Figure 26-2. Biological attachment to a dental implant. There is no insertion of connective tissue fibers into the implant surface.

four to six fixtures for proper support.[12] The precise number of implants depends on the local anatomy and the quantity and quality of available bone. More fixtures may be needed in the maxilla or in areas of poor quality bone (Figs. 26-5 through 26-7).

Although the original Brånemark cases involved only completely edentulous jaws, the concepts and techniques of osseointegration have expanded to include partially edentulous jaws and single-tooth replacements. Implant-supported restorations are indicated: (1) when there is an unfavorable number or location, or both, of potential abutments in the residual dentition; (2) to avoid involving neighboring teeth as abutments; and (3) to alleviate the need to maintain teeth with questionable prognoses as potential abutments for fixed restorations (Box 26-3).

In addition, it appears that the use of endosseous dental implants may help to maintain alveolar bone volume after tooth extraction.[13] This may be one of the most important

long-term benefits of dental implants and should be considered when discussing tooth replacement options.

Limiting Factors

Systemic

Most implant success studies have been conducted following strict guidelines and in controlled research settings. Thus the results may not apply directly to everyday clinical practice situations.[4-8,14] Implant success rates may depend on the expertise of the surgical/restorative team and on patient-related factors.

Failures can be classified relative to the time of occurrence. Early failures occur before implant loading and can be caused by tissue damage during surgery, infection, premature loading, or instability of the implant. Late failures, which occur after prosthetic loading, involve pathologic insults to a previously osseointegrated implant.

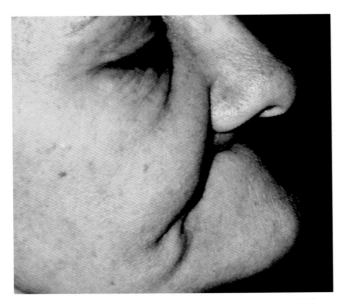

Figure 26-3. Clinical appearance of patient with "witch's chin." These characteristics are the typical result of edentulism and advanced loss of alveolar and muscular support.

This can include disturbances in the biomechanical equilibrium of the implant or overload, and alterations of the host—parasite balance.

The etiology of implant failure as either bacterial infection or occlusal overload has been well established.[15-18] Many implant failures, however, cluster around specific patient groups. This suggests there may be an underlying "patient" factor that modulates implant outcomes, leading to multiple implants being lost in the same patient.[8,19] The underlying host susceptibility to the punitive agents may play an important role in the final outcome of implant treatment. Meticulous screening and patient selection can help reduce the risk of failure or potential complications during implant treatment.

In Brånemark's classic text *Tissue-Integrated Prostheses,* the authors state: "It is possible to treat virtually all patients via the osseointegration technique, as long as the patients fulfill general requirements for surgery.

Box 26-1   Anatomical Changes Related to Edentulism

- Decreased height and width of supporting and basal bone
- Increased prominence of mylohyoid ridge, and superior genial tubercles
- Increased prominence of mandibular canal
- Relative prominence of mylohyoid and buccinator muscles
- Relative increase in the size of the tongue
- Decrease in the quantity and quality of attached keratinized mucosa

---

Box 26-2   Esthetic Deformities Related to Edentulism

- Prognathic appearance to the face
- Decrease in horizontal labial angle
- Thinning of the lips (especially in the maxilla)
- Deepening of the nasolabial groove
- Increase in depth of associated vertical lines
- Increase in columella-philtral angle
- Ptosis of the muscles (witch's chin)

Moreover, age and most chronic health conditions rarely influence patient selection."[2] Nonetheless, certain precautions must be taken.

Age is a consideration because dental implants are considered to be ankylosed elements that do not "develop" along with a growing child. Dental implant placement should not be considered until a child has fully developed and stopped growing, because placement may restrict normal growth of the jaws.

In general, any disease that alters the body's ability to fight infection or to heal after surgery may, in theory, contribute to implant failure. Implants can be considered in patients who have systemic diseases under control. For example, although diabetes mellitus may interfere with wound healing, there are reports that well controlled diabetes does not complicate healing after surgery.[19,20]

There also is no scientific evidence suggesting that an immunocompromised status is an absolute contraindication to implant surgery. In a large-scale study, Glick and colleagues[21] demonstrated that only 1% of patients with $CD4^+$ levels less than 200 per mm^3 experience postoperative complications such as excessive bleeding or poor healing after dental surgery. Although no large-scale studies have yet evaluated the success rate of dental implants in patients with human immunodeficiency virus (HIV), it is proposed that unless the surgery itself represents a major risk from a systemic point of view, patients with HIV can benefit both dentally and psychologically from dental implant treatment.

Because of the greater implant failure rate in poor quality bone,[22] osteoporosis has received much attention. This skeletal disorder involves a decrease in bone density and bone mass without significant change in the chemical composition of the bone (see Chapter 31). It is especially prevalent in postmenopausal women with estrogen deficiency, but also occurs in people with gastrointestinal absorption problems or nutritional deficiencies. Interpreting the literature in this area is difficult because of a variety of methods used to assess osteoporosis and oral bone loss, as well as to define treatment outcomes. The issue remains controversial, but currently there are no scientific data to contraindicate the use of osseointegrated implants in patients with osteoporosis.[23-25]

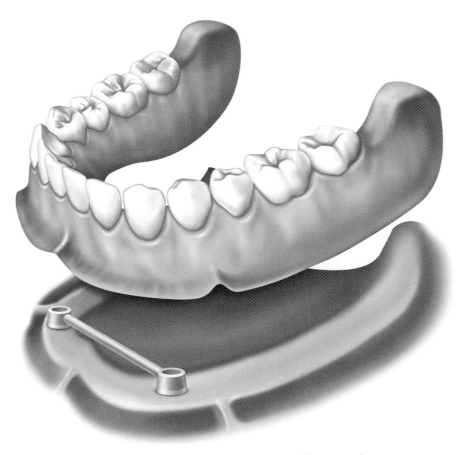

Figure 26-4. Bar and clip overdenture supported by two implants.

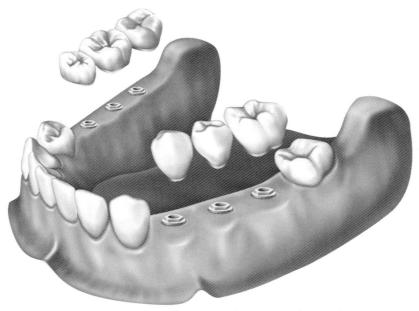

Figure 26-5. Partially edentulous implant supported restorations.

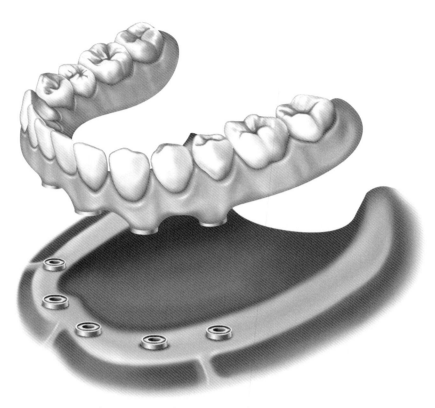

Figure 26-6. Implant-supported full-arch restoration.

Cigarette smoking has been documented as a detriment to implant success.[26-29] It is a potentially controllable risk factor that compromises wound healing through several mechanisms. Nicotine can reduce gingival circulation, increase platelet aggregation, compromise polymorphonuclear neutrophil function, and increase blood viscosity. Not surprisingly, when analyzing comparable bone quality and fixture length, the risk for implant failure in smokers is twice as high as in nonsmokers.[26,28] The risk is greater in the maxilla compared with the mandible[8,26] and with shorter implants compared with longer ones.[28]

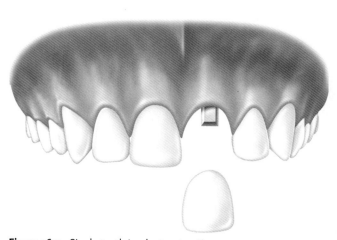

Figure 26-7. Single-tooth implant restoration.

Box 26-3	Indications for Implant Treatment

Indications for implant-assisted overdentures

- Replacement of lost hard tissue
- Replacement of lost soft tissue
- The presence of an unfavorable ridge morphology
- The presence of unfavorably oriented or inclined implants
- Expressed desire for removable prosthesis
- Economic constraints

Indications for implant-supported fixed restorations

- Unfavorable number and location of potential abutments in the residual dentition
- Avoid need to involve neighboring teeth as abutments
- Alleviate need to maintain teeth with questionable prognosis as potential abutments for fixed restorations
- Maintain bone volume after tooth extraction

Bain suggests that to reduce the risk for implant failures, patients should cease smoking at least 1 week before surgery to allow reversal of greater levels of platelet aggregation and blood viscosity.[28] The patient should continue to avoid tobacco for at least 2 months after implant placement, when osseointegration should be established. To increase patient compliance, this information should be clearly disclosed as part of the presurgical consent agreement.

Local

Osseous anatomy in three dimensions. The quality, quantity, and contour of bone will determine the size and position of the fixture to be placed.[2] Ultimately, this affects the prosthetic design and, consequently, the implant's success. For treatment planning and risk assessment purposes, it is convenient to classify the shape of the residual jaw relative to the amount of bone resorption (bone quantity) and the quality of bone relative to the amount of cortical and trabecular bone.

The bone quality (Box 26-4, Fig. 26-8) changes with the area of implantation and systemic modulators such as osteoporosis. Bone types I, II, and III offer good strength and are ideal for implant success. Type IV bone, often encountered in the maxillary posterior sextants, has a thin cortex and poor medullary strength with low trabecular

---

Box 26-4   Classification of the Shape of the Residual Jaw and the Quality of Bone

Quality of bone

  Type I: Almost the entire jaw comprises homogenous cortical bone.
  Type II: A thick layer of cortical bone surrounds a core of dense trabecular bone.
  Type III: A thin layer of cortical bone surrounds a core of dense trabecular bone of favorable strength.
  Type IV: A thin layer of cortical bone surrounds a core of low density trabecular bone.

Quantity of bone

  A: Most of the alveolar ridge is present.
  B: Moderate residual ridge resorption has occurred.
  C: Advanced residual ridge resorption has occurred and only basal bone remains.
  D: Minimal to moderate resorption of the basal bone has occurred.
  E: Extreme resorption of the basal bone has occurred.

Adapted from Brånemark P-I, Zarb GA, Albrektsson T: Tissue-integrated prostheses: osseointegration in clinical dentistry, Chicago, 1985, Quintessence Publishing.
See Figure 26-8.

---

density. It corresponds to the poorest implant success rates. In a study by Jaffin and Berman,[22] fixtures placed in type IV bone had a 35% failure rate. It is postulated that bone quality may be a better determinant for implant prognosis than the degree of resorption in the upper jaw.[30] Therefore, when poor bone quality compromises the stability of the implant, rough-surface, long, and wide-diameter implants are preferred to increase the potential surface area of osseointegration. When cortical bone is the only source of primary stability, implant placement is frequently performed without countersinking. This leaves the head of the implant in a supracrestal, or nonsubmerged, position and may place the implant at greater risk for transmucosal loading and micromovement, which can be detrimental to achieving osseointegration.[2] To avoid premature transmucosal loading of a nonsubmerged implant, the patient should refrain from wearing a removable prosthesis during the initial healing period (3 to 4 weeks). Another concern with nonsubmerged implants is the resulting coronal placement of the implant–abutment interface. This can reduce the amount of vertical (interarch) space available for the restorative components. Not only would this limit the restorative options, but it also could adversely affect the esthetics of the final restoration by not allowing sufficient room for the emergence profile of the artificial crown.

The available bone quantity (Box 26-4, Fig. 26-8) can be affected by the progression of periodontal disease or by tooth loss. Careful extraction techniques are fundamental to preserve the bony architecture around a socket. Several authors have suggested the use of bone grafts and barrier membranes in extraction sockets to help maintain the volume of bone after tooth loss.[31-34] Some have recommended immediate implant placement to preserve the facial osseous plate and to ensure a more pleasing emergence profile.[31,35]

To maintain the viability of bone, a minimum of 1.0 mm of bone is required around each aspect of the implant at the time of placement. Therefore, for a standard 3.75-mm diameter implant, at least 6.0 mm of bone is required in the faciolingual and mesiodistal dimensions. Smaller bone volumes will necessitate osseous reconstruction either before or at the time of implant placement.

For an esthetic and functional restoration, the bone morphology in three dimensions must mimic that found in the natural dentition. Biomechanical compensation may increase the cantilever effect, provide nonaxial loading (stresses the bone–implant interface), and diminish the esthetic results. If there is adequate bone volume for implant placement, it must be determined whether the available bone is properly located relative to the needs of the final restoration.[36] This process can be facilitated by a diagnostic wax-up of the final restoration. The diagnostic wax-up also can be used to fabricate a radiographic template, which helps the clinician to relate the existing

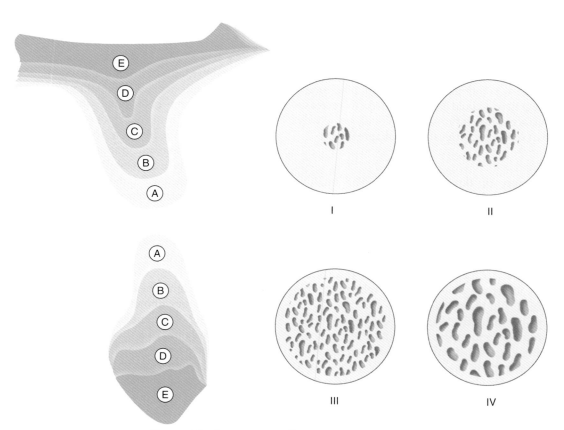

Figure 26-8. Categorization of bone quantity and quality.

volume of bone to the desired prosthetic design and can provide information to determine the need for reconstructive surgical procedures.

Implant positioning. The buccolingual position of the implant affects the biomechanics and emergence profile of the restoration. As the alveolar ridge resorbs palatally and apically in the maxillary anterior region, the resultant palatally placed implant necessitates a ridge lap restoration that can compromise function, oral hygiene, and esthetics. Bone grafting before implant placement allows the implant to be placed in the proper restorative position. Attempting to compensate for palatal implant positioning by angulating the implant to the buccal aspect creates a significant restorative challenge that may necessitate the use of custom abutments or a cemented restoration, or both, to avoid buccal screw access holes (Fig. 26-9).

Angulation of the implant in relation to the occlusal plane influences the mechanics and esthetic outcomes of the implant restoration.[37] If the fixture is placed perpendicular to the occlusal plane, the palatal positioning of the fixture often necessitates a ridge lap restoration. If the fixture is placed at a 45-degree angle to the occlusal plane, the facial positioning usually creates the optimal esthetic result (Fig. 26-10).[37]

The mesiodistal position of the implant determines the shape of the interproximal embrasures. Implants come in a wide variety of diameters and shapes. A standard diameter implant (3.75-mm diameter body, 4.1-mm diameter fixture table) being placed for a single-tooth restoration between two natural teeth requires at least 6.6 mm of interproximal space. At least 1.0 mm of bone should be present on either side of the implant, and an extra 0.5 mm to compensate for the periodontal ligament of each of the adjacent teeth. Violating this dimension can result in an implant that impinges on the natural tooth's periodontal ligament, encroaches on the interproximal papillae, and jeopardizes the esthetics of the restoration. When implants are to be placed adjacent to one another, at least 3 mm of bone is desirable between implants. Narrower diameter implants may be useful in areas of limited interproximal space (Fig. 26-11).

The apicocoronal position of the fixture also influences the function and esthetics of the restoration. In two-piece implant systems, positioning the fixture table (fixture-abutment connection point) 2.0 to 3.0 mm apical to the adjacent tooth's cementoenamel junction (CEJ) is sufficient. This allows enough room for the emergence of the restoration to mimic the profile of a natural tooth.

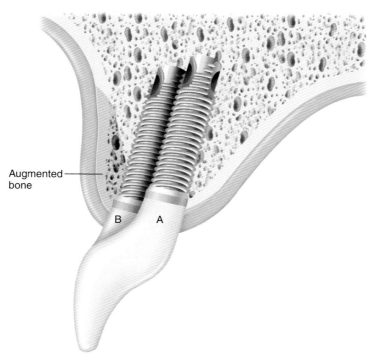

Figure 26-9. Importance of labiopalatal position of an implant. As the bone resorbs superiorly and posteriorly, implant placement becomes more palatal if implants are placed where the bone is located (**A**). The palatal positioning necessitates a buccal cantilever on the final restoration. This can be avoided if the site is prepared by augmenting the bone and placing the implant in a more labial position (**B**).

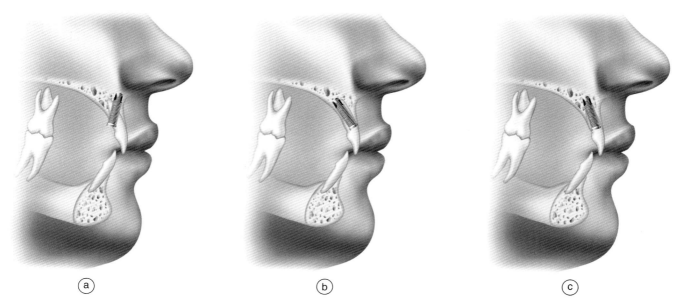

Figure 26-10. Daftary's demonstration of how the angulation of the implant can affect the restorative results.[37] Figure shows an anterior implant placed perpendicular to the occlusal plane (**A**). This can result in an extreme buccal cantilever. Excessive buccal angulation (**B**) can result in buccally located access openings and excessive off-axis implant loading. The best restorative result would be obtained with the implant placed at a 45-degree angle to the occlusal plane (**C**).

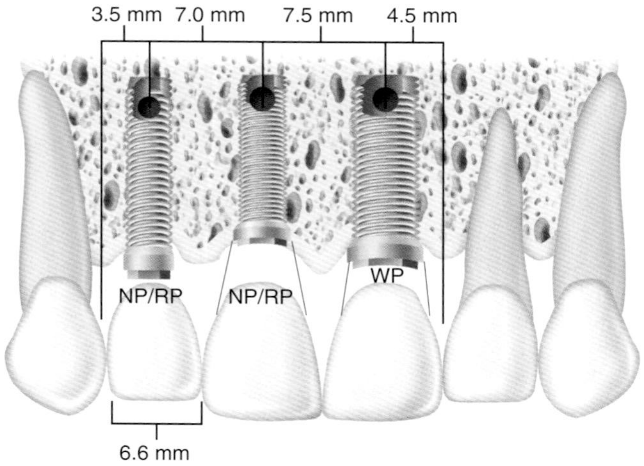

Figure 26-11. The mesiodistal position of the implant will affect the shape of the interproximal papillae and the esthetics of the restoration. The apicocoronal position of the implant can affect the emergence profile and esthetics of the restoration. Diagram illustrates the approximate minimal distances between implants for restorative simplicity, taking abutment width into consideration.

When replacing wide-diameter teeth, however, fixtures frequently need to be positioned further apically into the bone to increase the distance for establishing a proper emergence profile. This apical placement results in increased probing depths adjacent to the final restored implant, and it may reduce access for oral hygiene and compromise crown-to-implant ratio. Therefore, if the osseous volume is sufficient, wider diameter implants may help to deter some of these potential problems, because a flatter emergence profile can be used as the restoration emerges from the fixture (Fig. 26-11).

Periodontal biotypes. Ochsenbein and Ross[38] categorized healthy periodontal tissues into thin scalloped and thick flat biotypes. Jansen and Weisgold[39] further defined them and noted the different ways the tissue types react to irritation. Olsson and Lindhe[40] reported on their observations associating periodontium, tooth form, and susceptibility to gingival recession. Understanding these characteristics is essential to developing an esthetic implant restoration, especially in the periodontally compromised patient. The sequence and characteristics of disease progression are distinctive in these two periodontal tissue "biotypes" and must be considered when planning surgical reconstruction of the soft and hard tissue. The ultimate goal is to be sure that the quality, quantity, and contour of the gingiva around an implant within the esthetic zone corresponds to that of the adjacent natural teeth.[39]

The thin scalloped periodontium is characterized by the pronounced parabolic difference between the midfacial and the interproximal crests of the gingiva and underlying bone that parallels the scalloping of the gingiva and the CEJ. Fenestrations and dehiscences are commonly seen in the thin bony plates. The amount of keratinized mucosa is usually quite small both quantitatively and qualitatively, and the tissues have a tendency to be delicate and friable, reacting to injury by recession.

From a labial view the anatomic crowns of the thin scalloped periodontium are generally triangular, resulting in small contact areas in the incisal or occlusal third. The root forms in the thin scalloped type are generally thin and tapered. This results in a good deal of bony expanse between the roots of adjacent teeth. As this type of periodontium is prone to recession both facially and interproximally, there is a tendency to develop large interproximal spacing ("black triangles"). Faced with this situation, the restorative dentist is forced to make wider, squarer teeth to mask the black triangles. This periodontal biotype is sensitive to insult and may become an esthetic nightmare without proper planning and care.

In the thick flat periodontium, the root form is usually wider mesiodistally and does not taper as much as it proceeds apically. Because there is not as much mesiodistal breadth of bone between the roots, mild interproximal recession rarely causes noticeable black triangles. The crowns of the teeth are basically square, therefore the restorative dentist is not faced with making significant alterations in crown form. Also, the interproximal contact point is usually wider and is in a more apical position. The location of the contact in relation to the crest of bone may determine the presence of the interproximal papillae. Tarnow and colleagues[41] noted that when the distance between the apical extent of the interproximal contact point and the crest of bone was 5.0 mm, a papilla filling the entire space was present 100% of the time; at 6.0 mm, a papilla was present 56% of the time; and at 7.0 or more mm, the papilla was only present 27% of the time.

The gingiva in the thick flat periodontium is denser and more fibrotic, mimicking the flatter and thicker underlying osseous architecture. These characteristics contribute to the thick flat periodontium being more resistant to injury. The periodontium benefits from more ample keratinized gingiva, which is generally preferred but not required around dental implants. Stable long-term results have been observed in implants surrounded by "passive" movable mucosa, but movable soft tissue can increase the risk for plaque and foreign particle entrapment, which may necessitate gingival grafting.

Periodontal prosthesis. The functional demands of rehabilitating the completely edentulous patient with endosseous dental implants have been well documented in the literature.[4,14,42,43] More recently, progress has been made in reconstructing the partially edentulous patient with implant-supported restorations. The functional and esthetic demands of the modern era, however, provide even further challenges. Currently, we have the ability to do more than simply place implants where teeth are missing and bone is present. The current protocol is to strategically plan and develop the potential implant site to optimize and restore oral health and esthetics.

Disease progression and prolonged retention of periodontally hopeless teeth can result in anatomic deformities that, combined with the condition and location of the natural teeth, often make it difficult to develop an esthetic implant-supported reconstruction. To achieve our goals, emphasis must be placed on careful treatment planning, precise sequence of therapy, proper prosthetic design, and a well monitored maintenance program.[44,45] Primary to this end is understanding the anatomy of the hard and soft tissues and their relation to the natural teeth.

In 1974, Amsterdam recognized that the challenge in restoring the periodontally compromised patient is "the correction or modification of the deformities created by disease."[46] The loss of attachment apparatus results in architectural deformities such as: (1) loss of attached gingiva, (2) osseous deformities, (3) reverse contour of the hard and soft tissue architecture, (4) altered embrasure spaces and root proximity, and (5) exposure of cemental and dentinal surfaces on the root. Ultimately, all of these deficiencies can result in a quantitatively and qualitatively inadequate alveolar housing for the tooth, frequently resulting in secondary occlusal trauma.[46] Many of these same challenges confront the clinician contemplating the placement of implants in the periodontally involved partially edentulous patient.

The clinician must carefully and deliberately examine the edentulous areas where implants will be placed and address the following questions: (1) what type of tooth form and periodontium are present?; (2) what is the tooth position and angulation? (these will dictate embrasure forms); and (3) what are the faciolingual and incisoapical osseous dimensions?

Particularly challenging in restoring the implant-supported periodontal patient is the difference between the morphology of the implants and the natural teeth. In fact, for an esthetic result, the cross-sectional emergence profile of the prosthesis must resemble the adjacent natural teeth. This is difficult because the diameter of the head of many standard fixtures is usually narrower than the natural tooth at the CEJ. The Brånemark standard fixture, for example, has a coronal diameter of 4.1 mm and is round in cross-section, whereas the average maxillary central incisor is triangular in cross-sectional shape at the CEJ with dimensions of 7.0 × 6.0 mm. Positioning the fixture apically within the osseous tissue allows for a restoration with an emergence profile that can mimic

the natural root form. If a wider diameter fixture is used, less apical positioning of the fixture is required, because the round form and dimensions of the fixture more closely resemble that of the natural root.

When analyzing the root form at a more apical level, as would be found in cases of advanced attachment loss, the cross-sectional diameter of the root is smaller and the root is rounder. At this level, the standard fixture more closely resembles the root. The emergence profile of the prosthesis, therefore, can be developed similarly from the implant and the natural root.

The mandibular incisors present a different problem because their cross-sectional diameter is usually smaller than the standard implant. The ridge form in the mandibular incisor area often is very thin faciolingually, necessitating the use of a reduced-diameter implant.

When adequate bone quantity is available, wide-diameter implants can used in the posterior sextants. The total surface area of the wide-body implant approximates the multirooted teeth. In addition, the wide-body implants can facilitate the development of a molar-like emergence profile.

The treatment plan must include the long-term prognosis of the natural teeth and their ability to help in restoring the case. The position of the tooth in the arch will determine the morphology of the interproximal bone and the soft tissue papillae. Orthodontic treatment must be considered when drifting, tipping, tilting, rotation, or extrusion occur, because they can compromise implant placement and the final restorative result.

Special considerations relative to the area of implantation. Generally accepted implant survival rates are relative to the location of implantation. The maxilla generally has less dense, poorer quality bone and lower implant survival rates.[22] In a Swedish multicenter study of 8139 consecutively inserted machined titanium implants, the success rate of implants placed in the mandible was 99.1%, whereas in the maxilla it was 84.9%.[14] Each region of the mouth offers unique treatment challenges.

The maxillary anterior region generally presents with adequate bone quality, but the bone configuration may present a challenge to implant placement. Furthermore, esthetic considerations are critical in this region of the mouth, and it is important to consider the proposed position of the anterior teeth in relation to the lip, the smile line, and the opposing dentition. After tooth loss in the maxillary anterior region, the alveolar ridge resorbs in a palatal and posterior direction (Fig. 26-8). The resulting alveolar ridge is thin labiopalatally, with an overall reduction in the amount of available bone for ideal implant placement. Bone grafting may be required, either before or at the time of implant placement. To create the desired occlusal scheme and arch form, implants often must be placed more palatally and apically, resulting in a poor crown-to-implant ratio, buccal cantilever, and unfavorable off-axis loading (Fig. 26-9).[47]

An additional concern in the maxillary anterior region is the existence of the incisive foramen and canal. These anatomic landmarks may be quite large and can interfere with implant placement, thus requiring the removal and possible grafting of the neurovascular bundle in the incisive canal. Furthermore, the relative location of the nasal floor must be assessed to avoid a potential complication. In a study by Block and Kent,[48] 9 of 73 implants placed in the anterior maxilla engaged and most likely perforated the nasal floor. Perforation can lead to episodes of nose bleeding and may jeopardize the outcomes of implant treatment.

The maxillary posterior sextants present different challenges. In this area, implant failure rates are usually greater because of the poor bone quality often encountered.[22,49] The pneumatization of the maxillary sinus results in less available height of crestal bone, limiting the length of implants that can be inserted. Also, the increased occlusal forces encountered in the posterior regions of the mouth further jeopardize implant success. Because of these concerns, it is recommended that in the posterior maxilla at least one implant be placed to replace each missing tooth. Wider implants and shorter cantilevers also are recommended. To maximize the use of available bone by placing longer implants, some surgeons avoid countersinking the implant when using two-piece implant systems. This leaves the coronal extent of the fixture table at or slightly coronal to the osseous crest, rather than apical to the crest as occurs when countersinking is performed.

The mandibular anterior sextant usually has greater bone density and, therefore, better implant survival rates. Because of the narrow diameter of the mandibular anterior roots, interdental space may be limited in a mesiodistal dimension, and narrow-diameter implants may be indicated.

When placing implants in the vicinity of the mental foramen, the soft tissue must be carefully dissected to allow full visualization of the foramen and neurovascular bundle. Studies reveal that the inferior alveolar nerve can have an anterior loop that extends up to 4.0 mm anterior to the mental foramen.[50] To reduce the risk for nerve damage, implants should be placed at a safe distance of 4.0 mm from the mental foramen.

High success rates are documented in the mandibular posterior sextants.[6] Of concern in this region is the location of the mandibular canal and the inferior alveolar nerve. The vertical height of bone may be limited if the mandibular canal is located near the crestal bone or if vertical bone resorption has occurred. Multiple, wider, or root-shaped implants may help compensate for the diminished vertical bone dimension.

Diagnosis and Treatment Planning

Medical history

A thorough medical history is fundamental in preparation for dental implant treatment. Understanding the patient's medical status can make the difference as it relates to implant success and failure, as well as to the patient's health and well-being. Factors that may affect the patient's ability to withstand a surgical procedure should be ruled out. Such factors include but are not limited to history of angina, myocardial infarction, arrhythmias, compromised immune system, prolonged use of steroids, leukocyte dysfunction and deficiencies, neoplastic diseases requiring radiation or chemotherapy, renal failure, uncontrolled endocrine disorders, alcoholism, drug abuse, and excessive smoking. The most important part of collecting the medical history is to identify factors that potentially pose a risk to the patient during the course of periodontal, reconstructive, and implant surgery. The patient's medical health care provider should always be contacted for consultation when indicated.

Dental history

Understanding the patient's dental history is essential to implant treatment success. The timing of and reason for previous dental extractions will determine whether there has been adequate time for bone healing and whether there may be resultant osseous deformities. For example, if the teeth require removal as a result of a fracture or infection, the resultant osseous defect will more likely require correction. In addition, it is important to know how the extraction socket was treated at the time of extraction. It is currently recommended in many cases that the extraction socket be grafted at the time of tooth removal to preserve a site for future implant placement.[31-34] A dental history of treatment for occlusal problems or habits such as bruxism can be important in planning the potential implant case. Finally, understanding the patient's compliance with recommended dental care is necessary because maintenance is crucial for long-term implant success.

Oral examination

A comprehensive examination of the oral environment helps to minimize treatment complications. The examination should include a detailed dental and soft tissue evaluation that rules out infection, pathology, deformities and other potential areas of concern. The following information should be highlighted:

- Periodontal status and prognosis
- Endodontic integrity and vitality
- Integrity of existing restorations
- Caries detection
- Occlusal analysis and identification of parafunctional habits

- Tooth mobility
- Crown-to-root ratio
- Amount of interocclusal space
- Position of teeth: tipping, tilting, drifting
- Root configuration and space availability
- Ridge morphology, width, undercuts
- Esthetics

Although studies have shown that similar bacteria are associated with failing implants and periodontally involved teeth,[19] implant survival rates are comparable in recalcitrant periodontal patients compared with periodontally healthy patients.[51] Currently, there is no scientific evidence to support the theory that treated periodontal patients have a greater risk for implant failure or for development of periimplant disease. But active or potential oral infection, of any source, must be eliminated before considering dental implant treatment.

The oral examination also must include the study of articulated casts. These help in diagnosing arch form and arch relationship (horizontal and vertical overlap), as well as in determining the ideal implant sites in relation to the remaining teeth. Advanced or complex cases may also require the use of a facebow transfer, interocclusal registration, and custom incisal table. A diagnostic wax-up of the final restoration can help in finalizing the treatment plan and in determining the position and number of implants necessary to achieve the desired restoration. This wax-up can then be used to fabricate a diagnostic radiographic and surgical template.

The template can be made of polymethyl methacrylate resin, visible light-cured resin, or vacuum-formed material. Barium, gutta-percha, steel balls, or any other radiopaque markers can be used to represent proposed tooth position relative to the potential implant sites. When adapting the template for surgical use, holes are created in the template to accommodate the various drills used in preparing the implant osteotomy. When properly used, the surgical template ensures proper implant angulation and positioning relative to adjacent teeth or implants. The surgical template should have a stable fit, with either tooth or soft tissue support, and should fit passively after surgical flap reflection (Figs. 26-12 through 26-14).

Radiographic examination

The final decisions as to the feasibility of using potential sites for implant placement and the number, length, and width of implants to be placed to accommodate the prosthetic design are made with the aid of radiographs. Panoramic radiographs are helpful in giving an overview as to the relative positions of teeth to anatomic landmarks and in identifying significant pathology. Depending on the location, panographs are magnified 1.2 to 1.3 times and should not be used as definitive diagnostic tools. For example, panoramic radiographs accurately locate

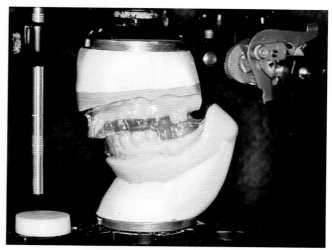

Figure 26-12. Articulated casts can be used to aid in diagnosing and treatment planning at the therapeutic vertical dimension. Acrylic shells of proposed restoration can be used to fabricate a radiographic and surgical stent.

the mandibular canal to within 1.0 mm of the anatomic position only 17% of the time, obviously not sufficiently accurate for implant procedures.[52] Periapical radiographs are more accurate in identifying the position of the mandibular canal to within 1.0 mm of the anatomic position 53% of the time.[52] Although periapical radiographs can give a fairly accurate estimate of the bone quantity in an apicocoronal dimension, they may be deceiving in evaluating bone quality. Often, the quality of the bone is determined when the osteotomy site is being prepared.

A computerized tomography scan, such as a Dentascan (GE Medical Systems; Waukesha, WI), can provide an accurate three-dimensional representation of the maxillary and mandibular jawbones. In addition to the quality and quantity of bone, the position of the mandibular canal can be identified within 1.0 mm of the anatomic landmark 94% of the time.[52] The Houncefield units used

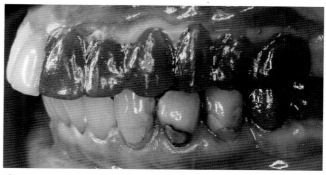

Figure 26-13. Barium-coated acrylic stent fitted in patient's mouth for use in radiographic evaluation.

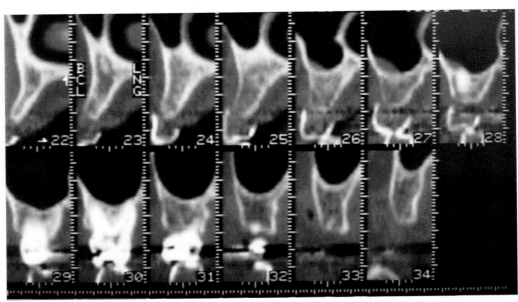

Figure 26-14. Maxillary Dentascan (GE Medical Systems) with barium-coated acrylic stent. Note the radiographic representation of the proposed restoration designated by the barium tooth outline (visible in slices 24-28).

in computed tomography (CT) scans can improve the diagnosis of bone quality by providing radiologic densitometric readings of bone. This information also can be used to accurately measure bone loss or gain over time, and it provides normative data to track osteoporosis risks.

With the Dentascan, axial scans are obtained parallel to the occlusal plane at 1.0-mm intervals through either the maxilla or the mandible. The software program then produces sequential oblique cross-sections every 2.0 or 3.0 mm around the entire curvature of the alveolar ridge. Each of the cross-sections is sequentially numbered and matched to tick marks on the axial views. Panoramic views also are available to complete accurate three-dimensional diagnosis and treatment planning.

As mentioned earlier, a template with radiopaque markers can relate the position of the existing bone to the proposed prosthetic location. The resulting information also helps to determine the need for reconstructive surgical procedures. When used appropriately, CT Dentascans relieve much of the dentist's preoperative guesswork in planning the position, angulation, and size of the implants (Figs. 26-14 through 26-17).

Implant Design and Terminology

There are numerous implant systems and manufacturers available worldwide, each providing a different design, shape, and surface characteristic. Although osseointegrated implants are chiefly composed of titanium, the implants' surfaces may differ. The first Brånemark implants were composed of machined surfaced titanium. Lately, the trend has been toward adding roughness to the implant surfaces through various subtractive or additive processes. There is microenhanced pure titanium, etched titanium, plasma-sprayed titanium, and plasma-sprayed hydroxyapatite. Textured surfaces on implants are believed to accelerate the initial healing phase and facilitate tissue growth, and they require increased torque forces for removal.[53] Torque is the energy that must be delivered to an implant to overcome the resistance provided by bone.

Implant systems also can be categorized as either the traditional two-stage (submerged) or one-stage (nonsubmerged) variety. The submerged system was designed to help protect the dental implant from inadvertent functional loading forces during the early healing period. Without exposure to the oral environment during early healing, submerged implants have less exposure to the oral epithelium and microorganisms. Subsequently, they may be preferable when guided bone regeneration (GBR) is necessary.

Submerged implant treatment is done in two stages. When the implant is placed, it is covered with soft tissue and allowed to be osseointegrated subgingivally for approximately 3 months in the mandible and 6 months in the maxilla (the differences are because of the different quality of bone encountered in the two jaws). In the second-stage surgical procedure, the implant is exposed to the oral environment by using a temporary healing abutment. The healing abutment is later replaced by the prosthetic abutment that connects the implant to the prosthetic device (Fig. 26-18). With the submerged system, the prosthetic abutment and implant interface occurs at the crest of the bone.

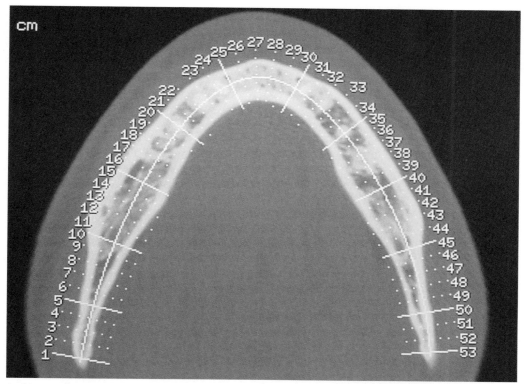

Figure 26-15. Sagittal image of Dentascan (GE Medical Systems). Oblique images were formatted 3.0 mm apart starting with number 1 on the right side. Panorex images were formatted 1.0 mm apart.

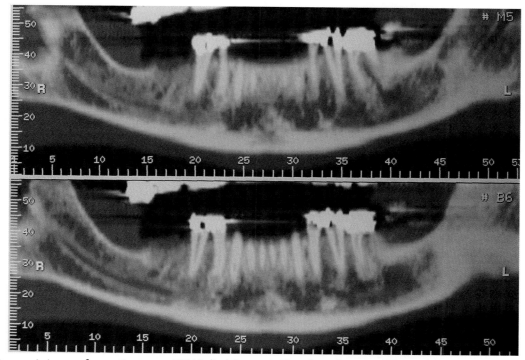

Figure 26-16. Panoramic image of same Dentascan (GE Medical Systems). The relative location of the mandibular canal can be followed on the patient's right side at approximately 10 mm below the crest of bone.

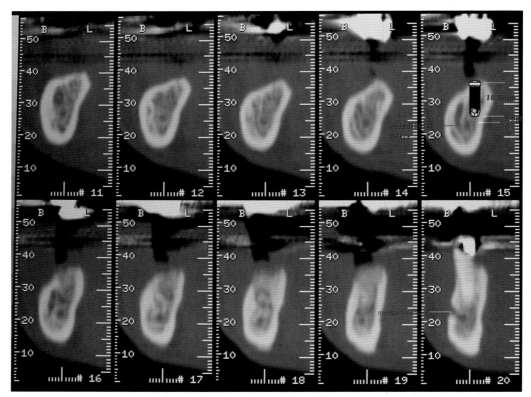

Figure 26-17. Oblique images of mandibular Dentascan (GE Medical Systems). Note the location of the mandibular foramen in image #20. The location of the mandibular canal can be followed distally to image #11 at approximately 12.0 mm below the crest of bone. After allowing a 2.0-mm "safety zone" on top of the mandibular canal, a 10.0-mm implant could be accommodated in this area. These oblique images also can reveal a lingual inclination of the alveolar process. These images can be used to determine the optimal implant length and inclination relative to teeth in the maxilla.

The one-stage, or nonsubmerged, implants have a polished collar that extends through the oral mucosa and attaches to the prosthetic components at a supragingival or slightly subgingival location. The prosthetic abutment and implant interface occurs at a supraosseous location. The major advantage of one-stage systems is that only one surgical procedure is involved and, therefore, fewer patient visits and potential discomfort. The ITI (International Team for Implantology) was the first one-stage implant developed.[54] Many implant manufacturers currently offer one-stage implant systems. The advantages of a single-stage surgery have led many clinicians to place the classic two-stage implant systems in a single-stage technique. Rather than submerging the implant at the time of placement and later uncovering the implant and placing a healing abutment transmucosally (Fig. 26-19), the healing abutment is placed at same time the implant is placed. After osseointegration has occurred, the healing abutment can be replaced with a prosthetic abutment without the need for a second surgical procedure.[55]

Implant designs also differ in shape and size. The Brånemark system is based on a screw-shape design.

Cylinder-shaped implants and tapered, or "root form"–shaped, implants also are available. Some implants connect to the prosthetic components through an external hexagonal connection, and others through an internal connection. Brånemark implants (Nobel Biocare, Gothenburg, Sweden) are available in three widths and corresponding platforms that relate to the implant-to-abutment interface (Table 26-1):

1. Regular platform (RP) implants are the most commonly used of the Brånemark system. They have a 4.1-mm diameter platform and 2.7-mm hex, and correspond to the 3.75- and 4.0-mm body diameter implants.

2. Wide-platform (WP) implants have a 5.1-mm diameter platform and a corresponding 5.0-mm fixture body. The hex diameter is 3.4 mm. They are recommended for posterior areas where additional occlusal loading is anticipated and for the restoration of molar-size crowns. They also are useful in areas of softer or poorer quality bone where the additional implant diameter may increase the implant–bone contact area and the implant's

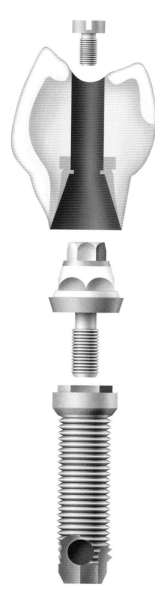

primary stability. Wide-platform implants also are useful "rescue" implants when regular platform implants lack initial primary stability.

3. Narrow-platform (NP) implants are for areas of limited space, either because of tooth proximity or a narrow ridge. The platform diameter is 3.5 mm corresponding to a 3.3-mm diameter implant body. The implant hex is 2.4 mm. Narrow platform implants should be used judiciously because of their decreased ability to withstand mechanical forces.

There are advantages and disadvantages to each implant system and design. The clinician learning to place and restore dental implants will encounter a wide array of possible companies, designs, and instrumentation choices. An inclusive review of all available options is beyond the scope of this text. For simplicity, the discussion in this chapter uses the terminology and describes the surgical technique for the Brånemark system. The Brånemark system is the most extensively researched system, with long-term prospective data dating back more than 30 years.[14] Many variations have evolved from the original protocol. The techniques described in this chapter reflect the conventional wisdom of current implant protocol.

Surgical Protocol

Surgical techniques are dependent on the implant system used. The manufacturer's instructions should be followed as recommended. The techniques may vary according to the implant's design, length, and width. Most implant companies have regional representatives who provide both training and support.

After assessing the patient's eligibility for implant treatment and completing the presurgical diagnostic and treatment planning procedures described earlier in this chapter, the patient should be prepared for surgery. To confirm that the patient understands the risks, possible complications, benefits, and alternative treatment to implant therapy, it is recommended that a comprehensive consent form be carefully read

Figure 26-18. Diagram of implant components starting with the fixture at the bottom, followed by the prosthetic abutment (which screws into the fixture), the crown (fabricated on a cylinder, which fits over the prosthetic abutment), and the prosthetic screw.

TABLE 26-1	Brånemark Implant (Nobel Biocare, Gothenburg, Sweden) Varieties, Specifications, and Indications for Use			
IMPLANT PLATFORM	PLATFORM DIAMETER, mm	HEX DIAMETER, mm	BODY DIAMETER, mm	INDICATIONS
• Regular platform	4.1	2.7	3.75, 4.0	Standard implant with most versatile applications
• Wide platform	5.1	3.4	5.0	Molar-size crowns, extreme occlusal loading, poor bone quality, as "rescue" implants
• Narrow platform	3.5	2.4	3.3	Limited space, narrow ridges

and thoroughly understood before the patient signs the form.

The original Brånemark protocol required that implant surgery be performed with sterile operating room conditions, but more recent evidence does not justify such a high degree of sterility. In a 1993 retrospective study, Scharf and Tarnow[56] demonstrated a high degree of clinical success when implants were placed in "sterile," as well as "clean," conditions. Currently, many surgeons elect to place implants in a conventional dental operatory. This has reduced treatment cost and increased access to patient care.

To avoid wound contamination or infection, preprocedural antimicrobial rinsing with chlorhexidine often is recommended. Many clinicians recommend systemic antibiotic therapy in conjunction with implant placement, although there is little evidence suggesting that such treatment improves implant success rates. Antibiotic therapy often begins presurgically. There is no consensus regarding recommendations for antibiotic prophylaxis, although penicillin or its derivatives are a reasonable option.

Once the patient has been prepared for surgery, the surgical site is anesthetized with local anesthesia. To benefit from the proprioceptive response that can be attained from the pressure of being in close proximity to the mandibular alveolar nerve, infiltration anesthesia often is recommended for mandibular implant placement, rather than use of a mandibular block. A local anesthetic with a vasoconstrictor is recommended unless it is medically contraindicated. For added comfort, some patients may prefer oral or intravenous conscious sedation (see Chapter 19).

Surgical incision and flap reflection

Soft tissue flap design depends on the need to completely visualize the surgical site, the location of anatomic landmarks, and the access required to accommodate a bone graft and membrane placement. Although remote incisions were originally recommended by the Brånemark protocol, crestal incisions on keratinized gingiva currently are generally preferred.[57] Crestal incisions tend to cause less postoperative bleeding, swelling, and discomfort and facilitate proper suturing. When exposure of the implants by dehiscence of the incision is of concern, a more palatal or facial incision may be indicated. A full-thickness mucoperiosteal flap is reflected beyond the mucogingival junction, ensuring adequate blood supply to the gingival flap. This facilitates flap movement and advancement, thus allowing for tension-free suturing. If needed to assist in flap reflection, vertical incisions should be kept at least one tooth width away from the proposed implant sites, when possible. This allows for adequate flap reflection and prevents exposure of any membrane

used. Finally, if implant placement is planned around the area of the mental foramen, incisions and flap reflection should proceed carefully until the mental foramen and neurovascular bundle are visualized.

After flap reflection, the crest of the alveolar bone should be contoured and prepared by removing all soft tissue and creating a smooth, level surface. Crestal bone chips that are removed should be placed with saline in a sterile receptacle for bone grafting if it is required.

Fixture site preparation

One of the most important considerations in preparing the implant osteotomy site is the preservation of bone vitality. A temperature of 47.0° C for 1 minute is generally accepted as the threshold temperature at which bone cells begin to loose vitality.[58,59] The use of sharp drills and copious irrigation helps to avoid deleterious heat production. Brånemark's long-term studies of high implant success rates suggest that external irrigation is acceptable for implant site preparation. A "pumping" or "up-and-down" drilling action also is recommended to help expel bone chips while cooling the bone. Bone being removed from the osteotomy site can be collected for use should a bone graft be required after implant placement.

Although variations exist amongst implant manufacturers, the general principles of implant site preparation are comparable. The Brånemark system uses a guide drill (round bur) for initial penetration of the cortical plate (Fig. 26-19). The penetrations should be spaced to allow at least 1.0 mm of bone around the circumference of each implant. In addition, to facilitate restorative procedures, at least 3.0 mm of bone are recommended between implants. These space requirements were developed to allow room for prosthetic components and the formation of proper interproximal embrasure spaces that permit adequate oral hygiene procedures. As such, the centers of the standard diameter implants (4.1-mm platform) should be no less than 7.0 mm from each other, or 3.5 mm from the adjacent tooth (Fig. 26-11). Compensations should be made for wider or narrower diameter implants. The surgical guide can be used to aid in making the guide drill perforations.

The guide drill is followed by a series of drills designed to widen the osteotomy site at the desired length. The 2.0-mm twist drill is used first. The marks on the drills are in millimeters and correspond to the implant lengths, when placed such that the fixture table is 1.0 mm subcrestal. That is, the drills are marked to allow placement of the implant platform in a subcrestal position, 1.0 mm apical to the bony crest, with the cover screw subsequently placed flush with the crestal bone (Fig. 26-20). This means that the 10-mm "mark" on the drill is actually more than 10 mm from the tip of the drill. In addition, the "V"-shape area at the tip of the drill accounts for

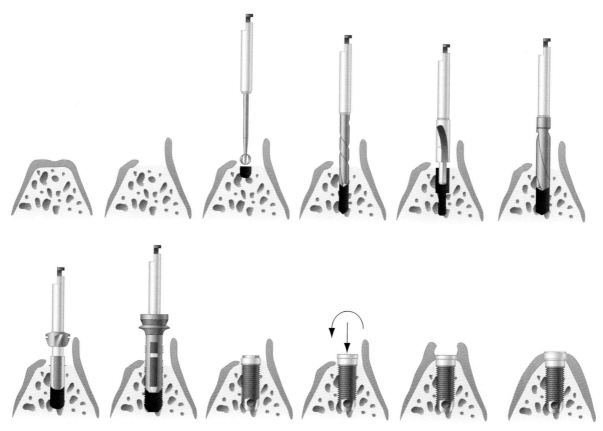

Figure 26-19. Drill sequence for preparation of standard-platform implant osteotomy. The guide drill is used to penetrate the cortical plate of bone after gingival flap reflection and preparation of the bone surface. This is followed by the 2.0-mm twist drill, the pilot drill, and the 3.0-mm twist drill. If necessary, implant site preparation can be completed with the use of the countersink and tap drills. The implant can then be inserted according to the manufacturer's instructions. The cover screw is seated on the implant and the gingival flap is reapproximated. If the clinician prefers to use a single-stage surgical approach, a healing abutment can be seated instead of the cover screw and the gingival tissues sutured around the healing abutment (see *lower right diagram*).

an additional 1.0 mm of preparation, which must be considered when estimating the amount of available bone. Thus, although the marking on the drill may correspond to a 10.0-mm implant, the actual preparation into the bone is almost 12.0 mm (10.0-mm implant length from the end of the implant to the fixture table, plus 1.0 mm for subcrestal placement of the fixture table, plus almost 1.0 mm for the tapered end of the drill) (Fig. 26-20). If the clinician wishes to place the fixture table at the level of the bony crest, rather than subcrestally, then the implant site does not need to be drilled all the way to the marking on the drill. Instead, the site can be drilled to a depth 1.0 mm "short" of the marking on the drill.

Caution must be exercised to prevent overdrilling around vital anatomic landmarks. Drilling is done at high speed (1500 to 2000 rpm) with copious irrigation. A "pumping," or up-and-down, drilling technique helps to ensure that the coolant reaches the bottom of the drill and that bony remnants are expelled from the site.

A drill extension may be required when adjacent natural teeth prevent the drill from reaching the desired length. It is critical that the clinician knows the exact drilling recommendations for every implant system used. Each implant company marks their drills differently. For example, the 10-mm mark on some companies' implant drills are actually 10 mm from the tip of the drill, whereas on others (as described earlier), the 10-mm mark is actually closer to 12 mm from the tip. When drilling close to important anatomic structures, such seemingly minimal differences can have dramatic consequences.

The surgical template can be a helpful tool for implant site preparation. If a template is not available, appropriate location and angulation must be guided by the position of the adjacent and opposing teeth and at the correct occlusal vertical dimension. Such placement often is not as accurate as that allowed when a surgical template is used. Implants placed for screw-retained restorations should have an axial orientation that allows the screw

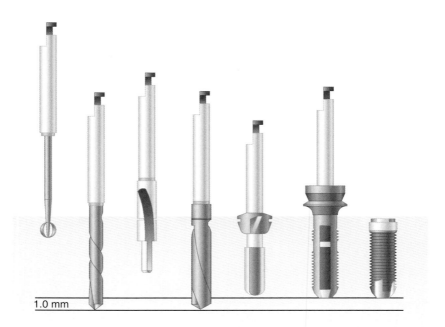

1.0 mm

Figure 26-20. The millimeter gradations on the twist drills and depth gauge represent the height of the corresponding fixture with cover screw. These marks do not indicate actual millimeter lengths. Twist drill preparation is deeper than the final position of the implant apex. The "V"-shaped end of the drill deepens the site approximately 1.0 mm more than the depth marker indicates.

access hole to penetrate through the cingulum of the anterior teeth and through the occlusal table of the posterior teeth. If cemented restorations are planned, the implant's axial orientation should allow for the eventual access hole to be through the incisal edge of the anterior teeth and the occlusal table of the posterior teeth.

The twist drills should be used with caution to prevent perforation of the axial walls (fenestration or dehiscence). If direct visualization is not possible, it is recommended that a small instrument, such as a probe, be placed parallel to the axial wall of bone to help assess the angulation. If an axial wall perforation occurs, bone grafting and membrane-assisted GBR may be required. The decision to graft the perforated site depends on the size and location of the perforation, the density of the bone, and the occlusal force to be placed on the implant. If contiguous bone surrounding the implant is adequate to sustain occlusal forces, a small lateral perforation may not require further treatment. Larger perforations that are closer to the labial aspect of maxillary implants will most likely require grafting to prevent implant surface exposure and an esthetic compromise.

After the 2.0-mm twist drill is used, the direction indicator can be used to assess initial implant position and angulation. Minor changes in angulation or position can be made before expanding the osteotomy site. Periapical radiographs, taken with either a direction indicator or the twist drill as radiopaque markers, may also be helpful to evaluate the length and mesiodistal angulation of the implant preparation.

Next, a pilot drill is used to expand the osteotomy site to accept the 3.0-mm twist drill (Fig. 26-19). The 3.0-mm twist drill enlarges the osteotomy at the desired length of the implant. Direction indicators are used to help guide the site preparations.

Variations in the drilling sequence may be needed depending on the bone density and the diameter of the intended implant. When the bone is very dense, a 3.15-mm twist drill may be necessary to expand the osteotomy site further. For wide-diameter implants, a pilot drill and another twist drill (4.3-mm diameter) are used after the 3.0-mm twist drill. For narrow-diameter implants, a 2.7- or 2.85-mm twist drill is used instead of the 3.0-mm twist drill.

The countersink drill is designed to prepare the site for the head of the implant and allows the seating of the implant with the cover screw to be level with or just below the crest of bone. This permits the implant to heal without being influenced by transmucosal loading forces (Fig. 26-19).

In areas where the bone is less dense and adequate interarch space is present to allow for the prosthetic components, limited or no countersinking is recommended. This allows the implant collar to engage the cortical layer of bone at the alveolar surface and increases initial implant stability. Also, because the measurements in the drill guides account for the countersink, a longer implant fixture can be placed in the same amount of vertical bone. Adequate interarch space may also allow the clinician to place the fixture table at the level of the bony crest (rather than subcrestally), with the cover screw in a supracrestal location. Countersinking is not performed when such an implant position is desired. Many clinicians prefer to place the fixture table at or slightly coronal to the bony crest, rather than subcrestally as originally recommended in the Brånemark protocol. This may prevent crestal bone loss during initial healing, because the junction between the fixture table and the abutment will be supracrestal, providing for some "biologic width" at the junction.[3]

Even when using self-tapped fixtures, prethreading the bone with a screw tap may be necessary in areas of dense cortical bone (Fig. 26-19). Limited tapping occasionally is required when a thick, dense cortical plate with softer trabecular bone exists. Tapping with copious irrigation is accomplished at lower speeds and higher torque (e.g., 25 rpm and 40 N-cm, respectively). In dense bone, the screw tap stops automatically if it is misdirected or reaches the apical aspect of the osteotomy site. If the angulation needs to be corrected, the tap drill should be reversed and redirected to its proper position.

Fixture installation

The implant length is determined by measuring the distance from the end of the bone preparation to the most apical marginal bone level. The implant fixture is installed at low speed and high torque (e.g., 20 to 50 N-cm depending on the bone quality). To avoid fixture contamination, the fixture must not come into contact with any instruments or oral tissues. Furthermore, it is recommended that irrigation be withheld until the fixture is inserted past the horizontal hole at its apical end. Profuse irrigation should follow. Like the screw tap, the fixture may stop automatically in dense bone when it reaches the end of the preparation or if it is misdirected. Again, if angulation needs to be corrected, the fixture should be removed in reverse speed along the same axis as insertion and then redirected. Once fully seated, a cylinder wrench can be used for final tightening of the fixture. At this point, the fixture should feel tight and stable (Fig. 26-19).

Primary stability is the implant's ability to resist movement when challenged manually. The more stable an implant is at the time of insertion, the greater the likelihood of its clinical success. If the fixture is tight, the fixture mount can be removed and the cover screw tightened. The cover screw will prevent bone from penetrating inside the fixture head during healing. If a single-stage surgical approach is used, the healing abutment would be placed instead of the cover screw. The length of the healing abutment will be determined by the height and thickness of the soft tissue (Fig. 26-19).

Fixtures demonstrating mobility and a lack of primary stability at the time of placement should be removed. When possible, wider diameter fixtures may be used as "rescue" fixtures to immediately replace loose fixtures. Otherwise, the site will require grafting with fixture placement reattempted in 4 to 6 months.

Soft tissue readaptation and suturing

Before reapproximating the gingival flaps, all nonsupporting or sharp bony edges should be removed. To evert the edges of the flap and obtain more predictable closure, horizontal or vertical mattress sutures are recommended. They should be reinforced by single interrupted or continuous sutures. Either resorbable or nonresorbable sutures may be used. Long-term success studies of one-stage implant systems indicate that complete soft tissue coverage of the implant is not required for osseointegration.[54] Clinical expertise has shown, however, that soft tissue coverage is advantageous to bone formation, especially in the case of GBR. If healing abutments are placed at the time of implant insertion, the flaps are closely approximated around the healing abutments in a way similar to adaptation around teeth.

Written postoperative instructions should be clearly explained and given to all patients. Failure to adhere to the postoperative protocol could result in failure of osseointegration. To help prevent infection of the implant and surgical site, postoperative antibiotics may be recommended for 7 to 10 days. The surgical site also should be kept as clean as possible and debrided twice daily; 0.12% chlorhexidine rinses are recommended. Rinsing should continue until after the sutures are removed and the patient is able to resume normal oral hygiene procedures. Analgesics can be dispensed before surgery and continued after surgery. Nonsteroidal antiinflammatory medication is usually satisfactory to control postoperative discomfort, but in certain cases, a narcotic analgesic may be required.

Removable prosthetic devices should be adjusted to prevent injury to the wound. Special consideration should be taken to avoid transmucosal implant loading forces that could result in micromovement of the implant and failure of osseointegration.[60] To prevent this complication, it is suggested that fully edentulous patients refrain from wearing a removable prosthesis for 2 to 3 weeks after surgery. At that time, the prosthesis should be carefully relined to prevent transmucosal implant loading. Alternative treatment plans should be considered for patients who refuse to go without a provisional removable prosthesis. (Some alternatives are described later in this chapter in the section detailing provisional restorations.)

Patients are usually seen 7 to 10 days after implant placement for suture removal and wound debridement. During the initial healing period, the patient may experience facial discoloration and swelling as part of the normal healing process. Patients should be informed that swelling may peak 48 to 72 hours after surgery.

The patient should be examined every 3 to 4 weeks during the healing period. In most cases, sufficient osseointegration occurs after 3 months in the mandible and 4 to 6 months in the maxilla. Healing time in the maxilla is longer because of the quality of bone (less dense and more trabecular). Longer healing periods may be required in poor quality bone or after bone grafting procedures. Some manufacturers have shown that early or even immediate loading of implants can be successful.

Abutment connection

If the implants were submerged under the soft tissues at the time of placement, a second surgical procedure is required before restoration. After the gingiva is anesthetized with local infiltration, a crestal incision is made to expose the fixture and cover screw. Alternatively, if there is ample keratinized gingiva, a soft tissue punch may be used to expose the implant. After removing the excess hard and soft tissues, the cover screw can be removed. Bone mills are available to help remove excess tissue around the implant head. A gauge can be used to measure the soft tissue thickness and select the appropriate healing abutment. The healing abutment helps to maintain the opening from the oral cavity to the implant through the soft tissue and allows for the formation of a sulcus. Ideally, it should be approximately 1.0 to 2.0 mm longer than the height of the soft tissue. For esthetic cases, anatomic healing abutments are available that mimic the shape of a natural root and selectively enlarge the transgingival space.

Once the healing abutment is placed, a radiograph is taken to confirm the proper fit of the abutment. Occasionally, it may be necessary to reshape the bone around the implant to accommodate the healing abutment. This should be done with extreme caution to prevent damaging the titanium implant surface.

After the abutment fit is confirmed, the soft tissue flaps are approximated and sutured with single interrupted sutures. This may require thinning or trimming of the flaps before suturing. Also, to assure a passive fit, the provisional restoration may need to be adjusted and relined to accommodate the healing abutment.

Temporary transitional implants

Temporary transitional implants were developed to address the need for uninterrupted healing and premature transmucosal forces caused by removable dentures, as well as to accommodate patient demands for immediate functional and esthetic fixed restorations. These can be used in conjunction with conventional implants and serve as abutments for a provisional fixed prosthesis during the osseointegration of the permanent implants. Temporary transitional implants can be placed in the mandible or the maxilla and are suitable for partially or fully edentulous patients.[61,62]

As opposed to conventional implants, transitional implants are not expected to be osseointegrated. In fact, because of their smaller diameter and if used for long-term loading, these implants are susceptible to structural fatigue and fracture. They are removed once the conventional implants have osseointegrated. As with conventional implants, the success of temporary implant treatment requires careful patient selection and treatment planning.[2,45] After soft tissue flap reflection and site preparation, the conventional implants are placed in the ideal position to satisfy the needs of the final restoration. Required bone augmentation procedures can then be performed if necessary. The transitional implants are placed at a minimum distance of 2.0 to 3.0 mm from the conventional implants or from natural teeth. As many temporary implants as possible should be positioned and distributed anteroposteriorly to support the temporary prosthesis.

To prepare for the placement of temporary implants, the cortical crestal bone is penetrated with the twist drill and prepared to the desired length. The transitional implants are then placed according to the manufacturer's instructions. To achieve primary implant stability at the time of placement, the transitional implants must engage the cortical crestal bone. Paralleling pins can help the clinician visualize implant angulation and ensure the path of insertion for the temporary restoration. Once the transitional implants are placed, the tissues are sutured, leaving the abutment portion of the transitional implants exposed. If necessary, small corrections in angulation can be made with bending tools. The temporary restoration can be fabricated at chairside (direct technique) or in the laboratory (indirect technique) with the same methodology used for conventional implants (Figs. 26-21 through 26-24).

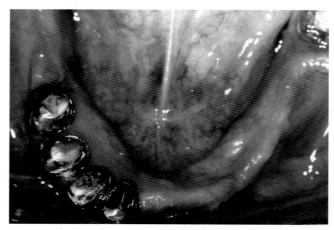

Figure 26-21. This patient had an insufficient number of natural abutments on the mandibular left quadrant to hold a fixed provisional restoration during the osseointegration of conventional implants.

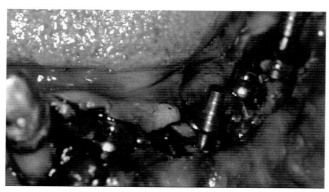

Figure 26-22. Five conventional implants were placed to satisfy the requirements of the final restoration. Two temporary implants were placed 2 to 3 mm from the conventional implants to help support the provisional restoration during healing.

Depending on the system used, transitional implants require at least 7.0 mm of vertical bone and are otherwise contraindicated. In addition, because the prosthetic abutment is incorporated in the implant design, the amount of interocclusal space should be at least 6.0 to 7.0 mm (4.0 mm for the abutment component and 2.0 mm for the coping and restorative material).

To ensure initial stabilization of the transitional implant, good bone quality (type I or type II bone) and sufficient crestal cortical bone are needed to engage the implant. Temporary implants are contraindicated if a sufficient number cannot be placed to adequately support the desired temporary prosthesis.

As with all implant treatments, routine clinical and radiographic follow-up should be done to evaluate the ongoing bone and soft tissue health. If there are signs of implant failure, mobility, fracture, or infection, the

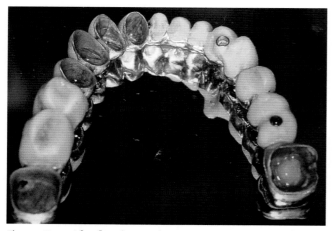

Figure 26-23. After flap closure, the existing restoration was relined to include the temporary implants as abutments for the left side. The access holes for the transitional implants are visible in the intaglio surfaces of the molar and canine.

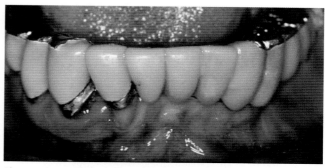

Figure 26-24. The provisional restoration remained in function for 6 months during the osseointegration of the conventional implants.

implants must be removed as soon as possible and the site treated accordingly. When the transitional implants are no longer needed, they can be removed with minimal discomfort to the patient. They are unscrewed by applying torque in a counter-clockwise direction. Any granulation tissue must be removed with curettage, and the area will heal similar to a tooth extraction site.

Provisionalization

The interim prosthesis (either fixed or removable) will provide invaluable data as to tooth relations in the centric and excursive positions, anterior esthetics, and phonetics. Although the provisional restoration is important, it often is neglected with resultant untoward complications. Depending on the patient's needs and desires, the restorative treatment plan, and the number and location of implants placed, there are several provisionalization options. Before implant uncovering, a removable interim prosthesis, a fixed bridge supported by retained natural teeth, or resin-bonded temporary restorations may be used. Methods for immediate or early loading of either interim or conventional implants are described later in this chapter.

For provisionalization after implant uncovering, the restoration may be delivered the day of uncovering if the implant has been indexed at the time of placement. Indexing is performed by recording the implant position and relation to the adjacent and opposing dentition at the time of implant placement. This can be accomplished with a conventional impression or by using indexing aids available through the implant manufacturers.

Temporary cylinders and abutments are used to fabricate a provisional restoration that fits on the selected abutment or directly on the implant platform. A laboratory-processed acrylic shell or the patient's modified existing denture can be adapted for use as a temporary restoration. For durability, it is recommended that these provisional restorations be reinforced with fibers, orthodontic wire, or a metal undercasting.

As with all implant treatment, temporary restorations must fit passively on the implant components. The occlusion should be evaluated to prevent excessive loading forces and the patient should be instructed in proper maintenance techniques.

Prosthetic Considerations

After soft tissue healing has occurred, definitive restorative procedures should commence. The position of the implant can be transferred to a cast for laboratory procedures either through an implant-level impression (transfer of the fixture position) or an abutment-level impression (transfer of the position of the abutment already placed on the implant). The implant-level impression is the recommended option.[63] Selecting the prosthetic abutment on a laboratory cast allows for enhanced visualization of the soft tissue profile, the interarch dimensions, and the alignment and angulation of the implant (Fig. 26-25).

After the temporary healing abutment is removed, the impression is made with a heavy-body elastomeric material injected around each impression coping and the impression tray. Either a tapered or a square impression coping can be used, matching the platform diameter of the implant. Tapered impression copings remain on the implant when the impression is removed and must be taken off the implant and reseated on the impression before pouring the cast. Otherwise, square impression copings are separated from the implant while the impression is still in the mouth (with a screw that protrudes through the impression tray). They remain in the impression and do not require reseating into the impression material. They are, therefore, considered to be more accurate. The use of square impression coping is limited in the posterior sextants when there is minimal interocclusal space and access for loosening the impression coping screw (Figs. 26-26 through 26-29).

In the laboratory, the implant replica is attached to the impression coping, and soft tissue material is injected around the replica to simulate the gingiva. Type IV die stone is poured into the impression. The casts are then articulated at the proper vertical dimension before the laboratory procedures are finalized, and the accuracy of the laboratory replicas are clinically verified.

Abutment selection

Selecting the restorative abutment is one of the most important steps in implant prosthodontics. Choosing the appropriate abutment depends on the restorative option desired, the position and angulation of the implants, the amount of interarch space available, the soft tissue dimensions, and the esthetic demands of the case. There are three basic abutment classifications, depending on the type of restoration: overdentures, screw-retained restorations, and cemented restorations.

Overdentures. Some overdentures are individual attachments that fit directly on fixtures. Others are attachments that are incorporated on gold cast-bars that interconnect two or more fixtures together. The requirements of the

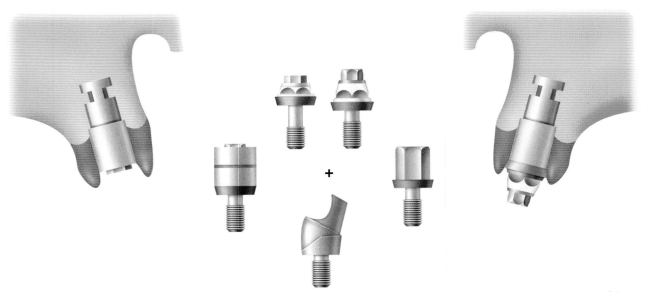

Figure 26-25. Abutment selection can be performed on laboratory replicas, mounted at the appropriate vertical dimension. The choice of the appropriate abutment depends on the restorative option desired, the position and angulation of the implants, the amount of interarch space available, the soft tissue dimensions, and the esthetic demands of the case. The abutments shown here are (clockwise from the top) multiunit abutments (two different height abutments shown), single-unit abutment, angulated abutment, and standard abutment.

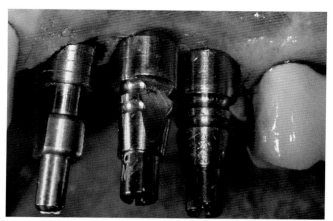

Figure 26-26. Square impression copings seated on one standard and two wide-platform implants.

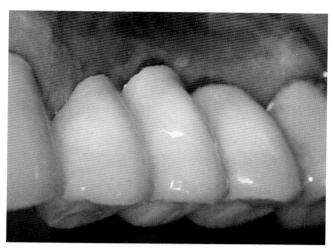

Figure 26-28. Provisional restoration delivered the day the custom fabricated abutments were seated.

final prosthesis dictate the category and the specific type of attachment to be used.

Screw-retained restorations. Screw-retained restorations offer easy retrievability for maintenance procedures (Fig. 26-18). In all screw-retained abutment systems, the prosthetic screw is designed to be the weakest link. Loosening or fracture of this replaceable gold screw occurs before breakage or fatigue of any other implant components.

The conventional abutments were the original transmucosal elements designed for the fabrication of fixed restorations in edentulous arches (Fig. 26-25). They are made of pure titanium in varying lengths and diameters to fit the different implant platforms. The height of the gingiva as it relates to the implant platform determines the length of the abutment selected. They connect directly to the implant with a corresponding titanium abutment screw. Conventional abutments are rounded at the base and do not have an antirotational effect. Thus, they are

only recommended for multiple implant restorations. Because the conventional abutment is designed to have the junction of the restoration and the abutment in a supragingival location, this abutment is rarely used in esthetic areas.

The multiunit abutment (Fig. 26-25) was designed for use in partially edentulous arches where esthetics is a concern. With this abutment design, the restoration may start closer to the implant fixture, in a subgingival location, and appear as if the teeth are emerging directly through the soft tissue. The different sizes relate to the height

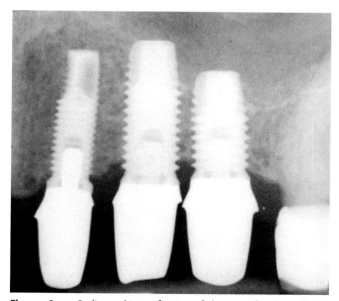

Figure 26-29. Radiographic verification of abutment fit. There should be no radiographically visible junction (radiolucent line) at the fixture–abutment interface.

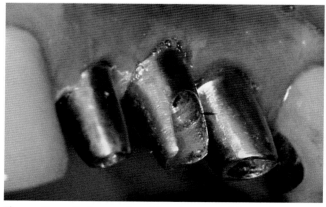

Figure 26-27. Custom-made gold copings were fabricated to correct the excessive buccal angulation of the center implant.

of the cuff at the base of the abutment (1.0 to 5.0 mm). A taller cuff is chosen when the soft tissues are thick, and a shorter cuff for thinner tissues. Each size has its own abutment screw. Like the conventional abutments, the Estheticone abutment (Nobel Biocare) was designed for use in multiple implant restorations and lacks a built-in antirotational device for use in single-tooth restorations (Figs. 26-18, 26-30 through 26-32).

Angulated multiunit abutments (Fig. 26-25) may be used when the implants have a significant axial divergence or convergence or to redirect the gold screw access hole when the implants are angled facially. These abutments are available in multiple angulations (17-degree and 30-degree angulations available from Nobel Biocare), but generally the greater the degree of angulation, the larger the requirement for interocclusal space.

Nonsegmented abutments, also called "UCLA abutments" (Fig. 26-25), were designed to omit the transmucosal element. They are available for single-unit or multiunit restorations. The castable retentive element is incorporated into the restoration and connects directly to the implant platform. This allows for a more esthetic and anatomic emergence profile through the soft tissue. Because these abutments are incorporated in the restoration, they require less vertical space and are recommended when there is limited interocclusal room.

Cemented restorations. Single-unit or multiunit restorations can be cemented to conical or Esthetic abutments (Nobel BioCare), which are available in straight and angulated versions. These abutments are available in metallic or ceramic materials. The ceramic variety often is preferred to improve translucency in esthetic cases. Customized or personalized abutments also can be fabricated to help solve implant angulation discrepancies. Once inserted, these conical abutments can be treated and prepared as natural teeth and restored with conventional crown and bridge procedures. Because the crowns on

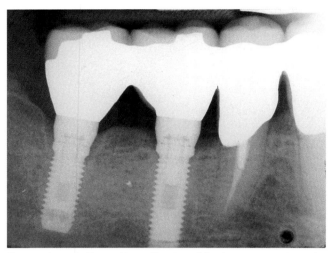

Figure 26-31. Radiographic verification of final restoration. Note the smooth emergence profile from the implant to the abutment to the restoration.

these abutments are cemented and may not be easily retrieved, the abutment must be tightened to 35 N-cm to prevent loosening after crown cementation. Using temporary cement can help to improve retrievability of the cemented restoration.

Completion of Restorative Procedures

Once the selected abutment is seated on the laboratory implant replica, standard laboratory procedures can proceed to fabricate the desired restoration. On completion of the restoration, both the implant abutment and the

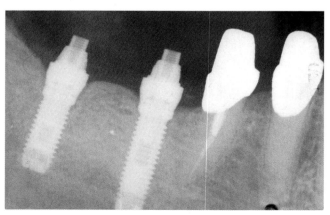

Figure 26-30. Radiograph of Estheticone (Nobel Biocare, Gothenburg, Sweden) abutments seated on two implants.

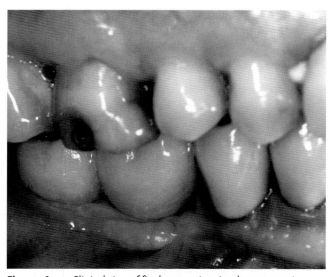

Figure 26-32. Clinical view of final restoration. Implant restoration was screw retained. The junction of the restoration and the abutment is located subgingivally, providing excellent esthetics.

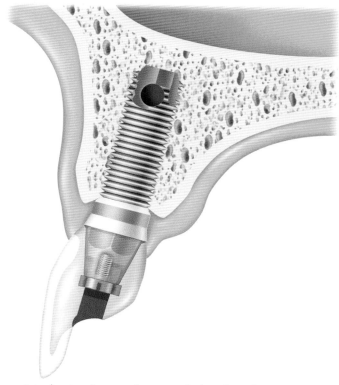

Figure 26-33. Diagram of final screw-retained restoration seated on a standard implant. The access opening is in the region of the cingulum.

restoration are transferred to the oral cavity. All components must fit passively and be verified both clinically and radiographically (Fig. 26-33). Ideally, occlusal forces are directed parallel to the long axis of the implant, and the occlusion is evaluated and adjusted to minimize occlusal trauma.

ADVANCED CONCEPTS IN IMPLANT THERAPY

Periodontal disease, tooth extraction, long-term use of removable appliances, and traumatic injuries typically result in advanced alveolar bone loss that prevents the placement of implants in an optimal prosthetic position. Fortunately, innovations in surgical techniques, together with advances in the biologic understanding of bone and soft tissue regeneration, have increased the predictability of reconstructing alveolar ridge deformities. The most critical aspect of creating an esthetic, functional restoration is the surgical placement of the implant in a prosthetically driven position, which should emulate the natural emergence of a tooth from soft tissue. This section focuses on bone and soft tissue augmentation procedures used to correct anatomic deficiencies for the optimal placement of dental implants.

Preservation of Alveolar Bone

Periodontal disease and other dental infections contribute to alveolar bone loss because of local biochemical factors that result in inflammatory bone resorption. Some of these factors, such as endotoxins, cytokines, and osteoclastic activity, may still be present even after tooth extraction and socket debridement. Systemic factors, such as malnutrition, avitaminosis, calcium deficiency, diabetes mellitus, osteoporosis, and steroid use also influence the eventual quality and quantity of residual alveolar bone. Although the loading characteristics of the mandible and maxilla are poorly understood, external pressure of the mucoperiosteum also is believed to result in bone resorption.[64]

To optimize implant placement, bone volume must be preserved. Failing teeth should be extracted early to avoid additional bone loss. After tooth extraction (or tooth loss), the alveolar ridge resorbs and may result in a significant osseous deformity. Most bone loss after extraction occurs in the first 6 to 24 months. Recent studies propose treating an extraction site with complete flap closure and formation of a stable clot to help preserve the bone volume after tooth loss.[33,65]

Atraumatic tooth removal

An important step to maintaining alveolar bone is to avoid tissue loss at the time of tooth removal. This should be given the highest priority because it may eliminate the need for later bone regeneration or grafting. Every effort should be made to minimize an esthetic deformity.

There are many reasons a tooth should be surgically removed. They include endodontically treated teeth, a severely dilacerated root, and a fractured tooth with little remaining coronal tooth structure. Appropriate instruments and surgical techniques ensure the best possible outcome. The proper surgical procedure for tooth extraction is as follows:

1. Do not reflect the interdental papilla, especially in the esthetic zone.
2. Focus on controlling the process of tooth removal. The use of a thin elevator (periotome) will reduce trauma to the bone. Luxation and controlled force or sectioning of the tooth will help to prevent bone loss.
3. Once the tooth is removed from the socket, eliminate all soft tissue fragments and pathology.
4. Ensure that a stable blood clot forms to initiate the first stages of bone healing and proper bone fill.

If the tooth to be extracted has sufficient bone support on all surfaces, the extraction site can be expected to fill with bone without any additional augmentation procedures. If the bony walls of the socket are compromised, however, it may be necessary to support the socket walls with a grafting material.

It is important to carefully evaluate the type of bone defect that exists immediately after the extraction, because this will dictate the treatment required to preserve or reconstruct the alveolar ridge. An easy way to categorize the defect is to determine the number of bony walls that remain after extraction. Each of these requires a specific approach to alveolar ridge preservation and may be treated differently.[66]

Five-wall socket. Most recent extraction sites that have all five walls intact (buccal, lingual, mesial, distal, and apical) and thick bony walls can accommodate implant placement without adjunctive procedures. However, grafting may be indicated at the time of tooth removal if the bony walls are thin. The bone graft material should be loosely condensed and should completely fill the socket. Many clinicians completely cover the graft with a tension-free flap or soft tissue autograft. To enhance regeneration, a membrane also should be considered when using bone grafting material. Some clinicians cover the graft with a membrane but do not attempt to obtain primary flap closure. This is usually done to avoid flap reflection beyond the mucogingival junction, which is required to coronally advance a flap to cover a socket. After socket grafting, the patient must then wait 3 to 6 months before implant placement, depending on the graft material used.[66] If no graft material is used, the implant may be placed after 3 to 4 months; however, the bone will not be fully mature and the implant will need to be placed into bone apical to the previous socket to establish primary implant stability.

Four- and three-wall sockets. For a tooth that has one or two bony walls missing, bone grafting is usually necessary before implant placement. The alveolar bone typically narrows, leaving an inadequate width for implant placement. To help restore the osseous dimensions, it may be necessary to place a bone graft in conjunction with a barrier membrane that helps prevent the ingrowth of soft tissue (Fig. 26-34).[66]

Two- and one-wall sockets. Some patients exhibit a long-standing osseous defect characterized by a knife-edged alveolar ridge. These are considered chronic one- or two-wall defects and may require a two-stage procedure involving bone grafting and then implant placement. Depending on the defect's severity, a monocortical block graft, as opposed to a particulate material, may be preferred. This type of graft requires careful surgical planning and is described in further detail later in this chapter.

To predictably maintain the maximum amount of alveolar bone immediately after extraction, the socket should be grafted. Autogenous, allogenic, or xenogenic bone have been used with varying rates of success (Fig. 26-35). A good blood supply and the formation of a stable blood clot are essential to graft success. To increase the amount of blood supply to the graft, it may be necessary to penetrate the socket walls with a small bur to induce bleeding. This provides a source of osteoprogenitor cells (see Chapter 25).

When primary closure cannot be achieved, the socket may be covered with a collagen material or a soft tissue graft. This will minimize soft tissue ingrowth, improve bony apposition, and aid in alveolar ridge preservation. The implants can be placed once bone has been regenerated (Fig. 26-36).

The optimal time to place implants into treated sockets has not been determined. Depending on the quantity and quality of existing bone and the clinician's preference, the implant placement after tooth extraction can be immediate, delayed, or staged. By definition, immediate implant placement occurs at the time of extraction. Delayed implant placement is performed approximately 2 months after extraction to allow for soft tissue healing. Staged implant placement allows for substantial bone regeneration and healing within the extraction site. This frequently requires 4 to 6 months.

Immediate implant placement

When the implant can be located in an ideal position with sufficient bone volume to achieve initial stabilization, it is

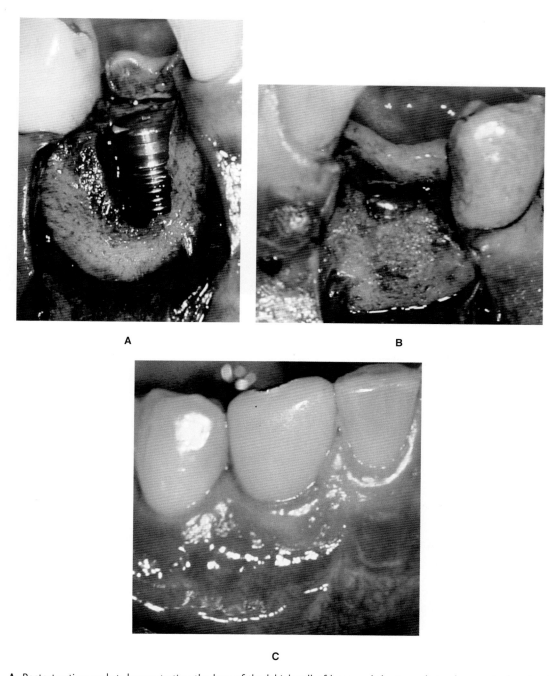

Figure 26-34. A, Postextraction socket demonstrating the loss of the labial wall of bone and the immediate placement of an implant. Note the exposed threads. **B,** Bovine bone and a nonresorbable membrane were used to regenerate the bone necessary to totally cover the implant. **C,** A 10-year postoperative view of the restored implant.

feasible to place the implant and the graft concurrently. When the implant is placed at the time of extraction, osseointegration begins immediately (Fig. 26-37).

The primary advantages of immediate implant placement are reduced healing time and only one surgical procedure. Because of the discrepancy in size and shape of the socket and the implant, a space often exists around the implant.[35] If there is insufficient soft tissue to cover the implant site, the outcomes may be compromised. The flap design may need to be modified, or a soft tissue autograft or regenerative membrane may be necessary to completely cover the implant.

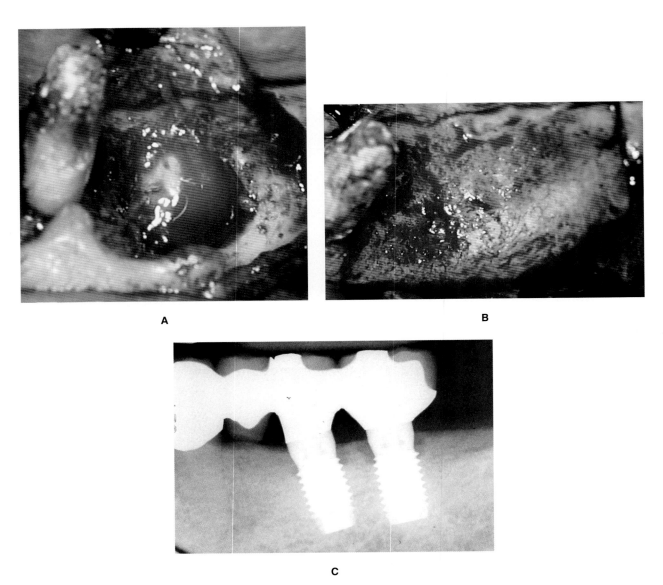

Figure 26-35. A, An infected tooth that created a significant loss of bone was extracted. After total debridement, freeze-dried demineralized bone and a nonresorbable membrane were used to develop the site. **B,** Five months after extraction, the defect has been reconstructed with new bone. **C,** A 12-year postoperative radiograph demonstrates a successful implant restoration. Note the marginal bone loss in the region of the fixture–abutment connection and around the first implant thread. This is a common finding when the implant is placed subcrestally, with the fixture–abutment connection apical to the bony crest.

Primary closure is difficult but possible to achieve. Bowers and Donahue[67] described a technique using a periosteal releasing incision and vertical incisions to achieve sufficient mobility and advancement of the buccal flap in a palatal direction. The disadvantage of this technique is that a discrepancy is created between the mucogingival junction of the treated site and the adjacent site. This may require correction at a later stage to prevent an esthetic compromise.

In 1995, Edel[68] described the use of an autogenous connective tissue graft to achieve primary closure over an occlusive membrane that covered an implant placed in an extraction socket. This method eliminates the need to reposition coronally the existing marginal gingiva and does not disturb the normal relation of the existing surrounding tissues. With this technique, the connective tissue graft is not placed on the periosteum but directly on the avascular membrane, and it is overlapped by the buccal and palatal replaced flaps. Consequently, any collateral circulation may arise only from the overlying flaps. Therefore, every effort should be made to ensure that the connective tissue graft is of an adequate dimension

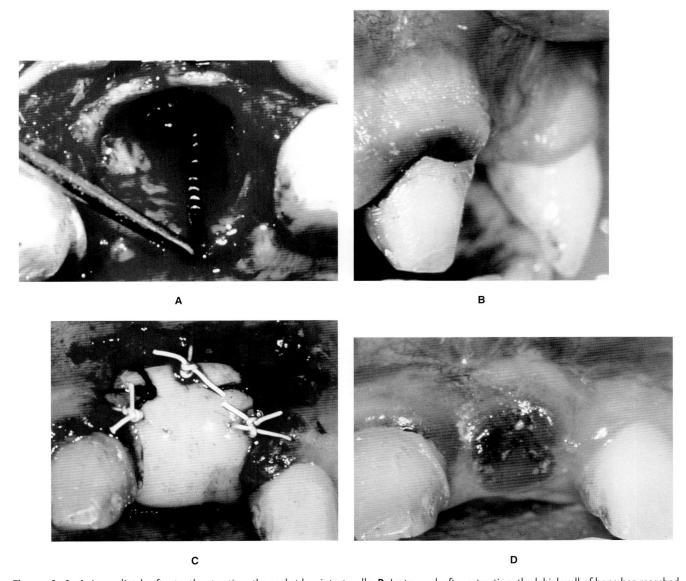

A   B

C   D

Figure 26-36. **A,** Immediately after tooth extraction, the socket has intact walls. **B,** Just 1 week after extraction, the labial wall of bone has resorbed, creating a major esthetic deformity. **C,** To correct the deformity, a bovine bone xenograft and an epithelialized thick soft tissue onlay autograft were used. **D,** Six months after surgical reconstruction of the ridge deformity.

to extend as far as possible under these flap margins. Closure of the surrounding flaps should be done without introducing tension and with adequate overlap of the graft so that any postsurgical edema does not result in wound dehiscence.

Delayed implant placement

Unlike immediate implant placement, which may be compromised by lack of soft tissue for complete coverage, the delayed implant placement technique allows time for soft tissue healing.[69] The "hole" in the gingiva left by extraction of the tooth has time to completely heal. Thus,

there is usually no need to coronally advance flaps to gain primary flap closure. In addition, because bone formation is active within the first few months after tooth extraction, this technique may facilitate more bone formation and osseointegration around the implant. The implant is placed into a socket in which osteogenic activity is occurring. Another advantage of delayed implant placement is that it provides extra time to resolve any residual infection that may have been present within the extraction site. The disadvantage to the patient is the longer treatment period because two surgical procedures are required (Fig. 26-38).

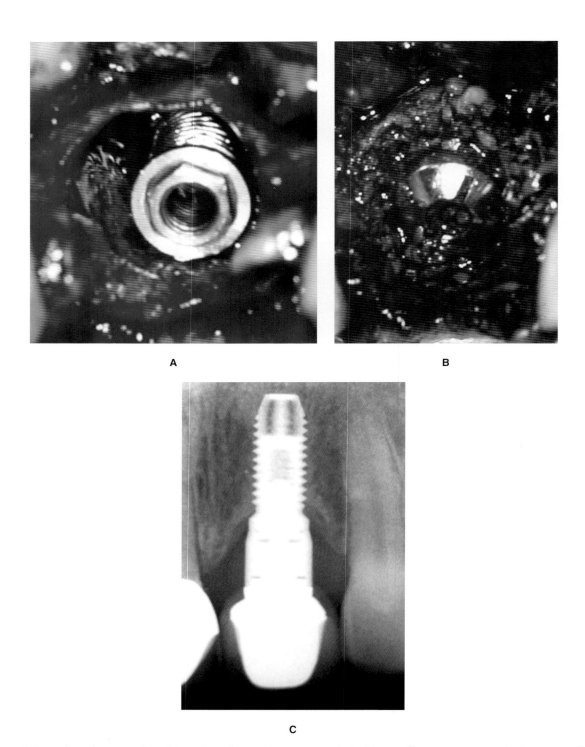

Figure 26-37. A, Immediate placement of a stable implant after tooth extraction in which all bony walls were intact. Note the discrepancy of the diameter of the socket and implant. **B,** Autogenous bone particles were placed into the socket to eliminate the space between the surface of the implant and the wall of the socket. **C,** Radiograph shows the restoration 12 years after implant placement. The restoration was attached to a standard abutment. Newer abutments allow more anatomically correct emergence profiles extending coronally from the fixture table.

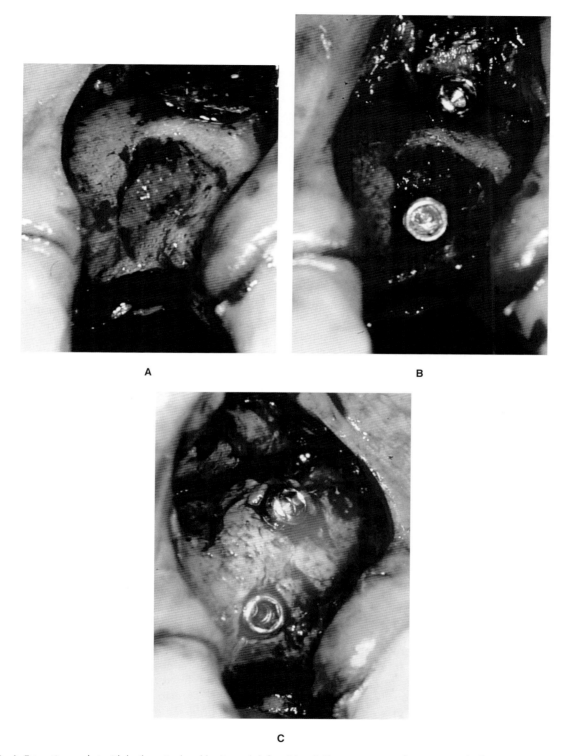

A

B

C

Figure 26-38. **A,** Extraction socket with both vertical and horizontal deformities. **B,** To regenerate and reconstruct the bone, supporting mini-screws were used to create a space between the barrier membrane and the host bone. No bone graft material was used. The cortical plate and socket walls were perforated with a small round bur to stimulate bleeding under the membrane. **C,** Four months after surgery, the site demonstrates horizontal and vertical bone regeneration. Note that the newly formed bone is at the same level as the head of both supporting mini-screws.

Staged implant placement

Staged implant placement allows for complete bone and soft tissue healing and permits the placement of implants into an ideal position, thereby enhancing the restorative result. This frequently eliminates the need for mucogingival flap advancement, allows for the resolution of preexisting infections, prevents soft tissue invasion, and provides time for maximum bone regeneration. The extended healing period also allows the grafted bone to become well vascularized. Bone grafts performed simultaneously with implant placement continue to heal, mature, and contour, causing a change in morphology and volume around the implant, which can compromise the success of osseointegration. The primary disadvantages of staged implant placement are the length of time required for bone healing and the two surgical procedures needed.

Site Enhancement Procedures

At one time, if an implant was used to replace a missing tooth or teeth, the implant was placed into whatever bone was present at the site. Because of bone resorptive patterns, this often resulted in implants being placed in less than ideal positions from a restorative standpoint. Currently, implant placement is no longer limited only to where there is bone. Implants should be placed and positioned with an eye toward achieving the desired restoration. Restoratively driven implant placement frequently necessitates developing an adequate volume of bone to support a properly positioned implant. Also, periodontal plastic and reconstructive surgical procedures may be necessary to create an esthetic recipient site.

The emergence of an implant-supported restoration from the gingiva should mimic three-dimensionally the profile of the soft tissues around the adjacent teeth. Because treatment planning for such a restoration must address both esthetic and functional needs, a successful outcome is best accomplished with an interdisciplinary team approach.[70]

Guided bone regeneration

The amount of bone needed for placement of a standard 3.75-mm diameter implant is at least 6 mm horizontally and 7 mm vertically. After tooth loss, however, alveolar ridge resorption often results in much smaller dimensions. When this occurs, implant placement with traditional techniques is not possible because of the discrepancy between the thickness of the ridge and the diameter of the implant, or between the vertical height of available bone and the length of the desired implant. For such cases, GBR techniques have been successfully introduced for preimplant ridge augmentation.[71-73] Various studies support the use of GBR for patients with unfavorable anatomic conditions.[71-74]

The advent of GBR with barrier membranes made bone regeneration possible by preventing the ingrowth of fibrous scar tissue and encouraging new bone formation to correct the osseous deficiency.

Barrier membranes

The membranes used for GBR should be bioinert and designed to protect the blood clot and allow osteogenic cells to populate the site, while at the same time exclude epithelial and connective-tissue from migrating into the bone defect. Membranes have been manufactured from biocompatible materials that are either nonresorbable (requiring removal) or resorbable. The ideal properties to consider when selecting a membrane include biocompatibility, space maintenance, cell exclusion, handling properties, and resorbability (see Chapter 25).

The size and shape of the membrane used should be based on the severity and morphology of the osseous defect. It should be contoured to completely cover the osseous deformity and extend 3 to 4 mm beyond the margins. The stabilization of the membrane is critical to the success of bone augmentation. This may be accomplished by securing the membrane with the cover screw of the implant or by using mini-screws to secure the membrane to surrounding bone. Occasionally, the membrane can be stabilized by positioning it beneath the periosteum. The membrane then adheres to the underlying blood clot or bone graft, promoting excellent adaptation.

Bone grafting

One of the most common reasons for failure of bone regeneration when using a membrane is the collapse of the membrane against the surface of the bone and the implant as a result of pressure from the overlying soft tissue.[75,76] To prevent this problem, clinicians and researchers have suggested placing various graft materials under the membrane to maintain the space necessary for new bone regeneration. Also, graft resorption can occur when a removable prosthesis is worn immediately after the surgical procedure. Transmucosal forces can be minimized by not inserting the prosthesis for at least 3 weeks after surgery. In addition, the removable restoration should be relined to stabilize the forces and eliminate undue pressure to the graft (Fig. 26-39). Alternatively, a tooth-borne removable prosthesis can be fabricated, if remaining teeth are present.

Many grafting materials are considered osteoconductive because of their ability to act as a scaffold for bone regeneration.[77] In some cases, they are thought to be osteoinductive—that is, they contain growth factors that induce new bone formation at the site. Autogenous bone grafts may also be osteogenic, incorporating vital cells with osteogenic capacity in the bone matrix.[78]

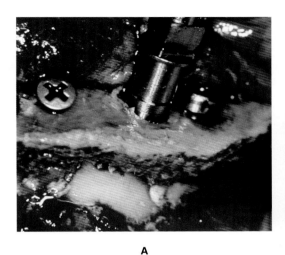

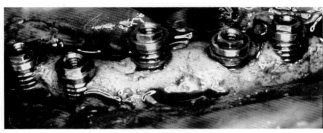

A   B

Figure 26-39. A, Simultaneous placement of an autogenous monocortical graft harvested from the medial aspect of the iliac crest and the implants. **B,** Six months after surgery. The patient insisted on wearing a poorly fitting removable denture 1 week after surgery, creating premature transmucosal forces on the bone graft and the implants. Note the degree of bone resorption.

The most widely used graft materials in association with GBR are autogenous bone, human freeze-dried bone allografts, and bovine bone xenografts. The rapid ingrowth of blood vessels (revascularization), greater number of osteoconductive surfaces, more exposure of osteoconductive growth factors, and easier biologic remodeling are some of the advantages of particulate bone grafts over block grafts (Fig. 26-40).

Autogenous bone grafts can be harvested from a number of intraoral sites, most commonly the ramus, the anterior mandible, or the tuberosity. When taking bone from the ascending ramus or the external oblique ridge, care must be taken to avoid the inferior alveolar neurovascular bundle. Also, the lingual nerve must be protected when removing bone from the anterior medial aspect of the ascending ramus.

The anterior mandible (symphysis) can be the source of a considerable amount of bone. The bone is harvested from approximately 5 mm beneath the apices of the anterior teeth to approximately 5 mm above the inferior border. The graft should include the labial cortex and the medullary bone, leaving the lingual cortex intact. This donor block is outlined with a fine fissure bur or wheel saw with copious irrigation. It is best elevated and removed with a single beveled, curved osteotome (Fig. 26-41).

The maxillary tuberosity is an excellent donor site for bone grafting. A considerable amount of soft cancellous bone exists with varying degrees of inductive capacity. End-cutting bone rongeurs are useful instruments for collecting tuberosity bone.

The iliac crest is considered the best donor site for grafting when a large quantity of bone is needed to correct an osseous deficiency. The graft is rich in cancellous bone and contains the necessary biologic factors for graft incorporation. The bone graft taken from the iliac crest is usually harvested from the anteromedial, anterolateral, and posterior locations. The anteromedial approach is generally safe, easily accessible, and usually free of complications as long as bone removal is limited to the medial cortex and its associated cancellous bone (Fig. 26-42).

The advantages of autogenous bone grafts are their biocompatibility, long-lasting space-maintaining potential, and the possibility of being completely resorbed and substituted with the normal turnover of native bone. The amount of bone that can be harvested from the oral cavity, however, may be insufficient for major augmentations.

Soft tissue flap management

When GBR is performed, the flap design should ensure generous access to the osseous defect with minimal trauma to the soft tissue. The flap must be able to completely cover the bone graft and barrier membrane during the entire healing period. Exposure of the graft or membrane will increase the possibility of infection and bone necrosis, ultimately compromising the success of the graft.

A conventional crestal incision may be used as long as periosteal releasing incisions and coronal advancement of the flap can be achieved with tension-free closure.[79,80] The site should be thoroughly prepared by meticulously removing all granulation tissue. Complete primary closure is recommended when membranes are used. This can be accomplished by mobilizing the

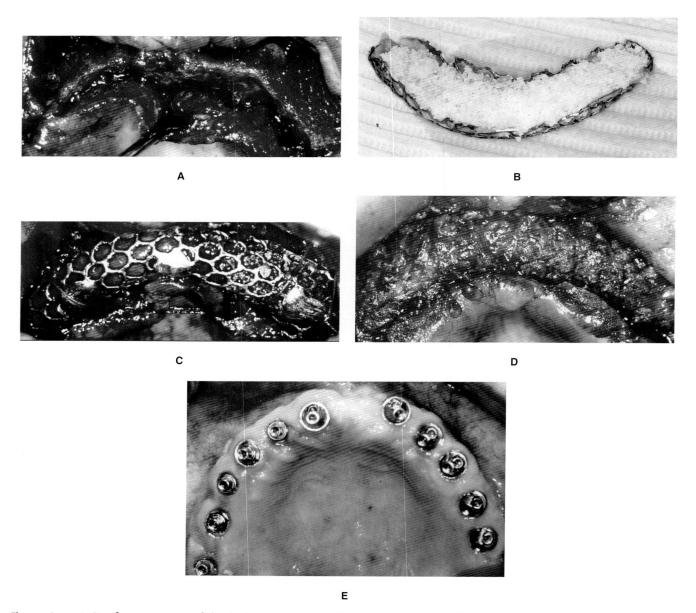

Figure 26-40. A, Significant resorption of alveolar bone creating a "knife edge" ridge. **B,** A metal framework was cast and lined with a resorbable membrane, then filled with bovine bone. **C,** The metal framework with the graft was positioned and stabilized with sutures. **D,** Six months after surgery the metal framework was removed. The clinical photograph demonstrates regeneration and reconstruction of the alveolar ridge in both a horizontal and vertical dimension. **E,** The reconstructed alveolar ridge allowed for proper placement and an adequate number of implants.

buccal flap and advancing it coronally to cover the grafted site. Releasing incisions within the periosteum may be required to obtain tension-free closure of the flap. Interrupted horizontal mattress sutures often are used to close the crestal incision, and interrupted sutures are interspersed to stabilize the flap. Removable prostheses should not be inserted for 2 to 3 weeks after surgery to avoid pressure on the wound during the early healing period. Sutures are removed approximately 10 to 14 days after surgery.

When performing a ridge augmentation, the following principles for flap management should be considered:
1. Full mucoperiosteal flap elevation at least 5 mm beyond the lateral edges and the most apical aspects of the bone defect is desirable.
2. The use of vertical incisions, although often required for surgical access, should be minimized whenever possible.
3. If vertical incisions are needed, they should be made at least one tooth away from the site to be grafted.

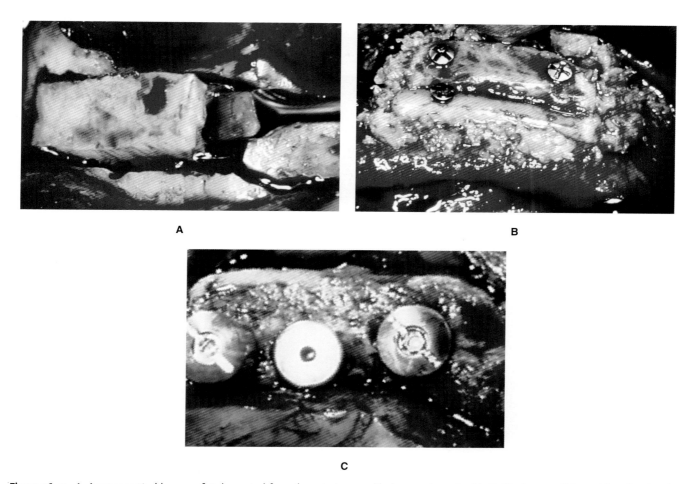

A

B

C

Figure 26-41. A, A monocortical bone graft is harvested from the anterior mandibular area (symphysis). **B,** The bone graft is positioned and stabilized with fixation screws on the facial surface of the alveolar ridge. **C,** Six months after surgery, the ridge has sufficient horizontal bone augmentation to properly place the implants.

4. Use of periosteal releasing incisions to give the flap elasticity and permit tension-free suturing is critical. This allows for complete closure without undue stress on the wound margins.

5. Postoperative trauma to the surgical site, particularly transmucosal forces caused by removable appliances, should be avoided.

Alveolar Bone Augmentation

The surgical reconstructive procedures for the preparation and placement of dental implants depend on the size and shape of the osseous deficiency. These augmentation procedures are classified according to the morphology of the existing bone as either horizontal or vertical procedures. The biologic mechanisms and properties of the various bone grafting materials are discussed in Chapter 25.

Horizontal ridge augmentation

A small deformity in the horizontal dimension of bone may be managed simultaneously with implant placement because most of the implant will be covered and stabilized by native bone. Conversely, if the horizontal deficiency is large and the implant fixture is significantly exposed, it may be more appropriate to reconstruct the bone before implant placement (staged implant placement).

Dehiscences and fenestrations. Dehiscence of the alveolus associated with the buccal/labial aspect of an implant is commonly seen in the maxilla, especially with narrow, deformed ridges (Fig. 26-43). If the morphology of the dehiscence allows for space when a membrane is placed over the area to be regenerated, the membrane frequently can be used without a bone graft. The membrane is contoured and adapted to the margin of the surrounding bone, allowing 3 to 4 mm of membrane to overlap the bone.

If space cannot be maintained between the exposed implant surface and the membrane by placing a membrane alone, a suitable bone graft or bone substitute can be used to create space and separate the membrane from the implant. In certain cases, mini-screws may be

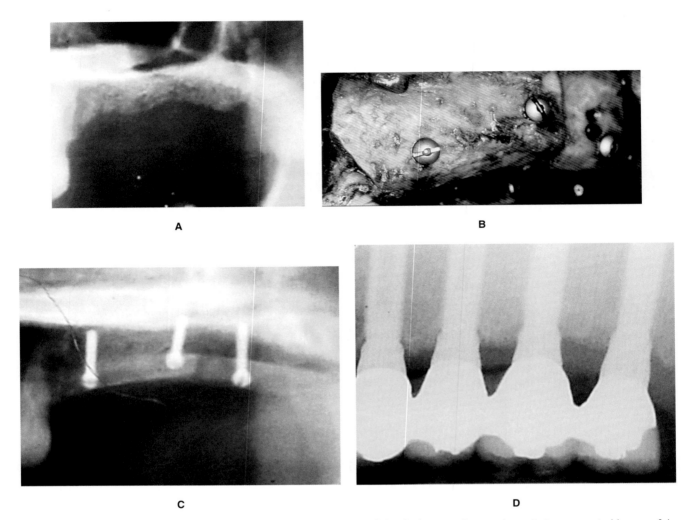

Figure 26-42. **A,** The panograph demonstrates insufficient height and width of alveolar bone to place implants. **B,** A monocortical bone graft harvested from the medial aspect of the iliac crest is contoured and stabilized in a position to increase both the horizontal and vertical dimension of the ridge. **C,** The panograph demonstrates the bone graft and fixation screws 6 months after surgery. **D,** The periapical radiograph 12 years after surgery.

used to secure and stabilize the membrane. Complete tension-free flap closure must be achieved.

Fenestrations of the maxillary alveolus usually occur when endosseous implants are placed in bone with resorptive deficiencies (Fig. 26-44). Small fenestrations that are more than 5 mm apical to the coronal margin of the implant sometimes do not require treatment. In many such cases, however, clinicians will place a small amount of bone graft material over the exposed implant, with a resorbable membrane over the graft. If the fenestration is larger (encompasses at least half of the circumference, or a third to half of the length of the implant), it must be treated. Again, a membrane alone or with bone grafting material is necessary to achieve an acceptable outcome.

Monocortical block graft. The use of autogenous bone grafts has been proposed for horizontal ridge augmentation.[75,76,81] The objective is to increase the alveolar

ridge width to correct the osseous deformity and to provide sufficient bone for ideal implant placement. Extensive alveolar deficiencies are frequently reconstructed by using monocortical block grafts. The bone is harvested from either an intraoral site (ramus, symphysis) or extraoral site (iliac crest, tibia). When the bone deficiency is extensive, the extraoral donor site may be preferable because a larger quantity of bone can be obtained.

The graft must be properly contoured, stabilized, and fixated to the host bone with fixation screws. A membrane covering the graft is usually recommended to minimize bone resorption. The mucoperiosteal flap must completely cover the graft site with tension-free closure of the wound. At one time, it was thought that healing and maturation of the bone graft required approximately 6 months or longer. However, more recent clinical trends point toward implant placement as early as 3 to 4 months

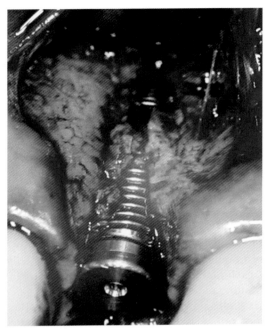

Figure 26-43. The clinical photograph demonstrates a dehiscence that can occur when an implant is properly positioned, but the anatomy of the bone has a facial deformity and insufficient horizontal dimension.

at grafted sites. Such early placement reduces the risk for bony resorption on the external surface of the block graft. At the time of implant placement, fixation screws and nonresorbable membranes should be removed and the implants placed. Most resorbable membranes will no longer be present by the time of implant placement.

The disadvantage of the monocortical block graft technique is the biologic limitation on revascularizing large blocks of bone. It is, therefore, crucial to have sufficient osteogenic cells in the residual surface of the monocortical

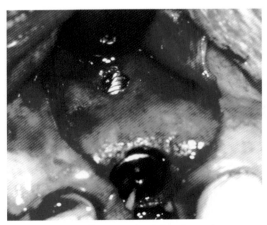

Figure 26-44. Because of a resorptive deformity such as a concavity in the alveolar bone, the placement of an implant may perforate, forming a fenestration.

graft and in the surrounding recipient bone. Perforating the bone at the recipient site with a round bur before securing the block graft is recommended to induce bleeding and to enhance graft revascularization (Fig. 26-45).

Ridge expansion (ridge splitting)

Autogenous bone grafts were once thought to be the only predictable procedure to address advanced alveolar bone atrophy that would otherwise deter implant placement. An alternative procedure that may be used for attempting to increase the horizontal dimension of the alveolar bone is called ridge expansion. Two ridge expansion procedures described in the literature are considered less invasive than bone grafting and are clinically predictable when attempting to simultaneously place implants in an alveolar ridge with a dramatically resorbed width.

In 1992, Simion and colleagues[75] reported the use of a "split-crest" technique in patients receiving immediate implant placement in alveolar ridges that had significantly reduced widths. After local anesthesia was administered, a full-thickness mucoperiosteal flap was elevated buccally

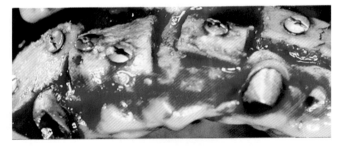

A

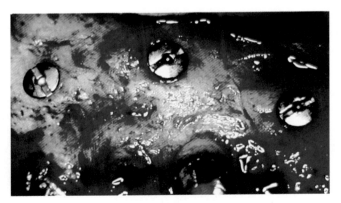

B

Figure 26-45. A, The alveolar ridge was deficient in a horizontal and vertical dimension. Bilateral sinus augmentation procedures and monocortical veneer grafts were performed to reconstruct the ridge. The bone was harvested from the iliac crest. **B,** Six months after surgery, bone augmentation has occurred. Note that the bone is level with the head of the fixation screw confirming the lack of graft resorption.

and lingually to expose the alveolar ridge. The cortical bone was curetted to remove all residual connective tissue and periosteum. Before implant placement, the alveolar ridge was split longitudinally in two parts, creating a greenstick fracture. This was accomplished by using a small chisel (Beaver blade #62). The chisel (3.5 mm in diameter) was gently tapped with a mallet to create a shallow incision longitudinally to the crest of bone. This was then used as a lever to spread the two cortical plates. The surgical fracture was extended to a depth of 5 to 7 mm. At least 3 to 4 mm of intact bone was left apical to the fracture to allow proper implant site preparation and to achieve primary stabilization of the implants. As is imperative with this procedure, care was taken to avoid sharp and complete vertical or horizontal fractures of the buccal, palatal, or lingual bone plates. The implants were covered with a nonresorbable barrier membrane that was contoured to extend 3 to 4 mm over the bone margin of the defects.

Releasing incisions in the periosteum at the base of the flap were made to advance the flap to achieve complete tension-free closure. The membranes were removed at the abutment-connection surgery (stage 2) after 6 months of healing.

In the study by Simion and colleagues,[75] there was a gain in ridge width of 1 to 4 mm. The maxillary alveolar ridge revealed a greater amount of increased ridge width (3 to 4 mm) than the mandibular alveolar ridge sites (1 to 1.5 mm). Histologic evaluation of the bone biopsy specimen in one patient showed regeneration of normal bone tissue between the two portions of the split crest (Fig. 26-46).

In 1994, Scipioni and colleagues[82] reported the clinical results of a similar surgical technique used to expand a narrow ridge involving a buccolingual width that precluded the placement of dental implants. In 170 patients, 329 implants were placed in sites treated with the edentulous ridge expansion procedure (ridge-splitting). The technique involved reflection of a partial-thickness flap, crestal and vertical intraosseous incisions into the ridge, and buccal displacement of the buccal cortical plate, including a portion of the underlying spongiosa. Implants in this study were placed in the expanded ridge

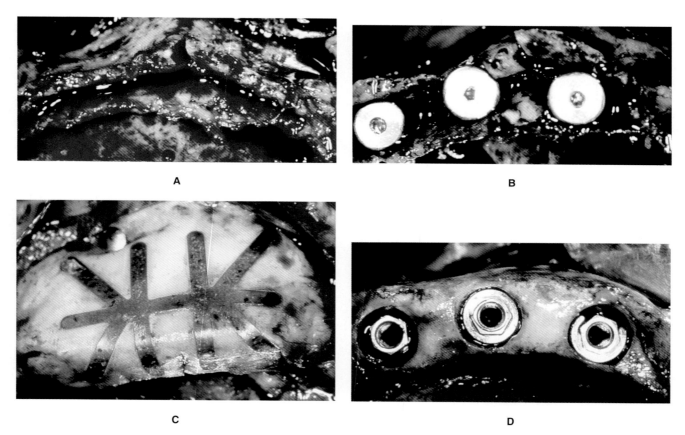

A

B

C

D

Figure 26-46. **A,** An atrophic alveolar ridge deficient in the height and width of bone needed to place implants. **B,** The alveolar crest is split longitudinally and spread buccolingually. **C,** Three implants are placed into the expanded ridge and a nonresorbable membrane is placed over the implants. **D,** Six months after surgery the implants are exposed. Dense bone has regenerated and filled in and around the implants. (*Courtesy Dr. Massimo Simion; Milan, Italy; private practice.*)

and were allowed to heal for 4 to 5 months. The implants were exposed during a second-stage surgery to allow visualization of the implant sites. Occlusal loading was applied during the following 3 to 5 months with a provisional fixed restoration. The final phase was the placement of the permanent prostheses. The results yielded a success rate of 98.8%.

The essential feature of this technique is use of a partial-thickness flap, retaining the undisturbed periosteum on the bony surface. In such procedures, the blood supply must be kept intact on the facial aspect of the radicular bone to ensure optimal healing and preservation of the thin bone that covers the implant. The partial-thickness flap also helps to immobilize the displaced buccal cortical plate. In addition, the integrity of the periosteum must be maintained so that fenestrations, dehiscences, or necrosis of the buccal plate are avoided during the implant placement and healing phases. It should be noted that this technique, as opposed to Simion's technique, is accomplished without the use of a membrane or a greenstick fracture.

Vertical ridge augmentation

Various studies during the last decade have reported good results using vertical bone augmentation techniques with bone graft materials, membranes, or both. However, vertical augmentation may be less predictable than horizontal augmentation.

In 1994, Scipioni and colleagues[82] demonstrated that up to 4 mm of vertical bone augmentation can be predictably regenerated in patients with atrophic edentulous ridges. The surgical protocol included the use of a membrane reinforced with a titanium structure (Fig. 26-46C). This membrane can be shaped to maintain the desired form, thereby creating and preserving sufficient space between the membrane and the bone defect.

The surgical technique used in this study incorporated a full-thickness flap with a crestal incision. Once exposed, the cortical bone was curetted with a back-action chisel to remove all residual connective tissue and the periosteum.

At the time of placement, the implants were left to protrude 4 to 7 mm coronal to the crest of bone. A pure titanium mini-screw (1.3 mm in diameter and 10 mm in length) was positioned distal to the implants in each surgical site to serve as a "tent pole" for the membrane. The mini-screws also were left to protrude from the bone at a level of 3 to 4 mm. Before the membrane was placed, the cortical bone was perforated with a round bur to expose the underlying cancellous bone and encourage bleeding. The titanium membranes extended at least 4 to 5 mm beyond the defect margins. Once positioned in the surgical site, the membranes were affixed to the bone with fixation screws. Releasing incisions were made in the periosteum at the base of the buccal flaps to enhance

elasticity of the flaps and achieve tension-free adaptation at closure.

Membranes were removed at the second stage of surgery after 9 months of healing. The pure titanium mini-screws were removed with a small trephine in such a way that a small biopsy specimen of preexisting and newly formed tissue was collected from each site. The specimens were processed for histologic examination.

This study data show that it is possible to obtain up to 4 mm of vertical bone augmentation with a high degree of predictability. When the most coronal aspect of the implants was left to protrude more than 4 mm from the bone crest, it was always covered with dense fibrous connective tissue. The apical portion of the bone in contact with the screws showed an advanced stage of bone maturation, whereas the most coronal bone showed bone-forming activity. This observation substantiates the hypothesis that bone regeneration was still in progress at the time of membrane removal.

In this study, vertical bone augmentation has been limited to a maximum of 4 mm. This may be because of one or more of the following scenarios:

- Poor adaptation of the membrane, causing folds at the borders that hinder complete bone regeneration.
- A large blood clot under the membrane causing shrinkage. It is possible that a bone-filling material could assist in stabilizing the blood clot and increase the vertical bone augmentation.[83]
- The blood supply in the most coronal portion of the space—under the membrane—might be insufficient to allow osteogenic activity.
- More time may be necessary to achieve additional bone regeneration. These study findings indicated that the regenerative process was still in progress when the membranes were removed after 9 months. Further research is needed to evaluate the load-bearing capability and the long-term results of the bone regenerated with this vertical ridge reconstruction technique.

Another study evaluating vertical bone augmentation used Scipioni's[82] surgical technique with the addition of demineralized freeze-dried bone allograft (DFDBA) or autogenous bone chips under the nonresorbable titanium-reinforced expanded polytetrafluoroethylene (e-PTFE) membrane[84] (Fig. 26-47). Twenty partially edentulous patients with vertical bone deficiencies were divided into 2 groups of 10. The 10 patients in group A received a total of 26 machined titanium implants in 10 surgical sites. The 10 patients in group B received a total of 32 implants in 12 surgical sites. Pure titanium mini-screws (1.3 × 10 mm) were positioned distally to the implant, protruding 3 to 7 mm from the crest of bone. Titanium-reinforced e-PTFE membranes were used to cover the implants. Before complete membrane fixation, DFDBA

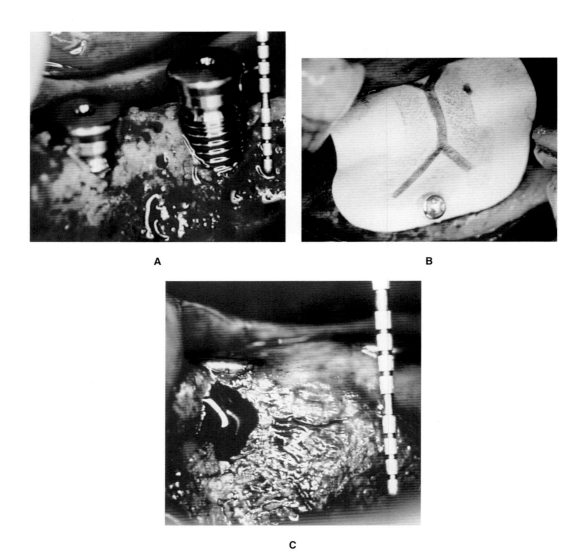

Figure 26-47. A, Two implants are placed in mandibular alveolar bone and are protruding above the crest of bone because of insufficient bone height. **B,** A titanium-reinforced membrane was used to cover the implants and create a space between the host bone and the top of the implant. The membrane was stabilized with fixation screws. **C,** Nine months after surgery the implants are exposed and the membrane is removed. Regenerated bone with a thin covering of connected tissue is noted. (Courtesy Dr. Massimo Simion, Milan, Italy, private practice.)

particles were condensed under the membrane in group A, whereas autogenous bone chips were used in group B.

At reentry, after 7 to 11 months, the membranes were removed and small biopsies, which encompassed the mini-screws, were collected from 11 sites. The clinical measurements from group A demonstrated a mean vertical bone gain of 3.1 mm with a mean percentage bone gain of 124%. The measurements from group B showed a mean vertical bone gain of 5.02 mm with a mean percentage bone gain of 95%.

Histomorphometric analysis clearly demonstrated a direct correlation between the density of the preexisting bone and the density of the regenerated bone. The mean percentage of new bone–titanium contact was between 39.1% and 63.2%, depending on the quality of the native bone. Both the clinical and histologic results of this study demonstrated that vertical ridge augmentation procedures, using DFDBA or autogenous bone particles, in addition to the membrane technique, can be obtained.

Maxillary sinus bone augmentation

Insertion of endosseous implants into an atrophic edentulous posterior maxilla often is challenging because of inadequate alveolar bone height. This is because of severe alveolar bone resorption or excessive pneumatization of the maxillary sinuses, or both. Maxillary sinus bone augmentation is a relatively predictable surgical procedure for altering the morphology of the posterior maxilla and creating sufficient bone to accommodate endosseous implants. More research is needed, however, to fully elucidate the risks versus benefits of this procedure and to evaluate the specific techniques and graft materials typically used.[85]

As a general rule, if less than 4 to 5 mm of vertical bone remains between the antral floor and the residual bone crest of the ridge, the sinus bone augmentation procedure is performed 4 to 6 months before implant placement ("staged approach" or "two-step procedure"). If more than 4 to 5 mm of vertical bone remains to provide initial implant stabilization, implants may be placed during the same surgical procedure ("simultaneous approach" or "one-step procedure").

The maxillary sinus bone augmentation procedure was described by Boyne and colleagues[86] in 1985 and Tatum[87] in 1986. The procedure is performed with some variations in technique and different bone filling materials. The limitations or contraindications for maxillary sinus bone augmentation include: (1) existing pathology, including chronic sinusitis; (2) history of sinus surgery that may limit the ability to perform maxillary sinus bone augmentation; (3) anatomic limitations, such as multiple septae dividing the sinus cavity; and (4) perforation of the sinus membrane requiring either repair (small perforations) or aborting of the procedure (large perforations).

Lateral-wall technique. According to a metaanalysis reported by the American Academy of Periodontology,[88] the lateral window technique for sinus bone augmentation is quite useful for regenerating sufficient bone for implant placement. The data, on the basis of 34 studies including 5267 implants, indicated an implant survival rate for these cases of more than 90%. This survival rate is similar to implants placed in native bone.[88]

To begin the lateral wall procedure, an incision is made palatal to the crest of the alveolar ridge and completely through the mucoperiosteal tissue. A vertical-releasing incision is needed in the premolar or canine region, and it may be required in the posterior tuberosity region to reflect the flap adequately to expose the lateral bone surface of the maxilla. Dissection is usually carried superiorly to achieve adequate access and visibility. An oral osteotomy is made through the cortical bone of the lateral wall of the maxilla using a round bur with copious irrigation (Fig. 26-48). The cortical bone is carefully removed until the translucence of the sinus membrane is visualized.

The sinus membrane is gently reflected from the inner aspect of the sinus wall, with the osseous window remaining attached to the membrane. This window will be inverted medially and superiorly to become the floor of the newly created sinus cavity. With the sinus membrane elevated from its inferior and lateral position, sufficient room is created for the graft materials. The graft may

include a variety of substances, such as autogenous bone, freeze-dried cancellous bone allograft (demineralized or nondemineralized), or bovine bone xenograft. Each can be used alone or in combination (e.g., autogenous bone and bovine bone). Small amounts of the graft are carried incrementally to the sinus recipient site and packed into position in a rather tight configuration, starting at the most medial and posterior aspect of the sinus to the most lateral and anterior position, and they are contoured to the outermost confines of the lateral aspect of the maxilla.

A barrier membrane is trimmed and contoured to fit over the lateral window between the mucoperiosteal flap and the underlying osseous surface and bone graft. The placement of a membrane was found to increase bone formation in the grafted sinus and to improve bony healing.[89,90] The mucoperiosteal flap is repositioned and sutured. Primary tension-free closure is important to prevent contamination of the graft from the oral environment.

According to the metaanalysis mentioned earlier,[88] evidence indicates that the following factors increase implant survival when performing lateral-wall sinus bone augmentation procedures:

- Membrane coverage of the lateral window (93.6% survival rate) compared with no membrane coverage (88.7% survival rate)
- Particulate bone grafts (92.3% survival rate) rather than block grafts (83.3% survival rate)
- Rough surface implants (94.6% survival rate) compared with machine surface implants (90.0% survival rate)

This metaanalysis also recommended the following areas of research be undertaken to individually evaluate the success of sinus bone augmentation techniques and the success of implants placed in augmented sinuses:

1. One area is research studies designed to identify the success rate of implants as it specifically relates to minimal crestal bone height. Currently, there are limited data regarding the variable of residual crestal bone height. These studies should ideally use a bilateral sinus mode.

2. Although no absolute contraindications exist in the literature, it would be beneficial to evaluate implant success as it relates to potential risk factors, such as Schneiderian membrane perforations, initial implant stability, postoperative sinus infections, smoking, periodontal disease, sinus pathology, and other systemic and behavioral factors.

3. Studies are warranted to evaluate tissue-engineering techniques (e.g., molecular, cellular, and genetic) that may reduce the time required before prosthesis delivery and may enhance bone quality and quantity. These studies ideally should use a bilateral sinus model.

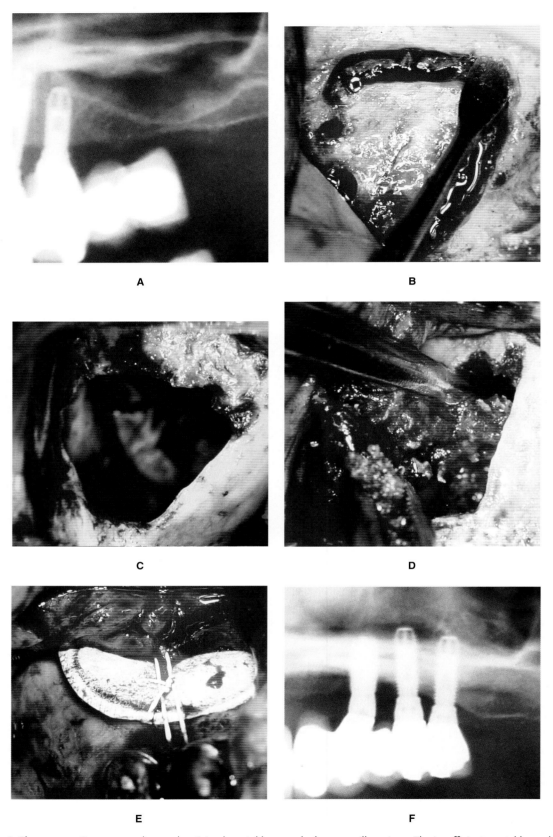

Figure 26-48. A, The preoperative panograph records minimal crestal bone and a large maxillary sinus. The insufficient crestal bone does not allow for placement of implants. **B,** After elevation of a mucoperiosteal flap, the lateral wall of the maxillary sinus is clearly visualized. An osteotomy is made into the cortical bone being sure that the Schneiderian membrane is not perforated. **C,** Once the wall of cortical bone is moveable and the membrane is visible, the sinus membrane is gently released from the inner aspect of the sinus. The window of bone is then carefully "infractured" medially and superiorly. The lateral wall ultimately becomes the floor of the newly created sinus. **D,** Cancellous bone harvested from the iliac crest is gently inserted into the sinus. **E,** A barrier membrane is used to protect the grafted sinus from any soft tissue invasion and to enhance the bone regeneration. **F,** The postoperative panograph demonstrates significant sinus bone augmentation allowing for proper placement of implants.

4. More studies are recommended to evaluate the efficacy of alternative sinus bone augmentation techniques (e.g., osteotome, localized management of the sinus floor, and crestal core elevation).

Osteotome techniques. A more conservative and less invasive approach to the conventional sinus elevation surgery can be achieved using osteotomes. With this technique, the osteotomy on the lateral sinus wall is avoided and the sinus is elevated by a crestal approach. Osteotomes of increasing diameter are used in a consecutive manner to create a site for implant placement and simultaneously to elevate the sinus floor[91] (Fig. 26-49). With this technique, minimal drilling is performed. The bone is condensed to the periphery of the site and in an apical direction by the osteotomes to enhance bone density (Fig. 26-50). In addition, placing small increments of particulate bone in the osteotomy site to further elevate the sinus floor is recommended. The grafting material acts as a buffer to prevent perforation of the sinus membrane. Also, the osteotomes cause the graft material and fluids to exert pressure on the sinus floor in all directions so that the sinus floor is elevated over an area wider than the diameter of the osteotomy itself (see Fig. 26-50).

After site preparation with the osteotomes and elevation of the sinus floor, implants can be placed immediately in the same surgical site.[91] This procedure is useful because it not only elevates the membrane and the floor of the maxillary sinus but also increases bone density at the implant site. The success rate of implants placed in this way may depend on the preexisting crestal bone height, which provides primary stabilization of the implant. Survival rate diminishes when 4 mm or less of crestal bone height exists.[92]

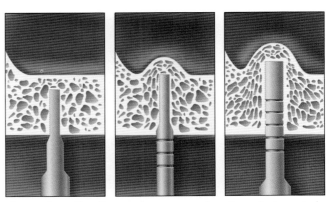

Figure 26-50. The diagram demonstrates how the osteotome technique increases the bone density of type IV bone by condensing the bone laterally, and also how it can elevate the sinus membrane to assist in placing stable implants appropriate in size and position.

In 1996, Lazzara[93] proposed a new sequence of surgery on the basis of the combined use of osteotomes, drills, and screw-type implants with a rough surface. This technique is indicated where the crestal height of bone is equal to or greater than 5 mm (Fig. 26-51). At no time during this procedure should any instrument (osteotome/drill) penetrate the sinus cavity. The positioning of the implant is carried out with a round bur, and the preparation of the site begins with a 2-mm twist drill. The 2-mm twist drill is used to prepare an osteotomy that ends just inferior to the floor of the sinus. A radiograph of the area is taken at this stage using a direction indicator or twist drill in the osteotomy site to aid orientation. This also will confirm the integrity of the subsinus cortex. It is important to remember that no instrument must penetrate the cavity of the sinus at any time. The 3-mm twist drill completes the preparation of the implant site for a standard-diameter implant. Again, drilling is stopped just inferior to the floor of the sinus.

Autogenous, allogeneic, or xenogeneic graft material is introduced into the osteotomy site before using the first osteotome.[92,93] The osteotome is then placed in the osteotomy and gently tapped superiorly. The graft material serves as a shock absorber to gently fracture the sinus floor inward. The osteotome is removed and another increment of bone graft material is placed in the osteotomy. The grafting material is progressively condensed using the osteotomes without penetrating the sinus cavity. The use of a countersink drill is optional and is indicated only in the presence of a thick cortical plate or when a temporary removable denture will be used.

The modified osteotome technique provides several advantages, including the following:

1. It offers a less invasive technique than a lateral window sinus augmentation for reconstructing the resorbed posterior edentulous maxilla.
2. It enables placement of implants 10 mm or longer.

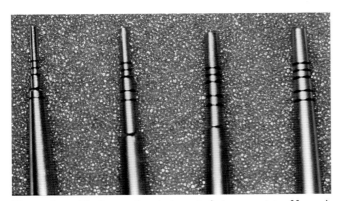

Figure 26-49. The Summer's osteotome technique consists of four calibrated osteotomes. Each consecutive osteotome increases in diameter. The tip of the instrument is concave, thereby advancing and condensing the bone in an apical and lateral direction. This is accomplished by gently tapping the instruments into the existing bone to create the osteotomy.

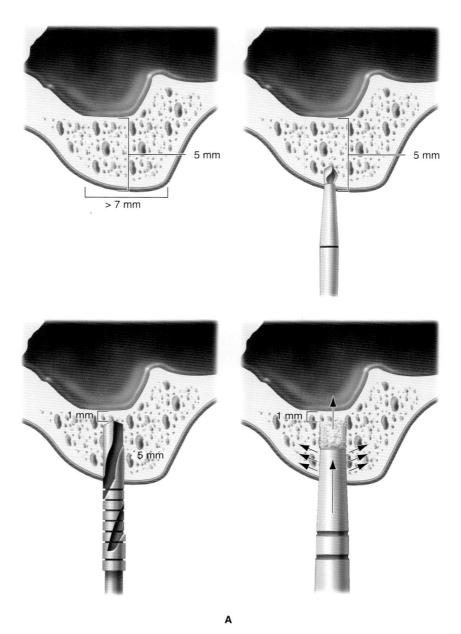

A

Figure 26-51. A, The modified osteotome technique is suggested if 5 mm or more of crestal bone exists below the sinus. A round bur is used to access the cortical bone. Then a 2-mm twist drill initiates the preparation of the osteotomy stopping 1 mm short of the sinus floor. Grafting material is inserted into the osteotomy and an osteotome advances the bone graft through the prepared site. The grafting material acts as a buffer to carefully infracture the sinus floor without perforating the membrane.

Continued

3. It allows implants to be placed at the same time as the sinus surgery (simultaneous approach).
4. It reduces operative time compared with lateral-wall sinus augmentation procedures.
5. It reduces postoperative discomfort.
6. It improves periimplant bone density.
7. It preserves the integrity of the sinus cavity (no instrument penetration).

Alveolar distraction osteogenesis

Modern distraction osteogenesis evolved primarily from the work of Gavriel Ilizarov. During the 1960s, in a clinic in Kurgan, Siberia, Ilizarov conceptualized the basis of this reconstructive technique. He had many patients with difficult traumatic and developmental limb deformities. These included complicated nonunions, malunions, and nonhealing wounds that had been difficult to manage

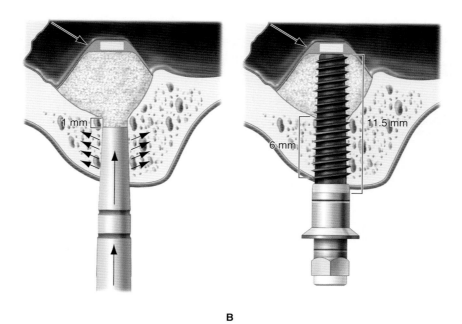

B

Figure 26-51. cont'd B, By gently tapping the osteotome, additional grafting material is used to fill the osteotomy, advance the bone, and raise the membrane to place an implant of sufficient height and stability.

even in the most sophisticated medical facility. Ilizarov responded to this challenge by developing a new system of reconstructive surgery, known as distraction osteogenesis.

Currently, distraction osteogenesis surgery for managing orthopedic disorders is available worldwide. Achievement of stable, functional rehabilitation of combined osseous and soft tissue deformities represents a major achievement in reconstructive surgery.

The process of alveolar distraction osteogenesis involves mobilization, transport, and fixation of a healthy segment of bone adjacent to the deficient or deformed site. A mechanical alveolar distraction device is used to provide gradual, controlled transport of a mobilized alveolar segment. When the desired repositioning of the bone segment is achieved, the distraction device is left in a static mode to act as a fixation tool. Displacement of the osseous segment results in positioning of a healthy portion of bone into a previously deficient site. Because the soft tissue is left attached to the transport segment, the movement of the bone also results in expansion of soft tissue adjacent to the bone segment. A regeneration chamber, which has a natural capacity to heal by filling with bone, is left at the original location of the segment. This propensity of the regeneration chamber to heal by filling with bone instead of fibrous tissue is a function of the surrounding healthy cancellous bone walls within the skeletal functional matrix. As a result of the distraction process, the volume of bone and soft tissue increases.

The reconstructed site is then suitable for further rehabilitation with osseointegrated implants, prosthetic pontic placement, or movement of a tooth with orthodontics (Fig. 26-52).

The distraction process may not produce the anatomic objective in a single step. Maxillofacial skeletal deformities are most often complex and three-dimensional in nature. The distraction process alone rarely results in an alveolar ridge of an ideal shape and size. Additional osteoplasty usually is indicated.

Soft Tissue Augmentation

Implant dentistry is seldom as challenging to the clinician as when an esthetic area requires treatment. A deformed ridge, insufficient in bone and soft tissue, will compromise the esthetic outcome of an implant restoration. At the completion of the restoration, most patients expect harmony, balance, and continuity of form between the teeth and the soft tissue. The challenge is magnified if the patient also has a high smile line. Before initiating any reconstruction procedures, the dentist and the patient must be aware of all biologic and anatomic limitations. Unrealistic expectations are a pathway to failure.

The challenge is to develop criteria to integrate fixture placement, abutment selection, and hard and soft tissue augmentation. The goal is an esthetic, functional restoration. This section discusses periimplant soft tissue considerations within the "esthetic zone."

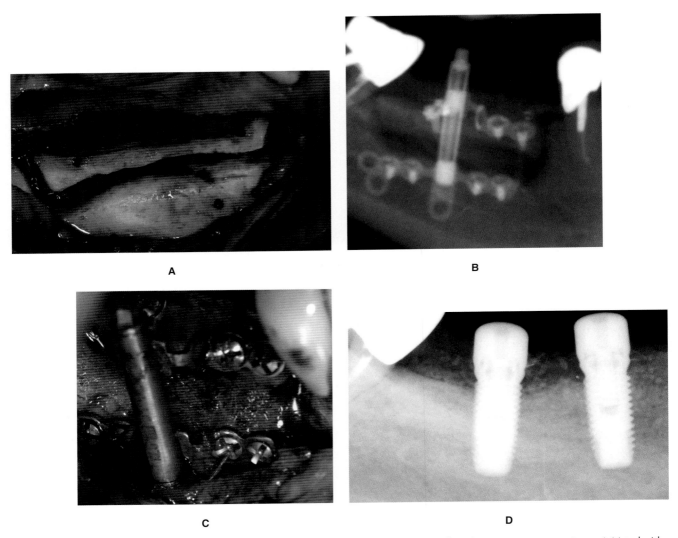

A, **B**, **C**, **D**

Figure 26-52. **A,** Six millimeters of alveolar bone existed above the inferior alveolar nerve. Therefore, distraction osteogenesis was initiated with an extraosseous distractor. Figure depicts the completed horizontal and vertical osteotomies just before final device fixation. **B,** After a 1-week latency healing period, the distraction phase was initiated at a rate of approximately 0.75 mm/day. The panoramic radiograph shows the case at the completion of 5 mm of distraction. **C,** After a 4-month consolidation healing phase, the distractor was removed and two 10-mm-long implants were placed. Photograph demonstrates several millimeters of newly regenerated bone between the device plates. **D,** Radiograph shows the integrated implants 3 months after placement. (Courtesy Dr. Bradley S. McAllister, Tigard, Oregon, private practice.)

The position of the implant contributes to the esthetic outcome of the restoration by establishing a proper emergence profile and soft tissue contour. To aid in this endeavor, the implant platform should always be placed subgingivally, regardless of whether a one-stage or two-stage implant system is being used. As a general rule, the implant head should be placed approximately 3 mm apical to the position of the intended gingival margin.[94-98] The application of this concept in recent years, as it relates to esthetic treatment planning for both teeth and implants, has enabled practitioners to develop more

coherent treatment protocols to enhance implant position relative to the gingival tissue in the esthetic zone.

Preservation of soft tissue

The most predictable way to ensure a sufficient amount of keratinized tissue around an implant is to preserve the keratinized tissue when designing the soft tissue flap at the time of surgery and any regenerative reconstructive surgical procedures. Although keratinized tissue is not absolutely essential to maintain healthy bone and gingiva around teeth and implants, most clinicians agree that this tissue allows the patient to comfortably and thoroughly perform oral hygiene procedures. However, the appearance of the soft tissue and comfort as perceived by the patient has a dramatic impact on whether the implant is a success or failure (Fig. 26-53).

Surgical enhancement of soft tissue

Soft tissue reconstructive surgery to augment and enhance the quality and quantity of the tissue requires the clinician to accurately delineate the specific defect and to recognize the criteria necessary to restore the contour and anatomy. Surgical procedures commonly recommended include a modified soft tissue flap design, soft tissue onlay grafts, and free autogenous subepithelial connective tissue grafts.

The surgical techniques for these procedures are described in Chapter 21. The criteria and objectives of soft tissue procedures around teeth are similar with implants. Sufficient gingiva to establish and maintain soft tissue health, including contour, color, and symmetry around teeth and implants must be achieved. Therefore, some essential principles should be considered when attempting to enhance the esthetic and functional aspects of the soft tissue around implants. The horizontal incision should include a sufficient amount of keratinized

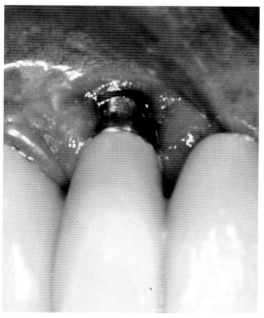

Figure 26-53. Inadequate keratinized gingiva surrounds the cervical facial surface of this maxillary anterior implant. Gingival recession, inflammation, and bleeding on probing are present. The patient complains of tenderness when brushing this area. The implant is osseointegrated and the restoration is functional, but the case is esthetically compromised.

gingiva, but should not include the papilla on the adjacent teeth. Currently, regeneration of an interproximal papilla is not a clinically predictable procedure especially when related to implant-supported restorations. It is much easier to preserve the interproximal papilla than to regenerate it, although adhering to specific parameters may enhance the success of regenerating papilla.[98,99] Therefore, every effort should be made to preserve the papilla when planning treatment and executing a surgical procedure. For that reason, surgical flap design generally should not include the interproximal papilla.

Choquet and co-workers[98] reported on criteria that can be applied successfully to situations where there are teeth present adjacent to an implant site (i.e., a single-tooth implant). It is possible to regenerate or to maintain a papilla if the distance between the crest of the interdental bone to the apical aspect of the contact area between the teeth is 5 mm or less. In essence, the height of the papilla is dependent on the height of the interproximal bone on the adjacent teeth. Therefore, every effort must be made to retain the bone as close to the CEJ as possible on teeth adjacent to implant sites. To preserve the soft tissue papilla, the vertical level of the bony crest around the implant should be approximately 2 mm apical to the CEJ of the adjacent teeth. The height of interproximal bone can be determined by comprehensive radiographic analysis and a clinical assessment by probing the level of the soft tissue attachment.

Also, a minimum horizontal distance of 1.5 mm is necessary between an implant and the adjacent tooth to preserve the height of interproximal bone.[98,99] If the clinician is placing multiple implants, at least 3 mm are necessary between adjacent implants to maintain interproximal bone height and to regenerate the papilla. The danger of placing the implants closer to each other or to adjacent teeth is that bone loss will be more pronounced, both vertically and horizontally, causing loss of the interproximal bone support for the papilla. The presurgical findings should support the diagnosis, and therefore contribute to establishing an appropriate treatment plan.

Soft tissue flap design. To enhance flap management, when attempting to completely cover the surgical site and establish tension-free closure, it may be necessary to use vertical-releasing incisions. These incisions are best made at least one tooth away from the surgical site. The advantage to a vertical incision is the ability to enhance visibility and access. The disadvantage is the involvement of soft tissue around the adjacent teeth, resulting in possible gingival recession and esthetic compromise. This can be prevented with appropriate incision design.

In addition, the undersurface of the labial or buccal flap may require further dissection using periosteal incisions in a mesiodistal direction. This will enable the flap to be advanced coronally, allowing for complete tension-free closure.

Soft tissue grafts. Three-dimensional soft tissue defects with a vertical and horizontal deficiency should be corrected either before or at the time of implant placement. A successful result requires stability and thorough vascularization of the graft. Consequently, any material such as barrier membranes, titanium screws, or abutments may compromise a successful outcome. Two-dimensional soft tissue defects (faciopalatal deformities) are more predictable and can be addressed during any phase of treatment. Often, a subepithelial connective tissue graft or an epithelialized autogenous soft tissue graft can be used (Fig. 26-54) (see Chapter 21 for a detailed discussion of various soft tissue grafting techniques). The disadvantages to the onlay palatal graft include difference in tissue color between the graft and the adjacent gingiva, as well as visible incision lines and scarring, which may compromise the esthetic result. When there is insufficient donor connective tissue to reconstruct the ridge, an acellular dermal connective allograft derived from donated human skin may be used. The acellular dermal connective tissue graft eliminates the need for an additional surgical procedure to harvest the tissue, and the quantity of tissue is not a limitation. The recipient site is prepared similar to the subepithelial connective tissue graft, and the graft

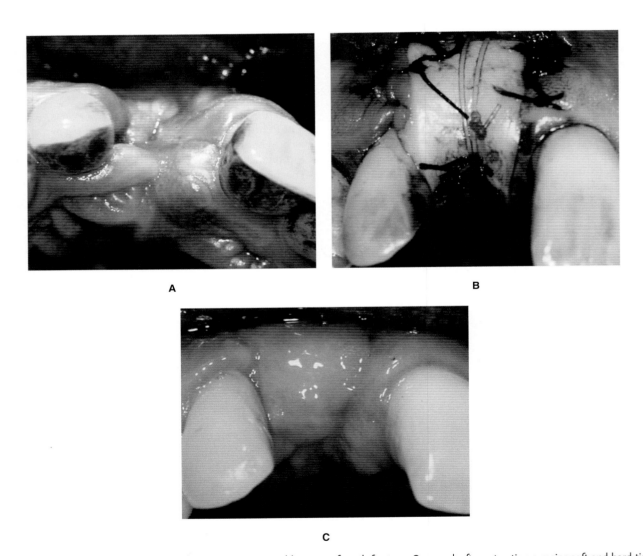

A

B

C

Figure 26-54. A, The maxillary right central incisor was extracted because of tooth fracture. One week after extraction a major soft and hard tissue deformity is present in the esthetic zone. The entire facial wall of bone has resorbed and, therefore, will require an autogenous bone graft. **B,** Because there is insufficient soft tissue to completely cover a bone graft, the soft tissue deformity was corrected first. Because of the quantity of tissue required, a full-thickness epithelialized soft tissue onlay graft was used rather than a subepithelial connective tissue graft. **C,** This is a 6-month postoperative result. The bone graft can now be performed with adequate soft tissue coverage.

material must be totally covered by the soft tissue flap. Any graft exposure will not adequately vascularize and will subsequently necrose.

Restorative enhancement of soft tissue (guided gingival regeneration)

Guided gingival regeneration is a nonsurgical approach to promoting gingival tissue regeneration around the abutments of a provisional (temporary) restoration. The objective is to influence the height and form of the interdental papilla and surrounding gingiva, establishing an harmonious appearance of the soft tissue and esthetic emergence profile of the implant restoration as it relates to the natural teeth.

The patient wears the provisional restoration for approximately 3 to 6 months, depending on the rate of papilla regeneration. During this time, the restoration is altered by the dentist to enhance the final result. The emergence profile of the provisional restoration is used to guide re-formation of the papillae, which generally involves a combination of overcontouring and undercontouring the profile to achieve the desired result. The aggressive use of interdental cleaners or stimulus during this phase of treatment is contraindicated. Trauma to the soft tissues may interfere with the regenerative process.

To maximize the results of guided gingival regeneration, five basic criteria must be considered:

1. Favorable emergence profile as it relates to adjacent teeth
2. Presence of keratinized tissue
3. Titanium provisional abutment
4. An atraumatic provisional restoration
5. Realistic goals of 1 to 4 mm of increased gingival height

Orthodontic enhancement of soft tissue and bone

Orthodontics also can be helpful in positioning natural teeth to create sufficient space to place implants (see Chapter 28). Uprighting teeth, moving teeth bodily, orthodontically extracting teeth (forced eruption), and establishing a physiologic occlusion are some ways that orthodontists become an essential member of the implant team.

Orthodontics is a nonsurgical approach to enhancing hard and soft tissue volume and height before the placement of an implant. Through controlled movement of hopeless teeth, the orthodontist can establish an environment that will ultimately house a functional, esthetic restoration. Forced eruption can be used not only as a means of atraumatically extracting hopeless teeth, but of "carrying" the surrounding bone and soft tissue into a more coronal position. This facilitates immediate implant placement after tooth extraction because an increased volume of periimplant bone and soft tissue are available.

Immediate Placement and Loading of Implants

The increased level of predictability and success with current implant therapy has encouraged a reevaluation of every aspect of traditional treatment planning protocols to better assimilate the benefits of osseointegration into clinical practice. These protocols are being updated to incorporate new regenerative modalities for treating patients with inadequate dimensions of bone and soft tissue to achieve a successful functional implant outcome.

Implants placed immediately after tooth extraction can be as successful as implants placed into healed sites, with a success rate of greater than 95%.[100-103] The need for a period of unloaded healing after implant placement, as originally described by Brånemark, also has been questioned. In some cases, implants may be loaded either immediately after placement or within a period of a few days to weeks. Such immediate loading techniques are successful in achieving clinically and histologically defined osseointegration.[104-107]

Numerous studies or case reports have been reported examining immediate implant loading for the edentulous arch and for partially edentulous and single-tooth replacement cases.[108,109] The single-tooth replacement, however, does not usually represent true immediate functional loading because clinicians often eliminate any function (force) on the temporary restoration. This type of restoration is frequently classified as "immediate temporization." True functional loading has been predominantly studied in cross-arch stabilized restorations for treatment of fully edentulous cases[108,109] (Fig. 26-55). As research continues to show excellent success rates for immediately loaded implant restorations, their use can be expected to increase. The concept is particularly appealing to the patient because a restoration can be fabricated within 24 hours of implant placement.

Schnitman and co-workers[110] placed implants in the mandible of 10 patients. The implants were immediately loaded and included natural teeth in 3 of the 10 restorations. Four of the 28 implants failed 3 to 4 months after loading and 1 implant failed after 21 months. The overall success rate was 84.7%. The 4 implants that failed were the most distal abutments in the restoration. Tarnow and colleagues[111] treated 10 edentulous cases (4 maxilla, 6 mandible) and reported their 1- to 5-year data. They immediately loaded a minimum of 4 implants in the mandible and a minimum of 6 implants in the maxilla. Two of 69 immediately loaded implants failed, both in the mandible. The implant success rate was 97.1%.

In 2001, Grunder[112] published a study in which 5 maxillae and 5 mandibles were treated with a total of 91 implants. Of these, 66 were placed immediately

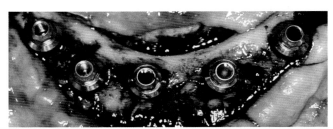

Figure 26-55. A, Five ITI (International Team for Implantology) fixtures with octabutments placed in mandibular anterior region. **B,** Transfer copings placed on octabutments. **C,** Surgical template used to transfer fixture position and occlusal registration. **D,** Laboratory-processed mandibular provisional restoration delivered 1 week after fixture placement. Such cross-arch stabilized prostheses may lend themselves to loading soon after implant placement. **E,** Gold and acrylic prosthesis, after 1 year in function.

after tooth extraction into the extraction sockets, and all implants were immediately loaded. In all 66 immediate implant sites, no bone substitutes or barrier membranes were used, despite several cases involving gaps between the implant and the bone of the extraction socket. Immediate functional loading of implants placed imme-

diately after extraction, without the use of any bone substitutes or barrier membranes, for fixed complete arch reconstructions was successful over a 2-year observation period.

Any deviation from the standard protocol of delayed loading may only be undertaken with the understanding of the inherent risks to the important development of the bone–implant interface. A reexamination of the concept of immediate loading, therefore, would need to address two main concerns. For obvious functional demands, immediately loaded implants must forsake one of the original prerequisites for osseointegration—namely, a submerged healing phase.[113] The findings of research using ITI implants (Institut Straumann, Waldenburg, Switzerland), however, have challenged this tenet by demonstrating highly predictable osseointegration with a one-stage nonsubmergence protocol.[114-116]

A second, but much more pivotal concern, regarding immediate loading pertains to shielding the bone–implant interface from functional overload during the early remodeling phase (Fig. 26-56). Toward that end, criteria must be identified to sufficiently stabilize the interface against micromovement, even in an immediately loaded environment.

Guidelines for immediate loading of implants

The following should be considered before treatment planning immediately loaded implants:

1. Comprehensive informed patient consent must be secured.
2. Bone quality and quantity is critical.
3. Implants with macrointerlock properties should be used. Screw-shaped implants provide the strongest immediate mechanical retention after placement.[117]
4. Implants with microinterlock properties also should be considered. Rough implant surfaces promote faster direct contact with bone than do smooth-surfaced implants.[115] It also has been demonstrated histologically that this contact can occur in as few as 7 days.[118]
5. Bicortical initial stabilization should be maximized (i.e., minimal counter-sinking).

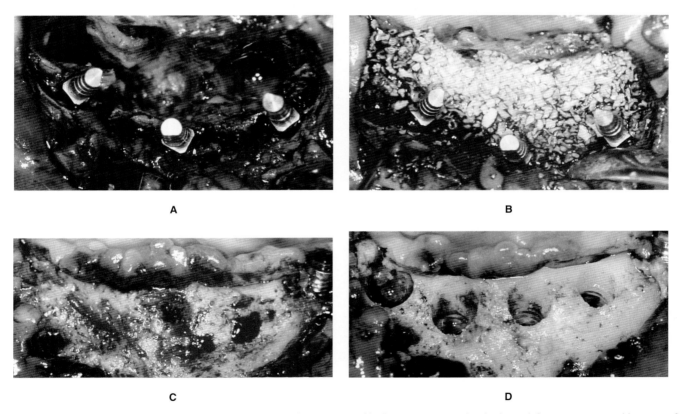

A   B

C   D

Figure 26-56. A, This is an 80-year-old man who was unable to have a removable denture. A major alveolar bone deformity was created because of the failure within 6 weeks of six implants that were immediately loaded with a removable prosthesis. The implants were removed and the treatment plan was to first place a bone graft, wait 4 to 6 months, and place implants that would be immediately loaded using a cross-arch stabilized fixed provisional prosthesis. Temporary mini-implants, plus the one implant that remained from the first surgery, were used to stabilize a provisional fixed restoration. **B,** The graft material used was bovine bone that was covered with nonresorbable membrane. **C,** Six months after surgery, the membrane was removed. The defect was totally reconstructed with regenerated bone. **D,** The bone was dense and allowed for the placement of five implants that were immediately loaded.

6. Cantilevers should be avoided or minimized in the provisional restoration.[119-121]

7. Provisional restorations should be fabricated with a rigid framework to prevent flexure.

8. An occlusal scheme that emphasizes axial loading and minimizes horizontal stress must be designed.[122]

9. A Hawley bite plane type of nighttime appliance can be used to minimize the effects of parafunctional habits.

Complications and Failures of Implants

Failures must be considered on the basis of when they occur in the sequence of therapy. There are two major phases in the "life" of a dental implant. Phase 1 is after surgical placement and before the implant is loaded. Phase 2 is after exposure of the implant to the oral environment and functional loading.

Early implant failures (phase 1)

Early implant failures occur after implant placement but before the implant is loaded. Failure during this period usually results in the complete loss of the implant because of infection, uncontrolled and/or undiagnosed systemic disease, transmucosal overloading, smoking, or excessive surgical trauma.

Infection. In the past, concerns regarding infection in the immediate perioperative period led to surgical protocols requiring absolute sterility.[123] A study by Scharf and Tarnow,[56] however, showed that implants placed under surgically "clean" conditions have the same statistical success rate as those placed under sterile conditions. Therefore, infection probably occurs infrequently, unless surgical conditions are contaminated either by the external environment or by an existing infection at the implant site.

If plaque accumulates on the implant surface, the subepithelial connective tissue becomes infiltrated by large numbers of inflammatory cells, and the epithelium appears ulcerated and loosely adherent. When the plaque continues to migrate apically, the clinical and radiographic signs of tissue destruction are seen around implants and teeth. Studies suggest that plaque-associated soft tissue inflammation around implants may have more serious implications than marginal inflammation around teeth and the periodontal ligaments. One reason for the increased inflammation around an implant may be the low vascularity of the periimplant soft tissue band and the difference in collagen-to-fibroblast ratio of gingival tissue. These affect the defense mechanisms around an implant as compared with those of the tissue around natural teeth with periodontal ligaments.[124-126] Also, various implant surface characteristics influence the amount of periimplant tissue breakdown and inflammation.[127-129]

Subgingival bacterial flora associated with clinically inflamed implant sites is quite different than that seen around healthy implants. These microbial shifts are similar to those occurring around natural teeth, and the bacterial flora in chronic periodontitis and periimplantitis are quite similar.[130-135]

Osseointegrated dental implants typically have a well documented high success rate. When failures occur, the sequelae can be distressing to the patient and create therapeutic difficulties for the clinician. Pathologic alterations of the periimplant tissues can be placed in the general category of periimplant disease.[136] Inflammatory alterations, which are confined to the soft tissue surrounding the implant, are diagnosed as periimplant mucositis.[136] Complications, conversely, may occur in patients who have highly unrealistic esthetic expectations and less than optimal implant placement and restorative treatment outcomes. When recommending a treatment plan for a patient, the dentist must consider biologic and anatomic limitations.

Clinical data demonstrate that after significant periods of implant function, bone loss can develop and even progress around the implant to levels that increase the risk for failure. The design and surface characteristics of the implant may influence the amount of periimplant bone loss.[129,137] Implants with a polished, coronal titanium surface and nonsplinted maxillary implants have shown increased periimplant bone loss during function.[137] Notably, crestal bone around an implant resorbs an average of 0.9 to 1.66 mm during the first year of implant function. In the follow-up years, mean annual rates of bone loss are 0.05 to 0.13 mm.[85,138,139]

The severity of the periimplant bone loss and the morphology of the bone defect, as well as the implant surface, will determine the procedure needed to treat a compromised implant and prevent it from total failure. It is possible to arrest the disease progression and to regenerate the lost periodontal tissues. Periimplant mucositis (soft tissue infection) and hyperplasia were noted in 21% to 28% of the jaws during the early period of clinical experience with osseointegration,[140] but this rate significantly decreased in future years. The improvement is attributed to better oral hygiene techniques and prosthesis changes.

Treatment of periimplantitis. As long as the implant surface is contaminated with soft tissue cells, bacteria, or bacterial byproducts, wound healing is compromised.[124,125,141] The nonsurgical treatment for periimplant bacterial infection involves removing plaque deposits with plastic instruments to avoid damaging the implant surface and polishing all accessible surfaces with pumice. The patient also is treated with subgingival irrigation with 0.12% chlorhexidine and encouraged to improve home oral hygiene practice if needed. The initial phase of therapy may be sufficient to reestablish gingival health. If not, a surgical procedure may be needed. If regeneration of new bone and osseointegration are to occur, the defect must first be debrided and the contaminated implant surface prepared. This can only be done with a surgical approach.

The surgical techniques currently advocated for controlling periimplant lesions are modifications of techniques used to treat bone defects around teeth. The type and size of bone defects must be identified before deciding on the appropriate treatment modality. This determines whether the implant should be removed or a regenerative procedure undertaken. Regenerative therapy is used to reduce pockets, but with the ultimate goal of regenerating lost bone tissue. Also, systemic antibiotics have been advocated as a supportive regimen during the treatment phase of periimplant disease.[142-144]

For implant surface preparation, mechanical devices and chemotherapeutics have been evaluated *in vitro* and *in vivo*.[144,145] Conventional and ultrasonic instruments are not suitable for preparing and detoxifying the implant surface. Mechanical instrumentation may damage the implant surface if performed with metal instruments harder than titanium. The method of choice involves a high-pressure, air-powered abrasive comprising a mixture of sodium bicarbonate and water. This method completely removes microbial deposits from titanium surfaces, does not significantly change the surface topography, and does not adversely affect cell adhesion.[140,146]

Systemic disorders. Implant candidates often present no signs, systems, or history of systemic disorders. These are usually discovered only after an unexpected poor response to therapy when suspicions are raised and a medical work-up is performed. This highlights the importance of eliciting a comprehensive medical history before any surgical procedure.

Patients with medical disorders that compromise their immune system or wound healing ability are frequently more susceptible to infection and heal poorly. If the medical disorder is undiagnosed before implant placement, the patient may experience "cluster failures," meaning the loss of multiple implants at one point in the healing process. For example, an undiagnosed patient with diabetes may present with multiple failed implants and no clear reason for such failures. The medical work-up would need to address the signs, symptoms, and laboratory evaluation of possible diabetes.

Transmucosal overloading. In patients who wear complete or removable partial dentures, implants should not be subjected to transmucosal loading during the healing period. Such transmucosal loading may occur when a removable, tissue-borne prosthesis is worn too soon after implant placement. It is imperative that the clinician relieves the internal aspect of a removable transitional prosthesis and relines it with a soft material. Reline materials must be replaced frequently because they tend to harden over time. The patient must be cautioned to eat a softer diet while the removable transitional prosthesis is worn (Fig. 26-57).

Smoking. Clinicians have long suspected that patients who smoke have a more compromised outcome after surgery than do nonsmokers. In a retrospective study of 2194 Brånemark implants placed in 540 patients over a 6-year period, smokers had a much greater failure rate than nonsmokers.[147] Overall failure rates were 5.92%, yet nonsmokers had a failure rate of only 4.76%, whereas smokers had a failure rate of 11.28%. In a metaanalysis of several studies with almost 5000 implants, there were no significant differences in overall implant failure rate between smokers and nonsmokers.[148] However, machined surface implants showed a greater difference in failure rate (greater rate for smokers) than did rough surface implants. Most studies are in agreement that differences between smokers and nonsmokers are found predominantly for maxillary implants, whereas mandibular implants have similar success rates in smokers and nonsmokers. It is incumbent on the clinician to warn patients who smoke of their risk for implant failure if they continue to smoke during the postoperative period. This recommendation should be included in the informed consent signed by the patient.

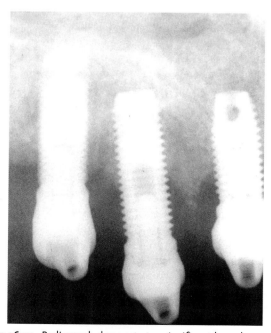

Figure 26-57. Radiograph demonstrates significant bone loss around the implants because of early transmucosal loading. The patient was noncompliant and wore a poorly fitting removable denture 2 weeks after implant placement.

Surgical trauma. An atraumatic surgical technique is a prerequisite for achieving osseointegration. This includes the use of slowly rotating drilling equipment, sharp drills, and copious irrigation. Overzealous or incorrect preparation can lead to overheating the bone at the osteotomy site and increasing hemorrhage with concomitant hematoma formation, swelling, and infection. The ultimate consequence of poor surgical technique is loss of the implant.

Late implant failures (phase 2)

The most vexing of implant failures are those that occur after the implant is loaded. The assumption is made by the patient, and by many clinicians, that achieving osseointegration is the difficult part of the implant experience. However, osseointegration is a predictable and readily achievable therapeutic outcome. Problems that occur after implant loading often are harder to solve because a final restoration may have been completed and the patient's expectations left unmet.

Essentially, there are three types of failures after loading. The first is an esthetic failure. The implant and prosthesis are intact, but the patient's esthetic needs have not been met. The second type of failure results in the complete loss of the implant because of failure at the bone–implant interface. The third prosthetic failure includes loosening of screws and fracture of the setscrew, abutment, implant, porcelain, or solder joint.

Biomechanical forces. Infection occurring after an implant is loaded does not appear to be a common cause of implant failure. Overloading contributes to prosthetic failure, to the loss of osseointegration, and, ultimately, to the loss of the implant. It is imperative that the clinician understands which types of forces are within physiologic tolerance and which are destructive and cause overload. Axial forces are best tolerated by osseointegrated implants, whereas off-axis forces induce bending moments at the osseous crest and are the most destructive.[149-151] Other equally destructive forces can be generated by the restorative process and are created by screwing in a framework that does not fit passively.

Experimental and clinical evidence supports the concept that excessive biomechanical forces may lead to high stress or microfractures in the coronal bone–implant contact, leading to loss of osseointegration around the neck of the implant.[152] Although overload is clinically difficult to define and measure, the role of overloading is likely to increase in four clinical situations:

1. The implant is placed in poor quality bone.
2. The implant position, or the total portion of the implant placed in bone, does not favor ideal load transmission over the implant surface.
3. The patient has a pattern of heavy occlusal function associated with parafunctional habits (Fig. 26-58).
4. The restoration does not precisely fit the implant.

Notably, the cause of periimplant crestal bone loss can be multifactorial, and both bacterial infection and biomechanical factors may be implicated. Other etiologic factors, such as traumatic surgical technique, smoking, inadequate host bone (resulting in an exposed implant surface at the time of placement), and a compromised host response may be implicated as cofactors in the development of periimplant disease.

The nonpassive framework. The most careful case planning and occlusal scheme will contribute little to long-term success if the prosthesis does not fit passively. This is an inviolate concept.[153] The typical implant-borne prosthesis is composed of several different components. The abutment, the gold screws, the framework and its accompanying veneering material, and the bone–implant interface are placed under permanent strain when a screw-retained framework does not fit passively. The constant stress may manifest itself as crestal bone loss, fracture of the porcelain or metal components, or screw loosening.

Determining passivity of fit often is clinically difficult. When supragingival abutments are used, the fit of the retainer can be evaluated using the single-screw test. When subgingival abutments are used, visual inspection is not possible and radiographs provide limited information. One method that can be used with subgingival abutments is to evaluate the feel or tactile sense of each screw as it is being tightened. If a framework is passive, each screw should become tight immediately after resistance

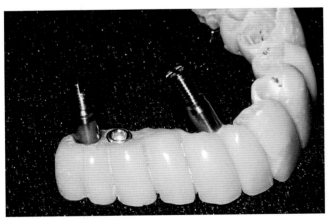

Figure 26-58. The patient has a history of significant parafunctional habits such as grinding and clenching. He had fractured porcelain and solder joints on previous restorations and could not wear a night guard appliance. Photograph shows an implant and tooth-supported restoration where two of the implants had fractured because of occlusal overload secondary to parafunctional forces.

to tightening is felt. If a screw becomes progressively tighter as it is turned, the implant and framework are actually being drawn together by the tightening screw. The framework must then be either sectioned or remade.

Implant anchorage unit disruption. The primary force reception unit in implantology is termed the *implant anchorage unit.*[149] It consists of the implant, the transmucosal abutment, the gold cylinder (and associated restoration), the abutment screw, and the prosthetic set screw (gold screw). This unit is responsible for transmitting all forces to the bone surrounding the implant. An analogous situation of the natural dentition is the "attachment apparatus." This consists of the bone lining the tooth socket, the fibers of the periodontal ligament, and the cementum covering the root. Forces delivered to the restoration have their primary effect on the implant anchorage unit and the attachment apparatus. The ability of the implant anchorage unit to adequately distribute applied force is controlled by a number of factors.

The location of the implant in the dental arch has a significant influence on the force applied to the bone and the screws in the implant anchorage unit. Implants should be placed along as large an arc as possible. When force is applied, implants are stressed in different directions, thereby distributing the force. When implants are placed in a straight line, any nonaxial directed force exerts a bending movement around each implant anchorage unit that can result in overloading of the implant. The greater the number and length of implants supporting the restoration, the better the system is able to distribute applied force.[154-156] The greater surface area of bone–implant contact and the greater number of abutments all contribute to the ability of the implant anchorage units to tolerate off-axis forces.

Even with the proper length, location, and number of implants, a traumatic occlusal scheme may cause failure because of overload. A therapeutic occlusion must be developed to ensure the proper distribution of applied forces.

Therapeutic occlusion. In the natural dentition, the therapeutic occlusion is conceived as a means to treat the pathologic occlusion.[46] A pathologic occlusion may be manifested by occlusal trauma (mobile teeth), retrograde wear, and myofascial pain-dysfunction syndrome. If occlusal trauma (overload of the attachment apparatus) is compared with implant failure after loading (overload of the implant anchorage unit), one significant difference is seen. In the natural dentition, the tooth responds to overloading by adaptation. There is bone loss in the walls of the socket, the periodontal ligament space widens, and the tooth becomes mobile. This is the tooth's attempt to move away from the traumatic force. If the traumatic force is controlled or removed, the situation will reverse itself and the tooth will once again become firm. With the implant anchorage unit, no such adaptation exists. When an overload situation develops, an irreversible failure will occur. Prosthetic failures can be repaired, but typically recur if the cause of overloading is not corrected. In the worst-case scenario, the overloading force is transmitted to the bone–implant interface, causing a loss of osseointegration and loss of the implant.

Occlusal vertical dimension. A proper occlusal vertical dimension (OVD) must provide for a functionally adequate freeway space. There is a range of acceptable OVDs. Establishing the OVD is a chair-side procedure. It cannot be arbitrarily chosen on an articulator. When fabricating an implant-borne restoration, the OVD has a profound impact on abutment selection, location of screw access holes, and the crown-to-implant ratio.

When surgeons are asked to place permanent, transmucosal abutments at the time of implant exposure, they are at a distinct disadvantage. The surgeon often is not aware of the OVD, which determines a specific implant abutment. Not until the restorative dentist chooses a therapeutic OVD can the distance from the top of the implant to the occlusal plane be measured. This is the space available for implant and restorative components. A change in OVD also can affect where screw access holes emerge. An increase in OVD will cause screw access holes to emerge facially rather than in the cingulum area of anterior teeth.

Anterior guidance. The greater the guidance is, the greater the horizontal component of force on the implant anchorage unit.[150] The therapeutic goal is to minimize horizontal forces because implants do not have the adaptive capacity inherent to the natural dentition. Practitioners do not have a reliable way to determine the optimum overbite in the implant-borne restoration. Therefore, the overbite must be minimized as much as possible without developing posterior interference during excursive movements of the mandible. If an excessive overbite is placed in a tooth-borne restoration, changes occur (e.g., tooth mobility) that will alert the clinician to intervene. It is extremely important that the occlusal table be as narrow as possible and placed over the long access of the implant. Failure to fulfill this requirement will result in a large bending moment and possible screw loosening, fracture, or both.[149]

Crown-to-implant ratio. The crown-to-implant ratio should be kept to a minimum. Changes in OVD can positively or negatively affect the crown-to-implant ratio. In severely resorbed jaws, an adverse crown-to-implant ratio is a particularly significant problem. Resorption of the alveolar process reduces the amount of bone available for implant placement, whereas it increases the length of the teeth. This poor crown-to-implant ratio in resorbed cases contributes to the poor prognosis of unsplinted implants under overdentures.

Clinicians must compensate for a poor crown-to-implant ratio in the same manner they compensate for a poor crown-to-root ratio in the natural dentition—by attempting to place a greater number of implants and considering bone grafting to allow use of longer implants. In addition, splinting may be necessary for mutual support.

Splinting. Splinting is an important treatment option in developing the therapeutic occlusion. It is indicated to control the adverse effects of an unfavorable crown-to-implant ratio, poor axial positioning of implants, and an insufficient number or length of implants to provide a freestanding quadrant or sextant restoration (Fig. 26-59). Although splinting is useful, it cannot substitute for an optimal occlusal scheme.

When splinting is required for an implant-borne restoration, the only abutments often available to splint to are natural teeth. Because implant components are considered rigid, it has been assumed that any natural tooth connected to an implant would not be loaded, but would instead function like a cantilever. However, in an *in vitro* study using an implant-abutment-gold cylinder component stack, Gunne and co-workers[157] showed that if the tooth abutment of a three-unit bridge was loaded, the screw joints of the implant abutment would open and close, providing flexibility in the implant component stack. The amount of deflection equaled the mobility of a periodontally sound tooth. The results of this study suggested that there is no biologic basis for the notion that implants and natural teeth should not be splinted. However, these three-unit fixed partial dentures had only a single implant abutment and a single tooth abutment. The authors acknowledge that the conclusions cannot be extrapolated to multiple implant restorations attached to natural teeth, because multiple implants form a more rigid unit. Also, the dentition opposing the implant-to-tooth fixed partial dentures in this study consisted of complete dentures, on which relatively small forces could be placed compared with a natural opposing dentition. Most problems associated with splinting implants and natural teeth are related to the need for retrievability for all or part of the restoration, rather than any inherent biologic concerns.

Retrievability. There are two methods for providing retrievability in a restoration that splints implants and natural teeth: one is to use screw-retention for implant abutments and the other is to use temporary cements for the natural tooth abutments. The major drawback of the latter approach is the possibility of unrecognized cement washout of the natural tooth abutments. Solutions to this problem have been to telescope the natural tooth abutment or to use semi-rigid attachments between the implant-borne component and the natural tooth-borne component. The telescope is cemented to the natural tooth permanently, and the overcase is temporarily cemented to the telescope. When using semi-rigid attachments, temporary cements are used to cement the crown directly to the natural tooth abutment. In each case, migration of the natural tooth–supported part of the restoration has been documented by investigators.[158,159] This generally manifests as intrusion of the natural tooth.

Various techniques may be used to prevent migration of natural tooth abutments. In the case of telescoped abutments, a set-screw may be placed to hold the tooth in position in case of cement washout. In the case of semi-rigid attachments, the clinician may place a screw or staple buccolingually through the attachment or arrange the attachment orientation so that intrusion of the natural tooth abutment cannot occur. Both approaches can be technically difficult and are not without problems.

A simpler answer to the problem is to avoid using screw retention when splinting teeth to implants. With implant abutments cemented to telescopes on the natural teeth, the clinician can temporarily cement the entire case and identify washouts by observing the movement of the restoration. It is then a simple maintenance task to tap off the restoration and recement it.

With careful planning and engineering of the implant-supported restoration, many failures can be prevented. By providing for retrievability, almost any problem that occurs after the restoration is completed can be handled with minimal inconvenience to both the patient and the practitioner. Many clinicians try to avoid these problem altogether by not splinting natural teeth to implants whenever they can place a fully implant-borne prosthesis instead.

Esthetic compromise. One of the most common causes of esthetic failure is loss of the interdental papilla or

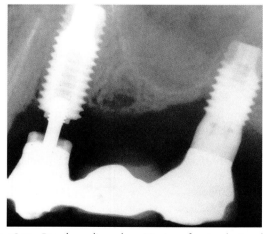

Figure 26-59. Poor buccolingual positioning of an implant and excessive occlusal forces contributed to this complication. Loosening of the abutment screw resulted in loss of rigidity, which allowed axial forces to act independently on the two implants. The result was loss of significant crestal bone.

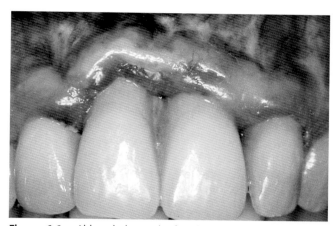

Figure 26-60. Although the result of implant treatment maybe a functional success, it can be an esthetic failure because of inaccurately diagnosing and treatment planning the problem. Regeneration and reconstruction of the bone and soft tissue before implant placement was not considered in this case, with resultant poor esthetic outcomes.

apical positioning of the facial gingival margin, or both, during postsurgical healing. Esthetically, this results in "black triangles" on either side of the implant-borne restoration and a gingival margin that is not in harmony with the rest of the dentition. This often is caused by the surgeon's failure to take into account the patient's soft tissue needs before or during surgery.

Implant placement in the esthetic zone requires precise three-dimensional tissue reconstruction and ideal implant placement. If crown form, dimension, shape, and gingival harmony around the implants are not ideal, the patient and dentist consider the implant restoration an esthetic failure because the result does not represent a natural profile (Fig. 26-60).

CONCLUSION

Successful implant restorations encompass both optimal function and esthetics. Osseointegration—once the sole focus of implant dentistry—is now a relatively predictable process given the plethora of research, the contemporary surgical and tissue reconstruction techniques, and the vast array of materials and implant systems introduced during the last 40 years. Cases that once seemed hopeless are now possible to treat with excellent and more predictable results. The added esthetic component means dentists also must meet patient demands for restorations that mimic the natural dentition in terms of performance, comfort, and appearance.

At its foundation, the successful implant restoration case involves a team approach with detailed communication between the various clinicians and technicians, as well as the patient. Thanks to the team concept the dental profession has embraced, complications have been minimized and therapeutic horizons have been expanded. Although further research is still needed to make successful implant dentistry a predictable procedure, the environment for success is better than ever.

REFERENCES

1. Carranza FA, Shklar G: Implant dentistry. In Carranza FA, Shklar G, editors: *History of periodontology*, Chicago, 2003, Quintessence.
2. Brånemark P-I, Zarb GA, Albrektsson T, editors: *Tissue-integrated prostheses: osseointegration in clinical dentistry*, Chicago, 1985, Quintessence.
3. Cochran DL, Herrmann JS, Schenk RK et al: Biologic width around titanium implants. A histometric analysis of the implanto-gingival junction around unloaded and loaded nonsubmerged implants in the canine mandible, *J Periodontol* 68:186-198, 1997.
4. Adell R, Eriksson B, Lekholm U et al: Long-term follow-up study of osseointegrated implants in the treatment of totally edentulous jaws, *Int J Oral Maxillofac Implants* 5:347-359, 1990.
5. Zarb G, Schmitt A: The longitudinal clinical effectiveness of osseointegrated dental implants in anterior partially edentulous patients, *Int J Prosthodont* 6:180-188, 1993.
6. Zarb G, Schmitt A: The longitudinal clinical effectiveness of osseointegrated dental implants in posterior partially edentulous patients, *Int J Prosthodont* 6:189-196, 1993.
7. Schmitt A, Zarb G: The longitudinal clinical effectiveness of osseointegrated dental implants for single-tooth replacement, *Int J Prosthodont* 6:197-202, 1993.
8. Minsk L, Polson AM, Weisgold A et al: Outcome failures of endosseous implants from a clinical training center, *Compend Contin Educ Dent* 17:848-859, 1996.
9. Schnitman PA, Schulman LB: Recommendations of the consensus development conference on dental implants, *J Am Dent Assoc* 98:373-377, 1979.
10. Albrektsson T, Zarb G, Worthington P, Eriksson AR: The long-term efficacy of currently used dental implants: a review and proposed criteria of success, *Int J Oral Maxillofac Implants* 1:11-25, 1986.
11. Smith DE, Zarb GA: Criteria for success of osseointegrated endosseous implants, *J Prosthet Dent* 2:567-572, 1989.
12. Brånemark P-I: Osseointegration and its experimental background, *J Prosthet Dent* 50:399-410, 1983.
13. Reddy MS, Geurs NC, Wang IC et al: Mandibular growth following implant restoration: does Wolff's law apply to residual ridge resorption?, *Int J Periodontics Restorative Dent* 22:315-321, 2002.
14. Albrektsson T, Dahl E, Enbom L et al: Osseointegrated oral implants. A Swedish multicenter study of 8139 consecutively inserted Nobelpharma implants, *J Periodontol* 59:287-296, 1988.

15. Rams TE, Link CC: Microbiology of failing dental implants in humans: electron microscopic observations, *J Oral Implantol* 11:93-100, 1983.

16. Becker W, Becker B, Newman M, Nyman S: Clinical and microbiologic findings that may contribute to dental implant failure, *Int J Oral Maxillofac Implants* 5:31-38, 1990.

17. Jemt T, Linden B, Lekholm U: Failures and complications in 127 consecutively placed fixed partial prostheses supported by Branemark implants: from prosthetic treatment to first annual checkup, *Int J Oral Maxillofac Implants* 7:40-44, 1992.

18. McGlumphy E, Robinson D, Mendel D: Implant superstructures: a comparison of ultimate failure force, *Int J Oral Maxillofac Implants* 7:35-39, 1992.

19. Mombelli A: Microbiology of the dental implant, *Adv Dent Res* 7(2):202-206, 1993.

20. Smith RA, Berger R, Dodson TB: Risk factors associated with dental implants in healthy and medically compromised patients, *Int J Oral Maxillofac Implants* 7:367-372, 1992.

21. Glick M, Abel SN, Muzyka BC, DeLorenzo M: Dental complications after treating patients with AIDS, *J Am Dent Assoc* 125:296-301, 1994.

22. Jaffin R, Berman C: The excessive loss of Branemark fixtures in type IV bone: a 5-year analysis, *J Periodontol* 62:2-4, 1991.

23. Dao TTT, Anderson JD, Zarb GA: Is osteoporosis a risk factor for osseointegration of dental implants?, *Int J Oral Maxillofac Implants* 8:137-144, 1993.

24. Baxter JC, Fattore LD: Osteoporosis and osseointegration of implants, *J Prosthodont* 2(2):120-125, 1993.

25. Fujimoto T, Niimi A, Naka H, Ueda M: Ossointegrated implants in a patient with osteoporosis: a case report, *Int J Oral Maxillofac Implants* 11:539-542, 1996.

26. De Bruyn H, Collaert B: The effect of smoking on early implant failure, *Clin Oral Implants Res* 5(4):260-264, 1994.

27. Gorman LM, Lambert PM, Morris HF et al: The effect of smoking on implant survival at second-stage surgery: DICRG Interim Report No. 5. Dental Implant Clinical Research Group, *Implant Dent* 3(3):165-168, 1994.

28. Bain CA: Smoking and implant failure—benefits of a smoking cessation protocol. *Int J Oral Maxillofac Implants* 11:756-759, 1996.

29. Jones JK, Triplett RG: The relationship of cigarette smoking to impaired intraoral wound healing: a review of evidence and implications for patient care, *J Oral Maxillofac Surg* 50(3):237-240, 1992.

30. van Steenberghe D: A retrospective multicenter evaluation of the survival rate of osseointegrated fixtures supporting fixed partial prostheses in the treatment of partial edentulism, *J Prosthet Dent* 61:217-223, 1989.

31. Becker W, Becker B: Guided tissue regeneration for implants placed into extraction sockets and for implant dehiscences: surgical techniques and case report, *Int J Periodontics Restorative Dent* 10:377-391, 1990.

32. Becker W, Becker B, Handelsman M et al: Guided tissue regeneration for implants placed into extraction sockets: a study in dogs, *J Periodontol* 62:703-709, 1991.

33. Becker W, Dahlin C, Becker B et al: The use of e-PTFE barrier membranes for bone promotion around titanium implants placed into extraction sockets: a prospective multicenter study, *Int J Oral Maxillofac Implants* 9:31-40, 1994.

34. Lekholm U, Becker W, Dahlin C et al: The role of early versus late removal of GTAM membranes on bone formation at oral implants placed into immediate extraction sockets—an experimental study in dogs, *Clin Oral Implants Res* 4:121-129, 1993.

35. Lazzara RJ: Immediate implant placement into extraction sites: surgical and restorative advantages, *Int J Periodontics Restorative Dent* 9:333-343, 1989.

36. Williams MY, Mealey BL, Hallmon WW: The role of computerized tomography in dental implantology, *Int J Oral Maxillofac Implants* 7(3):373-380, 1992.

37. Daftary F: Natural esthetics with implant prostheses, *J Esthet Dent* 7(1):9-17, 1995.

38. Ochsenbein C, Ross S: A concept of osseous surgery and its clinical applications. In Ward HL, Chas C, editors: *A periodontal point of view: A practical expression of current problems integrating basic science with clinical data.* Charles C. Thomas Publishing Co.: Springfield, Ill, 1973.

39. Jansen CE, Weisgold A: Presurgical treatment planning for the anterior single-tooth implant restoration, *Compend Contin Educ Dent* 16:746-762, 1995.

40. Olsson M, Lindhe J: Periodontal characteristics in individuals with varying forms of the upper central incisors, *J Clin Periodontol* 18:78-82, 1991.

41. Tarnow DP, Magner AW, Fletcher P: The effect of the distance from the contact point to the crest of bone on the presence or absence of the interproximal dental papilla, *J Periodontol* 63:995-996, 1992.

42. Adell R, Lekholm U, Rockler B, Brånemark P-I: A 15-year study of osseointegrated implants in the treatment of the edentulous jaw, *Int J Oral Surg* 10:387-416, 1981.

43. Jemt T, Book K, Linden B, Urde G: Failures and complications in 92 consecutively inserted overdentures supported by Branemark implants in severely resorbed edentulous maxillae: a study from prosthetic treatment to first annual check-up, *Int J Oral Maxillofac Implants* 7:162-167, 1992.

44. Bahat O: Surgical planning, *J Calif Dent Assoc* 20:31-46, 1992.

45. Rose LF, Salama H, Bahat O, Minsk L: Treatment planning and site development for the implant-assisted periodontal reconstruction, *Compend Contin Educ Dent* 16:726-742, 1995.

46. Amsterdam M: Periodontal prosthesis: twenty-five years in retrospect, *Alpha Omegan* 67(3):8-52, 1974.

47. Rangert B, Sennerby L, Meredith N, Brunski JB: Design, maintenance and biomechanical considerations in implant placement, *Dent Update* 24:416-420, 1997.

48. Block MS, Kent JN: Factors associated with soft- and hard-tissue compromise of endosseous implants, *J Oral Maxillofac Surg* 48:1153-1160, 1990.

49. Bass SL, Triplett RG: The effects of preoperative resorption and jaw anatomy on implant success, *Clin Oral Implants Res* 2:193-198, 1991.

50. Kuzmanovic DV, Payne AG, Kieser JA, Dias GJ: Anterior loop of the mental nerve: a morphological and radiographic study, *Clin Oral Implants Res* 14:464-471, 2003.

51. Nevins M, Langer B: The successful use of osseointegrated implants for the treatment of the recalcitrant periodontal patient, *J Periodontol* 66:150-157, 1995.

52. Klinge B, Petersson A, Maly P: Location of the mandibular canal: comparison of macroscopic findings, conventional radiography, and computed tomography, *Int J Oral Maxillofac Implants* 4:327-332, 1989.

53. Quirynen M, Bollen CM, Papaioannou W et al: The influence of titanium abutment surface roughness on plaque accumulation and gingivitis: short-term observations, *Int J Oral Maxillofac Implants* 11:169-178, 1996.

54. Buser D, Weber H, Bragger U, Balsiger C: Tissue integration of one-stage ITI implants: 3-year results of a longitudinal study with Hollow-Cylinder and Hollow-Screw implants, *Int J Oral Maxillofac Implants* 6:405-412, 1991.

55. Becker W, Becker BE, Ricci A et al: A prospective multicenter clinical trial comparing one- and two-stage titanium screw-shaped fixtures with one-stage plasma-sprayed solid-screw fixtures, *Clin Implant Dent Relat Res* 2:159-165, 2000.

56. Scharf DR, Tarnow DP: Success rates of osseointegration for implants placed under sterile versus clean conditions, *J Periodontol* 64:954-956, 1993.

57. Casino A, Harrison P, Tarnow DP et al: The influence of type of incision on the success rate of implant integration at stage II uncovering surgery, *J Oral Maxillofac Surg* 12(5):31-37, 1997.

58. Eriksson AR, Albrektsson T: Temperature threshold levels for heat-induced bone tissue injury: a vital-microscopic study in the rabbit, *J Prosthet Dent* 50:101-107, 1983.

59. Ericksson R, Adell R: Temperatures during drilling for the placement of implants using the osseointegration technique, *J Oral Maxillofac Surg* 44:4-7, 1986.

60. Brunski JB, Moccia AF, Soloman RP: The influence of functional use of endosseous dental implants on the tissue-implant interface. I. Histological aspects, *J Dent Res* 58:1953, 1965.

61. Froum S, Emtiaz S, Bloom MJ et al: The use of transitional implants for immediate fixed temporary prostheses in cases of implant restorations, *Pract Periodontics Aesthet Dent* 10:737-746, 1998.

62. Zubery Y, Bichacho N, Moses O, Tal H: Immediate loading of modular transitional implants: a histological and histomorphometric study in dogs, *Int J Periodontics Restorative Dent* 19:343-353, 1999.

63. Baumgarten HS, Salama H, Nelson A: Abutment head selection as a prosthetic discipline, *Compend Contin Educ Dent* 12:942-947, 1991.

64. Atwood D: Bone loss of edentulous alveolar ridges, *J Periodontol* 50:11-21, 1979.

65. Shanaman RH: A comparative study of 237 sites treated consecutively with guided tissue regeneration, *Int J Periodontics Restorative Dent* 14:292, 1994.

66. American Academy of Oral and Maxillofacial Surgery update: Preserving the alveolar ridge, *American Academy of Oral and Maxillofacial Surgery Update* 16(1):1-8, 2003.

67. Bowers M, Donahue J: A technique for submerging vital roots with associated intrabony defects, *Int J Periodontics Restorative Dent* 8(6):34-51, 1988.

68. Edel A: The use of a connective tissue graft for closure over an immediate implant covered with an occlusive membrane, *Clin Oral Implants Res* 6:60-65, 1995.

69. Schropp L, Kostopoulos L, Wenzel A: Bone healing following immediate versus delayed placement of titanium implants into extraction sockets: a prospective clinical study, *Int J Oral Maxillofac Implants* 18(2):189-199, 2003.

70. Garber D, Belser U: Restoration-driven implant placement with restoration-generated site development, *Compend Contin Educ Dent* 16:796-804, 1995.

71. Strub JR, Gaberthuel T, Grunder U: The role of attached gingiva in the health of periimplant tissue in dogs. Part 1 clinical findings, *Int J Periodontics Restorative Dent* 11:317, 1991.

72. Seibert J, Nyman S: Localized ridge augmentation in dogs: a pilot study using membranes and hydroxyapatite, *J Periodontol* 61:157-165, 1990.

73. Buser D, Bragger U, Lang N et al: Regeneration and enlargement of jaw bone using guided tissue regeneration, *Clin Oral Implants Res* 1:22-32, 1990.

74. Nyman S, Lang N, Buser D, Bragger U: Bone regeneration adjacent to titanium dental implants using guided tissue regeneration: a report of two cases, *Int J Oral Maxillofac Implants* 5:9-14, 1990.

75. Simion M, Baldoni M, Zaffe D: Jawbone enlargement using immediate placement associated with a split-crestal technique and guided tissue regeneration, *Int J Periodontics Restorative Dent* 12:463-473, 1992.

76. Lekholm U, Ericsson I, Adell R et al: The condition of the soft tissues at tooth and fixture abutments supporting fixed bridges. A microbiological and histological study, *J Clin Periodontol* 13:558, 1986.

77. Schenk RK, Buser D, Hardwick WR, Dahlin C: Healing pattern of bone regeneration in membrane-protected defects: a histologic study in the canine mandible, *Int J Oral Maxillofac Implants* 9:13-29, 1994.

78. Cushing M: Autogenous red marrow grafts: potential for induction of osteogenesis, *J Periodontol* 40:492-497, 2003.

79. Landsberg CJ: The reversed crestal flap: a surgical modification in endosseous implant procedures, *Quintessence Int* 25:229-232, 1994.

80. Buser D, Dula K, Belser UC et al: Localized ridge augmentation using guided bone regeneration. II. Surgical procedure in the mandible. *Int J Periodontics Restorative Dent* 15:11-29, 1995.

81. Jovanovic SA, Spiekermann H, Richter EJ: Bone regeneration around titanium dental implants in dehisced defect sites, a clinical study. *Int J Oral Maxillofac Implants* 7:233-245, 1992.

82. Scipioni A, Bruschi G, Calesini G: The edentulous ridge expansion technique: a five-year study, *Int J Periodontics Restorative Dent* 14:451-459, 1994.

83. Simion M, Dahlin C, Tiisi P, Pylant T: A qualitative and quantitative comparative study on different filling materials used for bone tissue regeneration, *Int J Periodontics Restorative Dent* 14:199-215, 1994.

84. Simion M, Jovanovic SA, Trisi P et al: A vertical ridge augmentation around dental implants using a membrane technique and bone auto or allograft in humans, *Int J Periodontics Restorative Dent* 18:9-23, 1998.

85. Simion M, Tiisi P, Pylant T: Vertical ridge augmentation using a membrane technique associated with osseointegrated implants, *Int J Periodontics Restorative Dent* 14:496-511, 1994.

86. Boyne P, Cole MD, Stringer D et al: A technique for osseous restoration of deficient edentulous maxillary ridges, *J Oral Maxillofac Surg* 45:87-91, 1985.

87. Tatum H: Maxillary and sinus implant reconstructions, *Dent Clin North Am* 30:207-229, 1986.

88. Wallace SS, Froum SJ: Effect of maxillary sinus augmentation on the survival of endosseous dental implants. A systematic literature review. American Academy of Periodontology 2003 Workshop on Contemporary Science in Clinical Periodontics. *Ann Periodontol* 8:328-343, 2003.

89. Tarnow DP, Wallace SS, Froum S et al: Histological and clinical comparison of bilateral sinus elevations with and without barrier membrane placed on 12 patients. Part 3 of an ongoing study, *Int J Periodontics Restorative Dent* 20:117-125, 2000.

90. Tawil G, Mawla M: Sinus floor elevation using a bovine bone mineral (Bio-Oss) with or without the concomitant use of a bilayered collagen barrier (Bio Gide): a clinical report of immediate and delayed implant placement, *Int J Oral Maxillofac Implants* 16:713-721, 2001.

91. Summers RB: Sinus floor elevation with osteotomes, *J Esthet Dent* 10:164-171, 1998.

92. Rosen PS, Summers RB, Mellado JR et al: Bone added osteotome sinus floor elevation technique: multicenter retrospective report of consecutively treated patients, *Int J Oral Maxillofac Implants* 14:853-858, 1999.

93. Lazzara RJ: The sinus elevation procedure in endosseous implant therapy, *Curr Opin Periodontol* 3:178-183, 1996.

94. Saadoun AP, LeGall M, Triplett RG: Selection and ideal tridimensional implant position for soft tissue aesthetics, *Pract Periodontics Aesthet Dent* 12:1063-1072, 1999.

95. Grunder U: Stability of the mucosal topography around single-tooth implants and adjacent teeth: 1 yr. results, *Int J Periodontics Restorative Dent* 20:11-17, 2000.

96. Small PN, Tarnow DP: Gingival recession around implants: a 1 year longitudinal prospective study, *Int J Oral Maxillofac Implants* 15:527-532, 2000.

97. Holt RL, Rosenberg MM, Zinser PJ, Ganeles J: A concept for a biologically derived, parabolic implant design, *Int J Periodontics Restorative Dent* 22:473-481, 2002.

98. Choquet V, Hermans M, Adriaenssens P et al: Clinical and radiographic evaluation of the papilla level adjacent to single tooth dental implants. A retrospective study in the maxillary anterior region, *J Periodontol* 72:1364-1371, 2001.

99. Tarnow DP, Cho SC, Wallace SS: The effect of inter-implant distance on the height of inter-implant bone crest, *J Periodontol* 71:546-549, 2000.

100. Gelb DA: Immediate implant surgery: three-year retrospective evaluation of 50 consecutive cases, *Int J Oral Maxillofac Implants* 8:388-399, 1993.

101. Mensdorff-Pouilly N, Haas R, Mailath G, Watzek G: The immediate implant. A retrospective study comparing the different types of immediate implantation, *Int J Oral Maxillofac Implants* 9:571-578, 1994.

102. Rosenquist B, Grenthe B: Immediate placement of implants into extraction sockets: implant survival, *Int J Oral Maxillofac Implants* 11:205-209, 1996.

103. Grunder U, Polizzi G, Goene R et al: A 3 year prospective multicenter follow-up report on the immediate and delayed immediate placement of implants, *Int J Oral Maxillofac Implants* 14:210-216, 1999.

104. Babbush CA, Kent JN, Misiek DJ: Titanium plasma-sprayed screw implants for the reconstruction of the edentulous mandible, *J Oral Maxillofac Surg* 44:274-282, 1986.

105. Schnitman PA, Wohrle PS, Rubenstein JE, et al: 10-year results for Branemark implants immediately loaded with fixed prosthesis at implant placement. *Int J Oral Maxillofac Implants* 12:495-503, 1997.

106. Lum LB, Beirne OR, Curtis DA: Histologic evaluation of HA coated versus uncoated titanium blade implants in delayed and immediately loaded applications, *Int J Oral Maxillofac Implants* 6:456-462, 1991.

107. Sagara M, Yasumasa A, Hiromasa N, Hiromichi T: The effects of early occlusal loading on one-stage titanium alloy implants in beagle dogs, *J Prosthet Dent* 69:281-288, 1993.

108. Wohrle PS: Single-tooth replacement in the aesthetic zone with immediate provisionalization: fourteen consecutive case reports, *Pract Periodontics Aesthet Dent* 10:1107-1114, 1998.

109. Ericsson I, Nilson H, Lindh T et al: Immediate functional loading of Branemark single tooth implants. An 18 month clinical pilot follow-up study, *Clin Oral Implants Res* 11:26-33, 2000.

110. Schnitman PA, Wohrle PS, Rubenstein JE et al: Ten year results for Branemark implants immediately loaded with fixed prostheses at implant placement, *Int J Oral Maxillofac Implants* 12:495-503, 1997.

111. Tarnow DP, Emitiaz S, Classi A: Immediate loading of threaded implants at stage 1 surgery in edentulous arches: ten consecutive case reports with 1 to 5 year data, *Int J Oral Maxillofac Implants* 12:319-324, 1997.

112. Grunder U: Immediate functional loading of immediate implants in edentulous arches: two-year results, *Int J Periodontics Restorative Dent* 21:545-551, 2001.

113. Brånemark PI, Breine U, Lindstrom J et al: Intra-osseous anchorage of dental prostheses. I. Experimental studies, *Scand J Plastic Reconstructive Surg* 3:81-100, 1969.

114. Schroeder A, van der Zypen E, Stich H, Sutter F: The reaction of bone, connective tissue and epithelium to endosteal implants with sprayed titanium surfaces, *J Oral Maxillofac Surg* 9:15-25, 1981.

115. Buser D, Schroeder A, Sutter F, Lang N: The new concept of ITI hollow-cylinder and hollow-screw implants: part 2. Clinical aspects, indications and early clinical results, *Int J Oral Maxillofac Implants* 3:173-181, 1988.

116. Buser D, Weber H, Lang NP: Tissue integration of non-submerged implants. 1-year results of a prospective study with 100 hollow-cylinder and hollow-screw implants, *Clin Oral Implants Res* 1:33-40, 1990.

117. Brunski J: Biomechanical factors affecting the bone-dental implant interface, *Clin Mater* 10:153-201, 1992.

118. Kirsch A, Donath K: Tier-experimentelle untersuchungen zur bedeutung der mikromorphologie titaniumplantataberflachen, *Fortschr Zahnarztl Implantol* 1:35-40, 1984.

119. Misch CE: Density of bone: effect on treatment plans, surgical approach, healing, and progressive loading, *Int J Oral Maxillofac Implants* 6:23-31, 1990.

120. Skolak R: Aspects of biomechanical considerations. In Branemark PI, Zarb G, Albrektsson T, editors: *Tissue integrated prosthesis: Osseointegration in clinical dentistry*, Chicago, Quintessence Publishing, pp. 117-128, 1985.

121. Brunski J, Skolak R: Biomechanics of osseointegration and dental prostheses. In Naert I, van Steenberghe D, Worthington P, editors: *Osseointegration and oral rehabilitation: an introductory textbook*, Chicago, Quintessence Publishing, pp. 133-156, 1993.

122. Roberts WG, Garetto L, DeCastro R: Remodeling of devitalized bone threatens periosteal margin integrity of endosseous titanium implants with threaded or smooth surfaces: indications for provisional loading and axially directed occlusion, *J Indiana Dent Assoc* 68(4):19-24, 1989.

123. Baumgarten H, Chiche G: Diagnosis and evaluation of complications and failures associated with osseointegrated implants, *Compend Contin Educ Dent* 16:814-822, 1995.

124. Jovanovic SA: Plaque induced periimplant bone loss in mongrel dogs. A clinical, microbial, radiographic and histological study, Los Angeles, Calif, 1994, University of California, Los Angeles (Master's thesis).

125. Lindhe J, Berglundh T, Ericsson I et al: Experimental breakdown of peri-implant and periodontal tissues—a study in the beagle dog, *Clin Oral Implants Res* 3:9-16, 1992.

126. Sanz M, Newman M, Nachnani S et al: Characterization of the subgingival microbial flora around endosteal dental implants in partially edentulous patients, *Int J Oral Maxillofac Implants* 5:247-253, 1990.

127. Golec TS, Krauser JT: Long-term retrospective studies on hydroxyapatite-coated endosteal and subperiosteal implants, *Dent Clin North Am* 36:39-65, 1992.

128. Johnson B: HA-coated dental implants: long term consequences, *J Calif Dent Assoc* 20:33, 1992.

129. Jovanovic SA, Kenney EB, Carranza FA, Donath K: The regenerative potential of plaque-induced periimplant bone defects treated by a submerged membrane technique. An experimental study, *Int J Oral Maxillofac Implants* 8:13-18, 1993.

130. Mombelli A: Microbiology of the dental implant, *Adv Dent Res* 7:202-206, 1993.

131. Jovanovic SA, James RA, Lessard G: Bacterial morphotypes and PGE2 levels from the perigingival site of dental implants with intact and compromised bone support, *J Dent Res* 67:28, 1988.

132. Lekholm U, Ericsson I, Adell R et al: The condition of the soft tissues at tooth and fixture abutments supporting fixed bridges. A microbiological and histological study, *J Clin Periodontol* 13:558, 1986.

133. Mombelli A, Marxer M, Gaberthuel T et al: The microbiota of osseointegrated implants in patients with a history of periodontal disease, *J Clin Periodontol* 22:124, 1995.

134. Naert I, Quirynen M, van Steenberghe D, Darius P: A study of 589 consecutive implants supporting complete fixed prosthesis. Part II: prosthetic aspects, *J Prosthet Dent* 68:949-956, 1992.

135. Quirynen M, van Steenberghe D, Jacobs R et al: The reliability of pocket probing around screw-type implants, *Clin Oral Implants Res* 2:186-192, 1991.

136. Lang N, Karring T: *Proceedings of the 1st European Workshop on Periodontology*, London, 1994, Quintessence Publishing.

137. Quirynen M, Marechal M, Busscher HJ et al: The influence of surface free energy and surface roughness on early plaque formation, *J Clin Periodontol* 17:138-144, 1990.

138. Polson AM, Sharkey D, Minsk L et al: Two-year alveolar bone levels of dental implants after immediate loading. International Association for Dental Research, April 2000, Washington, D.C.

139. Salama H, Rose LF, Betts NJ: Immediate loading of bilaterally splinted titanium root-form implants in fixed prosthodontics: a technique re-examined. Two case reports, *Int J Periodontics Restorative Dent* 15:345-361, 1995.

140. Thompson-Neal D, Evans G, Meffert RM: Effects of various prophylactic treatments on titanium, sapphire, and hydroxyapatite coated implants. An SEM study, *Int J Periodontics Restorative Dent* 9:300-311, 1989.

141. Krauser JT, Berthold P, Tamery I et al: A SEM study of failed endosseous root formed dental implants, *J Dent Res* 70:274, 1991.

142. Jovanovic SA, Spiekermann H, Richter EJ et al: Guided tissue regeneration around titanium dental implants. In Laney WR, Tolmen DE, editors: *Tissue integration in oral, orthopedic and maxillofacial reconstruction*, Chicago, 1992, Quintessence.

143. Lehmann B, Bragger U, Hammerle CH et al: Treatment of an early implant failure according to the principles of guided tissue regeneration, *Clin Oral Implants Res* 3(1):42-48, 1992.

144. Meffert RM: Treatment of the ailing, failing implants, *J Calif Dent Assoc* 20:42, 1992.

145. Newman M, Flemmig T: Periodontal considerations of implants and implant associated microbiota, *Int J Oral Implantol* 5:737-744, 1988.

146. Dennison DK, Huerzeler MB, Quinones C, Caffesse RG: Contaminated implant surfaces: an in vitro comparison of implant surface coating and treatment modalities for decontamination. *J Periodontol* 65:942-948, 1994.

147. Bain CA, Moy PK: The association between the failure of dental implants and cigarette smoking, *Int J Oral Maxillofac Implants* 8:609-615, 1993.

148. Bain CA, Weng D, Meltzer A et al: A meta-analysis evaluating the risk for implant failure in patients who smoke. *Compend Contin Educ Dent* 23:695-699, 702, 704, 2002.

149. Rangert B, Jemt T, Jorneus L: Forces and moments on Branemark implants, *Int J Oral Maxillofac Implants* 4:241-247, 1989.

150. Weinberg LA: The biomechanics of force distribution on implant supported prostheses, *Int J Oral Maxillofac Implants* 8:19-31, 1993.

151. Brunski J: Biomechanics of oral implants: future research directions, *J Dent Educ* 52:775-787, 1988.

152. Hadeen G, Ismail Y, Garrana H et al: Three dimensional finite element stress analysis of Nobelpharma and Core-Vent implants and their supporting structures, *J Dent Res* 67:286, 1998.

153. Waskewics GA, Ostrowski JS, Parks VJ: Photoelastic analysis of stress distribution transmitted from a fixed prosthesis attached to osseointegrated implants, *Int J Oral Maxillofac Implants* 9:405-411, 1994.

154. Pylant T, Triplett RG, Key MC, Brunsvold MA: A retrospective evaluation of endosseous titanium implants in the partially edentulous patient, *Int J Oral Maxillofac Implants* 7:195-202, 1992.

155. Jemt T, Lekholm U: Oral implant treatment in posterior partially edentulous jaws: a 5-year follow-up report, *Int J Oral Maxillofac Implants* 8:635-640, 1993.

156. Bahat O: Treatment planning and placement of implants in the posterior maxillae: report of 732 consecutive Nobelpharma Implants, *Int J Oral Maxillofac Implants* 8:151-161, 1993.

157. Gunne J, Rangert B, Glantz PO, Svensson A: Functional loads on freestanding and connected implants in three-unit mandibular prostheses opposing complete dentures: an in vivo study, *Int J Oral Maxillofac Implants* 12:335-341, 1997.

158. Sheets C, Earthmann J: Natural tooth intrusion and reversal in implant-assisted prosthesis: evidence of and a hypothesis for the occurrence, *J Prosthet Dent* 70:513-520, 1993.

159. English C: Root intrusion in tooth-implant combination cases, *Implant Dent* 2:79-85, 1993.

Part IV

Multidisciplinary Care

John Kois, Louis F. Rose, and Brian L. Mealey

27

Restoration of the Periodontally Compromised Dentition

Arnold S. Weisgold and Neil L. Starr

Portions of this chapter are from Starr NL: Treatment planning and treatment sequencing with and without endosseous implants: a comprehensive therapeutic approach to the partially edentulous patient, *Seattle Study Club Journal* 1:1, 21-34, 1995.

The term *periodontal prosthesis*[1,2] was coined by Amsterdam about 50 years ago. He defined periodontal prostheses as "those restorative and prosthetic endeavors that are absolutely essential in the treatment of advanced periodontal disease." New, more sophisticated techniques are currently available, and with the advent of endosseous implants[3] many patients can avoid wearing a removable prosthesis, or at least have one that is extremely stable. Nevertheless, the concepts of identifying the etiologic risk factors, establishing an accurate diagnosis and prognosis, formulating an interdisciplinary treatment plan, and developing a logical sequence of therapy hold as true today as they did five decades ago. In this new millennium, the philosophy of periodontal prosthesis has gained universal acceptance as the foundation of interdisciplinary dental therapeutics.

NATURAL DENTITION

The major goal of the dentist is the preservation and maintenance of the natural dentition in a state of health. With increased use of the endosseous implant, it appears at times that some in the profession have lost sight of this *major* responsibility. In the past, teeth with a poor or guarded prognosis were frequently maintained, whereas today there is an option to extract them and replace them with dental implants. The concern, however, is knowing when to save or extract a tooth. In light of the observations of many astute clinicians, developing a treatment plan that will provide the best long-term prognosis is a challenge in the advanced periodontally involved dentition. If anything has been learned from the retention of these severely compromised teeth, it has been the healing potential of the periodontium once the known etiologic risk factors are eliminated or controlled.[4]

IMPACT OF ESTHETICS

Esthetics and osseointegration were developing on parallel paths during the mid-1980s to early 1990s and have emphasized the importance of the integrated team approach to achieve the ultimate periodontal and restorative result. Maintaining the papilla between two teeth is somewhat predictable,[5] but between a tooth and an adjacent implant is less predictable.[6,7] Concern for the loss of or reduction in height of the papilla between two adjacent implants has created a new esthetic concern.[8] Therefore, the concepts of selective extraction of teeth, socket preservation, and augmentation at the time of tooth extraction appear to be invaluable in the restoration of form, function, and esthetics[9-14] (see Chapter 26).

Esthetics play a major role in our diagnostic and therapeutic endeavors. However, long-term clinical assessments have shown that its real value will play out optimally when it is achieved in concert with all the functional needs of the dentition.

PERIODONTAL BIOTYPES

Ochsenbein and Ross,[15] Weisgold,[16] and Olsson and Lindhe[17] suggested two distinct types of periodontium found in humans. Becker and colleagues[18] reported that there are three periodontal biotypes: flat, scalloped, and pronounced scalloped. Measuring from the height of the bone interproximally to the height at the direct midfacial, their findings were as follows: flat = 2.1 mm; scalloped = 2.8 mm; and pronounced scalloped = 4.1 mm. *Note that the distance in the pronounced scalloped is approximately twice as great as in the flat type.* Normally, the distance from the cementoenamel junction (CEJ) to the crest of bone on the direct facial in a healthy periodontium of a young adult is approximately 2 mm, with the gingival margin being located on the enamel (slightly coronal to the CEJ). However, in the pronounced scalloped type, the distance between CEJ and the bone on the direct facial is usually 3 to 4 mm. This results in the gingival margin being located at the CEJ, or quite often, on the cementum—that is, in the pronounced scalloped type, the gingival margin is, in a sense, located on the root in health. This type of periodontium, because of its thinness and friability, is more likely to recede than the flat type. There is no question that the most favorable gingival and esthetic results occur in the flat type, not the pronounced scalloped type (Fig. 27-1; Boxes 27-1 and 27-2).

Tarnow and colleagues[5] observed that in healthy mouths the gingival papilla filled the space between teeth 100% of the time when the distance from the contact point of adjacent teeth to the interproximal crest of bone was 5 mm or less. When the distance was 6 mm, the papilla did not fill the space completely in approximately 50% of the patients, and when it was 7 mm or more, it did not fill the space in about 75% of the cases. The pronounced scalloped periodontal biotype (because of its triangular-shaped tooth) usually has a distance between 6 and 7 mm. Hence, under normal conditions, this is the tissue type that usually has some interproximal recession with the formation of "black triangles". Further clinical insults to soft tissue, such as tooth preparation, excessively rapid orthodontic tooth movement, tooth extraction, scaling and root planing, and injudicious retraction of soft tissue may increase the gingival recession, thus further compromising the esthetic result (Fig. 27-2).

The extraction of an anterior tooth usually results in resorption of bone on the facial and interproximal surface (Fig. 27-3). In addition, a decrease in the faciolingual dimension of the interproximal areas is not uncommon. These findings are more obvious in the scalloped type of periodontium, and even more so, in the pronounced

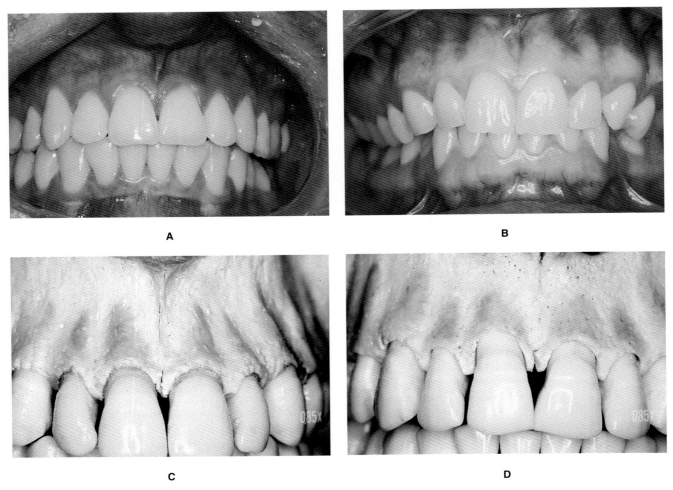

Figure 27-1. A, Thin-scalloped periodontal biotype. **B,** Thick-flat periodontal biotype. **C,** Thick-flat skull material. **D,** Thin-scalloped skull material. (*Courtesy Dr. Clifford Ochsenbein, Dallas, Tx.*)

Box 27-1 | Description of Thin/Scalloped Periodontal Biotype

- Distinct disparity between height of gingival margin on direct facial and that interproximally
- Delicate and friable soft tissue curtain
- Underlying osseous form scalloped, dehiscences and fenestrations often present
- Small amount of attached masticatory mucosa (quantitative and qualitative)
- Reacts to insult by recession
- Subtle, diminutive convexities in cervical thirds of facial surfaces
- Contact areas of adjacent teeth located decidedly toward the incisal or occlusal thirds
- Teeth "triangular" in shape
- Contact areas of adjacent teeth small faciolingually and incisogingivally
- Steeper posterior cusps

Box 27-2 | Description of Thick/Flat Periodontal Biotype

- Not as great a disparity between height of gingival margin on direct facial and that interproximally
- Denser, more fibrotic soft tissue curtain
- Underlying osseous form flatter and thicker
- Larger amount of attached masticatory mucosa (quantitative and qualitative)
- Reacts to insult by increased pocket depth
- More prominent, bulbous convexities in cervical thirds of facial surfaces
- Contact areas of adjacent teeth located more toward the apical
- Teeth "square" in shape
- Contact areas of adjacent teeth larger faciolingually and incisogingivally
- Flatter posterior cusps

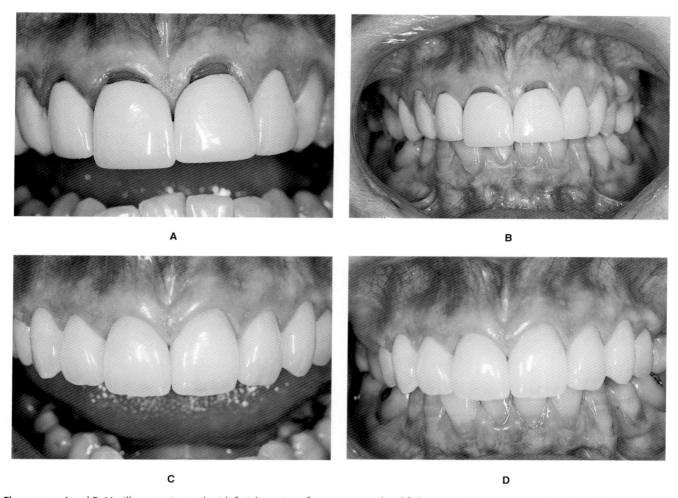

A   B

C   D

Figure 27-2. **A** and **B,** Maxillary anterior teeth with facial margins of crowns exposed and failing composite restorations. **C** and **D,** All ceramic crowns for maxillary anterior teeth, respecting the gingiva and harmonizing with the gingival topography.

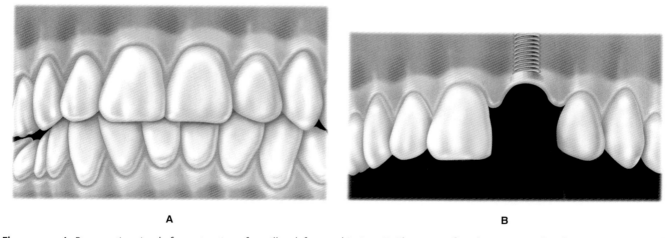

A   B

Figure 27-3. **A,** Preoperative view before extraction of maxillary left central incisor. **B,** Placement of implant at 2 months after extraction. Note the recession of the interproximal papillae.

Continued

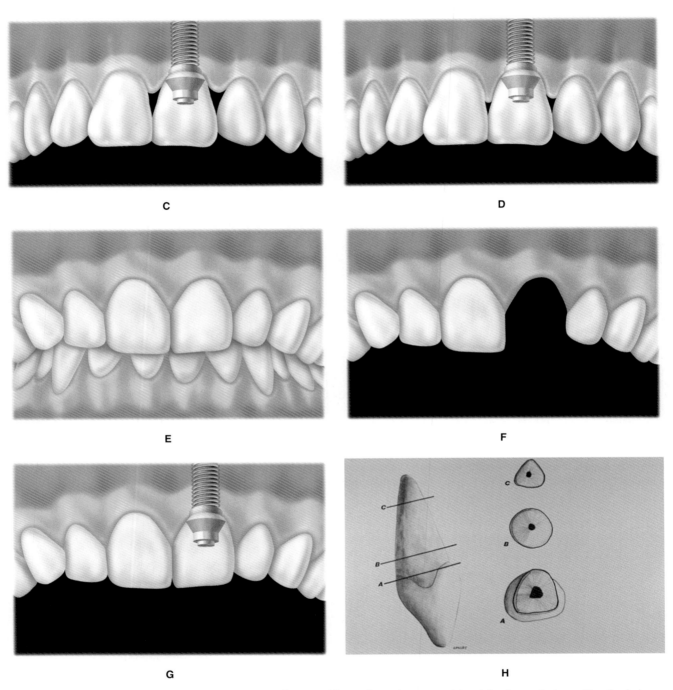

Figure 27-3. cont'd C, Insertion of final crown ("black" triangles). **D,** Addition of porcelain on mesial and distal—results in masking the dark areas, but also a wider crown. **E,** Preoperative view before extraction of maxillary left central incisor. **F,** Two months after extraction. Note there is little to no papillary recession. **G,** Placement of final crown. Note that esthetic result compares favorably to preextraction **(E). H,** Diagram illustrating the cross-sectional forms of a maxillary central incisor. Note it is triangular at the cementoenamel junction.

Continued

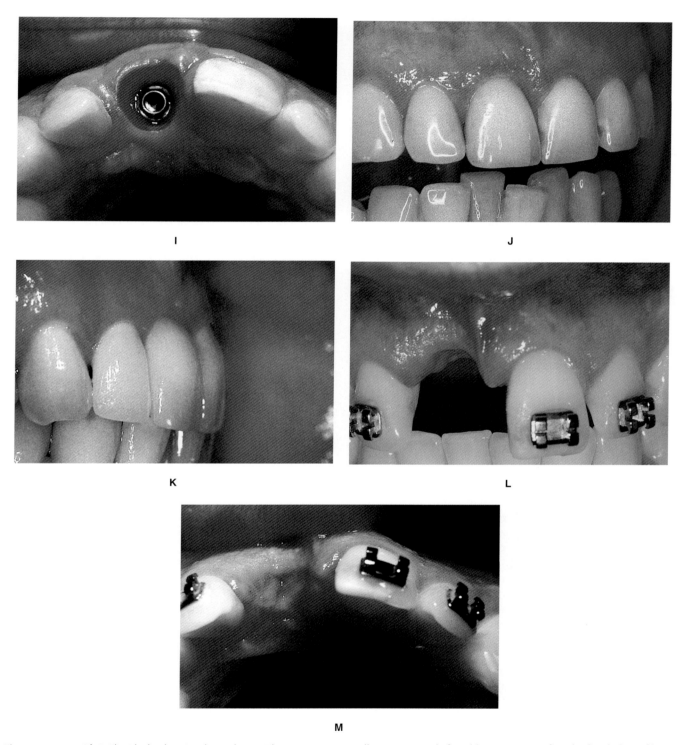

Figure 27-3. cont'd **I,** The ideal sulcus/implant relation. This situation is usually not commonly found because most often the facial plate of bone and interproximal areas resorb somewhat. **J,** Maxillary right central incisor. The ideal artificial crown/implant/periodontal relationship. **K,** Maxillary right central incisor. Note there are ceramo-metal crowns on the right lateral incisor and left central incisor natural tooth. The right central incisor crown is on an implant. Note the slight "ridge lap" in cervical because ridge is slightly resorbed on the facial surface and out of necessity the implant is placed toward the palatal area. **L,** Facial view showing resorbed ridge in maxillary right central incisor area. Note vertical deficiency. **M,** Incisal view of the same area. Note deficiency faciopalatally.

scalloped type. This may create an esthetic dilemma for both the patient and the dentist. Complicating the matter is that the morphology of the roots of the anterior teeth is usually more tapered, both faciolingually and mesiodistally than those found in the flat type periodontium. The end result of extracting an anterior tooth with a scalloped type periodontium is: (1) Greater loss of interproximal hard and soft tissues; (2) the interproximal papillae are positioned more palatally; and (3) a wider mesiodistal dimension between the adjacent teeth (because of the taper of their roots). The outcome is a large noticeable "black triangle," which is often treated by closing the space with a wider crown or laminate[19] placed on the adjacent teeth, or the use of pink porcelain to simulate the lost gingiva. Often these options are not satisfactory.

ROLE OF OCCLUSION

Success in occlusal therapy depends on controlling the etiologic factors that cause the problem (see Chapter 29). Unfortunately, occlusal disorders, at times, originate from a host of seemingly disparate, random factors. This led us to rely often on inadequate data and unproven techniques. Compounding the problem is the tendency to "mix vocabularies"—that is, giving different definitions for the same thing—and to commonly use different terminology (e.g., centric relation, centric occlusal relation, maximum intercuspal position, retruded contact position, and so on).

Occlusal trauma is injury to the attachment apparatus resulting from tooth-to-tooth contact, oral musculature activities, or foreign object to tooth contacts. *It is the failure of the supporting structure to resist or to adapt to these forces.*[20] Clinically, the most common finding is tooth mobility, and, radiographically, widened periodontal ligament spaces of the involved teeth are often seen.

Primary occlusal trauma can occur in a healthy mouth or one affected by periodontal disease. It is caused by forces greater than those that occur during normal function. It is usually caused by a parafunctional habit (i.e., bruxism, clenching, and other habits).[1,2,21] It is thought that mastication is not a source of primary trauma because of the minimal amount of time devoted to this activity, subsequently minimizing tooth contact, and the buffering capability of the periodontal ligament. Removal or controlling of the forces should result in the reversal of the effects of primary traumatism.

Secondary occlusal trauma is usually associated with a periodontally compromised dentition that has resulted in severe bone loss and teeth with adverse crown-to-root ratios. Usually, the teeth are very mobile; therefore, the teeth are subjected to continued injury with normal forces such as mastication or deglutition, or both. It is

here where periodontal prosthesis is usually indicated. The splinting of teeth with partial or full coverage crowns is indicated in most cases.[1,2,22] Successful management of periodontal disease and occlusal trauma is the goal of periodontal prosthetics.

Posterior bite collapse is the result of the loss of one or more posterior teeth, with drifting of adjacent teeth, extrusion of opposing teeth, and the creation of uneven marginal ridge relations and adjacent CEJ levels, and concomitant unleveled bony crests. These events establish an environment where the self-protective capacity of the teeth is compromised; resulting in the development of angular bony crests frequently predisposing to infrabony pocket formation and posterior interproximal caries. The occlusal vertical dimension is supported by the posterior occlusion but with posterior tooth loss, the forces of occlusion are on the remaining anterior teeth. In addition, the remaining anterior teeth must provide anterior guidance, disarticulating the posterior teeth through excursive movements of the mandible. This will have a significant impact on their long-term function and viability.[23]

When posterior bite collapse has occurred, the restoration of form and function is more difficult to accomplish. Posterior occlusion must be reestablished, the occlusal vertical dimension restored and the anterior incisal guidance developed in concert with the posterior cusp height. This should allow for disarticulation of the posterior teeth during excursive movements of the mandible.

Given the abundance of research data and good clinical documentation,[24-33] important questions relative to occlusal etiology and the effects that trauma has on the progression of existing periodontal disease may be answered. Ultimately, this will establish a more "outcome-based" approach to occlusal therapy. For example, when the patient is periodontally susceptible and the posterior teeth in the same arch are seriously compromised or missing, the remaining anterior teeth may be stressed unfavorably, demonstrating varying degrees of mobility.[23] Placing posterior implants with fixed/splinted crown and bridgework is the preferred treatment for this patient type.[23] The restoration of the posterior occlusion at the correct occlusal vertical dimension can significantly decrease or eliminate the mobility patterns present in the anterior teeth and thereby help to stabilize them.

One must not downplay the role of occlusion evidenced by the manifestation of occlusal trauma on the endosseous implant prosthesis and its component parts. This is often a more common observance than damage to the surrounding bone or the implant. Without the cushioning effect of the periodontal ligament, the forces have a greater potential to cause breakage of the prosthetic parts, or of the implant to bone contact itself.[34]

TREATMENT PLANNING AND TREATMENT SEQUENCING WITH AND WITHOUT ENDOSSEOUS IMPLANTS: A COMPREHENSIVE THERAPEUTIC APPROACH TO THE PARTIALLY EDENTULOUS PATIENT

The ultimate therapeutic goal is to achieve maximum health, masticatory function, speech, aesthetics, and comfort for the patients.[35]

The treatment can be divided into three levels:

1. Emergency care for relief of pain or sudden dysfunction
2. Removal of the causative factors of the disease processes
3. Removal of the consequences of the disease or traumatic insult

Level one, emergency treatment, must be accomplished before any other level of therapy is instituted (Table 27-1).

The purpose of the second level is to control infection. A basic tenet of periodontal therapy is the debridement of all accretions adherent to the clinical crowns and roots of teeth or restorative materials, both supragingivally and subgingivally. This is accomplished by scaling and root planing procedures in concert with oral hygiene instruction. If dental caries is present, the early placement of "direct-filling" restorations prevents the need for more extensive intervention later. In addition, the control of adverse occlusal forces should be managed at this level.

The third level of care is the focus of this chapter: attempting to correct alterations in form and function because of the effects of periodontal infections and traumatic injury to the teeth and their supporting tissues.

Diagnostic Evaluation

Diagnosis, treatment planning, and treatment sequencing continue to be significant challenges for the general dentist and specialist in the management of the partially edentulous patient. A comprehensive dental/periodontal examination must first be performed. This will ensure that all members of the treating team have addressed each problem area and have collated their respective treatments into the overall therapeutic program.

The clinical evaluation consists of caries, periodontal, endodontic, orthodontic, orthognathic, occlusal and temporomandibular joint exams, as well as a comprehensive physical evaluation or medical history (Box 27-3). To facilitate this diagnostic evaluation, a full-mouth series of periapical radiographs of teeth and residual ridges must be obtained. A panoramic radiograph, a cephalometric radiograph, and a dental computed axial tomography (CAT) scan[36] are suggested if there is a need to help assess the bone quality and quantity, and supplement conventional dental radiography.

Impressions should be taken and models correctly articulated. In most situations, it is suggested that two sets of the original casts be obtained—one to be kept as a permanent record and the other to be used as part of the treatment planning. After gathering the necessary data, the information must be collated into a comprehensive treatment program.

Amsterdam[1,2] has stated that although the situation truly requiring periodontal prosthesis traditionally has been one of advanced dental disease, it became apparent that with certain modifications, its philosophy, concepts, principles, and techniques could be applied to any therapeutic endeavor involving the natural dentition.

Esthetic Treatment Approach

When a patient's needs are primarily restoratively focused, such as veneering or crowning one or more teeth (Fig. 27-4), gingival aesthetic guidelines (Fig. 27-5) will be a significant component of the overall effort. In order to properly address the esthetic requirements of the patient, it is necessary to envision the desired outcome before performing the procedure.[37]

Esthetics is fundamentally about tooth form, and it is therefore most predictably realized with the assistance of an intraoral diagnostic "mock-up" to improve incisal form, lip line esthetics, and gingival topography (Fig. 27-6). The outcome is the development of an intraoral esthetic

TABLE 27-1	Emergency Treatments	
PROBLEM	**TREATMENT CATEGORY**	**TREATMENT**
• Deep/extensive caries	• Sedative restorations	• "Direct-filling" or temporary crowns
• Occlusal trauma or myofascial pain syndrome	• Occlusal therapy	• Selective adjustment, appliance therapy, antiinflammatory medication
• Large circumscribing periodontal/periapical lesions	• Extraction of hopeless teeth	• Interim fixed or removable restoration as necessary
• Broken appliances	• Prosthetic repair	• Reestablish masticatory function and esthetics

Box 27-3   Diagnosis

Caries

- Supragingival
- Subgingival
- Insufficient clinical crown height

Endodontic Considerations

- Symptomatic teeth
- Separated endodontic instruments
- Dystrophic calcifications
- Fractured roots
- Apical and lateral zones of osseous rarefaction
- Status of existing posts/cores

Esthetics

- Smile analysis
- Lip line analysis
- Gingival topography assessment
- Incisal plane assessment

Malocclusion

- Loss of occlusal vertical dimension

Missing teeth

- Without replacement
- With delayed replacement

Occlusal Trauma

- Primary
  - Bruxism
  - Clenching
  - Retrograde wear
- Secondary
- Temporomandibular joint considerations

Orthodontics

- Tooth drifting or bite collapse

Periodontal Disease[107]

- Degree of bone loss
- Topography of alveolar defect (potential impact of bone loss on adjacent teeth)
- Classification of periodontal biotypes

Size and Shape of Residual Deformed Bony Ridge Areas

- The degree of resorption will influence the surgical and restorative ventures

Medical Status

- Systemic disorders
- Psychologic concerns

Traumatic Injury

- Clinical crown deformity
- Soft and hard tissue deformities
- Facial deformity

Developmental/Acquired Deformities

- Cleft palate, cleft lip
- Amelogenesis imperfecta, other deformities

---

blueprint. This results in dentist verification, improved laboratory communication, and patient affirmation. Molds of the improved intraoral anatomic form of the teeth should be poured in stone, and then enhanced further in the dental laboratory with the application of wax. Silicone impressions are fabricated by the laboratory and then returned to the clinician to be used to verify proper tooth reduction.[37]

The incorporation of one single-tooth implant and crown, together with a series of all ceramic crowns or veneers for the adjacent natural teeth, creates a great challenge for the clinician and dental ceramist.[9] Endosseous implant installation requires careful staging, in accordance with the healing time frames associated with tissue maturation. The addition of bone and soft tissue at or after tooth extraction, or tooth lengthening by restorative and/or surgical measures to achieve esthetic outcomes, requires even greater interdisciplinary planning (Box 27-4).

DENTAL THERAPEUTICS: WITHOUT IMPLANTS

Amsterdam[1,2] has stated that "the correction or modification of the deformities created by the disease may be much more complicated in therapy than the treatment of the active disease process."

To establish a diagnosis in more compromised situations, it is important to ascertain the patient's history of tooth loss. A host of etiologic factors may have contributed to tooth loss, such as caries, subsequent endodontic complications, traumatic injuries to teeth (and/or alveolus), periodontal disease, occlusal trauma, and iatrogenic dentistry.

Many teeth may serve as strong viable abutments. However, teeth substantially affected by periodontal disease, caries, or endodontic problems must be identified early because they may have minimal value as abutments for either individual crowns or splinted restorations. These

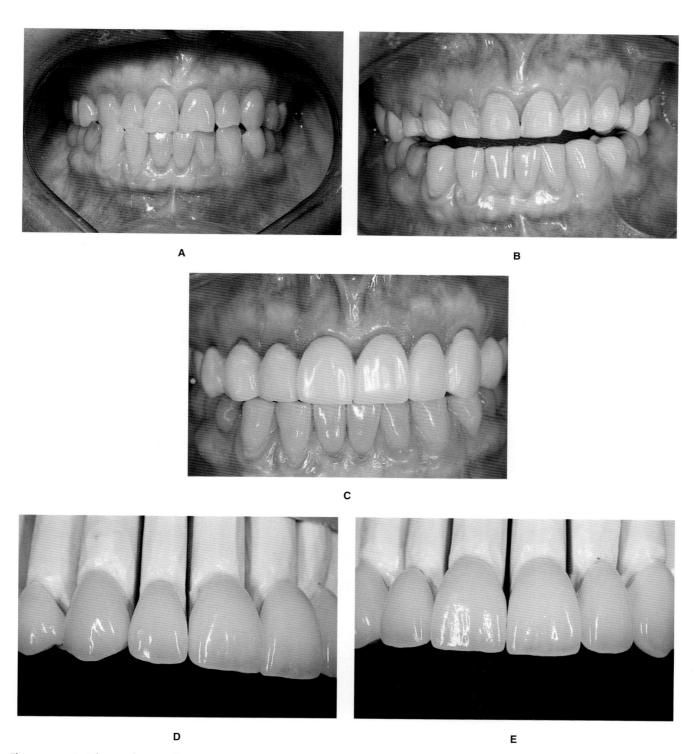

Figure 27-4. A, Edge-to-edge maxillary incisor relation with crossbite at teeth #26, #27, and #28, demonstrating marked incisal wear. The dentoskeletal Class III arrangement (with thin lip form) exaggerates the flat facial profile. **B,** After performing a diagnostic composite mock-up, directed at creating anterior guidance, building out the teeth to enhance the facial profile, and improving the incisal edge relation to the lower lip, the maxillary teeth were prepared to receive ceramic veneers. The incisal edges of the mandibular teeth were reshaped by odontoplasty to create the proper overbite–overjet relation. **C,** Interim provisional acrylic veneer restorations. **D-F,** All ceramic veneers are on master stone model.

Continued

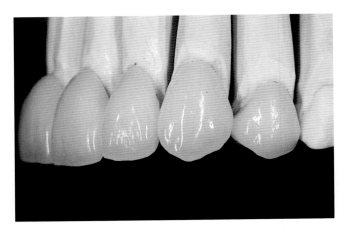

F

G

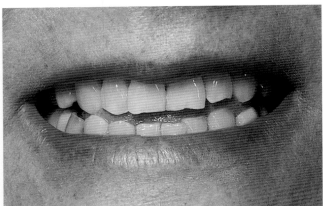

H

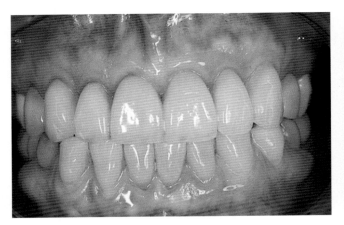

I

Figure 27-4. cont'd G, Final ceramic veneers for the maxillary teeth, with restored occlusal function and improved dental esthetics and facial aesthetics. **H,** Preoperative smile profile. **I,** Final ceramic veneers with smile profile.

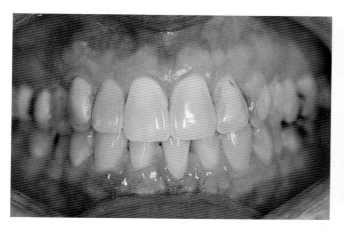

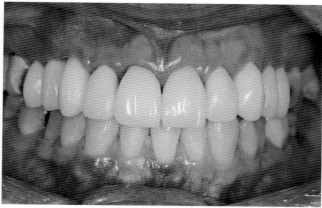

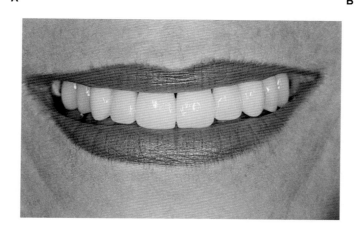

Figure 27-5. A, Mottled enamel with marked discoloration and recurrent caries. **B,** Provisional acrylic restorations to restore form, function, and esthetics for the involved maxillary teeth. **C,** Smile photograph of the provisional acrylic restorations, creating both gingival and incisal balance with patient's lips and facial form.

teeth also may represent a serious periodontal liability to adjacent teeth.

When sophisticated dental therapy can be managed without the use of endosseous implants, the approach to treatment can be subdivided into periodontal, orthodontic/orthognathic surgery, occlusal, and restorative phases. These phases are interdependent, even if one may initially have precedence over another, or if two or more of the phases are initiated concurrently (Box 27-5).

The objective of periodontal therapy is directed toward eliminating the inflammatory process and establishing bone and soft tissue healing. Amsterdam[1,2] has noted that this is most predictably accomplished for teeth of normal anatomic root lengths with probing depths not exceeding 4 to 7 mm as measured from the CEJ (Fig. 27-7). The added advantage with this osseous surgical approach has been to increase the clinical crown length, thereby pro-

viding a final crown design with sufficient biomechanical retention/resistance.

When teeth require subgingival preparation to be treated with full coverage restorations, it is important to evaluate the mucogingival environment and determine the value of re-creating or enhancing the gingival tissues. Autogenous gingival grafts, subepithelial connective tissue grafts, and repositioning of an existing gingival complex are procedures commonly used.

The orthodontic phase strives to improve tooth alignment, to erupt fractured or impacted teeth, or to facilitate the extrusion of teeth with infrabony defects.[38] With these cases, it is prudent to consider a mucogingival procedure before tooth movement if a minimal zone of attached gingiva exists on the facial or lingual surface. This eliminates the concern regarding recession during orthodontic treatment.

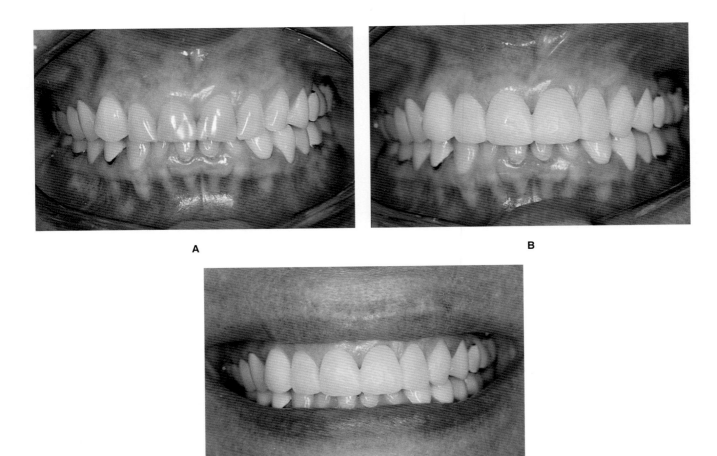

Figure 27-6. **A,** Preoperative worn dentition. **B,** Full view of composite mock-up. **C,** Composite mock-up of lip line smile.

Box 27-4 | Esthetic Considerations and Ceramic Restorations

I. Emergency Treatment

A. Restore Anatomic/Clinical Crowns
- Fabrication of provisional acrylic restorations or application of composite bonding to restore form

B. Endodontic Treatment
- Fractured teeth
- Pulpal involvement
- Periapical infection

II. Initial Therapy
- Debridement of plaque and calculus deposits adherent to clinical crowns and roots of teeth or restorative materials both supra and subgingivally
- Oral hygiene instruction

III. Intraoral Digital Imaging and Diagnostic Mock Up[37]

Enables the clinician, patient, and laboratory technician to evaluate:
- The three dimensional appearance, form, and function of teeth
- The actual size, shape, and form of teeth

Box 27-4 | **Esthetic Considerations and Ceramic Restorations—cont'd**

- Incisal length and incisal plane relative to lip profile[108]
- Location and form of the gingival topography to compliment tooth form relative to smile profile

IV. In Anticipation of Endosseous Implant Placement

- Placement into recently or immediately extracted tooth root(s) sites
- Augment the volume of bone and soft tissue before placing the implant

V. Restorative Tooth Lengthening

- Fabrication of post/cores for teeth with insufficient tooth length/retention

VI. Surgical Tooth Lengthening

- To improve the tooth's biomechanical profile
- To enhance retention and resistance
- To improve esthetic profile and length of tooth form

VII. Installation of Endosseous Implants

- To create an individual clinical crown
- After tissue healing associated with clinical tooth lengthening
- Use of surgical template to provide correct implant location and angulation
- At time of tooth extraction, with immediate placement of the provisional restoration (without opposing tooth contact)

VIII. Uncovering of Endosseous Implants: "Two-Stage" Protocol

- Mucogingival therapy as needed

IX. Fabrication of Implant-Supported Provisional Restoration

X. Tooth Preparation and Impression

- Performed using an index of the form of the teeth. On the basis of the diagnostic mock-up, the preparation of the teeth can be accurately performed; followed by a master impression technique that is predictable for the clinician.

XI. Fabrication of Interim Provisional Restoration

- From Bis-GMA or acrylic materials
- To restore tooth form, function, and esthetics on an interim basis

XII. Try-in/Insertion of Ceramic Restorations:

- Check the individual and collective fit of the restorations. Adjust the contact point or contact areas, and then use radiographic verification of seating of the restorations, to help ensure successful luting, long-term function, and maintenance of the restorations.

XIII. Adjustment and Installation of an Occlusal Guard or Bite Platform Appliance

- When deemed necessary

When orthodontic intervention is indicated, it generally precedes the provisional restorative phase. If the sequence is reversed, the clinical team may be involved with additional repairs and recementations. Cement washout places teeth at greater risk for development of caries, and the patient often may require a new provisional restoration before the impression phase of therapy.

After the provisional restorations are fabricated and tooth stability is achieved, the restorations can be removed to better access the surgical field for correction of any hard and soft tissue reconstruction. Once tissue maturation has occurred and after the prognosis is established for all remaining teeth on both an individual and collective basis, subgingival preparation can be finalized and the provisional restorations relined. This is followed by completion of the fixed or fixed-removable prosthesis (Fig. 27-8).

The resective periodontal surgical approach is a predictable one. However, experimental and clinical research has shifted the focus of periodontics toward

---

Box 27-5   Dental Therapy Without Implants

I. Emergency Treatments: (see Table 27-1)

II. Scaling, Root Planing, Oral Hygiene Instruction

Closed or open flap debridement
- Mechanical debridement of calculus and plaque deposits adherent to clinical crowns and roots of teeth or restorative materials both supragingivally and subgingivally
- Removal of all chronic granulation tissue

III. Operative Dentistry
- Conservative control of dental caries

IV. Orthodontic Treatment (Partial or Full Therapy)
- Level and align teeth
- Erupt fractured or impacted teeth
- Extrude teeth to correct infrabony defects and augment the bone and soft tissue topography
- To support orthognathic correction

V. Fabrication of Interim Provisional Restorations

Guidelines[51]
- Replace missing, or recently extracted teeth, or both
- Maintain or reestablish interarch and intraarch harmony
- Assess adequacy of tooth reduction
- Determine the clinical crown profiles
- Develop therapeutic occlusal arrangement
- Control occlusal forces and assess function

VI. Periodontal Surgical Treatments

A. Osseous Therapy
- Regeneration and augmentation
  - Regeneration of attachment apparatus of teeth
  - Regeneration and augmentation of ridge deformities
- Ostectomy/osteoplasty
  - Improve bone morphology
  - Reduce pocket depth

B. Mucogingival Therapy
- Enhance the gingival complex around teeth and implants
- Grafting procedures (e.g., subepithelial connective tissue grafts, allogenic dermal grafts, and others)

VII. Reevaluation

A. Establish the Prognosis of the Remaining Teeth
- Function and esthetics
- Occlusion
- Phonetics
- Mucogingival considerations
- Emergence profiles

VIII. Final Prosthetic Treatment
- Fixed prosthesis
- Fixed-removable prosthesis
- Fabrication of an occlusal appliance after installation of the final prosthesis, when deemed necessary

IX. Maintenance

---

increased use of guided tissue membrane techniques to regenerate desired attachment apparatus circumscribing the periodontally compromised root. This newer era of "regeneration" therapeutics represents a positive shift in treatment strategy.[39]

DENTAL THERAPEUTICS: WITH IMPLANTS

Based on longitudinal studies, the viability[40-46] of endosseous implants becomes an integral part of periodontal prosthesis. Implant stability and load-bearing capacity, when secured in alveolar bone, adequate in quality and quantity, will result in a functional fixed restoration. The damage associated with primary and secondary occlusal trauma on many teeth often can be reversed. Teeth that appear to have a guarded prognosis may be able to assume a useful role in the final prosthesis.

During the past decade, implant restorations were reasonably acceptable from an esthetic perspective. However, in cases of advanced periodontal disease, the resorption of alveolar bone creates a significant challenge to achieve an esthetic, functional restoration. Placing implants in resorbed bone often results in long, unesthetic teeth with an adverse crown-to-implant ratio. Implant positioning is critical from faciolingual, mesiodistal, and incisoapical perspectives. It was quickly determined that the type of periodontium, whether thick-flat or thin-scalloped, significantly affects the esthetic outcome. The thin-scalloped type, with its friable gingival and osseous morphology, often results in tissue recession, ultimately exposing metal at the gingival crown margins.

Therefore, biologic and anatomic limitations such as insufficient bone, location of the maxillary sinus and the

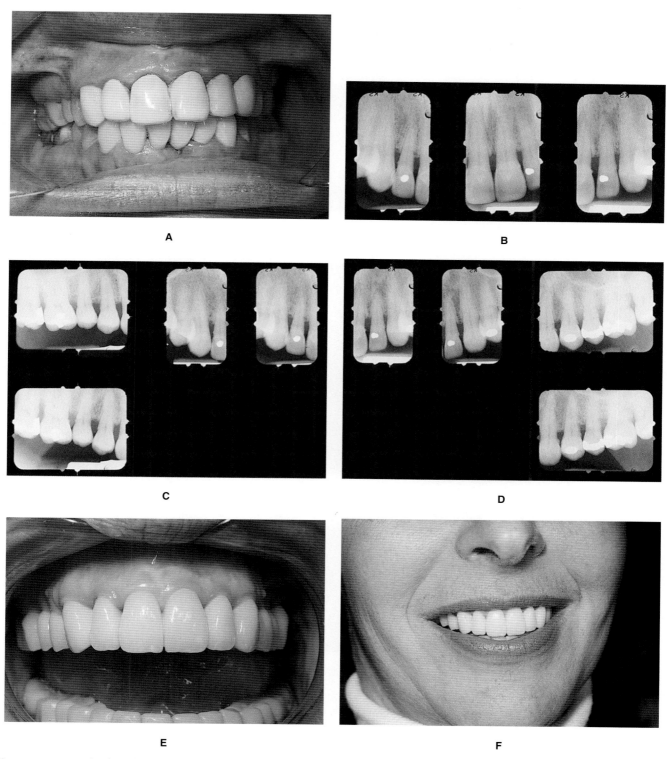

Figure 27-7. **A,** Poorly adapted composite veneers for maxillary anterior teeth, with marked gingival inflammation and generalized probing depth in the 5- to 6-mm range. **B-D,** Radiographic evidence of subgingival calculus accumulations and inconsistent bony margins. Resultant increase in crown-to-root ratios of maxillary anterior group of teeth. **E** and **F,** Splinted ceramo-gold-metal restorations, after healing from apically positioned muco-periosteal flap surgery to eliminate the periodontal disease and create normal topographic form, with minimal probing depth throughout. (Periodontal surgical therapy performed by Dr. Garry Miller.)

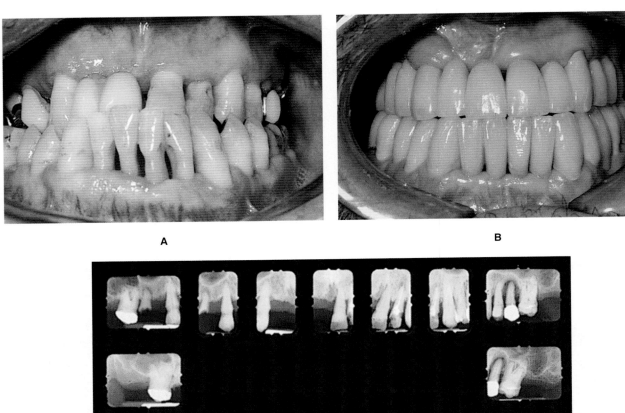

Figure 27-8. **A** and **B,** Class III malocclusion with severe periodontitis and occlusal trauma, as evidenced by significant loss of alveolar bone circumscribing many maxillary and mandibular teeth and associated widened ligament spaces and mobility patterns. **C,** Final ceramo-gold–splinted crownwork, restoring normal form, function, and esthetics.

Continued

alveolar nerve, and various bone and soft-tissue deformities, must be properly diagnosed before establishing a realistic treatment plan.[47-50] This requires effective communication between the periodontal surgeon, the restorative dentist, and the lab technician. The dental team must try to anticipate the size and shape of the deformity that will be created by removal of the involved teeth.[51]

Patients with advanced periodontal disorders may have compromised teeth that can be retained to offer short-term function with an interim fixed provisional

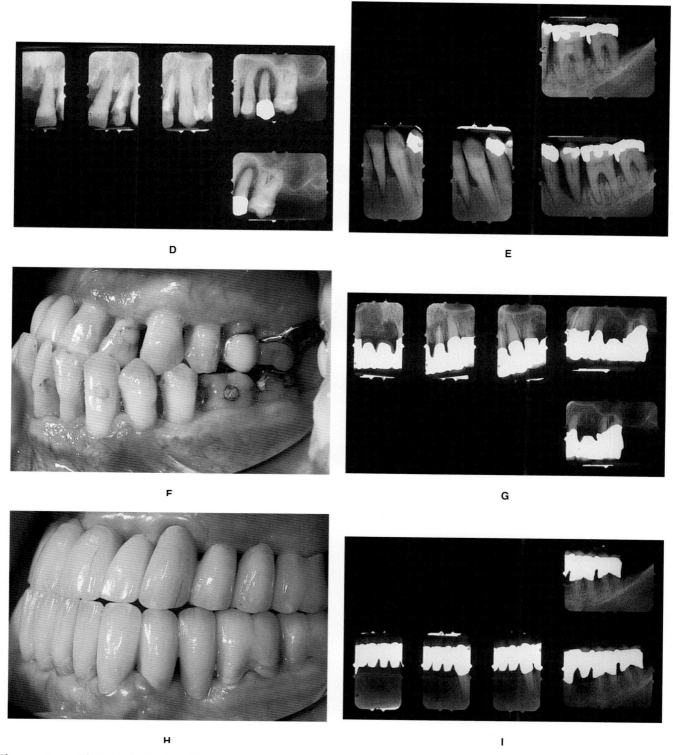

D

E

F

G

H

I

Figure 27-8. cont'd D-F, Left side view of dentition pretreatment with radiographic evidence of severe periodontal destruction. **G-I,** Final ceramo-gold restorations with postoperative radiographs. (Periodontal therapy performed by Dr. Michael Stiglitz.)

prosthesis rather than forcing them to rely on a removable denture. In this way, the risk for prematurely loading the implant and inducing micromotion during the initial stages of healing is reduced.[52] A well-designed and well-constructed interim provisional restoration is most important because the surgical procedures needed to establish the proper environment for the placement of implants increases the amount of time the patient needs to function with the provisional restoration.[53-63] (Box 27-6).

The compromised teeth that remain may be removed at a later stage in favor of additional endosseous implant support, as dictated by the biomechanical needs of the final restoration. Appropriate periodontal therapy is performed for all teeth that have a favorable prognosis. Either regenerative approaches[38] or pocket reduction[64-66]

Box 27-6 Dental Therapy with Implants

I. Emergency Treatments (see Table 27-1)

II. Scaling, Root Planing, Oral Hygiene Instruction

Closed, Open Flap Procedures
- Mechanical debridement of calculus and plaque deposits adherent to clinical crowns and roots of teeth or restorative materials both supragingivally and subgingivally
- Removal of all chronic granulation tissue

III. Operative Dentistry
- Conservative control of dental caries

IV. Orthodontic Treatment
- Level and align teeth—improve tooth position
- Erupt fractured or impacted teeth—rebuild/reposition bony complex
- Extrude teeth to correct infrabony defects and augment the hard and soft tissue topography
- To support orthognathic correction

V. Fabrication of Interim Provisional Restoration

Guidelines
- Allow for extraction of hopeless teeth
- Maintain or reestablish interarch and intraarch harmony
- Assess adequacy of tooth reduction
- Determine the clinical crown profiles
- Develop therapeutic occlusal arrangement
- Control occlusal forces and assess function
- Allow for fabrication of "Diagnostic Template" with markers for radiographic analysis

VI. Periodontal Surgical Treatments

A. Osseous Therapy
- Regeneration and augmentation
  - Regeneration of the attachment apparatus of teeth and bone augmentation of deformed alveolar ridges
- Ostectomy/osteoplasty
  - Improve bone morphology
  - Reduce pocket depth

B. Mucogingival Therapy
- Enhance the gingival complex around teeth and implants
- Grafting procedures (e.g., subepithelial connective tissue grafts, allogenic dermal grafts, and others)

VII. Bone Grafting, Sinus Bone Augmentation Procedures
- Dictated by the need to properly place implants

VIII. Fabrication of Surgical Template
- To guide implant placement—based on clinical and radiographic interpretation

Box 27-6 | **Dental Therapy with Implants—cont'd**

IX. Implant Placement

- Existing alveolar bone sites or healed extraction sites
- Bone augmentation sites (e.g., sinus, alveolar ridges)
- Fresh extraction sites

X. Interim Maintenance (to Facilitate Healing)

A. Surgical Sites

- Continue to evaluate the healing and treat any complications (e.g., exposed membranes, incision dehiscence, loose cover screws)
- Interim provisional prosthesis
- Repair broken acrylic joints
- Replace soft reline materials
- Maintain and monitor transitional implants

XI. Transitional Implant-Assisted/Supported Restoration

- Placement of transepithelial healing components at the second-stage procedure
- Selection of implant abutments
- Conversion of existing provisional to implant-assisted/supported restoration
- Fabrication of new implant provisional restoration or new implant and tooth-assisted provisional restoration

XII. Reevaluation

- Stability of implants and remaining teeth
- Occlusal vertical dimension
- Phonetics
- Esthetics
- Proper emergence profiles of crowns for teeth and implants

XIII. Prosthetic Treatment

- Implant-assisted
  - Fixed prosthesis
  - Fixed-removable prosthesis
- Implant-supported
  - Fixed prosthesis
  - Fixed-removable prosthesis
  - Fabrication of an occlusal appliance after the final prosthesis is installed, if deemed necessary

XIV. Maintenance

and clinical crown exposure procedures should be rendered before endosseous implant installation.

Orthodontic treatment may be necessary to establish adequate space before placing an implant. Therefore, tooth movement should be initiated during the early stages of treatment. In some situations, with flared maxillary anterior teeth and few posterior teeth, implants may be placed first and used as an anchorage mechanism to retract and align the remaining teeth. One must not minimize the value of orthodontics. After complete debridement of the root surface(s) adjacent to periodontal bony defects, mechanotherapy may help to reduce and to modify the size and shape of angular osseous deformities, often through eruption/extrusion.[67-69] The improvement in hard and soft

tissue topography allows the newly regenerated bone to successfully receive endosseous implants. Forced eruption of hopeless teeth is currently used to alter the soft and hard tissues before placing implants. Also, orthodontic extrusion is used to recreate lost interproximal papillae (see Chapter 28).

Outcome-Based Planning

Interim provisional restoration

The interim restoration may be designed in several different ways. One approach is to modify an existing bridge or splint, reline the crowns on selected natural teeth, and convert other crowns to pontics as necessary. With a paucity of strong, well distributed natural teeth, the existing rigid metal framework can better resist normal occlusal forces and help to prevent prosthesis fracture.

The removable interim prosthesis is less desirable for preserving masticatory function. It should be used when the support provided by the remaining teeth is compromised and the number and distribution of teeth is insufficient to allow for the use of a fixed prosthesis. If a removable prosthesis must be used, it is imperative that the restorative dentist evaluates the edentulous areas frequently and replaces the soft liner material when it becomes hard or brittle or precipitates a pressure ulceration of the soft tissue. Currently, there are "temporary" implant systems that preclude the use of the removable appliance. It allows the clinician to use a fixed "mini-implant" supported restoration throughout the phase of implant osteointegration.[70-75]

Ideally, a fixed provisional restoration should be made from a diagnostic wax-up, incorporating all of the esthetic and functional characteristics. Any preexisting limitations should be corrected to allow the prosthesis to serve as a blueprint of the final prosthesis. (Fig. 27-9)

With advanced periodontal disease, the maxilla generally resorbs apically and palatally; therefore, the mandible appears to be much larger than the maxilla. When all the maxillary teeth are eventually lost and the edentulous cast is mounted on an articulator, it appears as if the patient has a prognathic relationship. However, this is not a true prognathic arch profile, but rather a result of the bone resorption of the maxilla. And if the patient desires implants and a fixed restoration this[76] becomes a surgical and restorative challenge. The clinician(s) must know before the implants are placed how this occlusal disparity will be corrected in the final prosthesis. In this situation, the volume of available bone is significant to the long-term survival of implants because of the exaggerated anterior–posterior discrepancy.

It is wise and judicious to fabricate a temporary appliance simulating the final restoration before any surgical procedures. This is essential when the clinician is contemplating a change in the occlusal vertical dimension. This alteration will change the faciopalatal relationship of the mandible as it relates to the maxilla.

The lip line esthetic diagnosis, as well as the lip support, will influence the decision to fabricate a fixed or removable prosthesis. A simple and effective way to make a reasonable esthetic appraisal of the final prosthesis is

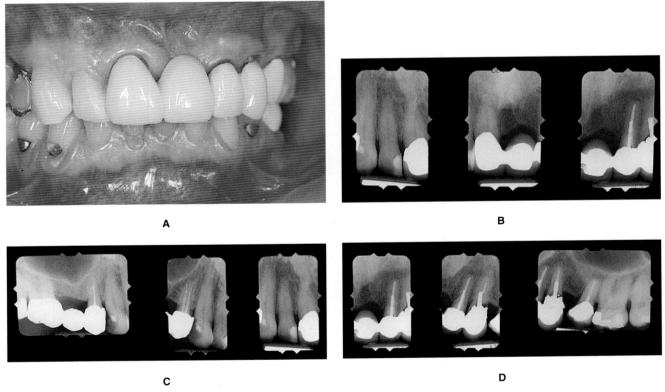

A

B

C

D

Figure 27-9. A, Pretreatment Class II, division I malocclusion with failing crown and bridgework—a result of caries, post/core failures, and periodontitis. **B-D,** Pretreatment radiographs.

Continued

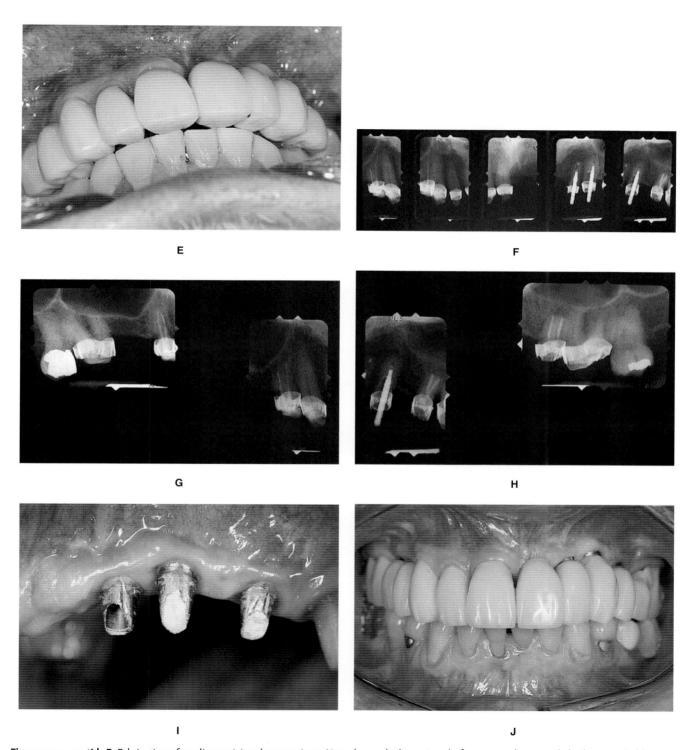

E

F

G

H

I

J

Figure 27-9. cont'd E, Fabrication of acrylic provisional restorations. Note the marked anterior platform created to provide both centric holding area and necessary anterior guidance (socket preservation by Dr. Karl A. Rose). **F-H,** Radiographs of tooth preparations after fabrication of provisional restorations. Tooth preparations and temporary transitional implant abutments. **I,** After second stage surgical implant exposure, temporary titanium implant abutments are machined and connected to the implant bodies, followed by relining of the existing provisional restoration (socket preservation and subsequent implant placement performed by Dr. Karl A. Rose). **J,** Transitional acrylic provisional restorations supported by teeth and implant abutments.

Continued

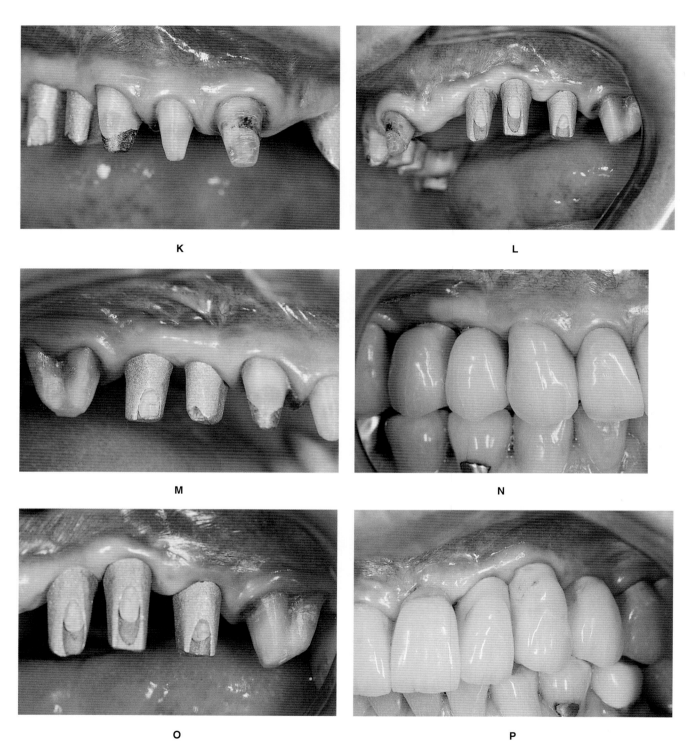

Figure 27-9. cont'd K and **L,** Gold implant abutments screw-retained and sealed with gutta percha. **M,** Final gold implant abutments at former tooth sites #4 and #5. **N,** Ceramo-gold implant crowns and their relation to the implant abutments. **O,** Final gold implant abutments at former tooth sites #10, #11, and #12. **P,** The implant crowns at former tooth sites #10, #11, and #12 have been created with ceramic root form to address the loss of residual ridge height. The final prosthetic replacement of both the anatomic crown and anatomic root is classified by Misch as the FPII[109] prosthesis.

Continued

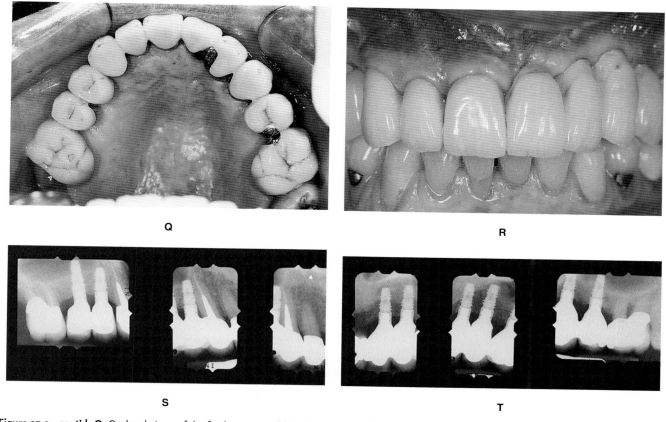

Figure 27-9. cont'd Q, Occlusal views of the final ceramo-gold implant-supported and tooth-supported restorations. **R,** Final ceramo-gold implant-supported and tooth-supported crownwork. **S** and **T,** Final radiographic appearance of completed maxillary restoration.

to evaluate the appearance of the patient's existing prosthesis. Assuming that it is acceptable to the patient and the dentist, it is wise to duplicate the existing prosthesis and evaluate the patient's profile. If the appearance is the same as the original restoration, it can be assumed that the teeth are supporting the lip. In this situation, it is likely that an acceptable fixed restoration can be made. Conversely, if the lip "collapses in", the final prosthesis will likely require some form of labial support, often necessitating a removable prosthesis. A fixed restoration would likely be unsatisfactory.

The trends that have brought dentistry to its current level of esthetic sophistication require the clinician to predict the outcome before implants are placed. If the esthetic evaluation is inaccurate, the final result will be less than desirable to the patient and the dentist.

Diagnostic and Surgical Templates

A diagnostic template with radiographic markers, like the surgical template, may be fabricated to assist the surgeon and restorative dentist in analyzing the available bone to place the implants. This is accomplished by using CAT radiography before implant surgery.[77]

The surgical template, a guide to surgical implant placement, is fabricated from either a diagnostic wax-up or, preferably, a stone model of the functioning provisional restoration.

After placing the provisional restoration intraorally, impressions are made of both the prosthesis and the underlying edentulous ridges and tooth preparations. Stone models are made and an acrylic shell of the restoration is cured on a model of the remaining prepared or unprepared teeth, or both. Locations and axial alignments are carefully planned with the surgeon and are carved into the acrylic template to anticipate implant placement.

Although a lingual or palatal approach is commonly used to design the surgical guide, a facial approach also may be considered. This will provide the surgeon with an accurate visualization of the ideal implant sites, the desired path of abutment emergence, and the axis orientation in relation to the final prosthesis. The ability to perform surgical procedures demands direct access, which is provided by removal of the provisional interim restoration. The surgeon can orient the surgical template by securing it to the existing teeth, and prepare the osteotomy to properly position the implants.

Significant progress in biotechnology, radiology, and computer technology have allowed for more accurate diagnosis and treatment planning. This has recently resulted in the construction of three-dimensional bone models, stereolithography[78] and navigational surgery to position endosseous implants with greater precision (Fig. 27-10).

Considerations at the Surgical Phase

The well-organized treatment plan may require various scenarios to place endosseous implants into bone where teeth still exist in areas of ridge deformity.

Where implant placement is anticipated, the teeth to be extracted usually are removed when the provisional restoration is inserted. The newly formed bone in the recent extraction sites is considered to be an excellent source of pluripotential cells to promote successful osseointegration. Simultaneous extraction of the tooth and placement of the implant shortens the duration of treatment.

In an effort to more precisely determine the quality of the alveolar bone for immediate implant placement and to minimize the overall maturation phase, the teeth may be sectioned horizontally at their gingival margins or at the height of the alveolus.[79] The pulps should be extirpated, the canals medicated and sealed, and provisional restorations fabricated leaving these tooth roots for the surgeon to extract at the time of implant installation. This avoids interference with early socket healing and precludes the risk for additional crestal bone resorption of the healing socket.[80] The surgeon will decide whether to extract and immediately place an implant into the socket. However, the surgeon may prefer to extract the

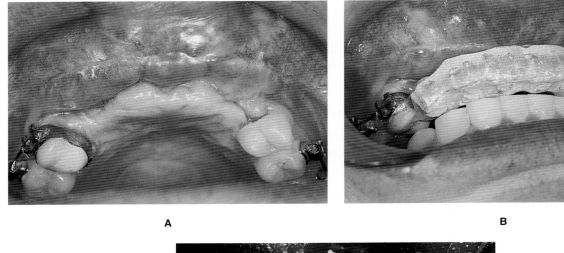

A   B

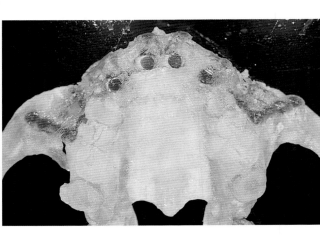

C

Figure 27-10. A, Premaxilla after LeFort I osteotomy, with inlay graft increasing ridge height by 7 mm. **B,** Diagnostic template using gutta percha markers and barium sulfate to locate endosseous implants in premaxillary region. **C** and **D,** Simulation of endosseous implant installation into four available premaxillary sites, as determined by evidence of bone on the computed axial tomography (CAT) scan images.

Continued

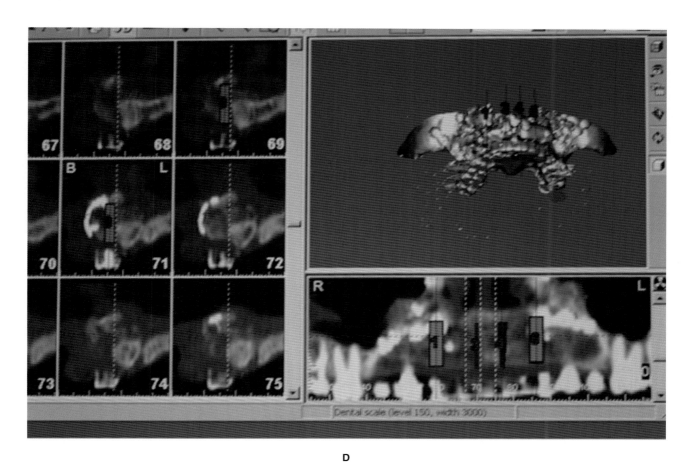

D

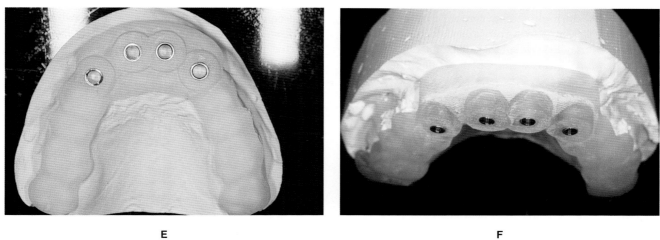

E **F**

Figure 27-10. cont'd E, Creation of three-dimensional maxillary bone model from CAT scan imaging. **F,** Surgical template with titanium cylinders to locate the implant sites with surgical precision.

Continued

tooth, place a bone graft and membrane, and allow it to heal 3 to 4 months before placing an implant.

If an edentulous ridge is modestly deformed and the site has been planned for implant placement, the surgeon may elect to position the implants at an angle that corresponds to the ideal final restoration. If a dehiscence or fenestration occurs, it can be corrected by placing a bone graft and barrier membrane.[81]

Dental implant placement in the atrophic or deformed alveolar ridge can be a surgical challenge (see Chapter 26).

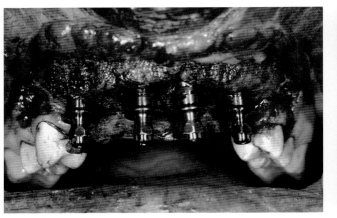

G

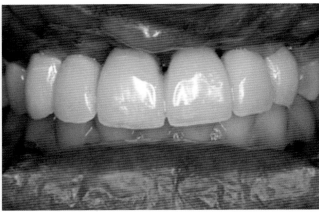

H

Figure 27-10. cont'd G and H, Surgical endosseous implant placement based on CAT scan technology and stereolithography.

Alveolar bone augmentation is currently accomplished with guided bone regeneration techniques,[63,82,83] sinus bone augmentation,[84] bone grafting,[85-87] and alveolar distraction osteogenesis.[88] Two or more surgical interventions are frequently required to correct a major ridge deformity.[63,82,83] First, the ridge must be reconstructed to a more normal anatomic form and size,[77] followed by implant placement and soft tissue augmentation[89,90] (Fig. 27-11).

Depending on the extent of the original ridge deformity, the surgical bone augmentation procedure can be relatively successful at restoring the bony contour to the following levels: Class I, 1 mm to 2 mm apical to the cementoenamel junction (CEJ) level of the adjacent teeth; Class II, 3 mm to 4 mm apical to the CEJ level of the adjacent teeth; Class III, 5 mm or greater, apical to the CEJ level of the adjacent teeth.[77]

In reconstructing the deformed ridge to a Class I bone level, a normal overlying soft-tissue profile will often be created. For the Class II bone level, where there is still some horizontal and vertical deficiency, soft-tissue augmentation by means of connective tissue grafts,[89,90] autogenous grafts (free or pedicle), or repositioning of the gingival complex, may mask the bony deficiency and create the appearance of normal topography.[77]

For the Class III level defect, prosthetic materials are frequently required to restore the hard-tissue and soft-tissue deformities and simulate the Class I reconstructed profile, which otherwise may be compromised in both height and width[77] (Fig. 27-12).

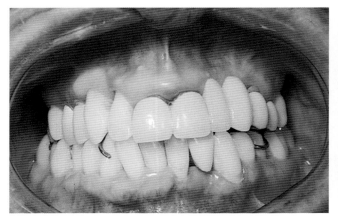

A

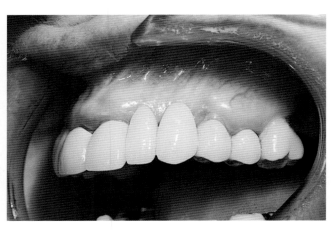

B

Figure 27-11. A, Clinical preoperative view. B-D, Preoperative views and radiographs reveal severe loss of periodontal support with ridge deformities and deep infrabony defects.

Continued

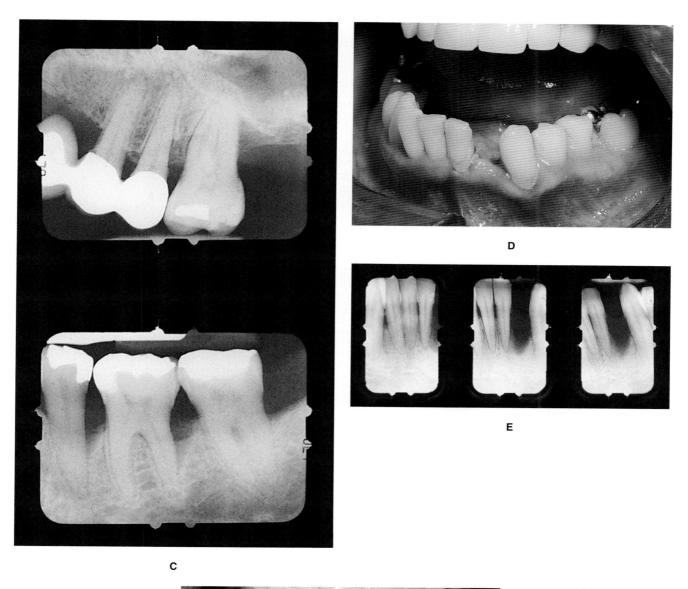

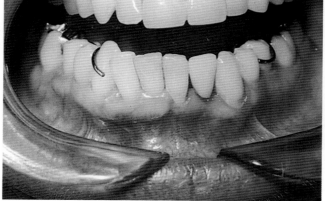

Figure 27-11. cont'd E and **F,** Preoperative view and radiographs show severe loss of periodontal support with ridge deformities.

Continued

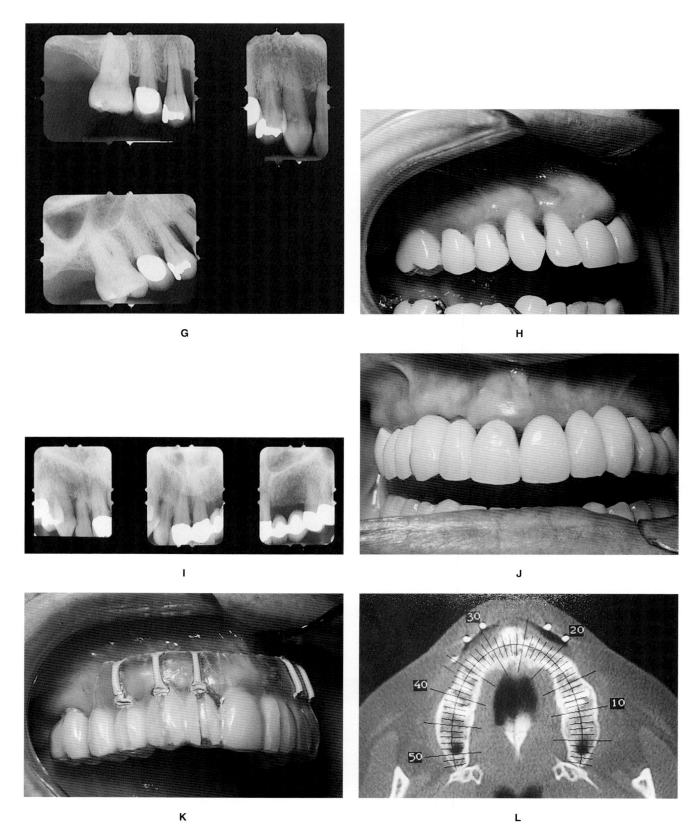

Figure 27-11. cont'd G-I, Preoperative views and radiographs show severely periodontally compromised teeth #5, #6, and #7. **J,** Fabrication of maxillary provisional acrylic restorations simultaneous with extraction of teeth #5, #6, #7, #9, and #13. **K,** Diagnostic template with gutta percha markers for CAT scan. **L,** Diagnostic template demonstrates the lack of available bone for endosseous implant placements, as evidenced by the voids on the stone model in the premaxilla and on the radiographic CAT scan.

Continued

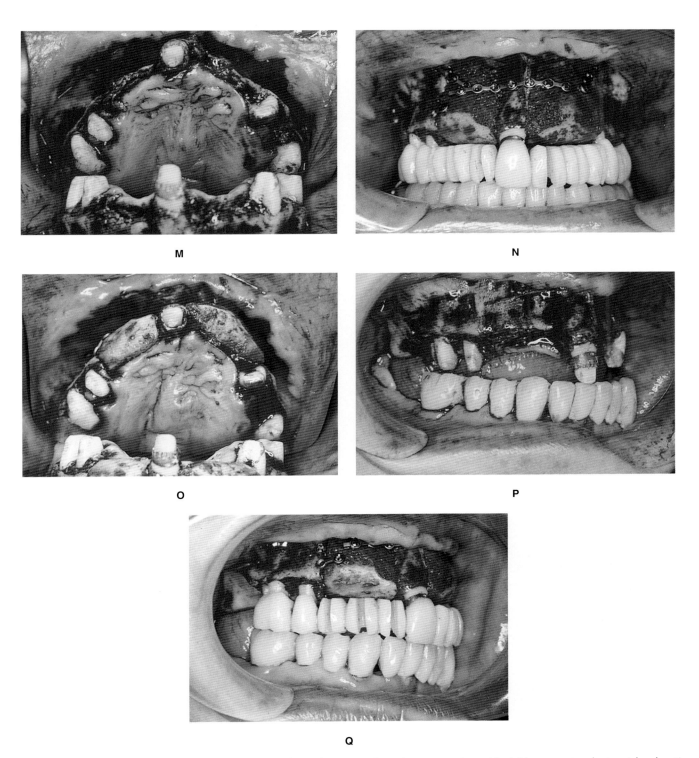

M

N

O

P

Q

Figure 27-11. cont'd M-O, Iliac crest bone grafting, mortised into the upper right and upper anterior residual ridges to restore horizontal and vertical component of bone loss (performed by Dr. Jeffrey Posnick). **P** and **Q,** Views of onlay graft of upper right side with fixation (performed by Dr. Jeffrey Posnick).

Continued

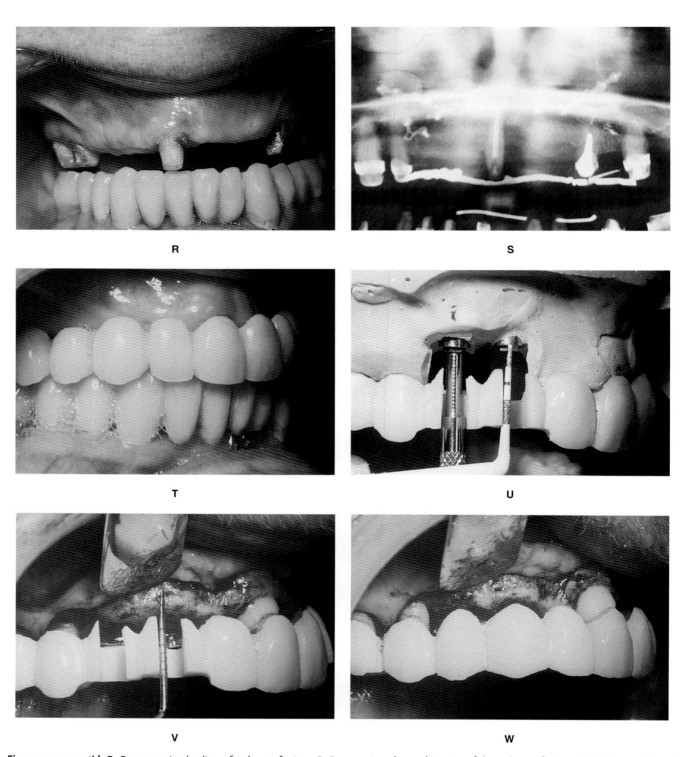

R

S

T

U

V

W

Figure 27-11. cont'd R, Postoperative healing of onlay graft sites. **S,** Panoramic radiographic view of the onlay graft sites. **T,** Interim provisional restoration. **U,** Vertical relation of endosseous implants to surgical template. **V** and **W,** Preparation of onlay graft site to install endosseous implants. First, the surgical template is installed. Measurements taken relative to the template will locate the implants vertically in the onlay-grafted bone, relative to the cementoenamel junction of the adjacent teeth. Note the use of the second surgical template to define the rise and fall of the bony topography, relative to the vertical depth to which each implant is positioned. Implants installed to proper mesiodistal, buccopalatal, and vertical positions (performed by Dr. Garry Miller).

Continued

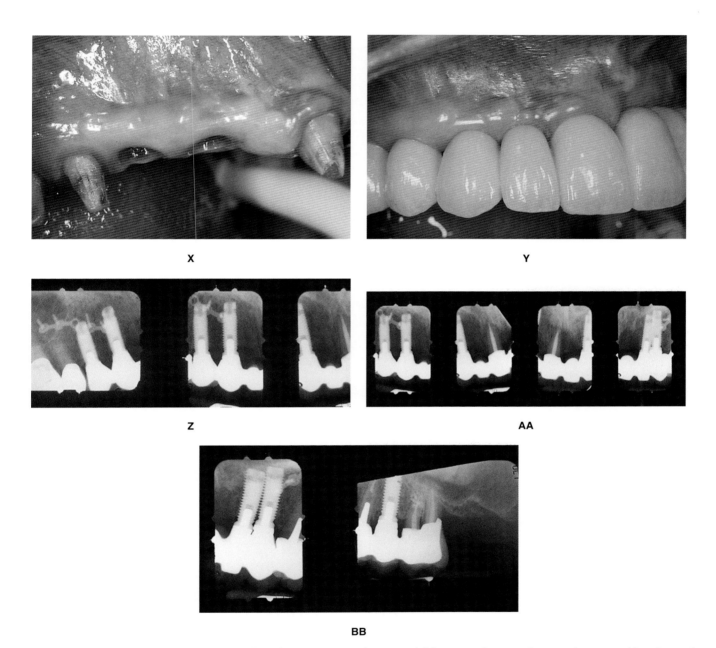

X, Soft tissue topography without demonstrating modest rise and fall to gingival topography. Y, Final ceramo-gold implant and tooth-supported restoration. Z-BB, Final maxillary radiographic images.

Figure 27-11. cont'd **X,** Soft tissue topography without demonstrating modest rise and fall to gingival topography. **Y,** Final ceramo-gold implant and tooth-supported restoration. **Z-BB,** Final maxillary radiographic images.

Continued

After the bony ridge has been reconstructed and the endosseous implants installed, a sufficient healing period must be observed to ensure a satisfactory "take." Bone remodeling adjacent to implant fixtures occurs over a period of at least a year, leading to more mature bone (compact lamellar bone) within which the implant can better tolerate the forces of occlusion.[91]

The essential criteria for alveolar ridge reconstruction and successful implant placement are the following:

(1) appropriate quantity of horizontal and vertical bone and adequate quality of bone; (2) sufficient keratinized tissue overlying the bony crest; and (3) adequate distance between implants.[8]

Transitional Implant-Assisted Restoration

It is important to coordinate the schedules of the surgeon and the restorative dentist to begin the process of restoring the implants after an established healing period.

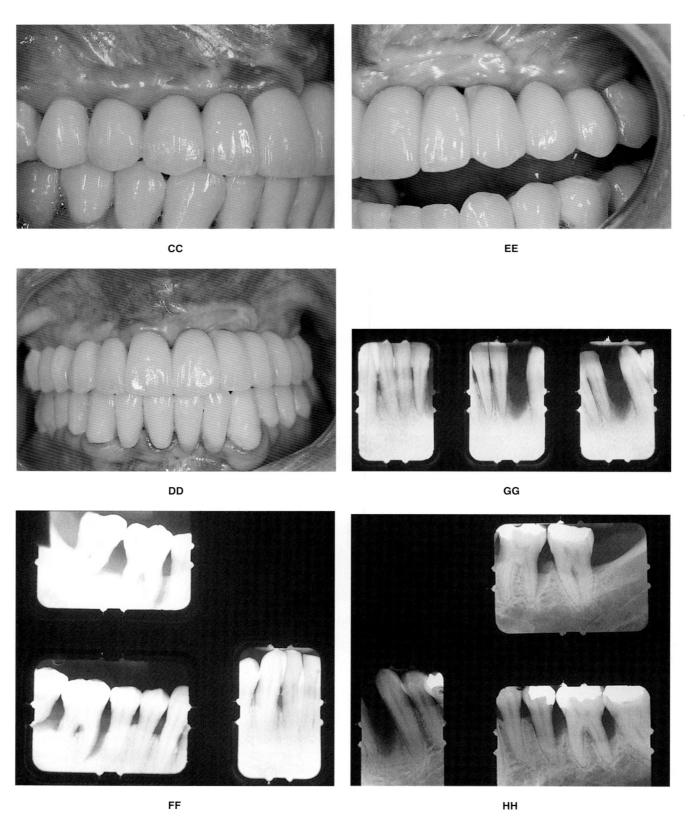

CC

EE

DD

GG

FF

HH

Figure 27-11. cont'd CC-EE, Final ceramo-gold restorations demonstrating reasonably normal soft tissue topography. The adjacent endosseous implants minimize the potential to preserve the height of the interproximal papilla (as described by Tarnow and colleagues[8]). **FF-HH,** Preoperative mandibular radiographs.

Continued

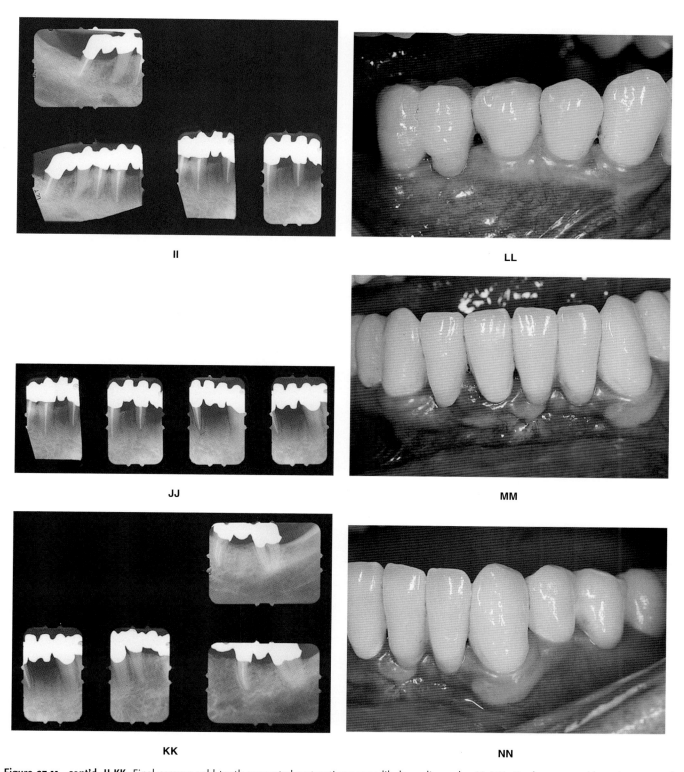

Figure 27-11. cont'd II-KK, Final ceramo-gold tooth-supported restorations: mandibular radiographs. **LL-NN,** Final ceramo-gold tooth-supported mandibular restoration with root resected molars and extraction of hopeless teeth.

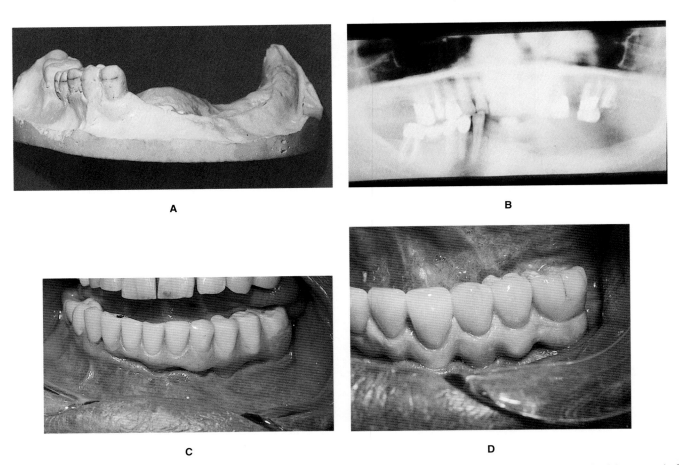

Figure 27-12. A, Preoperative model view of residual ridge extending from former tooth site #17 through #26 inclusive—a result of the removal of a squamous cell carcinoma. **B,** Panoramic view of residual ridge extending from former tooth #17 through #26 inclusive. **C,** Provisional implant-supported restoration. **D,** Implant-supported (×5), fixed, ceramo-gold restorations, replacing the anatomic crown, root, and gingiva—the Misch FPIII[109] classification for fixed implant prostheses (implant placement by Dr. Karl A. Rose).

The surgeon will perform a small gingival punch procedure to expose the head of the implant or a muco-periosteal flap procedure to reposition the gingival complex around the implants. A transepithelial healing component is then secured to the implant. After soft tissue maturation,[8,92-95] a high or low profile transepithelial abutment may be selected depending on the biologic dimension of tissues,[96] and a provisional restoration is fabricated to restore form and function. For "one-stage" implants, the restorative dentist can begin the provisional restoration at the appropriate scheduled time.

When multiple implants are exposed and angulation is a concern, it may be beneficial to take an impression that records the orientation of the fixture heads after early soft tissue healing. A new provisional restoration is then fabricated in the laboratory (Fig. 27-5), using temporary cylinders that are designed to mate directly with the implant body.[97]

Frequently at the second stage, the existing interim provisional prosthesis is modified by shortening the undersurface of the pontics to provide room for the healing components. Later these components are removed, abutments of proper height are screwed into position and temporary crown cylinders are seated, shortened to contact the opposing occlusion, and incorporated into the existing provisional restoration.

If there is any doubt as to the feasibility of accomplishing functional and esthetic alignment of the implant abutments, temporary crown cylinders are available from most implant manufacturers. They ensure an intimate fit to the titanium abutment or fixture head and allow the clinician to start developing the anticipated contours. Should the form require modification, the acrylic offers ample opportunity to make any modifications without jeopardizing the accuracy of the fit.

Chiche and colleagues[98] have pointed out that as a result of "surgical and anatomic limitations, implant placement may not correspond to the initial expectation set at the presurgical phase, and over-contouring the final restoration could create aesthetic and functional liabilities." They continue their explanation, stating that "the path of emergence of the fastening screw through the prosthesis may compromise part of the facial or occlusal morphology, especially if it passes through a primary centric occlusal contact, an interproximal embrasure" or the facial veneer. "Even minor discrepancies between an implant and crown axis may result in eccentric screws, since such deviations are magnified at the level of the occlusion." Here the transitional prosthesis is invaluable in diagnosing these prosthetic limitations. With this early awareness, a plan can be better anticipated involving the use of angled abutments, custom-angled abutments, the fabrication of an auxiliary substructure, and the application of pink ceramic to facilitate the prosthetic result by the dental laboratory. Some have conjectured that the implant-assisted provisional restoration may provide a shock-dampening effect that may be beneficial during the first year of bone maturation adjacent to the implant fixtures.

At this stage, a radiographic and clinical evaluation of the stability of the implant fixtures is made. The compromised teeth that were retained to support the interim prosthesis are extracted at this time.[52] Some of the natural teeth may be removed in favor of additional implants or retained as indirect retainers in situations in which fewer implants are used in the overall support of the prosthesis. If a new transitional prosthesis has recently been fabricated, there may have been a change in the occlusal vertical dimension or the esthetic form, both of which would require further modification. In addition, it may be necessary to consider mucogingival treatment to enhance the complex of attached masticatory mucosa around selected teeth or implants.[99]

A transepithelial collar of minimal height, shallow sulcus depth, and a circumscribed border of bound-down keratinized tissue are essential for conventional plaque-control measures around implant crowns.

Final Prosthetic Phase of Treatment

Now that the final prognoses for all teeth and implants have been established, the restorative dentist can use crown and bridge techniques to construct the final prosthesis. The dentist may proceed with final impressions of the natural teeth, relate them to the proper position of the implant fixtures or abutments, and fabricate a master model. To initiate the laboratory procedures, the case is carefully mounted on an appropriate articulator by means of a series of occlusal registrations.

On the master model, a soft tissue marginal profile should be fashioned around each natural tooth die and implant analogue to simulate the gingival condition in the oral cavity. This allows for predictable abutment head selection in terms of proper height, angulation, and emergence profile. Technical choices are made concerning case design, case construction, the use of telescopic copings on retained natural teeth, or the use of precision "dovetail" slide attachments to interlock sections of teeth and implants, when indicated. When fixed implant-supported prostheses in combination with a removable partial denture are used, "stress-relieving" attachments may be considered.

The primary substructure is fabricated and examined relative to the gingival margin placement; the fit of the copings is tested individually then collectively soldered, and the final ceramo-metal restoration is completed. Today it is possible for the computer to be used as a complementary or alternative technique to conventional impressions. Photogrammetry with digitized images, and laser/optical scanners can support computer-assisted design/computer-assisted manufacturing and computer-milling techniques in the fabrication of titanium-implant frameworks and ceramic and zirconium-oxide implant frameworks.[100] On delivery of the final prosthesis, a strong cement is used to secure the crowns on the remaining teeth. The fixture-assisted dental reconstruction is then seated with a temporary cement to create a hermetic seal at the interface of the abutment and superstructure. Retention and resistance to displacement may be enhanced by securing the prosthesis with set screws.[101] Using carefully machined/milled abutments, the practitioner may choose to cement the prosthesis in lieu of screw retention.[102]

Long-Term Maintenance/Professional Care

The completed prosthesis and its supporting components (teeth and implants) are carefully monitored with a maintenance program, alternating visitations between the surgeon and the restorative dentist (Fig. 27-13). Any tissue changes or prosthetic problems can be detected early and addressed efficiently.[35,103,104] Periapical and panoramic radiographs are taken at appropriate intervals to ascertain any changes that may haven taken place at the bone/implant interface and around natural teeth.

Mechanical failures (such as breakage of porcelain, solder joints, components, and implants) may occur long after the placement of the prosthesis, sometimes between 5 and 10 years.[105] According to Wiskott and colleagues,[106] fatigue failure is a "result of the development of microscopic cracks in areas of stress concentration." Continual loadings result in the cracks fusing to an ever-growing fissure that insidiously weakens the restoration. Eventually catastrophic failure results from a final loading cycle that exceeds the mechanical capacity of the remaining sound portion of the material. Based on the occlusal indicators, there may be great value in fitting the patient's dentition

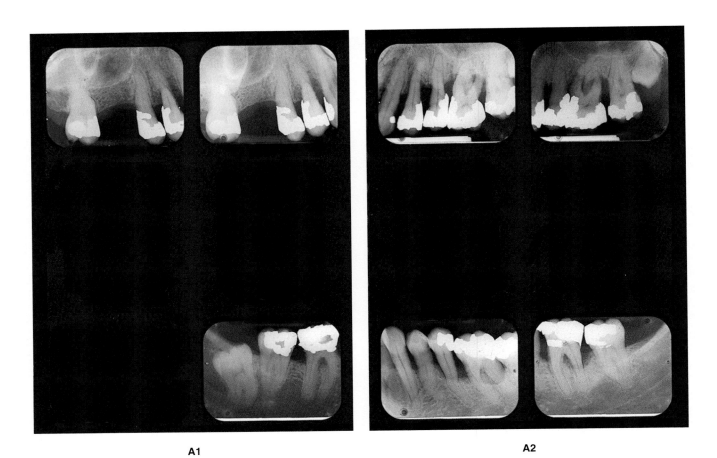

A1

A2

A3

Figure 27-13. A, Pretreatment full-mouth radiographic series (year 2/1967) demonstrating missing teeth, severe periodontitis with furcation invasions, and marked areas of alveolar bone destruction around many maxillary and mandibular teeth.

Continued

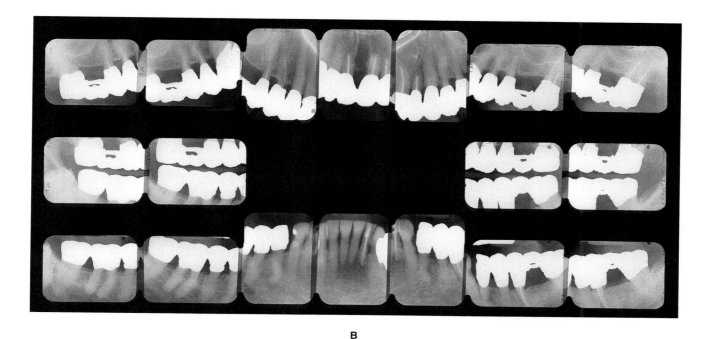

B

Figure 27-13. cont'd B, Posttreatment full-mouth radiographic series (year 9/1997) demonstrating 30 years of clinical and radiographic follow-up. Note the long-term success and maintenance of the supporting teeth of the fixed splinted periodontal prosthesis (periodontal prosthetic treatment performed by Dr. Jeffrey Ingber).

with an occlusal appliance as part of the long-term preservation of the prosthesis.

CONCLUSION

The field of periodontal prosthesis has contributed much to our understanding of dental diseases and the methods of treating these problems. Periodontal prosthesis has truly been the hallmark of interdisciplinary care. Its future lies in all disciplines acting in concert to expand and enhance the accomplishments made during the last 50 years.

ACKNOWLEDGMENTS

This chapter is dedicated to Dr. Morton Amsterdam, the father of Periodontal Prosthesis. Any errors in omission or commission are not his, but are attributable to us, the authors. Additional thanks go to Sylvie Rupple-Bozilov for her technical assistance in the preparation of this manuscript.

The authors thank the Seattle Study Club and Dr. Michael Cohen specifically, for allowing us to update and reprint much of the article Starr, N.L., "Treatment Planning and Treatment Sequencing With and Without Endosseous Implants; A Comprehensive Therapeutic Approach to the Partially Edentulous Patient", Seattle Study Club Journal; 1995; 1:1, 21-34.

REFERENCES

1. Amsterdam M: Periodontal prosthesis—twenty-five years in retrospect, *Alpha Omegan* 67:8-52, 1974.
2. Amsterdam M, Abrams L: Periodontal prosthesis. In Goldman HM, Cohen DW, editors: *Periodontal therapy*, St. Louis, 1973, CV Mosby Company, pp 977-1013.
3. Adell R, Lekholm U, Rocklen B, Branemark PJ: A 15-year study of osseointegrated implants in the treatment of the edentulous jaw, *Int J Oral Surg* 10:387-416, 1981.
4. Amsterdam M, Weisgold AS: Periodontal prosthesis: a 50-year perspective, *Alpha Omegan* 93:23-30, 2000.
5. Tarnow DP, Magner AW, Fletcher P: The effect of the distance from the contact point to the crest of bone on the presence or absence of the interproximal dental papilla, *J Periodontol* 63:995-996, 1992.
6. Choquet V, Hermans M, Adrianssens P et al: Clinical and radiographic evaluation of the papilla level adjacent to single-tooth dental implants. A retrospective study in the maxillary anterior region, *J Periodontol* 72:1364-1371, 2001.
7. Salama H, Salama M, Garber D, Adar P: The interproximal height of bone. A guidepost to predictable aesthetic strategies and soft tissue contours in anterior tooth replacement, *Pract Periodontics Aesthet Dent* 10:1131-1141, 1998.
8. Tarnow D, Cho SC, Wallace SS: The effect of inter-implant distance on the height of inter-implant bone crest, *J Periodontol* 4:546-549, 2000.

9. Garber D: The esthetic dental implant: letting the restoration be the guide, *J Am Dent Assoc* 126:319-325, 1995.

10. Kois JC: Predictable single tooth peri-implant esthetics: five diagnostic keys, *Compend Contin Educ Dent* 22:199-206, 2001.

11. Salama H, Salama M, Garber D et al: Developing optimal peri-implant papillae within the esthetic zone; guided soft tissue augmentation, *J Esthet Dent* 7:125-129, 1995.

12. Phillips K, Kois JC: Aesthetic peri-implant site development—the restorative connection, *Dent Clin North Am* 42:57-70, 1998.

13. Jansen C, Weisgold AS: Presurgical treatment planning for the anterior single tooth implant restoration, *Compend Contin Educ Dent* 16:746-761, 1995.

14. Weisgold AS, Arnoux J-P, Lu J: The single tooth anterior implant: a word of caution, part I, *J Esthet Dent* 9:225-233, 1998.

15. Ochsenbein C, Ross S: A concept of osseous surgery and its clinical applications. In Ward HL, Chas C, editors: *CDS. A periodontal point of view.* Springfield, Ill, 1973, Charles C. Thomas.

16. Weisgold AS: Contours of the full crown restoration, *Alpha Omegan* 10:77-89, 1977.

17. Olsson M, Lindhe J: Periodontal characteristics in individuals with varying forms of the upper central incisors, *J Clin Periodontol* 18:78-82, 1991.

18. Becker W, Ochsenbein C, Tibbetts L, Becker BE: Alveolar bone anatomic profiles as measured from dry skulls. Clinical ramifications, *J Clin Periodontol* 24:727-731, 1997.

19. Magne P, Douglas WH: Additive contour of porcelain veneers: a key element in enamel preservation, adhesion, and esthetics for aging dentition, *J Adhes Dent* 1(1):81-92, 1999.

20. Svanberg G, Lindhe J: Experimental tooth hypermobility in the dog: a methodological study, *Odontol Revy* 24:269-282, 1973.

21. Kantor M, Polson AM, Zander H: Alveolar bone regeneration after removal of inflammatory and traumatic factors, *J Periodontol* 47:687-695, 1976.

22. Lindhe J, Nyman S: The role of occlusion in periodontal disease and the biological rationale for splinting in treatment of periodontitis, *Oral Sci Rev* 10:11-43, 1977.

23. Starr NL: The distal extension case: an alternative restorative design for implant prosthetics, *Int J Periodontics Restorative Dent* 21:1, 61-67, 2001.

24. Lindhe J, Svanberg G: Influence of trauma from occlusion on progression of experimental periodontitis in the beagle dog, *J Clin Periodontol* 1:3-14, 1974.

25. Lindhe J, Svanberg G: Vascular reactions in the periodontal ligament incident to trauma from occlusion, *J Clin Periodontol* 1:58-69, 1974.

26. Lindhe J, Ericcson I: Influence of trauma from occlusion on reduced but healthy periodontal tissues in dogs, *J Clin Periodontol* 3:110-122, 1976.

27. Ericcson I, Lindhe J: Lack of effect of trauma from occlusion on the recurrence of experimental periodontitis, *J Clin Periodontol* 4:115-127, 1977.

28. Lindhe J, Nyman S: The role of occlusion in periodontal disease and the biological rationale for splinting in treatment of periodontitis, *Oral Sci Rev* 10:11-43, 1977.

29. Nyman S, Lindhe J, Ericcson I: The effect of progressive tooth mobility on destructive periodontitis in the dog, *J Clin Periodontol* 5:213-225, 1978.

30. Waerhaug J: The infrabony pocket and its relationship to trauma from occlusion and subgingival plaque, *J Periodontol* 50:355-365, 1979.

31. Ericcson I, Lindhe J: Effect of longstanding jiggling on experimental marginal periodontitis in the beagle dog, *J Clin Periodontol* 9:497-503, 1982.

32. Lindhe J, Ericcson I: Effect of elimination of the jiggling forces on periodontally exposed teeth in the dog, *J Periodontol* 53:562-567, 1982.

33. Philstom BL, Anderson KA, Aeppli D, Schaffer EM: Association between signs of trauma from occlusion and periodontitis, *J Periodontol* 57:1-6, 1986.

34. Rangert B, Jemt T, Jorneus L: Forces and moments on Branemark implants, *Int J Oral Maxillofac Implants* 4:241-247, 1989.

35. Starr NL: Treatment planning and treatment sequencing with and without endosseous implants: a comprehensive therapeutic approach to the partially edentulous patient, *Seattle Study Club Journal* 1:1, 21-34, 1995.

36. Israelson H, Plemons JM, Watkins P, Sony C: Barium-coated surgical stents and computer-assisted tomography in the preoperative assessment of dental implant patients, *Int J Periodontics Restorative Dent* 12:53-61, 1992.

37. Gurel G: Predictable, precise, and repeatable tooth preparation for porcelain laminate veneers, *Pract Proced Aesthet Dent* 15(1):17-24, 2003.

38. Marks MH: Tooth movement in periodontal therapy. In Goldman HM, Cohen DW, editors: *Periodontal therapy*, St. Louis, 1973, CV Mosby Company, pp 533-537.

39. Nyman S, Lindhe J, Karring T: Reattachment—new attachment. In Lindhe J, editor: *Textbook of clinical periodontology*, Copenhagen, 1989, Munksgaard, pp 450-476.

40. Lekholm U, Zarb GA, editors: *Tissue-integrated prostheses: osseointegration in clinical dentistry*. Chicago, 1985, Quintessence Publishing Company, pp 199-209.

41. Alberektsson T, Zarb GA, Worthington P, Eriksson AR: The long-term efficacy of currently used dental implants: a review and proposed criteria of success, *Int J Oral Maxillofac Implants* 1:11-25, 1986.

42. Zarb GA, Schmitt A: The longitudinal clinical effectiveness of osseointegrated dental implants. The Toronto Study. Part I: surgical results, *J Prosthet Dent* 62:451-457, 1989.

43. Zarb GA, Schmitt A: The longitudinal clinical effectiveness of osseointegrated dental implants. The Toronto

Study. Part II: the prosthetic results, *J Prosthet Dent* 64:53-61, 1989.

44. Zarb GA, Schmitt A: The longitudinal clinical effectiveness of osseointegrated dental implants. The Toronto Study. Part III: problems and complications encountered, *J Prosthet Dent* 64:185-194, 1989.

45. Friberg B, Jemt T, Lekholm U: Early failures in 4,641 consecutively placed Branemark dental implants: a study from stage I surgery to the connection of the completed prostheses, *Int J Oral Maxillofac Implants* 6:142-146, 1991.

46. Lekholm U, Adell R, Lindhe J et al: Marginal tissue reactions at osseointegrated titanium fixtures. (II) A cross-sectional retrospective study, *Int J Oral Maxillofac Surg* 15:53-61, 1986.

47. Nevins M, Mellonig JT: Enhancement of the damaged edentulous ridge to receive dental implants: a combination of allograft and the Gore-Tex membrane, *Int J Periodontics Restorative Dent* 12:97-111, 1992.

48. Misch CM, Misch CE, Resnick RR, Ismail YH: Reconstruction of maxillary alveolar defects with mandibular symphysis grafts for dental implants: a preliminary procedural report, *Int J Oral Maxillofac Implants* 3:360-366, 1992.

49. Hirsch JM, Ericsson I: Maxillary sinus augmentation using mandibular bone grafts and simultaneous installation of implants. A surgical technique, *Clin Oral Implants Res* 2:91-96, 1991.

50. Hurzeler MB, Kirsch A, Ackermann K-L, Quinones CR: Reconstruction of the severely resorbed maxilla with dental implants in the augmented maxillary sinus: a 5-year clinical investigation, *Int J Oral Maxillofac Implants* 11:466-475, 1996.

51. Amsterdam M, Fox I: Provisional splinting—principles and techniques, *Dent Clin North Am* 3:73, 1959.

52. Langer B, Sullivan DY: Osseointegration: its impact on the interrelationship of periodontics and restorative dentistry. Part III, *Int J Periodontics Restorative Dent* 4:241-261, 1989.

53. Ericsson I, Lekholm U, Branemark PI et al: A clinical evaluation of fixed bridge restorations supported by the combination of teeth and osseointegrated implants, *J Clin Periodontol* 13:307-312, 1986.

54. Ericsson I, Glantz PO, Branemark PI: Use of implants in restorative therapy in patients with reduced periodontal tissue support, *Quintessence Int* 19:801-807, 1988.

55. Van Steenberghe D: A retrospective multicenter evaluation of the survival rate of osseointegrated fixtures supporting fixed partial prostheses in the treatment of partial edentulism, *J Prosthet Dent* 61:217-223, 1989.

56. Van Steenberghe D, Lekholm U, Bolender C et al: The applicability of osseointegrated oral implants in the rehabilitation of partial edentulism: a prospective multicenter study of 558 fixtures, *Int J Oral Maxillofac Implants* 5:272-281, 1990.

57. Jemt T, Lekholm U, Adell R: Osseointegrated implants in the treatment of partially edentulous patients: a preliminary study on 876 consecutively placed fixtures, *Int J Oral Maxillofac Implants* 4:211-217, 1989.

58. Klinge B: Implants in relation to natural teeth, *J Clin Periodontol* 18:482-487, 1991.

59. Astrand P, Borg K, Gunne J, Olsson M: Combination of natural teeth and osseointegrated implants as prosthesis abutments: a 2-year longitudinal study, *Int J Oral Maxillofac Implants* 3:305-312, 1991.

60. Gunne J, Astrand P, Ahlen K et al: Implants in partially edentulous patients: a longitudinal study of bridges supported by both implants and natural teeth, *Clin Oral Implants Res* 2:49-56, 1992.

61. Pylant T, Triplett RG, Brunsvold MA: A retrospective evaluation of endosseous titanium implants in the partially edentulous patient, *Int J Oral Maxillofac Implants* 7:195-202, 1992.

62. Buser D, Bragger U, Lang NP, Nyman S: Regeneration and enlargement of jaw bone using guided tissue regeneration, *Clin Oral Implants Res* 1:22-32, 1990.

63. Jovanovic SA, Nevins M: Bone-formation utilizing titanium-reinforced barrier membranes, *Int J Periodontics Restorative Dent* 15:1, 1995.

64. Schluger S: Osseous resection—a basic principle in periodontal surgery, *Oral Surg Oral Med Oral Pathol* 2:316, 1949.

65. Ochsenbein C: Osseous resection in periodontal therapy, *J Periodontol* 29:15, 1958.

66. Friedman N: Periodontal osseous surgery, osteoplasty, osteoectomy, *J Periodontol* 26:257, 1955.

67. Salama H, Salama M: The role of orthodontic extrusive remodeling in the enhancement of soft and hard tissue profiles prior to implant placement: a systemic approach to the management of extraction site defects, *Int J Periodontics Restorative Dent* 13:312-333, 1993.

68. Ingber JS: Forced eruption, I. A method of treating isolated one and two wall infrabony osseous defects—rationale and case report, *J Periodontol* 45:199-206, 1974.

69. Ingber JS: Forced eruption, II. A method of treating isolated one and two wall infrabony osseous defects—rationale and case report, *J Periodontol* 47:203-216, 1976.

70. Schnitman P, Wohrle P, Rubenstein J: Immediate fixed interim prosthesis supported by two stage threaded implants: methodology and results, *J Oral Implants* 16:96-105, 1990.

71. Wong KM, Youdelis RA, Heindl H: Aesthetic tooth replacement using osseointegrated implants: pontics and immediate implant site development, *Pract Proced Aesthet Dent* 15:45-47, 2003.

72. Proussaefs P: Histologic evaluation of an immediately loaded titanium provisional implant retrieved after functioning for 18 months: a clinical report, *J Prosthet Dent* 89:331-334, 2003.

73. Froum S, Emtiaz S, Bloom M et al: The use of transitional implants for immediate fixed temporary prosthesis in cases of implant restorations, *Pract Periodontics Aesthet Dent* 10:737-746, 1998.

74. Bohsali K, Simon H, Kan J, Redd M: Modular transitional implants to support the interim maxillary overdenture, *Compen Contin Educ Dent* 20:975-978, 980, 982-983, 1999.

75. Zubery Y, Bichacho N, Moses O, Tal H: Immediate loading of Modular transitional implants: a histologic and histomorphometric study in dogs, *Int J Periodontics Restorative Dent* 19:343-353, 1999.

76. Zitman N, Marinello G: Treatment plan for restoring the edentulous maxilla with implant-supported restorations: removable overdenture versus fixed partial denture design, *J Prosthet Dent* 82:188-196, 1999.

77. Starr NL, Miller GM: Implant placement in the vertically enhanced ridge, *Compend Contin Educ Dent* 22:13-22.

78. Sarment DP, Al-Shammari K, Kazor CE: Stereolithographic surgical templates for placement of dental implants in complex cases, *Int J Periodontics Restorative Dent* 23:287-295, 2003.

79. Langer B: Spontaneous in situ gingival augmentation, *Int J Periodontics Restorative Dent* 14:525-535, 1994.

80. Lazzara RJ: Immediate implant placement into extraction sites: surgical and restorative advantages, *Int J Periodontics Restorative Dent* 9:333-343, 1989.

81. Shanaman RH: The use of guided tissue regeneration to facilitate ideal prosthetic placement of implants, *Int J Periodontics Restorative Dent* 12:257-265, 1992.

82. Simion M, Trisi P, Piattelli A: Vertical ridge augmentation using a membrane technique associated with osseointegrated implants, *Int J Periodontics Restorative Dent* 14:496-511, 1994.

83. Buser D, Dula K, Hirt HP et al: Localized ridge augmentation using guided bone regeneration. In Buser D, Dahlin C, Schenk RK, editors: *Guided bone regeneration in implant dentistry*, Chicago, 1994, Quintessence, pp 189-233.

84. Froum SJ, Tarnow DP, Wallace SS et al: Sinus floor elevation using anorganic bovine bone matrix (Osteograf/N) with and without autogenous bone: a clinical, histologic, radiographic, and histomorphometric analysis—Part 2 of an ongoing prospective study, *Int J Periodontics Restorative Dent* 18:528-543, 1998.

85. Collins TA, Brown GK, Johnson N et al: Team management of atrophic edentulism with autogenous inlay, veneer, and split grafts and endosseous implants: case reports, *Quintessence Int* 26:79-93, 1995.

86. Keller EE, Tolman DE, Eckert S: Surgical-prosthodontic reconstruction of advanced maxillary bone compromise with autogenous onlay block bone grafts and osseointegrated endosseous implants: a 12-year study of 32 consecutive patients, *Int J Oral Maxillofac Implants* 14:197-209, 1999.

87. Keller EE, Van Roekel NB, Desjardins RP et al: Prosthetic-surgical reconstruction of the severely resorbed maxilla with iliac bone grafting and tissue-integrated prostheses, *Int J Oral Maxillofac Implants* 3:155-165, 1987.

88. Chin M, Toth BA: Distraction osteogenesis in maxillofacial surgery using internal devices: review of five cases, *J Oral Maxillofac Surg* 54:45-53, 1996.

89. Siebert JS: Reconstruction of deformed, partially edentulous ridges, using full thickness onlay grafts. Part I. Technique and wound healing, *Compend Contin Educ Dent* 4:437-453, 1983.

90. Seibert JS, Louis JV: Soft-tissue ridge augmentation utilizing a combination onlay-interpositional graft procedure: a case report, *Int J Periodontics Restorative Dent* 16:310-321, 1996.

91. Roberts WE, Turley PK, Brezniak N, Fielder PJ: Implants: bone physiology and metabolism, *CDA J* 15:54-61, 1987.

92. Bengazi F, Wennstrom JL, Lekholm U: Recession of the soft tissue margin at oral implants. A 2-year longitudinal prospective study, *Clin Oral Implant Res* 7:303-310, 1996.

93. Small PN, Tarnow DP: Gingival recession around implants: a 1-year longitudinal prospective study, *Int J Oral Maxillofac Implants* 15:527-532, 2000.

94. Grunder U: Stability of the mucosal topography around single-tooth implants and adjacent teeth: 1-year results, *Int J Periodontics Restorative Dent* 20:11-17, 2000.

95. Small P-N, Tarnow DP, Cho S-C: Gingival recession around wide-diameter versus standard-diameter implants: a 3- to 5-year longitudinal prospective study, *Pract Periodontics Aesthet Dent* 13:143-146, 2001.

96. Berglundh T, Lindhe J: Dimension of the peri-implant mucosa. Biological width revisited, *J Clin Periodontol* 23:971-973, 1996.

97. Binon P: Provisionalization in implant prosthodontics for partially edentulous arch, *Dent Implantol Update* 6(8):57-61, 1995.

98. Chiche G, Weaver C, Pinault A, Elliot R: Auxiliary substructure for screw-retained prostheses, *Int J Prosthodont* 5:407-412, 1989.

99. Krekeler G, Schilli W, Diemer J: Should the exit of the artificial abutment tooth be positioned in the region of the attached gingiva? *Int J Oral Surg* 14:504-508, 1985.

100. Lang LA, Hoffensburger M, Wang R-F et al: The universal acceptance of a CAD/CAM created abutment by six implant systems. University of Michigan on line: Available at www.umich.edu/~nbumictr/

101. Rangert B, Gunne J, Sullivan DY: Mechanical aspects of a Branemark implant connected to a natural tooth: an in vitro study, *Int J Oral Maxillofac Implants* 6:177-186, 1991.

102. Hebel K, Gajjar R: Cement-retained versus screw-retained implant restorations: achieving optimal occlusion and esthetics in implant dentistry, *J Prosthet Dent* 77:28-35, 1997.

103. Van Steenberghe D: Periodontal aspects of osseointegrated oral implants ad modum Branemark, *Dent Clin North Am* 32:355-370, 1988.

104. Lekholm U, Ericsson I, Adell R, Slots J: The condition of soft tissues at tooth and fixture abutments supporting fixed bridges: a microbiological and histological study, *J Clin Periodontol* 13:558-562, 1986.

105. Baumgarten H, Chiche G: Diagnosis and evaluation of complications and failures associated with osseointegrated implants, *Compend Contin Educ Dent* 16:814-823, 1995.

106. Wiskott H, Nicholls J, Belser U: Stress fatigue: basic principles and prosthodontics implications, *Int J Prosthet* 8:105-116, 1995.

107. Armitage GC: Development of a classification system of periodontal disease and conditions, *Ann Periodontol* 4:1-6, 1999.

108. Pinault A, Chiche GJ: *Esthetics of anterior fixed prosthodontics.* Carol Stream, Ill, 1994, Quintessence Publishing.

109. Misch C: *Contemporary implant dentistry.* St. Louis, 1999, Mosby.

28 Orthodontic Therapy for the Periodontal-Restorative Patient

Vincent G. Kokich and Vincent O. Kokich

Orthodontic tooth movement may be a substantial benefit to the adult periorestorative patient. Many adults who seek routine restorative dentistry have problems with tooth malposition that compromise their ability to clean and maintain their dentitions. If these individuals also are susceptible to periodontal disease, tooth malposition could be an exacerbating factor that could cause premature loss of specific teeth. Orthodontic appliances have become smaller, less noticeable, and easier to maintain during orthodontic therapy. Many adults are seeking orthodontic therapy to improve the esthetics of their smile. If these individuals also have underlying gingival or osseous defects, these problem areas often can be improved during orthodontic therapy. In addition, implants have now become a primary method of tooth replacement for patients with congenitally absent, previously extracted, or hopeless teeth. In some of these situations, there is insufficient bone to support the implant. In other situations, adjacent teeth may have drifted into the implant space preventing proper placement of the implant. Orthodontic therapy not only can create sufficient space for the implant, but strategic tooth movement can result in implant site development to create sufficient bone for the implant and to avoid surgical ridge augmentation. However, the orthodontist must be aware of these situations and design the appropriate tooth movement for all of these adjunctive procedures. The purpose of this chapter is to illustrate how orthodontic therapy can enhance the periodontal health and restorability of teeth and implants.

ORTHODONTIC MANAGEMENT OF GINGIVAL DISCREPANCIES

Uneven Gingival Margins

The relative level of the gingival margins of the six maxillary anterior teeth plays an important role in the esthetic appearance of the crowns.[1,2] Four characteristics contribute to ideal gingival form. First, the gingival margins of the two central incisors should be at the same level or within 1 mm of the same level. Research has shown that lay people will regard a 1.5-mm discrepancy between central incisors as unesthetic.[3] Second, the gingival margins of the central incisors should be positioned more apically than the lateral incisors and should be at the same level as the canines.[4] Third, the contour of the labial gingival margins should mimic the contour of the cementoenamel junctions (CEJs) of the teeth. Last, there should be a papilla between each tooth, and the height of the tip of the papilla is usually halfway between the incisal edge and the labial gingival height of contour over the center of each anterior tooth. Therefore, the gingival papilla occupies half of the interproximal contact space, and the adjacent teeth form the other half of the contact.

However, some patients may have gingival margin discrepancies between adjacent teeth (Figs. 28-1 and 28-2). These discrepancies could be caused by abrasion of the incisal edges or delayed migration of the gingival margins. When gingival margin discrepancies are present, the clinician must determine the proper solution for the problem: orthodontic movement to reposition the gingival margins or surgical correction of gingival margin discrepancies.

To make the correct decision, it is necessary to evaluate four criteria.[5] First, the relation between the gingival margin of the maxillary central incisors and the patient's lip line should be assessed when the patient smiles. If a gingival margin discrepancy exists, but the patient's lip does not move upward to expose the discrepancy, it often does not require correction. If a gingival margin discrepancy is apparent, the next step is to evaluate the labial sulcular depths of the two central incisors. If the shorter tooth has a deeper sulcus, excisional gingivectomy may be appropriate to move the gingival margin of the shorter tooth apically (Fig. 28-1). However, if the sulcular depths of the short and long incisors are equivalent, and the CEJ is at the depth of the sulcus, gingival surgery may not be appropriate, because it could expose the cementum of the shorter tooth.

The third step is to evaluate the relation between the shortest central incisor and the adjacent lateral incisors. If the shortest central incisor is still longer than the lateral incisors, the other possibility is to extrude the longer central incisor and equilibrate the incisal edge. This will move the gingival margin coronally and eliminate the gingival margin discrepancy. However, if the shortest central were shorter than the lateral incisors (Fig. 28-2), this technique would produce an unesthetic relation between the gingival margins of the central and lateral incisors.

The fourth step is to determine if the incisal edges have been abraded. This is best appreciated by evaluating the teeth from an incisal perspective. If one incisal edge is thicker labiolingually than the adjacent tooth, this may indicate that it has been abraded and the tooth has overerupted. In addition, if the incisal edge has a yellow or brown central region, this could indicate abrasion into the dentin of the tooth. In these situations, the best method of correcting the gingival margin discrepancy is to intrude the short central incisor (Fig. 28-2). This method will move the gingival margin apically and allow restoration of the incisal edges. The intrusion should be accomplished at least 6 months before appliance removal. This allows reorientation of the principal fibers of the periodontium and avoids reextrusion of the central incisor(s) after appliance removal.[6]

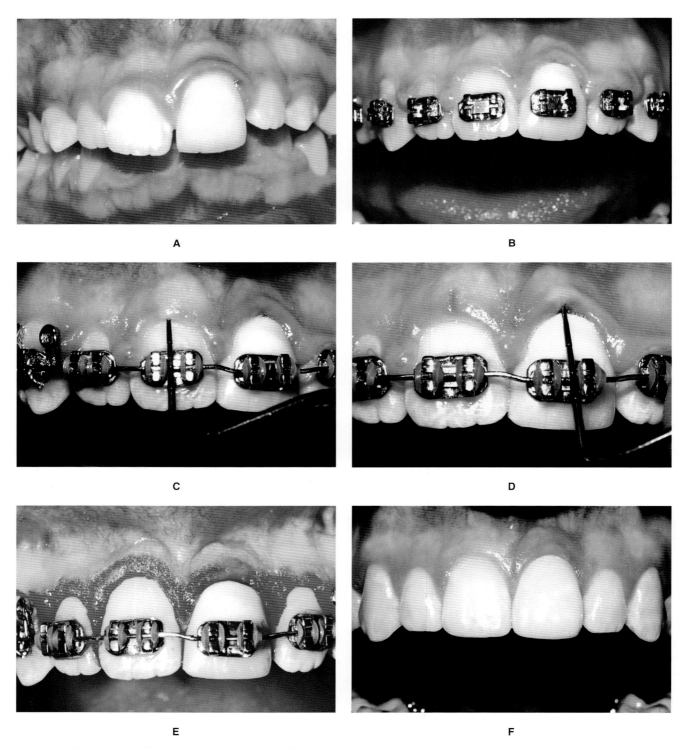

A   **B**

C   **D**

E   **F**

Figure 28-1. This patient had fallen and injured the maxillary left central incisor. Root canal therapy was performed and a crown had been placed on the tooth (**A**). The original discrepancy in crown lengths between right and left central incisors (**A** and **B**) did not improve during orthodontic alignment. Periodontal probing showed that the sulcus depth over the right central incisor (**C**) was greater than over the left central (**D**). The diagnosis was altered passive eruption, and gingivectomy was performed to level the margins (**E**). The final crown on the left central now matches the length of the nonrestored right central incisor. Enameloplasty was performed on teeth #7, 8, and 10 (**F**). A gingivectomy approach was possible in this case because the distance from the cementoenamel junction to the crest of the bone was 3 mm on all incisors; thus, use of a gingivectomy did not violate the biologic width.

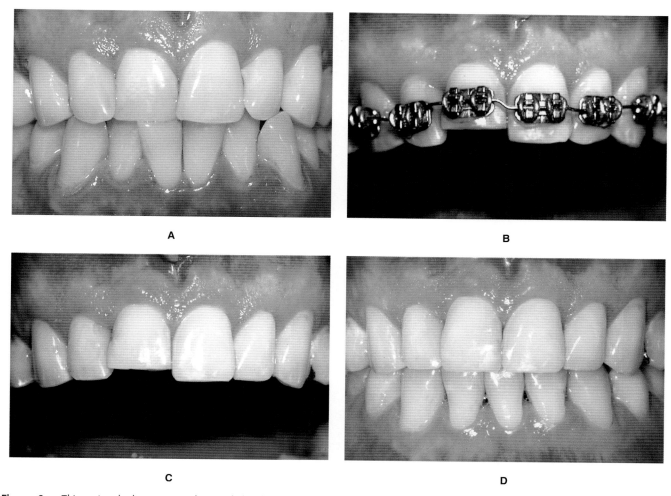

Figure 28-2. This patient had a protrusive bruxing habit that had resulted in abrasion and overeruption of the maxillary right central incisor (**A**). The objective was to level the gingival margins during orthodontic therapy. Although gingival surgery was a possibility, the labial sulcular depth of the maxillary right central incisor was only 1 mm, and the cementoenamel junction was located at the bottom of the sulcus. Therefore, the best solution involved positioning the orthodontic brackets to facilitate intrusion of the right central incisor (**B**). The right central incisor has been intruded (**C**), permitting the restorative dentist to restore the portion of the tooth that the patient had abraded (**D**), resulting in the correct gingival margin levels and crown lengths at the end of treatment.

Significant Abrasion and Overeruption

Occasionally, patients will have destructive dental habits such as a protrusive bruxing habit that could result in significant wear of the maxillary and mandibular incisors (Fig. 28-3) and compensatory overeruption of these teeth. When the restorative dentist contemplates restoration of these abraded teeth, it is often impossible, because of the lack of crown length, to achieve adequate retention and resistance form for the crown preparations.[5] Two options are available. One option is extensive crown lengthening by elevating a flap, removing sufficient bone, and apically positioning the flap to expose adequate tooth length for crown preparation. However, this type of procedure is contraindicated in the patient with short tapered roots,

because it could adversely affect the final root-to-crown ratio, and it could potentially result in "black triangles" or open gingival embrasures between the anterior teeth.

The other option for improving the restorability of these short abraded teeth is to orthodontically intrude the teeth and move the gingival margins apically (Fig. 28-3). It is possible for the orthodontist to intrude as many as four maxillary incisors by using the posterior teeth as anchorage during the intrusion process. This process is accomplished by placing the orthodontic brackets as close to the incisal edges of the maxillary incisors as possible. The brackets are placed in their normal position on the canines and remaining posterior teeth. The patient's posterior occlusion will resist the eruption of the posterior

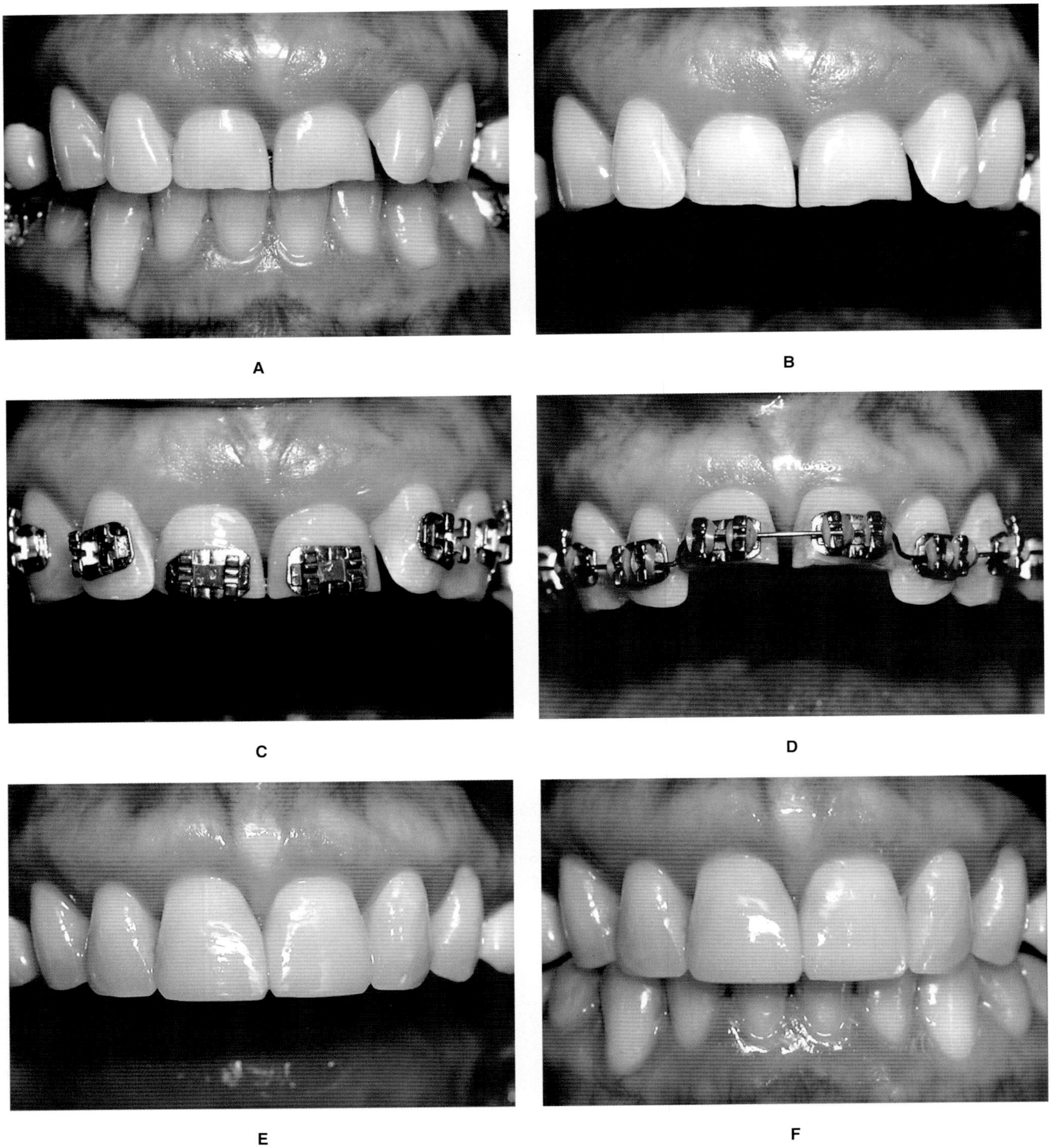

Figure 28-3. This patient had a protrusive bruxing habit that had caused severe abrasion of both maxillary central incisors, resulting in loss of more than half of the crown length of these teeth (**A** and **B**). Two possible options existed for gaining crown length to restore the central incisors. One possibility was an apically positioned flap with osseous recontouring, which would expose the roots of the teeth. The less invasive option was to intrude the central incisors orthodontically, level the gingival margins (**C** and **D**), and allow the dentist to restore the abraded incisal edges (**E** and **F**). The orthodontic option was clearly successful and desirable in this patient.

teeth, and the incisors will gradually intrude and move the gingival margins and the crowns apically. This creates the restorative space necessary to temporarily restore the incisal edges of these teeth (Fig. 28-3) and to eventually place the final crowns.

When abraded teeth are intruded significantly, it is necessary to hold these teeth for at least 6 months in the intruded position with the orthodontic brackets and/or archwires, or some sort of bonded retainer. The principal fibers of the periodontium must accommodate to the new intruded position,[6] and this process could take a minimum of 6 months in most adult patients. Orthodontic intrusion of severely abraded and overerupted teeth is usually a distinct advantage over periodontal crown lengthening, unless the patient has extremely long and broad roots or has had extensive horizontal bone loss.

Open Gingival Embrasures

The presence of a papilla between the maxillary central incisors is a key esthetic factor in any individual.[7,8] Occasionally, adults will have open gingival embrasures or black triangles between their central incisors. These unsightly areas often are difficult to resolve with periodontal therapy. However, orthodontic treatment can correct many of these open gingival embrasures, even in some adult periodontal patients. This space is usually due to one of three factors: tooth shape, root angulation, or periodontal bone loss.[9]

The interproximal contact between the maxillary central incisors consists of two parts: one portion is the tooth contact, and the other portion is the papilla. The papilla-to-contact ratio is about 1:1; in other words, half the space is occupied by papilla and half is formed by the tooth contact.[8] If the patient has an open embrasure, the first aspect that the clinician should evaluate is whether the problem is caused by the papilla or the tooth contact. If the papilla is the problem, then the cause is usually a lack of bone support caused by an underlying periodontal osseous defect.

In some situations, a deficient papilla can be lengthened slightly with orthodontic treatment. By closing open contacts, the orthodontist can squeeze the interproximal gingiva and move it incisally. This type of movement can help to create a more esthetic papilla between two teeth despite alveolar bone loss. Another possibility is to erupt adjacent teeth when the interproximal bone level is positioned apically.

Most open embrasures between the central incisors are caused by problems with tooth contact. The first step in the diagnosis of this problem is to evaluate a periapical radiograph of the central incisors. If the root angulation is divergent (Fig. 28-4), then the brackets should be repositioned so the root position can be corrected. In these situations, the incisal edges may be uneven and require restoration with either composite or porcelain restorations.

If the periapical radiograph shows that the roots are in their correct relation, then the open gingival embrasure is because of triangular tooth shape.

If the shape of the tooth is the problem, two solutions are possible: one possibility is to restore the open gingival embrasure; the other option is to reshape the tooth (Fig. 28-5), by flattening the incisal contact and then closing the space orthodontically. This will result in lengthening of the contact until it meets the papilla. In addition, if the embrasure space is large, closing the space will squeeze the papilla between the central incisors. This will help to create a 1:1 relation between the contact and papilla, and will restore uniformity to the heights between the midline and adjacent papillae.

ORTHODONTICS AND THE IMPLANT PATIENT

Implants are routinely used in dentistry. In some situations, orthodontic intervention could be advantageous to enhance the outcome of implant therapy. Three situations could require interaction between the orthodontist and the implant surgeon. First, implants are used commonly to replace congenitally missing teeth in adolescent orthodontic patients. In some of these patients, there is insufficient space for the implant, and the orthodontist must create the appropriate space for the surgeon. Second, there may be insufficient thickness of alveolar bone to house the implant. These situations could require alveolar bone grafting to create enough buccolingual width for the implant. However, strategic orthodontic movement of adjacent teeth also could create the necessary thickness of the alveolar ridge. Third, implants could be used as abutments for orthodontic anchorage. The orthodontist and implant surgeon must collaborate not only on the precise placement of the implant, but also the timing of implant placement.

Congenitally Missing Second Premolars

Often adolescent patients are congenitally missing mandibular second premolars. If the patient does not have an arch length deficiency with a satisfactory profile, extraction of teeth and space closure may be disadvantageous. In these situations, the space from the congenitally missing premolars must be maintained and restored with either a bridge or an implant.

If an implant is planned for the congenitally missing mandibular second premolar, the space and bone support must be monitored and maintained.[10] It is ideal to allow the mandibular primary molar to remain in position as long as possible to maintain the bone support. However, the primary molar may be too wide (mesiodistally) to occlude properly with the opposing dentition (Fig. 28-6). In this situation, it may be advantageous to reduce the width of the primary molar so it approximates the width of a second premolar (Fig. 28-6).

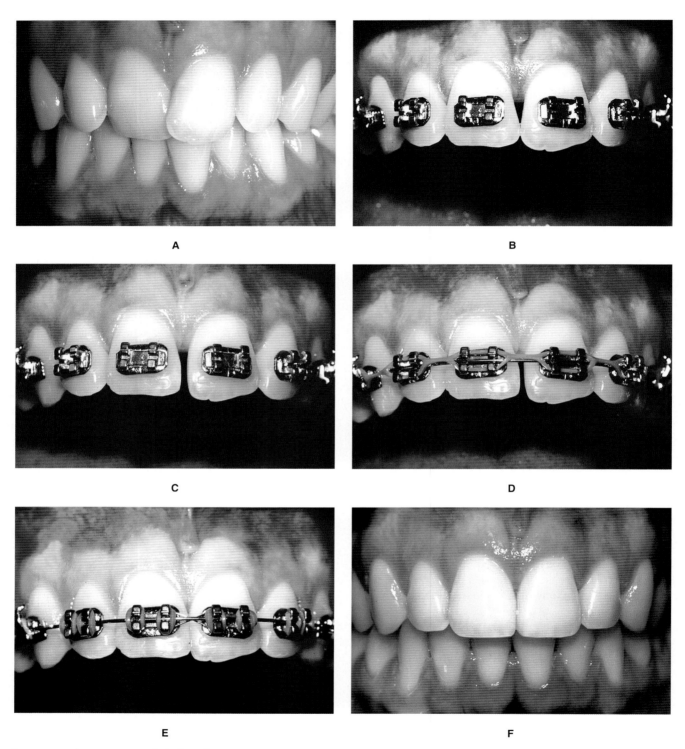

A

B

C

D

E

F

Figure 28-4. This patient initially had overlapped maxillary central incisors (**A**), and after initial orthodontic alignment of the teeth, an open gingival embrasure appeared between the central incisors (**B**). Because the roots had been aligned already, the correct option for closing the open gingival embrasure was to reshape the mesial surfaces of the central incisors (**C**). This created a diastema between these teeth (**D**), which was closed orthodontically (**E**). Because the incisal edges of these teeth had worn unevenly before orthodontics, they required restoration after orthodontics (**F**).

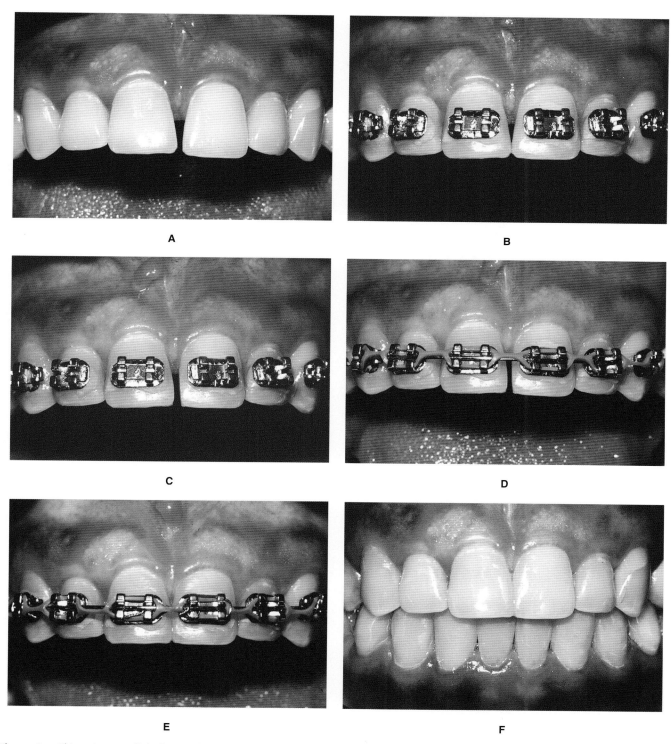

Figure 28-5. This patient initially had triangular-shaped central incisors (**A**), which produced an open gingival embrasure after orthodontic alignment (**B**). Because the roots of the central incisors were parallel with one another, the appropriate solution for the open gingival embrasure was to recontour the mesial surfaces of the central incisors (**C**). As the diastema was closed (**D** and **E**), the tooth contact moved gingivally, and the papilla moved incisally, resulting in the elimination of the open gingival embrasure (**F**).

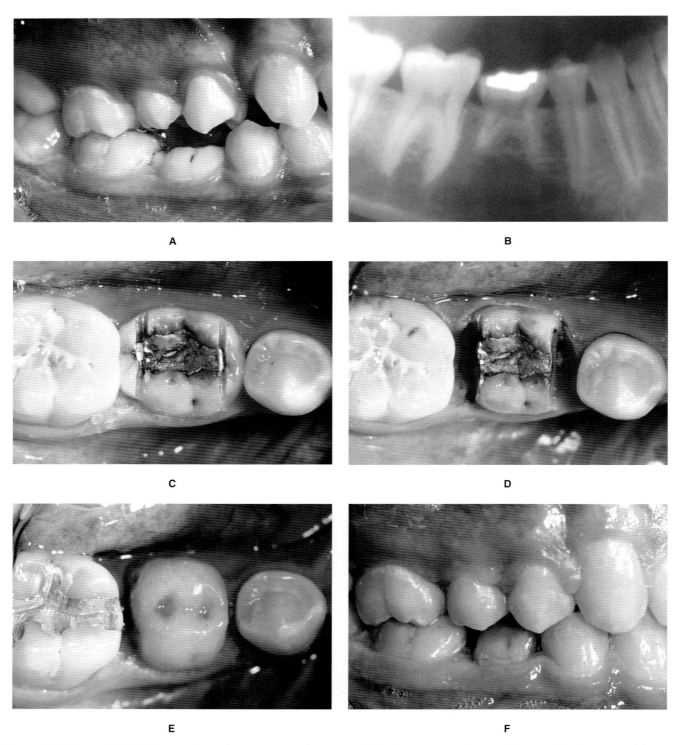

Figure 28-6. The mandibular right second premolar was congenitally missing (**A**), but the primary molar was still present (**B**). This young adolescent patient would eventually receive an implant after she completed facial growth, but the mesiodistal width of the primary molar was much larger than the missing premolar. Therefore, the primary molar crown was reduced in width to approximate the size of a premolar (**C** and **D**). To cover the exposed dentin, the primary molar was restored with a composite buildup approximately the size of a premolar crown (**E**). With the reduction in mesiodistal width, the primary molar could be fit into the correct occlusal relation with the maxillary arch (**F**) and remain in position and maintain the alveolar bone until facial growth is complete and the implant can be placed.

After reduction of the primary molar, it is advantageous to cover the exposed dentin on the mesial and distal surfaces. This can be accomplished with a light-cured composite (Fig. 28-6). Then the composite restoration may be trimmed to simulate the shape and size of a mandibular premolar. In this way, the primary molar may be bracketed and remain in position to maintain the alveolar bone before implant placement.

The age for implant placement in adolescent boys and girls is completely dependent on the completion of facial growth.[11] As the mandibular ramus continues to grow, the posterior teeth erupt. If an implant is placed too early, before growth is completed, it will mimic an ankylosed tooth and become submerged in the alveolus. This could cause a periodontal defect between the implant and adjacent teeth. The most precise method for determining if facial or ramal growth is completed is to superimpose sequential cephalometric radiographs. If growth is continuing, the distance between nasion and menton will continue to increase, indicating that it is too early to place the implant. The implant should not be placed until there is no change in facial vertical dimension taken on two head films 1 year apart. In general, implants should not be placed in boys until after 21 years of age and in girls until after 17 years of age.[11]

If an ankylosed primary molar is not extracted early, and a vertical ridge defect is produced, an option to improve the implant site and eliminate the defect is to move the mandibular first premolar into the second premolar position[10] and to place the implant in the first premolar position (Fig. 28-7). Previous studies have shown that it is possible, within limits, to move a tooth into a narrower edentulous ridge[12,13] to create an implant site. The bone that is created behind the moving tooth typically will be the width of the root of the tooth that was moved.[10] This type of orthodontic movement may eliminate the need for a bone graft in the edentulous site. This type of tooth movement is called orthodontic implant site development.

Congenitally Missing Lateral Incisors

Another common congenitally missing tooth is the maxillary lateral incisor. A primary factor that the orthodontist must be aware of is the amount of mesiodistal space that should be created for the lateral incisor implant.[10] First, if a contralateral incisor is present, the space for the missing lateral incisor crown should match the width of the natural lateral incisor. In general, this space should be at least 5.5 mm in width. If the contralateral lateral incisor is malformed or peg-shaped and is smaller than 5.5 mm, then the crown should be built up to a width that is 67% to 75% the width of the central incisor. The width of most central incisors ranges from 8 to 10 mm. Therefore, the width of the lateral incisor implant crown should range from about 5.5 to 7.0 mm.

The width of the edentulous space should allow at least 1 mm between the implant and the adjacent teeth. If the distance between implant and tooth is less than 1 mm, the interproximal bone could be jeopardized,[14,15] and the space for the papilla between the implant crown and the adjacent teeth will be constricted and could appear much shorter than the contralateral papillae.[10] This will make the implant crown more obvious and appear less esthetic.

The space between the roots of the adjacent central incisor and canine must be sufficient to permit placement of the implant (Fig. 28-8). As space is created between a central incisor and canine by pushing the crowns apart, the roots tend to move toward one another. This root proximity must be corrected before implant placement. This type of tooth movement is accomplished by progressively bending the archwires to move the apices of the roots in opposite directions.

The labiolingual dimension of the alveolar ridge must be wide enough to place the implant in its proper position. If insufficient ridge width exists, a bone graft may be necessary before or during implant placement. However, a bone graft can be avoided if the central incisor and canine erupt adjacent to one another (Fig. 28-9). As the space is opened orthodontically for the future implant, bone is laid down along fiber tracks of the periodontal membrane. The labiolingual width of the alveolar ridge formed in this manner is generally stable over time. Therefore, if implant placement is delayed until an adolescent has completed facial growth, the ridge will not become narrower.

Implant Anchorage during Orthodontics

Occasionally, adult orthodontic patients may be missing several teeth. This could be a problem for the orthodontist, because adjacent teeth are necessary to provide the reciprocal anchorage necessary for orthodontic tooth movement. In these situations, if implants will be used to restore the edentulous spaces anyway, the implants could be placed before orthodontics[16,17] and used initially as an anchor to facilitate tooth movement, and then as a restorative abutment to restore the edentulous space (Fig. 28-10). In this situation, careful planning and collaboration are necessary between the orthodontist and implant surgeon to position the implant properly. A diagnostic wax-up is mandatory, because the implant is placed before orthodontic procedures are begun. The orthodontist must construct the set-up using specific guidelines that will simulate the eventual tooth movement. Then a plastic placement guide is constructed from the wax-up to provide the surgeon with the precise location of the implant. By locating the implant in this manner, it will be in the correct position not only for the orthodontist, but also for the restorative dentist.

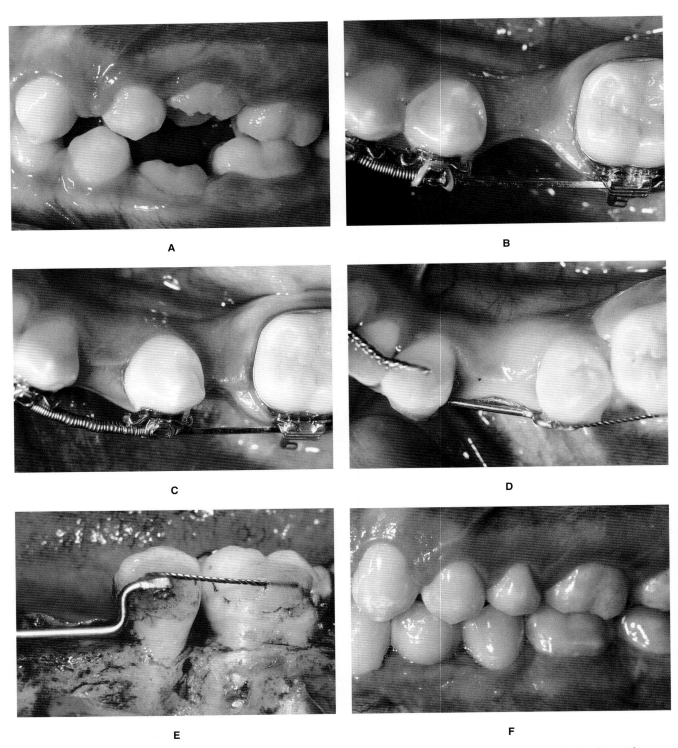

Figure 28-7. The mandibular left second premolar was congenitally missing, and the primary molar was ankylosed and submerged (**A**). After extraction of the primary second molar, the alveolar ridge narrowed significantly (**B**), and there was insufficient thickness of bone for an implant. To increase the ridge thickness and avoid a bone graft, the mandibular first premolar was moved distally (**C** and **D**). When a flap was elevated to place an implant, there was adequate bone in the implant site and also over the root of the first premolar (**E**), which permitted placement of the implant without the need for a bone graft (**F**).

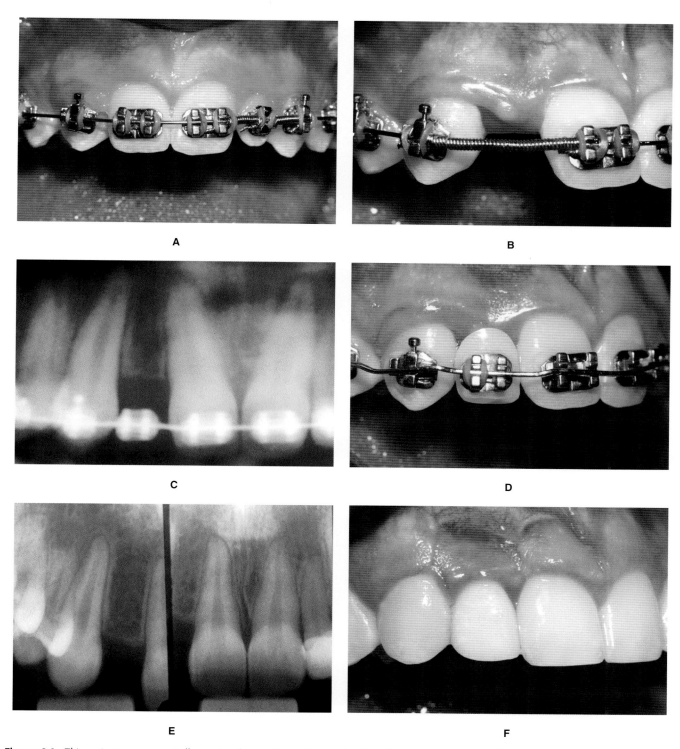

Figure 28-8. This patient was congenitally missing the maxillary right lateral incisor (**A**). As space was opened for the missing tooth, the roots moved toward one another as the crowns moved apart (**B** and **C**). The arch wire was adjusted to tip the roots apart (**D**) to create space for the implant (**E**). When sufficient space exists for an implant, gingival esthetics will be enhanced around the implant (**F**).

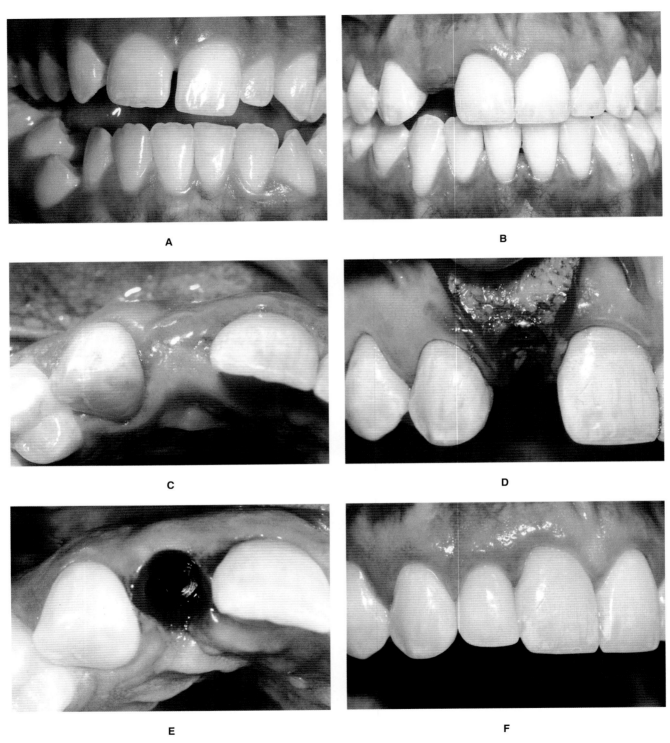

Figure 28-9. Implant site development is a method of creating alveolar bone in which to place an implant. This is especially important in the esthetic zone. This patient is congenitally missing the maxillary right lateral incisor, but fortunately the canine erupted into the lateral position (**A**). This is ideal, because as the orthodontist moves the central incisor and canine apart (**B**) to open space for the lateral incisor implant, alveolar bone is created in the path of the tooth movement (**C**). This provides an ideal ridge in which to position the implant (**D** and **E**), to maximize the esthetic result when the crown is seated on the implant (**F**).

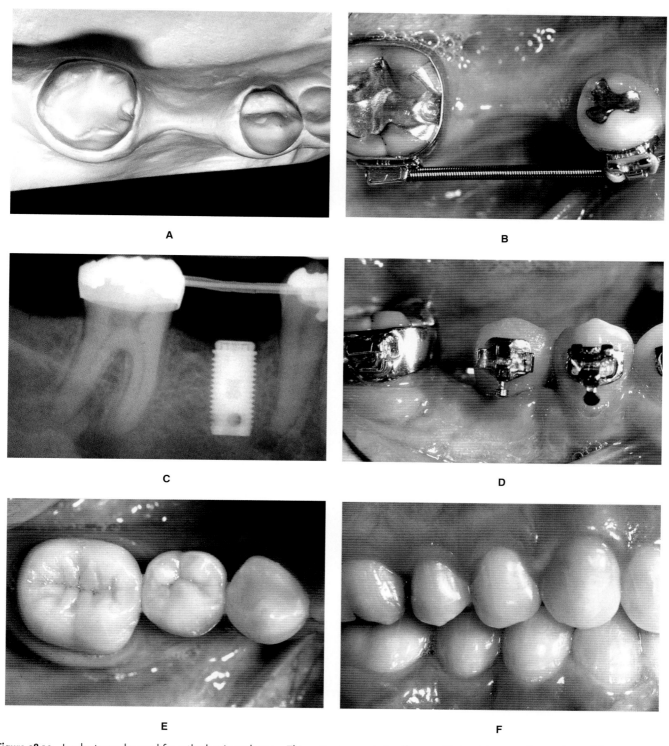

Figure 28-10. Implants can be used for orthodontic anchorage. This patient was missing the mandibular right second premolar and first molar (**A**). Part of the space had closed. There was not enough space for two teeth, and too much space for a one-tooth prosthesis. Because implants were chosen as the method of restoration, the teeth were initially aligned (**B**), and an implant was placed in the position of the future second premolar (**C**). Then a provisional crown and bracket were placed on the implant (**D**). The implant was used as an anchor to drag the second molar mesially, without affecting the position of the first premolar. After orthodontic treatment, the same implant was restored as a second premolar (**E** and **F**).

ORTHODONTIC MANAGEMENT OF OSSEOUS DEFECTS

Hemiseptal Defects

Hemiseptal defects are one-wall osseous defects. Often these are found around mesially tipped teeth (Fig. 28-11) or teeth that have supraerupted. Usually these defects can be eliminated with the appropriate orthodontic treatment. In the case of the tipped tooth, uprighting[18,19] and eruption of the tooth will level the bony defect (Fig. 28-11). In the case of the supraerupted tooth, intrusion and leveling of the adjacent CEJs can help to level the osseous defect.

It is imperative that periodontal inflammation be controlled before orthodontic treatment. This usually can be achieved with initial debridement and rarely requires any preorthodontic surgery. After the completion of orthodontic treatment, these teeth should be stabilized for at least 6 months and reassessed periodontally. Often the pocket has been reduced or eliminated and no further periodontal treatment is needed. It would be injudicious to do preorthodontic osseous corrective surgery in lesions such as these if orthodontics is a part of the overall treatment plan.

In the periodontally healthy patient, orthodontic brackets are positioned on the posterior teeth relative to the marginal ridges and cusps. However, some adult patients may have marginal ridge discrepancies caused by uneven tooth eruption during orthodontic treatment. When the orthodontist encounters marginal ridge discrepancies, the decision where to place the bracket or band is not determined by the anatomy of the tooth. In these situations, it is important for the orthodontist to assess bitewing or

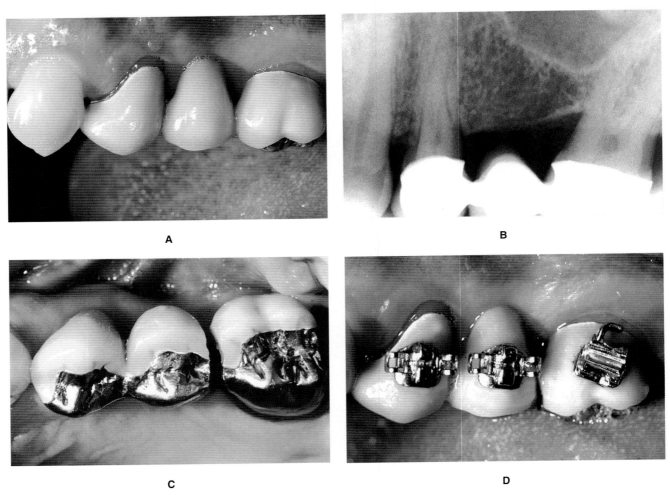

Figure 28-11. This patient was missing the maxillary left second premolar and first molar. The second molar on that side had tipped mesially and had been used as a fixed partial denture abutment connecting the first premolar and second molar (**A**). A radiograph (**B**) confirmed the hemiseptal periodontal defect on the mesial of the second molar abutment, which was associated with a 7 mm pocket. Orthodontics was used to erupt this tooth and eliminate the defect. The pontic was sectioned (**C**), and a bracket was placed at an angle on the tipped molar abutment (**D**).

Continued

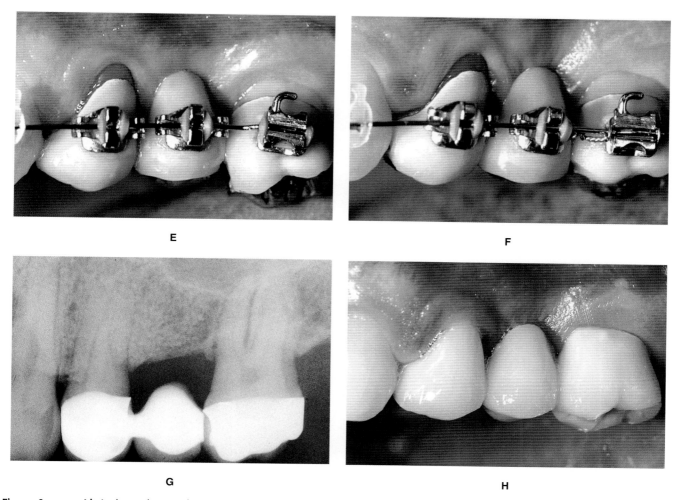

Figure 28-11. cont'd As the tooth erupted (**E**), the mesial marginal ridge of the second molar extended coronal to the occlusal plane. The marginal ridge was equilibrated (**F**). The radiograph shows the positive effect that orthodontics has on leveling the periodontal defect (**G**), and providing for a better fixed partial denture restoration for the patient (**H**).

periapical radiographs of these teeth to determine the interproximal bone level.[20]

If the bone level is oriented in the same direction as the marginal ridge discrepancy, then leveling the marginal ridges will level the bone. However, if the bone level is flat between adjacent teeth, and the marginal ridges are at significantly different levels, correction of the marginal ridge discrepancy orthodontically will produce a hemiseptal defect in the bone. This could cause a periodontal pocket between the two teeth.

If the bone is flat and a marginal ridge discrepancy is present (Fig. 28-12), the orthodontist should not level the marginal ridges orthodontically. In these situations, it may be necessary to equilibrate the crown of the tooth. For some patients, the latter technique may require endodontic therapy and restoration of the tooth because of the amount of reduction of the length of the crown that is required. This

approach is acceptable if the treatment results in a more favorable bone contour between the teeth.

In some patients, a discrepancy may exist between both the marginal ridges and the bony levels between two teeth. However, these discrepancies may not be of equal magnitude. In these patients, orthodontic leveling of the bone may still leave a discrepancy in the marginal ridges. In these situations, the clinician should not use the crowns of the teeth as a guide for completing orthodontic therapy. The clinician should level the bone orthodontically and equilibrate any remaining discrepancies between the marginal ridges. This method will produce the best occlusal result and will improve the periodontal health.

In some patients, accidental or iatrogenic dental trauma may cause an osseous defect adjacent to the affected tooth (Fig. 28-13). In these situations, surgical

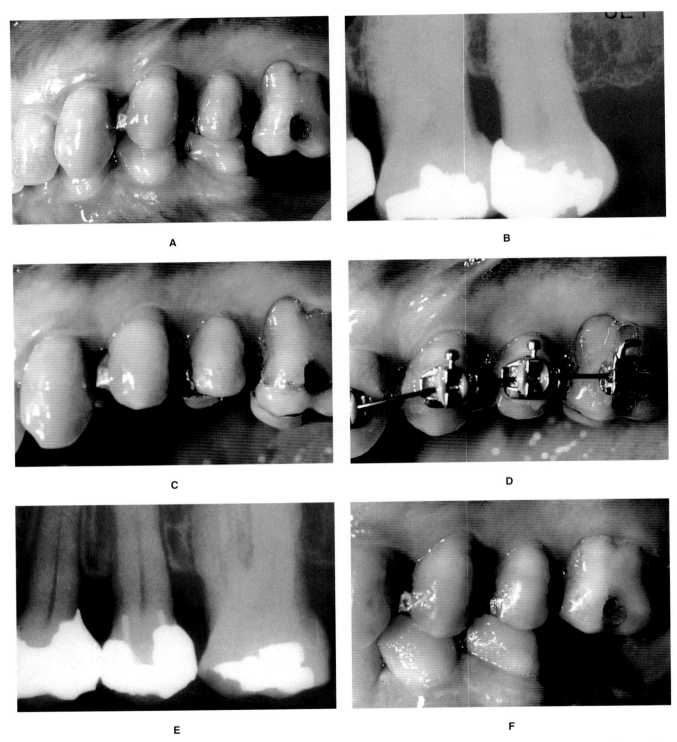

Figure 28-12. This patient had overeruption of the maxillary left first molar and second molars and a marginal ridge defect between the second premolar and first molar (**A**). A pretreatment periapical radiograph (**B**) showed that the interproximal bone was flat. The second molar was extracted. To avoid creating a hemiseptal defect between the first molar and second premolar, the occlusal surface of the first molar was equilibrated (**C** and **D**) and the malocclusion was corrected orthodontically (**E** and **F**). The opposing arch was subsequently restored.

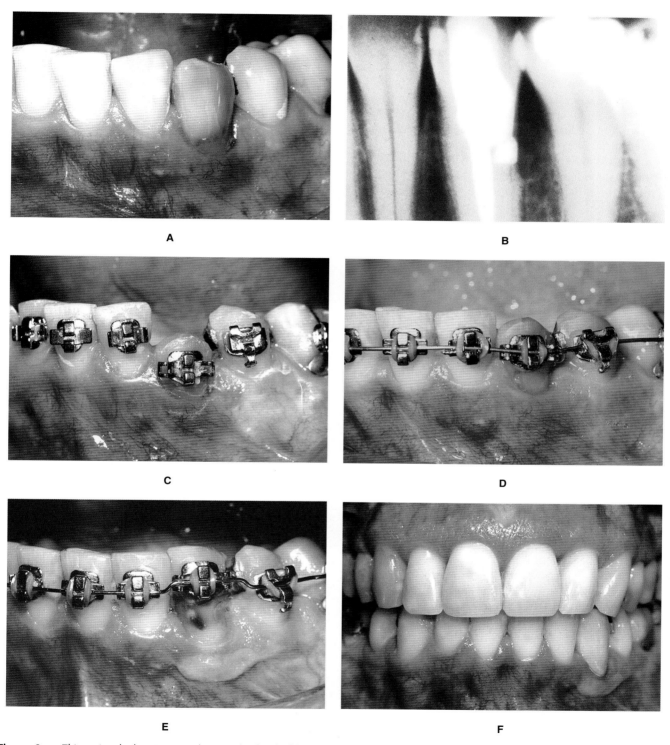

Figure 28-13. This patient had an 8-mm probing on the distal of the mandibular left canine (**A**), which was caused by a perforation on the root surface during previous endodontic therapy (**B**). This produced a two-wall defect, with loss of the labial and distal walls. To correct this defect, the orthodontic brackets were placed gingivally and the cusp tip was equilibrated (**C**). This permitted eruption of the tooth to level the distal defect (**D**). However, to eliminate the mesial and lingual bone level discrepancies created by the eruption, an apically positioned flap was performed. Also, a free epithelialized soft-tissue graft was used to correct the lack of sufficient keratinized tissue (**E**). This allowed the restorative dentist to maintain and restore this previously difficult endodontic/periodontic situation (**F**).

correction of the osseous defect could require significant removal of bone from the adjacent healthy tooth to create an interproximal osseous relation that the patient can maintain. The other alternative in this situation is to erupt the tooth with the osseous defect to eliminate the vertical discrepancy in bone levels. If this were a two-wall defect, periodontal crown lengthening may be necessary after eruption, to level the bone on the nonperiodontally involved surfaces of the affected tooth (Fig. 28-13).

During orthodontic treatment, when teeth are being extruded to level hemiseptal defects, the patient should be monitored regularly by the dentist or periodontist. Initially, the hemiseptal defect will have a greater sulcular depth and will be more difficult for the patient to clean. As the defect is ameliorated through tooth extrusion, interproximal cleaning becomes easier. The dentist or periodontist should recall the patient every 2 to 3 months during the leveling process to control inflammation in the interproximal region.

Advanced Horizontal Bone Loss

After orthodontic treatment has been planned, one of the most important factors that determine the outcome of orthodontic therapy is the location of the bands and brackets on the teeth. In a periodontally healthy individual, the position of the brackets is usually determined by the anatomy of the crowns of the teeth. Anterior brackets should be positioned relative to the incisal edges. Posterior bands or brackets are positioned relative to the marginal ridges. If the incisal edges and marginal ridges are at the correct level, the CEJs also will be at the same level. This relation will create a flat bony contour between the teeth. However, if a patient has underlying periodontal problems and significant alveolar bone loss around certain teeth, using the anatomy of the crown to determine bracket placement is not appropriate.

In a patient with advanced horizontal bone loss, the bone level may have resorbed several millimeters from the CEJ. As this occurs, the crown-to-root ratio will become less favorable. By aligning the crowns of the teeth, the clinician may perpetuate tooth mobility by maintaining an unfavorable crown-to-root ratio. In addition, by aligning the crowns of the teeth and disregarding the bone level, there will be significant bone discrepancies between healthy and periodontally diseased roots. This could require periodontal surgery to ameliorate the discrepancies.

The orthodontist can correct many of these problems by using the bone level as a guide to position the brackets on the teeth (Fig. 28-14). In these situations, the crowns of the teeth may require considerable equilibration. If the tooth is vital, the equilibration should be performed gradually to allow the pulp to form secondary dentin and insulate the tooth during the equilibration process.[21] The goal of equilibration and creative bracket placement is to provide a more favorable bony architecture and a more favorable crown-to-root ratio. In some of these patients, the periodontal defects that were apparent initially may not require periodontal surgery after orthodontic treatment.

Furcation Defects

Furcation defects can be classified as incipient (Class I), moderate (Class II), and advanced (Class III). These lesions require special attention in the patient undergoing orthodontic treatment. Often the molars will require bands with tubes and other attachments that will impede the patient's access to the buccal furcation for home care and instrumentation at the time of recall.

Class I defects are amenable to osseous surgical correction with a good prognosis. Class II furcation defects can be treated with grafting or regenerative therapy with barrier membranes, or both. Class III furcation defects are more difficult to treat, and use of grafting and membranes in these lesions is not as predictable. Treatment of Class III furcation lesions in the lower arch can range from open-flap curettage to create a through-and-through furcation for easier cleaning, to hemisection (Fig. 28-15), or even extraction and replacement[22] with an implant (Fig. 28-16). In the upper arch, Class II and III furcations can sometimes be treated with root resection. The most favorable root to remove is the distobuccal root of an upper molar. This treatment has a good prognosis. The disadvantage of root resection is that it requires endodontic therapy and a full-coverage restoration. Detailed discussion of furcation treatment is found in Chapter 24.

Furcation lesions need special attention because they are the most difficult lesions to maintain and can worsen during orthodontic therapy. These patients will need to be maintained on a 2- to 3-month recall schedule. Detailed instrumentation of these furcations will help to minimize further periodontal breakdown.

Regenerative therapy using membranes, bone grafting, or both has been successful in Class I and II furcations. However, in Class III furcations, the use of membranes has not produced consistently satisfactory results. Therefore, another method of treatment must be used for orthodontic patients with Class III furcations in the mandibular arch.

If a patient with a Class III furcation defect will be undergoing orthodontic treatment, a possible method for treating the furcation is to eliminate it by hemisecting the crown and root of the tooth. This procedure, however, will require endodontic, periodontal, and restorative treatment. If the patient will be undergoing orthodontic treatment, it is advisable to perform the orthodontic treatment first. This is especially true if the roots of the teeth will not be separated or moved apart. In these patients, the molar

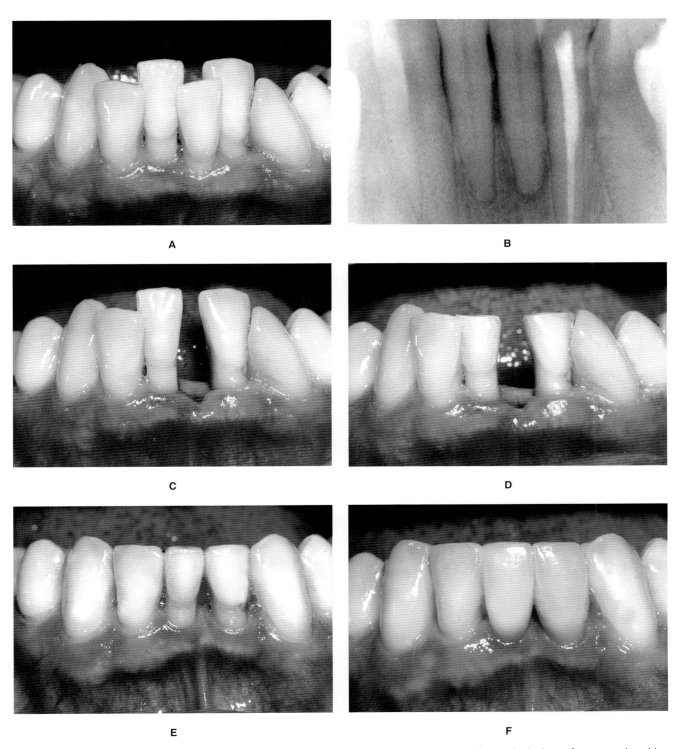

Figure 28-14. This patient had severe crowding and overeruption of the mandibular incisors (**A**). In addition, she had significant periodontal bone loss around the mandibular anterior teeth, but the bone level was flat between these teeth (**B**). To align the teeth, a diagnostic set-up showed that a mandibular incisor extraction (**C**) would produce a good occlusion. To maintain the flat bone levels and to improve the unfavorable crown-to-root ratio, the incisal edges of the overerupted teeth were reduced (**D**). In this way, after orthodontic treatment (**E**), porcelain veneer restorations were able to improve the unesthetic shape of the mandibular incisors (**F**).

to be hemisected remains intact during orthodontics. These patients would require 2- or 3-month recall visits with the periodontist to ensure that the furcation defect does not lose bone during orthodontic treatment. By keeping the tooth intact during the orthodontic treatment, it simplifies the finishing and tooth movement for the orthodontist.

After orthodontic treatment, endodontic therapy must be performed on both roots of the tooth. Then, periodontal surgery is necessary to divide the tooth. Sulcular incisions are made, a flap is elevated buccal and lingual to the molar, and a fissure bur is used to divide the crown and roots of the teeth. In some situations, the process is more difficult if the furcation is positioned toward the apices of the tooth. After the tooth has been divided, the bone is recontoured around each of the roots and the tissue is allowed to heal. If the roots are short and tapered, the

crowns that restore the two halves of the tooth could be splinted together. If the solder joint of the splinted teeth is positioned toward the occlusal, the patient can clean interproximally in the area of the previous furcation.

In some patients requiring hemisection of a mandibular molar with a Class III furcation, it may be advantageous to push the roots apart during orthodontic treatment (Fig. 28-15). If the hemisected molar will be used as an abutment for a fixed partial denture after orthodontics, moving the roots apart orthodontically will permit more favorable restoration and splinting across the adjacent edentulous spaces.[23]

In the latter situation, hemisecting the tooth, endodontic therapy, and periodontal surgery must be completed before the start of orthodontic treatment. After these procedures have been completed, the orthodontist may place bands or brackets on the root fragments and use a coil

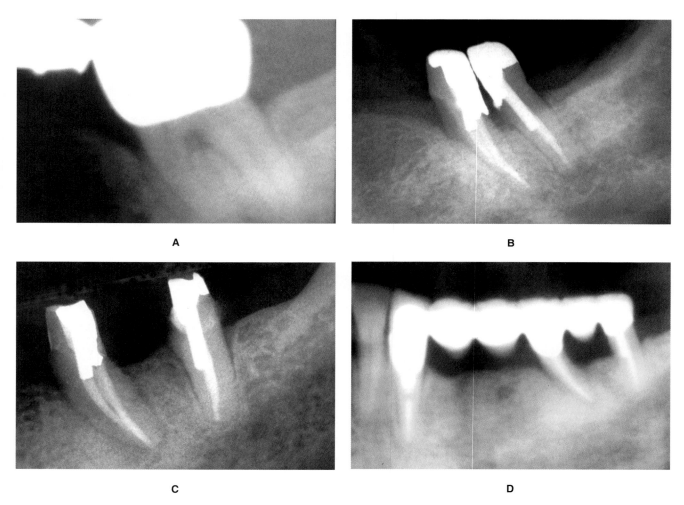

Figure 28-15. Before orthodontic treatment, this patient had a Class III furcation defect in the mandibular left second molar (**A**). Because the patient had an edentulous space mesial to the molar, the tooth was hemisected (**B**), and the root fragments were separated orthodontically (**C**). After orthodontic treatment, the root fragments were used as abutments to stabilize a multiunit posterior fixed partial denture (**D**).

spring to separate the roots. The amount of separation is determined by the adjacent edentulous spaces and the occlusion in the opposing arch. About 7 or 8 mm may be created between the roots of the hemisected molar (Fig. 28-15). This process eliminates the original furcation problem and allows the patient to clean the area with greater efficiency.

In some molars with Class III furcation defects, the tooth will have short roots, advanced bone loss, fused roots, or some other problem that prevents hemisection and crowning of the fragments. In these patients, it may be more advisable to extract the tooth with a furcation defect and place an osseointegrated implant (Fig. 28-16). If this type of plan were adopted, the timing of the extraction and placement of the implant could occur at any time relative to the orthodontic treatment. In some situations,

the implant could be used as an anchor to facilitate pre-restorative orthodontic treatment.

Root Proximity

When roots of posterior teeth are in close proximity, the ability to maintain periodontal health and accessibility for restoration of adjacent teeth may be compromised.[7] However, if the patient is undergoing orthodontic therapy, the roots can be moved apart and bone will be laid down between the adjacent roots. This will open the embrasure beneath the tooth contact, provide additional bone support, and enhance the patient's access to the interproximal region. This generally improves the periodontal health of this area.

If orthodontic treatment will be used to move roots apart, the orthodontist must be aware of this plan before

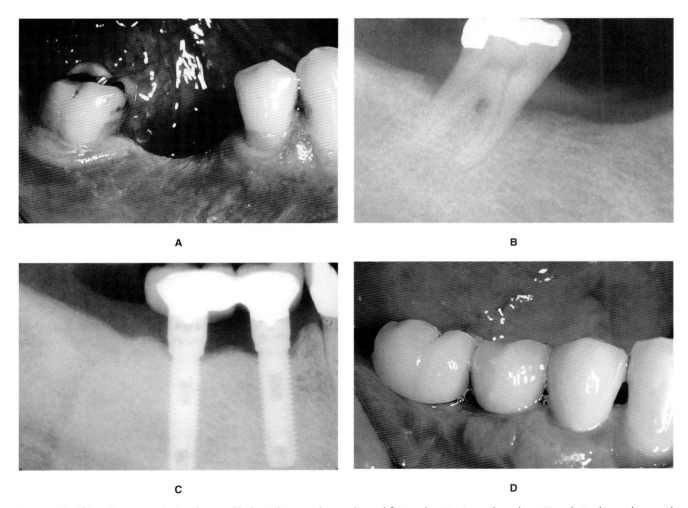

A

B

C

D

Figure 28-16. This patient was missing the mandibular right second premolar and first molar (**A**). Severe bone loss (**B**) and attachment loss on the second molar prevented its use as an abutment. Also, a Class III furcation invasion was present. Therefore, the second premolar and first molar were restored with an implant-supported fixed partial denture (**C, D**).

bracket placement. It is advantageous to place the brackets so the orthodontic movement to separate the roots will begin with the initial archwires (Fig. 28-17). Therefore, brackets must be placed obliquely to facilitate this process. To determine the progress of orthodontic root separation, radiographs will be needed to monitor the status. Generally, 2 to 3 mm of root separation will provide adequate bone and embrasure space to improve periodontal health. During this time, the patient should be maintained by the restorative dentist or periodontist to ensure that a favorable bone response will occur as the roots are moved apart. In addition, these patients will need occasional occlusal adjustment to recontour the crown, as the roots are moving apart (Fig. 28-17). As this happens, the crowns may develop an unusual occlusal contact with the opposing arch. This should be equilibrated to improve the occlusion.

Fractured Teeth/Forced Eruption

Occasionally, an individual will traumatically injure a tooth. If the injury is minor and results in a small fracture of enamel, the tooth can be restored with light-cured composite or a porcelain veneer. However, in some situations, the fracture may extend beneath the level of the gingival margin and terminate at the level of the alveolar ridge. In these situations, restoration of the fractured crown is impossible, because the tooth preparation would extend to the level of the bone. This overextension could result in an invasion of the biologic width of the tooth and cause persistent inflammation of the marginal gingiva (Fig. 28-18).

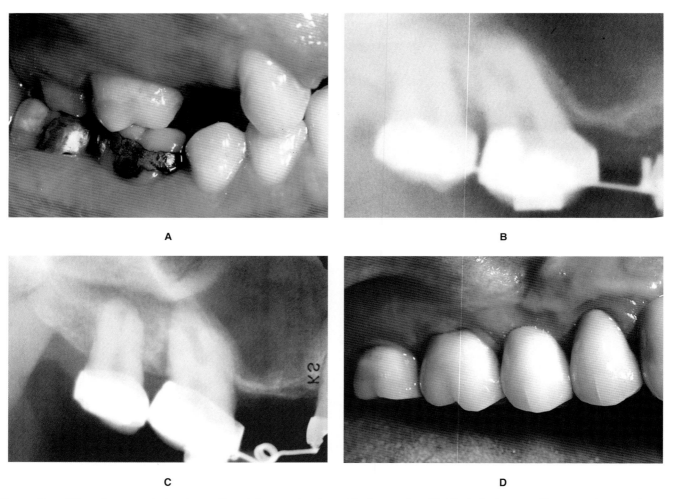

A

B

C

D

Figure 28-17. This patient was missing the maxillary right second molar and both premolars (**A**). She had a large maxillary sinus, because the premolars were congenitally missing. The restorative treatment plan was a fixed prosthesis with the abutments on the first and third molars soldered together. However, the patient had root proximity and little bone between the first and third molar roots (**B**). Therefore, orthodontics was used to tip the roots of the first molar mesially (**C**), so when they were splinted together (**D**) there would be sufficient embrasure space apical to the soldered contact for the patient to maintain this area.

In these situations, it may be beneficial to erupt the fractured root out of the bone and move the fracture margin coronally, so that it can be restored without creating gingival inflammation.[23] However, in some situations, if the fracture is too severe, it may be better to extract the tooth and replace it with an implant or fixed partial denture. The orthodontist, restorative dentist, and periodontist should evaluate six criteria to determine if the tooth should be erupted or extracted.

The first criterion is root length. Is the root long enough so that a crown-to-root ratio of 1:1 will be preserved after the root has been erupted? To determine the answer to this question, the clinician must know how far to erupt the root. If a tooth fracture extends to the level of the bone, it must be erupted 4 mm. The first 2.5 mm will move the fracture margin far enough away from the bone to prevent a biologic width problem. The other 1.5 mm

will provide the proper amount of ferrule for adequate resistance form of the crown preparation. Therefore, if the root is fractured to the bone level and must be erupted 4 mm, the clinician must evaluate a periapical radiograph and subtract 4 mm from the end of the fractured tooth root (Fig. 28-18). Then the length of the residual root should be compared with the length of the eventual crown on this tooth. The crown-to-root ratio should be about 1:1. If the ratio is greater than 1:1, too little root may remain in the bone for stability. In this situation, it may be more prudent to extract the root and place a fixed partial denture or implant.

Root form is the second criterion that determines whether forced eruption is feasible. The shape of the root should be broad and nontapering rather than thin and tapered (Fig. 28-18). A thin, tapered root will provide a narrower cervical region after the tooth has been erupted

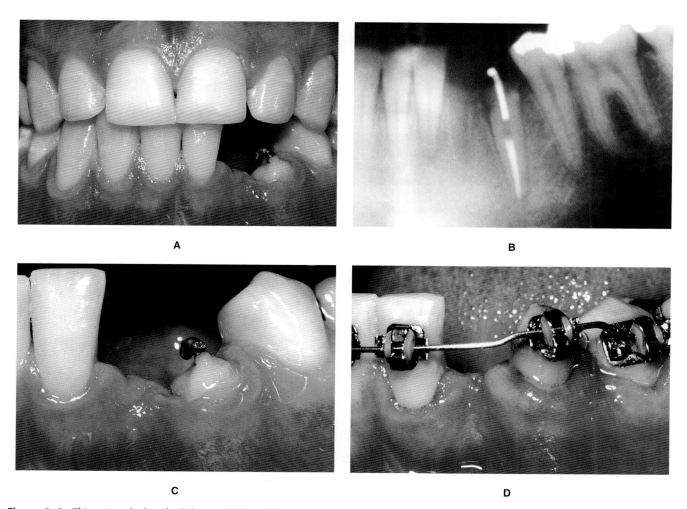

A

B

C

D

Figure 28-18. This patient had avulsed the mandibular left lateral incisor and had a severe fracture of the mandibular left canine (**A**) that extended apical to the level of the alveolar crest on the mesial (**B**). To restore the tooth adequately and avoid impinging on the periodontium, the fractured root was extruded (**C**). As the tooth erupted, the gingival margin followed the tooth (**D**).

Continued

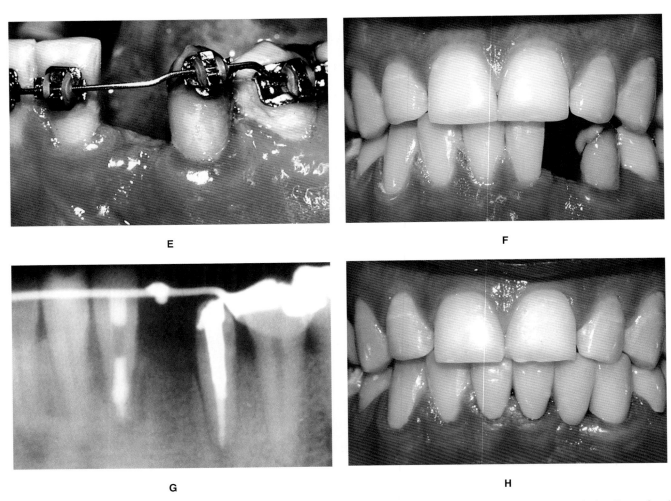

E

F

G

H

Figure 28-18. cont'd Gingival surgery was required to lengthen the crown of the canine (**E-G**) so that the final restoration (**H**) had sufficient ferrule for resistance and retention.

4 mm. This could compromise the esthetic appearance of the final restoration. The internal root form also is important. If the root canal is wide, the distance between the external root surface and root canal filling will be narrow. In these situations, the walls of the crown preparation will be thin, which could result in early fracture of the restored root. The root canal should not be more than a third of the overall width of the root (Fig. 28-18, *B*). In this way, the root could still provide adequate strength for the final restoration.

A third criterion that determines whether a fractured root should be erupted is the level of the fracture. If the entire crown is fractured 2 to 3 mm apical to the level of the alveolar bone, it is difficult if not impossible to attach to the root to erupt it. The fourth criterion is the relative importance of the tooth. If the patient were 70 years of age, and both adjacent teeth had prosthetic crowns, then

it might be more prudent to simply construct a fixed partial denture attaching to the crowned teeth. However, if the patient were 15 years of age, and the adjacent teeth were not restored, then forced eruption would be much more conservative and appropriate.

The fifth criterion to evaluate before beginning forced eruption of a fractured root is esthetics. If the patient has a high lip line and shows 2 to 3 mm of gingiva when smiling, then any type of restoration in this area will be more obvious. In this situation, keeping the patient's own tooth would provide much better esthetic results than any type of implant or prosthetic replacement. The sixth and final criterion to determine whether a tooth should be erupted is the endodontic/periodontal prognosis. If the tooth has a significant periodontal defect, it may not be possible to salvage the root. In addition, if the tooth root has a vertical fracture, then it is hopeless and must be extracted.

If all of these factors are favorable, then forced eruption of the fractured root is indicated (Fig. 28-18). The orthodontic mechanics necessary to erupt the tooth can vary from elastic traction to orthodontic banding and bracketing. If a large portion of the tooth is still present, then orthodontic bracketing will be necessary. If the entire crown has fractured leaving only the root, then elastic traction from a bonded bar may be possible. The tooth root may be erupted rapidly or slowly. If the movement is performed rapidly, the alveolar bone will be left behind temporarily, and a circumferential fiberotomy may be performed to prevent bone from following the erupted root.[24] However, if the root is erupted slowly, the bone will follow the tooth. In this situation, the erupted root will require crown lengthening and an apically positioned flap to expose the correct amount of tooth to create the proper ferrule, resistance form, and retention for the final restoration.

After the tooth root has been erupted, it must be stabilized to prevent it from intruding back into the alveolus. The reason for reintrusion is the orientation of the principal fibers of the periodontium. During forced eruption, the periodontal fibers become oriented obliquely and stretched as the tooth root moves coronally.[6] These fibers eventually will reorient themselves after about 6 months. Before this time, the tooth root can reintrude significantly. Therefore, if this type of treatment is performed, an adequate period of stabilization is necessary to avoid significant relapse and reintrusion of the root.

As the root erupts, the gingiva will move coronally with the tooth (Fig. 28-18, C). As a result, the clinical crown length will become shorter after extrusion. In addition, the gingival margin may be positioned more incisally than adjacent teeth. In these situations, gingival surgery is necessary to create ideal gingival margin heights.[25,26] The type of surgery varies depending on whether bone removal will be necessary. If bone has followed the root during eruption, the surgeon will elevate a flap and remove the appropriate amount of bone to match the bone height of the adjacent teeth. If the bone level is flat between adjacent teeth and adequate biologic width will remain, a simple excisional gingivectomy will correct the gingival margin discrepancy.

After gingival surgery, an open gingival embrasure may exist between the erupted root and adjacent teeth. This space occurs because the narrower root portion of the erupted tooth has been moved into the oral cavity. This space may be closed in one of two ways[9]: one method involves overcontouring of the replacement restoration, and the other method involves reshaping of the crown of the tooth and movement of the root to close the space. This latter method often helps to improve the overall shape of the final crown on the restored tooth.

Hopeless Teeth

Patients with moderate to advanced periodontal disease may have specific teeth that are deemed hopeless and normally would be extracted before orthodontic treatment. However, these teeth can be useful for orthodontic anchorage, if the periodontal inflammation can be controlled. In moderate to advanced cases, some periodontal surgery will be necessary around a hopeless tooth. When the flaps are reflected, debridement of the roots of the hopeless tooth may be all that is necessary to control inflammation during the orthodontic process. The important factor is to maintain the health of the bone around the adjacent teeth. Rigidly enforced 3-month periodontal recall is imperative during the process.

After orthodontic treatment, there is a 6-month period of stabilization before reevaluating the periodontal status. Occasionally, the hopeless tooth may be so improved after orthodontic treatment that it is retained. However, most of the time, the hopeless tooth will require extraction, especially if other restorations are planned in the segment. Again, these decisions need to be negotiated among the specialists, restorative dentist, and the patient.

CONCLUSION

This chapter has discussed and illustrated the benefits of integrating orthodontics and periodontics in the management of restorative patients with underlying periodontal defects. The key to treating these types of patients is communication and proper diagnosis before orthodontic therapy, as well as continued dialogue during orthodontic treatment. Not all periodontal problems are treated in the same way. Hopefully, this discussion of horizontal bone loss, intrabony defects, hemiseptal defects, furcation problems, root proximity, fractured teeth, uneven gingival levels, open gingival embrasures, periodontally hopeless teeth, single-tooth implants, and implant anchorage provides the clinician with a framework that will be helpful in treating these situations.

REFERENCES

1. Kokich VG, Spear F, Kokich VO: Maximizing anterior esthetics: an interdisciplinary approach. In McNamara JA Jr, editor: *Frontiers in dental and facial esthetics, craniofacial growth series*, Ann Arbor, Mich, 2001, University of Michigan, Needham Press.
2. Kokich V: Esthetics and vertical tooth position: the orthodontic possibilities, *Compend Cont Educ Dent* 18:1225-1231, 1997.

3. Kokich VO, Kiyak HA, Shapiro PA: Comparing the perception of dentists and lay people to altered dental esthetics, *J Esthet Dent* 11:311-324, 1999.

4. Kokich V, Nappen D, Shapiro P: Gingival contour and clinical crown length: their effects on the esthetic appearance of maxillary anterior teeth, *Am J Orthod* 86:89-94, 1984.

5. Kokich VG, Spear F: Guidelines for managing the orthodontic-restorative patient, *Semin Orthod* 3:3-20, 1997.

6. Reitan K: Clinical and histological observations of tooth movement during and after orthodontic treatment, *Am J Orthod* 53:721-745, 1967.

7. Rufenacht C: Structural esthetic rules. In Rufenacht C, editor: *Fundamentals of esthetics*, Chicago, 1990, Quintessence.

8. Kurth JR, Kokich VG: Open gingival embrasures after orthodontic treatment in adults. Prevalence and etiology, *Am J Orthod Dentofacial Orthop* 120:116-123, 2001.

9. Kokich V: Esthetics: the orthodontic-periodontic-restorative connection, *Semin Orthod* 2:21-30, 1996.

10. Spear F, Mathews D, Kokich VG: Interdisciplinary management of single-tooth implants, *Semin Orthod* 3:35-74, 1997.

11. Fudalej P: Determining the cessation of facial growth to facilitate implant placement, Master's Thesis, Seattle, Wash, 1998, University of Washington.

12. Stepovich M: A clinical study of closing edentulous spaces in the mandible, *Angle Orthod* 49:277-283, 1979.

13. Hom B, Turley P: The effects of space closure on the mandibular first molar area in adults, *Am J Orthod* 85:475-489, 1984.

14. Esposito M: Radiological evaluation of marginal bone loss at tooth surfaces facing single-tooth implants, *Clin Oral Implant Res* 4:151-157, 1993.

15. Thilander B: Osseointegrated implants in adolescents. An alternative to replacing missing teeth?, *Eur J Orthod* 16:84-95, 1994.

16. Kokich VG: Management of complex orthodontic problems: the use of implants for orthodontic anchorage, *Semin Orthod* 2:27-35, 1996.

17. Kokich VG: Comprehensive management of implant anchorage in the multidisciplinary patient. In Higuchi KW, editor: *Orthodontic applications of osseointegrated implants*, Chicago, 2000, Quintessence.

18. Ingber J: Forced eruption: Part I. A method of treating isolated one and two wall infrabony osseous defects—rationale and case report, *J Periodontol* 45:199-206, 1974.

19. Brown IA: The effect of orthodontic therapy on certain types of periodontal defects. I. Clinical findings, *J Periodontol* 44:742-756, 1973.

20. Mathews D, Kokich VG: Managing treatment for the orthodontic patient with periodontal problems, *Semin Orthod* 3:21-38, 1997.

21. Zachrisson B, Mjor I: Remodeling of teeth by grinding, *Am J Orthod* 68:543-553, 1975.

22. Kramer GM: Surgical alternatives in regenerative therapy of the periodontium, *Int J Periodontics Restorative Dent* 12:11-21, 1992.

23. Kokich V: Enhancing restorative, esthetic and periodontal results with orthodontic therapy. In Schluger S, Youdelis R, Page R et al, editors: *Periodontal therapy*, Philadelphia, 1990, Lea and Febiger.

24. Pontoriero A, Celenza F: Rapid extrusion with fiber resection: a combined orthodontic-periodontic treatment modality, *Int J Periodontics Restorative Dent* 5:31-43, 1987.

25. Kokich V: Anterior dental esthetics: an orthodontic perspective I. Crown length. *J Esthet Dent* 5:19-23, 1993.

26. Chiche G, Kokich V, Caudill R: Diagnosis and treatment planning of esthetic problems. In Pinault A, Chiche G, editors: *Esthetics in fixed prosthodontics*, Chicago, 1994, Quintessence.

29 Role of Occlusion in Periodontal Therapy

Leonard Abrams, Stephen R. Potashnick, Edwin S. Rosenberg, and Cyril I. Evian

Occlusal analysis and therapy have been a part of periodontal treatment since the turn of the twentieth century when Karolyi[1] postulated that there was a relation between occlusal stress and periodontitis. The relation of occlusion to the pathogenesis of periodontal lesions and to periodontal therapy, however, was not clear until more recently, and several theories were proposed to explain this relation. For example, early workers believed that excessive occlusal load on the dentition was a primary etiologic factor leading to pocket formation, gingival changes, and osseous and connective tissue destruction.[2,3] These authors believed that occlusal trauma was, therefore, integral to periodontitis. Still others thought that occlusal stress led to angular bony defects or infrabony pockets by altering the pathway or spread of plaque-induced inflammation, and, therefore, that occlusal trauma was an aggravating factor in periodontal disease.[4,5] A third concept, proposed by Waerhaug,[6] considered that excessive occlusal forces resulted in changes distinct from periodontitis and that there was little or no relation between occlusal trauma and the changes associated with inflammatory plaque-associated periodontitis. According to this school of thought there was no rationale for treating occlusion as part of the management of periodontal disease. Research has put much of this controversy to rest and we now have a clearer understanding of the effects that occlusal forces have on the periodontium and the relation of these periodontal changes to plaque-induced inflammatory periodontitis.

CHANGES IN THE PERIODONTIUM FROM OCCLUSAL TRAUMA

Occlusal trauma is defined as an "injury resulting in tissue changes within the attachment apparatus as a result of occlusal forces"[7] (Box 29-1). The periodontal attachment apparatus is the target for occlusal trauma and manifests clinical, radiographic, and histologic changes when excessive occlusal loads are placed on the attachment apparatus.[8] Tooth mobility is a clinical hallmark of occlusal trauma. Excessive occlusal forces may result in radiographic changes, including widening of the periodontal ligament space, especially at the alveolar crest, which often is described as crestal funneling, alteration in furcation bone quality, and variations in the appearance of the lamina dura (Fig. 29-1). Clinical mobility depends on several factors. For example, it is affected by the height of the remaining alveolar bone around the tooth, the integrity of the surrounding tissues, and the level and repetitiveness of the force applied to the tooth. The shape of the tooth crown and the length, shape, and number of roots dictate crown-to-root ratios and, therefore, the mechanical resistance of the tooth to applied force.

When subjected to a force on the occlusal surface, the tooth moves about a fulcrum point or rotational axis that is located within the clinical root and is determined by the height of the remaining supporting alveolar bone (Fig. 29-2). Within the periodontal ligament space, zones of pressure and tension are created. A tooth can move, however, only as far as the width of the ligament space allows, and then actual bone and possibly even tooth deformation occur. When occlusal forces become excessive because of their duration, magnitude, direction, distribution, or frequency, they may overwhelm the physical limitations of the periodontal ligament, which becomes traumatized.

The periodontal ligament is highly vascularized with many vessels aligning themselves parallel to the long axis of the root and freely anastomosing with the blood vessels of the trabecular spaces (see Chapter 1). When the occlusal forces on a tooth exceed the ability of the principal fibers of the periodontal ligament to stretch, the tooth can actually create sufficient pressure on the ligament in the pressure zone to deform the alveolar crest.

When injury occurs there is, at first, vascular embarrassment in the form of transient hemorrhage, edema, and thrombosis. This is followed by an increase in vascularization, with increased vascular permeability and

Box 29-1	Definitions of Occlusal Trauma[7]	
Occlusal trauma	•	Injury resulting in tissue changes within the attachment apparatus as a result of occlusal force(s).
Primary occlusal trauma	•	Injury resulting in tissue changes from excessive occlusal forces applied to a tooth or teeth with normal support. It occurs in the presence of (1) normal bone levels, (2) normal attachment levels, and (3) excessive occlusal force(s).
Secondary occlusal trauma	•	Injury resulting in tissue changes from normal or excessive occlusal forces applied to a tooth or teeth with reduced support. It occurs in the presence of (1) bone loss, (2) attachment loss, and (3) "normal"/excessive occlusal force(s).

From 1999 International Workshop for a Classification of Periodontal Diseases and Conditions. Consensus Report: Occlusal trauma. Ann Periodontol 4:108, 1999.

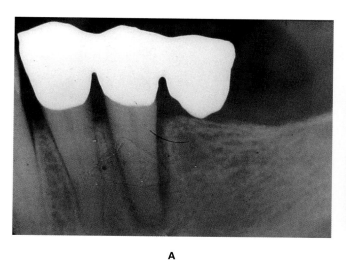

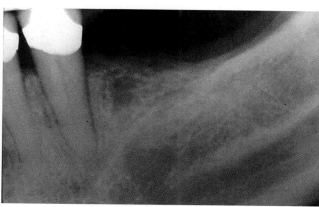

A

B

Figure 29-1. A, Radiograph of a patient with discomfort and awareness of mobility around a three-unit cantilever fixed partial denture. The patient was undergoing emotional stress and was aware of a bruxing habit. **B,** Radiographic appearance 4 months after clinical presentation. Treatment consisted of immediate removal of the cantilever unit followed by scaling and replacement of the fixed partial denture with two individual crowns. Note dramatic narrowing of periodontal ligature space. (*Courtesy Dr. Richard Yamada, Chicago, Ill.; S. Potashnick, Chicago, Ill; and Leonard Abrams, Philadelphia, Pa.*)

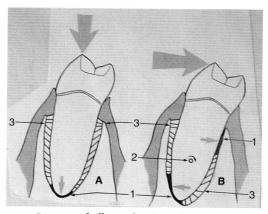

Figure 29-2. Diagram of effects of occlusal forces. **A,** The tooth with vertical occlusal forces has a small area of periodontal ligament pressure (*1*) and an increased area of periodontal ligament tension (*3*). **B,** Horizontal occlusal force causes the tooth to rotate about an axis (*2*) and demonstrates an increase in area of periodontal ligament pressure (*1*) and a reduced area of ligament tension (*3*). Horizontal occlusal force causes a tipping motion and rotation around the rotational axis, with increased tension forces at the apex on the side opposite the force and at the crestal region on the same side as the force. The horizontal force causes periodontal ligament pressure at the crest on the side opposite the force and at the apex on the same side as the force.

extravasation of vascular elements. In addition, periodontal ligament fiber bundles become disorganized, collagen is destroyed, and there is an increased number of osteoclasts with resorptive bony areas within the ligament space and the marrow spaces (Fig. 29-3). These changes

are seen in the pressure zone and result in widening of the periodontal ligament space at the expense of the socket wall. Occasionally, cemental resorption along the root surfaces also can be seen. The alterations in the periodontal tissues often are described as an adaptive response, with widening of the socket and periodontal ligament space, allowing movement of the tooth away from the excessive occlusal forces (Fig. 29-4).

The bone resorption can occur on the surface of the bony socket (called frontal resorption or direct bone resorption) or deeper in the marrow spaces behind the socket wall (called rear resorption or indirect bone resorption) (Fig. 29-5). Rear resorption probably occurs during extreme forces and is seen if the force is great enough to create necrosis of the periodontal ligament. During necrosis, hyalinization of the principal fibers occurs and there is disintegration of fiber matrix and cells. The rear resorption continues until it reaches the hyalinized tissue and the adjacent cells replace the damaged tissue. When orthodontic or occlusal forces create tipping movements, there are distinct areas of pressure and tension within the periodontal ligament (Fig. 29-2). Bone resorption occurs in the pressure zone, whereas the tension zone is accompanied by the deposition of new bone as if to reestablish the periodontal ligament space (Fig. 29-6).

In the clinical situation of jiggling type ("back-and-forth") trauma caused by occlusal forces, the socket wall is usually destroyed in a "funnel-like" shape and there is no distinct tension or pressure side within the periodontal ligament (Fig. 29-7). Therefore, changes associated with both tension and pressure often are seen.

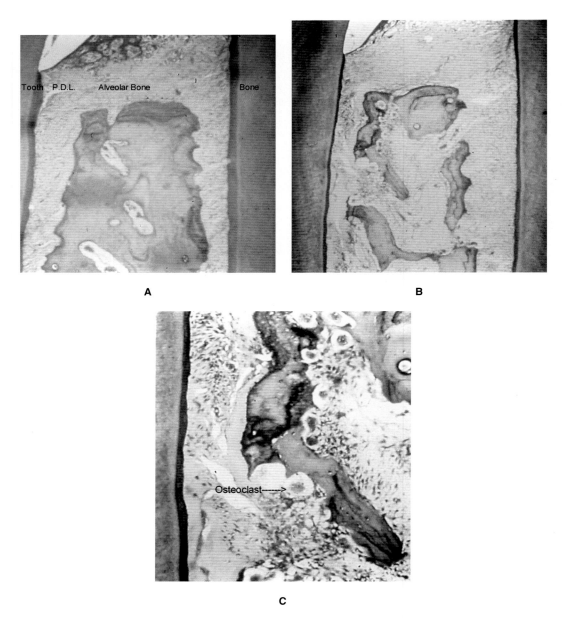

Figure 29-3. A, Normal periodontal ligament seen in squirrel monkey. The periodontal ligament (*PDL*) is intact and the alveolar bone is free of resorptive areas on the socket surface and within the marrow spaces. (*Courtesy of Dr. Alan Polson, Philadelphia, Pa.*) **B,** The result of jiggling trauma in the squirrel monkey periodontium. There is a loss of bone volume with resorptive areas on the surface of the socket and in the marrow spaces. Note the disruption of the principal fibers and a loss of cellularity. (*Courtesy of Dr. Alan Polson, Philadelphia, Pa.*) **C,** Greater magnification of Figure 29-3B shows the large number of osteoclasts and altered periodontal ligament.

With increased occlusal forces, a process of physiologic adaptation occurs within the periodontium. The adaptive response is the widening of the socket and periodontal ligament, allowing movement of the tooth out of trauma and a "cushioning" of the occlusal forces. When this occurs, there is no permanent vascular embarrassment to the ligament tissues. When traumatic forces are present, the tooth and the tissues of the attachment apparatus come to a level of accommodation that adapts to the chronic occlusal stress. Vasculitis resolves and osteoclastic activity returns to within normal limits. Mobility of the tooth remains, and the ligament is widened; however, mobility

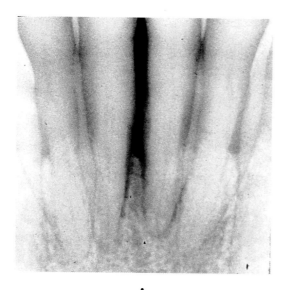

A

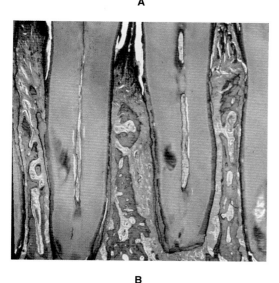

B

Figure 29-4. A, Example of adaptation to trauma made possible by the widened periodontal ligament space. Radiograph showing reduced osseous support in the mandibular central incisors and increased periodontal ligament space width. **B,** Autopsy section of the same individual showing a histologic picture of adaptation. The periodontal ligament is much wider on the central incisor to the reader's right than the other teeth, but is otherwise normal with no evidence of active tissue destruction. The surface of the bone is devoid of resorptive areas. *(Courtesy of Dr. Jay Siebert, deceased.)*

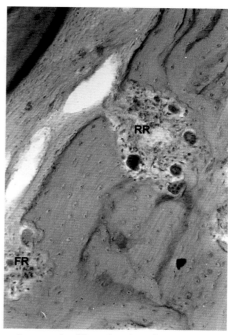

Figure 29-5. An example of frontal or direct bone resorption (*FR*) along the surface of the socket and rear or indirect bone resorption (*RR*) deeper in the marrow spaces. *(Courtesy of Dr. D.W. Cohen, Philadelphia, Pa.)*

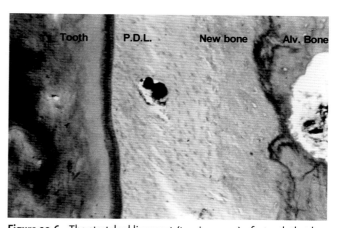

Figure 29-6. The stretched ligament (tension zone) of a tooth that has received unilateral force. The periodontal ligament space is widened and newly formed bone is noted along the surface of preexisting alveolar bone. *(Courtesy of Dr. D.W. Cohen, Philadelphia, Pa.)*

RESEARCH IN OCCLUSAL TRAUMA

does not grow progressively worse. The tooth may be displaced within its socket without additional damage to the tissues of the periodontal ligament at this point (see Fig. 29-4B). If the degree or duration of occlusal forces is greater than the adaptive capacity of the periodontium, progressive destructive changes are seen.

Wentz and coworkers[9] demonstrated in monkeys that excessive occlusal forces caused the periodontal ligament space to widen up to three times the width of that seen in teeth without excessive forces. They stated, "at one point the damaging effect of jiggling trauma was nullified by the extreme width of the periodontal space and no future

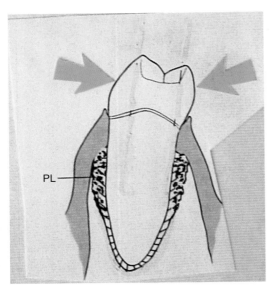

Figure 29-7. In jiggling trauma the direction of forces are multidirectional and the bony area of breakdown will be "funnel" shaped as the periodontal ligament (*PL*) widens on both sides of the tooth. This differs from changes seen in unidirectional orthodontic forces.

resorption occurred." The supracrestal tissues were unaffected and there was no apical migration of the sulcular epithelium.

There are two major research groups that performed extensive animal research during the 1970s and 1980s in the area of occlusal trauma: "the Gothenberg School" in Sweden and the "American Group" in Rochester, New York. The results of their research clarified many of the controversies surrounding the impact of occlusal forces on the periodontal tissues and on the pathogenesis of inflammatory periodontal diseases.

A result similar to Wentz and coworkers[9] was obtained by Svanberg and Lindhe,[10] who demonstrated that jiggling-type trauma applied to premolars in dogs created changes in the periodontal ligament including increased tooth mobility, widening of the periodontal ligament space, loss of crestal bone height, and a series of cellular alterations. The observed histologic alterations included vascular changes such as thrombosis, hemorrhage, and increased vascular permeability; destruction of collagen; and increased number of osteoclasts with bone resorption. If the dogs' mouths were kept clean by frequent plaque removal, the supracrestal tissues were free of inflammation. The changes in the periodontium occurred during the first 60 days of the experiment, after which all of the findings associated with occlusal force ceased, except for increased tooth mobility and periodontal ligament width, which remained constant. That is, in the absence of plaque-induced inflammation, excessive occlusal forces caused physiologic adaptation within the periodontium.

Progressive destructive changes did not occur. Importantly, when plaque-induced inflammation was prevented, no loss of connective tissue attachment took place.

A second Swedish study by Lindhe and Svanberg[11] examined the ability for this physiologic adaptation to take place in the presence of plaque-induced experimental periodontitis. In animals with periodontal inflammation, superimposed on jiggling-type trauma, the process of physiologic adaptation did not occur. Instead, there were progressively increasing tooth mobility, bone destruction, and vascular changes. The inference that can be drawn from this work is that the attachment apparatus may be inhibited in its ability to adapt to jiggling-type trauma in the presence of supracrestal plaque-induced inflammation. The same study also indicated that "...trauma from occlusion combined with experimental periodontitis accelerated periodontal breakdown characterized by continuous periodontal pocket formation and loss of fiber attachment."[11] The periodontal pockets that formed were of an infrabony type, which may have been influenced by the tremendous intrusive forces that were applied by the hyperoccluded restorations used to induce occlusal trauma.

In a study in which the periodontal attachment level of teeth in beagle dogs was reduced before the onset of jiggling-type trauma, researchers were able to demonstrate that jiggling-type trauma in a severely reduced periodontium that is free of plaque-induced inflammation will not cause further deterioration of the periodontal support.[12] Thus, physiologic adaptation is independent of the level of bony support and attachment; it is dependent primarily on an absence of plaque-induced inflammation.

One of the most important questions answered by animal research is: "Do occlusal forces increase the rate or degree of periodontal destruction during periodontitis?" Nyman and coworkers[13] compared the degree of attachment loss caused by experimental periodontitis alone to the degree of loss caused by a combination of experimental periodontitis and excessive occlusal forces. Experimental periodontitis was induced in both test teeth and control teeth, and jiggling-type trauma was then applied only to the test teeth. A greater degree of attachment loss was seen in 80% of the test teeth compared with control teeth. Thus, excessive occlusal forces were shown to have the potential to increase the degree of periodontal destruction. The mechanism by which the jiggling forces increased apical migration of the infiltrated connective tissue and pocket epithelium is not known, especially because the distance between the apical border of the plaque and the apical border of the infiltrated connective tissue was the same in control and test sites.

Increased tooth mobility, a hallmark of occlusal trauma, may be associated with changes in tissue resistance to periodontal probing. In one study, jiggling-type trauma was induced on the test teeth of dogs that also received frequent plaque removal.[14] Control teeth had plaque removed, but no jiggling forces were induced. After approximately 90 days, the periodontal ligament of the test teeth became wider and tooth mobility increased. Some bone was lost at the crest. These changes were not progressive, indicating that physiologic adaptation had taken place. The test and control teeth were free of plaque and had the same histologic connective tissue attachment levels. However, the supracrestal gingival tissue subjacent to the sulcular and junctional epithelium differed in that the test teeth contained less collagen and more cellular elements than did the gingiva of control teeth. The histologic distance from the cementoenamel junction (CEJ) to the bony crest was greater in test teeth because crestal bone loss had occurred. This resulted in a longer supracrestal connective tissue attachment area (distance from most coronal point of connective tissue attachment to the bony crest) in the test teeth than in control teeth because part of the supracrestal connective tissue in the test teeth included an area that was previously occupied by the periodontal ligament and crestal bone. Importantly, probing depths were approximately 0.5 mm greater in test teeth than in control teeth, despite a constant force on the probe. The increased probing depth was likely the result of less tissue resistance to probing force, caused by the increased supracrestal connective tissue attachment area and the decreased collagen content within this tissue.

Using a monkey model, the U.S. group led by Polson and coworkers[15,16] demonstrated many of the same findings that the Swedish group identified in dogs. When traumatic forces were introduced in the premolars of squirrel monkeys without periodontal inflammation, characteristic changes occurred in the attachment apparatus: widening of the periodontal ligament space, increased tooth mobility, and loss of crestal bone height and bone volume (density). These changes ceased to progress once the process of physiologic adaptation was complete. No loss of connective tissue attachment occurred. After the traumatic forces were withdrawn and time was allowed for healing, much of the lost bone volume was restored, the width of the periodontal ligament decreased, and mobility diminished. Conversely, if plaque-retentive ligatures were placed and plaque-induced inflammation was permitted to take hold, there was no restoration of bone volume after the removal of traumatic forces. Bone volume was only restored when removal of occlusal forces was combined with elimination of plaque and inflammation.

In one major area of research, findings from the U.S. group differed from those of the Swedish group. Whereas occlusal forces superimposed on plaque-induced experimental periodontitis had been shown to increase the degree of connective tissue attachment loss in dogs when compared with periodontitis alone, this was not true in the monkey model. In monkeys, there was no difference in connective tissue attachment loss between animals having experimental periodontitis alone and those having both periodontitis and excessive occlusal forces.[17]

PRIMARY AND SECONDARY OCCLUSAL TRAUMA

Occlusal trauma is defined as being either primary or secondary[7] (Box 29-1). The term *occlusal trauma* is generally used as a diagnosis, whereas the term *traumatogenic occlusion* refers to the cause (etiology) and is defined as "an occlusion that produces forces that cause an injury to the attachment apparatus."[7]

A tooth subject to excessive occlusal forces but otherwise exhibiting intact periodontal support and no loss of bone or connective tissue attachment is classically described as a tooth having primary occlusal trauma. In Figure 29-1, a tooth with primary occlusal trauma can be seen while traumatic forces are present (Fig. 29-1A) and after they have been removed (Fig. 29-1B). Teeth with primary occlusal trauma may reach a state of stability in which mobility is no longer increasing and the clinical, radiographic, and histologic changes do not worsen over time. This occurs through the adaptive remodeling process.

The clinical signs of occlusal trauma, which include mobility, widening of the radiographic PDL space, and migration of teeth, can be reversible when the forces are removed or modified. Likewise, symptoms of occlusal trauma such as pain on mastication and sensitivity to cold stimuli also can be reversed when the forces are removed. Parafunctional activity is likely the main culprit in many cases of primary occlusal trauma. Other cases have an iatrogenic cause, such as placement of a "high" restoration (Fig. 29-8). Parafunctional habits can be classified according to what contacts the teeth[18] (Box 29-2). Habits such as bruxism and clenching cause occlusal trauma mainly because of the increased duration of forces on the teeth. In people without such habits, actual tooth contact is limited to periods of chewing and swallowing. Conversely, in those with the habits of bruxism or clenching, the duration of tooth contact is greatly increased. In addition, the degree (magnitude) of force placed on the teeth during bruxism is much greater than during normal daily function. Some parafunctional habits are factitial injuries caused by biting on objects such as pipe stems (Fig. 29-9), pens or pencils, and fingernails (Fig. 29-10). These forces are generally localized to a few teeth, whereas bruxism and clenching often involve many or most of the teeth. Parafunctional habits are difficult to control and many tooth-to-tooth

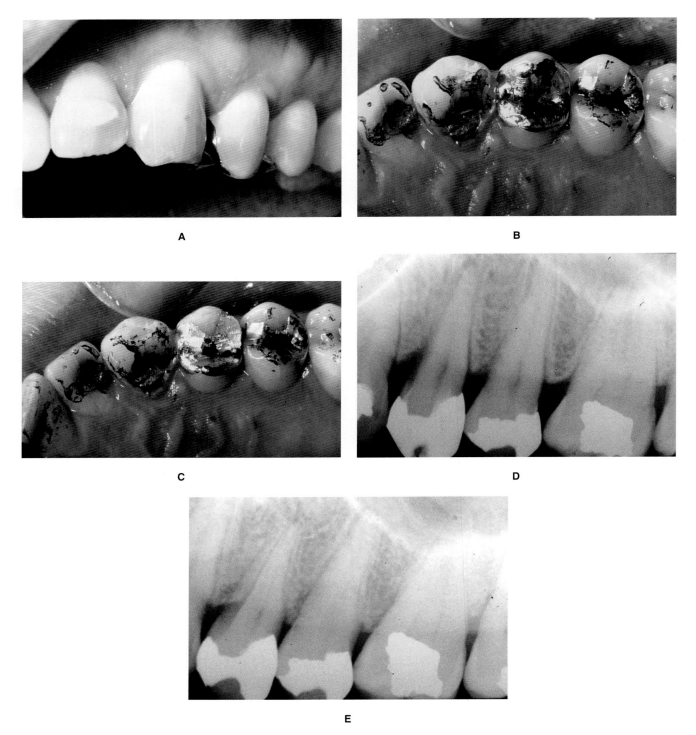

A

B

C

D

E

Figure 29-8. A, Presenting appearance of a patient with a recently placed gold onlay on first premolar. Tooth was temperature sensitive and patient was aware of parafunctional action of the teeth. Note wear facet on canine and length of buccal cusp of first premolar. The tooth had increased mobility compared with ipsilateral second premolar and contralateral first and second premolars. **B,** Occlusal examination revealed working and balancing contacts. Onlay has "locked" tooth into position. **C,** After occlusal adjustment by selective grinding of first premolar, working and balancing contacts have been removed and centric contacts are present in central fossa, marginal ridge, and palatal cusp tip. Tooth is freed in lateral contacting movements while maintaining axially directed contact in maximum intercuspation. **D,** At initial presentation, depth of onlay on first premolar and widening at apex may easily be mistaken for changes of pulpal origin. However, the tooth was vital. Note widened ligament space at apex and at crestal region on distal aspect of first premolar. What appears to be a mesial vertical bony defect probes within normal limits. There is no attachment loss, despite crestal bone loss. **E,** Eight months after occlusal adjustment, on first premolar note narrowing of ligament space, resolution of apical widening, and change in crestal morphology. (*From Potashnick SR, Abrams L: The significance of occlusal adjustment in periodontal therapy,* Alpha Omegan *78:25-46, 1985.*)

Box 29-2	Classification of Parafunctional Habits on the Basis of Objects Touching the Teeth

- Tooth to tooth
  - Bruxism
  - Clenching
- Oral musculature to tooth
  - Lip biting
  - Tongue thrusting
- Foreign object to tooth
  - Fingernail biting
  - Pipe or cigar biting
  - Other objects

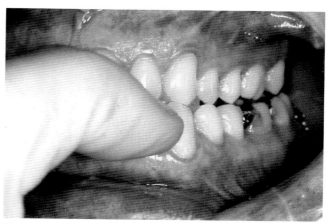

Figure 29-10. Foreign object to tooth habit in the form of fingernail biting. Occlusal trauma limited to site of fingernail habit.

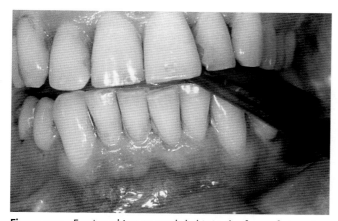

Figure 29-9. Foreign object to tooth habit in the form of pipe stem biting. Occlusal trauma limited to site of pipe stem.

habits are best handled with occlusal appliances (occlusal splints, night guards). Factitial injuries must be identified by the clinician, and the patient should be strongly encouraged to eliminate the habit.

Before undertaking treatment it is necessary to distinguish between the periodontium that is in a state of adaptation and one that is in trauma. Teeth that have adapted to occlusal stress and are mobile but do not experience increasing mobility over time may not necessarily require treatment—that is, mobility itself can be accepted if there are no symptoms or if the tooth does not increase in mobility and the patient can function properly with the dentition. The changes of primary occlusal trauma, occurring in a healthy periodontium, are reversible when the trauma is removed.

Secondary occlusal trauma is defined as occurring on a tooth having reduced periodontal support (Box 29-1; Fig. 29-11). The tooth often can be displaced in the remaining alveolus by any force applied to it, which might include the force of the tongue or lips or chewing food. Secondary occlusal trauma may occur with active periodontitis or may persist after the inflammatory periodontitis

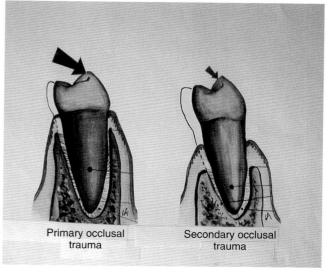

Primary occlusal trauma   Secondary occlusal trauma

Figure 29-11. Diagram of primary and secondary occlusal trauma. *Primary occlusal trauma*: A large nonaxial occlusal force causes the tooth to move and zones of pressure and tension to be created within the periodontal ligament. The tooth can only move a distance equal to the width of the periodontal ligament at the level of the osseous crest. Mobility is recorded by movement observed at the crown level. *Secondary occlusal trauma*: A smaller nonaxial occlusal force causes the tooth to move the same horizontal distance at the level of the osseous crest. However, the axis of rotation on the tooth has moved apically as the periodontal support has moved apically. Horizontal movement, therefore, will be greater at the crown level, and the mobility recording will be greater in teeth with reduced attachment levels. Because one has a different expectation of mobility for teeth with reduced support, it is helpful to record the approximate percentage of radiographic bone remaining.

has been resolved—that is, the clinician could encounter secondary occlusal trauma at the time a diagnosis of chronic periodontitis is made and before treatment has begun. Likewise, secondary occlusal trauma might be diagnosed after periodontitis has been treated and periodontal health reestablished, but with diminished support for the tooth or teeth. Again, the seriousness of the occlusal trauma depends on whether progressive changes are detected—that is, progressively increasing mobility, bone loss, or widening of the periodontal ligament. In many cases of secondary occlusal trauma, especially when periodontal support is markedly reduced, splinting of the remaining teeth may be indicated if the teeth are to be retained (Fig. 29-12).

OCCLUSAL TRAUMA AND PLAQUE-INDUCED INFLAMMATORY PERIODONTITIS

Excessive occlusal forces placed on a noninfected periodontium do not initiate gingival connective tissue attachment loss or pocket formation. Occlusal trauma, as described earlier, results in widening of the periodontal ligament space with loss of alveolar bone volume. Because the maximum compressive stress occurs just apical to the alveolar crest as the tooth is intruded into the socket, there may be loss of alveolar crestal height. Because the tooth is similar in shape to a truncated cone, pressure would be greatest at the rim of the alveolar socket. This often leads to the development of an angular bony defect noted on the radiograph. However, clinically, there is no pocket because there is no loss of connective tissue attachment or apical migration of the junctional or sulcular epithelium. The widening of the periodontal ligament space and vertical alveolar crestal bone loss (funnel-shaped lesion) are completely reversible once the excessive occlusal stress has been removed. The lesion of the periodontal ligament associated with primary occlusal trauma in the absence of inflammatory periodontitis does not cause changes in the

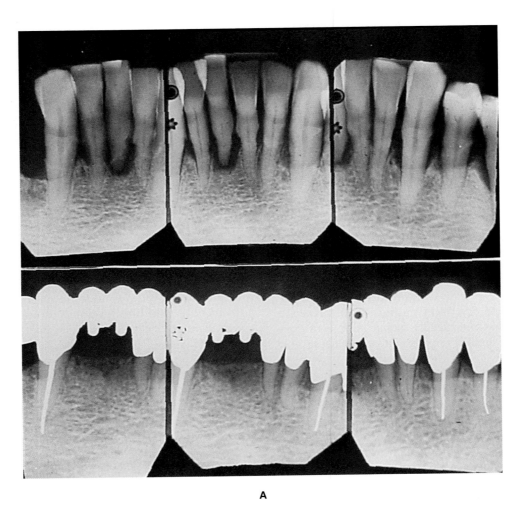

A

Figure 29-12. **A,** Preoperative (*top*) and postoperative (*bottom*) radiographs of a patient with secondary occlusal trauma requiring splinting of the remaining mandibular teeth.

Continued

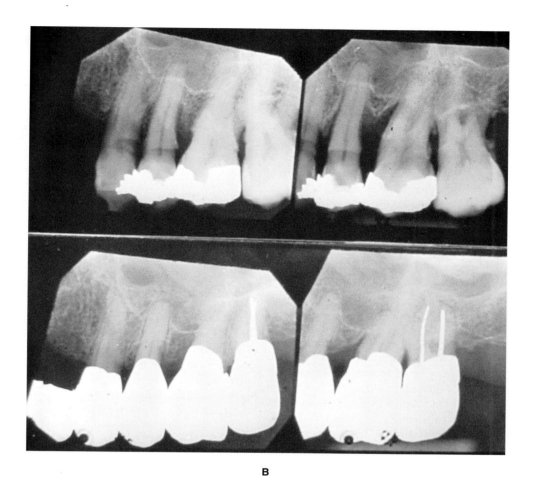

B

Figure 29-12. cont'd B, Preoperative *(top)* and postoperative *(bottom)* radiographs of the maxillary right posterior sextant in the same patient.

gingival connective tissue or the epithelium, probably because there is structural and functional independence of the periodontal and gingival blood circulation.[19]

Is a tooth in occlusal trauma more susceptible to inflammatory periodontitis? It is clear that a tooth that is free of periodontal infection and has a widened periodontal ligament and alveolar crestal bone loss caused by occlusal forces is *not more susceptible* to plaque-induced inflammation and attachment loss. Connective tissue attachment loss around teeth with widened periodontal ligament spaces progresses at a rate that is independent of the mobility of the teeth and is unrelated to periodontal ligament width.[20] Another way of stating this is that the loss of connective tissue attachment is not related to the absence or presence of the bony component of the periodontium.[21] When a tooth with occlusal trauma loses bone *in the absence of plaque-induced inflammation,* the base of the sulcus remains in the same location on the tooth. This increases the dimension of the supracrestal connective tissue attachment area, because the bone has resorbed but the pocket has not deepened.[14,21]

Furthermore, teeth that have lost supporting tissues because of previous periodontitis, but are currently free of inflammation, respond to occlusal forces in the same way as teeth with normal support—that is, physiologic adaptation may result in a widened periodontal ligament, tooth mobility, and crestal bone loss, but there is no additional loss of attachment.[12] Indeed, it has been estimated that the reduction of alveolar bone height may have little effect on the degree of periodontal ligament stress until as much as 60% of the bone support has been lost.[22]

Periodontitis is an inflammatory disease caused by bacterial infection of the subgingival area. The tissue loss in inflammatory periodontitis is seen mainly in the supraalveolar soft connective tissue, with loss of gingival connective tissue attachment to the tooth and migration of the junctional and sulcular epithelium apical to the CEJ (see Chapter 1). Histologically, the supraalveolar connective tissue is infiltrated primarily by inflammatory cells, collagen is destroyed, and the epithelium migrates, proliferates, and often ulcerates, forming a pocket wall. The resultant region of inflammation subadjacent to the subgingival plaque is separate and distinct from the underlying lesion of occlusal trauma. The two lesions often are divided by a cell-poor, collagen-rich zone of connective tissue at or near the alveolar crest.

When occlusal trauma is superimposed on plaque-induced inflammatory periodontitis, accommodation and adaptation of the vascular and connective tissue elements of the attachment apparatus do not occur.[11,23] In this case, vascularity and osteoclastic activity remain increased, and tooth mobility and periodontal ligament width continue to increase without approaching a stable plateau. There is an enhanced loss of alveolar bone height and volume as compared with inflammatory periodontitis alone. There also may be an increase in the degree of connective tissue attachment loss; this was demonstrated in the dog model,[11] but not in the monkey model.[17] Because such experimental studies would be unethical in humans, it is unknown whether superimposition of plaque-induced periodontitis and occlusal forces increase attachment loss in humans.

Inflammation from the region of the periodontal pocket extends into the bone primarily along perivascular routes. Thus, the inflammatory process extends primarily toward the periosteal side of the bone, rather than apically into the periodontal ligament. When excessive occlusal forces are placed on the teeth, there is evidence that, occasionally, the inflammatory disease is exaggerated. This is the reason that occlusal trauma has been called a "codestructive" factor in the pathogenesis of periodontal destruction.[5] One of the hallmarks of the codestructive process was considered to be the formation of infrabony pockets—that is, vertical bony defects. These defects supposedly formed because inflammatory cells migrated directly into the periodontal ligament, causing bone resorption along the ligament side. In fact, angular bony defects seen on the radiograph were considered the *sine qua non* of the codestructive lesion.[4,24] The codestructive progress and the formation of intrabony defects remains a controversial topic.

Human autopsy studies by Waerhaug[6] called this concept into question when they revealed that angular bony defects were just as common adjacent to teeth without excessive occlusal forces as they were adjacent to teeth with these forces. Instead of being related to occlusal forces, angular bony defects were directly associated with the apical extension of bacterial plaque. Waerhaug[6] stated that an angular defect forms when the subgingival plaque front on one tooth surface in an interproximal region advances further apically than does the plaque front on the adjacent tooth. The clinician also should recall that the appearance of angular bony defects on radiographs must be related to the position of the CEJ on adjacent teeth, because the bony crest in health follows a line running parallel to adjacent CEJs[25] (Fig. 29-13) (see Chapter 9).

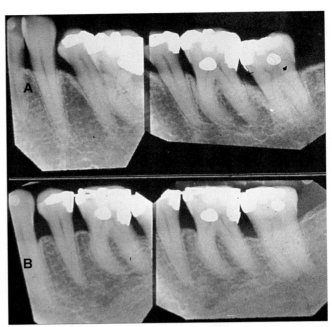

Figure 29-13. A, Apparent angular bony defects are noted on the mesial of the second premolar and second molar. The defect angle parallels a line running from the cementoenamel junction (CEJ) of one tooth to the CEJ of the adjacent teeth. **B,** After orthodontic correction, the radiographic bony defects are eliminated.

Several studies have shown that infrabony defects can exhibit osseous repair in the presence of hypermobility after removing only the plaque-induced inflammation, but not altering the occlusal forces.[26,27] This suggests that the occlusal forces were not a primary etiologic factor in the initiation of the infrabony pockets. Despite the capacity of mobile teeth to exhibit periodontal repair, an 8-year longitudinal study on 1974 teeth that received periodontal therapy showed a statistically significant relation between original tooth mobility before treatment and the change in clinical attachment level after treatment.[28] Mobile teeth had less favorable probing depth and attachment level changes than did nonmobile teeth. The study concluded that mobile teeth do not respond as well to periodontal treatment. An important difference in these studies was the frequency of professional plaque control procedures. In studies where mobile teeth responded favorably to treatment, subjects received professional prophylaxis every 2 weeks,[26,27] whereas patients in the study with less favorable treatment responses on mobile teeth had cleanings only once every 3 months.[28] Despite their differences, all of these studies concluded that mobile teeth have the potential to respond favorably to periodontal treatment.

Stahl's[29] human biopsy results were unique in that he had the opportunity to physically examine the dentition of four individuals for evidence of occlusal stress and gingival inflammation before the removal of block sections because of oral malignancy. Stahl[29] observed that in most cases the inflammatory exudates spread from the connective tissue region subjacent to the apical plaque front into the crestal bony septum and not into the periodontal ligament space, even though the ligament space was altered because of occlusal forces. He concluded that the "prediction of altered pathology resulting from the combined periodontal insults is limited."[29]

That there is contradictory evidence on the effect of occlusal trauma on the inflammatory pathway does not mean that there is no relation between the two destructive processes. Indeed, whether plaque-induced inflammation is present or absent, vascular permeability is increased in the supraaveolar connective tissue when trauma is present and tooth mobility is increasing.[10,30] The extent to which vascular metabolic changes in the supraalveolar connective tissue during occlusal trauma affect adaptation or periodontal ligament lesions is unclear. However, clinical experience suggests that a small number of patients are highly susceptible to the destructive capacity of plaque-induced infection combined with excessive occlusal forces. Further research is needed to resolve this issue and to find means of identifying these susceptible patients.

OCCLUSAL THERAPY AND PERIODONTAL INFLAMMATION

When occlusal trauma is controlled in the presence of continued inflammation, a reduction in mobility often is noted. This occurs without restoration of lost alveolar bone volume or accommodation of the periodontal ligament. Removal of occlusal interferences and the subsequent reduction in mobility without control of periodontal inflammation will not, however, improve the level of attachment.[27] It is clear that the presence of gingival inflammation inhibits the potential for alveolar bone regeneration, and that connective tissue attachment levels will remain unchanged unless the plaque-induced inflammatory lesion is treated. In experimental animal model systems, bone regeneration restoring volume and height of bone of the combined lesion (i.e., the lesion caused by occlusal trauma and periodontitis) does not occur when inflammation remains uncontrolled.[31]

Repair of the periodontal ligament and alveolar bone regeneration can occur when both marginal infection and traumatogenic occlusal forces are controlled. This regeneration often does not result in complete restoration of the original height of the attachment; however, the periodontal ligament space of the remaining periodontium may return to within normal limits. Maximum repair of periodontal tissue is most likely to occur with the resolution of both inflammatory periodontitis and

occlusal trauma in a patient *proven to be susceptible* to the combined effects of both processes (Fig. 29-14).

The following are six reasonable occlusal assumptions:

1. Supracrestal plaque-induced inflammation may inhibit the restoration of bone volume after the removal of jiggling forces.[27]
2. Supracrestal plaque-induced inflammation may prevent adaptation to ongoing jiggling forces.[11]
3. Infrabony pocket formation does not automatically imply occlusal trauma.[6]
4. Healing of periodontal tissues (including infrabony pockets) can occur in the presence of hypermobility.[26,27]
5. The true etiologic role of traumatogenic occlusion cannot be determined until plaque-induced inflammation has been eliminated.[27]
6. In those instances where both traumatogenic occlusion and plaque-induced inflammation are operating in concert, the capacity for periodontal destruction can be greatly magnified in some patients.[13]

In the past, during routine periodontal therapy, mobility was almost automatically addressed by some form of occlusal intervention. Currently, however, the belief is strongly held that correcting the existing occlusion should be done only if there is reasonable evidence that the given occlusal arrangement is a causative agent in the disease process. To determine this, the following questions must be answered:

1. Is the mobility increased or increasing?
2. Can the examiner show that the teeth in question are jiggled by the opposing teeth (positive fremitus or functional mobility)?
3. Is there a rational method within reasonable cost–benefit ratios to correct the situation?
4. Does the mobility interfere with the patient's comfort, function, level of esthetic satisfaction, or stability of the arch?

A number of studies have attempted to clarify the relation between occlusal discrepancies and periodontal status. In some of these studies, teeth with nonworking contacts had deeper probing depths, greater tooth mobility, and greater bone loss than did teeth without nonworking contacts.[32-34] In other studies, the periodontal status was similar in teeth with occlusal discrepancies compared with those without discrepancies.[35,36] This has led to some confusion as to the role that occlusal discrepancies play in periodontal destruction and the need, or lack of need, for elimination of such discrepancies.

In the most recent of these studies, recordings were made of the periodontal status of teeth that had or did not have occlusal discrepancies.[34,37] Some of the patients who had occlusal discrepancies received occlusal adjustment as part of their periodontal treatment, whereas other

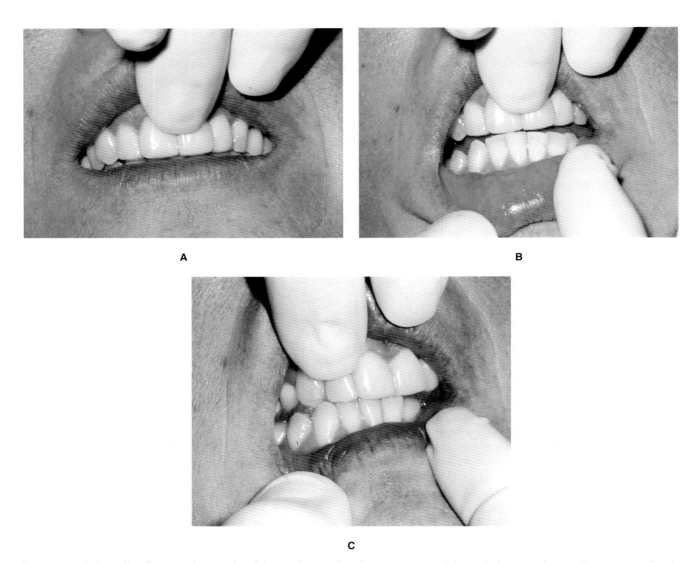

Figure 29-14. **A,** Recording fremitus (functional mobility). Palpating the vibratory patterns of the teeth during occlusion. The patient is closed in the maximum intercuspal position and the teeth are palpated as the patient taps the teeth together. **B,** Assessing fremitus as the patient makes protrusive contacting movement. **C,** Assessing fremitus during working contacting movement.

patients did not have adjustments. The patients were followed over time to determine the effects of periodontal therapy. Teeth with untreated occlusal discrepancies had a small but significant increase in probing depth over time, when averaged on an annual basis. Teeth with treated occlusal discrepancies or without discrepancies at all had no significant increase in probing depth over time. The results of these studies suggest that treatment of occlusal discrepancies as part of the periodontal treatment plan may have beneficial long-term effects. However, the clinician may question the need to correct all occlusal discrepancies simply because they exist. Many studies have been conducted to show that occlusal discrepancies

are widespread in the population.[38-40] In fact, in some studies, more than half of the patients and half of all molar teeth had nonworking contacts.[32,35] Clearly not all of these teeth require occlusal adjustment. Unless one can tie the occlusal discrepancies directly to the signs or symptoms in question, there is no rational periodontal therapeutic reason for adjusting them.

Burgett and coworkers conducted a randomized trial of occlusal adjustment in the treatment of periodontitis.[41] Of 50 patients who received hygienic therapy, 22 received occlusal adjustment. Selective grinding was performed to create stable contacts in centric relation with smooth gliding contacts in eccentric movements and the elimination of balancing interferences. All of the 50 patients were then subjected to surgical (modified Widman) and nonsurgical (scaling and root planing) therapy in a split-mouth design. The 22 patients with occlusal adjustment demonstrated a slightly (average, 0.4 mm) greater gain in clinical attachment level when compared with the nonadjusted subjects. There was no difference in probing depth reduction between the adjusted and nonadjusted patients. This study suggests that prophylactic occlusal adjustment is of little benefit as part of the periodontal treatment plan in most patients. Therefore, each patient must be evaluated individually to determine the presence of occlusal trauma, the role of traumatogenic occlusion in the pathogenesis of periodontitis, and the need for treatment of the occlusal relations.

CLINICAL AND RADIOGRAPHIC SIGNS OF OCCLUSAL TRAUMA

In examining the periodontal patient, clinical and radiographic parameters are evaluated to assess the role of occlusion in the patient's condition. Mobility, fremitus, the presence of plaque-induced inflammation, the quantity of remaining support, and the radiographic signs of occlusal trauma are assessed.

Mobility

Mobility is a measurement of horizontal and vertical tooth displacement created by the examiner's force. Blunt ends of two dental instruments are placed approximately at the buccal and lingual height of contour of the tooth, and forces are applied in the buccolingual direction (see Chapter 8). Mobility also should be assessed in a mesiodistal direction when possible (e.g., terminal teeth in the arch; teeth with no adjacent tooth present). The horizontal mobility is assessed by comparing a fixed point on the tooth against a fixed point on the adjacent tooth. It is designated as Class I, II, or III as follows:

Class I: The tooth can be moved less than 1 mm in a buccolingual or mesiodistal direction.

Class II: The tooth can be moved 1 mm or more in a buccolingual or mesiodistal direction, but it does not exhibit abnormal mobility in an occlusoapical direction.

Class III: The tooth can be moved 1 mm or more in a buccolingual or mesiodistal direction **and** it exhibits abnormal mobility in an occlusoapical direction (i.e., it is depressible in the socket).

Some mobility classification systems use the terms *degree 1, 2, and 3, Class 1, 2, and 3,* or *grade 1, 2, and 3,* rather than *Class I, II, and III,* and some of the parameters used to categorize teeth into the individual mobility categories differ. The clinician must determine which classification scheme he or she will use in practice and must ensure

that referring and consulting dentists are familiar with that system so that all practitioners are "speaking the same language" when managing patients.

Fremitus (Functional Mobility)

Assessment of fremitus involves measurement of the vibratory patterns of the teeth when the teeth are placed in contacting positions and movements (Fig. 29-14). To measure fremitus, a finger is placed along the buccal and labial surfaces of the maxillary teeth. The patient is asked to tap the teeth together in the maximum intercuspal position and then grind systematically in lateral, protrusive, and lateral-protrusive contacting movements. The teeth that are displaced by the patient in these jaw positions are then identified by palpation. Assessment of fremitus is relatively straightforward on the maxillary teeth; however, in cases of edge-to-edge occlusion or when there is little overlap of the teeth, mandibular teeth also can be assessed. The following classification system is used[38]:

Class I fremitus: Mild vibration detected

Class II fremitus: Easily palpable vibration but no visible movement

Class III fremitus: Movement visible with the naked eye

Fremitus differs from mobility in that fremitus is tooth displacement created by the patient's own occlusal force. Therefore, the amount of force varies greatly from patient to patient, unlike mobility, wherein the force with which it is measured tends to be similar for each examiner. Fremitus is a guide to the ability of the patient to displace and traumatize the teeth. If there is mobility but not fremitus, it is unlikely that there is sufficient movement of the tooth in the alveolus under occlusal loading to create the vascular embarrassment and other findings typical of occlusal trauma.

Radiographic Assessment

The clinician should assess the degree of bone loss relative to the length of the root (CEJ to apex). The width of the periodontal ligament space should be examined around each tooth. Crestal bone patterns should be assessed for angular bony defects. Not every tooth with a widened periodontal ligament space or an angular bony defect necessarily has occlusal trauma; however, the presence of these radiographic findings should lead the examiner to closely evaluate occlusal patterns and forces.

Mobility and fremitus should be correlated with radiographic bone levels. As discussed earlier, teeth with reduced levels of bone support can be expected to exhibit a greater degree of mobility and fremitus with a given force than would a similar tooth with normal bone support. This is true because the tooth with reduced support has a fulcrum point located further apically, and therefore a greater degree of tooth deflection will occur when subjected to occlusal forces (Fig. 29-11).

Occlusal Summary Chart

When fremitus and mobility are correlated in both location and degree, there is reason to believe that the existing occlusal arrangement may be contributing a destructive role and that occlusal trauma is present. If fremitus does not correlate, either by location or degree, with mobility or with occlusal discrepancies, trauma from occlusion is less likely. When fremitus and mobility correspond, but they are both less severe than expected, occlusal trauma may still exist. In this situation, the percentage of remaining alveolar bone must be evaluated. Although radiographic signs may suggest an adverse response to occlusal forces, without fremitus it is impossible to indict occlusal contact as a causative agent.

An occlusal summary chart (Fig. 29-15) is beneficial during initial occlusal assessment, because it provides a baseline from which future treatment decisions and responses to therapy can be determined.[42] The summary chart is not intended to be a laborious exercise; rather, the clinician records the minimum amount of information needed to allow an assessment of the potential relation between occlusal forces and the periodontal status of the individual patient being evaluated (Fig. 29-16; Fig. 29-17).

EFFECTS OF ANTIINFECTIVE PERIODONTAL THERAPY ON TOOTH MOBILITY

The decision as to the presence of occlusal trauma, either primary or secondary, in a periodontal patient is not readily done in one appointment. It requires reevaluation after a sequence of initial therapeutic procedures. For example, mobility must be evaluated so that a distinction can be made between *increased* mobility and *increasing* mobility. Teeth that are mobile in the presence of plaque-associated inflammation often exhibit decreased mobility once the infection is resolved and inflammation decreases. This occurs without any occlusal adjustment (Fig. 29-18). The response of a patient to an appropriate sequence of therapy helps to distinguish between primary and secondary occlusal trauma and to determine the diagnosis and subsequent treatment needs. Unless there is overwhelming evidence of occlusal disease, such as tooth displacement or pain with an obvious occlusal discrepancy, there is no need for aggressive occlusal management during the early stages of periodontal therapy. Also, it is not reasonable to establish a diagnosis of secondary occlusal trauma and subsequent need to splint on the basis of some arbitrary hypothetical rule of percentage of alveolar bone remaining (Fig. 29-19; Fig. 29-20).

Active assessment of the role of occlusion and whether it threatens the dentition cannot be determined in the presence of plaque-induced inflammation. Control of plaque-induced periodontitis begins with patient personal plaque control instruction and nonsurgical therapy (see Chapters 13 and 14). After this course of therapy, with resolution of inflammation and elimination or reduction of the pathogenic microbial challenge, reexamination of the occlusion is necessary because often there is marked reduction in fremitus and mobility (see Fig. 29-18). Other factors that may be contributing excess forces on the teeth also must be considered. For example, parafunctional habits or factitial injuries must be addressed (Fig. 29-21; Fig. 29-22).

Surgical therapy generally should be avoided in the early stages of the treatment plan if occlusal trauma is suspected. Flap reflection and debridement may remove soft tissues just coronal to the crest of resorbed bone, where the periodontal ligament space is widened. These tissues may have osteogenic potential after elimination of excessive occlusal forces; removing the tissues through surgical debridement may reduce the potential for new bone formation. If after resolution of the plaque-induced inflammation and reevaluation of the occlusion there is still doubt as to the role the occlusal forces play, further occlusal analysis and longitudinal monitoring are indicated. At this stage, the clinician can begin to determine whether the mobility found at the baseline examination is stable or is progressively increasing. Fremitus, mobility, the degree of plaque-induced inflammation, and radiographic signs of trauma are recorded over a period of months, and possibly up to a year, to allow for full healing. This longitudinal record allows better evaluation of the role of trauma, if any, on the dentition.

PHYSIOLOGIC AND PATHOLOGIC OCCLUSION

Once a diagnosis of occlusal trauma is made, an evaluation of the occlusal arrangement is performed. Is it physiologic or pathologic? A *physiologic occlusion* is one that has demonstrated the ability to survive despite anatomic aberrations from the hypothetical normal or preconceived "ideal form" of occlusion and function. A physiologic occlusion may be an anatomic malocclusion, but it is a masticatory system functioning free of occlusally induced disease.

Pathologic occlusions, however, show evidence of disease attributable to occlusal activity. A pathologic occlusion is a dentition that often requires therapeutic alteration of the existing occlusion. This diagnosis is made only after careful documentation of the signs and symptoms of occlusal disease. If occlusal trauma is documented, treatment of the intact dentition is directed toward the elimination of occlusal interferences, creation of a stable interarch

Tooth #	Probing Depth*		Mobility	Fremitus†		Bone Remaining,‡ %	Other
	M	D		MIP	EM		
1							
2							
3							
4							
5							
6							
7							
8							
9							
10							
11							
12							
13							
14							
15							
16							
17							
18							
19							
20							
21							
22							
23							
24							
25							
26							
27							
28							
29							
30							
31							
32							

The object of the charting is to record the least amount of information necessary to allow a reasonable judgment as to the relation between occlusal forces and periodontal disease progression.

*Record deepest probing depth in millimeters for mesial (mesiolingual or mesiofacial) and distal (distolingual or distofacial) surfaces.

†Record fremitus in the maximal intercuspal position (MIP) and in eccentric movements (EC).

‡Record radiographic amount (%) of bone remaining, relative to entire root length.

Figure 29-15. Sample Occlusal Summary Chart.

Tooth #	Probing Depth M	D	Mobility	Fremitus MIP	EM	Bone Remaining, %	Other
1	Missing						
2	8	7	III	III	III	70	Class I B&L furcation
3	Missing						
4	7	5	III	III	III	80	
5	8	5	III	III	III	90	
6	5	5	I	I	III	90	
7	6	5	II	I	III	50	
8	5	5	III	I	III	80	
9	5	5	II	I	III	80	
10	5	6	II	I	III	50	
11	6	5		I	III	80	
12	7	8	III	III	III	60	
13	5	8		I	III	80	
14	Missing						
15	6	7	III	III	III	60	Class I M furcation
16	5	7		III	III	50	Class I B furcation
17	Missing						
18	11	8	III			60	Class II B furcation
19	Missing						
20	5	5	III			40	Blunted root
21	8	10	II			70	
22	5	5	I			70	
23	5	5	I			60	
24	5	5	I			50	
25	5	5	I			50	
26	5	5	I			60	
27	5	5	I			90	
28	5	5	III			60	
29	Missing						
30	Missing						
31	Missing						
32	7	8	III			70	Class II B furcation

The chart for this patient suggests that traumatogenic occlusion is part of the disease process. There is increased mobility and increased fremitus, and the location and the amount of mobility and fremitus are correlated.

Figure 29-16. Occlusal Summary Chart for patient depicted in Figure 29-17.

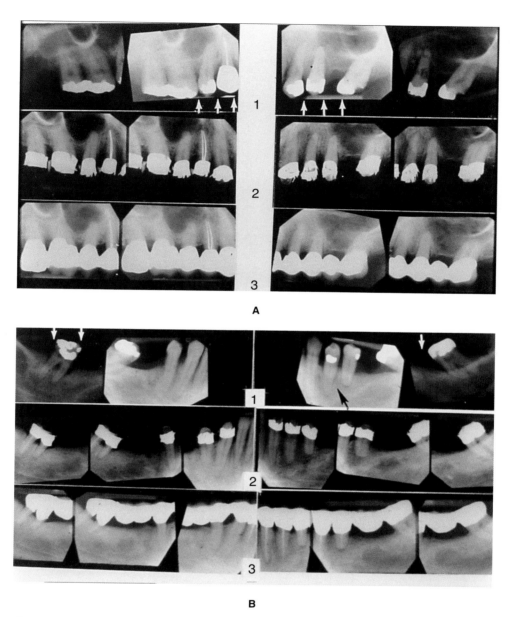

Figure 29-17. A, Maxillary posterior teeth of patient whose occlusal summary chart is shown in Table 29-2. The radiographs are mounted with the patient's right side on the reader's *right. 1,* Preoperative posterior maxillary radiographs. *Arrows* indicate location of infrabony pockets. *2,* The same area after scaling, root planing, minor tooth movement, major occlusal adjustment, and splinted provisional restorations. Note the radiographic improvement of the angular bony defects. *3,* After final restoration in which teeth were splinted for stabilization. **B,** Mandibular posterior teeth of patient whose occlusal summary chart is shown in Table 29-2. The radiographs are mounted with the patient's right side on the reader's *right. 1,* Preoperative radiographs of mandibular posterior teeth. *Arrows* indicate location of infrabony pockets. *2,* Splinted provisional restorations were placed after scaling, root planing, minor tooth movement, and major occlusal adjustment. *3,* After final restoration in which the teeth were splinted for stabilization.

relation, and axial loading of forces over a favorable distribution of teeth. Furthermore, the establishment of nonrestrictive mandibular movements with acceptable tooth guidance patterns that reduce and minimize fremitus is desirable. In a patient with previous periodontal disease, axial direction of force over a reasonable number of teeth is extremely important. The majority of the principal fibers of the periodontal ligament are obliquely oriented, and these fibers are best able to resist forces that are directed parallel to the long axis of the tooth.

JUNE 2000

Tooth #	Probing Depth M	D	Mobility	Fremitus MIP	EM	Bone Remaining, %
1	Missing					
2	5	4	I	I		90
3	7	7	II	II		50
4	4	4	I	I		60
5		8	II	II		70
6						
7	5		I	I		60
8			I	I		
9		5	I	I		
10	6		I	I		60
11		5		I	I	
12	7	7		I	I	80
13			I			
14	5	8	I	I		
15	7	6	I			90
16	Missing					

DECEMBER 2001

Tooth #	Probing Depth M	D	Mobility	Fremitus MIP	EM	Bone Remaining, %
1						
2	5	4	I			90
3	5	6	I	I		50
4	4					60
5		6	I	I		70
6						
7	5					60
8			I			
9			I			
10	4					60
11						
12	5					80
13						
14						
15	6	4				90
16						

The follow-up charting was made 18 months after the initial charting. No occlusal adjustment was done. Note the decrease in mobility that accompanied reduced inflammation and probing depth reduction.

Figure 29-18. Occlusal Summary Charts for maxillary arch before and after multiple scaling and root planing procedures in a patient with plaque-induced periodontitis.

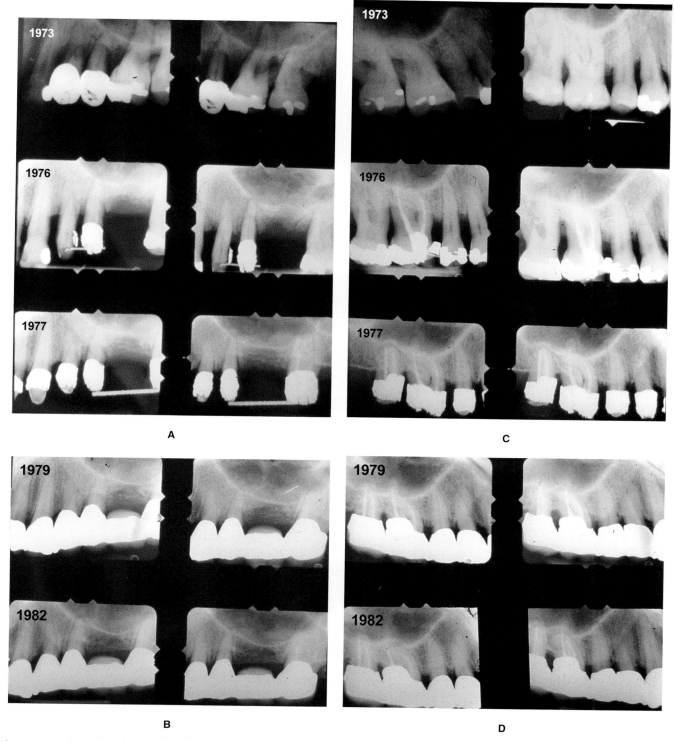

Figure 29-19. A, Patient whose occlusal trauma is confirmed by a longitudinal analysis. Initial occlusal summary and follow-up summary chart 16 months later can be seen in Table 29-4. Maxillary right posterior radiographs at initial periodontal evaluation (1973); after periodontal evaluation, nonsurgical therapy, and a period of periodontal maintenance (1976); and at the time of provisionalization (1977). After nonsurgical therapy and maintenance, mobility and fremitus did not resolve and continued to increase. The diagnosis was secondary occlusal trauma. Major occlusal adjustment was done and splinting was performed with fixed partial dentures. The patient remained in provisional restorations for more than 12 months. **B,** Maxillary right posterior radiographs at the time of final restoration (1979). Follow-up radiographs 3 years after restoration (1982). Compared with initial radiographs 9 years earlier (**A**), note the improved bone levels. **C,** Maxillary left posterior radiographs at initial periodontal evaluation (1973), after periodontal evaluation, nonsurgical therapy and a period of periodontal maintenance (1976), and at the time of provisionalization (1977). Therapy was the same as that in **A**. **D,** Maxillary left posterior radiographs at the time of final restoration (1979). Follow-up radiographs 3 years after restoration (1982). Compared with initial radiographs (**C**), note the improved bone levels.

OCTOBER 1973

Tooth #	Probing Depth M	Probing Depth D	Mobility	Fremitus MIP	Fremitus EM	Bone Remaining, %
1	Missing					
2	5	8	II			40
3	7	10	I	I	II	50
4	5	6	III	II	II	50
5	5	8	I	II	II	50
6	5	5	I	I	II	70
7	8	3	II	II	II	60
8	3	7	III	II	II	60
9	8	3	II	II	II	50
10	3	3	I	I	II	80
11	2	2		I	I	80
12	5	8	III	II	III	30
13	5	9	IIII	II	III	40
14	8	8	I	II	II	40
15	3	5	I	I	I	40
16	Missing					

JUNE 1976

Tooth #	Probing Depth M	Probing Depth D	Mobility	Fremitus MIP	Fremitus EM	Bone Remaining, %
1	Missing					
2	2	3	II			40
3	2	3	II	II	II	50
4	3	2	III	II	III	50
5	2	3	III	II	III	50
6	2	2	II	II	II	70
7	2	2	III	II	III	60
8	2	2	III	II	III	60
9	3	2	III	II	II	50
10	2	2	I	II	II	80
11	2	2	II	II	II	80
12	3	2	III	III	III	40
13	3	3	III	III	III	30
14	Missing					
15	3	3	II	II	II	40
16	Missing					

Nonsurgical therapy was performed, resulting in dramatic improvement in probing depth and reduction in inflammation; however, mobility and fremitus continued to increase. A diagnosis of secondary occlusal trauma was made. Occlusal adjustment and splinting were then performed.

Figure 29-20. Occlusal Summary Charts for maxillary arch for patient depicted in Figure 29-19.

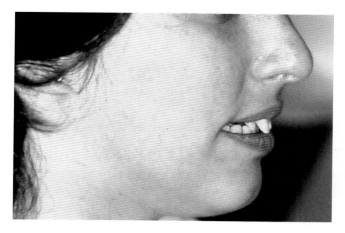

A

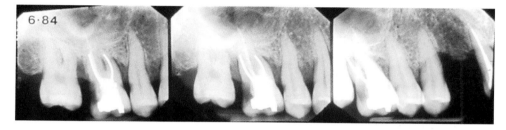

B

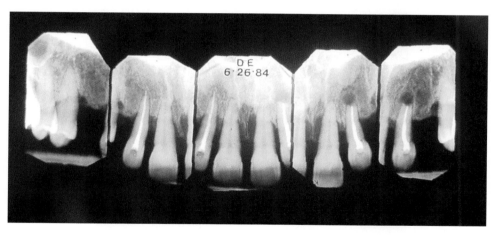

C

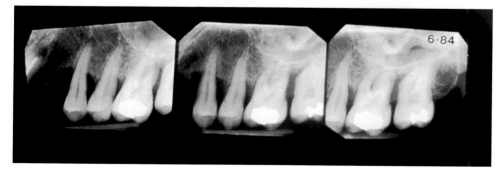

D

Figure 29-21. A, A 30-year-old woman with generalized aggressive periodontitis. Preoperative photograph showing the lower lip being trapped under the maxillary teeth. Patient has Class II malocclusion. The maxillary incisors have Class III mobility. Although they do not exhibit fremitus in maximal intercuspal position because of severity of overjet, incisors have Class III fremitus caused by the trapped lip. The occlusal summary charting can be seen in Table 29-5. **B,** Pretreatment radiographs of maxillary left posterior sextant. Note severe bone loss. **C,** Pretreatment radiographs of maxillary anterior sextant. Note severe bone loss. **D,** Pretreatment radiographs of maxillary right posterior sextant. Note severe bone loss.

Continued

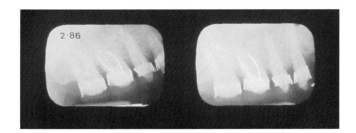

E

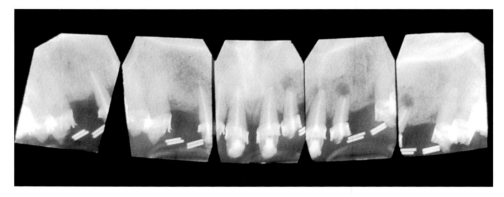

F

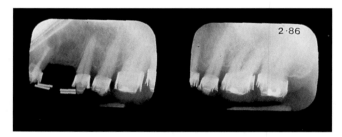

G

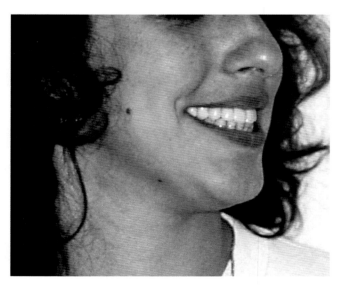

H

Figure 29-21. cont'd E, Posttreatment radiographs of maxillary left posterior sextant after scaling, root planing, systemic antibiotic therapy, orthodontic correction of malocclusion, and splinted provisional restorations. Note the improvement in bone levels. **F,** Posttreatment radiographs of maxillary anterior sextant. Significant bone loss is still present, but correction of malocclusion and trapped lip has eliminated fremitus. Apical scar can be seen on tooth #7. **G,** Posttreatment radiographs of maxillary right posterior sextant. Note the improvement in bone levels, especially between the molars and on #5 mesial. **H,** Posttreatment clinical view demonstrating correction of lip trap and improvement in esthetic appearance.

Tooth #	Probing Depth		Mobility	Fremitus		Bone Remaining, %	Other
	M	D		MIP	EM		
1	Missing						
2	6		I			75	
3	5	8				65	
4	5	6			I	75	
5	9	7	I		I	70	
6	Missing						
7	5	5	III	III (lip)		45	Lip trap
8	5	7	III	III (lip)		55	Lip trap
9	8	9	III	III (lip)		60	Lip trap
10	8	7	III	III (lip)		55	Lip trap
11	Missing						
12	8	7	I		I	70	
13	5	5			I	80	
14	10	9	I			60	
15	6	6	I			70	
16	Missing						

The 30-year-old patient had generalized aggressive periodontitis with severe bone loss and occlusal trauma from a "trapped lip" (seen in Figure 29-17a). The maxillary incisors had no fremitus in maximum intercuspal position, but did have Class III fremitus when the patient closed her jaws because of pressure on the teeth from a trapped lower lip (Class II malocclusion). The posterior teeth had practically no fremitus despite an occlusion that was locked by steep posterior cuspal anatomy.

Figure 29-22. Occlusal Summary Charts for maxillary arch in patient whose radiographs are seen in Figures 29-21 B and G.

After establishing a stable maxillomandibular relation with axial loading and maximum distribution of force, excursive movements of the mandible must be evaluated and modified if necessary. Fremitus is an essential guide to the amount of correction necessary and to the distribution of force in contacting movements. The occlusal adjustment techniques used to modify guidance in contacting movements should reduce fremitus as much as allowed by the mechanical limitations of the dentition. It is not necessary to establish a predetermined occlusal pattern of cuspal anatomy. Anterior guidance in contacting movements with posterior disarticulation of the teeth is desirable. However, orthodontic malocclusions, missing anterior teeth, severely weakened anterior teeth, the need to reduce anterior crown-to-root ratios, or generalized fremitus patterns may require that patterns of group function in lateral contacting movements on the working side be modified. Cross-tooth working contacts and cross-arch balancing contacts are mechanically complicating and are to be avoided or eliminated. In addition to elimination of occlusal interferences, creation of a stable interarch relation and axial loading of forces over a favorable distribution of teeth, a major goal of occlusal intervention is to preserve or improve the esthetics, phonetics, and masticatory function of the patient. If successful, occlusal intervention will result in reduced mobility, with a narrowing of the periodontal ligament space and increased stability of the tooth. If secondary occlusal trauma is the diagnosis made after successful antiinfective treatment, then splinting often is necessary. Patients with parafunctional tooth habits may require occlusal night guards or splints to control force.

Constant evaluation and reevaluation is required throughout treatment, and adequate time must be allowed for the attachment apparatus to respond before irreversible procedures are undertaken. Often, repair can be seen within the first several weeks; however, it is more reasonable to evaluate the occlusion after several months to determine whether changes are stable or transient. Before making major changes in the occlusal arrangement on the basis of perceived necessity for splinting, the clinician should be certain that occlusal trauma is indeed present and that the patient will respond to the splinting in a desirable fashion.

Briefly then, occlusal trauma and plaque-induced inflammatory periodontitis often occur in the same patient. Control of both conditions is necessary for maximum resolution of the disease. Careful study is needed to determine if the two processes are interacting to determine the need for occlusal therapy. In those patients in whom the two processes are acting in concert, a rational approach involving evaluation of antiinfective therapy and evaluation of occlusal therapy is necessary in determining if the occlusal trauma is leading to a deteriorating situation. This concept can best be summarized by paraphrasing Nyman and coworkers[43]: The tooth or tooth segment with *increased* mobility can be tolerated as long as the mobility does not interfere with patient comfort, function, or esthetic satisfaction. When there is *increasing* mobility, however, it cannot be tolerated without a reliable judgment of an end-point to the increasing mobility.

REFERENCES

1. Karolyi M: Beobachtungen uber pyorrhea alveolaris. Oster-relchisch-vngarische viertel, *Jahresschrift fur zahnheilkunde* 17:279, 1901.
2. Stillman PR: What is traumatic occlusion and how can it be diagnosed? *J Am Dent Assoc* 12:1330-1338, 1925.
3. Box HK: Experimental traumatogenic occlusion in sheep, *Oral Health* 29:9-15, 1935.
4. Macapanpan LC, Weinmann JP: The influence of injury to the periodontal membrane on the spread of gingival inflammation, *J Dent Res* 33:263-272, 1954.
5. Glickman I: Inflammation and trauma from occlusion, co-destructive factors in chronic periodontal disease. *J Periodontol* 34:5-10, 1963.
6. Waerhaug J: The angular bone defect and its relationship to trauma from occlusion and down growth of subgingival plaque, *J Clin Periodontol* 6:61-82, 1979.
7. Hallmon WW: Occlusal trauma: effect and impact on the periodontium. Consensus report: occlusal trauma. American Academy of Periodontology. 1999 International Workshop for a Classification of Periodontal Diseases and Conditions. *Ann Periodontol* 4:102-108, 1999.
8. Goldman H, Cohen DW: *Periodontal therapy*, ed 6, St. Louis, 1980, CV Mosby.
9. Wentz FM, Jarabak J, Orban B: Experimental occlusal trauma imitating cuspal interferences, *J Periodontol* 29:117-127, 1958.
10. Svanberg GK, Lindhe J: Vascular reactions in the periodontal ligament incident to trauma from occlusion, *J Clin Periodontol* 1:58-69, 1975.
11. Lindhe J, Svanberg GK: Influence of trauma from occlusion on progression of experimental periodontitis in the beagle dog, *J Clin Periodontol* 1:3-14, 1974.
12. Lindhe J, Ericsson I: The influence of trauma from occlusion on reduced but healthy periodontal tissues in dogs, *J Clin Periodontol* 3:110-122, 1976.
13. Nyman S, Lindhe J, Ericsson I: The effect of progressive tooth mobility on destructive periodontitis in the dog, *J Clin Periodontol* 7:351-360, 1978.
14. Neiderud AM, Ericsson I, Lindhe J: Probing pocket depth at mobile/non mobile teeth, *J Clin Periodontol* 19:754-759, 1992.
15. Polson AM, Meitner SW, Zander HA: Trauma and progression of marginal periodontitis in squirrel monkeys. III. Adaption of interproximal alveolar bone to repetitive injury, *J Periodont Res* 11:279-289, 1976.
16. Polson AM, Meitner SW, Zander HA: Trauma and progression of periodontitis in squirrel monkeys. IV. Reversibility of bone loss due to trauma alone and trauma superimposed upon periodontitis, *J Periodont Res* 11:290, 1976.
17. Polson AM, Zander HA: Effect of periodontal trauma upon intrabony pockets, *J Periodontol* 54:586-591, 1983.
18. Abrams L, Coslet G: Occlusal adjustment by selective grinding. In Goldman H, Schluger S, Fox L, Cohen DW, editors: *Periodontal therapy*, St. Louis, 1967, CV Mosby.
19. Gaengler P, Merte K: Effects of force application on periodontal blood circulation, *J Periodont Res* 18:86-92, 1983.
20. Ericsson I, Lindhe J: Lack of significance of increased tooth mobility in experimental periodontitis, *J Periodontol* 55:447-452, 1984.
21. Nyman S, Ericsson I, Runstad L, Karring T: The significance of alveolar bone in periodontal disease. An experimental study in the dog, *J Periodont Res* 19:520-525, 1984.
22. Reinhardt RA, Pao YC, Krejcii RF: Periodontal ligament stresses in the initiation of occlusal traumatism, *J Periodont Res* 19:238-246, 1984.
23. Lindhe J, Nyman S: The role of occlusion in periodontal disease and the biologic rationale for splinting in treatment of periodontitis, *Oral Sci Rev* 10:11-43, 1977.
24. Glickman I, Smulow JB: Alterations in the pathway of gingival inflammation to the underlying tissues induced by excessive occlusal forces, *J Periodontol* 33:7-13, 1962.
25. Ritchey B, Orban B: The crests of interdental alveolar septa, *J Periodontol* 24:75-87, 1953.
26. Rosling B, Nyman S, Lindhe J: The effect of systematic plaque control on bone regeneration in infrabony pockets, *J Clin Periodontol* 3:38-53, 1976.
27. Polson AM, Adams RA, Zander HA: Osseous repair in the presence of active tooth hypermobility, *J Clin Periodontol* 10:370-379, 1983.
28. Fleszar TJ, Knowles JW, Morrison EC et al: Tooth mobility and periodontal therapy, *J Clin Periodontol* 7:495-505, 1980.
29. Stahl SS: The responses of the periodontium to combined gingival inflammation and occluso-functional stresses in four human surgical specimens, *Periodontics* 6:14-22, 1968.

30. Simmons TA, Avery JK, Svanberg GK: Periodontal collagen formation in jiggling beagle dog teeth, *J Dent Res* 58(A):328, 1979.

31. Kantor M, Ramfjord SP, Zander HA: Alveolar bone regeneration after removal of inflammatory and traumatic factors, *J Periodontol* 47:687-695, 1976.

32. Youdelis RA, Mann WV: The prevalence and possible role of nonworking contacts in periodontal disease. *Periodontics* 3:219-223, 1965.

33. Pihlstrom BL, Anderson KA, Aeppli D, Schaffer DM: Associations between signs of trauma from occlusion and periodontitis. *J Periodontol* 57:1-6, 1986.

34. Nunn ME, Harrel SK: The effects of occlusal discrepancies on periodontitis. I. Relationship of initial occlusal discrepancies to initial clinical parameters, *J Periodontol* 72:485-494, 2001.

35. Shefter GJ, McFall Jr WT: Occlusal relations and periodontal status in human adults, *J Periodontol* 55:364-374, 1984.

36. Jin LJ, Cao CF: Clinical diagnosis of trauma from occlusion and its relation with severe periodontitis, *J Clin Periodontol* 19:92-97, 1992.

37. Harrel SK, Nunn ME: The effects of occlusal discrepancies on periodontitis. II. Relationship of occlusal treatment to the progression of periodontal disease, *J Periodontol* 72:495-505, 2001.

38. Ingervall B: Tooth contacts on the functional and non functional side in children and young adults, *Arch Oral Biol* 17:191-200, 1972.

39. Ingervall B, Harrel SK, Kessis S: Pattern of teeth contacts in eccentric mandibular positions in young adults, *J Prosthet Dent* 66:160-176, 1991.

40. Yaffe A, Ehrlich J: The functional range of tooth contact in lateral gliding movements, *J Prosthet Dent* 57:730-733, 1987.

41. Burgett FG, Ramford SP, Nissle RR et al: A randomized trial of occlusal adjustment in the treatment of periodontitis patients, *J Clin Periodontol* 19:381-387, 1992.

42. Potashnick SR, Abrams L: The significance of occlusal adjustment in periodontal therapy, *Alpha Omegan* 78:25-46, 1985.

43. Nyman S, Lindhe J, Lundgren D: The role of occlusion for the stability of fixed bridges in patients with reduced periodontal tissue support, *J Clin Periodontol* 2:53-66, 1975.

30 Endodontic–Periodontal Considerations

Louis E. Rossman

The effects of pulpal disease on the periodontium, the effects of periodontal diseases on the pulp, classification of periodontal/endodontic problems, and their sequelae, diagnosis, and treatment are presented in this chapter.

Inflammation of the supporting tissues with deep pockets along the side of the root, suppuration from these pockets, swelling and bleeding of the gingiva, fistula formation, tenderness to percussion, increased tooth mobility, and angular bone loss are most often associated with periodontitis, which begins at the margin of the gingiva and proceeds apically. However, these same signs and symptoms may be caused by pulpal infections that have entered the periodontal ligament either through the apical foramen, through the lateral canals, or through the dentinal tubules. Pulpal irritants and infections cause lesions that are often difficult to distinguish from those caused by marginal periodontal infections. Differentiation of pulpal infections is possible, because pulpal infections can be diagnosed through careful evaluation, testing, and diagnosis. In addition, radiographic changes or severe pain are usually localized to the tooth. Symptoms of plaque-associated periodontitis are usually nonexistent or minor, and signs of disease are confined to the marginal periodontium. When these lesions occur as combined lesions (i.e., pulpal infection proceeding to periodontal infection), they are more difficult to diagnose. Furthermore, periodontal disease and periodontal treatment may cause pulpal changes, and proper diagnosis of these is also important.

DIAGNOSIS

There are several signs and symptoms of pulpal and periodontal lesions that allow them to be distinguished. These include pain; swelling; periodontal probing; tooth mobility; percussion on palpation; pulp tests, including thermal, electric, and preparation of the test cavity; and radiographic interpretation.

Pain

Pain of endodontic origin is usually acute in onset and severe. It can occur spontaneously during the early stages of pulpal inflammation when there is poor localization, and the pain may be referred to other sites. Pain intensifies and localizes once the inflammation spreads to the periodontal ligament and surrounding osseous structures. Often, potent analgesics are not adequate to control endodontic pain, which can at times awaken the person from sleep. Endodontic pain often can be eliminated only by root canal treatment.

Pain of periodontal origin is chronic and usually mild or moderate, responding to mild analgesics. If an acute flare-up occurs, creating a periodontal abscess, pain can be severe. This severe pain often regresses after drainage. It usually does not awaken a patient from sleep.

Combined pulpal–periodontal infections usually exhibit minimal pain. Enough periodontal tissue loss occurs to open an avenue of drainage through the gingival sulcus, thereby minimizing pressure and pain.

Swelling

Swelling caused by endodontic infections often occurs in the mucobuccal fold or spreads to the fascial planes. Muscle attachments and root length determine the route of drainage. Swelling associated with periodontal problems is characteristically found in the attached gingiva and rarely spreads beyond the mucogingival line, and most often no facial swelling is involved.

Probing

The presence of a sinus tract often allows a diagnosis of the problem. A radiograph taken with a gutta-percha point or fine wire threaded into the orifice of the tract reveals the source. When the tracing goes to the apex of the tooth, the tract is usually of endodontic origin (Fig. 30-1). When the traced sinus tract goes to the midroot, furcation, or any other portion of the tooth, a lateral canal or periodontal problem is diagnosed[1,2] (Fig. 30-2).

When endodontic problems develop into a periapical abscess, an escape route is made through a sinus tract or fistula. If the sinus tract occurs within the sulcus or periodontal pocket (Fig. 30-1), probing alone cannot clearly determine the origin of the tract, because periodontitis may also result in deep probing depths. Periodontal problems may cause progressive bone loss from the margin to the apex, creating periodontal attachment loss that may allow probing to the apex. Periodontal probing to the apex hence may not indicate a pulpal lesion. The results of pulp testing are necessary to diagnose the origin of such lesions, because if the lesion is periodontal in origin, the pulp is most often vital.

Mobility

When mobility is present around one isolated tooth, the source of the problem can be endodontic, periodontal, or occlusal. In the acute stage of an endodontic infection, mobility involves a single tooth. Generalized mobility, however, involving many teeth suggests periodontal or occlusal origin.

Clinical Tests

Percussion and Palpation

Results of percussion and palpation tests are usually negative in an individual tooth with a periodontal problem. When a periodontal abscess is present, these clinical entities may be positive; however, other tests indicate

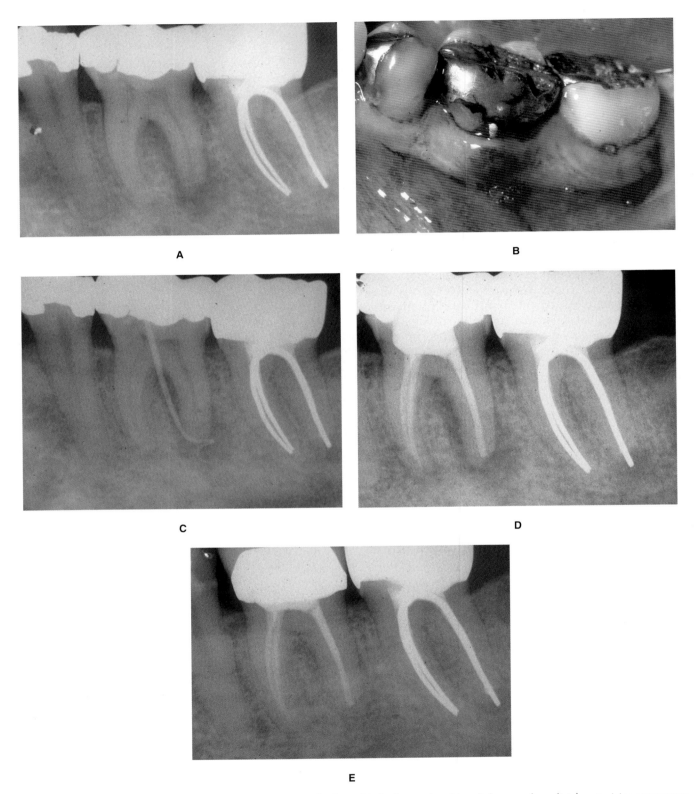

Figure 30-1. Primary endodontic lesion. **A,** Preoperative radiograph of mandibular first molar with radiolucency along distal root, giving appearance of periodontal disease with osseous breakdown in furcation. **B,** Fine gutta-percha point placed into deep periodontal pocket on direct buccal aspect, which was the only probeable tract. Thermal tests and test cavity confirmed necrotic pulp. **C,** Radiograph of fine gutta-percha point revealing root canal as source of draining abscess. Note that osseous destruction involves only this one tooth. **D,** Posttreatment radiograph. Periodontal pocket was completely resolved. No root planing was performed. **E,** View at 5 year recall after endodontic therapy only. Furcation and surrounding osseous structures about distal root have regenerated. (*Restorative therapy by Dr. H. Silverstein.*)

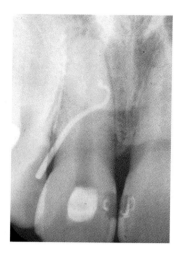

A

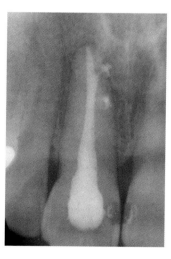

B

Figure 30-2. Primary endodontic lesion. **A,** Preoperative radiograph of maxillary central incisor with fine gutta-percha point tracing a sinus tract. Note origin of sinus tract is at midpoint of root. No significant periodontal probing was observed. Vitality tests confirmed a necrotic pulp. **B,** Posttreatment radiograph. Note bifurcated root canal and presence of lateral canal at midpoint of root junction of apical and middle thirds of the root. Root canal filling material now occupies apparent source of the sinus tract. Healing is complete.

a vital pulp. A tooth with an endodontic problem usually produces definite tenderness and pain on percussion and palpation.

Cold

The normal response of a healthy pulp to cold testing is immediate and disappears when the stimulus is removed. If there is no response or the pain lingers once the stimulus is removed, the pulp is necrotic or irreversibly

inflamed. This is a one-time test because the pulp requires time to recover before it will respond again. 1,1,1,2-tetrafluoroethane (Frigi-dent: Ellman International; Hewlett, NY) should be used because it creates rapid fluid movement in the dentinal tubules better than any other cold substance.[3] This modality can also be used on teeth with metal crowns and often is effective with porcelain crowns.[4]

Electric

The electric pulp test is viewed as a "yes" or "no" response: there is vitality or there is no vitality. It does not indicate the status of the pulp. If there is no response, the pulp is necrotic and root canal therapy is required. However, one should not rely on only one pulp test. Rubber gloves will not allow the passage of current, and the circuit will not be completed; hence electric pulp tests should be carried out with an ungloved hand or with the patient holding the device to complete the circuit.[5]

Heat

The normal response of a healthy pulp to heat is pain that increases in intensity until the stimulus is removed. Once the heat is removed, the pain disappears immediately. Lingering pain indicates an irreversibly inflamed pulp. When pain persists after removal of the heat stimulus from periodontally involved teeth, a pulpitis should be suspected. Hot gutta-percha should be applied to the tooth coated with petroleum jelly to prevent the material from sticking to the tooth surface. If a crown is present, a rotating rubber prophylaxis cup can be run on a dried tooth to create heat.

Test cavity

Preparation of a test cavity should be done without anesthesia. A small access preparation is made through a crown or through the enamel to determine whether vitality is present in the pulp. No response indicates necrosis of the pulp. This test does not give information as to the status of the pulp other than whether it is vital. These results are similar to the results obtained with the electric pulp test.

Radiographs

Periodontal and endodontic problems can radiographically mimic each other; therefore pulp testing and periodontal probing must be used along with the radiograph. If bone loss exists around one tooth in an otherwise periodontally healthy patient and pulp tests are negative (i.e., nonvital), then this loss of bone may be of endodontic origin. The prognosis is excellent for regeneration of these structures after endodontic therapy. If there is periapical radiolucency and results of the pulp tests show necrosis, then the lesion may also be of endodontic origin.

Periodontally susceptible patients may exhibit lesions that appear to be of pulpal origin but are not. When bone loss exists in this situation and pulp test results are normal, the lesion is of periodontal origin. Periapical radiographic lesions can sometimes be of periodontal origin. These may occur on teeth that have deep radicular grooves that provide a channel for apical downgrowth of plaque. Lesions of occlusal trauma can also be observed as radiolucencies around the apex of the tooth. The pulpal tissue in these teeth will usually prove to be vital.

Radiographs are also helpful in determining the quality of a previous root canal treatment. If the etiology is questionable and there is any doubt as to the quality of previous root canal treatment, then re-treatment should be considered.

EFFECTS OF PULPAL DISEASES ON THE PERIODONTIUM

The functions of the dental pulp include formative, protective, and reparative responses. The protective response is mediated by the neural and vascular elements of the pulp. The best root canal filling is healthy pulp tissue, and every effort should be made to preserve its integrity and to avoid unnecessary endodontic procedures.[6]

Sinus Tract

A sinus tract is nature's way of allowing pus to escape when chronic apical or lateral periodontitis is present. Pus seeks the easiest way out of the bone, with the resulting sinus tract usually appearing on either the buccal or lingual mucosa. The tract often cannot be detected radiographically, because its path parallels the x-ray beam. When, however, the tract occurs along the periodontal ligament, the radiographic appearance may mimic an infrabony defect or furcation involvement because the osseous lesion, created by the bone erosion that is not masked by the root, is perpendicular to the x-ray beam (Fig. 30-1).[7]

Pain is usually absent in the presence of a sinus tract, because the tract provides drainage. The diagnosis of its source can be aided by tracing the tract with a gutta-percha point, fine orthodontic wire, or a silver point (Figs. 30-1 and 30-2).[8] A radiograph taken with the traced sinus tract reveals the source of the abscess. When the tract is traced to the radiographic apex, the endodontic etiology can be confirmed by failure of the tooth to respond to electric or cold test procedures. When the fistula is traced to the midroot, periodontal etiology or pulp necrosis in a lateral canal must be considered in the differential diagnosis (Fig. 30-2).[1,2] When root canal treatment has already been performed, an incomplete root fracture or a perforation must be suspected.[9] The latter suspicion is aroused when there is overzealous instrumentation with marked enlargement of the root canal or a large post.

Periodontal abscesses can also drain through the gingival sulcus or periodontal pocket as a sinus tract. Tracing a tract of periodontal origin usually demonstrates that the apex of the tooth is not involved. A positive response to pulp testing usually indicates vitality.[3,10]

Dentinal Tubules

Dentinal tubules contain cytoplasmic extensions, the odontoblastic processes, which extend from the odontoblasts at the pulpal–dentin border to the dentinoenamel junction or dentinocementum junction. When dentin is cut, either by a bur or a curette, it reacts in the same manner as any other tissue in the body. There is an initial injury followed by an inflammatory response, concluding with a healing phase. Communication through dentinal tubules has been demonstrated in dogs and monkeys, in which peri-radicular changes in the periodontium were found after pulpotomy and placement of caustic agents in the pulp chamber.[11] Communication in the other direction is demonstrated by the inflammatory reaction of the pulp to exposure of dentinal tubules after the protective layer of enamel or cementum has been removed with a bur or a curette.[12] The effect of periodontal disease on the dental pulp was first described by Turner and Drew in 1919.[13] In 1927, Cahn[14] described the presence of communicating channels, and these channels continue to be actively studied.

A pathologic condition that illustrates this intercommunication between the pulp and the periodontal tissues is inflammatory root resorption. This occurs after avulsion or replantation of the tooth because of injury to the periodontal ligament and necrosis of the pulp with the presence of bacteria in the root canal system.[15] The result is quickly developing, large resorptive lacunae along the lateral aspect of the root despite the protection from the cementum. In immature teeth, with their wide dentinal tubules, removal of cementum facilitates rapid movement of bacterial products from the necrotic pulp to the periodontal ligament, resulting in inflammatory root resorption. In mature teeth, the tubules are much narrower. If cementum is experimentally removed, a new cementum layer can be formed.[16]

The effect of direct dentinal communication can also be observed after free autogenous soft tissue grafts. In animal models, the graft failure rate was greater when grafts were placed over untreated teeth with necrotic pulps than when they were placed over teeth with vital pulps or after successful root canal therapy.[17] The bacteria and their toxins in the root canal system most likely adversely affect the ability of the soft tissue to reattach to the root surface. Therefore careful assessment of pulpal status is critical for successful periodontal therapy.

Another vivid example of the importance of dentinal tubules is hypersensitivity, in which the patient experiences pain to various stimuli such as cold and sweets. The use of a topical application of potassium oxylate solution causes crystal formation within the dentinal tubules, thereby clogging these channels to prevent fluid movement, which excites the sensory terminal nerve endings within the dentin–predentin region.[18] Calcium hydroxide burnished on the root surface produces the same result. Varnish can also be used, but it is governed by time until it wears off or is physically removed through brushing.

Reducing the neuronal response to dentin hypersensitivity appears to be most effective to the chief compliant of cold. An application of 0.717% tin (II) fluoride (SnF2) works well.[19] In addition, in a majority of cases, potassium nitrate–containing dentifrices appear to be effective to reduce cold sensitivity. In a review of the literature, potassium nitrate–containing dentifrices were successful 60% of the time.[20]

Lateral Canals

The terms *lateral canal* and *accessory canal* are often used interchangeably. The glossary of the American Association of Endodontics[21] makes the distinction that lateral canals run perpendicular to the main canal, whereas accessory canals are any branch of the canal or chamber that communicates with the root surface. Lateral canals are most often found in the apical third of the root and in the furcation area of multirooted teeth. Obliteration of these canals occurs naturally as part of the aging process as dentin and cementum are produced.

A large number of lateral canals exist in human teeth, and inflammation of the periodontal ligament can affect the dental pulp by way of these lateral canals.[22] Lateral canals rarely cause endodontic therapy failure.[23] Indeed, if the lateral canal contains vital tissue, it will not appear on the post endodontic radiograph. It is sometimes possible to force cement or a filling material into a lateral canal if the tissue in the canal has become necrotic and large enough to allow penetration of filling material (Fig. 30-2, *B*).

When the concentration of contaminants in a necrotic lateral canal is great enough, pain or radiographic evidence of breakdown on the lateral surface of the root can occur (Fig. 30-3). When the pulp tests indicate necrosis and a sinus tract can be traced to the lateral portion of the root, a lateral canal might be the cause of an endodontic–periodontal lesion.[1] It is advisable to keep post preparations away from areas with demonstrated lateral canals to reduce the chance of leakage and contamination.

Lateral canals in the floor of the furcation are found in up to 28% of multirooted teeth.[24] These canals can supply much of the circulation to the pulp. Some clinicians have found when caustic compounds are placed in the chamber complete destruction of the furcation occurs. This stresses the importance of sealing the floor of the pulp chamber after root canal therapy.

EFFECTS OF PERIODONTAL DISEASES ON THE PULP

Bender and Seltzer[25] found that periodontally involved human teeth have a much greater incidence of pulpal inflammation and degeneration than intact human teeth with no periodontal disease. This correlation has not been noted in animal studies, most likely because they lack lateral canals.[10,26] The teeth of rice rats and some monkeys, for example, do not demonstrate any lateral canals.

Atrophic Changes

Teeth with caries or restorations that also have periodontal disease have more atrophic pulps than teeth with caries or restorations but no periodontal disease.[25] A larger collagen content in the pulp, with more dentin and dystrophic calcification, is found in teeth with periodontal disease, and the canal space may be markedly narrowed.[15] The cause of these atrophic changes is the disruption of blood flow through the lateral canals, which leads to localized areas of coagulation necrosis in the pulp. These areas eventually are walled off from the healthy pulp tissue by collagen and dystrophic mineralization.

Root planing may have the same effect on the dental pulp and has been shown to increase the rate of reparative dentinogenesis.[27] One possible explanation for this is that blood vessels leading into lateral canals are severed, causing localized areas of pulpal necrosis. Another explanation is that the removal of the protective layer of cementum exposes dentinal tubules, providing an avenue for pulpal irritation with subsequent reparative dentin deposition.

In cases of slowly advancing periodontal disease, cementum deposition may act to obliterate a lateral canal before pulpal irritation occurs. This, along with the absence of lateral canals, may explain why not all periodontally involved teeth demonstrate pulpal atrophy and canal narrowing.

MICROBIOLOGY OF PULPAL DISEASES

Just as in other protected connective tissues, the enclosed, healthy, vital dental pulp is sterile. Thus infections of the pulp are almost always secondary to other tooth infections, iatrogenic causes, or in some rare cases, traumatic occlusion. This contrasts markedly with the other major dental infections, caries, and periodontal disease that are directly associated with dental plaque. Because of

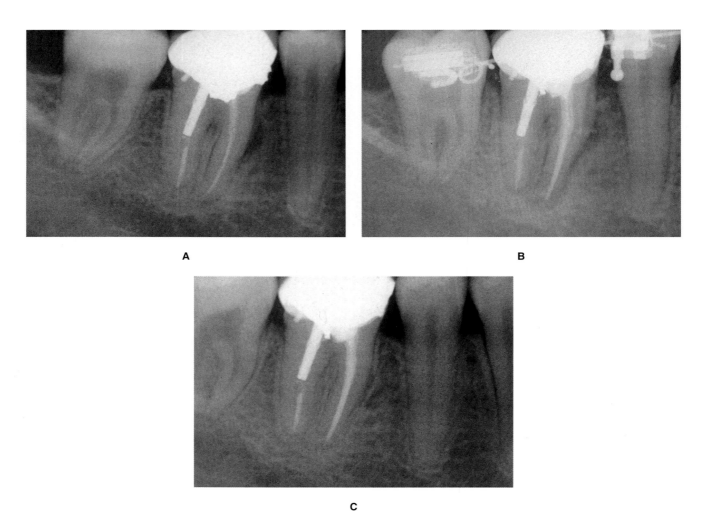

Figure 30-3. Mandibular first molar with lateral canal. **A,** Pretreatment radiograph. A previous dentist performed endodontic therapy 3 years earlier. Note radiolucency on lateral aspect of mesial root, amalgam in chamber, post in distal canal, and inadequate biomechanical instrumentation of root canals. **B,** Posttreatment radiograph with root canal filling material forced into a lateral canal because tissue had become necrotic and created osseous breakdown. Distal canal was not retreated conventionally, because of post. **C,** View at 6-year recall demonstrating complete regeneration of previous radiolucency.

this, the organisms that are the direct antecedent of the inflammatory process associated with pulp infections are endogenous oral bacteria (bacteria normally present in the oral cavity) that gain access to the pulpal connective tissues. This hospitable environment provides them with the nutrition that allows them to multiply. More often than not, these bacteria lack or cannot express properties that can initiate invasion in their normal environment, and therefore they are usually considered of low virulence.[28] Their "virulence" is usually only expressed when they gain access to the connective tissues such as the dental pulp. For this reason they are called "opportunistic pathogens" and the infections they cause are called endogenous opportunistic infections.

Among the factors affecting the kinds of bacteria that are isolated from root canal infection are the route of infection (e.g., extension of caries), mechanical exposure, trauma, and association with periodontal disease. The invasion of the pulp as a result of direct extension of dental caries is probably one of the most common routes of infection, particularly in younger patients. Studies in which samples have been obtained immediately after a "mechanical exposure" of a root canal indicate that the majority of organisms are nonhemolytic streptococci, the most prevalent organisms in the oral cavity. In patients with periodontal disease, accessory canals on the lateral surfaces of the tooth may become exposed to the plaque bacteria. These organisms can multiply in accessory canals resulting in inflammation and necrosis; eventually these organisms spread to infect the pulp chamber. Again proving that this avenue is an important source of infection is problematic, but it remains a real possibility. Certainly infection of accessory canals often is a cause of apparent failure of root canal therapy.[1]

In addition to gram-positive streptococci, pulp infections have been associated with gram-negative organisms such as species of *Neisseria, Bacteroides, Fusobacterium*, and coliforms. Spirochetes were often observed in bacterial smears but at the time these studies were done, these strictly anaerobic organisms could not be grown in the laboratory. More recent studies have used sampling and growth methods that allow a better enumeration of the species originally present. Deepening periodontal pockets and infected pulpal tissues appear to favor anaerobic growth. The source of each of these infections is the same—the more than 400 bacterial species that are present in the oral cavity.[29]

An organism that seems to be closely associated with root canal infection is *Porphyromonas endodontalis*.[30] Originally described as a black-pigmented *Bacteroides*, it is believed to have pathogenic potential similar to those described for *Porphyromonas gingivalis*. Since its original isolation from root canals, the organism has been found in other ecologic niches within the oral cavity, suggesting that its appearance in the root canal again reflects a selective mechanism that allows this opportunist to grow. This organism is often found in acute suppurative infections of the root apex.

Trowbridge[12] has described inflammation of the dental pulp caused by bacterial products and toxins. When caries is removed, dead tracts that have been formed are sealed off by the remaining vital odontoblasts by elaborating reparative dentin. The dead tracts are not as highly mineralized as sclerotic dentin. In the presence of dead tracts, caries progresses more rapidly.

Given the right combination of periodontal and cariogenic pathogens, root caries develops, often rapidly. Endodontic complications with root caries include calcification at the level of the caries, thereby blocking access into the canal, and an inability to isolate the tooth and create a sterile operating environment. The most difficult problems occur when an acute or chronic apical periodontitis occurs as a result of pulpal necrosis from root caries.

Asymptomatic periapical areas around teeth with root caries are also often difficult to manage. Initiation of endodontic therapy can trigger an acute exacerbation of a chronic apical periodontitis, with pain and swelling. These abscesses are known as a recrudescent or "phoenix" abscess. The loss of pulpal vitality allows invading bacteria to penetrate the root canal and freely develop a periapical abscess.

PERIODONTAL–ENDODONTIC PROBLEMS

Different systems have been developed for classification of endodontic and periodontal problems.[30-37] When examining and treating the combined or individual problems in endodontics and periodontics, one must bear in mind that teeth are often in their terminal stage and that successful treatment depends on a correct diagnosis.[38] Diagnosis and treatment methods are presented below.

Primary Endodontic Lesion

Sequelae

A primary endodontic lesion is one that manifests a necrotic pulp with a chronic apical periodontitis and a draining sinus tract (Figs. 30-4, *A* and *B*, and 30-5). The sinus tract in these cases drains through the periodontal ligament or the gingival sulcus. Usually the radiograph reveals an isolated periodontal problem around an individual tooth. There is usually no associated generalized periodontal disease, and osseous destruction involves this one tooth only. If a buccal or lingual swelling appears, a lateral canal should be considered. Swelling in the mucobuccal fold is pathognomonic for endodontic disease.

Tests

Confirmation of the diagnosis comes from negative pulp vitality tests. The electric pulp test, thermal tests, and test cavity usually reveal no response. Periodontal probing is within normal limits throughout the patient's mouth. This type of lesion develops rapidly and presents a dramatic change, sometimes within a short period, even between regular dental appointments. Probing the gingival sulcus with a flexible probe, gutta-percha point, or fine silver point or wire often reveals the presence of a sinus tract. When the sinus tract is of endodontic origin, generally only one wire can be inserted, whereas if the lesion is of periodontal origin, multiple wires or diagnostic probes can be inserted. Conventional periodontal probes for this diagnosis are of limited value. Tracing the fistula often reveals that the origin is at the apex of the tooth. It also may go to the midroot, and a lateral canal may be involved.

Treatment

Treatment consists of conservative or conventional root canal therapy. Root canal therapy should be performed with multiple appointments so that a reevaluation of the healing process between the completion of root canal debridement and obturation visits can be made. A sinus tract usually heals after instrumentation and irrigation of the root canal. The closure of the tract and the elimination

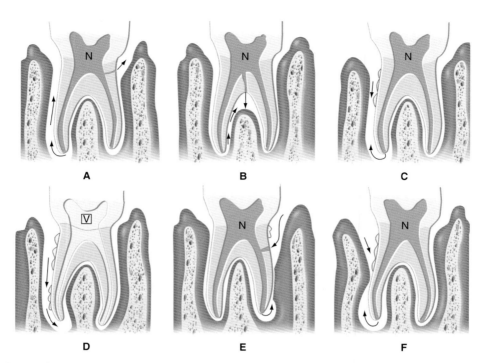

Figure 30-4. Potential routes for development of endodontic–periodontal lesions. **A,** Endodontic lesion. The pathway of communication is evident through the periodontal ligament from the apex or a lateral canal. **B,** Communication through the apex or a lateral canal may cause bifurcation involvement. **C,** Primary endodontic lesion with secondary periodontal involvement. The existing pathway as in **A** is shown, but with the passage of time periodontitis with calculus formation begins at the cervical area. **D,** Periodontal lesion. The progression of periodontitis is toward the apex. Note the vital pulp (V). **E,** Primary periodontal lesion with secondary endodontic involvement, showing the primary periodontal lesion at the cervical margin and the resultant pulpal necrosis once the lateral canal is exposed to the oral environment. **F,** "True" combined lesion. The two separate lesions are heading to coalescence, which forms the "true" combined lesion. N, Necrotic pulp. (*Redrawn from Simon JH, Glick DH, Frank AL: The relationship of endodontic-periodontic lesions,* J Periodontol *43:202, 1972.*)

of probing depth indicate that the root canal has been properly cleansed, and the prognosis is excellent.

No root planing should be done when the sinus tract is along the periodontal ligament. It is important to preserve these fibers so that reattachment can occur. If root planing and curettage are performed, the likelihood of a good prognosis may be greatly reduced.

Prognosis

The prognosis is excellent. The radiographic and clinical healing that occurs is rapid and quite spectacular. Healing is usually accomplished within 3 to 6 months.

Primary Endodontic Lesion with Secondary Periodontal Involvement

Sequelae

If the primary endodontic lesion with a sinus tract is not diagnosed and treated early, plaque and calculus often form in the draining sinus tract, creating a secondary periodontal problem (Fig. 30-4, *C*). This usually appears when healing with closure of the sinus tract does not take place.

Tests

Pulp vitality tests are negative. There is no response to the electric or thermal pulp test or test cavity. Probing the sinus tract reveals the presence of plaque and calculus in the pocket. Usually the coronal portion of the tract resembles a more chronic periodontal problem such as is observed in a periodontal pocket.

Treatment

Good, conservative endodontics must be performed. Periodontal therapy is necessary, usually in the form of root planing to eliminate the calculus and pathogenic flora. Root planing, however, should not be initiated until complete debridement of the root canal system has been performed. This will allow for maximal reattachment, and any remaining probing depth is usually a result of the periodontal flora and can be treated periodontally.

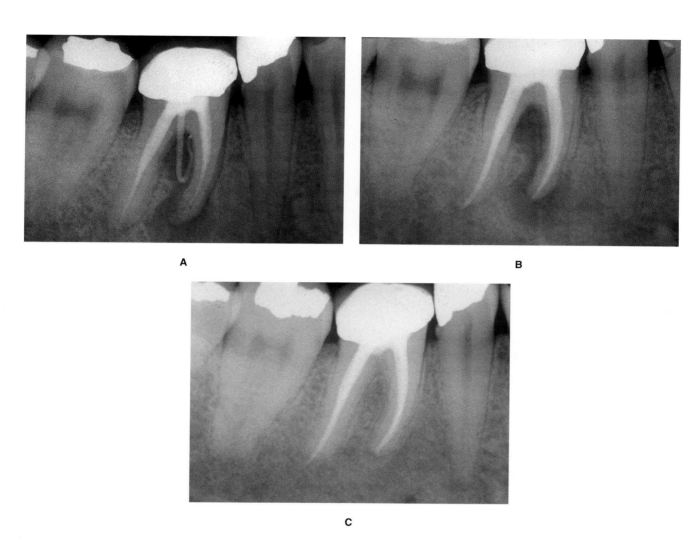

Figure 30-5.   Primary endodontic lesion. **A,** Preoperative radiograph of mandibular first molar with radiolucency at apex of mesial root and along distal aspect of mesial root, giving appearance of periodontal disease with osseous breakdown in furcation. A fine gutta-percha point placed into only probeable tract, a deep periodontal pocket on direct buccal aspect indicates the source root canal, fracture, or perforation. Note that osseous destruction involves only this one tooth. **B,** Posttreatment radiographs. Periodontal pocket completely resolved following instrumentation of the canals and prior to obturation. No root planing was performed. **C,** View at 25-year recall after endodontic therapy only. Furcation and surrounding osseous structures about distal root have regenerated.

Prognosis

The prognosis of the endodontic component is excellent, and regeneration of the attachment apparatus is limited by the periodontal prognosis. If root canal therapy alone is performed, only a limited healing capacity should be expected, because the periodontal component of the lesion will not have been treated adequately.

Primary Periodontal Lesion

Sequelae

Primary periodontal lesions can sometimes mimic an endodontic problem both clinically and radiographically.[39]

This problem, however, develops over a longer period. Periodontal problems that are chronic in nature can also often be observed on *other* teeth, as opposed to endodontic problems, which are isolated to individual teeth. The former lesion is usually observed as a progressive periodontal problem extending to the root apex (Fig. 30-4, *D*). The borders of this lesion are usually wider at the gingival margin, whereas the endodontic lesion is usually wider at the root apex and narrower at the gingival margin. Minimal or no pain is usually experienced by the patient with periodontal disease.

When pain is experienced, a coronal fracture that extends into the periodontal ligament can not be ruled out. Microscopic examination and diagnosis using a bite stick will help to determine the diagnosis.

Tests

Periodontal probing may reach the apex of an involved tooth. The differential diagnosis is made when the results of thermal and electric pulp testing of these teeth are within normal limits. The pulp invariably manifests vitality.

Treatment

Periodontal therapy is indicated. Root canal therapy is not indicated, unless pulp vitality test results change. Reevaluation must be performed periodically after therapy to check for possible retrograde endodontic problems.

Prognosis

The prognosis is entirely dependent on the periodontal therapy. Most teeth with periodontitis resulting in attachment loss to the apex do not have a favorable prognosis.

Primary Periodontal Lesion with Secondary Endodontic Involvement

Sequelae

When periodontal involvement extends to the apex of the tooth, retroinfection of the pulp tissue may occur, and the patient can sometimes experience severe pain. Infection of the pulp can also follow the path through a lateral canal (Fig. 30-4, *E*). Dental abrasions and root planing can also contribute to the death of the pulp.

Tests

The tests are similar to those used in primary endodontic and secondary periodontal lesions. The patient often has generalized periodontitis. Pulp vitality test results can sometimes be mixed. The pulp can be necrotic, or there may be partial necrosis with one or more vital canals, especially in multirooted teeth. When the original diagnosis is strictly periodontal disease and therapy produces no healing, pulp vitality tests should be repeated. Cold is the preferred test for vitality. There should be little if any response as compared with control teeth. When the pulp is inflamed, the application of cold produces an immediate response followed by a prolonged recovery phase. However, when the pulp is necrotic, there is no response.

Treatment

Conservative root canal therapy is indicated. Periodontal therapy should already have been initiated and can proceed in conjunction with the endodontics.

Prognosis

The prognosis is dependent on the periodontal therapy. The healing response of the periapical lesion is not predictable, because of the periodontal communication. A favorable endodontic prognosis is obtained only when the tooth is in a closed and protected environment.[40] The periodontal problem that exists in these cases allows for a direct communication with the oral environment. Failures also occur when a periodontal problem develops along a cementoenamel groove or fused roots in posterior teeth. These areas become a haven for the accumulation of plaque and calculus and reduce the possibility for reattachment.

True Combined Lesion

Sequelae

True combined endodontic–periodontal lesions usually have significant periodontal involvement. The lesion is formed when pulpal and periodontal pathoses develop independently and unite (Figs. 30-4, *F*, and 30-6). This problem is similar to the previously described secondary endodontic involvement on a preexisting primary periodontal lesion.

Differential diagnosis must include a vertical root fracture.[41-43] Perforations and resorptive perforations can produce this true combined lesion. Aggressive instrumentation of the root canal can create perforation along the root canal, and this may initially mimic a lateral canal. If a perforation is created near the gingival sulcus, such as the furcation area, physical disruption of the periodontal ligament and adjacent alveolar bone results in an inflammatory response. Sulcular epithelium may migrate to this area, developing communication between the periodontal inflammation and the oral environment.[44-46] The most severe reactions occur when perforations are not sealed, and the worst prognosis exists with perforations in the furcation region.[47] These should be sealed as quickly as possible.

Tests

In the combined lesion, pulp testing gives negative results. The tooth in question will have periodontal probing depths at numerous sites. Confirmation of the periodontal involvement of the apex of the tooth can be demonstrated with radiographs by placing a periodontal probe, multiple gutta-percha points, or silver points into the sulcus and tracing them to the apex. If the probes are traced to any other area besides the apex, then it is possible that resorption, a perforation, or vertical root fracture is the source of the periodontal communication.

A vertical root fracture can produce a "halo" effect around the tooth radiographically. Examination of the root surface should be done with a sharp explorer held perpendicular to the root surface to feel for any cracks. The fractured root can mimic the lesion of occlusal trauma, with localized loss of lamina dura, altered trabecular pattern, and widened periodontal ligament.[6]

Treatment

Treatment must not be initiated until the patient understands limitations of the prognosis. Good conservative endodontic treatment is performed to reduce the critical concentration of contaminants in the combined lesion. Periodontal therapy can be performed before, during, or immediately after the endodontic treatment.

A number of periodontal and endodontic clinical approaches may be required, including hemisection or root resection.[48,49] Advanced endodontic surgical intervention may also be indicated.[50,51] Any tissue that is surgically removed should be examined histologically.[52]

Internal resorption, if detected radiographically, must be treated immediately by extirpating the pulpal tissue. The multinucleated giant cells must be removed before the resorptive process perforates the canal wall and establishes communication with the periodontal ligament. The prognosis worsens significantly if this communication is established. Treatment then involves the use of long-term calcium hydroxide therapy.[53] External root resorption is a completely different clinical entity. It is usually not implicated in the combined lesion.[54] Differential diagnosis is made in two ways. First by changing the horizontal radiographic views, and secondly by examining the lesion in the radiograph. If the outline of the lesion is continuous with the canal walls, internal resorption exists. If the resorptive lesion is superimposed over the root canal, external resorption exists.

Fractures and complete bone loss are the two entities that condemn a tooth to extraction. Confirmation of the fracture can often be made through surgical exploration.[9] In addition, a vertical root fracture often mimics occlusal trauma. Occlusal trauma is identified on the radiograph when there is a widened periodontal ligament, often with vertical bone loss adjacent to the root surface. There may also be a loss of the lamina dura and an altered trabecular pattern. Vertical root fractures may exhibit the same radiographic changes. Periodontal probing with a vertical root fracture exists along the fracture line from the gingival sulcus to the apical extent of the fracture, usually the apex of the tooth.

If the fracture line does not travel through the epithelial attachment at the base of the gingival sulcus and does not communicate with the oral environment, then surgical removal of the fractured segment may produce a good prognosis. This can be observed with oblique and apical fractures.

Root perforations must be sealed immediately; various locations require different approaches. The important factor is to close off the perforation as quickly as possible and leave options open, treating this as a weak link. The location of the perforation and its size and duration often dictate the material of choice. Cavit, amalgam, guttapercha, calcium hydroxide, and glass ionomer cements have all been used.

Prognosis

The prognosis for the combined endodontic and periodontal problem is dependent on the periodontal

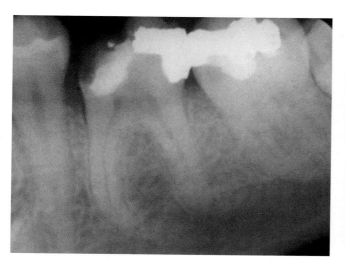
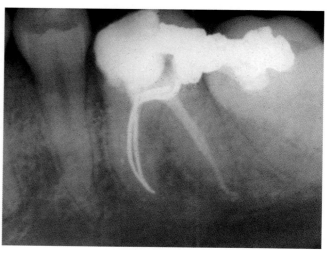

A   **B**

Figure 30-6. True combined lesion. **A,** Preoperative radiograph of mandibular first molar with caries necessitating endodontic therapy. **B,** Root canal therapy was performed using silver points in mesial canals and gutta-percha in distal canal.

Continued

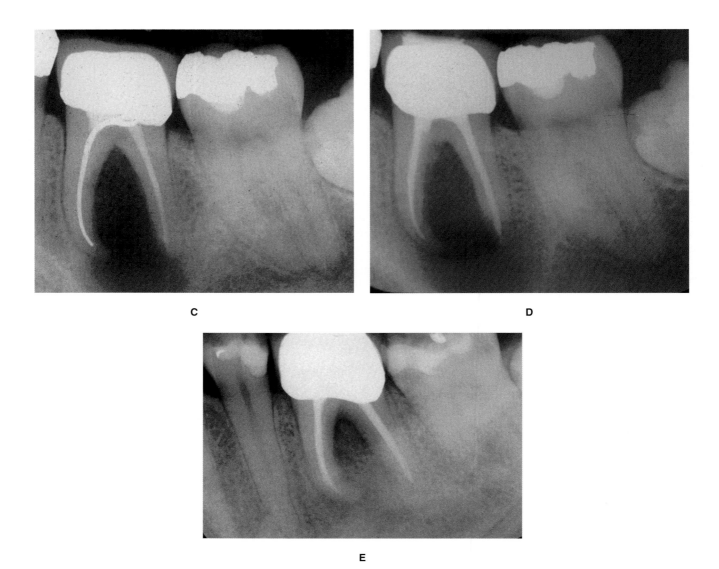

Figure 30-6. cont'd C, View at 10-year recall demonstrating severe periodontal and periapical breakdown. A primary endodontic lesion was suspected; however, no reduction in gingival probing was observed after root canal debridement. A silver point probe could still be placed anywhere along buccal or lingual surfaces after complete instrumentation, however, the probe did not go directly to root apex. Deep periodontal probings were present along the entire buccal and lingual surfaces. **D,** Posttreatment radiograph after re-treatment obturation of canals with gutta-percha. The area was accessed surgically and thorough root debridement was performed to remove all plaque and calculus. **E,** Radiograph at 20-year recall demonstrating excellent regeneration of osseous structures. (*Periodontal therapy by Dr. D.W. Cohen.*)

therapy. Obviously, the root canal therapy cannot be performed with any deviation from accepted standards. The greater the periodontal involvement, the poorer the prognosis is. Patients cannot be promised a favorable prognosis. As long as they understand this and are willing to undergo these procedures with the possibility of failure, advanced procedures can be tried (Fig. 30-7).

CLINICAL CONSIDERATIONS WITH COMBINED ENDODONTIC–PERIODONTAL THERAPY

Endodontics has a success rate that exceeds 96%, with both vital and nonvital pulps showing no periapical radiolucency. Conversely, only 86% of endodontic cases with pulp necrosis and periapical radiolucency show apical healing.[55] Re-treatment of previous root canal therapy has

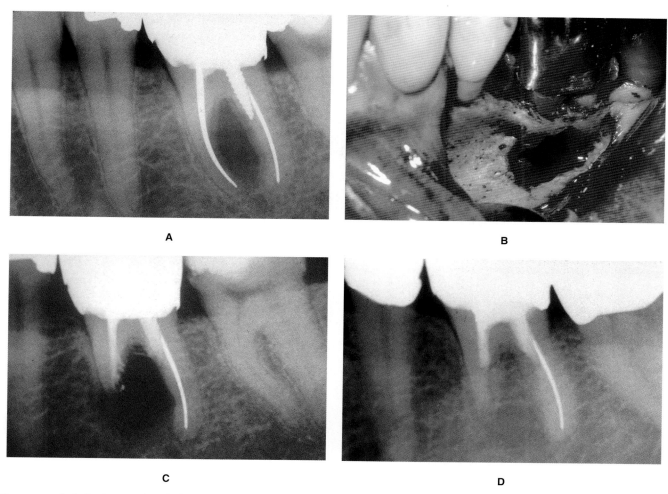

A

B

C

D

Figure 30-7. Endodontic–periodontal advanced procedures. **A,** Radiograph of mandibular first molar. Previous root canal therapy was inadequately performed using silver points. Large screw-type post appears to have perforated mesial surface of distal root. Note apical resorption of distal surface of mesial root and severe osseous destruction. *No significant periodontal probing was obtained.* Complete debridement of root canals and calcium hydroxide therapy was attempted with no success and no reduction of lesion over 6 months. **B,** A full-thickness flap revealed almost complete loss of buccal bone. Remaining crestal bone indicated that success was possible. **C,** Postsurgical radiograph after removal of partially resorbed apical half of mesial root. **D,** View at 12-year recall shows excellent regeneration of surrounding osseous structures. Maintenance and preservation of arch integrity have been obtained. Removal of only a portion of the mesial root was possible because the marginal periodontium was intact and the furcation lesion had no communication with the sulcus. Had such communication been present, treatment options would include complete root resection, hemisection with removal of the mesial half of the tooth, or extraction of the tooth.

a much lower success rate, which is closer to 60%.[55] Therefore early diagnosis and treatment are paramount to success. There have been numerous recent advances in endodontic research, and development of new instruments has improved the quality of endodontic therapy. One of these instruments is the surgical operating microscope. Areas that could not be visualized or were not clinically obtainable are a thing of the past. Procedures and access to areas such as the apex, perforations, and extra canals are routinely achieved using this instrument.

The importance of bacteria in the root canal system cannot be overemphasized. There is no question that bacteria play a role in root canal infection, necrosis, periapical pathosis, and endodontic failure. Infection of the root canal system reduces the success rate for endodontic treatment.[55] Therefore every effort to completely eliminate bacteria from the root canal system must be made. This cannot be obtained in a one visit treatment because it is not possible to eradicate all infection from the root canal without the support of an interappointment antimicrobial dressing.[56] If the root canal system is sterile, a single appointment endodontic procedure is acceptable. When endodontic failure is the diagnosis, re-treatment of the root canal system must be paramount in the development of a treatment plan and prognosis. The microbial flora in canals after failed endodontic therapy differs greatly from the flora of untreated teeth.[57] Therefore every effort should be instituted to re-treat a failing root canal treatment.

Failing root canal treatment occurs because of leakage. This leaking of bacteria into the filled root canal space can occur from the dentinal tubules, lateral canals, an inadequately debrided or sealed root canal, or a failing restoration. If gutta-percha is exposed to the oral environment for 1 week, dye studies have shown leakage throughout the root canal.[58] Restorative dentists and endodontists alike have seen clinical examples of gutta-percha fillings exposed to the oral environment for extended periods. Re-treatment of these teeth is not always necessary. Diagnosis of coronal and periapical ends can help make the decision whether to retreat. The surgical operating microscope can allow visualization of the gutta-percha to detect for staining secondary to leakage. If the root canal filling was performed with silver points, then exposure to the oral environment commits it to re-treatment. This is because of the oxidative potential and corrosion of silver points.

The quality of the coronal restoration adds to the success of endodontics. When 1010 teeth were studied, those with a poor restoration and good endodontics showed a greater percentage of failure.[59] If the root canal treatment and the coronal restoration were each poorly executed, then the greatest rate of failure was seen. Many of the newer bonding technique advocates blame the failure of the restoration on the eugenol used in the root canal sealer. This has not been demonstrated to be true. Studies show that pure eugenol and eugenol-containing cements do not affect the bond strength and shearing strength of composite to enamel or dentin.[60,61]

Although endodontics is predictable, scientific and clinical development of implants has allowed the clinician to offer an alternative in those severely compromised periodontal situations. The prognosis of the endodontic–periodontal lesion worsens as the periodontal component increases. Consequently, to preserve the alveolar bone, those procedures that were once performed years ago might not be currently used. There are some patients that require a treatment plan designed to maintain their natural dentition. Their expectations are to keep their natural teeth as long as possible. These values may have been learned from parents or developed from personal desires. The emotional need to maintain the natural dentition should not be underestimated. For these patients, advanced endodontic and periodontal procedures may be indicated to retain a strategic tooth, even if the prognosis

is less than favorable. However, in many cases, extraction of the involved tooth and placement of a dental implant may a more predictable procedure, and may be the best choice of therapy.[62] (See Chapter 26.)

Endodontics is predictable and if the endodontic–periodontal problem has a good prognosis, all efforts should be directed toward saving the natural dentition. Different problems call for different solutions, which may include surgery, root resection, or intentional replantation. If the natural tooth is saved through diagnosis and treatment, then restorative, periodontal, and endodontic misadventures can be minimized. There are some situations in which a tooth should be saved at any cost. A tooth with a thin scalloped periodontium may not provide the optimum esthetic result if an implant must be placed.[63] Therefore, with this tissue type, every effort should be attempted to save the natural dentition.

The percentage of success is always dependent on the expertise of the clinician. Molar teeth risk progression of periodontal disease more than any other tooth in the mouth. When these teeth are affected, the furcation may break down, creating a treatment dilemma as to whether a root resection will improve the prognosis or have the opposite effect. In some instances, implant therapy may be more predictable.

CONCLUSION

The endodontic–periodontal lesion often presents a diagnostic and treatment dilemma. Once periodontal disease progresses to involve the pulp, careful diagnosis and classification help determine the outcome and subsequent prognosis. Those teeth that appear to have a periodontal problem of endodontic origin have an excellent prognosis. As the periodontal disease progresses and becomes more chronic, the success rates decrease. In some cases, only endodontic therapy or periodontal treatment alone is indicated. In other cases, a combined approach is required. If the prognosis is questionable or poor even with good periodontal and endodontic treatment, extraction of the affected tooth may be indicated. The treatment rendered, and the subsequent success or failure of that treatment, is directly dependent on making an accurate diagnosis of the lesion.

REFERENCES

1. Rossman LE, Rossman SR, Garber DA: The endodontic-periodontic fistula, *Oral Surg* 53:78, 1982.
2. Fuss Z, Bender IB, Rickoff BD: An unusual periodontal abscess, *Oral Surg* 12:116, 1986.
3. Fuss Z, Trowbridge H, Bender IB et al: Assessment of reliability of electric and thermal pulp testing procedures, *J Endod* 12:301, 1986.

4. Augsburger RA, Peters DD: In vitro effects of ice, skin refrigerant, and CO_2 snow on intrapulpal temperature, *J Endod* 7:110, 1981.

5. Cooley RL, Stilley J, Lubow RM: Evaluation of a digital pulp tester, *Oral Surg* 58:437, 1984.

6. Amsterdam M: Periodontal prosthesis: twenty-five years in retrospect, *Alpha Omegan* 67:7, 1974.

7. Bender IB: Factors influencing the radiographic appearance of bony lesions, *J Endod* 8:161, 1982.

8. Bender IB, Seltzer S: The oral fistula-its diagnosis and treatment, *Oral Surg* 14:1367, 1961.

9. Rossman LE, Rossman SR: Endodontic surgery: diagnosis, considerations and technique, *Compend Contin Educ Dent* 2:18, 1981.

10. Rutherford B: Interrelationship of pulpal and periodontal disease. In Hargreaves KM, Goodis HE, editors: *Seltzer and Bender's dental pulp*, Chicago, 2002, Quintessence.

11. Seltzer S, Bender IB, Azimov H, Sinai I: Pulpitis induced interradicular periodontal changes in experimental animals, *J Periodontol* 38:124, 1967.

12. Trowbridge HO: Pathogenesis of pulpitis resulting from dental caries, *J Endod* 7:52, 1981.

13. Turner JH, Drew AH: Experimental injury into bacteriology of pyorrhea, *Proc R Soc Med (Odontol)* 12:104, 1919.

14. Cahn L: Pathology of pulps found in pyorrhetic teeth, *Dent Items Interest* 49:598, 1927.

15. Andreasen JO: Relationship between surface and inflammatory root resorption and changes in the pulp after replantation of permanent incisors in monkeys, *J Endod* 7:294, 1981.

16. Andreasen JO: Cementum repair after apicoectomy in humans, *Acta Odontol Scand* 31:211, 1973.

17. Perlmutter S, Tagger M, Tagger E, Abram M: Effect of the endodontic status of the tooth on experimental periodontal reattachment in baboons: a preliminary investigation, *Oral Surg* 63:232, 1987.

18. Pashley DH: Smear layer: physiological considerations, *Oper Dent* 3:13, 1984.

19. Thrash W, Dodds M, Jones D: The effect of stannous fluoride on dentinal hypersensitvity, *Int Dent J* 44(Suppl 1):107-118, 1994.

20. Orchardson R, Gillam D: The efficacy of potassium salts as agents for treating dentin hypersensitivity, *J Orofacial Pain* 14:9-19, 2000.

21. American Association of Endodontics: *An annotated glossary of terms used in endodontics*, ed 7, Chicago, 2003, The Association.

22. Rubach WC, Mitchell DF: Periodontal disease, accessory canals and pulp pathosis, *J Periodontol* 36:34, 1965.

23. Weine FS: The enigma of the lateral canal, *Dent Clin North Am* 28:833, 1984.

24. Gutmann J: Prevalence, location and patency of accessory canals in the furcation region of permanent molars, *J Periodontol* 49:21-26, 1978.

25. Bender IB, Seltzer S: The effect of periodontal disease on the dental pulp, *Oral Surg* 33:458, 1972.

26. Seltzer S, Bender IB, Ziontz M: The inter-relationship of pulp and periodontal disease, *Oral Surg* 16:1474, 1963.

27. Hattler AB, Listgarten MA: Pulpal response to root planing in a rat model, *J Endod* 10:471, 1984.

28. Rosan B, Rossman L: Endodontic microbiology. In Lamont RJ, Burne RA, Lantz M, LeBlanc DJ, editors: *Oral microbiology and immunology*, Washington, DC, 2004, ASM Press.

29. Zehnder M, Gold SI, Hasselgren G: Pathologic interactions in pulpal and periodontal tissues, *J Clin Periodontol* 29:663, 2002.

30. Nissan R, Makkar SR, Sela MN, Stevens R: Whole genomic DNA probe for detection of *Porphyromonas endodontalis*, *J Endod* 26:217-220, 2000.

31. Oliet S, Pollock S: Classification and treatment of endoperio involved teeth, *Bull Phila Cty Dent Soc* 34:12, 1968.

32. Simon JH, Glick DH, Frank AL: The relationship of endodontic-periodontic lesions, *J Periodontol* 43:202, 1972.

33. Guldener PHA: The relationship between periodontal and pulpal disease, *Int Endod J* 18:41, 1985.

34. Mori K: Diagnosis and treatment of the dental pulp, *Quintessence Int* 6:43, 1987.

35. Whyman RA: Endodontic-periodontic lesions. 1. Prevalence, aetiology, and diagnosis, *NZ Dent J* 84:74, 1988.

36. Whyman RA: Endodontic-periodontic lesions. 2. Management, *N Z Dent J* 84:109, 1988.

37. Paul BF, Hutter JW: The endodontic-periodontal continuum revisted: new insights into etiology, diagnosis and treatment, *J Am Dent Assoc* 128:1541, 1997.

38. Goldman HM, Schilder H: Regeneration of attachment apparatus lost due to disease of endodontic origin, *J Periodontol* 59:609, 1988.

39. Gold SI, Moskow BS: Periodontal repair of periapical lesions: the borderland between pulpal and periodontal disease, *J Clin Periodontol* 14:251, 1987.

40. Evian C, Rosenberg ES, Rossman LE, Lerner SA: The effect of submerging roots with periodontal defects, *Compend Contin Educ Dent* 4:37, 1983.

41. Bender IB, Freedland JB: Adult root fractures, *J Am Dent Assoc* 107:413, 1983.

42. Rivera EM, Williamson A: Diagnosis and treatment planning: cracked tooth, *Tex Dent J* 120:278, 2003.

43. Luebke R: Vertical crown-root fractures in posterior teeth, *Dent Clin North Am* 28:883, 1984.

44. Seltzer S, Sinai I, August D: Periodontal effects of root perforations before and during endodontic procedures, *J Dent Res* 49:332, 1970.

45. Petersson K, Hasselgren G, Tronstad L: Endodontic treatment of experimental root perforations in dog teeth, *Endod Dent Traumatol* 1:22, 1985.

46. Beavers RA, Bergenholtz G, Cox CF: Periodontal wound healing following intentional root perforations in permanent teeth of Macaca mulatta, *Int Endod J* 19:36, 1986.

47. Stromberg T, Hasselgren G, Bergstedt H: Endodontic treatment of traumatic root perforations in man, *Swed Dent J* 65:457, 1972.

48. Abrams L, Trachtenberg DI: Hemisection-technique and restoration, *Dent Clin North Am* 18:415, 1974.

49. Eastman JR, Backmeyer J: A review of the periodontal, endodontic and the prosthetic considerations in odontogenous resection procedures, *Int J Periodontics Restorative Dent* 6:34, 1986.

50. Rossman S, Kaplowitz B, Baldinger SR: Therapy of the endodontically and periodontally involved tooth, *Oral Surg* 13:361, 1960.

51. Skoglund A, Persson G: A follow-up of apicoectomized teeth with total loss of the buccal bone plate, *Oral Surg* 59:78, 1985.

52. Baumann E, Rossman SR: Clinical, roentgenologic and histopathologic findings in teeth with apical radiolucent areas, *Oral Surg* 9:1330, 1956.

53. Frank A, Weine F: Nonsurgical therapy for perforative defect of internal resorption, *J Am Dent Assoc* 87:863, 1973.

54. Andreasen JO: External root resorption: its implications in dental traumatology, paedodontics, periodontics, orthodontics, and endodontics, *Int Endod J* 18:109, 1985.

55. Sjogren U, Hagglund D, Sundqvist G, Wing K: Factors affecting the long-term results of endodontic treatment, *J Endod* 16:498-504, 1990.

56. Sjogren U, Figdor D, Persson S, Sundqvist G: Influence of infection at the time of root filling on the outcome of endodontic treatment of teeth with apical periodontitis, *Int Endod J* 31:297-306, 1997.

57. Sundqvist G, Figdor D, Persson S, Sjogren U: Microbiologic analysis of teeth with failed endodontic treatment and the outcomes of conservative re-treatment, *Oral Surg* 85:86-93, 1998.

58. Madison S, Wilcox L: An evaluation of coronal microleakage in endodontically treated teeth. Part III. In vivo study, *J Endod* 14:455-458, 1988.

59. Ray H, Trope M: Periapical status of endodontically treated teeth in relation to the technical quality of the root filling and the coronal restoration, *Int Endod J* 28:12-18, 1995.

60. Ganss C, Jung M: Effect of eugenol-containing temporary cements on bond strength of composite to dentin, *Oper Dent* 23:55-62, 1998.

61. Jung M, Ganss C, Senger S: Effect of eugenol-containing temporary cements on bond strength of composite to enamel, *Oper Dent* 63:63-68, 1998.

62. Kinsel RP, Lamb RE, Ho D: The treatment dilemma of the furcated molar: root resection versus single-tooth implant restoration. A literature review, *Int J Oral Maxillofac Implants* 13:322-332, 1998.

63. Weisgold A, Arnoux JP, Lu J: Single-tooth anterior implant: a word of caution, part I, *J Esthet Dent* 9:225-233, 1997.

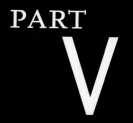

PART

V

PERIODONTAL
MEDICINE

Brian L. Mealey and Louis F. Rose

31 Systemic Factors Impacting the Periodontium

Brian L. Mealey, Terry D. Rees, Louis F. Rose, and Sara G. Grossi

The impact of systemic diseases and conditions on oral health is well recognized. The periodontium is an end-organ similar in many ways to other end-organs such as the skin and the glomerulus of the kidney. In this regard, conditions commonly affecting various end-organs throughout the body may also influence the periodontium. Other systemic disorders may affect the host immunoinflammatory response to oral pathogens, exacerbating certain periodontal conditions. Some systemic diseases increase the risk for gingivitis and periodontitis, or alter their presentation, progression, or severity. This chapter reviews the effects of systemic conditions on the periodontium.

HORMONAL CONSIDERATIONS

A number of hormonal conditions affect the periodontal tissues, including diabetes mellitus and fluctuations in female sex hormones associated with puberty, pregnancy, and menopause. Changes in corticosteroid and thyroid hormone homeostasis may also affect the oral cavity. Hormonal changes may directly alter the periodontal tissues or may change the way the host responds to accumulation of local factors such as plaque and calculus. In addition, the presence of certain hormonal conditions may require alterations in dental treatment.

Diabetes Mellitus

Epidemiology and Classification

Diabetes mellitus is a hormonal disease characterized by changes in carbohydrate, protein, and lipid metabolism.[1] The main feature of diabetes is an increase in blood glucose levels (hyperglycemia), which results from either a defect in insulin secretion from the pancreas, a change in insulin action, or both. A number of hormones affect glycemic homeostasis, but only one decreases blood glucose: insulin (Box 31-1). Insulin is required for transport of glucose from the bloodstream into the cells, where glucose is used for energy (Fig. 31-1). Quantitative decreases in insulin production or qualitative reduction in

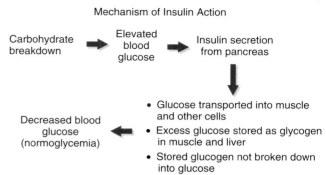

Mechanism of Insulin Action

Figure 31-1. Mechanism of insulin action. Carbohydrate is broken down in the gut after meals into glucose molecules, which are then absorbed into the bloodstream. The increase in blood glucose triggers the pancreas to release insulin. Insulin facilitates the transport of glucose into cells, especially muscle, where it is used for energy. Insulin also allows excess glucose to be stored in muscle and in the liver in the form of glycogen. Finally, insulin prevents the breakdown of stored glycogen into glucose. The net effect of insulin action is to decrease blood glucose levels.

insulin action results in an inability or diminished capacity to transport glucose into cells. Glucose is retained within the bloodstream, causing hyperglycemia. Sustained hyperglycemia affects almost all tissues in the body and is associated with significant complications of multiple organ systems including the eyes, nerves, kidneys, and blood vessels (Box 31-2). The periodontium is also a target for diabetic damage, and periodontal disease has been suggested to be the sixth classic complication of diabetes.[2]

Diabetes is a huge public health problem in the United States and in other regions of the world. Approximately 16 million people in the United States (i.e., 7% of the population) have diabetes.[3] Almost half of these individuals are unaware that they have the disease, and therefore are

---

Box 31-1   Hormones Affecting Blood Glucose

Glucose decreasing hormone:
  • Insulin
Glucose increasing hormones:
  • Glucagon
  • Catecholamines
  • Glucocorticoids
  • Growth hormone
  • Thyroid hormone

Box 31-2   Complications of Diabetes Mellitus

Five "Classic" Complications:
  • Retinopathy
  • Nephropathy
  • Neuropathy
    • Sensory
    • Autonomic
  • Macrovascular disease
    • Cerebrovascular
    • Cardiovascular
    • Peripheral vascular
  • Altered wound healing

Proposed "Sixth" Complication:
  • Periodontal diseases

unable to do what is needed to prevent long-term complications. The prevalence of diabetes increases every year, as do the costs associated with its management and complications. In 1997, the health care costs associated with diabetes were estimated at $98 billion.[4] The high prevalence of diabetes ensures that oral health care providers will frequently treat patients with this disease in their practices.

The most commonly encountered types of diabetes are type 1, type 2, and gestational diabetes, although others exist[5] (Box 31-3). Type 1 diabetes is caused by autoimmune destruction of the beta cells in the pancreatic islets of Langerhans. These cells normally produce insulin, and their autoimmune destruction renders the patient incapable of producing endogenous insulin. Type 1 diabetes most often occurs in children and young adults, hence its previous classification as "juvenile" diabetes. Only about 5% to 10% of all patients with diabetes have type 1. Because these patients lack the ability to produce insulin, they must inject exogenous insulin to maintain normal blood glucose levels. Poor glucose control may result in sustained hyperglycemia. During these conditions, patients with type 1 diabetes are highly prone to development of diabetic ketoacidosis, or DKA. In the absence of adequate insulin levels, glucose in the bloodstream cannot be transported into cells properly, leading to cellular starvation. This results in the breakdown of body fat through lipolysis, releasing large quantities of free fatty acids that accumulate in the bloodstream and are converted to ketones. Increased blood ketone levels result in their excretion, along with large volumes of water, causing dehydration. Accumulation of ketones in body fluids, dehydration and loss of electrolytes in urine, and changes in the bicarbonate buffering system lead to diabetic ketoacidosis. This life-threatening condition may result in coma or death if not treated immediately. Patients with type 1 diabetes are absolutely dependent on injection of exogenous insulin for survival; this is why type 1 was once called "insulin-dependent" diabetes. Patients with type 1 diabetes often demonstrate the classic symptoms associated with undiagnosed or poorly controlled diabetes: polydipsia (excessive thirst), polyuria (frequent urination), and polyphagia (excessive feeling of hunger).

In contrast to type 1, type 2 diabetes usually occurs in adults, and was once called "adult-onset diabetes." Because type 2 constitutes about 90% of all diabetic cases, it is the form most commonly encountered in the dental office.[5] Type 1 is more common in white individuals, and type 2 occurs more frequently in Hispanic, American Indian, African American, and Pacific islander populations. Unlike type 1, which has a sudden onset, type 2 diabetes may remain undiagnosed for years. In fact, dental health care providers may be the first to recognize signs and symptoms of undiagnosed type 2 diabetes. Until the past decade, type 2 was rarely seen in children. Unfortunately, the incidence of type 2 in children and teenagers has increased dramatically.[3] Type 2 diabetes is closely associated with obesity.[6,7] As the prevalence of obesity among young individuals in the United States has increased, so has the incidence of type 2 diabetes. Unlike type 1, where patients no longer produce insulin, patients with type 2 diabetes retain an ability to make insulin, although insulin production decreases as the duration of diabetes increases. Type 2 is characterized by increased glucose production in the liver, peripheral resistance to insulin, especially in muscle, and impaired insulin secretion. These changes lead to sustained hyperglycemia, with its accompanying complications. Diabetic ketoacidosis, a common threat in type 1 diabetes, is uncommon in patients with type 2 diabetes because their endogenous insulin production is sufficient to suppress ketone formation.

The mainstays of type 2 diabetes management are weight loss and exercise, both of which improve insulin sensitivity (decrease insulin resistance) in peripheral tissues.[1] Medications are often used to improve carbohydrate metabolism, increase pancreatic insulin production, or decrease insulin resistance (see Chapter 37). Although patients with type 2 diabetes are not dependent on insulin injection for survival, they may inject exogenous insulin, especially if pancreatic insulin production has decreased significantly. Use of insulin injections alone does not

---

Box 31-3   Diagnosis and Classification of Diabetes Mellitus

Type 1 diabetes (formerly insulin-dependent diabetes)
Type 2 diabetes (formerly noninsulin-dependent diabetes)
Gestational diabetes
Other types of diabetes
  • Genetic defects in pancreatic β cell function
  • Genetic defects in insulin action
  • Pancreatic diseases or injuries
    • Pancreatitis, neoplasia, cystic fibrosis, trauma, pancreatectomy
  • Infections
    • Cytomegalovirus, congenital rubella
  • Drug-induced or chemical-induced diabetes
    • Glucocorticoids, thyroid hormone
  • Endocrinopathies
    • Glucagonoma, pheochromocytoma, hyperthyroidism, Cushing syndrome, acromegaly
  • Other genetic syndromes with associated diabetes

From the American Diabetes Association: Report of the expert committee on the diagnosis and classification of diabetes mellitus, Diabetes Care 24(suppl 1):s5-s20, 2001.

mean that a patient has type 1 diabetes. Patients with type 1 diabetes always take insulin because their survival is dependent on it. Conversely, patients with type 2 diabetes may take insulin to improve their glycemic state, especially when other medications have not been completely effective. Because type 2 diabetes is also closely associated with hypertension and hyperlipidemia, these patients are often taking multiple medications, many of which may affect the way dental treatment is provided.

Gestational diabetes occurs in approximately 7% of pregnancies in the United States, resulting in more than 200,000 cases annually.[8] It usually develops during the third trimester and significantly increases the risk for perinatal morbidity and mortality. Proper diagnosis and management of gestational diabetes improves pregnancy outcomes.[9] Like type 2 diabetes, the pathophysiology of gestational diabetes is associated with increased insulin resistance. Most patients with gestational diabetes return to a normoglycemic state after parturition; however, type 2 diabetes will develop within 10 years in about 30% to 50% of women with a history of gestational diabetes.

The conditions known as impaired glucose tolerance (IGT) and impaired fasting glucose (IFG) represent metabolic states lying between diabetes and normoglycemia.[5] People with IFG have increased fasting blood glucose levels, but glucose levels are usually normal after food consumption. Those with IGT are normoglycemic most of the time, but can become hyperglycemic after large glucose loads. IGT and IFG are not considered to be clinical entities; rather, they are risk factors for future diabetes. The pathophysiology of IFG and IGT is related primarily to increased insulin resistance; endogenous insulin secretion from the pancreas is normal in most patients. Type 2 diabetes will develop in approximately 30% to 40% of individuals with IGT or IFG within 10 years after onset.

Systemic Complications of Diabetes

The major cause of the high morbidity and mortality rates associated with diabetes is a group of microvascular and macrovascular complications affecting multiple organ systems (Box 31-2). People with diabetes have a greatly increased risk for blindness, kidney failure, myocardial infarction, stroke, limb amputation, and a host of other maladies. Sustained hyperglycemia is strongly associated with the onset and progression of these complications.[1] The incidence and severity of complications increase as the duration of diabetes increases. In addition to genetic predisposing factors, other disorders commonly seen in people with diabetes, such as hypertension and dyslipidemia, increase the risk for microvascular and macrovascular complications. In large blood vessels, diabetes is associated with an increase in lipid deposition, thickness

of arterial walls, and atheroma formation. Microvascular damage results from proliferation of endothelial cells, alterations in endothelial basement membranes, and changes in endothelial cell function.

The pathophysiology of diabetic complications is highly complex. Hyperglycemia plays a major role in both microvascular and macrovascular disease. Hyperglycemia dramatically alters the function of multiple cell types and their extracellular matrices, resulting in structural and functional changes in affected tissues. Research has focused on lipoprotein metabolism and on glycation of proteins, lipids, and nucleic acids as possible common links between the various diabetic complications.[10-12]

The function of cell membranes is determined in large part by their phospholipid bilayer; thus changes in lipid metabolism can have major effects on cell function. Oxidation of circulating low-density lipoprotein in individuals with hyperglycemia increases oxidant stress within the vasculature.[11] This induces chemotaxis of monocytes and macrophages into the vessel walls, where oxidized low-density lipoprotein causes changes in cellular adhesion and increased production of cytokines and growth factors. Stimulation of smooth muscle cell proliferation increases vessel wall thickness. Other changes include increased atheroma formation and development of microthrombi in large blood vessels, and alterations in vascular permeability and endothelial cell function in small vessels.

Hyperglycemia also results in the glycation of proteins, lipids, and nucleic acids. Deposits of glycated proteins called advanced glycation end-products (AGEs) accumulate in the walls of large vessels and in the microvasculature of the retina, renal glomerulus, and endoneurial areas.[12] Although all people form AGEs, their accumulation is much greater in individuals with diabetes, especially when the diabetic state is poorly controlled. AGE formation alters the structural and functional properties of the affected tissues. For example, AGE formation on collagen macromolecules impairs their normal homeostatic turnover. In the walls of the large blood vessels, AGE-modified collagen accumulates, thickening the vessel wall and narrowing the lumen. AGE-modified arterial collagen immobilizes circulating low-density lipoprotein, contributing to atheroma formation. AGE accumulation causes increased basement membrane thickness in the microvasculature of the retina and around the nerves, and increased thickness of the mesangial matrix in the glomerulus. The cumulative effect of these changes is progressive narrowing of the vessel lumen and decreased perfusion of affected tissues.

AGE formation also has major effects at the cellular level, causing modifications in extracellular matrix components and changes in cell-to-matrix and matrix-to-matrix interactions.[10,13] Binding of AGEs to specific cellular receptors on the surface of smooth muscle cells, endothelial cells, neurons, monocytes, and macrophages results in increased vascular permeability and thrombus formation, proliferation of smooth muscle in vessel walls, and phenotypic alteration in monocytes and macrophages. The latter effect causes hyperresponsiveness of monocytes and macrophages on stimulation, with resultant increases in production of proinflammatory cytokines and certain growth factors. These cytokines and growth factors contribute to the chronic inflammatory process in the formation of atherosclerotic lesions. They also significantly alter wound healing events. Increased production of proinflammatory mediators results in increased tissue destruction in response to antigens such as the bacteria that cause periodontal disease.

These changes in protein and lipid metabolism, induced by the increased plasma glucose levels characteristic of diabetes, may thus provide a common connection between the various diabetic complications, including those in the periodontium.[14]

Oral Manifestations of Diabetes

Oral conditions often associated with diabetes include burning mouth, altered wound healing, and increased incidence of infection.[1] Enlargement of the parotid glands and xerostomia can occur. The frequency or severity of these conditions may be related to the overall level of glycemic control. People with diabetes often take medications not only for diabetes, but for other related or unrelated systemic conditions. These medications may have significant xerostomic effects; therefore the xerostomia seen in patients with diabetes may result more from medications than from diabetes itself.

One of the classic complications of diabetes is neuropathy. Although this disorder usually affects the sensory nervous system, neuropathy of the autonomic system may cause changes in salivary secretion, because salivary flow is controlled by the sympathetic and parasympathetic pathways.[15] Dry mucosal surfaces are easily irritated, and they are associated with burning mouth syndrome. They also provide a favorable ecologic niche for growth of fungal organisms. Some studies have shown an increased incidence of oral candidiasis in patients with diabetes, whereas other studies have not.[16,17]

The effect of diabetes on dental caries is unclear. Some studies indicate increased caries in diabetes, which has been associated with xerostomia or increased gingival crevicular fluid glucose levels.[18] Increased caries rates may be associated with poor glycemic control. Other studies have shown similar or decreased caries rates in patients with diabetes compared with individuals without diabetes.[19] Because most people with diabetes limit their intake of fermentable carbohydrates, their less cariogenic diet may serve to decrease caries incidence. In some studies of subjects with and without diabetes, no differences were seen in salivary flow rates, organic constituents of saliva, salivary counts of acidogenic bacteria (*Streptococcus mutans* and lactobacilli), or salivary counts of fungal organisms.[15,20] Furthermore, coronal and root caries rates were the same for diabetic and nondiabetic study groups. These findings suggest that patients with diabetes as a group are similar to individuals without diabetes with regard to these oral conditions.

Evidence suggests that diabetes is a risk factor for increased prevalence and severity of gingivitis.[21-23] Diabetes is associated with increased gingival inflammation in response to bacterial plaque, but the degree of glycemic control is an important variable in this relationship. In general, patients with well controlled diabetes have a similar degree of gingivitis as individuals without diabetes who have the same level of plaque. Conversely, patients with poorly controlled diabetes have significantly increased gingival redness, swelling, or bleeding compared with both individuals without diabetes and patients with well controlled diabetes.[24,25]

The risk for periodontitis is also increased when diabetes is present.[21,23] In 21 studies of children, adolescents, or adults with type 1 diabetes since 1968, 20 studies found a greater prevalence, extent, or severity of periodontal disease parameters in patients with diabetes compared with nondiabetic control subjects.[23] In large epidemiologic studies, type 2 diabetes increased the risk for attachment loss and alveolar bone loss by approximately threefold compared with nondiabetic control subjects.[26,27] Diabetes increases not only the prevalence and severity of periodontitis, but also the progression of bone loss and attachment loss over time. In fact, subjects with type 2 diabetes were shown to have a fourfold increased risk for progressive destruction compared with individuals without diabetes.[28]

Periodontitis is similar to the classic complications of diabetes in its variation among individuals. Just as retinopathy, nephropathy, and neuropathy are more likely to be seen in patients with poorly controlled diabetes, progressive destructive periodontitis is more common in those with poor control. However, significant periodontal destruction does not develop in some patients with poorly controlled diabetes, just as the classic diabetic complications do not develop in some patients. Conversely, good metabolic control of diabetes decreases the risk for periodontal disease, to a level similar to that for individuals without diabetes. Yet, patients with well controlled diabetes may still experience periodontitis, just as individuals without diabetes may. Other risk factors for periodontitis such as poor oral hygiene and smoking play similar deleterious roles in individuals with or without diabetes. Clearly, the presence of diabetes increases the risk for periodontal disease; furthermore, as glycemic control worsens, the adverse effects of diabetes on the periodontium increase. That a patient has diabetes should increase the dental professional's index of suspicion, and should prompt him or her to carefully examine the patient's periodontium for signs of destructive disease.

Likewise, a degree of periodontal destruction that is not commensurate with the level of local factors is often a clue to the presence of underlying systemic diseases such as diabetes (Figs. 31-2 and 31-3). Patients with poorly controlled or previously undiagnosed diabetes may have multiple periodontal abscesses, exophytic tissue extending

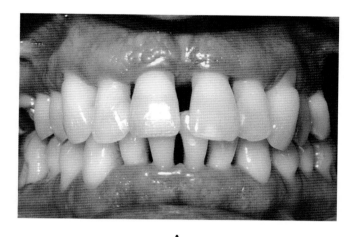

A

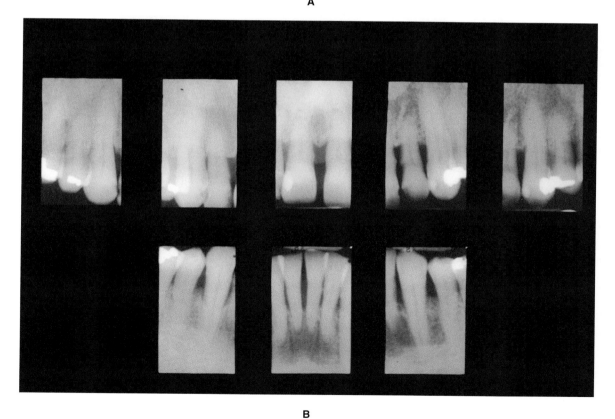

B

Figure 31-2. **A,** Clinical view of maxillary/mandibular anterior region in a 46-year-old man. The patient has minimal local factors, slight plaque accumulation, relatively healthy gingival tissues, and generalized recession. **B,** Radiographs of maxillary/mandibular anterior region in the same patient. Clinical examination revealed severe bone and attachment loss. The patient had undiagnosed type 2 diabetes mellitus.

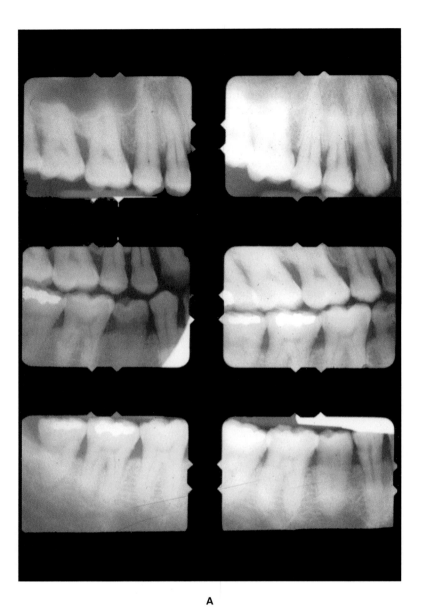

A

Figure 31-3. A, Radiographs of right posterior sextants in a 45-year-old Hispanic man with generalized slight chronic periodontitis and generalized calculus visible on radiographs. The patient received scaling and root planing, but did not return for reevaluation.

Continued

from the periodontal pocket, mobile or displaced teeth, and severe bone loss (Fig. 31-4).

Pathogenic Mechanisms: Diabetes and Periodontal Diseases

The mechanisms by which diabetes influences the periodontium are similar in many respects to the pathophysiology of the classic diabetic complications. Early research focused on potential differences in the subgingival bacterial flora in people with diabetes as a likely explanation for increased periodontal destruction. However, the preponderance of research shows few differences in the subgingival microbiota between patients with periodontitis who have or do not have diabetes.[29,30] This lack of significant differences in the primary bacteriologic agents of periodontal disease suggests that differences in host response may play a primary role in the increased prevalence and severity of periodontal destruction seen in patients with diabetes.

Because gingival crevicular fluid is a serum transudate or exudate, hyperglycemia results in increased gingival crevicular fluid glucose levels.[31] Increased gingival

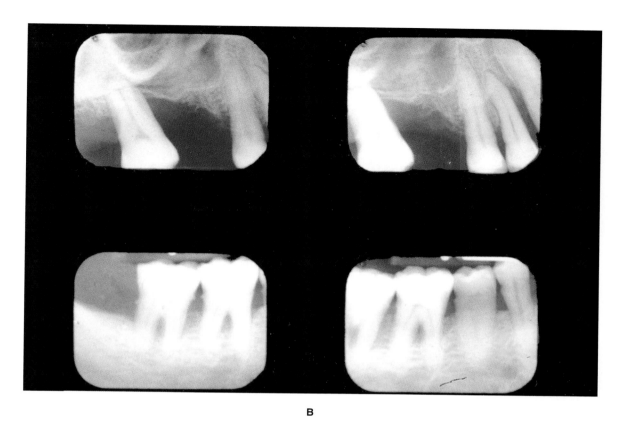

B

Figure 31-3. cont'd B, Same patient as in **A** 5 years later, demonstrating severe bone loss in both maxillary and mandibular sextants. Teeth #1 and #3 had been extracted. The patient had undiagnosed type 2 diabetes mellitus.

crevicular fluid glucose may significantly alter periodontal wound healing events by changing the interaction between cells and their extracellular matrix within the periodontium.[32]

Vascular changes seen in the retina, glomerulus, and perineural areas also occur in the periodontium.[33,34] Formation of AGEs results in collagen accumulation in the periodontal capillary basement membranes, causing membrane thickening.[35] AGE-stimulated smooth muscle proliferation increases the thickness of vessel walls. These changes decrease periodontal tissue perfusion and oxygenation. AGE-modified collagen in gingival blood vessel walls binds circulating low-density lipoprotein, which is frequently increased in diabetes, resulting in atheroma formation and further narrowing of the vessel lumen.[11] These changes in the periodontium may alter the tissue response to periodontal pathogens, resulting in increased tissue destruction and diminished repair potential.

Diabetes has dramatic effects on the function of host defense cells, such as polymorphonuclear leukocytes, monocytes, and macrophages.[11] An intact host immunoinflammatory response is critical to establishment and maintenance of periodontal health. In diabetes,

polymorphonuclear leukocyte adherence, chemotaxis, and phagocytosis are impaired. Defects in this first line of defense against periodontopathic microorganisms may decrease bacterial killing, allowing proliferation of pathogenic bacteria and increased periodontal destruction. Another major cell line necessary for effective periodontal defense mechanisms is the monocytes/macrophage line. In individuals with diabetes these cells may be hyperresponsive to bacterial antigens.[36] This up-regulation results in significantly increased production of proinflammatory cytokines and mediators, and it is likely related to the interaction between AGEs in the periodontium and cellular receptors on the surface of monocytes and macrophages. In response to endotoxin from *Porphyromonas gingivalis*, monocytes from patients with diabetes produce up to 32 times greater levels of the inflammatory mediator tumor necrosis factor-α compared with monocytes from individuals without diabetes.[37] The proinflammatory mediators IL-1β and prostaglandin E_2 are also increased in patients with diabetes.[38] Thus the patient with diabetes may have a decreased ability for polymorphonuclear leukocytes to kill periodontal pathogens, resulting in their proliferation, combined with an exuberant proinflammatory and destructive

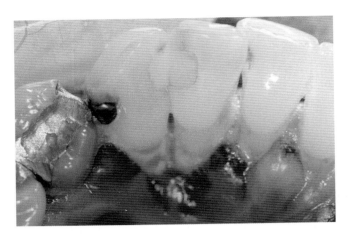

A

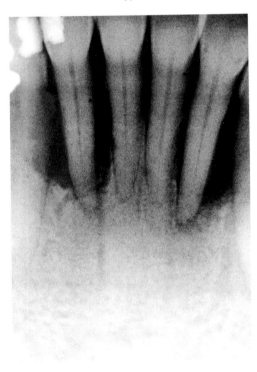

B

Figure 31-4. A, Clinical view of lingual mandibular anterior region in a 65-year-old African American woman with poorly controlled type 2 diabetes (HbA1c = 13.7%). She had four periodontal abscesses. Teeth #21 to #24 show enlarged, hemorrhagic gingival tissues with probing depths of 8 to 10 mm. **B,** Radiograph of mandibular anterior teeth reveals severe bone loss. Radiograph from 5 years previously showed no significant bone loss in this area.

monocyte/macrophage response that produces severe local damage to periodontal tissues. The net clinical effect of these host defense alterations is an increase in periodontal inflammation, attachment loss, and bone loss.

Collagen is the primary structural protein in the periodontium. Changes in collagen metabolism in patients with diabetes contribute to wound healing alterations and periodontal destruction. Production of matrix metalloproteinases, such as collagenase, increases in many patients with diabetes.[39] Increased collagenase production readily degrades the newly formed collagen that is critical to healing of the periodontium. At the same time, AGE modification of existing collagen decreases its solubility. The net results of these changes in collagen metabolism are a combination of rapid dissolution of recently synthesized collagen by host collagenase and accumulation of older, AGE-modified collagen. Thus diabetes induces a shift in the normal homeostatic mechanism by which collagen is formed, stabilized, and eventually turned over, a shift that alters wound healing responses to physical or microbial wounding of the periodontium.

Tetracycline antibiotics and chemically modified tetracycline agents reduce host collagenase production and collagen degradation through mechanisms that are independent of their antimicrobial activity.[40] These drugs may have benefits in managing conditions such as periodontitis, arthritis, diabetes, osteoporosis, and others in which collagen metabolism is altered. (The periodontal management of patients with diabetes is discussed in Chapter 37.)

Female Sex Hormones

Sex steroid hormones (androgens, estrogens, and progestin) have modulatory effects on all periodontal tissues. However, female sex hormones exert the most clinically recognizable effects on periodontal tissues. The levels of female sex hormones and balance between them have been implicated as a modifying factor in the pathogenesis of periodontal disease. A relation has been observed between altered levels of sex hormones and variations in the degree of gingival inflammation. Women comprise at least half of the patients seen by the general dentist and even a larger percentage of those who are treated by the periodontist. Therefore clinicians should be aware and able to recognize the characteristic female sex hormone–associated changes in oral tissues. The effects of female sex hormones in periodontal tissues are examined here in different stages of the female life cycle—that is, puberty, menstruation cycle and oral contraceptive use, pregnancy, and menopause.

Notably, the gingival changes associated with increased female sex hormone levels may appear similar to one another—that is, puberty gingivitis may appear similar to pregnancy gingivitis or gingival inflammation associated with oral contraceptives. The difference tends to be one of degree. These conditions associated with increased sex hormone levels differ from those associated with the diminished level of hormones seen in menopause.

Puberty

Secretion of gonadotropin (follicle-stimulating and leuteinizing) hormones by the anterior pituitary gland stimulates the ovaries to begin the cyclical production and secretion of female sex hormones (estrogen and progesterone). With the onset of estrogen production, development of sexual characteristics and maturation of reproductive organs takes place. Progesterone works synergistically with estrogen, contributing to maturation of breast tissue and the cyclical changes in the cervix and vagina. Female sex hormones also have effects on a number of other organ systems, including the oral cavity. A large body of evidence including in vitro and human studies suggests the periodontium is a target tissue for female sex hormones. Receptors for both estrogen and progesterone have been demonstrated in human gingiva,[41,42] gingival fibroblasts,[43] and periodontal ligament fibroblasts.[44] In addition, inflammatory cytokines may alter the expression of steroid hormones, modulating the metabolism of circulating steroids and their effects on target tissues.[45,46] Thus the effect of female sex hormones on periodontal tissues may be magnified by the inflammatory response to bacteria in dental plaque, resulting in greater hormone-related changes in all periodontal tissues. Classical clinical examples of this interaction are seen in puberty and pregnancy gingivitis.

Gingivitis is virtually nonexistent in young children. With the onset of puberty there is a dramatic increase in the incidence and severity of gingivitis.[47] Steroid hormones increase the permeability of blood vessels, thereby contributing to inflammation. In addition, dramatic changes in subgingival microbiota during puberty are also responsible for the sudden increase in gingivitis during this period. Longitudinal studies have examined the transformation of subgingival flora from prepuberty to puberty and have demonstrated a significant increase in the frequency of *Eikenella corrodens*, *Prevotella intermedia*, *Bacteriodes melaninogenicus*, *Prevotella nigrescens*, and other species commonly associated with gingivitis and gingival bleeding.[48-50] It has been suggested that hormonal changes during puberty support growth of this emerging microbiota. Subgingival microorganisms appear to react to increased availability of hormones in oral fluids, especially crevicular fluid. Estradiol and progesterone may be used by certain bacterial species, such as *Bacteroides*, as a substitute for menadione (vitamin K), an important growth factor for black-pigmented *Bacteroides*.[51] Thus it appears that the increase in circulating sex hormones during puberty has a modulatory effect in subgingival flora, favoring gram-negative anaerobic organisms associated with gingival inflammation. This transformation in subgingival flora mimics the transformation in vaginal bacterial flora from a facultative to a strict anaerobic gram-negative flora seen during puberty.

Gingival tissues respond to the increased levels of circulating hormones and the related shift in subgingival flora with a greater degree of inflammation and gingival bleeding.[47,50] The classical clinical presentation for puberty gingivitis is increased gingivitis and tendency for gingival bleeding in the presence of small amounts of plaque (Fig. 31-5, *A*). If plaque control is poor, these changes can be dramatic, resulting in spontaneous bleeding and severe inflammation (Fig. 31-5, *B*). The effects on gingival tissue from increased hormone levels during puberty are transient, suggesting that as sexual development progresses and hormonal levels stabilize so does the response of periodontal tissues to bacterial plaque.[52]

Menstrual Cycle and Oral Contraceptives

The cyclical pattern of hormonal fluctuation associated with the menstrual cycle has been associated with changes in gingiva and oral mucosa, such as increased gingival bleeding and presentation of aphthous ulcers. Despite a number of reports and multiple clinical observations of this association, dramatic inflammatory changes in gingival tissue associated with the menstrual cycle are rather infrequent. Most women experience virtually no variations in gingival status as a result of menstruation. On the contrary, gingival changes associated with the menstrual cycle include more subtle changes, such as an increase in gingival crevicular fluid that often occurs during ovulation.[53] Female patients with irregular menstrual cycles may experience increased severity of gingivitis and tendency for gingival bleeding. The degree of gingival inflammation associated with hormonal imbalances appears incommensurate with the amount of dental plaque, although local plaque retentive factors may play a role. The clinical manifestations of gingivitis associated with hormonal imbalance generally present as bright red marginal gingivitis with excessive tendency in gingival bleeding.

Oral contraceptives include the use of gestational hormones at a concentration to mimic pregnancy to prevent ovulation. Early studies report increased gingival inflammation associated with use of oral contraceptives.[54,55] The dose of steroids in these early contraceptive formulations was quite high. A recent experimental gingivitis study in women using oral contraceptives did not demonstrate an effect of oral contraceptive in plaque accumulation, gingival inflammation, or gingival fluid volume.[56] The substantially lower concentration of hormones in the most current formulations of oral contraceptives was proposed as a cause for the lack of effect on gingival tissues. However, the clinician will encounter women with marginal gingival inflammation that does not respond to debridement and home care (Fig. 31-5, *A*). In these cases, the clinician should question the patient about the use of oral contraceptives.

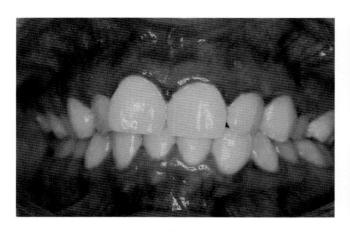

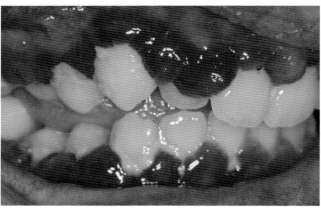

A

B

Figure 31-5. A, Typical appearance of puberty gingivitis. Marginal and papillary gingival inflammation noted in presence of minimal plaque (most visible in #8 to #10 and #22 to #23 regions). This same clinical presentation may occur in women taking oral contraceptives. In these women, gingival inflammation is often persistent even after scaling and polishing and tends to subside only with cessation of the oral contraceptive agent. A similar mild appearance also may be noted in pregnant women or in women with menstruation-associated gingivitis. **B,** More severe case of puberty gingivitis. The patient is a 13-year-old girl with poor oral hygiene and large accumulations of plaque and calculus. A similar severe presentation may be seen in pregnancy, but would rarely be associated with oral contraceptive use or menstruation.

Pregnancy

The landmark study by Löe and Silness in 1963[57] describes one of the most widely used clinical indexes in dental research, the gingival index, and describes for the first time the condition defined as "pregnancy gingivitis." Elegant in its simplicity, this study shows that gingivitis increases progressively during pregnancy, independent of dental plaque accumulation, and returns to normal levels postpartum. This suggests that the gingival inflammatory response during pregnancy follows the hormonal cycle, increasing with increasing gonadotropin levels, maintaining high levels from 4 to 9 months as estrogen and progesterone levels continue to increase, and returning to prepregnancy levels as hormone secretion suddenly decreases at the end of pregnancy. Several cross-sectional and longitudinal studies report a prevalence rate for pregnancy gingivitis ranging from 30% to 70%.[57-59] Consistent findings from all these studies indicate that the prevalence and severity of gingivitis is increased during pregnancy compared with after pregnancy, even though plaque scores are not increased, suggesting that the gingival inflammatory response to bacterial plaque is accentuated during pregnancy as a result of increased hormone levels. Notwithstanding the severity of gingivitis during pregnancy, in the absence of pocketing and attachment loss the condition is self-limiting and reversible when hormonal balance is achieved (Fig. 31-6). However, bleeding on probing and gingival crevicular fluid are increased during pregnancy. Therefore thorough

periodontal treatment and monitoring is absolutely important for all female patients during pregnancy, especially if they exhibit pregnancy gingivitis. Recent reports of periodontal disease being an important risk factor for preterm labor and low birth weight underscore the importance and relevance of oral and periodontal care as an essential component of prenatal care.[60] (See Chapter 32.)

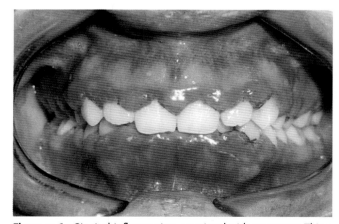

Figure 31-6. Gingival inflammation associated with pregnancy. This a relatively severe case of pregnancy gingivitis, with generalized gingival enlargement, edema, and spontaneous bleeding. Most women with pregnancy gingivitis have more subtle changes. Pregnancy also may result in formation of pyogenic granulomas (see Chapter 35).

The underlying mechanisms for the enhanced inflammatory response during pregnancy are varied. Increased progesterone levels increase membrane permeability, contributing to vascular permeability and edema of the gingival tissues.[61] The severity of gingival inflammation correlates with the levels of estrogen and progesterone during pregnancy. In addition, a shift in subgingival flora from aerobic to strict anaerobic, with a 55-fold increase in proportions of *P. intermedia*, has been reported during pregnancy.[62,63] A significant increase in the proportion of *P. intermedia* was observed during the fourth month of pregnancy, correlating with increasing levels of estradiol and progesterone in saliva.[64] Gingival inflammation and bleeding on probing increased concomitantly. Levels of hormones in saliva peaked at the ninth month of pregnancy. Thereafter, the proportion of *P. intermedia* decreased. *P. intermedia* and other *Bacteroides* species are able to substitute progesterone and estrogen for vitamin K, an essential growth factor.[51] Increased progesterone levels, therefore, may play a major role in the microbial shift seen during pregnancy. Thus the increased levels of hormones in the gingiva combined with the microbial shift favoring an anaerobic flora dominated by *P. intermedia* are partly responsible for the exaggerated response to bacterial plaque in pregnancy.

Immunoreactivity to periodontal disease–related microorganisms is also altered during pregnancy.[65] An association has been reported between gingival response to dental plaque in pregnancy and components of the fibrinolytic system in gingival crevicular fluid. Plasminogen activator activates the fibrinolytic system, enabling connective tissue breakdown and spread of inflammation. Plasminogen activator inhibitor (PAI) attenuates this response. Lower plasminogen activator inhibitor (PAI-2) response in women with greater gingival inflammatory reactions during pregnancy has been reported, providing additional mechanisms to explain the basis of pregnancy gingivitis.[66]

Menopause/Osteoporosis

Menopause is defined by the complete cessation of menstrual flow (amenorrhea) for 1 year as a result of cessation in ovarian secretion of estrogen and progesterone. It usually begins when women reach their forties, with a mean age of 50 years, unless accelerated by hysterectomy or ovariectomy, and the average woman can expect to live one third of her life after her last menstrual period. At this stage, there is a dramatic decrease in circulating female sex hormones as ovarian function begins to fail. Progressive decrease in estrogen may lead to neuroendocrinal changes, urogenital atrophy, skin and hair changes, osteoporosis, and increased risk for cardiovascular disease. Menopause is also associated with adverse changes in oral and periodontal tissues.

Postmenopausal women have decreased unstimulated saliva flow, which has been associated with increased dental caries and alterations in taste.[67] Postmenopausal women may also experience a distinct change in gingival condition, almost of an atrophic nature, characterized by pale, shiny gingiva with absence of stippling (Fig. 31-7). Gingival recession and a general thinning of gingiva and oral mucosa are also frequent in postmenopausal women. These atrophic changes are likely related to the estrogen-deficient state associated with menopause. Management of these friable tissues may present a challenge during periodontal treatment, especially during surgical procedures and implant placement.

Osteoporosis and increased risk for fractures is likely the most prevalent condition associated with the estrogen deficiency seen during menopause. This is demonstrated by evidence that women treated with supplemental estrogen experience less osteopenia and osteoporosis and a decreased risk for fractures. Whether the incidence and rate of progression of periodontal disease also increases after menopause has not been definitively established. However, several pieces of evidence suggest that this is the case. In other words, in a manner similar to systemic osteopenia and osteoporosis, estrogen deficiency increases the risk for mandibular bone loss and periodontal disease. Several studies have examined directly the relation between estrogen status/deficiency and periodontal disease. Less attachment loss and less gingival bleeding have been reported in postmenopausal women receiving estrogen replacement therapy (ERT) compared with estrogen-deficient postmenopausal women.[68] A longitudinal study of women with surgical or natural menopause receiving ERT compared lumbar spine bone mineral density with mandibular bone mass and observed a significant correlation between mandibular and lumbar spine bone mass.[69] ERT after surgical or natural menopause had a positive effect on bone mass not only of the lumbar spine but the

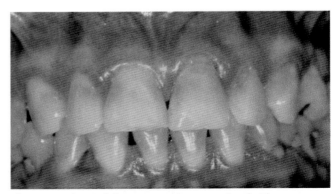

Figure 31-7. Gingival changes sometimes associated with menopause. Note the marginal tissue recession, thinning, and pallor of the gingival tissues.

mandible as well. In a longitudinal study, postmenopausal women who were not taking ERT had an overall decrease in alveolar bone density, whereas women taking ERT had a net gain in bone density.[70] These results suggest that estrogen deficiency plays an important role in oral bone loss and may be an important factor in modifying the severity of periodontal disease in postmenopausal women.

Several studies have examined the relation between osteopenia, osteoporosis, and periodontal disease. Kribbs and colleagues[71] found that mandibular bone density correlated with radial and vertebral bone mass in postmenopausal women. Cortical thickness at the gonion was correlated with the number of remaining teeth. In addition, subjects with greater mandibular bone mass retained more teeth with deeper pockets. In a subsequent study, the same authors found that osteoporotic postmenopausal patients had less mandibular bone mass and density, thinner cortex at the gonion, and fewer teeth than a nonosteoporotic group of comparable age.[72] However, there were no differences between osteoporotic and nonosteoporotic groups regarding periodontal attachment loss. This study concluded that osteoporosis had an adverse effect on mandibular bone mass and density.

Wactawkski-Wende and colleagues[73] report a significant relation between alveolar crestal height and skeletal osteopenia (femur and lumbar spine) in postmenopausal women controlling for dental plaque, years of menopause, and smoking. In addition, there was a relation between femoral osteopenia and probing attachment loss in this same group. Similarly, von Wowern and associates[74] report significantly greater periodontal attachment loss in women with osteoporosis compared with healthy women. They found that women with osteoporosis had less mandibular bone mineral content compared with the healthy women. These studies collectively support an association between osteopenia, osteoporosis, and periodontal disease, which may be explained in part by estrogen deficiency.[75]

An association also exists between estrogen status and tooth loss. In several longitudinal studies, the use of ERT has been associated with a decreased risk for tooth loss.[76-78] In some of these studies, the risk for tooth loss decreased with increasing duration of ERT treatment, suggesting that long-term estrogen replacement therapy confers protection against tooth loss and reduces the risk for edentulism.

Adrenal Insufficiency/Corticosteroids

The clinical syndrome of glucocorticoid deficiency in humans is caused by inadequate production of a single hormone: cortisol. When this results from disorders involving destruction of the adrenal glands, such as granulomatous diseases, the disorder is termed primary adrenal failure, hypoadrenocorticism, or Addison's disease.

If, however, the deficiency is caused by failure of adrenocorticotrophic hormone (ACTH) to stimulate cortisol production, the resulting syndrome is termed secondary adrenal failure. Two important distinctions between primary and secondary adrenal failure are noteworthy:

1. Addison's disease, because it is caused by actual destruction of the adrenal gland, is commonly associated with loss of adrenal steroids other than cortisol. In particular, aldosterone production is reduced or absent; by contrast, secondary adrenal failure is not associated with aldosterone deficiency.
2. Primary adrenal failure is accompanied by markedly increased levels of plasma ACTH as a physiologic feedback consequence of cortisol deficiency; conversely, plasma ACTH is low or undetectable in secondary adrenal failure.

Adrenal failure occurs as either an acute or a chronic syndrome. The predominant feature of acute adrenal failure is hypotension (Box 31-4). Sudden, unexpected shock may be the only finding that prompts suspicion of the diagnosis. This commonly occurs during the course of a serious illness or other major physical/emotional stress. In Addison's disease, a lack of aldosterone, which normally mediates extracellular fluid volume and sodium concentration, leads to hypovolemia, hyperkalemia, and acidosis.

Chronic adrenal failure develops progressively over months to years, the course being variable in duration and severity, depending on the destructive process. Weakness is a universal complaint, noted initially as easy fatigue, but increasing in time to profound exhaustion that limits normal activity. Weight loss is also a regular occurrence, usually accompanied by a poor appetite and sometimes by episodes of nausea and vomiting. Hypotension, particularly with upright posture, is frequently noted. Occasionally this is symptomatic, with episodes of dizziness occurring after standing.

Hyperpigmentation is the single most characteristic clinical finding of primary adrenal failure. This pigmentation results from melanocyte stimulation induced by high levels of ACTH, and thus is absent in secondary adrenal failure. The skin darkening is generalized but is

---

Box 31-4   Signs and Symptoms of Acute Adrenal Insufficiency

- Hypotension
- Headache
- Lethargy, weakness
- Confusion, mental fatigue
- Nausea and/or vomiting
- Syncope
- Severe abdominal pain
- Vascular collapse and shock
- Loss of consciousness

most intense in sun-exposed areas, sometimes described as a summer tan that never fades. Other involved areas, particularly in white individuals, reveal bluish black mottling of the lips, gingiva, buccal mucosa, palate, and ventral surface of the tongue. On the skin freckles and moles become more intense, the nipple areolae darken, recent scars are heavily pigmented, and the palmar and finger creases of the hand acquire pigmentation. Linear pigmented lines may appear on the fingernails, and the exterior (pressure) surfaces of the extremities, such as the elbows and knees, acquire a dirty brown color.

Oral pigmentations appear as irregular spots that may vary in color and intensity, ranging from pale brown to gray or even black. They occur most frequently on the buccal mucosa but may be found on the gingiva, palate, tongue, or lips.

Administration of corticosteroids is the usual treatment for Addison's disease and often leads to suppression of the individual's immune response. Consequently, patients receiving steroid therapy are more prone to development of bacterial, viral, and fungal infections. These infections may be difficult to treat with conventional therapy. Controlled clinical studies suggest that exogenous steroid use decreases clinical signs of gingival inflammation. Patients taking steroids do not appear to be at increased risk for periodontal disease.[79,80] However, steroid use is clearly associated with osteopenia and osteoporosis in the systemic skeleton, and the clinician should be aware of this potential in the maxilla and mandible.[81,82]

Dental management is similar for patients with primary or secondary adrenal insufficiency. Patients who have been taking exogenous steroids present two potential problems: an increased susceptibility to infection and the possibility of adrenal crisis. Dental patients taking corticosteroids may be at increased risk for development of severe dental infection, because corticosteroids alter the host's normal inflammatory response. The chance of infection can be minimized by using atraumatic and aseptic techniques and by adequate antimicrobial therapy. Stress induced by infection, trauma, surgery, and anesthesia may lead to adrenal crisis in any patient with adrenal insufficiency.

In a healthy patient, stress activates the hypothalamic–pituitary–adrenal axis, resulting in an increased secretion of cortisol by the adrenal glands. Although cortisol is normally produced at a rate of 15 to 30 mg/day, during acute stress the rate increases up to 300 mg/day. Patients with primary or secondary adrenal insufficiency are unable to respond to stress with increased endogenous cortisol production, creating the potential for acute adrenal crisis. These individuals may require increased dosages of exogenous steroids during times of physical or emotional stress. Secondary adrenal insufficiency frequently occurs after administration of exogenous steroids

to treat a variety of endocrine, autoimmune, respiratory, joint, intestinal, neurologic, renal, skin, liver, or connective tissue diseases. The degree of adrenal suppression depends on the dosage and duration of steroid use (Box 31-5).

It has been common practice to administer prophylactic systemic steroids before dental treatment for patients who are taking or have recently taken exogenous steroids. However, such steroid supplementation may not be required for many procedures in patients with secondary adrenal insufficiency.[83] Patients taking 5 to 20 mg/day prednisone may maintain some adrenal reserve after termination of steroid therapy.[84] Higher doses may suppress the adrenal glands to a greater degree. At one organ transplant center with patients receiving long-term steroid therapy, oral surgical procedures were performed without steroid supplementation for 3 years without a single case of adrenal crisis.[85] In a study of organ transplant patients taking a maintenance dose of 5 to 1o mg prednisolone daily, gingivectomies were performed either with or without steroid supplementation.[86] No signs or symptoms of adrenocortical suppression were seen in any subject, either with or without steroid supplementation. Although exogenous steroids may suppress normal adrenal cortisol secretion for an extended period, the ability of the adrenal gland to respond to acute stress may return quickly after termination of steroid therapy. However, complete restoration of normal adrenal function may take a year or longer.

The severe consequences of adrenal crisis suggest caution in patient management. People with primary adrenal insufficiency have no adrenal reserve, and thus have absolutely no means of increasing circulating cortisol levels for stressful situations other than by increasing exogenous steroid dosages. Before treating patients with a history of recent or current steroid use, physician consultation is indicated to determine whether the patient's dental needs and proposed treatment require

Box 31-5 | **Exogenous Corticosteroid Equivalent Doses (Equivalencies to 2o mg Cortisol)**

Corticosteroid Agent	Equivalent Dose (mg)
Cortisone	25
Hydrocortisone	20
Prednisone	5
Prednisolone	5
Methylprednisone	5
Methylprednisolone	4
Triamcinolone	4
Dexamethasone	0.75
Betamethasone	0.6

supplemental steroids. A laboratory assay is available to determine the degree of adrenal reserve by measurement of serum cortisol levels 30 and 60 minutes after intravenous administration of synthetic corticotrophin.[85] Use of a stress reduction protocol and profound local anesthesia may help minimize the physical and psychological stress associated with therapy and may reduce the risk for acute adrenal crisis.

Despite all precautions, an acute adrenal crisis may occur, and the dentist should be able to recognize and initially manage the condition. Signs and symptoms of crisis include hypotension, weakness, nausea, vomiting, diarrhea, dehydration, severe abdominal cramping, progressive irritability, headache, and fever. Acute adrenal crisis is life-threatening, and immediate treatment consists of 100 mg hydrocortisone administered intravenously or intramuscularly. The patient should be transferred to a hospital facility as soon as possible.

Hyperparathyroidism

Parathyroid hormone affects both osteoblastic and osteoclastic activity, depending on its secretion level.[87] When present in low levels, it can stimulate bone formation. However, the primary effect at physiologic or greater levels is to suppress bone formation and to increase bone resorption. In patients with hyperparathyroidism, increased bone resorption can occur rapidly and to a severe degree. Primary hyperparathyroidism is usually the result of a benign or malignant lesion in the parathyroid gland. Excess parathyroid hormone secretion releases calcium from bone during osteoclasis; multiple skeletal sites are often affected. The resorbed bone is replaced with fibrous tissue, a condition known as osteitis fibrosa cystica. The fibrous tissue is accompanied by numerous multinucleated giant cells.

When hyperparathyroidism affects the maxilla and mandible, radiographs may demonstrate multilocular radiolucencies, the so-called brown tumors of hyperparathyroidism. The lesions can be mistaken for periapical pathology of endodontic origin; however, the teeth remain vital (Fig. 31-8). These lesions are actually giant cell granulomas, rather than tumors, and they may be associated with soft tissue swelling. The alveolar bone may also develop a "ground glass" appearance, with fine, closely compacted trabeculae; however, this radiographic appearance is not always present. The lamina dura may be lost around the teeth, although this finding is also inconsistent.

Secondary hyperparathyroidism usually results when kidney disease allows excess excretion of calcium in the urine. A feedback mechanism stimulates parathyroid hormone secretion in an attempt to maintain normal serum calcium levels. Oral lesions are identical to those in primary hyperparathyroidism, but they are a late finding in both forms of the disease.

HEMATOLOGIC CONDITIONS

Red and white blood cells are the cornerstones of systemic health, and disorders of these cells may have profound effects on all organ systems. In the periodontium, red blood cells carry oxygen and nutrients to the tissues. Platelets are critical for hemostasis and for production of critical immunoinflammatory mediators. White blood cells protect the periodontium and oral mucosa from bacterial, viral, and fungal pathogens. These cells exist in an exquisite homeostatic balance. Disorders that disturb this balance may manifest within the periodontium or on other mucosal surfaces. Oral signs and symptoms may be the first clinical evidence of underlying blood disorders, and the dental health practitioner must pay careful attention to possible indicators of occult disease.

Leukocyte Disorders

The importance of an intact host immunoinflammatory response in maintaining periodontal health underscores the changes that may occur when patients have leukocyte disorders. The neutrophil or polymorphonuclear leukocyte is the first line of defense against periodontal pathogens. A defect in this cell line has clear negative consequences, often resulting in severe periodontal destruction at an early age. Although the clinician will not encounter these disorders on a routine basis, the severe periodontal destruction associated with neutrophil disorders can be overwhelming for both the patient and the provider.

Neutrophils circulate within the bloodstream and must pass out of the vessels and into the tissues to defend against periodontal pathogens. Pathogens and host cells produce chemotactic agents that signal neutrophils to enter an area of infection. To be fully functional, neutrophils must be able to do the following:

1. Slow down their flow within the vasculature—a process involving cell surface glycoproteins known as selectins on the surface of neutrophils and endothelial cells lining the blood vessels. Up-regulation of these selectins results in "rolling" of the neutrophils along the endothelial lining of the vessel.
2. Adhere to the endothelial cells—a process involving interaction between receptors called integrins on the surface of neutrophils and receptors on the endothelial cell surface.
3. Pass between the intercellular spaces of the endothelial lining to exit the vessel and to enter the perivascular tissues—a process known as diapedesis.
4. Move toward the pathogens that they will attack—a process involving locomotion (movement) of the

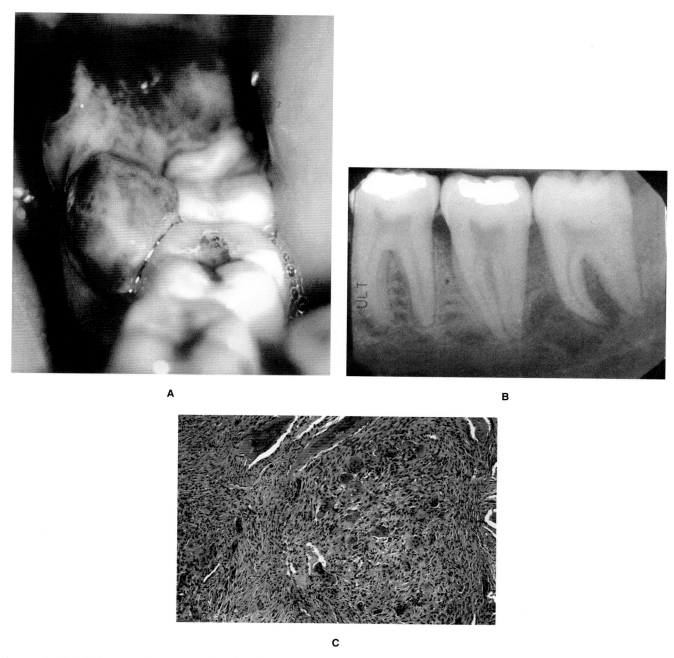

Figure 31-8. A, Soft tissue swelling associated with teeth #17 and #18 in a 22-year-old man. Teeth were vital. **B,** Radiograph revealed periradicular radiolucency associated with the mesial root of #17, with loss of trabeculation in the alveolar crest distal to #17 and between #17 and #18. **C,** Biopsy revealed numerous giant cells in fibrous stroma, features of a classic giant cell granuloma. Systemic work-up disclosed hyperparathyroid state. (*Courtesy Dr. Richard Day, Private Practice, Wasilla, Alaska; and Dr. Craig Fowler, Wilford Hall Medical Center, Lackland Air Force Base, TX.*)

neutrophil toward the bacteria or host cells that are producing factors called chemoattractants. This is the process of chemotaxis (directed movement toward a chemoattractant).

5. Bind to the pathogens, engulf them, and move them into the intracellular environment of the neutrophil—a process known as phagocytosis.

6. Kill the offending pathogen—a process called degranulation, involving enzyme release from intracellular granules. Another method of killing involves release of free oxygen radicals. This process not only kills the offending pathogen but may result in host tissue damage, especially if the response is exuberant.

Defects in the response of neutrophils to pathogens can occur at any step along this pathway.[88] This results in an inability to clear a bacterial infection and allows bacteria and their products to continue to destroy host tissues. The clinical effect is usually a rapid loss of alveolar bone and attachment.

Leukocyte Adhesion Deficiency

Leukocyte adhesion deficiency (LAD) is an inherited disorder that follows an autosomal recessive pattern. There have been just more than 600 cases described, each identified shortly after birth. More than 75% of children will die before the age of 5 years if they do not receive a bone marrow transplant. Leukocyte adhesion deficiency is caused by a deficiency in cell surface integrins that prevents the neutrophil from adhering to the vessel wall at the site of an infection. Neutrophils are unable to migrate into the affected tissues and remain within the vasculature. This prevents them from attacking bacterial pathogens. Patients have early loss of teeth, severe alveolar bone loss and attachment loss, and severely inflamed gingival tissues, often with ulceration and necrosis (Fig. 31-9). Both

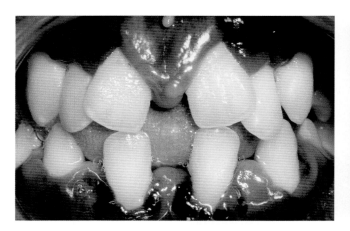

A

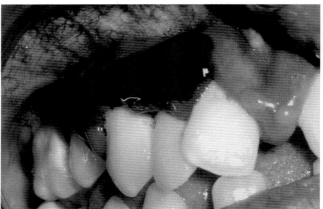

B

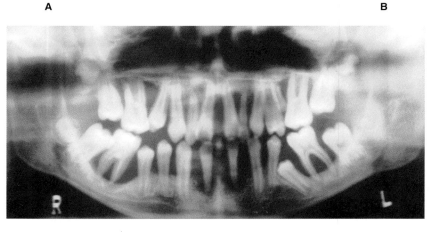

C

Figure 31-9. Patient with generalized aggressive periodontitis. **A,** Clinical appearance of a 12-year-old boy with generalized aggressive periodontitis resulting from leukocyte adhesion deficiency (LAD). **B,** Gingival tissues are fiery red, painful to touch, and bleed profusely on stimulation. **C,** Panoramic radiograph reveals severe bone loss at age 12 years affecting all permanent teeth. Teeth #23 and #26 exfoliated spontaneously.

primary and permanent teeth are affected.[89] Treatment is difficult, involving mechanical debridement, topical antimicrobials, and systemic antibiotics. Unfortunately, treatment rarely results in long-term retention of teeth.

Chediak–Higashi Syndrome

Chediak–Higashi syndrome is a rare autosomal recessive disorder that primarily affects neutrophils.[88] The average lifespan for children with Chediak–Higashi syndrome is only 6 years, although some patients live into early adulthood. The syndrome becomes clinically evident early in life, resulting in frequent pyogenic infections and lymphadenopathy. Abnormalities of pigmentation, recurrent infections, and bleeding tendencies also occur. Albinism may affect the skin, eyes, and hair. Hair color is usually metallic silver, the skin color white to gray because of defective melanosomes, and the eyes demonstrate reduced pigmentation of the retina and iris. Infections usually present as skin abscesses, pneumonitis, otitis media, and sinusitis. Bleeding problems arise because of platelet abnormalities that inhibit normal clot formation. Oral findings include severe gingivitis, ulcerations of the tongue and buccal mucosa, and early-onset periodontitis. Bone loss is usually generalized and severe. Patients do not respond to periodontal therapy, leading to premature loss of both deciduous and permanent dentitions.

The hallmark of Chediak–Higashi syndrome is the presence of large azurophilic inclusions within the cytoplasm of neutrophils. These large inclusions hinder neutrophil migration and their ability to phagocytize and digest microbes. A mutation in the LYST (lysosome trafficking regulation) gene—the only gene known to cause Chediak–Higashi syndrome—may be responsible for this phenomenon.[90,91] Bone marrow transplantation appears to be the most effective treatment for correcting these neutrophil abnormalities.

Chronic Neutropenia

The normal adult absolute neutrophil count (ANC) is between 1800 to 8000 cells/μl. Neutropenia (low ANC) is considered clinically significant when the ANC decreases to less than 1000 cells/μl. Chronic neutropenia is defined as a low ANC for greater than 6 months. The risk for infection caused by neutropenia is inversely proportional to the ANC. When the ANC is less than 500 cells/μl, control of endogenous microbiota is often impaired and the risk for serious infection increases. An ANC less than 200 cells/μl results in an inability to mount an inflammatory response.

Chronic benign neutropenia (CBN) is characterized by a prolonged noncyclic neutropenia as the sole abnormality. The neutropenia is not associated with any underlying disease.[92] CBN is the most common form of neutropenia in infants and children younger than 4 years.

The clinical presentation is variable, ranging from benign to life-threatening; however, most people with CBN live a normal lifespan. An increased incidence of recurrent oral ulcerations, upper respiratory infections, otitis media, cellulitis, lymphadenopathy, pneumonia, and sepsis occurs as a result of the decreased neutrophil response. The risk for infection appears to decrease with age. Oral manifestations of CBN may include hyperplastic, edematous, and fiery red gingiva with areas of desquamation, although not all patients with CBN are similarly affected. Severe pocketing and bone loss may occur. Ulceration, chronic gingivitis, and chronic periodontitis also have been reported.[93] Within the periodontal tissues, the chronic lack of neutrophils may be counterbalanced by increased antibacterial activity from monocytes. This may explain the milder periodontal findings in some patients with CBN.

Cyclic neutropenia is characterized by periodic recurring symptoms of fever, malaise, mucosal ulcers, and possibly life-threatening infections related to cyclical fluctuations in the number of neutrophils.[94] This disorder usually presents before age 10 years with episodes of fever, malaise, mood swings, and oral ulcerations that can last 3 to 6 days and recur approximately every 3 weeks. The interval between neutropenic episodes is not always clinically evident and may require frequent laboratory studies to identify. A complete blood count performed twice weekly for 6 weeks generally provides an accurate picture of the cycle. For most patients, the cycle is approximately 21 days, with a 3- to 10-day period of severe neutropenia.

Cyclic neutropenia tends to improve with age. Its clinical presentation may vary widely among individuals. Although usually not fatal, death can occur due to pneumonia, cellulitis, gangrene, or peritonitis. Oral conditions associated with cyclic neutropenia may include recurrent severe gingivitis and oral ulcerations. Periodontitis may progress more rapidly than expected because of periodic diminishment of the neutrophil response. Unfortunately, even with the best of professional and home care, teeth are often lost because of advancing periodontal disease. Treatment to increase neutrophil levels has been successful using recombinant human granulocyte colony-stimulating factor (G-CSF) given three times per week.[93] G-CSF is a hematopoietic growth factor that simulates the proliferation and differentiation of neutrophils. It has been widely successful in correcting chemotherapy-induced neutropenia in patients with cancer, greatly decreasing the risk for life-threatening infections during periods of immunosuppression.

Congenital neutropenia, also known as Kostmann syndrome, is an inherited disorder manifesting in infancy and characterized by severe bacterial infections. Diminished ANC is the result of arrested neutrophil hematopoiesis. Oral symptoms are virtually universal in congenital neutropenia. Despite their young age, patient with this syndrome not only demonstrate severe gingivitis, but most also have periodontitis with significant alveolar bone loss.[95,96] In the past, most patients with congenital neutropenia died within the first year of life; however, aggressive antibiotic therapy has more recently prolonged the lifespan of these children. Congenital neutropenia is now treated with G-CSF, which is effective at increasing the ANC to more than 1000/μl in most patients. Although G-CSF treatment improves symptoms, it is not curative and most patients demonstrate cyclic improvements followed by relapses in neutrophil levels. Even with G-CSF treatment, most of these patients have persistent gingivitis, which tends to wax and wane depending on their ANC.

Agranulocytosis is characterized by a reduction or complete elimination of granular leukocytes (neutrophils, basophils, eosinophils). The decreased number of granulocytes can result from either a decreased production or an increased peripheral destruction of cells. Decreased production of granulocytes is often caused by bone marrow hypoplasia; however, it can also be the result of an idiosyncratic drug reaction. Patients with agranulocytosis are often febrile and may exhibit necrotizing nonpurulent lesions of mucous membranes, including oral, gastrointestinal, and vaginal membranes.[88] Oral signs and symptoms include generalized, painful stomatitis, spontaneous bleeding, and necrotic tissue. Severe gingivitis, rapidly progressive bone loss, and tooth loss may appear at an early age. Cases related to drug idiosyncrasy usually occur in adulthood.

Lazy leukocyte syndrome is a rare disorder characterized by quantitative and qualitative neutrophil defects.[97] Deficiency in neutrophil chemotaxis combined with systemic neutropenia results in recurrent infections. Impaired neutrophil motility inhibits their migration into tissue sites of inflammation. In the few reported cases of lazy leukocyte syndrome, all have had oral manifestations. In addition to systemic signs and symptoms such as high fever, cough, pneumonia, and purulent skin abscesses, oral manifestations include painful stomatitis, gingivitis, recurrent ulcerations of the buccal mucosa and tongue, rapidly progressive bone loss, and tooth loss at an early age.

Papillon–Lefèvre Syndrome

Papillon–Lefèvre syndrome (PLS) belongs to a heterogenous group of 19 different skin diseases characterized by hyperkeratosis of the palms of the hands and soles of the feet (palmar–plantar hyperkeratosis).[88,98] PLS is caused by mutations in the cathepsin C gene located on chromosome 11. Cathepsin C is a protease, normally found in high levels in epithelium and immune cells such as

neutrophils, which acts to degrade proteins and activate proenzymes in immune cells. Patients with PLS have little or no cathepsin C activity.

PLS differs from other members of this group of hyperkeratoses in that patients with PLS universally have generalized rapid destruction of the periodontal attachment apparatus resulting in premature loss of primary and permanent teeth. The presence of neutrophil defects in PLS is commonly noted. Diminished chemotaxis, phagocytosis, and intracellular killing of certain bacteria have been reported in some but not all cases. It is possible that neutrophil defects are not entirely responsible for the findings in PLS. Some authors have hypothesized that the hereditary defect in PLS is located in the epithelial barrier, which in the gingival sulcus may lead to a reduced defense against pathogenic bacteria.[99] Alterations in cementum, collagenolytic activity in the periodontal ligament, and osteoclastic activity have also been suggested in some patients with PLS. Taken together, these findings could explain the aggressive periodontal destruction seen in patients with PLS even in the absence of significant neutrophil abnormalities.

The periodontal condition in PLS is difficult to treat, and use of conventional mechanical debridement rarely has been successful. Systemic administration of synthetic retinoids, when combined with meticulous plaque control, debridement, topical antimicrobials such as chlorhexidine, and systemic antibiotic therapy, may give the best chance for preventing progression of periodontitis and retaining teeth.[100]

Down Syndrome

Down syndrome (DS) is one of the most common causes of mental retardation in children. Periodontal diseases are practically universal in this disorder. In the deciduous dentition, gingivitis is almost always present and is often severe. As the patient with DS reaches puberty, periodontitis is a common finding. The prevalence of periodontitis is greater in DS than in many other types of mental retardation and is often quite severe.[101] Plaque levels are greater in the DS population, yet the degree of periodontal destruction far exceeds that expected even with large accumulations of local factors. Endogenous factors may be involved in the pathogenesis of periodontitis in DS. The number of neutrophils in DS appears normal; however, neutrophil chemotaxis, phagocytosis, or intracellular killing may be inhibited. The release of tissue-destructive enzymes such as collagenase from salivary and gingival crevicular fluid neutrophils also may be increased.[102] The evidence suggests a range of qualitative neutrophil defects in patients with DS that may help to explain the prevalence and severity of periodontal diseases in these individuals.

Glycogen Storage Disease

Glycogen storage diseases include at least 18 inherited disorders caused by abnormalities of enzymes that control glycogen synthesis and degradation.[88] Glycogen storage disease type 1 b is usually diagnosed in infancy or early childhood and includes features such as a "doll-like" facial appearance, stunted growth, hypoglycemia, ketosis, lactic acidosis, hyperlipidemia, gout, and bleeding episodes brought on by impaired platelet function. Patients with glycogen storage disease type 1 b often have qualitative and quantitative neutrophil defects, leading to an increased susceptibility to infection. Neutropenia may be either constant or cyclic, and is often accompanied by defects in neutrophil migration, chemotaxis, and bacterial killing.[103] Oral disease, including mucosal ulceration, candidiasis, gingivitis, and periodontitis, is common in patients with glycogen storage disease type 1 b.[103,104] Periodontitis may be generalized and aggressive in some patients. There are few reports of the success or failure of periodontal treatment.

Anemias

Anemias are qualitative or quantitative deficiencies of the blood, usually resulting from a decrease in the number of circulating red blood cells (erythrocytes) or in the amount of hemoglobin, or from a qualitative change in erythrocytes. The major categories of anemias include the following:

- Normocytic–normochromic anemia
- Macrocytic hyperchromic anemia
- Microcytic hypochromic anemia
- Sickle cell anemia

Aplastic anemia is a form of normocytic–normochromic anemia that results from a lack of bone marrow production of erythrocytes and other blood cells. The disorder may be genetic or acquired. The acquired form usually follows exposure to certain drugs, toxic chemicals, or ionizing radiation. The severity of the clinical manifestations is directly dependent on the degree of pancytopenia. Because all bone marrow–derived cells are affected, including leukocytes and platelets, hemorrhage and infection are the major threats to patients with aplastic anemia. Oral manifestations include petechiae, gingival swelling and bleeding (often spontaneous), gingival overgrowth, and herpetic infections.[105] Rapid bone loss has been reported, and periodontal infections have led to severe, life-threatening systemic infection. *Fanconi's anemia* is a rare form of aplastic anemia in which chromosomes break and rearrange easily. Most patients with Fanconi's anemia have birth defects involving multiple organ systems, and early-onset periodontitis may be seen.[106] BMT may provide the best long-term outcome for individuals with aplastic anemia.

Pernicious anemia, a form of macrocytic hyperchromic anemia, is caused by a lack of intrinsic factor, normally produced by the gastric mucosa. Intrinsic factor is essential to the absorption of vitamin B_{12} and to the formation of erythrocytes. The condition can vary in its clinical severity. Like many anemias, the complexion may appear pale. Gingival pallor is also common. The tongue is affected in more than 75% of cases; atrophy of the papillae leaves the dorsal surface red, shiny, and smooth.[107] It is often painful to eat. Pernicious anemia is treated with vitamin B_{12} supplementation either orally or by injection.

Iron deficiency anemia, a microcytic hypochromic anemia, is the most common form of anemia. In addition to the presence of hypochromic, microcytic red blood cells, it is characterized by low iron stores, low serum iron concentration, and low hemoglobin concentration or hematocrit. Iron deficiency anemia may result from blood loss, such as an occult gastrointestinal bleed or excessive menstruation. Oral signs and symptoms are similar to pernicious anemia and primarily affect the tongue and gingiva. Iron deficiency anemia is present in a disorder known as Plummer–Vinson syndrome and warrants particular attention. This syndrome is characterized by the glossitis seen in other forms of iron deficiency anemia, combined with enlargement of the tongue, ulceration of the oral and esophageal mucosa, and dysphagia (difficulty swallowing).[108] Patients with Plummer–Vinson syndrome are at significantly increased risk for esophageal squamous cell carcinoma and should undergo frequent esophageal endoscopy.[109] Iron supplementation is the key to management of iron deficiency anemia and may relieve the dysphagia associated with Plummer–Vinson syndrome.

Sickle cell anemia is a hereditary hemolytic anemia that is found almost exclusively in black individuals. An abnormal hemoglobin gene is present. During conditions of decreased oxygen tension, the red blood cell changes shape and resembles a sickle. This can result in sickle cell crisis, in which the oxygen-carrying capacity of the erythrocytes is diminished and blood viscosity is increased. Sickle cell crisis is a life-threatening phenomenon. Sickle cell anemia may present with pallor of the gingiva and oral mucosa. Studies have not demonstrated an increased risk for gingivitis or periodontitis in individuals with sickle cell anemia.[110] However, it is important for the clinician to thoroughly examine the periodontium of these patients, because acute periodontal infection may precipitate sickle cell crisis.

Thrombocytopenia

Thrombocytopenic purpura is a blood dyscrasia associated with a decrease in circulating platelets. Thrombocytopenia of clinical significance exists when the whole blood platelet count is less than 150,000/mm³, although the precise limits for normal vary slightly among laboratories. Excessive hemorrhage during or after invasive dental treatment is often seen with platelet counts less than 50,000/mm³. The most common manifestation of thrombocytopenic purpura is spontaneous hemorrhage into the skin and mucous membranes. The disease is also characterized by prolonged bleeding. Two major forms of thrombocytopenic purpura—primary and secondary—have been described. *Primary (idiopathic) thrombocytopenic purpura (ITP)* is of unknown etiology. This is a relatively common form of the disease and may be seen at any age. *Secondary thrombocytopenia* is caused by a known etiologic factor such as chemicals or drugs.

Two forms of ITP are recognized: acute and chronic. Acute ITP is a self-limited disease that generally remits permanently without sequelae. The onset is usually sudden, with thrombocytopenia manifested by bruising, bleeding, and petechiae a few days to several weeks after an otherwise uneventful viral illness. Conversely, chronic ITP is usually a disease of adults and can be sudden or insidious in onset. It is more frequent in women than in men, and the course is characterized by remissions and exacerbations. In both acute and chronic ITP, thrombocytopenia and its manifestation are the only physical or laboratory abnormalities.

The oral manifestations of thrombocytopenia may be the first clinical signs of the disease. Purpura, the most common oral sign, is defined as any escape of blood into subcutaneous tissues. Purpura includes petechiae, ecchymoses, hemorrhagic vesicles, and hematomas. These may appear on any mucosal surface and are often seen on the tongue, lips, and occlusal line of the buccal mucosa secondary to minor trauma. Purpura may be differentiated from vascular lesions by applying pressure directly to the area. Because purpura results from blood extravasated into the tissues, these lesions will not blanch. Other oral signs include spontaneous gingival hemorrhage and prolonged bleeding after trauma, toothbrushing, extractions, or periodontal therapy. Similar purpuric findings are seen on the skin. The patient may have a positive history of epistaxis (bleeding from the nose), hematuria (blood in urine), melena (darkening of feces caused by blood pigments), and increased menstrual bleeding.

Good oral hygiene and complete removal of plaque and calculus help to minimize gingival inflammation and reduce gingival bleeding associated with thrombocytopenia. Gentle plaque control reduces the risk for bleeding. Periodontal therapy should be limited unless platelet counts exceed a minimum of 50,000/mm³, and surgery should be avoided until platelet counts are greater than 80,000/mm³. Any drug previously associated with the onset of thrombocytopenic episodes should be avoided. Aspirin and nonsteroidal antiinflammatory agents should also be avoided, because they may potentiate prolonged bleeding.

Leukemias

Leukemia is a neoplastic disorder of the blood-forming tissues, primarily affecting leukocytes. This heterogenous group of diseases arises from a neoplastic proliferation in the bone marrow. The replacement of normal bone marrow elements by leukemic cells causes decreased production of erythrocytes, normal white blood cells, and platelets. The clinical result is anemia, with weakness, fatigue, pallor of skin, and mucous membranes; thrombocytopenia with associated bleeding tendencies; and leukopenias resulting in increased susceptibility to infection. Leukemias are classified as either acute or chronic, depending on the presentation of the disease. They are further classified relative to the predominant cell affected as either lymphocytic or myelocytic.[111] Monocytic leukemias form a subgroup of myelocytic leukemia.

Oral involvement is common in leukemia and may represent the first sign of the disease. Dental professionals were responsible for initiating the diagnosis of leukemia in 25% to 33% of cases.[112] Overall, 15% to 80% of patients with leukemia have oral manifestations, with the acute forms presenting oral signs in approximately 65% of cases, compared with only 30% in chronic leukemias. Oral petechiae or bleeding, mucosal ulceration, and gingival enlargement are the most common signs.[113] Acute periodontal infection, pain, pharyngitis, and lymphadenopathy also may be seen.

Gingival enlargement may be localized or generalized and represents an infiltration of leukemic cells into the gingiva, and less frequently into bone (Fig. 31-10). Gingival

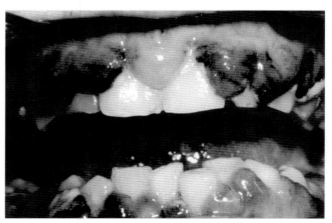

Figure 31-10. Leukemic gingival enlargement in 33-year-old man. Biopsy of gingiva revealed large leukemic infiltrate. (*Courtesy Dr. Craig Fowler, Wilford Hall Medical Center, Lackland Air Force Base, TX; and Dr. Robert Brannon, Louisiana State University School of Dentistry, New Orleans, LA.*)

enlargement is most common in acute monocytic leukemia (67% of cases), followed by acute myelomonocytic leukemia (18.5%), and acute myelocytic leukemia (4%).[114] The enlarged gingiva tends to be relatively firm in texture and most prominent in the interdental regions. The marginal tissues may be bluish-red or cyanotic. Gingival enlargement creates pseudopockets where plaque accumulates, stimulating a host response that may further exacerbate the swelling. Gingival bleeding is also common, and may be an early indicator of leukemia. Oral mucosal ulcers are a frequent finding in patients with leukemia. These lesions may result from bacterial invasion caused by severe leukopenia or from mucosal atrophy caused by a direct effect on epithelial cells of the chemotherapeutic drugs used to treat leukemia. Trauma from a dental prosthesis or teeth may result in large secondarily infected ulcers progressing to facial cellulitis and septicemia.

Treatment for leukemia may include chemotherapy, radiation therapy, and BMT, each of which has the potential to produce a wide range of oral complications. Mucositis, xerostomia, and secondary infection with a variety of bacterial, viral, and fungal agents may occur.[115,116] Candidiasis is almost universally seen in hospitalized patients with leukemia undergoing chemotherapy. Infections with unusual organisms (e.g., *Pseudomonas* and *Klebsiella* species) are common in this group of patients. Many drugs used for chemotherapy are neurotoxic and may cause intense oral pain, which is usually transient. These symptoms must be distinguished from pain of odontogenic origin. Patients undergoing BMT require special consideration because they receive very high-dose chemotherapy, often in combination with total body irradiation. The extreme immunosuppression experienced by patients with BMT predisposes to systemic spread of even mild infections. A large percentage of patients with BMT develop graft-versus-host disease, a condition where transplanted immunocompetent marrow cells recognize the host tissues as foreign and react against them, resulting in fever, mucosal ulcerations, skin erythema, and systemic involvement (Fig. 31-11).

It is critical that dental needs be assessed as soon as a definitive diagnosis of leukemia has been rendered and a decision is made to initiate a radiation, chemotherapy, or BMT protocol. Unfortunately, oral care has been overlooked in the past, but aggressive promotion of dental intervention as a part of leukemia treatment protocols in recent years has dramatically decreased the incidence of oral complications.[112]

During the acute phase of the disease only those procedures that are necessary to alleviate the discomfort and hemorrhaging should be performed. Conversely, during a period of remission every attempt should be made to achieve a state of periodontal health. The

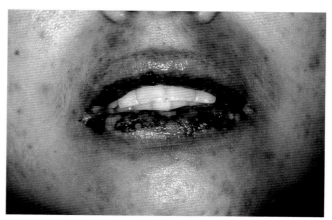

Figure 31-11. Ulcerations on lips of a female patient with graft-versus-host disease (GVHD) after bone marrow transplantation. Severe intraoral ulcerations also were present on the buccal mucosa, the floor of mouth, and the ventral surface of the tongue. The patient died within 1 month of this photograph. (*Courtesy Dr. Alex DePeralta, Wilford Hall Medical Center, Lackland Air Force Base, TX.*)

treatment should be conservative, consisting of the removal of all local irritants and instruction in good plaque control techniques. The distinct benefits of strict plaque control in severely granulocytopenic leukemia patients have been demonstrated: obtaining excellent gingival health and minimizing oral ulceration throughout chemotherapy.[118]

Severe gingival bleeding resulting from thrombocytopenia often can be managed successfully with localized treatment. The use of an absorbable gelatin sponge with topical thrombin or placement of microfibrillar collagen is often sufficient. Some authors report successful management of gingival bleeding with oral rinses of antifibrinolytic agents. If these measures are not successful in stopping blood flow from an oral site, platelet transfusions may be necessary.

Management of oral ulcers in patients with leukemia should be directed toward preventing the spread of localized infection and bacteremia, promoting healing of the lesion, and decreasing pain. Oral ulcers or extensive tissue sloughing may serve as the source of life-threatening septicemia in patients with leukemia (Fig. 31-12). Topical antibacterial and antifungal medication should be used. Chlorhexidine mouth rinses are effective in reducing the severity of oral ulcerations, primarily by minimizing secondary infection of these lesions.[119] Severe ulcers showing clinical signs of infection should be treated with a combination of topical medication and systemic antibiotics.

Patients with myelosuppressed leukemia are at risk for a variety of viral infections, most commonly herpes simplex, varicella zoster, and cytomegalovirus (CMV; Fig. 31-13).

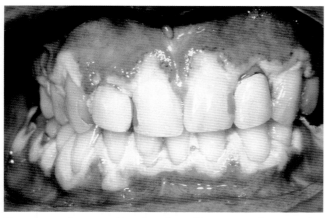

Figure 31-12. A 43-year-old male patient with severe myelosuppression secondary to immunosuppressive drug therapy. Sloughing of gingiva is apparent around all teeth and affects both marginal and papillary gingiva.

These infections may become severe and must be recognized early. Herpes simplex virus and varicella zoster virus respond well to systemic acyclovir or other antiviral agents, and many patients with leukemia undergoing chemotherapy are treated prophylactically to prevent infection.

Coagulation Disorders

The predominant inherited coagulation disorders are hemophilia A, hemophilia B, and von Willebrand disease. Coagulopathies may also be acquired. Liver disease affects coagulation because most of the clotting factors are synthesized in the liver; thus the clinician should be wary of coagulation disorders in alcohol abusers and patients with hepatitis. Vitamin K deficiency, usually associated with long-term antibiotic usage or with malabsorption syndromes, can result in coagulation problems.

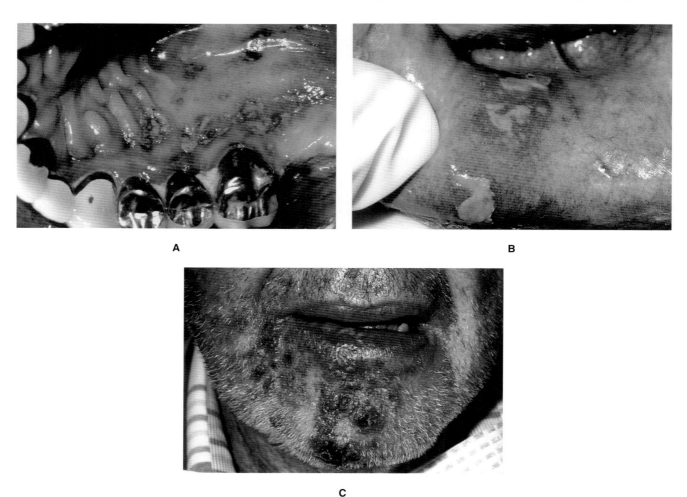

Figure 31-13. Herpes zoster. **A,** Unilateral right palatal ulcerations noted in 68-year-old man. Lesions were acutely painful. Patient had no history of trauma in this region. **B,** Ulcerations also noted on labial mucosa of lower lip. Again, lesions were confined to the patient's right side. A diagnosis of herpes zoster was made. **C,** Within 1 week, this patient had major skin ulcerations on the right side extending across the entire distribution of the trigeminal nerve. The patient was treated with systemic acyclovir. The lesions resolved but resulted in significant and prolonged postherpetic neuralgia.

Several of the clotting factors are dependent on vitamin K for their synthesis. The most common oral manifestation of coagulopathies, excessive bleeding, is generally associated with surgical therapy (see Chapter 37 for complete discussion). On occasion, a patient with a coagulation disorder will have spontaneous gingival bleeding. This is usually caused by accumulation of plaque, and its presence emphasizes the importance of excellent oral hygiene in these patients.

INFLUENCES OF NUTRITION

The relation between nutritional factors and maintenance of periodontal health, or the role of nutritional factors in the pathogenesis of periodontal disease, is controversial. Many practitioners are ardent supporters of the concept that nutrition not only influences the onset and progression of disease but is critical to proper periodontal therapy. Others decline to place much importance on the role of nutrition in either the pathogenesis of periodontal disease or its treatment. Most of the scientific evidence is derived from laboratory or animal studies. Because of inadequacies in study design, few controlled human studies exist on which to base conclusions about the effect of nutrition on periodontal health, disease, or treatment. Well designed population, observational, mechanistic, and intervention studies are needed to clarify this issue.[120] Although dental plaque is the major etiologic factor in periodontal disease, it is possible that inadequate nutrition may alter the host response to bacterial irritants and render the host more susceptible to establishment or progression of periodontal diseases.[121]

Nutritional disorders are not only the result of inadequate dietary intake but also may be caused by disturbances in absorption of nutrients, economic and educational limitations, self-imposed dietary restrictions, and geographic isolation from an adequate food supply. The impact of nutrition on periodontal, oral, and overall systemic health can best be seen by examining extreme nutritional deprivation. This situation is uncommon in the developed world, which may explain the paucity of useful human data in the area of nutritional influences on the periodontium.

Physical Dietary Factors

In animals, the physical characteristics of food play a role in plaque accumulation and development of gingivitis. Soft diets contribute to accumulation of plaque and calculus, whereas hard or fibrous foods have a physical cleansing that decreases plaque accumulation and gingival inflammation. In fact, experimental gingivitis is often enhanced by placing animals on a soft diet to foster plaque accumulation. The nutritional adequacy of the diet appears to have little impact on gingivitis in animals, whether the food is soft or hard. In contrast, plaque accumulation and gingivitis in humans appears unrelated to the physical characteristics of the diet. Hard or fibrous foods are not associated with decreased plaque accumulation.[122] The difference in the physical effects of foods between animals and humans may be related to differences in study design. In animal studies of dietary characteristics, the subjects can be fed an exclusively hard diet. Humans, conversely, cannot be fed an exclusively hard diet for any significant length of time.

Nutritional Deficiencies

Nutritional deficiencies are most common in underdeveloped parts of the world. It is estimated that more than 150 million children, primarily in sub-Saharan Africa and southern Asia, are malnourished.[123] In the United States and other developed countries, cases of malnutrition can be found primarily among the elderly, the poor, and abusers of alcohol and other drugs.

The interactions between nutrition, the immune system, and infection may be of significance in the oral cavity.[124] A vicious cycle may be present in some individuals when malnutrition suppresses the immune system, which may intensify infectious diseases; this may then lead to further malnourishment. In addition, there is evidence that malnutrition may increase the pathogenicity of certain infecting microorganisms, although this has not been demonstrated with periodontal pathogens.

The starkest example of an association between nutrition and oral health is the presence of necrotizing gingivitis and noma in malnourished African children. The prevalence rate of necrotizing gingivitis among children in some African villages is as great as 15% to 25%.[124] This disorder is uncommon in the developed world. Most of these children are malnourished, have poor oral hygiene, and have common tropical infections. Measles, a viral infection, often precedes development of necrotizing gingivitis and noma. Herpes viruses also have been associated with these maladies. A model has been proposed by which an initial viral infection cannot be eliminated by the immune system because of impaired host resistance derived from a malnourished state.[124] When combined with poor oral hygiene, the impairment in host resistance allows viral replication in the mouth, impairs the integrity of the oral mucosal barrier, promotes selective growth of pathogenic bacteria, reduces T-cell and neutrophil function, and leads to necrotizing gingivitis. This condition, if unresolved, can lead to necrotizing periodontitis and even to noma. Noma is a severe gangrenous process that destroys the bone and soft tissues of the mouth and face. Noma can lead to death.

The oral epithelial tissues are able to play a protective role by virtue of their capacity to replace cells rapidly and to act as a functional barrier. The epithelial lining of the gingival sulcus has one of the fastest turnover rates in the body and requires a continuous and adequate supply of nutrients. Dietary studies in experimental animals demonstrate that 70% to 80% calorie restriction or protein calorie malnutrition reduces mitotic activity in epithelial tissues, including the oral cavity.[125] The barrier function of the oral epithelium and its permeability depend on the cumulative integrity of an intraepithelial barrier: the basement membrane and the plasma membrane of the epithelial cells. Such a barrier serves to limit the passage of antigenic material, such as bacterial endotoxins and other metabolic byproducts, from the surface into the underlying connective tissue. An increase in oral mucosal permeability may occur with ascorbic acid, folate, and zinc deficiencies.

Inadequate nutrition may impair the host response to the bacterial etiology of periodontal diseases, thereby modifying the inflammatory process. The complex interactions among immune cells, cytokines, hormones, and other inflammatory mediators may be altered by nutritional deficiencies.[121] Both cellular and humoral immune responses to bacterial challenge can be suppressed, and chronically malnourished individuals may be at increased risk for more rapid and advanced periodontal destruction. Neutrophil function may be adversely affected by certain nutritional deficiencies, especially vitamin C deficiency, and could play a role in enhanced periodontal destruction. The properties of salivary defense include adequate flow rate, buffering capacity, and antimicrobial activity. The antimicrobial activity stems from salivary immunologic and nonimmunologic constituents, and it may be impaired by malnutrition. These proteins perform the vital task of inhibiting bacterial adherence, growth, and colonization.

The process of tissue repair, including repair of periodontal tissues, is influenced by several factors, notably integrity of the inflammatory immune response, hormones, and an adequate supply of nutrients, particularly immunoacids, ascorbate, riboflavin, folic acid, vitamin A, and zinc. The local nutrient requirement of the periodontal tissues may be considerably increased compared with other tissues. The gingival sulcus, because of the ever-present antigenic challenge, is in a state of continuous repair. It is conceivable that inadequate nutrient levels in this tissue may result in "end-organ" deficiency, causing impairment of the repair process and facilitating the progression of periodontal disease.

Protein Deficiency

Protein–energy malnutrition impairs cell-mediated immunity, the complement system, secretory antibody, phagocyte activity, and cytokine production.[126] Activity of helper and cytotoxic T cells is diminished. Serum cortisol levels are increased in protein–energy malnutrition, and

the normal diurnal variations in serum cortisol levels are abolished. This inhibits the normal homeostatic diurnal variation in immune activity that is critical to an intact host defense. Increased serum cortisol levels may also increase local cortisol levels in gingival crevicular fluid. This inhibits macrophage function and decreases production of major cytokines involved in the immunoinflammatory response. Cytokines have both beneficial and deleterious effects, therefore the net effect of nutrition on various cytokine profiles is difficult to delineate clearly. For example, malnutrition may decrease circulating levels of both the antiinflammatory cytokine transforming growth factor-β and the proinflammatory cytokines tumor necrosis factor-α and interleukin-1 (IL-1).[126,127] The acute-phase response also appears to be blunted in protein–energy malnutrition. The acute-phase response is a systemic response to infection characterized by release of acute-phase reactants such as fibrinogen and C-reactive protein from the liver. These reactants participate in immediate host defense against infection. Severe protein deficiency, known as kwashiorkor, may result in a shift to a more periodontopathic subgingival microbiota predominated by anaerobes not commonly seen in children, such as *P. gingivalis, P. intermedia, Fusobacterium* species, and spirochetes.[128] The prevalence of fungal organisms and oral candidiasis is also increased in these children.[129] Candidiasis is rare in children, except in cases of immunosuppression such as that seen during cancer chemotherapy. The high prevalence of candidiasis in malnourished children highlights the potential oral impact of severe protein deficiency.

In animal studies, protein deficiency has been reported to cause osteoporosis of alveolar bone and a narrowing of the periodontal ligament fibers. In addition, protein deprivation in animals has been known to retard the healing of wounds and the repair of local tissue irritation. It does not initiate any local inflammatory reaction in the absence of bacterial or mechanical injury. Protein deprivation in the presence of periodontal tissue injury can decrease the rate of connective tissue and bone repair and can cause a breakdown of the healing wound.[130]

In human studies, severe protein deficiency has been associated with a greater prevalence of chronic periodontitis, necrotizing gingivitis, and necrotizing periodontitis.[124] Combinations of protein supplementation and mechanical periodontal therapy are more effective than either approach alone in restoring periodontal health.[131]

Vitamin Deficiencies

Vitamins are essential for systemic and periodontal health. Vitamins are classified as either fat soluble (A, D, E, and K) or water soluble (B and C). Fat-soluble vitamins are stored in the body, whereas water-soluble vitamins are excreted, primarily in the urine.

Vitamin A is important in the synthesis and maintenance of epithelial cells in the skin and mucous membranes. It is also involved in synthesis of proteoglycans. Vitamin A deficiency may manifest in degenerative changes in epithelial tissues, with an alteration of the integrity of the barrier, and keratinization of normally nonkeratinizing cells. In animal studies, vitamin A deficiency results in hyperplasia and hyperkeratosis of the gingiva, proliferation of the junctional epithelium, and inhibition of gingival wound healing.[132] Resorption of cementum also may be increased. Deeper periodontal pockets may develop in vitamin A–deficient animals than in animals with normal vitamin A levels. There is little evidence available to evaluate the effect of vitamin A deficiency on the periodontium in humans.

Vitamin B is actually a complex of water-soluble vitamins that includes thiamin (B_1), riboflavin (B_2), niacin, pyridoxine (B_6), biotin, folic acid, and cobalamin (B_{12}). Deficiency in just one of the B-complex vitamins in not common, and oral manifestations generally reflect a deficiency of multiple B vitamins. In the United States, vitamin B deficiencies are most often seen in alcoholics and drug abusers. The most common oral signs of vitamin B deficiency include glossitis with loss of lingual papillae, glossodynia (painful tongue), gingivitis, angular cheilitis, and generalized mucositis. Gingivitis results primarily from plaque accumulation, but the vitamin deficiency may exacerbate the signs of inflammation.

Thiamin deficiency may lead to myelin degeneration in peripheral nerves and to a condition known as *beriberi*. Beriberi is characterized by peripheral paralysis and polyneuritis, cardiovascular changes, and loss of appetite. This disorder is more common in areas where rice is a diet staple and is uncommon in the United States. Oral manifestations of thiamin deficiency include generalized oral mucositis and small vesicular eruptions on the buccal mucosa, floor of mouth, and palate.

A deficiency of riboflavin is associated with angular cheilitis, glossitis, and oral mucosal ulcerations. Seborrheic dermatitis may also be present. The dorsal surface of the tongue often appears bald and purple. In animals, riboflavin deficiency may cause severe gingival inflammation and ulceration, which may progress to necrotizing periodontitis and noma. These findings have not been demonstrated in humans.

Severe deficiency of niacin results in *pellagra*, which was once common in some parts of the United States. People with pellagra usually have deficiencies of riboflavin and niacin. Pellagra is characterized by gastrointestinal symptoms such as loss of appetite, nausea, vomiting, and diarrhea; dermatitis presenting as thick, red, scaly skin, especially on the back of the hands and neck; and mental disturbances such as insomnia, anxiety, and depression. The oral signs of pellagra include glossitis, stomatitis,

and ulceration of the mucosa. In animals, gingival inflammation, pocketing, and bone destruction may be seen, as may tissue necrosis, depending on the severity of niacin deprivation. In humans, necrotizing gingivitis may be seen.

Long-term deficiencies in pyridoxine can result in anemia, dermatitis, and peripheral neuropathy. Like other B vitamin deficiencies, lack of pyridoxine can cause glossitis, stomatitis, and increased gingivitis.

Vitamin B_{12} deficiency is associated with pernicious anemia, which inhibits absorption of the vitamin from the gut (see earlier). Epithelial thinning and ulceration can occur in the oral cavity, and the tissues may be at greater risk for epithelial dysplasia.[133] Folic acid functions in concert with vitamin B_{12} and is critical to the proper formation of erythrocytes. Folic acid deficiency can lead to megaloblastic anemia, in addition to gastrointestinal changes causing diarrhea and malabsorption. In folate-deficient animals, necrosis of the gingival tissues and bone may occur. In humans, the most common oral changes are angular cheilitis, stomatitis, and glossitis with ulceration of the tongue. Folic acid supplements have been studied in humans to determine their effect on the periodontium. A reduction in gingival inflammation without a decrease in plaque accumulation has been seen after topical or systemic folate supplementation when compared with a placebo.[134,135] In pregnant women, topical folate rinses were associated with reduced gingivitis, whereas systemic folate was not.[136] Folic acid supplementation may also reduce the incidence and severity of phenytoin-induced gingival overgrowth, although not all studies demonstrate a significant effect.[135,137]

Vitamin C deficiency has long been associated with oral changes and has been studied in the dental community more than any other vitamin deficiency.[138] Vitamin C is required for collagen synthesis and cross-linking; therefore, deficiency of this vitamin can adversely affect the periodontal tissues, wound healing, and vascular integrity. Furthermore, vitamin C accumulates in neutrophils and is important to normal immune function. Severe or prolonged deprivation of vitamin C results in *scurvy*. Scurvy is uncommon in the developed world, where it is most likely seen in alcohol or drug abusers. Scurvy is accompanied by periodontal changes that can be severe. Gingivitis occurs as an early sign of the disease. The tissues become highly inflamed and bleed easily, sometimes spontaneously. Excessive swelling and bleeding is caused by increased permeability of the sulcular epithelium and capillary fragility. Neutrophil chemotaxis and phagocytosis are hindered, preventing proper elimination of offending bacteria. As scurvy progresses, increased destruction of the periodontal ligament and bone result in tooth mobility. Because collagen synthesis is impaired, proper wound healing, including new bone formation, does not occur. Notably, scurvy does not occur unless vitamin C deprivation is prolonged for months. There is little evidence suggesting that mild vitamin C deficiencies have a major effect on initiation or progression of periodontal diseases. An analysis of epidemiologic data from more than 12,000 adults in the United States demonstrated only a weak relation between reduced dietary vitamin C intake and the presence of periodontitis.[139] Although some clinicians suggest vitamin C supplements for their patients, there is little evidence that such supplementation significantly affects the risk for periodontal diseases.

Vitamin D is composed of a group of steroid hormones that have a major role in maintaining calcified tissues throughout the body. Vitamin D is required for the absorption of calcium from the gut and for maintenance of the calcium–phosphorous balance. Vitamin D_3 forms within the skin in response to ultraviolet rays from the sun. Vitamin D_3 concentrates in the liver and is converted in the kidneys to form the active hormones 1,25-vitamin D_3 and 24,25 vitamin D_3. These hormones regulate plasma calcium levels by promoting absorption from the gut, regulating calcium reabsorption in the kidneys, and (in conjunction with parathyroid hormone) controlling bone resorption and release of calcium from mineralized stores. Vitamin D deficiency alters normal bone homeostasis and turnover. Organic bone matrix is not properly mineralized, leading to fragility. This condition is called *rickets* when it occurs in children and *osteomalacia* in adults. Osteomalacia in older adults is generally caused by kidney or liver dysfunction. Rickets is characterized by defective formation of long bones and retarded skeletal development. The cortical plates of the maxilla and mandible may undergo thinning, and the trabecular pattern may be sparse.[140] Because teeth require normal calcium–phosphorous homeostasis for proper formation, dental anomalies are common. Enamel and cementum hypoplasia, enlarged pulp chambers, and delayed development of the permanent dentition are noted. Osteomalacia may be accompanied by resorption of alveolar bone with replacement of bone by fibrous tissue, destruction of the periodontal ligament, and narrowing of the periodontal ligament space. These changes are similar to those that occur in hyperparathyroidism (see earlier). This type of secondary osteoporosis, resulting from vitamin D deficiency or hyperparathyroidism, must be distinguished from the primary osteoporosis commonly associated with aging. Treatment of vitamin D deficiency involves vitamin D supplementation and increased exposure to sunlight.

Calcium metabolism is influenced not only by parathyroid hormone and vitamin D but by dietary calcium intake as well. In a large epidemiologic study of approximately 12,000 Americans, the risk for having clinical attachment loss was increased in men and women younger than 40 years who had a low dietary calcium intake compared with those with a normal recommended daily calcium intake (800 mg/day).[141] The lower the daily intake, the greater the risk for attachment loss. This suggests that patients should follow the recommended guidelines for dietary calcium intake and that dental providers should encourage this in their practices. In a longitudinal trial of elderly adults comparing daily calcium supplementation with placebo, those subjects consuming at least 1000 mg calcium per day had a significantly smaller risk for tooth loss than did those consuming lower calcium levels.[142] This suggests that calcium supplementation may have a beneficial effect on tooth retention; however, this study did not address the causes of tooth loss.

Vitamin E is an antioxidant that reduces free oxygen radicals—toxic substances that can cause DNA mutations, peroxidation of lipid membranes, and cell death. Free radicals are involved in a host of diseases affecting multiple organ systems, and antioxidant therapy may be useful in disease prevention, although the use of antioxidant supplementation remains controversial in the medical literature. Vitamin E deficiency has its primary deleterious effects on cell membranes. There is a paucity of scientific data regarding the relation between vitamin E and the periodontium.

Vitamin K is formed by bacteria present in the gut and is critical to the proper production of numerous clotting factors. Vitamin K deficiency usually results from disturbances of the normal gastrointestinal flora. This can be caused by malabsorption syndromes or long-term antibiotic usage. The result of vitamin K deficiency is an increased bleeding tendency that may be severe if dental surgery is performed. There is no evidence that vitamin K deficiency has a direct effect on the periodontium.

Impact of Nutrition on Periodontal Health

Published evidence related to the systemic influence of nutrition on the periodontium in health and disease has led to the following conclusions:

1. Animal studies have demonstrated inconclusively that when a large number of nutrients are either withheld from the diet or ingested in excessive amounts, a deleterious effect may be seen. Animal experiments reside at the bottom of the evidence chain. They may give us a clue as to what to study in humans, but we cannot make conclusions about the pathogenesis of human periodontal disease solely from results obtained from animal experiments.
2. Nutritional imbalance in humans does not cause periodontal disease without the presence of local factors. Deficiencies in nutrition appear to modify

the severity and extent of periodontal disease by altering the host immunoinflammatory response and the potential for repair of the affected tissues. To date, evidence to support nutritional disorders as a major factor in the initiation of periodontal disease is scant. Some nutritional deficiencies (e.g., calcium, vitamin C) have shown a weak to moderate association with the risk for periodontitis, but further research is indicated.

3. To date, intervention studies are lacking. Well-controlled nutritional studies in human subjects will be essential and helpful for definitive and valid assessment of the systemic role of nutrition in periodontal health and disease.

It is clear that periodontal disease is primarily an infectious process involving an inflammatory response to local factors (e.g., bacterial plaque). Current knowledge suggests that the response can be conditioned by nutritional factors. However, prevention or reversal of this disease by short-term nutritional therapy has not been demonstrated. Thus the fundamental basis for patient counseling relative to diet, nutrition, and periodontal disease rests with instructing the patient to ingest a nutritionally adequate diet in the long term. If periodontitis responds positively to plaque control and conventional modes of treatment, existing evidence does not warrant nutritional supplementation.

STRESS AND PSYCHOGENIC DISORDERS

Stress comes in physical, emotional, and psychological forms. Emotional or psychological stress within the social environment may arise during periods of bereavement, strain or failure of relationships, major work- or school-related events, and periods of financial difficulty, to name a few. Periodontal diseases occur in susceptible individuals when certain pathogens colonize the periodontal environment. These pathogens are necessary for disease but are not sufficient to cause disease in all individuals. Rather, other intrinsic (e.g., genetic predisposition) or extrinsic factors (e.g., systemic disease and smoking) exist that increase the risk that a disease will develop in a given individual. Stress may act as a factor to increase the susceptibility to periodontal diseases.

Stress/Depression

Physical and mental stress are known to alter immune responsiveness and may increase the susceptibility to periodontal infection.[143] Early case studies suggest a correlation between periodontal disease parameters and certain psychiatric disorders and major life event stressors. The most commonly studied periodontal disease in relation to stress is acute necrotizing ulcerative gingivitis

(NUG). The incidence of NUG has been shown to increase during periods of stress.[144,145] Stress has been suggested to be one of the greatest risk factors for NUG, especially in patients who smoke.

Case-control studies support a relation between chronic periodontitis, life events, and social demographics.[146] Individuals who were married, employed, and had few negative life events had less periodontitis compared with those who were unmarried, unemployed, and/or experienced negative life events. Other studies have confirmed that high work demands and low marital quality are associated with poorer periodontal status.[147] Rapidly progressive forms of periodontitis have been shown to be associated with increased depression and loneliness compared with either chronic periodontitis or periodontal health.[148]

A large epidemiologic study involving more than 1,400 subjects evaluated the relation between periodontitis and stress, but, importantly, also considered stress coping mechanisms.[149,150] People with high levels of financial strain had more attachment loss than did people with low financial strain. Among the people with high financial strain, however, those individuals who showed adequate coping mechanisms (problem-based coping) had no greater risk for attachment loss than did those with little financial strain. Conversely, those people with inadequate coping mechanisms (emotion-focused coping) who had high financial strain levels had the greatest risk for attachment loss and bone loss. Occupational stress also has been associated with greater progression of periodontal destruction longitudinally.[151] Over a 5-year period, people with low job satisfaction levels had greater loss of periodontal attachment than did those with high job satisfaction. When coping mechanisms were examined, subjects with an internal locus of control—those who believed that they had personal control over what happened to them—had less attachment loss than those who felt that their environment had more control than did they personally (external locus of control). The important conclusion of these studies is that one must consider not only the levels of stress and strain that a patient may experience but also the adequacy of their coping mechanisms in assessing the impact of stress on periodontal health.

Stress also may impact the outcome of periodontal therapy. In a study of 700 patients from a large health maintenance organization, individuals with clinical depression had a less favorable periodontal treatment outcome than did individuals without depression.[152] This study was only a review of records, therefore its conclusions must be viewed with caution. However, the mechanisms that may explain the influence of stress on the periodontium might also influence the results of periodontal therapy.

The effects of stress on the periodontium may be mediated through a number of pathways. Stress may simply increase other behaviors that negatively affect periodontal health. For example, people experiencing stress may have poorer oral hygiene, poorer compliance with dental care, and may smoke more than those individuals not under stress. Unlike recent studies,[149,150] older studies frequently did not adjust for these behavioral factors when examining the impact of stress. Stress appears to have adverse potential effects that go beyond what can be explained simply by associated changes in behavioral factors.

The central nervous system can influence the immune response through complex pathways that link the nervous, endocrine, and immune systems. The two main pathways that link the central nervous system and immune system are the hypothalamic–pituitary–adrenal axis and the direct neuronal connections from the autonomic nervous system.[153] Stress mediates multiple changes in the endocrine system. Stress increases cortisol production in the adrenal cortex by stimulating increased release of ACTH from the pituitary gland. Salivary cortisol levels may be increased by stress and poor coping mechanisms. Cortisol depresses the immune response including neutrophil activity and production of IgG and secretory IgA, all of which are critical in the host immunoinflammatory response to periodontal pathogens. Secretory IgA may decrease initial colonization by pathogens, and IgG opsonizes bacteria so they can be phagocytized and killed by neutrophils. Suppression of the immune response by increased stress-induced cortisol levels increases the potential for pathogen-related periodontal destruction.

Direct neural–immune interaction may also mediate the effects of stress on the periodontium. Neurotransmitters such as epinephrine, norepinephrine, neurokinin, and substance P that are released at neuroeffector junctions interact directly with cells of the immune system. Lymphocytes, neutrophils, monocytes, and macrophages all possess receptors for these neurotransmitters. Stress may increase neurotransmitter release, causing a shift in immune function from a protective response to a destructive one.[153] This results in decreased immune cell response to antigens and a decrease in T-cell activity and antibody production. Cytokine production also may be altered, with a reduction in antiinflammatory cytokines and a shift toward proinflammatory profiles. Substance P and neurokinin levels have been shown to be increased in gingival crevicular fluid of patients with periodontitis compared with healthy control subjects, suggesting that increased neuropeptide levels are associated with disease.[154] These physiologic changes in endocrine, nervous, and immune systems induced by stress may help explain the increased risk for periodontal diseases seen in many studies.

Psychosomatic Disorders/Self-Injury

Occasionally the clinician will encounter a patient with self-inflicted injury to the periodontium. This may involve habitual trauma induced by foreign objects (e.g., pencil, bobby pin, or pipes) or by fingers or fingernails, and is usually unintentional. Self-inflicted gingival injury has been described in children and adults. The lesions are usually isolated to one area of the mouth. These cases can be difficult to diagnose and the cause is usually found through the process of elimination. Treatment involves identification of the habit, patient education, and appropriate follow-up.

More serious psychological problems can lead to bizarre oral presentations as well. Munchausen syndrome is a psychiatric disorder in which the patient may inflict injury on himself or herself to attract attention and garner concern.[155] These patients often visit multiple practitioners or hospitals in search of provider concern. They may have a variety of symptoms and often have numerous scars and bruises. They may be willing to undergo multiple diagnostic procedures as the clinician searches for the cause of the patient's complaint. The self-inflicted injury may involve the periodontium. These cases are difficult to diagnose, which further satisfies the patient's desires because clinicians are likely to continue referring the patient to other practitioners in search of a diagnosis.

HUMAN IMMUNODEFICIENCY VIRUS/ ACQUIRED IMMUNE DEFICIENCY SYNDROME

An unexplained acquired immunodeficiency syndrome was first reported in 1981 and was believed to be limited to homosexual males. Subsequently, the syndrome was identified in heterosexuals, usually those who engaged in unprotected sexual activities or who used illicit injected drugs. A viral pathogen was long suspected as the etiologic agent and ultimately was identified in 1984.[156] By mutual agreement, scientists involved with this virus ultimately named it the *human immunodeficiency virus* (HIV). The debilitating and fatal condition the virus causes was designated as the *acquired immune deficiency syndrome* (AIDS). The virus attacks most cells in the human immune system, especially those that carry the CD4 cell surface receptor molecule. These cells include helper T lymphocytes, monocytes, macrophages, dendritic cells, and even neuronal and glial cells.[157] The virus survives and multiplies within the cells, is transmitted to other similar cells, and ultimately induces death of the host cell. This results in the gradual elimination of host resistance to a wide variety of infectious processes and malignant changes. B lymphocytes and neutrophils are not infected, but as the disease progresses, there is marked secondary dysregulation of their function. These factors render the HIV-infected individual more suscep-tible to disseminated infections, malignancy, and adverse drug reactions.

Epithelial cells of mucous membranes may become infected and allow access for the virus into the body. Available evidence, however, indicates that transmucosal viral entry primarily occurs through infection of circulating lymphocytes, macrophages, and dendritic cells.[159,160] In most instances, mild to severe traumatic injury or percutaneous penetration of mucosa is necessary for an exposed individual to become infected. HIV has been found in most body fluids including saliva and breast milk. However, the greatest quantities of virus are found in blood, semen, and cerebrospinal fluid. Transmission of the infection primarily occurs by sexual contact or by reuse of infected needles by users of illicit injectable drugs. Exposure to contaminated blood and blood products in the health care setting was initially a means of trans-mission to individuals who required transfusions. How-ever, blood banks in developed countries carefully screen blood donors and evaluate blood products and this risk has ceased to be of major concern. The problem, however, continues in undeveloped, third world countries.

Transmission of HIV from infected mothers to infants takes place by fetal infection, infection at time of delivery, or by breastfeeding. Recent evidence indicates, how-ever, that the risk for maternal transmission has been markedly reduced by early testing of expectant mothers and administration of antiretroviral drugs to the HIV-positive mother before and after parturition.[161]

In the United States 807,075 AIDS cases have been reported as of December 31, 2001.[162] Although the numbers of patients with AIDS continue to increase in developed countries, death from this infection has decreased. This is primarily the result of inception of highly active antiretroviral therapy (HAART) that com-bines the use of antiretroviral and protease inhibitor drugs.[163-165] The World Health Organization estimates that approximately 40 million individuals worldwide are infected by 1 of the 10 identified strains of HIV. The majority of these individuals are expected to die from lack of health care and unavailability of therapeutic drugs, complicated by nutritional deficiencies and the presence of other debilitating diseases. The AIDS epidemic consti-tutes the most severe medical crisis in world history.

Transmission of the virus from infected health care workers to patients has been reported on only three occasions.[166,167] One incident involved six patients who contracted the infection after treatment by one HIV-infected dentist.[166] Conversely, health care workers are at greater risk for seroconversion if injured while managing HIV-infected patients. The degree of risk appears to be directly related to high levels of plasma viral bioload in the patient being treated, and most events result from inadvertent exposure to infected blood. Deep penetration of the injury is a usual feature, although contact with large quantities of infected blood on mucous membranes may be another source of viral entry. To date, 103 docu-mented cases of HIV seroconversion because of occu-pational exposure have been reported in health care workers. No occupationally derived viral seroconver-sion has been documented among dental health care workers, although nine unconfirmed cases have been reported.[166,168] The reduced risk in the dental office may relate to the use of small-bore needles in dentistry and to the small amount of blood induced by most invasive dental procedures. Although injuries occur among dental workers, adherence to universal protective pre-cautions provides additional safety in dental practice. Nevertheless, every effort should be made to prevent occupational injury. All dental offices should have a standardized protocol of action in event of injury to a patient or dental worker.[169]

Human Immunodeficiency Virus/Acquired Immune Deficiency Syndrome Classification

Under current Centers for Disease Control (CDC) guide-lines, the presence of at least 1 of 25 specific clinical conditions constitute transition from HIV infection to AIDS[170] (Box 31-6). These conditions include plasma CD4-T lymphocytes less than 200/mm^3 or CD4-T lymphocyte percentage less than 14% of total lymphocytes. More recently, the level of the HIV plasma bioload has been determined to significantly influence the severity and frequency of HIV-related diseases and the ability of an infected individual to transmit the infection to others. With the advent of HAART, people with AIDS may obtain markedly increased T4 lymphocyte counts and markedly reduced viral loads. In some individuals, the T4 count may reach normal levels and viral bioload may decrease below the level of detection.[171] These individuals, how-ever, are still designated as patients with AIDS and may be infectious to others.[172] Despite the success of therapy, the virus is latent somewhere in the body and will return if medications are discontinued or if viral resistance develops.[173]

The acute phase of HIV infection occurs a few weeks to a few months after initial exposure. Although some individuals will not notice any symptoms, others will be affected by acute illness featuring malaise, fever, fatigue, myalgia, erythematous cutaneous eruptions, and possibly thrombocytopenia.[174] This phase may last for 1 to 2 weeks, but detectable seroconversion and antibody formation is delayed for 3 to 8 weeks or more.[175] The transition from HIV infection to outright AIDS signifies a gradual decrease in host immunity accompanied by increasing incidents of opportunistic infections. This transition has been markedly delayed with the advent of HAART and

Box 31-6   1993 CDC AIDS Surveillance Case Definition Conditions

- Candidiasis of esophagus, bronchi, trachea, or lungs
- Cervical cancer, invasive
- Coccidioidomycosis, disseminated or extrapulmonary
- Cryptococcosis, extrapulmonary
- Cryptosporidiosis, chronic intestinal (>1 month in duration)
- Cytomegalovirus disease (other than liver, spleen, or nodes)
- Cytomegalovirus retinitis (with loss of vision)
- Encephalopathy, HIV-related
- Herpes simplex: chronic ulcer(s) (>1 month in duration) or bronchitis, pneumonitis, or esophagitis
- Histoplasmosis, disseminated or extrapulmonary
- Isosporiasis, chronic intestinal (1 month in duration)
- Kaposi sarcoma
- Lymphoma, Burkitt's lymphoma, immunoblastic, primary of brain
- *Mycobacterium avium* complex, *Mycobacterium kansasii*, or other species, disseminated or extrapulmonary
- *Mycobacterium tuberculosis*, any site (pulmonary or extrapulmonary)
- *Pneumocystis carinii* pneumonia
- Pneumonia, recurrent
- Progressive multifocal leukoencephalopathy
- *Salmonella* septicemia, recurrent
- Toxoplasmosis of brain
- Wasting syndrome because of HIV

AIDS, Acquired immune deficiency syndrome; CDC, Centers for Disease Control; HIV, human immunodeficiency virus. Modified from the Centers for Disease Control: 1993 Revised classification system for HIV infection and expanded surveillance case definition for AIDS among adolescents and adults, MMWR 41:RR-17, December 18, 1992.

AIDS may not develop in many individuals for 15 or more years after initial infection.[176]

In the 1993 guidelines, the CDC established a surveillance case classification system on the basis of progressive loss of immunologic function.[170] This new classification is based on three ranges of CD4 cell counts (<200/mm^3, 200 to 499/mm^3, and ≥500/mm^3), combined with three clinical categories to produce a total of nine separate categories. AIDS is now defined objectively by a CD4 count less than 200/mm^3 or a CD4 percentage less than 14% of total lymphocytes. The AIDS definition based on CD4 percentage less than 14% was added to improve the accuracy of the classification system, because of the normal diurnal variation in raw numeric CD4 cell

counts that may cause differences in CD4 counts in blood samples taken at different times of the day (Table 31-1). Not all individuals pass progressively through these stages and the usefulness of the classification may have diminished with modern treatment methods. It is important to understand, however, that many AIDS treatment centers continue to follow these guidelines in determining when to initiate or to discontinue HAART. This is because of the severe adverse side effects sometimes associated with antiretroviral or protease inhibitor drugs.[177]

Oral Manifestations of Human Immunodeficiency Virus Infection

Oral lesions are common in HIV-positive individuals, and their presence may represent the first manifestation of HIV infection. Several reports have identified a strong correlation between HIV infection and oral candidiasis, certain malignancies (Kaposi sarcoma and non-Hodgkin's lymphoma), oral hairy leukoplakia (OHL), and some types of atypical periodontal diseases.[170,178-180] Other oral lesions found less commonly in HIV-infected individuals include mycobacterial infections, necrotizing stomatitis, oral ulcers of unknown origin, and viral infections such as herpes simplex, herpes zoster, and oral warts. There are also reports of a possible increase in incidence of recurrent aphthous stomatitis, bacillary angiomatosis (epithelioid angiomatosis), and less common viral infections such as CMV and molluscum contagiosum.[170,181,182] With the advent of HAART, the occurrence of oral manifestations has markedly diminished.[183-185] However, current HAART protocols delay the use of the drugs until immune suppression is relatively severe and discontinue their use once a satisfactory level of immune stability has been achieved. This new protocol suggests that orofacial opportunistic infections and other conditions related to decreasing immune competence may become more common than in the recent past. Therefore the dental practitioner must be aware of these lesions and their possible significance.

HAART drugs may induce significant adverse side effects including lipodystrophy, increased insulin resistance, gynecomastia, blood dyscrasias, exfoliative cheilitis, and possible increased incidence of oral warts.[186-188] Other side effects may include erythema multiforme, toxic epidermal necrolysis, oral lichenoid reactions, xerostomia, taste abnormalities, and perioral paresthesia.

Oral Candidiasis

Fungal infections of the oral cavity are common among HIV-infected individuals. On occasion, deep fungal infections may represent the first sign of HIV infection, but candidiasis is the most common lesion found in HIV-positive individuals.[188] Lesions may occur in the presence of only slight immunosuppression, but the incidence and

TABLE 31-1 **CDC Classification System for HIV Disease**

CD4 Lymphocyte Categories:

- Category 1:
- Category 2:
- Category 3:

- ≥500 cells/mm³
- 200-499 cells/mm³
- <200 cells/mm³

Clinical Categories:

Category A	One or more of the following: • Asymptomatic HIV infection • Persistent generalized lymphadenopathy • Acute (primary) HIV infection with accompanying illness or history of acute HIV infection
Category B	Conditions associated with cell-mediated immune defects such as: • Bacillary angiomatosis • Candidiasis: oropharyngeal (thrush); vulvovaginal; persistent, frequent, or poorly responsive to therapy • Cervical dysplasia (moderate or severe)/cervical carcinoma in situ • Constitutional symptoms, such as fever or diarrhea lasting ≥1 month • Herpes zoster (shingles), involving at least two distinct episodes or more than one dermatome • Idiopathic thrombocytopenic purpura • Listeriosis • Oral hairy leukoplakia • Pelvic inflammatory disease, particularly if complicated by tubo-ovarian abscess • Peripheral neuropathy
Category C	Patient has one or more of the conditions listed in CDC AIDS surveillance case definition (See Box 31-6)

AIDS, acquired immune deficiency syndrome; CDC, Centers for Disease Control; HIV, human immunodeficiency virus.
From the Centers for Disease Control: 1993 Revised classification system for HIV infection and expanded surveillance case definition for AIDS among adolescents and adults, MMWR 41:RR-17, December 18, 1992.

severity increases as the patient becomes more severely immunocompromised and viral bioload increases.[190] Candidal species are often found as normal commensal microorganisms in the oral cavity, and the organisms tend to overgrow in any circumstance in which host resistance is diminished. Candidiasis has been reported to be more prevalent in immunocompromised women than in men with similar viral bioload.[191,192] In HIV-positive individuals, the incidence and severity of candidal overgrowth tends to increase in direct proportion to the degree of immuno-suppression.[193] In most instances, *Candida albicans* is the causative organism. At least 11 species of *Candida* have been identified, however, and nonalbicans infections may be increasing. Candidal species such as *tropicalis, glabrata, krausei, kefyr, parapsilosis, inconspicua,* and *dubliniensis* may be more common in immunocompromised individuals.[194]

Candidal infection may occur in a variety of forms. Pseudomembranous candidiasis (thrush) is the form most often encountered in both HIV-positive and -negative individuals. Some evidence indicates that its presence and severity are closely associated with low CD4 lymphocyte counts in HIV-infected people.[195] It is characterized by the presence of creamy yellow-white, curdlike deposits that usually may be wiped away, leaving small punctate bleeding sites. It may occur anywhere in the oral cavity, and it may be asymptomatic (Fig. 31-14). On other occasions, patients may complain of burning discomfort or altered taste sensation.

Erythematous (atrophic) candidiasis is characterized by a generalized or patchy erythema. Its presence may be more closely related to high HIV bioload.[195] It may occur alone or simultaneously with the pseudomembranous form of the disease[196] (Fig. 31-15). It may affect the gingiva and may be clinically mistaken for desquamative gingivitis. On the tongue it may result in depapillation, and on occasion may be diagnosed as median rhomboid glossitis.

Hyperplastic candidiasis is also white, but the surface lesion usually does not rub away. It may be symptomatic or asymptomatic, and it may be mistaken for OHL if it occurs on the lateral borders of the tongue. In HIV-infected individuals, the hard and soft palate may be the most common sites of occurrence.

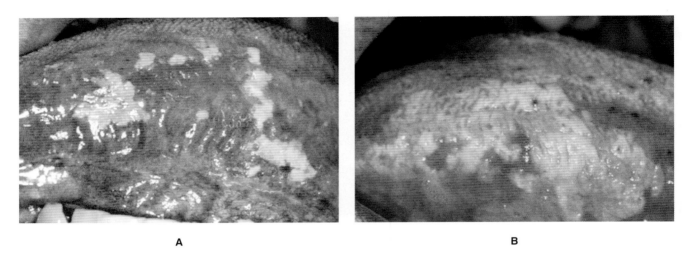

Figure 31-14. Pseudomembranous candidiasis on dorsum of tongue. **A,** The lesion may affect relatively small surface areas. This is a classic example of pseudomembranous candidiasis. **B,** A more widespread lesion of pseudomembranous candidiasis on the tongue.

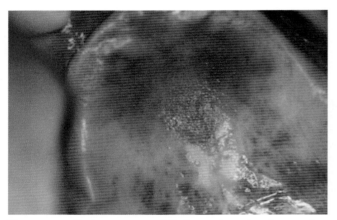

Figure 31-15. Erythematous candidiasis on the palate in a patient with human immunodeficiency virus who wore dentures. A smear was positive for *Candida*.

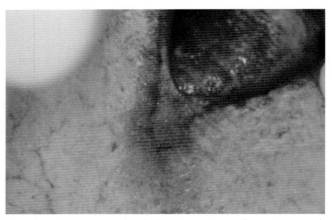

Figure 31-16. Severe angular cheilitis in a patient with xerostomia with acquired immune deficiency syndrome.

Angular cheilitis affects the commissure of the lips, and it is often caused by candidal infection (Fig. 31-16). Lesions may present as erythematous areas on perioral tissue but cracking and fissuring also may be a common feature. These lesions also tend to cause burning discomfort.

Diagnosis of oral candidiasis can be accomplished by culture, oral cytology, or biopsy. If available, cultures offer the advantage of speciation of the organisms present. Candidal hyphae and yeast forms may be identified in cytology and biopsy evaluation (Fig. 31-17). In most instances, however, a diagnostic method is not available to the clinician and diagnosis is based on the clinical features of the lesions.

Severe candidiasis may also occur in HIV-negative individuals in the presence of predisposing factors such as xerostomia, mouth breathing, wearing of removable dental appliances, recent use of antibiotics or topical or systemic immunosuppressant drugs, and general debilitation caused by underlying systemic disease. In HIV-infected individuals, esophageal candidiasis is diagnostic for AIDS.[170]

Therapy for oral candidiasis may include the use of topical antifungal agents such as nystatin oral suspension or clotrimazole lozenges. However, these agents contain sucrose, and patients who require long-term therapy may be better treated by dissolving vaginal tablets in the mouth. Itraconazole oral suspension contains saccharin as a substitute for sucrose. However, itraconazole is contraindicated if patients are taking a number of drugs, and careful medical review is indicated before it is prescribed. Amphotericin B oral suspension also may be effective. Chlorhexidine products have been reported to have some

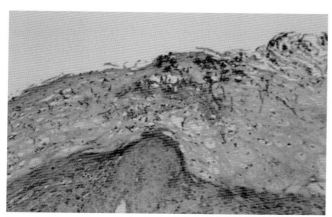

Figure 31-17. Microscopic view of candidiasis in biopsy specimen. Note penetration of candidal hyphae into the epithelial cell layer.

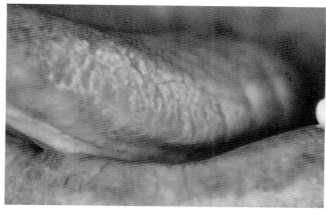

Figure 31-18. Oral hairy leukoplakia in a patient infected with human immunodeficiency virus. The lesions may be fairly subtle, such as in this example, or more fulminating in appearance.

antifungal properties, but those agents are probably best used for prevention rather than for treatment of established lesions. Systemic drugs useful in management of oral candidiasis include fluconazole, ketoconazole, itraconazole, and amphotericin B.[197] Candidal resistance to antifungal agents can be reduced by administering high dosages of the medications for a short time.[198] Although not all studies agree, some indicate that the advent of HAART has resulted in a decreased incidence of oropharyngeal candidiasis and resistance to antifungal agents.[184,199,200]

Oral Hairy Leukoplakia

OHL classically presents as painless white lesions found most often on the lateral borders of the tongue (Fig. 31-18). However, OHL also has been identified on the gingiva, floor of mouth, soft palate, and labial or buccal mucosa (Fig. 31-19).[201] The lesions may have a shaggy (hairy), corrugated appearance and they do not rub off. They are often secondarily infected with candidiasis. The etiologic agent for OHL has been identified as the Epstein–Barr virus, a member of the herpes virus group.[202]

Microscopically OHL presents with a hyperkeratotic surface and keratotic projections that resemble hairs. Beneath this surface, "balloon" cells resembling koilocytes are found. Koilocytes are most closely associated with infection by the human papillomavirus, and these "pseudo-koilocytes" created some initial confusion in identifying the causative agent. Acanthosis is also present but the inflammatory infiltrate is minimal.[203]

OHL was originally believed to occur exclusively in HIV-positive individuals and to represent a marker for impending transition to AIDS.[201,204] Later, OHL lesions were also identified in HIV-negative individuals who were

recipients of solid organ transplants and in others who were taking immunosuppressant drugs.[204] OHL has also been found on rare occasions in HIV-negative, immune competent individuals, and pseudo–hairy leukoplakia has been reported in individuals who do not have Epstein–Barr virus. Nonetheless, a histopathologic diagnosis of OHL warrants investigation of the patient's HIV status, if that is unknown.

OHL lesions are painless unless secondarily infected with candidiasis. Vigorous treatment is not necessary unless the lesion presents esthetic concerns. Lesions may be responsive to antiviral agents such as acyclovir, and some benefit has been reported with the use of topical podophyllin and possibly topically applied interferon. The condition tends to recur, however, if treatment is discontinued.

Most reports suggest that HAART has resulted in a markedly decreased incidence of OHL in individuals who are responsive to the drugs being used.[183,185] OHL

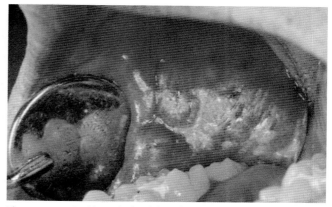

Figure 31-19. Oral hairy leukoplakia of right buccal mucosa.

that occurs despite HAART may signify either a severe immunodeficiency, a failure to take the prescribed medications, a declining dosage regimen of medications, or therapeutic failure.

Oral Malignancies

Kaposi Sarcoma. Kaposi sarcoma (KS) is an angiomatous malignant neoplasm that affects skin, mucosa, or internal organs (Fig. 31-20). By definition, an HIV-positive

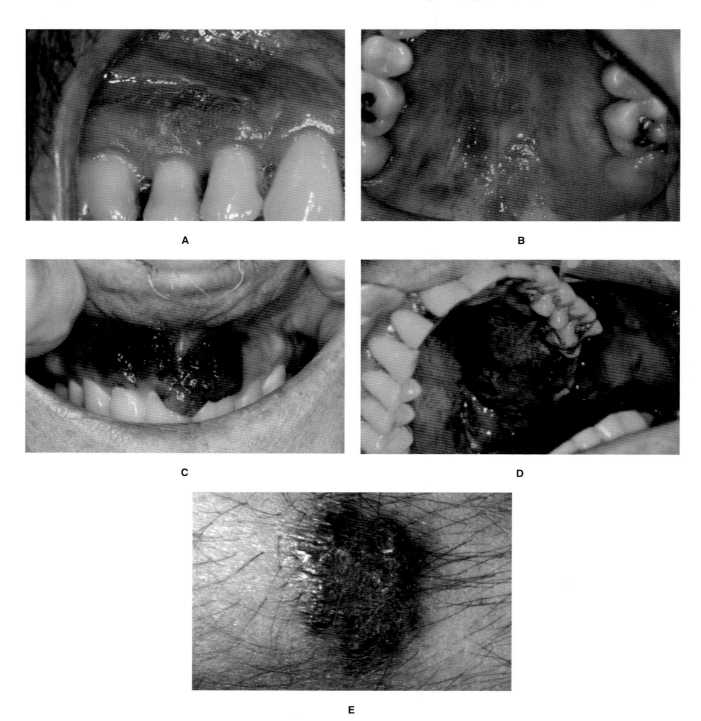

Figure 31-20. Kaposi sarcoma. **A,** Subtle appearance of oral Kaposi sarcoma on maxillary gingiva. **B,** Kaposi sarcoma of hard and soft palate. Note bluish-red discoloration. **C,** Large Kaposi sarcoma of labial gingiva in anterior maxillary region. **D,** Large Kaposi sarcoma affecting the palate and maxillary ridge. **E,** Kaposis sarcoma on the skin.

individual with KS is designated as having AIDS.[170,205] In recent years the presence of human herpes virus type 8 has been identified as necessary but not sufficient in itself to cause KS. Other factors, such as immunosuppression, play a major role.[205,206] The virus appears to be sexually transmitted but transmission from mother to infant has been reported.[207] KS is believed to be 7000-fold more likely to develop in HIV-infected individuals than in the general population.[208] Notably, however, approximately 30% of the HIV-negative adults in the United States may carry human herpes virus type 8 without complication unless the infected individual becomes immunocompromised.[209] KS has been reported in HIV-negative patients with lupus erythematosus, in renal transplant patients, and in other individuals receiving corticosteroid or cyclosporin therapy.[210]

Early oral lesions present as painless, flat, reddish purple mucosal macules, although occasionally the lesion may display normal pigmentation (Fig. 31-20). Lesions may subsequently become nodular in appearance and may mimic other vascular lesions such as hemangioma, hematoma, varicosity, or pyogenic granuloma. Diagnosis is based on histologic features.[211] When other oral conditions such as candidiasis exist in conjunction with KS, diagnosis may be more difficult.

With the advent of HAART the incidence of KS has been drastically reduced and existing lesions have been responsive to HAART therapy alone.[212] However, the lesions are still found in individuals who are unaware of their immunocompromised status, who have severe immunosuppression, or for whom HAART is failing. Systemic therapy with chemotherapy, radiotherapy, and/or immunotherapy may be necessary.

Localized oral lesions may require treatment if they are cosmetically troublesome or if they interfere with function. Therapy may include laser ablation, cryotherapy, radiation therapy, or intralesional injections with vinblastine or sclerosing agents.[212]

Non–Hodgkin's Lymphoma. Non–Hodgkin's lymphoma is also seen more frequently in immunocompromised individuals than in the general population, and its presence in an HIV-positive person places the individual in CDC Category C: AIDS.[170] The cause is unknown. The Epstein–Barr virus has been found in some types of non–Hodgkin's lymphoma, but an etiologic role for the virus has not been confirmed or supported by some studies.[213] Although HAART has resulted in a slight decline in incidence of the tumor, the decline is far less than that reported for KS.[214,215] However, the introduction of HAART has resulted in prolongation of overall survival rates among HIV-positive men even when the therapy is initiated after the diagnosis of a malignancy. Approximately 4% of individuals with non–Hodgkin's lymphoma will have oral lesions and, on occasion, the lesions are

confined entirely to the oral cavity. The lesion usually appears as a rapidly expanding, painful, fungating mass (Fig. 31-21). The gingiva and palate are common sites, and diagnosis is made on the basis of histopathologic features of the malignancy. Identification of oral non–Hodgkin's lymphoma should lead to immediate medical referral and an extensive search for lesions elsewhere in the body. Systemic treatment may include radiation therapy or chemotherapy, or both, and the dental practitioner should be prepared to assist in management of patients subjected to this type of therapy.

Squamous Cell Carcinoma. KS and non–Hodgkin's lymphoma represent approximately 95% of all neoplasms in patients with AIDS.[216] However, immunosuppressed individuals are at risk for developing other oral malignancies and there is evidence suggesting that the incidence of squamous cell carcinoma is increased in individuals with AIDS.[217] Oral squamous cell carcinoma comprises 2% to 3% of diagnosed malignancies in all patients in the United States, and evidence of an increased risk in patients with AIDS currently has not been confirmed.[218] Regardless, since the discovery of AIDS in 1981, there has been a progressive increase in the incidence of oral squamous cell carcinoma and anorectal carcinoma among homosexual men.[219] There are numerous case reports and case series suggesting atypical squamous cell carcinoma in immunocompromised individuals including those with HIV infection and AIDS. Lesions occur in significantly younger HIV-positive patients than in the general population.[220] To date, the effect of HAART on incidence of AIDS-associated squamous cell carcinoma is unknown.

Bacillary (Epithelioid) Angiomatosis. Bacillary (epithelioid) angiomatosis (BA) is an infectious vascular proliferative disease that closely mimics KS in both clinical and histopathologic features. The condition is caused by rickettsia-like organisms such as *Bartonellaceae henselae, Bartonellaceae quintana, Bartonellaceae bacilliformis,* or

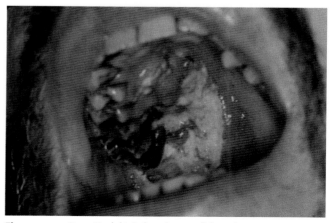

Figure 31-21. Non–Hodgkin's lymphoma of the palate.

others.[221,222] Gingival BA lesions may manifest as red, purple, or blue edematous soft tissue lesions capable of destroying the periodontal ligament and alveolar bone.[223,224] Differentiation of BA from KS is made on the basis of histopathologic appearance. Treatment with antirickettsial antibiotics may be effective, although BA lesions usually occur in individuals with very low CD4-T lymphocyte levels and high HIV bioloads.

Oral Hyperpigmentation. Oral or skin hyperpigmentation, or both, are relatively common in HIV-infected individuals, especially those receiving antiviral therapy.[225] Pigmented spots or striations may be found anywhere in the oral cavity, but the tongue may be most frequently involved (Fig. 31-22). Drugs such as azidothymidine, zidovudine, ketoconazole, or clofazimine are associated with hyperpigmentation.[226,227] Presence of these lesions should alert the clinician to the possibility that the HIV-positive patient may have developed adrenocortical insufficiency. This could occur as a result of infection with *Pneumocystis carinii* or various viruses, but drug therapy appears to be a common etiologic factor.[228,229]

Oral Ulcerations. Recurrent aphthous stomatitis has been described in HIV-positive individuals, possibly more frequently than in the general population.[230,231] However, data are lacking regarding incidence rates in the two groups.[181] Recurrent aphthous stomatitis lesions in immunocompromised individuals tend to be more severe and of longer duration, and they may require more vigorous treatment (Fig. 31-23). Proven successful methods of treatment include application of topical or intralesional corticosteroids, chlorhexidine or other antimicrobial rinses, oral tetracycline rinses, or topical amlexanox. On occasion, systemic corticosteroid therapy is necessary

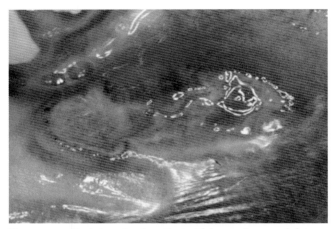

Figure 31-23. Oral ulceration in patient with human immunodeficiency virus. Lesions may be deeper and of longer duration in immunocompromised individuals.

to control the lesions and thalidomide has been reported to be successful in managing lesions resistant to other therapy.[231-233]

Atypical oral ulcerations may manifest as single, deeply cratered lesions of irregular shape and without the erythematous borders associated with recurrent aphthae. Available evidence suggests that these lesions are more common in severely immunocompromised individuals. They often are the result of CMV infection or coinfection with herpes simplex virus, Epstein–Barr virus, and CMV.[234,235] CMV is a member of the herpes family of viruses and at least one half of the general population is infected, but without clinical lesions. The outbreak of lesions appears to be associated with deterioration of immune competence. Extraoral sites of CMV lesions include the retina, colon, and esophagus. Diagnosis may require viral culture of a tissue biopsy, and treatment requires administration of potent antiviral agents such as valacyclovir, ganciclovir, foscarnet, or cidofovir.

The presence of persistent atypical oral ulcers should always increase the clinician's suspicions of squamous cell carcinoma, tuberculosis, actinomycosis, syphilis, deep fungal infections, or a variety of rare infectious diseases[236] (Fig. 31-24). Histoplasmosis and cryptococcosis are the most common deep fungal diseases. Oral lesions may occur on the gingiva, tongue or buccal mucosa and usually feature granulomatous, soft, boggy tissues that may or may not be ulcerated. Individuals with diseases of this nature require immediate medical attention and a search for extraoral lesions. HIV-associated neutropenia should be suspected if oral ulcers persist or symptoms suggestive of NUG do not improve with therapy.[237] Neutropenic ulcerations in HIV-positive individuals have been reported to be successfully treated using recombinant human G-CSF.

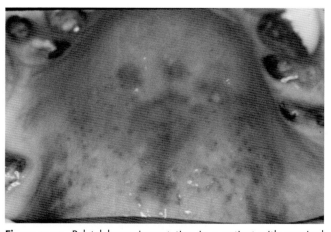

Figure 31-22. Palatal hyperpigmentation in a patient with acquired immune deficiency syndrome taking zidovudine. The lesions were similar to those seen in patients with adrenal insufficiency. The patient did not have Kaposi sarcoma.

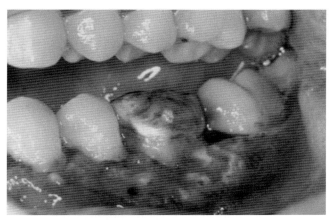

Figure 31-24. Gingival histoplasmosis in an individual who did not know his human immunodeficiency virus status until developing this deep fungal disease.

Oral ulcerations also may occur in association with infections by *Penicillium marneffei*, or enterobacterial microorganisms such as *Klebsiella pneumoniae, Enterobacter cloacae*, and *Escherichia coli*, although such infections are rare and are usually associated with systemic involvement.[224]

Herpes Simplex Virus Infection. Primary or recurrent herpes simplex viral infections are common in the general population and in immunocompromised individuals. Approximately 10% of HIV-positive patients may experience oral lesions. The infection may be caused by herpes simplex virus type 1 or type 2, and sexual transmission may occur. Primary herpes simplex virus infection may induce a severe, generalized, fiery red gingivitis, with small punctate ulcerations of the gingiva and other oral tissues. It is accompanied by lymphadenopathy and fever. Recurrent herpetic stomatitis features multiple, small vesicles that quickly rupture to form ulcerations. On occasion, these ulcerations may coalesce and give the appearance of other types of oral ulcers. The herpetic lesions may persist for months in immunocompromised patients, and the CDC HIV classification system designates mucocutaneous herpes of more than 1 month in duration as diagnostic of outright AIDS.[170]

Individuals who are severely immunocompromised may have larger, atypical herpetic lesions and viral culture is probably indicated for any ulcerative lesion occurring in an HIV-positive patient. Topical antiviral therapy for herpetic lesions of the lip may reduce the healing time, provided the medication is applied early in the onset of the lesions. Available topical drugs include acyclovir, penciclovir, or docosanol. Oral herpetic lesions are not responsive to topical therapy, and systemic antiviral agents such as acyclovir, valacyclovir, or famciclovir may be indicated.[238]

Adverse Drug Effects

A growing number of adverse effects have been reported related to the drugs used in management of patients with HIV infection. As mentioned earlier, oral and cutaneous hyperpigmentation is a common side effect of several drugs. Oral ulcerations have been reported in connection with use of foscarnet, interferon, and 2'-3'-dideoxycytidine. Didanosine has been associated with development of erythema multiforme, and zidovudine and ganciclovir may induce oral ulcers and mucositis secondary to leukopenia.[239] Other adverse drug reactions include: xerostomia, altered taste sensation, perioral paraesthesia, and lichenoid drug reactions.[186,240]

Adverse systemic drug reactions have become more common with the advent of HAART. Lipodystrophy is an abnormal distribution of body fat that often results in gaunt facial features and increased abdominal fat. The condition also may be associated with hyperlipidemia and may contribute to development of heart disease and hypertension. Drug-induced insulin resistance may contribute to development of diabetes. Other common effects include nausea, development of kidney stones, and enlarged breast size (gynecomastia) in male individuals. Multidrug therapy may also accelerate liver cirrhosis in individuals who are coinfected with hepatitis C and HIV.[241] Because of the many adverse effects associated with the newer recommended drug regimens, some physicians delay initiation of therapy until the HIV-positive patient begins to show signs and symptoms of significant immunosuppresstion.[164]

Exfoliative Cheilitis

Exfoliative cheilitis is an erythematous, edematous condition that affects the lips of some individuals with AIDS (Fig. 31-25). It features exfoliation of hyperkeratinized lip

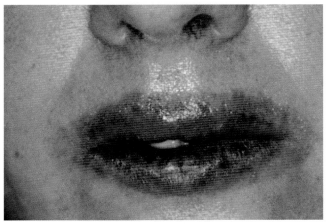

Figure 31-25. Exfoliative cheilitis, a newly identified perioral complication of highly active antiretroviral therapy (HAART).

epithelium, crater formation, fissuring, erosions, and the formation of papules, vesicles and blisters.[187] Perioral tissues also may be affected.

Exfoliative cheilitis has been reported as a factitious injury related to a habit of excessive licking of the lips, possibly complicated by secondary infection with *Candida* species.[242,243] It may be more common in individuals receiving chemotherapy or in those with AIDS, especially those being treated with HAART. It is highly likely that the condition is associated with drug-induced xerostomia and lip dryness, leading to chronic lip licking. No successful therapy has been described, but use of lip moisturizers and interruption of the licking habit could be of benefit.

Human Papillomavirus Lesions

More than 100 substrains of human papillomavirus have been identified and many of these substrains are associated with development of oral lesions in immune-deficient individuals. Epithelial papilloma, focal epithelial hyperplasia, and condyloma acuminatum are the most common disorders. Each features the development of single or multiple, elevated, wartlike lesions. Any area of the oral soft tissues may be affected (Fig. 31-26). Condyloma acuminatum is a sexually transmitted human papillomavirus infection that is associated with genital and perianal exophytic growths. Individuals who engage in unprotected oral/genital sex are susceptible to this infection in the oral cavity, and its eradication is one of the most perplexing problems in management of oral disease in immunocompromised individuals. Antiretroviral therapy is generally unsuccessful in controlling these lesions,

and available evidence indicates that HAART is associated with an increased incidence.[188]

Treatment usually consists of removal using laser ablation, cryotherapy, electrocautery, or intralesional bleomycin injections. However, the human papillomavirus is not eliminated from the oral tissues by removal of lesions and reactivation of latent virus is common. Recently, some long-term success has been reported using interferon either systemically or for intralesional injection, but the treatment is very expensive.[244] Periodic topical application of podophyllin appears to be beneficial in controlling genital and perirectal lesions, but the safety and efficacy of this drug in the oral cavity has not been adequately studied.[245] Topical cidofovir shows promise, but studies are limited.[246]

Salivary Gland Disease

Xerostomia is a frequent finding in immunocompromised individuals, in part because of anticholinergic side effects of many drugs used to manage HIV infection.[247] In the absence of normal salivary flow, oral tissues may be easily traumatized and candidiasis is prevalent. In one report, 29% of HIV-positive patients receiving medical treatment reported xerostomia. Individuals with a viral load greater than 100,000 cells/mm³ were 1.5 times more likely to experience dry mouth.[248] Thus it appears that HIV infection and its treatment may induce xerostomia and the condition may be irreversible.

Management of xerostomia is only partially successful but every effort should be made to alleviate HIV-associated oral dryness. Management principles include intake of copious amounts of water throughout the day. It may be

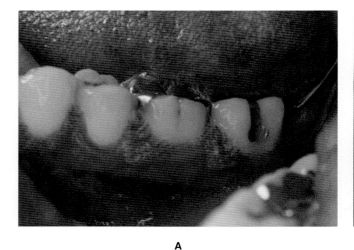

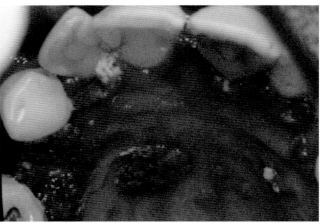

A   **B**

Figure 31-26. Human papillomavirus lesions. **A,** Lesions isolated to a few interproximal papillary areas. **B,** Lesions more widespread, affecting the maxillary gingiva and palatal mucosa.

possible to stimulate salivary flow by chewing sugarless gum and snacking on nonadherent foods such as raw carrots or celery. Systemic sialogogues such as pilocarpine or cevimeline may stimulate salivary flow, whereas artificial saliva substitutes may be of assistance to some individuals. Home and dental office use of topical fluorides is essential to prevent xerostomia-related dental caries.

Bilateral enlargement of major salivary glands has been reported in HIV-positive individuals, and the virus may have a direct adverse effect on the saliva-producing cells of the glands.[249] In addition, glandular enlargement is more common in patients receiving HAART.[248] The parotid salivary gland is most often involved. The significance of this phenomenon is not yet fully understood. The enlarged glands are painless, but the condition may interfere with salivary flow, causing xerostomia. Lacrimal, gastrointestinal, and lung secretions also may be diminished. Currently, there is no known treatment for glandular enlargement, but it is essential to thoroughly evaluate involved glands by biopsy or radiographic examination to rule out the possibility of other infections or neoplasms.

Delayed Wound Healing

Numerous reports suggest that patients infected with HIV may experience significantly delayed wound healing after invasive medical or dental procedures. This risk may be greater in those who are severely immunocompromised. However, postoperative complications appear relatively uncommon after most invasive dental procedures.[250-252] Currently, there are no reports of undue complications after periodontal procedures such as scaling and root planing, prophylaxis, periodontal surgery, or implant placement. Consequently, there appears to be no need for special precautions such as prophylactic antibiotic coverage on the basis of the patient's HIV status alone. However, the overall health status of each patient must be taken into consideration, and antibiotic coverage may be warranted when providing dental treatment for severely immunocompromised individuals.

Periodontal Diseases

Controversy exists over the relation of HIV infection to periodontal disease. Numerous studies suggest a correlation between the presence and severity of HIV infection and various forms of periodontal inflammation and disease. However, the majority of these studies do not take all confounding factors into consideration. Several reports have been based on findings in sexually transmitted disease clinics or dental institutions without HIV-negative control subjects. Other reports do not account for the varying degrees of immunodeficiency in the study population or for lifestyle factors such as intravenous drug use, poor oral hygiene, lack of dental care, nutritional deficiency, or tobacco smoking. In many instances, the oral diagnostic skills of examiners are subject to challenge and study participant selection is sometimes based on patient self-impressions of the presence of signs and symptoms of periodontal disease.[253] Therefore only a few studies provide evidence-based data regarding periodontal diseases in individuals with HIV/AIDS infection.

Chronic Periodontitis

Some controlled longitudinal or prevalence studies have report that chronic periodontitis is more common and/or severe among HIV-positive individuals.[254-257] However, the microbial flora found in periodontal pockets of HIV-positive individuals is consistent with the putative periodontal pathogens found in conventional periodontitis.[258,259] Accelerated periodontal pocket formation or attachment loss has been described by some, whereas others report the incidence and severity of chronic periodontitis to be similar in HIV-positive individuals and their HIV-negative control subjects.[260,261] However, several studies report increased gingival recession or clinical attachment loss, or both, in HIV-infected patients, suggesting that accelerated periodontis does occur in this patient population.[253,255-257,262]

On balance, the limited data available appear to affirm that periodontal destruction is more prevalent and somewhat more severe in HIV-positive individuals, and that this susceptibility may worsen as CD4-T cell counts decrease and as viral bioload increases.[263,264] There is ample evidence, however, that an individual with AIDS may maintain periodontal health throughout his or her lifetime. In addition, the incidence of chronic periodontitis may be decreasing with the advent of HAART.[265]

Human Immunodeficiency Virus–Associated Periodontal Diseases

In 1993, the European Community Clearing House on Oral Problems Related to HIV Infection published a widely accepted classification and diagnostic criteria for oral lesions seen in association with HIV infection.[181] Several periodontal conditions were among those reported to be strongly associated. These were linear gingival erythema (LGE), necrotizing (ulcerative) gingivitis, and necrotizing (ulcerative) periodontitis. Less commonly seen was necrotizing (ulcerative) stomatitis, a condition that may be an extension of the other necrotizing diseases. Notably, these conditions also occur in HIV-negative individuals with the same or greater frequency than in those who are HIV-positive. None of these periodontal diseases occurs exclusively in HIV-positive individuals regardless of their immune status or viral bioload and it is inappropriate to use terminology that gives this implication. The following discussion addresses these conditions.

Linear Gingival Erythema

LGE has been described as a linear, erythematous, sometimes painful gingivitis that may occur in three forms: (1) a linear pattern of erythema confined to the gingival margin, (2) punctate or diffuse erythema that extends into the attached gingiva, and (3) diffuse inflammation that extends from the gingival margin into the alveolar mucosa (Fig. 31-27). LGE may be found in the absence of normal quantities of bacterial plaque commonly associated with gingivitis, and a reduction in bleeding on probing has been reported.[266]

The etiology of LGE is unclear. The microbial flora may be consistent with plaque-related marginal gingivitis or may be more typical of periodontitis.[258] Recent evidence indicates that on most occasions various subspecies of *Candida* can be identified in LGE lesions, and case reports describe complete or partial remission after administration of systemic antifungal therapy.[267,268] In fact, the current classification system for periodontal diseases and conditions lists LGE as a gingival disease of fungal origin (see Chapter 2).

LGE may be more common in children and young adults and is often resistant to conventional periodontal therapy.[264] Conversely, it may undergo spontaneous remission.[269] The condition was originally believed to be a possible precursor to necrotizing gingivitis or periodontitis. There is little evidence, however, to suggest that it is any more harmful to the periodontal supporting structures than plaque-related gingivitis.[22,264,266]

Necrotizing Ulcerative Gingivitis

Existence of a painful, easily bleeding, erythematous, ulcerative gingivitis has been described occasionally throughout recorded history. The condition is believed to occur in individuals who have diminished host resistance caused by a variety of factors such as smoking, emotional or physical stress, poor oral hygiene, or underlying systemic disease. It is logical to assume that the incidence of NUG is greater in immunocompromised individuals and most, but not all evidence, supports this impression. However, some studies report NUG to be more frequent in individuals with normal or only slightly diminished CD4-T cell counts.[270,271]

Classically NUG involves destruction of interdental papillae but, if untreated, marginal gingiva may be affected as well (Fig. 31-28). The interdental area develops a "punched out" appearance and spontaneous bleeding may occur. It may be accompanied by fever, lymphadenopathy, and general malaise. The microbial flora includes fusiform bacilli, spirochetes, and putative periodontal pathogens such as *P. intermedia*.

Necrotizing Ulcerative Periodontitis

A necrotizing ulcerative form of periodontitis (NUP) has been described that features rapid, mild to severe destruction of gingival tissues and alveolar bone (Fig. 31-29). The condition may be generalized, but more commonly it is localized to a few sites in the dental arches. Some evidence indicates that NUP is an extension of NUG.[264] NUP usually begins in the interproximal areas and it has been described as exquisitely painful. In this event, immediate treatment is indicated. However, over time, individuals affected with NUP cease to have pain, and they sustain deep interproximal craters that may result in superimposition of conventional periodontitis in the NUP site.[266]

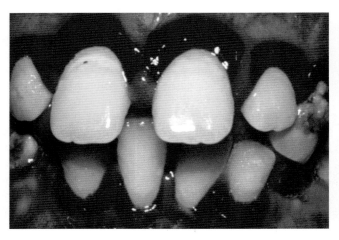

A

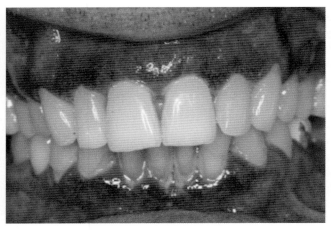

B

Figure 31-27. Linear gingival erythema. **A,** Intense, well defined, fiery red band of gingiva along the facial aspect of the incisors. **B,** More diffuse redness in maxillary gingiva, with linear pattern in mandibular incisor region.

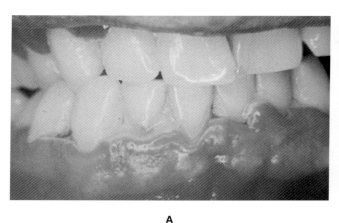
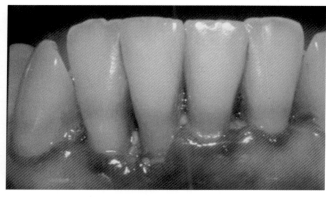

A   B

Figure 31-28. Necrotizing ulcerative gingivitis. **A,** Interproximal gingival necrosis noted in mandibular anterior region. **B,** More extensive necrosis with classic "punched out" interproximal papillae. If necrosis continues, patient will have necrotizing ulcerative periodontitis.

Several studies indicate that the microbial flora of NUP is consistent with that associated with chronic periodontitis.[270,272] Other studies, however, describe the presence of fuso-spirochetal microorganisms consistent with those found in NUG.[262] The condition may serve as a marker for increased immune suppression in HIV-positive individuals.[273] On occasion, it may be the first indication of the presence of an immunocompromising condition, and patients with NUP who are unaware of their HIV status should be encouraged to obtain serologic testing.

Necrotizing Ulcerative Stomatitis

Necrotizing ulcerative stomatitis is an acutely painful, severely destructive, fuso-spirochetal condition that has occasionally been reported in HIV-positive individuals or others who are severely debilitated. Soft and hard tissues of the oral cavity may undergo extensive damage that is not self-limiting. Histopathologic and immunochemical evaluation indicate that ulceration, necrosis, histocytic vasculitis, and other changes are present in a reproducible pattern.[274] Several case reports describe necrotizing ulcerative stomatitis as a continuation of NUG and NUP.[262,275] A similar condition (noma, cancrum oris) has been described in children living in sub-Saharan Africa and may represent the same ulceronecrotic disease. Predisposing factors in the African children include poverty, malnutrition, poor oral hygiene, and infectious diseases such as measles or those caused by herpesviridae.[124,276]

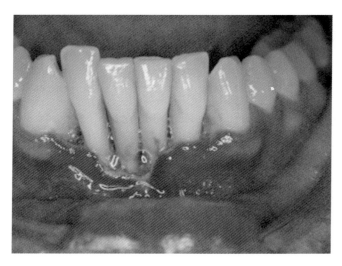

Figure 31-29. Necrotizing ulcerative periodontitis. Severe loss of bone and soft tissue.

OTHER CONDITIONS AFFECTING THE PERIODONTIUM

In addition to the conditions described earlier, a variety of other systemic disorders may impact the oral cavity, and particularly the periodontium. Most of these conditions have widespread systemic effects, and the periodontium is only one of many organs affected.

Paget's Disease of Bone (Osteitis Deformans)

Paget's disease of bone is a nonmalignant disease involving accelerated bone resorption followed by deposition of dense, chaotic, and ineffectively mineralized osseous matrix.[277] The affected, poorly mineralized bones are often distorted. The bones most commonly affected are the long bones of the legs, the lower spine, pelvis, and skull. The origin of the disease is unknown. Paget's disease is frequently asymptomatic; however, the patient may present with symptoms depending on the bones involved. The most common symptom is pain in the affected bone. Complications may affect vision, hearing, the nervous system, and the heart. The disease is usually diagnosed radiographically as an incidental finding during examination for other problems. The incidence of Paget's disease increases with age, and there is a slight predominance for the male sex. Pain may be present before radiographic changes, and the diagnosis at that time is often missed. The pain is aggravated by weight bearing if the lower extremity or spine is involved.

Headache, dizziness, and hearing loss result from Paget's disease in the skull. Cranial enlargement develops over many years. With marked involvement of the skull, patients may have cranial nerve compression. Other skeletal deformities can include distortion of the clavicles, multiple compression fractures, pagetic vertebrae resulting in severe kyphosis, and unexpected pathologic fractures. Patients who have one third or more of the skeleton involved can have increased cardiac output, only to increase vascularity of the bone lesions. This can ultimately lead to congestive heart failure.

Jaw involvement in Paget's disease is common, with the maxilla more commonly targeted. Jaw involvement is usually symmetric, although unilateral lesions may occur. There is a gradual enlargement of the maxilla or the mandible, or both. This osseous enlargement in the edentulous patient often causes an inability to wear existing dentures, which may be the initial presenting sign of underlying disease. In patients with teeth, the expansion of the jaws results in spreading, flaring, and mobility of the dentition and the production of an abnormal occlusal pattern.

The characteristic osteolytic, osteoblastic, and combined phases are evident in Paget's disease of the jaw. The initial demineralization is reflected by an increase in fine bony trabeculation and a ground glass appearance of bone. Radiolucent, ill-defined, demineralized areas also may be apparent. The osteoblastic and combined phases produce the well known "cotton wool appearance" associated with the disease. Bone during the final "burnout" stage is extremely dense and radiopaque.

A gradual encroachment by Paget's bone on the teeth is occasionally observed. Radiographic changes include a gradual loss of lamina dura, hypercementosis, and occasional calcification of pulp chambers. Increased periapical radiolucencies have been associated with involved teeth, with little or no differentiation between tooth and bone. Progressive root resorption may occur.

Bisphosphonates are the most common treatment for Paget's disease.[278] These drugs, such as alendronate and risedronate, concentrate selectively in the skeleton at active sites of Paget's disease and suppress osteoclastic bone resorption.

Hypophosphatasia

Hypophosphatasia is a rare familial disease caused by mutations in the alkaline phosphatase gene responsible for tissue nonspecific (liver, kidney, and bone) alkaline phosphatase production. The deficiency in this important enzyme results in abnormal mineralization of bone and cementum, resulting in skeletal abnormalities and cemental hypoplasia. The disease comes in a variety of forms, including a lethal form that is evident shortly after birth (congenital lethal hypophosphatasia), a severe form during infancy, and a milder form occurring later in childhood.[93] Cardinal features of the disease are rickets and/or osteomalacia of variable severity, with a low serum and bone alkaline phosphatase level and the excretion of excessive amounts of phosphoethanolamine in the urine.

Dental abnormalities are common in hypophosphatasia, the first clinical symptom of which is often the premature loss of primary teeth.[279] The teeth most frequently involved are the primary mandibular central and lateral incisors, followed by the maxillary incisors and, less commonly, the posterior teeth. Primary incisors are usually lost before 24 months of age. Permanent teeth may or may not be affected. The teeth are lost despite minimal signs of inflammation. Additional signs of hypophosphatasia include loss of alveolar bone, lack of periodontal ligament integrity, and reduced or complete absence of cementum. If the disorder affects the permanent dentition, the clinical presentation may be similar to localized aggressive periodontitis.

Radiographic evidence of hypophosphatasia affecting the teeth consists of enlarged pulp chambers and root canals, sometimes giving the tooth a "shell" appearance; reduction in the thickness of the dentin and irregular dentin formation with large dentinal tubules and many areas of interglobular dentin; enamel hypoplasia; and irregular calcifications and lesions in the alveolar bone. The histologic features of the jawbone are similar to those of rickets and osteomalacia.

Periodontal treatment in the primary dentition is usually futile; instead, extraction of mobile teeth should be performed to improve comfort. In the permanent dentition, more conventional periodontal therapy may be attempted. In one long-term study of three individuals who were diagnosed with hypophosphatasia as children and then managed over 15 years, the permanent teeth were all retained, despite poor oral hygiene.[280] Thus the periodontal manifestations of hypophosphatasia are limited to the primary dentition in most cases and are not as likely to be seen in adults.

Inflammatory Bowel Disease (Crohn's Disease and Ulcerative Colitis)

Inflammatory bowel disease (IBD) is an inflammatory disease of the small or large intestine consisting of two chronic clinical entities: Crohn's disease and ulcerative colitis. The inflammation involves all layers of the gut, thus the term transmural colitis has been used to describe this disease in the colon. Whereas ulcerative colitis is usually contiguous, beginning in the rectum and extending retrograde to involve various portions of the colon, Crohn's disease is usually segmental, and there is normal intestine between areas of inflammation. Most commonly, the terminal ileum and colon are involved. Lesions also have been reported in the esophagus, stomach, and duodenum. Gross examination may reveal mucosal ulceration, aphthous ulcers within mucosa that appears normal, deep ulcers within areas of swollen mucosa, and long linear ulcers. Serpiginous areas of mucosal hemorrhage may alternate with areas of gross hemorrhage.[281] Osteopenia and osteoporosis often are seen in Crohn's disease.[282]

Although the onset of symptoms is not totally understood, IBD is likely caused by a complex combination of genetic, environmental, and bacterial triggering events that activate immune and nonimmune systems within the intestine. Cell-mediated and humoral immune systems are involved and a combination of antibodies, cytokines, growth factors, prostaglandins, leukotrienes, reactive oxidative metabolites, nitric oxide, and proteolytic enzymes culminate in chronic inflammation and tissue damage. Crohn's disease tends to undergo periods of exacerbation and remission. In fact, the onset and progression of IBD and periodontal diseases share similar pathophysiologic mechanisms involving chronic exposure to bacterial antigens and a persistent immunoinflammatory response.[283]

Oral lesions have been found in approximately 6% to 20% of patients with Crohn's disease. They can occur at any time during the course of the disease and may be present before intestinal involvement is demonstrable. These lesions may recur in various forms in different locations in the same patient and may or may not be correlated with the exacerbation and remission of intestinal symptoms. Oral lesions occur more commonly in patients with disease involving the colon rather than those confined to the small bowel. Patients with extraintestinal manifestations of Crohn's disease, such as skin and joint lesions, have a greater chance of having oral manifestations.

The oral lesions seen in patients with Crohn's disease are either "specific" or "nonspecific," as differentiated by clinical and histologic features. "Specific" oral lesions are histologically similar to the intestinal lesions of the disease. They most commonly occur in the mucobuccal fold or buccal mucosa, where they are described as having a lobulated, hypertrophic, fissured appearance, with or without linear ulcerations. The diffuse buccal lesions have a "cobblestone" appearance that is characteristic of Crohn's disease. Lesions on vestibular and retromolar mucosa are indurated and polypoid, often resembling

denture granulomas (epulis fissuratum). Specific lesions of the gingiva, alveolar mucosa, and lips appear as areas of diffuse red swelling, sometimes accompanied by angular cheilitis. "Nonspecific" lesions are recurrent aphthous ulcers and are probably the most common oral sign of Crohn's disease. The onset of these ulcers, which are generally widespread and severe, may be concurrent with bowel symptoms. Oral lesions generally regress when intestinal symptoms are brought under control. Local steroids may reduce inflammation in some patients.

A number of reports of periodontal disease in patients with IBD have been published, but most have examined small numbers of patients.[284,285] Some of these reports suggest that more aggressive forms of periodontitis are seen in patients with IBD. Conversely, larger studies suggest no relation between IBD and periodontitis.[286]

A link between periodontitis and neutrophil defects in patients with IBD has been proposed. Some researchers have identified depressed neutrophil chemotaxis in patients with IBD.[287] Others have found neutrophil chemotaxis consistently suppressed in patients with periodontitis and ulcerative colitis, but not in those with periodontitis and Crohn's disease, or in patients with IBD without periodontitis.[285] Still other researchers suggest an exuberant neutrophil response in IBD, which may amplify the inflammatory response and increase tissue destruction.[281,284] Currently, the relation between IBD and periodontal diseases remains unclear.

Ehlers–Danlos Syndromes

The Ehlers–Danlos syndromes (EDS) are a group of connective tissue disorders characterized by hypermobility of joints, hyperextensibility of skin, and increased tissue friability. For many years the disorder was thought to be a single entity, but it has since been shown to exhibit extensive heterogeneity with at least 10 types classified on the basis of clinical presentation and inheritance pattern (Table 31-2).[93] Dental abnormalities could serve as important diagnostic clues when associated with other features of EDS. Both hard and soft oral tissues can be affected in this disorder. Excessive fragility of the gingival tissues is apparent. Dental hard tissue findings include hypoplastic enamel and structural changes associated with the dentinoenamel and cementodentinal junctions, irregular dentin formation, and increased tendency for development of pulp stones. Several of these developmental pulpal aberrations result in calcification of pulp tissue or malformed, stunted roots, or both. Hypermobility of the temporomandibular joint can result in repeated joint dislocation in some individuals.

The recognition of EDS is especially important in treating oral problems associated with wound healing.[288] Many patients with EDS have a history of excessive or prolonged bleeding; therefore, the clinician must obtain

TABLE 31-2   Classification of Ehlers–Danlos Syndrome Types

TYPE	INHERITANCE PATTERN	CLINICAL FEATURES	BASIC DEFECT
• I (Gravis)	• AD	• Generalized severe joint hypermobility; skin hyperextensibility; easy bruising; molluscoid pseudotumors; subcutaneous spheroids; poor wound healing; premature rupture of fetal membranes	• Unknown
• II (Mitis)	• AD	• Similar to ED I but milder; joint laxity limited to hands and feet; little cutaneous involvement and tissue friability	• Unknown
• III (Benign hypermobile)	• AD	• Severe hypermobility of all joints; minimal skin involvement	• Unknown
• IV (Sack's ecchymotic)	• AD/AR	• Spontaneous rupture of large arteries; perforation of bowel; thin skin with prominent underlying veins	• Reduced or absent synthesis of type III collagen
• V (X-linked)	• XL	• Marked hyperextensibility of skin; minimal joint hypermobility	• Possible deficiency of lysyl oxidase
• VI (Ocular)	• AR	• Severe scoliosis; moderate joint involvement; ocular fragility with scleral rupture or retinal detachment; hyperelastic skin	• Deficiency of lysyl hydroxylase
• VII (Arthrochalasis multiplex congenital)	• AD-AR	• Congenital hip dislocation; short stature; generalized joint hypermobility; hyperelastic, velvety skin	• Deficiency of procollagen peptidase (affects mainly type I collagen)
• VIII (Periodontitis)	• AD	• Periodontitis; mild to moderate skin hyperextensibility and joint hypermobility; marked skin friability	• Unknown
• IX (X-linked recessive skeletal)	• XL	• Mild skin hyperelasticity; widening and bowing of long bones; deformed clavicles; occipital exostoses	• Defective collagen cross-linking
• X (Dysfibronectinemia)	• AR	• Joint hypermobility; moderate skin hyperelasticity; defective platelet aggregation	• Dysfunction in plasma fibronectin

AD, Autosomal dominant; AR, autosomal recessive; ED, Ehlers–Danlos; XL, X-linked.

a thorough bleeding history. It is possible to perform intraoral surgical procedures on most patients with EDS without any untoward effects, although special precaution must be taken to prevent postoperative hemorrhage. In addition, because of tissue fragility great care should be exercised in placing sutures to minimize tissue tearing. Wound healing may be considerably impaired.[288]

EDS type VIII warrants specific discussion because the distinguishing feature of this disorder is aggressive early-onset periodontitis.[288] Skin hyperextensibility and fragility, tendency to bruising with minor trauma, tissue

scarring, and hyperextensible finger joints also may be present to varying degrees. In some cases, aggressive periodontitis is the first presenting sign of the underlying connective tissue disorder.[289] The literature reveals numerous case reports of patients with EDS with severe periodontal destruction, often at an early age. Some cases demonstrate less severe bone and attachment loss. EDS types VIII and IV may appear very similar clinically, except that periodontal involvement is not usually seen in type IV.[290] It is important for the clinician to distinguish between these two forms of the disease, because type IV has the potential to be life-threatening. In EDS type IV, there is a defect in formation of type III collagen, a major component of blood vessels and internal organs. This defect can lead to rupture of major blood vessels, the intestines, or the uterus. A skin biopsy to evaluate the structure and biosynthesis of collagen can help to distinguish EDS type IV from other phenotypically similar forms of the disease.[93]

Sturge–Weber Syndrome

Sturge–Weber syndrome, or encephalotrigeminal syndrome, consists of craniofacial angiomatosis and cerebral calcification.[291] The cutaneous vascular nevus, often called a *port wine stain*, varies in size and shape and is present at birth. It is usually located along the course of the superior and middle branches of the trigeminal nerve. There is an associated meningeal hemangioma on the same side, with calcification and cortical atrophy of adjacent brain tissue, often resulting in contralateral Jacksonian convulsions, paralysis, sensory deficit, and mental retardation. Although the nevus is usually unilateral with a sharp border, it may be bilateral or midline. The oral mucous membranes may be affected on the same side, and glaucoma may be present in the ipsilateral eye. The cause of the Sturge–Weber syndrome is unknown.

Characteristic calcification in the outer layer of the cerebral cortex may be seen in radiographs of the skull as sinuous, double-contoured lines ("tram lines") that follow the convolutions of the cerebral cortex on the affected side. It is demonstrated quite well with computed tomography scanning. Treatment is directed at the neurologic manifestations. Because the occurrence is sporadic and cannot be determined before birth, there are no preventive measures available. The diagnosis of Sturge–Weber syndrome should be suspected in all children with a typical facial nevus and neurologic symptoms.

In addition to angiomas of the face, mucosal involvement may be seen. Oral involvement, seen in about 40% of patients, consists of a bluish red lesion that blanches on pressure and is found most commonly on the buccal mucosa and lips. Occasionally seen are lesions involving the gingiva and palate. When present on the gingiva, the angioma often causes gingival enlargement, which may range from slight vascular hyperplasia to extremely large masses that make closure of the mouth impossible.[291,292] This complication of gingival enlargement may be caused by the increased vascular component or the phenytoin (Dilantin: Parke-Davis [Division of Warner-Lambert]; Morris Plains, NJ) therapy, or both, often used to manage the epileptic seizures common to the syndrome. The floor of the mouth and tongue are rarely involved. Alveolar bone changes rarely have been reported, although a few cases of bizarre bone resorption, widened bony trabeculation, and excessive tooth mobility may be seen.

Because the angiomas of Sturge–Weber syndrome may involve oral tissues, periodontal and oral surgical procedures in the affected area may be associated with severe and at times fatal hemorrhage. The clinician must take hemostatic precautions such as splints, pressure dressings, antifibrinolytic agents, and hospitalization. Treatment of gingival enlargement has been accomplished by means of complete surgical excision, injection of sclerosing solutions, radiation therapy, carbon dioxide snow, and electrodissection.

Wegener's Granulomatosis

Wegener's granulomatosis is a disseminated granulomatous necrotizing vasculitis of the small vessels of the upper and lower respiratory tract. In the generalized form, glomerulonephritis is an important component of the disease process. Although a localized, limited form confined to the airways has been described, this probably represents an early stage of generalized disease before the development of detectable renal disease. The histologic features characteristic of Wegener's granulomatosis include necrotizing vasculitis of small arteries and veins with coexistent granuloma formation.

The mean age at onset is 40 years. Early in the disease the clinical picture is dominated by upper respiratory tract signs, including rhinorrhea, paranasal discharge, septal perforations, saddle nose deformity, and otitis media. However, virtually any manifestation of the disease may be seen at the time of presentation. Patients frequently demonstrate persistent epistaxis (nosebleed) as an initial clinical presentation of the disease. Nonspecific pulmonary complaints may include cough, hemoptysis (bloody sputum), chest discomfort, and shortness of breath. It is not uncommon for asymptomatic pulmonary infiltrates to be seen on radiographs of the chest. Renal disease is characterized by focal and segmental glomerulonephritis. Virtually any organ system may be involved in Wegener's granulomatosis, but these manifestations are usually less dramatic in comparison with the respiratory tract and renal disease. Skin disease results from vasculitis with or without granuloma formation and is manifested in up to 50% of patients as petechiae, purpura, papules, vesicles, ulcerations, or subcutaneous nodules.

A variety of oral lesions have been described in association with Wegener's granulomatosis.[293] The most common is a distinctive hyperplastic gingivitis originating in the interdental papilla areas. The gingiva is generally described as granular and red to purple with many petechiae, and it has been termed *strawberry gingivitis*.[294] The lesions extend to the labial and buccal aspects, eventually involving the entire gingiva and periodontium, resulting in tooth mobility and loss of teeth.[295] Once the teeth are lost, extraction sites do not heal properly.

Oral and other mucosal membrane ulcerations also can occur. There have been reports of extensive ulcerative stomatitis. In many cases these lesions are the initial manifestation of the disease. On biopsy, the distinct histologic feature of the gingival lesion is the unusual combination of well formed multinucleated giant cells in the midst of an acute inflammatory infiltrate in the absence of a demonstrable pathogen.

Before the advent of chemotherapy, the prognosis was poor for patients with Wegener's granulomatosis. Early diagnosis and institution of treatment are important factors in determining survival. The gingival involvement diminishes after cytotoxic therapy in responsive patients. The dentist may play an important role in the early detection of Wegener's granulomatosis by associating the oral manifestations with other clinical signs and symptoms.

Heavy Metal Poisoning

Systemic absorption of certain heavy metals, such as mercury, bismuth, lead, and arsenic, can produce pigmentation or discoloration of oral mucosal surfaces, including the gingiva.[296] These metals may come from environmental exposure or from certain medications. Although uncommon, heavy metal poisoning must be ruled out if unusual pigmentation is noted by the clinician. Typically, these metals produce a black or bluish line in the gingiva that follows the gingival margin. This pigmentation is more likely to be seen in areas where marginal gingival inflammation exists. Metals that have been absorbed systemically are carried in the bloodstream and then precipitated into the tissues from the blood vessels. Therefore, when inflammation is present and vascular permeability increases, the metals are more likely to be deposited into the gingival tissues. Periodontal therapy aimed at reducing gingival inflammation may result in disappearance of the pigmentation, even without discontinuation of metal exposure.

REFERENCES

1. Mealey BL: Diabetes mellitus. In Rose LF, Genco RJ, Mealey BL, Cohen DW, editors: *Periodontal medicine*, Toronto, 2000, BC Decker Publishers.

2. Loe H: Periodontal disease. The sixth complication of diabetes mellitus, *Diabetes Care* 16(suppl 1):329-334, 1993.

3. Mokdad AH, Ford ES, Bowman BA et al: The continuing increase of diabetes in the U.S., *Diabetes Care* 24:412, 2001.

4. American Diabetes Association: Economic consequences of diabetes mellitus in the U.S. in 1997, *Diabetes Care* 21:296-309, 1998.

5. American Diabetes Association: Report of the expert committee on the diagnosis and classification of diabetes mellitus, *Diabetes Care* 26(suppl 1):s5-s20, 2003.

6. Ford ES, Williamson DF, Liu S: Weight change and diabetes incidence: findings from a national cohort of U.S. adults, *Am J Epidemiol* 146:214-222, 1997.

7. Resnick H, Valsania P, Halter J, Lin X: Relation of weight gain and weight loss on subsequent diabetes risk in overweight adults, *J Epidemiol Community Health* 54:596-602, 2000.

8. American Diabetes Association: Gestational diabetes mellitus, *Diabetes Care* 26(suppl 1):103-105, 2003.

9. Langer O, Rodriguez DA, Xenakis EMJ et al: Intensified versus conventional management of gestational diabetes, *Am J Obstet Gynecol* 170:1036-1047, 1994.

10. Vlassara H, Bucala R: Recent progress in advanced glycation and diabetic vascular disease: role of advanced glycation end product receptors, *Diabetes* 45(suppl 3): s65-s66, 1996.

11. Iacopino AM: Periodontitis and diabetes interrelationships: role of inflammation, *Ann Periodontol* 6:125-137, 2001.

12. Bierhaus A, Hofmann MA, Ziegler R, Nawroth PP: AGEs and their interaction with AGE-receptors in vascular disease and diabetes mellitus. I. The AGE concept, *Cardiovasc Res* 37:586-600, 1998.

13. Lalla E, Lamster IB, Stern DM, Schmidt AM: Receptor for advanced glycation end products, inflammation, and accelerated periodontal disease in diabetes: mechanisms and insights into therapeutic modalities, *Ann Periodontol* 6:113-118, 2001.

14. Lalla E, Lamster IB, Drury S et al: Hyperglycemia, glycoxidation and receptor for advanced glycation end products: potential mechanisms underlying diabetic complications, including diabetes-associated periodontitis, *Periodontology 2000* 23:50-62, 2000.

15. Meurman JH, Collin HL, Niskanen L et al: Saliva in non-insulin-dependent diabetic patients and control subjects. The role of the autonomic nervous system, *Oral Surg Oral Med Oral Pathol Oral Radiol Endod* 86:69-76, 1998.

16. Fisher BM, Lamey PJ, Samaranayake LP et al: Carriage of *Candida* species in the oral cavity in diabetic patients: relationship to glycaemic control, *J Oral Pathol* 16:282-284, 1987.

17. Phelan JA, Levin SM: A prevalence study of denture stomatitis in subjects with diabetes mellitus or elevated plasma glucose levels, *Oral Surg Oral Med Oral Pathol* 62:303-305, 1986.

18. Jones RB, McCallum RM, Kay EJ et al: Oral health and oral health behavior in a population of diabetic clinic attenders, *Community Dent Oral Epidemiol* 20:204-207, 1992.

19. Tavares M, DePaola P, Soparkar P, Joshipura K: Prevalence of root caries in a diabetic population, *J Dent Res* 70:979-983, 1991.

20. Collin HL, Uusitupa M, Niskanen L et al: Caries in patients with non-insulin-dependent diabetes mellitus, *Oral Surg Oral Med Oral Pathol Oral Radiol Endod* 85:680-685, 1998.

21. Papapanou PN: Periodontal diseases: epidemiology, *Ann Periodontol* 1:1-36, 1996.

22. Mealey BL: Periodontal implications: medically compromised patients, *Ann Periodontol* 1:256-321, 1996.

23. Taylor GW: Bidirectional interrelationships between diabetes and periodontal diseases: an epidemiologic perspective, *Ann Periodontol* 6:99-112, 2001.

24. Ervasti T, Knuuttila M, Pohjamo L, Haukipuro K: Relation between control of diabetes and gingival bleeding, *J Periodontol* 56:154-157, 1985.

25. Karjalainen KM, Knuuttila MLE: The onset of diabetes and poor metabolic control increases gingival bleeding in children and adolescents with insulin-dependent diabetes mellitus, *J Clin Periodontol* 23:1060-1067, 1996.

26. Shlossman M, Knowler WC, Pettitt DJ, Genco RJ: Type 2 diabetes mellitus and periodontal disease, *J Am Dent Assoc* 121:532-536, 1990.

27. Emrich LJ, Shlossman M, Genco RJ: Periodontal disease in non-insulin-dependent diabetes mellitus, *J Periodontol* 62:123-130, 1991.

28. Taylor GW, Burt BA, Becker MP et al: Non-insulin dependent diabetes mellitus and alveolar bone loss progression over 2 years, *J Periodontol* 69:76-83, 1998.

29. Sastrowijoto SH, Hillemans P, van Steenbergen TJ et al: Periodontal condition and microbiology of healthy and diseased periodontal pockets in type 1 diabetes mellitus patients, *J Clin Periodontol* 16:316-322, 1989.

30. Zambon JJ, Reynolds H, Fisher JG et al: Microbiological and immunological studies of adult periodontitis in patients with non-insulin dependent diabetes mellitus, *J Periodontol* 59:23-31, 1988.

31. Ficara AJ, Levin MP, Grower MF, Kramer GD: A comparison of the glucose and protein content of gingival crevicular fluid from diabetics and nondiabetics, *J Periodont Res* 10:171-175, 1975.

32. Nishimura F, Takahashi K, Kurihara M et al: Periodontal disease as a complication of diabetes mellitus, *Ann Periodontol* 3:20-29, 1998.

33. Frantzis TG, Reeve CM, Brown AL: The ultrastructure of capillary basement membranes in the attached gingiva of diabetic and non-diabetic patients with periodontal disease, *J Periodontol* 42:406-411, 1971.

34. Seppala B, Sorsa T, Ainamo J: Morphometric analysis of cellular and vascular changes in gingival connective tissue in long-term insulin-dependent diabetes, *J Periodontol* 68:1237-1245, 1997.

35. Schmidt AM, Weidman E, Lalla E et al: Advanced glycation endproducts (AGEs) induce oxidant stress in the gingiva: a potential mechanism underlying accelerated periodontal disease associated with diabetes, *J Periodont Res* 31:508-515, 1996.

36. Offenbacher S: Periodontal diseases: pathogenesis, *Ann Periodontol* 1:821-878, 1996.

37. Salvi GE, Collins JG, Yalda B et al: Monocytic TNF-α secretion patterns in IDDM patients with periodontal diseases, *J Clin Periodontol* 24:8-16, 1997.

38. Salvi GE, Yalda B, Collins JG et al: Inflammatory mediator response as a potential risk marker for periodontal diseases in insulin-dependent diabetes mellitus patients, *J Periodontol* 68:127-135, 1997.

39. Ryan ME, Ramamurthy NS, Golub LM: Matrix metalloproteinases and their inhibition in periodontal treatment, *Curr Opin Periodontol* 3:85-96, 1996.

40. Golub LM, Lee H-M, Ryan ME: Tetracyclines inhibit connective tissue breakdown by multiple non-antimicrobial mechanisms, *Adv Dent Res* 12:12-26, 1998.

41. Vittek J, Hernandez MR, Wennk EJ et al: Specific estrogen receptors in human gingiva, *J Clin Endocrinol Metab* 54:608-612, 1982.

42. Vittek J, Munnangi PR, Gordon GG et al: Progesterone "receptors" in human gingiva, *IRCS Med Sci* 10:381-384, 1982.

43. Tilakaratne A, Soory M: Modulation of androgen metabolism by estradiol-17beta and progesterone, alone and in combination, in human gingival fibroblasts in culture, *J Periodontol* 70:1017-1025, 1999.

44. Morishita M, Shimazu A, Iwamoto Y: Analysis of oestrogen receptor mRNA by reverse transcriptase-polimerase chain reaction in human periodontal ligament cells, *Arch Oral Biol* 44:781-783, 1999.

45. Morishita M, Miyagi M, Iwamoto Y: Effects of sex hormones on production of interleukin-1 by human peripheral monocytes, *J Periodontol* 70:757-760, 1999.

46. Lapp CA, Thomas ME, Lewis JB: Modulation by progesterone of interleukin-6 production by gingival fibroblasts, *J Periodontol* 66:279-284, 1995.

47. Mombelli M, Gusberti FA, van Oosten MAC, Lang NP: Gingival health and gingivitis development during puberty, *J Clin Periodontol* 16:451-456, 1989.

48. Gusberti FA, Mombelli A, Lang NP, Minder CE: Changes in subgingival microbiota during puberty. A 4-year longitudinal study, *J Clin Periodontol* 17:685-692, 1990.

49. Delaney JE, Ratzan SK, Kornman KS: Subgingival microbiota associated with the development of puberty gingivitis, *J Periodont Res* 8:331-338, 1990.

50. Nakagawa S, Fujii H, Machida Y, Okuda K: A longitudinal study from prepuberty to puberty of gingivitis. Correlation between the occurrence of Prevotella intermedia and sex hormones, *J Clin Periodontol* 21:658-665, 1994.

51. Kornman KS, Loesche WJ: Effects of estradiol and progesterone on *Bacteroides melaninogenicus*, *Infect Immun* 35:256-263, 1982.

52. Tiainen I, Asikainen S, Saxén L: Puberty-associated gingivitis, *Community Dent Oral Epidemiol* 20:87-89, 1992.

53. Holm-Pedersen P, Löe H: Flow of gingival exudates as related to menstruation and pregnancy, *J Periodont Res* 2:13-20, 1967.

54. Kalkwarf KI: Effect of oral contraceptive therapy on gingival inflammation in humans, *J Periodontol* 49:560-563, 1978.

55. Lindhe J, Bjorn AL: Influence of hormonal contraception on the gingiva of women, *J Periodont Res* 2:1-6, 1967.

56. Preshaw PM, Knutsen MA, Mariotti A: Experimental gingivitis in women using oral contraceptives, *J Dent Res* 80:2011-2015, 2001.

57. Löe H, Silness J: Periodontal disease in pregnancy I. Prevalence and severity, *Acta Odontol Scand* 21:533-551, 1963.

58. Löe H: Periodontal changes in pregnancy, *J Periodontol* 36:209-216, 1965.

59. Cohen DW, Shapiro J, Friedman L et al: A longitudinal investigation of the periodontal changes during pregnancy and fifteen months post-partum. II, *J Periodontol* 42:653-657, 1971.

60. Offenbacher S, Katz V, Fertik G et al: Periodontal disease as a possible risk factor for preterm low birth weight, *J Periodontol* 67(suppl):1103-1113, 1996.

61. O'Neil TCA: Plasma female sex-hormone levels and gingivitis in pregnancy, *J Periodontol* 50:279-282, 1979.

62. Kornman KS, Loesche WJ: The subgingival microflora during pregnancy, *J Periodont Res* 15:111-122, 1980.

63. Jansen J, Liljermark W, Bloomquist C: The effect of female sex hormones on subgingival plaque, *J Periodontol* 52:599-602, 1981.

64. Muramatsu Y, Takaesu Y: Oral health status related to subgingival bacterial flora and sex hormones in saliva during pregnancy, *Bull Tokyo Dent Coll* 35:139-151, 1994.

65. Lopatin DE, Kornman KS, Loesche WJ: Modulation of immunoreactivity to periodontal disease-associated microorganisms during pregnancy, *Infect Immun* 28:713-718, 1980.

66. Kinnby B, Matsson L, Astedt B: Aggravation of gingival inflammatory symptoms during pregnancy associated with the concentration of plasminogen activator inhibitor type 2 (PAI-2) in gingival fluid, *J Periodont Res* 31:271-277, 1996.

67. Friedlander A: The physiology, medical management and oral implications of menopause, *J Am Dent Assoc* 133:73-81, 2002.

68. Norderyd OM, Grossi SG, Machtei EE et al: Periodontal status of women taking postmenopausal estrogen supplementation, *J Periodontol* 64:957-962, 1993.

69. Jacobs R, Ghyselen J, Koninckx P, van Steenberghe D: Long-term bone mass evaluation of mandible and lumbar spine in a group of women receiving hormone replacement therapy, *Eur J Oral Sci* 104:10-16, 1996.

70. Payne JB, Zachs NR, Reinhardt RA et al: The association between estrogen status and alveolar bone density changes in postmenopausal women with a history of periodontitis, *J Periodontol* 68:24-31, 1997.

71. Kribbs PJ, Chesnut CH, Ott SM, Kilcoyne RF: Relationship between mandibular and skeletal bone in an osteoporotic population, *J Prosthet Dent* 62:703-707, 1989.

72. Kribbs PJ: Comparison of mandibular bone in normal and osteoporotic women, *J Prosthet Dent* 63:218-222, 1990.

73. Wactawski-Wende J, Grossi SG, Trevisan M et al: The role of osteopenia in periodontal disease, *J Periodontol* 67:1076-1084, 1996.

74. Von Wowern N, Klausen B, Kollerup G: Osteoporosis: a risk factor in periodontal disease, *J Periodontol* 65:1134-1138, 1994.

75. Jeffcoat MK: Osteoporosis: a possible modifying factor in oral bone loss, *Ann Periodontol* 3:312-321, 1998.

76. Paganini-Hill A: The benefits of estrogen replacement therapy on oral health, *Arch Intern Med* 155:2325-2329, 1995.

77. Grodstein F, Colditz GA, Stampfer MJ: Post-menopausal hormone use and tooth loss: a prospective study, *J Am Dent Assoc* 127:370-377, 1996.

78. Krall EA, Dawson-Hughes B, Hannan MT et al: Postmenopausal estrogen replacement and tooth retention, *Am J Med* 102:536-542, 1997.

79. Safkan B, Knuuttila M: Corticosteroid therapy and periodontal disease, *J Clin Periodontol* 11:515-522, 1984.

80. Markitziu A, Zafiropoulos G, Flores de Jacoby L, Pisanty S: Periodontal alterations in patients with pemphigus vulgaris taking steroids. A biannual assessment, *J Clin Periodontol* 17:228-232, 1990.

81. Dubois EF, Roder E, Dekhuijzen PN et al: Dual energy X-ray absorptiometry outcomes in male COPD patients after treatment with different glucocorticoid regimens, *Chest* 121:1456-1463, 2002.

82. Heinemann DF: Osteoporosis. An overview of the National Osteoporosis Foundation clinical practice guide, *Geriatrics* 55:31-36, 2000.

83. Glick M: Glucocorticosteroid replacement therapy: a literature review and suggested replacement therapy, *Oral Surg Oral Med Oral Pathol* 67:614-620, 1989.

84. Shapiro R, Carroll PB, Tzakis A et al: Adrenal reserve in renal transplant recipients with cyclosporine/azathioprine/ prednisone immunosuppression, *Transplantation* 49:1011-1013, 1990.

85. Ziccardi VB, Abubaker AO, Sotereanos GC, Patterson GT: Maxillofacial considerations in orthotopic liver transplantation, *Oral Surg Oral Med Oral Pathol* 71:21-26, 1991.

86. Thomason JM, Girdler NM, Kendall-Taylor P et al: An investigation into the need for supplementary steroids in organ transplant patients undergoing gingival surgery. A double-blind, split-mouth, cross-over study, *J Clin Periodontol* 26:577-582, 1999.

87. Howard GA, Bottemiller BL, Turner RT et al: Parathyroid hormone stimulates bone formation and resorption in organ culture: evidence for a coupling mechanism, *Proc Natl Acad Sci USA* 78:3204-3208, 1981.

88. Deas DE, Mackey SA, McDonnell HT: Systemic disease and periodontitis: manifestations of neutrophil dysfunction, *Periodontology 2000* 32:82-104, 2003.

89. Waldrop TC, Anderson DC, Hallmon WW et al: Periodontal manifestations of the heritable Mac-1, LFA-1, deficiency syndrome, *J Periodontol* 58:400-416, 1987.

90. Trigg ME, Schugar R: Chediak-Higashi syndrome: hematopoietic chimerism corrects genetic defect, *Bone Marrow Transplant* 27:1211-1213, 2001.

91. Introne W, Boissy RE, Gahl WA: Clinical, molecular, and cell biological aspects of Chediak-Higashi Syndrome, *Mol Genet Metab* 68:283-303, 1999.

92. Bernini J: Diagnosis and management of chronic neutropenia during childhood, *Pediatr Clin North Am* 43:773-792, 1996.

93. Meyle J, Gonzales JR: Influences of systemic diseases on periodontitis in children and adolescents, *Periodontology 2000* 26:92-112, 2001.

94. Lakshman R, Finn A: Neutrophil disorders and their management, *J Clin Pathol* 54:7-19, 2001.

95. Carlsson G, Fasth A: Infantile genetic agranulocytosis, morbus Kostmann: presentation of six cases from the original "Kostmann family" and a review, *Acta Paediatr* 90:757-764, 2001.

96. Defraaia E, Marinelli A: Oral manifestations of congenital neutropenia or Kostmann Syndrome, *J Clin Pediatr Dent* 26:99-102, 2001.

97. Miller ME, Oski FA, Harris MB: Lazy leukocyte syndrome. A new disorder, *Lancet* 1:665-669, 1971.

98. Hart TC, Shapira L: Papillon-Lefevre syndrome, *Periodontology 2000* 6:88-100, 1994.

99. Preus HR: Treatment of rapidly destructive periodontitis in Papillon-Lèfevre syndrome. Laboratory and clinical observations, *J Clin Periodontol* 15:639-643, 1988.

100. Lundgren T, Crossner CG, Tewtman S, Ullbro C: Systemic retinoid medication and periodontal health in patients with Papillon-Lefevre syndrome, *J Clin Periodontol* 23:176-179, 1996.

101. Barnett ML, Press KP, Friedman D, Sonnenberg EM: The prevalence of periodontitis and dental caries in a Down's syndrome population, *J Periodontol* 57:288-293, 1986.

102. Halinen S, Sorsa T, Ding Y et al: Characterization of matrix metalloproteinase (MMP-8 and 9) activities in the saliva and in gingival crevicular fluid of children with Down's syndrome, *J Periodontol* 67:748-754, 1996.

103. Visser G, Rake JP, Fernnandes J et al: Neutropenia, neutrophil dysfunction, and inflammatory bowel disease in glycogen storage disease type 1b: results of the European study on glycogen storage disease type 1, *J Pediatr* 137:187-191, 2000.

104. Salapata Y, Laskaris G, Drogari E et al: Oral manifestations of glycogen storage disease type 1b, *J Oral Pathol Med* 24:136-139, 1995.

105. Brennan MT, Sankar V, Baccaglini L et al: Oral manifestations in patients with aplastic anemia, *Oral Surg Oral Med Oral Pathol Oral Radiol Endod* 92:503-508, 2001.

106. Nowzari H, Jorgensen MG, Ta TT et al: Aggressive periodontitis associated with Fanconi's anemia. A case report, *J Periodontol* 72:1601-1606, 2001.

107. Field EA, Speechley JA, Rugman FR et al: Oral signs and symptoms in patients with undiagnosed vitamin B12 deficiency, *J Oral Pathol Med* 24:468-470, 1995.

108. Hoffman RM, Jaffe PE: Plummer-Vinson syndrome. A case report and literature review, *Arch Intern Med* 155:2008-2011, 1995.

109. Sanai FM, Mohamed AE, Al Karawi MA: Dysphagia caused by Plummer-Vinson syndrome, *Endoscopy* 33:470, 2001.

110. Crawford JM: Periodontal disease in sickle cell disease subjects, *J Periodontol* 59:164-169, 1988.

111. Krause JR: Morphology and classification of acute myeloid leukemias, *Clin Lab Med* 20:1-6, 2000.

112. Stafford R, Sonis S, Lockhart P, Sonis A: Oral pathoses as diagnostic indicators in leukemia, *Oral Surg Oral Med Oral Pathol* 50:134-139, 1980.

113. Childers NK, Stinnett EA, Wheeler P et al: Oral complications in children with cancer, *Oral Surg Oral Med Oral Pathol* 75:41-47, 1993.

114. Dreizen S, McCredie KB, Keating MJ, Luna MA: Malignant gingival and skin "infiltrates" in adult leukemia, *Oral Surg Oral Med Oral Pathol* 55:572-579, 1983.

115. Semba SE, Mealey BL, Hallmon WW: The head and neck radiotherapy patient: Part 1—oral manifestations of radiation therapy, *Compendium Contin Educ Dent* 15:250-260, 1994.

116. Mealey BL, Semba SE, Hallmon WW: Dentistry and the cancer patient: Part 1—oral manifestations and complications of chemotherapy, *Compendium Contin Educ Dent* 15:1252-1261, 1994.

117. Lizi EC: A case for a dental surgeon at regional radiotherapy centres, *Br Dent J* 173:24-26, 1992.

118. Ellegaard B, Bergmann OJ, Ellegaard J: Effect of plaque removal on patients with leukemia, *J Oral Pathol Med* 18:54-58, 1989.

119. Ferretti GA, Ash RC, Brown AT et al: Control of oral mucositis and candidiasis in marrow transplantation: a prospective, double-blind trial of chlorhexidine digluconate oral rinse, *Bone Marrow Transplant* 3:483-493, 1988.

120. Mangan DF: Nutrition and oral infectious diseases: connections and future research, *Compendium Contin Educ Dent* 23:416-422, 2002.

121. Enwonwu CO: Cellular and molecular effects of malnutrition and their relevance to periodontal diseases, *J Clin Periodontol* 21:643-657, 1994.

122. Alfano M: Controversies, perspectives, and clinical implications of nutrition in periodontal disease, *Dent Clin North Am* 20:569-584, 1976.

123. Tomkins A: Malnutrition, morbidity, and mortality in children and their mothers, *Proc Nutr Soc* 59:135-146, 2000.

124. Enwonwu CO, Phillips RS, Falkler Jr WA: Nutrition and oral infectious diseases: state of the science, *Compendium Contin Educ Dent* 23:431-446, 2002.

125. Alvares O, Worthington B, Enwonwu CO: Regional differences in the effects of protein calorie malnutrition on oral epithelium, *J Dent Res* 55(B):173, 1976.

126. Woodward B: Protein, calories, and immune defenses, *Nutr Rev* 56:s84-s92, 1998.

127. Grimble RF: Modification of inflammatory aspects of immune function by nutrients, *Nutr Res* 18:1297-1317, 1998.

128. Sawyer DR, Nwoku AL, Rotimi VO et al: Comparison of oral microflora between well-nourished and malnourished Nigerian children, *ASDC J Dent Child* 53:439-443, 1986.

129. Jabra-Rizk MA, Falkler WA, Enwonwu CO et al: Prevalence of yeast among children in Nigeria and the United States, *Oral Microbiol Immunol* 16:383-385, 2001.

130. Stahl SS, Tonna EA, Weiss R: Autoradiographic evaluation of gingival response to injury. V. Surgical trauma in low-protein fed mature rats, *J Dent Res* 49:537-545, 1970.

131. Cheraskin E, Ringsdorf WM, Setyaadmadja AT, Barrett RA: An ecologic analysis of gingiva state: effect of prophylaxis and protein supplementation, *J Periodontol* 39:316-321, 1968.

132. Dreizen S, Levy B, Bernick S: Studies on the biology of the periodontium of marmosets. XI. Histopathologic manifestations of spontaneous and induced vitamin A deficiency in the oral structures of adult marmosets, *J Dent Res* 52:803-809, 1973.

133. Theaker J, Porter S, Fleming K: Oral epithelial dysplasia in vitamin B_{12} deficiency, *Oral Surg Oral Med Oral Pathol* 67:81-83, 1989.

134. Vogel RI, Fink RA, Schneider LC et al: The effect of folic acid on gingival health, *J Periodontol* 47:667-668, 1976.

135. Vogel RI, Fink RA, Frank O, Baker H: The effect of topical application of folic acid on gingival health, *J Oral Med* 33:20-22, 1978.

136. Pack A, Thomson M: Effects of topical and systemic folic acid supplementation on gingivitis in pregnancy, *J Clin Periodontol* 7:402-414, 1980.

137. Poppell T, Keeling S, Collins J, Hassell T: Effect of folic acid on recurrence of phenytoin-induced gingival overgrowth following gingivectomy, *J Clin Periodontol* 18:134-139, 1991.

138. Woolfe SN, Hume WR, Kenney EB: Ascorbic acid and periodontal disease: a review of the literature, *J West Soc Periodontol Periodontal Abstr* 28:44-56, 1980.

139. Nishida M, Grossi SG, Dunford RG et al: Dietary vitamin C and the risk for periodontal disease, *J Periodontol* 71:1215-1223, 2000.

140. Bissada N, Demarco J: The effect of a hypocalcemic diet on the periodontal structure of the adult rat, *J Periodontol* 45:739-745, 1974.

141. Nishida M, Grossi SG, Dunford RG et al: Calcium and the risk for periodontal disease, *J Periodontol* 71:1057-1066, 2000.

142. Krall EA, Wehler C, Garcia RI et al: Calcium and vitamin D supplements reduce tooth loss in the elderly, *Am J Med* 111:452-456, 2001.

143. Ballieux RE: Impact of mental stress on the immune response, *J Clin Periodontol* 18:427-430, 1991.

144. Giddon DB, Goldhaber P, Dunning JM: Prevalence of reported cases of acute necrotizing ulcerative gingivitis in a university population, *J Periodontol* 34:66-70, 1963.

145. Shields WD: Acute necrotizing ulcerative gingivitis: a study of some of the contributing factors and their validity in an army population, *J Periodontol* 48:346-349, 1977.

146. Croucher R, Marcenes WS, Torres MC et al: The relationship between life events and periodontitis. A case control study, *J Clin Periodontol* 24:39-43, 1997.

147. Marcenes WS, Sheiham A: The relationship between work stress and oral health status, *Soc Sci Med* 35:1511-1520, 1992.

148. Monteiro da Silva AM, Oakley DA, Newman HN et al: Psychosocial factors and adult onset rapidly progressive periodontitis, *J Clin Periodontol* 23:789-794, 1996.

149. Genco RJ, Ho AW, Kopman J et al: Models to evaluate the role of stress in periodontal disease, *Ann Periodontol* 3:288-302, 1998.

150. Genco RJ, Ho AW, Grossi SG et al: Relationship of stress, distress, and inadequate coping behaviors to periodontal diseases, *J Periodontol* 70:711-732, 1999.

151. Linden GJ, Mullally BH, Freeman R: Stress and the progression of periodontal disease, *J Clin Periodontol* 23:675-680, 1996.

152. Elter JR, White BA, Gaynes BN, Bader JD: Relationship of clinical depression to periodontal treatment outcome, *J Periodontol* 73:441-449, 2002.

153. Rozlog LA, Kiecolt-Glaser JK, Marucha PT et al: Stress and immunity: implications for viral disease and wound healing, *J Periodontol* 70:786-792, 1999.

154. Linden GJ, McKinnell J, Shaw C, Lundy FT: Substance P and neurokinin A in gingival crevicular fluid in periodontal health and disease, *J Clin Periodontol* 24:799-803, 1997.

155. Asher R: Munchausen's syndrome, *Lancet* (i):339-341, 1959.

156. Relman AS: Pathogenic human retroviruses, *N Engl J Med* 318:243-246, 1988.

157. Fauci AS, Schnittman SM, Poli G et al: Immunopathogenic mechanisms in human immunodeficiency virus (HIV) infection, *Ann Intern Med* 114:678-693, 1993.

158. Jacobs DS, Piliero PJ, Kuperwaser MG et al: Acute uveitis associated with rifabutin use in patients with human

immunodeficiency virus infection, *Am J Ophthalmol* 118:716-722, 1994.

159. Baron S: Oral transmission of HIV, a rarity: emerging hypotheses, *J Dent Res* 80:1602-1604, 2001.

160. Challacombe SJ, Sweet SP: Oral mucosal immunity and HIV infection: current status, *Oral Dis* 8(suppl 2):55-62, 2002.

161. Ferrero S, Gotta G, Melica G et al: 162 HIV-1 infected pregnant women and vertical transmission. Results of a prospective study, *Minerva Ginecol* 54:373-385, 2002.

162. CDC-NCHSTP-DHAP: HIV/AIDS Surveillance Report, *Commentary* 13:1-3, 2002.

163. Kaplan JE, Masur H, Holmes KK: Guidelines for preventing opportunistic infection among HIV-infected persons—2002: recommendations of the U.S. Public Health Service and the Infectious Diseases Society of America, *MMWR Recomm Rep* 137:435-477, 2002.

164. Yeni PG, Hammer SM, Carpenter CC et al: Antiretroviral treatment for adult HIV infection in 2002. Updated recommendations of the International AIDS Society-USA Panel, *JAMA* 288:222-235, 2002.

165. Panel on Clinical Practices for the Treatment of HIV: Guidelines for using antiretroviral agents among HIV-infected adults and adolescents. Recommendations of the Panel on Clinical Practices for Treatment of HIV, *MMWR Recomm Rep* 51(RR-7):1-55, 2002.

166. McCarthy GM, Bednarsh H, Jorge J et al: Transmission of HIV in the dental clinic and elsewhere, *Oral Dis* 8 (suppl 2): 126-135, 2002.

167. Lot F, Seguier J-C, Fegueux S et al: Probable transmission of HIV from an orthopedic surgeon to a patient in France, *Ann Intern Med* 130:1-6, 1999.

168. Ippolito G, Puro V, Heptonstall J et al: Occupational human immunodeficiency virus infection in health care workers: worldwide cases through September 1997, *Clin Infect Dis* 28:365-383, 1999.

169. Centers for Disease Control: Updated U.S. Public Health Service guidelines for management of occupational exposures to HBV, HCV, and HIV and recommendations for postexposure prophylaxis, *MMWR Recomm Rep* 50(RR-11):1-42, 2001.

170. Centers for Disease Control: 1993 Revised classification system for HIV infection and expanded surveillance case definition for AIDS among adolescents and adults, *MMWR Recomm Rep* 41(RR-17), December 18, 1992.

171. Fleming PL, Ward JW, Karon JM et al: Declines in AIDS incidence and deaths in the USA: a signal change in the epidemic, *AIDS* 12 (suppl A):S55-S61, 1998.

172. Haase AT, Schacker TW: Potential for the transmission of HIV-1 despite highly active antiretroviral therapy, *N Engl J Med* Dec 17;339:1846-1847, 1998.

173. Blankson JN, Persuad D, Siliciano RF: The challenge of viral reservoirs in HIV-1 infection, *Annu Rev Med* 53:557-593, 2002.

174. Gaines H, Von Sydow M, Pehrson PO, Lundbergh P: Clinical picture of primary HIV infection presenting as a glandular-fever-like illness, *Br Med J* 97:1363-1368, 1988.

175. Vanhems P, Dassa C, Lambert J et al: Comprehensive classification of symptoms and signs reported among 218 patients with acute HIV-1 infection, *J Acquir Immune Defic Syndr* 21:99-106, 1999.

176. Veugelers PJ, Cornelisse PGA, Craib KJP et al: Models of survival in HIV infection and their use in the quantification of treatment benefits, *Am J Epidemiol* 148:487-496, 1998.

177. Carr A, Cooper DA: Adverse effects of antiretroviral therapy, *Lancet* 356:1423-1430, 2000.

178. Margiotta V, Campisi G, Mancuso S et al: HIV infection: oral lesions, CD4+ cell count and viral load in an Italian study population, *J Oral Pathol Med* 28:173-177, 1999.

179. Santos LC, Castro GF, de Souza IP, Oliveira RH: Oral manifestations related to immunosuppression degree in HIV-positive children, *Braz Dent J* 12:135-138, 2001.

180. Thompson SH, Charles GA, Craig DB: Correlation of oral disease with the Walter Reed staging scheme for HIV-1-seropositive patients, *Oral Surg Oral Med Oral Pathol* 73:289-292, 1992.

181. Classification and diagnostic criteria for oral lesions in HIV infection. EC-Clearinghouse on Oral Problems Related to HIV Infection and WHO Collaborating Centre on Oral Manifestations of the Immunodeficiency Virus. *J Oral Pathol Med* 22:289-291, 1993.

182. Patton LL, van der Horst C: Oral infections and other manifestations of HIV disease, *Infect Dis Clin North Am* 13:879-900, 1999.

183. Ceballos-Salobrena A, Gaitan-Cepeda LA, Ceballos-Garcia L, Lezama-Del Valle D: Oral lesions in HIV/AIDS patients undergoing highly active antiretroviral treatment including protease inhibitors: a new face of oral AIDS?, *AIDS Patient Care STDS* 14:627-635, 2000.

184. Patton LL, McKaig R, Stauss R et al: Changing prevalence of oral manifestations of human immunodeficiency virus in the era of protease inhibitor therapy, *Oral Surg Oral Med Oral Pathol Oral Radiol Endod* 89:299-304, 2000.

185. Tappuni AR, Fleming GJP: The effect of antiretroviral therapy on the prevalence of oral manifestations in HIV-infected patients: a UK study, *Oral Surg Oral Med Oral Pathol Oral Radiol Endod* 92:623-628, 2001.

186. Scully C, Diz Dios P: Orofacial effects of antiretroviral therapies, *Oral Dis* 7:205-210, 2001.

187. Casariego Z, Pombo T, Perez H, Patterson P: Eruptive cheilitis: a new adverse effect in reactive HIV-positive patients subjected to high activity antiretroviral therapy (HAART). Presentation of six clinical cases, *Med Oral* 6:19-30, 2001.

188. King MD, Reznik DA, O'Daniels CM et al: Human papillomavirus-associated oral warts among human immunodeficiency virus-seropositive patients in the era

of highly active antiretroviral therapy: an emerging infection, *Clin Infect Dis* 34:641-648, 2002.

189. Magalhaes MG, Bueno DF, Serra E, Goncalves R: Oral manifestations of HIV positive children, *J Clin Pediatr Dent* 25:103-106, 2001.

190. Campo J, Del Romero J, Castilla J et al: Oral candidiasis as a clinical marker related to viral load, CD4 lymphocyte count and CD4 lymphocyte percentage in HIV-infected patients, *J Oral Pathol Med* 31:5-10, 2002.

191. Campisi G, Pizzo G, Mancuso S, Margiotta V: Gender differences in human immunodeficiency virus-related oral lesions: an Italian study, *Oral Surg Oral Med Oral Pathol Oral Radiol Endod* 91:546-551, 2001.

192. Fernandez Feijoo J, Dios P: Oral candidiasis in human immunodeficiency virus-infected women, *Oral Surg Oral Med Oral Pathol Oral Radiol Endod* 93:219-220, 2002.

193. Fidel PI Jr: Immunity to candida, *Oral Dis* 8(suppl 2): 69-75, 2002.

194. Schuman P, Sobel JD, Ohmit SE et al: Mucosal candidal colonization and candidiasis in women with or without risk for human immunodeficiency virus infection, *Clin Infect Dis* 27:1161-1167, 1998.

195. McPhail LA, Komaroff E, Mario EA et al: Differences in risk factors among clinical types of oral candidiasis in the Women's Interagency HIV study, *Oral Surg Oral Med Oral Pathol Oral Radiol Endod* 93:45-53, 2002.

196. Patton LL: Sensitivity, specificity, and positive predictive value of oral opportunistic infections in adults with HIV/AIDS as markers of immune suppression and viral burden, *Oral Surg Oral Med Oral Pathol Oral Radiol Endod* 90:182-188, 2000.

197. Patton LL, Bonito AJ, Shugars DA: A systematic review of the effectiveness of antifungal drugs for the prevention and treatment of oropharyngeal candidiasis in HIV-positive patients, *Oral Surg Oral Med Oral Pathol Oral Radiol Endod* 92:170-179, 2001.

198. Samaranayake LP, Fidel PL, Naglik JR et al: Fungal infections associated with HIV infection, *Oral Dis* 8(suppl 2): 151-160, 2002.

199. Diz Dios P, Ocampo A, Miralles C et al: Frequency of oropharyngeal candidiasis in HIV-infected patients on protease inhibitor therapy, *Oral Surg Oral Med Oral Pathol Oral Radiol* Endod 87:437-441, 1999.

200. Martins MD, Lozano-Chiu M, Rex JH: Declining rates of oropharyngeal candidiasis and carriage of Candida albicans associated with trends toward reduced rates of carriage of fluconazole-resistant *C. albicans* in human immunodeficiency virus-infected patients, *Clin Infect Dis* 27:1291-1294, 1998.

201. Greenspan D, Conant M, Silverman S Jr et al: Oral hairy-leukoplakia in male homosexuals. Evidence of association with both papilloma virus and a herpes-group virus, *Lancet* 2:831-834, 1984.

202. Greenspan JS, Greenspan D, Lennette ET et al: Replication of Epstein-Barr virus within the epithelial cells of oral hairy leukoplakia, and AIDS associated lesion, *N Engl J Med* 313:1564-1571, 1985.

203. Schiodt M, Greenspan D, Daniels TE, Greenspan JS: Clinical and histologic spectrum of oral hairy leukoplakia, *Oral Surg Oral Med Oral Pathol* 64:716-720, 1987.

204. Greenspan D, Greenspan JS, de Souza Y et al: Oral hairy leukoplakia in an HIV-negative renal transplant recipient, *J Oral Pathol Med* 18:32-34, 1989.

205. Geraminejad P, Memar O, Aronson I et al: Kaposi's sarcoma and other manifestations of human herpesvirus 8, *J Am Acad Dermatol* 47:641-655, 2002.

206. Sirianni MC, Vincenzi L, Topino S et al: NK cell activity controls human herpesvirus 8 latent infection and is restored upon highly active antiretroviral therapy in AIDS patients with regressing Kaposi's sarcoma, *Eur J Immunol* 32:2711-2720, 2002.

207. Bourboulia D, Whitby D, Boshoff C et al: Serologic evidence for mother-to-child transmission of Kaposi sarcoma-associated herpesvirus infection, *JAMA* 20:31-32, 1998.

208. Jin Y-T, Tsai S-T, Yan J-J, et al: Presence of human herpesvirus-like DNA sequence in oral Kaposi's sarcoma, *Oral Surg Oral Med Oral Pathol Oral Radiol Endod* 81:442-444, 1996.

209. Jaffe HW, Pellett PE: Human Herpesvirus 8 and Kaposi's sarcoma-some answers, more questions, *N Engl J Med* 340:1912-1913, 1999.

210. Duman S, Toz H, Asci G et al: Successful treatment of post-transplant Kaposi's sarcoma by reduction of immunosuppression, *Nephrol Dial Transplant* 17:892-896, 2002.

211. Regezi JA, MacPhail LA, Daniels TE et al: Oral Kaposi's sarcoma: a 10-year retrospective histopathologic study, *J Oral Pathol Med* 22:292-297, 1993.

212. Cattelan AM, Trevenzoli M, Aversa SM: Recent advances in the treatment of AIDS-related Kaposi's sarcoma, *Am J Clin Dermatol* 3:451-462, 2002.

213. Solomides CC, Miller AS, Christman RA et al: Lymphomas of the oral cavity: histology, immunologic type and incidence of Epstein-Barr infection, *Hum Pathol* 33:153-157, 2002.

214. Gates AE, Kaplan LD: AIDS malignancies in the era of highly active antiretroviral therapy, *Oncology (Huntingt)* 16:657-665, 2002.

215. Eltom MA, Jemal A, Mbulaiteye SM et al: Trends in Kaposi's sarcoma and non-Hodgkin's lymphoma incidence in the United States from 1973 through 1998, *Natl Cancer Inst* 94:1204-1210, 2002.

216. Ficarra G, Eversole LE: HIV-related tumors of the oral cavity, *Crit Rev Oral Biol Med* 5:159-185, 1994.

217. O'Connor PG, Scadden DT: AIDS oncology, *Infect Dis Clin North Am* 14:945-965, 2000.

218. Casiglia J, Woo SB: A comprehensive review of oral cancer, *Gen Dent* 49:72-82, 2001.

219. Tirelli U, Vaccher E, Zagonel V et al: Malignant tumors other than lymphoma and Kaposi's sarcoma in association with HIV infection, *Cancer Detect Prev* 12:267-272, 1988.

220. Singh B, Sabin S, Rofim O et al: Alterations in head and neck cancer occurring in HIV-infected patients—results of a pilot, longitudinal, prospective study, *Acta Oncol* 38:1047-1050, 1999.

221. Braekeveld R, Verstraete K, Deprest K et al: Bacillary angiomatosis in a patient with AIDS, *JBR-BTR* 85:124-125, 2002.

222. Karem KL, Paddock CD, Regnery RL: Bartonella henselae, B. quintana, and B. bacilliformis: historical pathogens of emerging significance, *Microbes Infect* 2:1193-1205, 2000.

223. Mohle-Boetani JC, Koehler JE, Berger TG et al: Bacillary angiomatosis and bacillary peliosis in patients infected with human immunodeficiency virus: clinical characteristics in a case-control study, *Clin Infect Dis* 22:794-800, 1996.

224. Rivera-Hidalgo F, Stanford TW: Oral mucosal lesions caused by infective microorganisms. I. Viruses and bacteria, *Periodontol 2000* 21:106-124, 1999.

225. Langford A, Pohle HD, Gelderblum HR et al: Oral hyperpigmentation in HIV-infected patients, *Oral Surg Oral Med Oral Pathol* 67:301-307, 1989.

226. Granel F, Truchetet F, Grandidier M: Diffuse pigmentation (nail, mouth and skin) associated with HIV infection, *Ann Dermatol Venereol* 124:460-462, 1997.

227. Greenberg RG, Berger TG: Nail and mucocutaneous hyperpigmentation with azidothymidine therapy, *J Am Acad Dermatol* 22:327-330, 1990.

228. Hoshino Y, Nagata Y, Gatanaga H et al: Cytomegalovirus (CMV) retinitis and CMV antigenemia as a clue to impaired adrenocortical function in patients with AIDS, *AIDS* 11:1719-1724, 1997.

229. Piedrola G, Casado JL, Lopez E et al: Clinical features of adrenal insufficiency in patients with acquired immunodeficiency syndrome, *Clin Endocrinol (Oxf)* 45:97-101, 1996.

230. Phelan JA, Eisig S, Freedman PD et al: Major aphthous-like ulcers in patients with AIDS, *Oral Surg Oral Med Oral Pathol* 71:68-72, 1991.

231. Glick M, Muzyka BC: Alternative therapies for major aphthous ulcers in AIDS patients, *J Am Dent Assoc* 123:61-65, 1992.

232. Casiglia JM: Recurrent aphthous stomatitis: etiology, diagnosis, and treatment, *Gen Dent* 50:157-166, 2002.

233. Gorin I, Vilette B, Gehanno P, Escande P: Thalidomide in hyperalgic pharyngeal ulceration of AIDS, *Lancet* 335:1343, 1990.

234. Regezi JA, Eversole LR, Barker BF et al: Herpes simplex and cytomegalovirus coinfected oral ulcers in HIV-positive patients, *Oral Surg Oral Med Oral Pathol Oral Radiol Endod* 81:55-62, 1996.

235. Syrjanen S, Leimola-Virtanen R, Schmidt-Westhausen A, Reichart PA: Oral ulcers in AIDS patients frequently associated with cytomegalovirus (CMV) and Epstein-Barr virus (EBV) infection, *J Oral Pathol Med* 28:204-209, 1999.

236. Stanford TW, Rivera-Hidalgo F: Oral mucosal lesions caused by infective microorganisms. II. Fungi and parasites, *Periodontol 2000* 21:125-144, 1999.

237. Boxer L, Dale DC: Neutropenia: causes and consequences. *Semin Hematol* 39:75-81, 2002.

238. Amir J: Clinical aspects and antiviral therapy in primary herpetic gingivostomatitis, *Paediatr Drugs* 3:593-597, 2001.

239. Drugs for AIDS and associated infections, *Med Lett Drugs Ther* 35:79-86, 1993.

240. Bayard PJ, Berger TG, Jacobson MA: Drug hypersensitivity reactions and human immunodeficiency virus disease, *J Acquir Immune Defic Syndr* 5:1237-1257, 1992.

241. Martin-Carbonero L, Soriano V, Valencia E et al: Increasing impact of chronic viral hepatitis on hospital admissions and mortality among HIV-infected patients, *AIDS Res Hum Retroviruses* 1:1467-1471, 2001.

242. Daley TD, Gupta AK: Exfoliative cheilitis, *J Oral Pathol Med* 24:177-179, 1995.

243. Reichart PA, Weigel D, Schmidt-Westhausen A, Pohle HD: Exfoliative cheilitis (EC) in AIDS: association with candida infection, *J Oral Pathol Med* 26:290-293, 1997.

244. Lozada-Nur F, Glick M, Schubert M, Silverberg I: Use of intralesional interferon-alpha for the treatment of recalcitrant oral warts in patients with AIDS: a report of 4 cases, *Oral Surg Oral Med Oral Pathol Oral Radiol Endod* 92:617-622, 2001.

245. Wiley DJ, Douglas J, Beutner K et al: External genital warts: diagnosis, treatment and prevention, *Clin Infect Dis* 15(suppl 2):S210-S224, 2002.

246. Calista D: Resolution of recalcitrant human papillomavirus gingival infection with topical cidofovir, *Oral Surg Oral Med Oral Pathol Oral Radiol Endod* 90:713-715, 2000.

247. Navazesh M, Mulligan R, Komaroff E et al: The prevalence of xerostomia and salivary gland hypofunction in a cohort of HIV-positive and at-risk women, *J Dent Res* 79:1502-1507, 2000.

248. Younai FS, Marcus M, Freed JR et al: Self-reported oral dryness and HIV disease in a national sample of patients receiving medical care, *Oral Surg Oral Med Oral Pathol Oral Radiol Endod* 92:629-636, 2001.

249. Mulligan R, Navazesh M, Komaroff E et al: Salivary gland disease in human immunodeficiency virus-positive women from the WIHS study, *Oral Surg Oral Med Oral Pathol Oral Radiol Endod* 89:702-709, 2000.

250. Dodson TB: HIV status and the risk of post-extraction complications, *J Dent Res* 76:1644-1652, 1997.

251. Glick M, Abel SN, Muzyka BC, Delorenzo M: Dental complications after treating patients with AIDS, *J Am Dent Assoc* 125:296-301, 1994.

252. Patton LL, Shugars DA, Bonito AJ: A systematic review of complication risks for HIV-positive patients undergoing dental procedures, *J Am Dent Assoc* 133:195-203, 2002.

253. Robinson PG: The significance and management of periodontal lesions in HIV infection, *Oral Dis* 8(suppl 2):91-97, 2002.

254. Barr C, Lopez MR, Rua-Dobles A: Periodontal changes by HIV serostatus in a cohort of homosexual and bisexual men, *J Clin Periodontol* 19:794-801, 1992.

255. Yeung SCH, Stewart GJ, Cooper DA et al: Progression of periodontal disease in HIV seropositive patients, *J Periodontol* 64:651-657, 1993.

256. Robinson PG, Boulter A, Birnbaum W, Johnson NW: A controlled study of relative attachment loss in people with HIV infection, *J Clin Periodontol* 27:273-276, 2000.

257. McKaig RG, Thomas JC, Patton LL et al: Prevalence of HIV-associated peridontitis and chronic periodontitis in a southeastern U.S. study group, *J Public Health Dent* 58:294-300, 1998.

258. Gornitsky M, Clark DC, Siboo R et al: Clinical documentation and occurrence of putative periodontopathic bacteria in human immunodeficiency virus-associated periodontal disease, *J Periodontol* 62:576-585, 1991.

259. Moore LVH, Moore WEC, Riley C et al: Periodontal microflora of HIV-positive subjects with gingivitis or adult periodontitis, *J Periodontol* 64:48-56, 1993.

260. Ndiaye CF, Critchlow CW, Leggot PJ et al: Periodontal status of HIV1 and HIV2 seropositive female commercial sex workers in Senegal, *J Periodontol* 68:827-831, 1997.

261. Scheutz F, Matee MIN, Andsager L et al: Is there an association between periodontal condition and HIV infection? *J Clin Periodontol* 24:580-587, 1997.

262. Robinson PG, Sheiham A, Challacombe SJ et al: Gingival ulceration in HIV infection: a case series and case-controlled study, *J Clin Periodontol* 25:260-267, 1998.

263. Ryder MI: Periodontal management of HIV-infected patients, *Periodontol 2000* 23:85-93, 2000.

264. Robinson PG, Adegboye A, Rowland RW et al: Periodontal diseases and HIV infection, *Oral Dis* 8(suppl 2):144-150, 2002.

265. McKaig RG, Patton LL, Thomas JC et al: Factors associated with periodontitis in an HIV-infected southeast USA study, *Oral Dis* 6:158-165, 2000.

266. Glick M, Holmstrup P: HIV infection and periodontal diseases. In Rose LF, Genco RJ, Mealey BL, Cohen DW, editors: *Periodontal medicine*, Toronto, 2000, BC Decker Publishers.

267. Lamster IB, Begg MD, Mitchell-Lewis D et al: Oral manifestations of HIV infection in homosexual men and intravenous drug users, *Oral Surg Oral Med Oral Pathol* 78:163-174, 1994.

268. Velegraki A, Nicolatou O, Theodoridou M et al: Paediatric AIDS-related linear gingival erythema: a form of erythematous candidiasis? *J Oral Pathol Med* 28:178-182, 1999.

269. Murray PA: Periodontal diseases in patients infected by human immunodeficiency virus. *Periodontol 2000* 6:50-67, 1994.

270. Glick M, Muzyka BC, Salkin LM, Lurie D: Necrotizing ulcerative periodontitis: a marker for immune deterioration and a predictor for the diagnosis of AIDS. *J Periodontol* 65:393-397, 1994.

271. Horning GM, Cohen ME: Necrotizing ulcerative gingivitis, periodontitis and stomatitis: clinical staging and predisposing factors, *J Periodontol* 66:990-998, 1995.

272. Murray PA, Winkler JR, Peros WJ et al: DNA probe detection of periodontal pathogens in HIV-associated periodontal lesions, *Oral Microbial Immunol* 6:34-40, 1991.

273. Glick M, Muzyka BC, Lurie D, Salkin LM: Oral manifestations associated with HIV disease as markers for immune suppression and AIDS, *Oral Surg Oral Med Oral Pathol* 77:344-349, 1994.

274. Jones AC, Gulley ML, Freedman PD: Necrotizing ulcerative stomatitis in human immunodeficiency virus-seropositive individuals: a review of the histopathologic, immunochemical, and virologic characteristics of 18 cases, *Oral Surg Oral Med Oral Pathol Oral Radiol Endod* 89:323-332, 2000.

275. Patton LL, McKaig R: Rapid progression of bone loss in HIV-associated necrotizing ulcerative stomatitis, *J Periodontol* 69:710-716, 1998.

276. Enwonwu CO, Falkler WA, Idigbe EO: Oro-facial gangrene (noma/cancrum oris): pathogenic mechanisms, *Crit Rev Oral Biol Med* 11:159-171, 2001.

277. Schneider D, Hofmann MT, Peterson JA: Diagnosis and treatment of Paget's disease of bone, *Am Fam Physician* 65:2069-2072, 2002.

278. Cremers S, Dam Sv S, Vermeij P: Bisphosphonate (olpadronate) retention and its determinants in Paget's disease of bone, *Br J Clin Pharmacol* 53:544-545, 2002.

279. Baab DA, Page RC, Morton T: Studies of a family manifesting premature exfoliation of deciduous teeth, *J Periodontol* 56:403-409, 1985.

280. Lepe X, Rothwell BR, Banich S, Page RC: Absence of adult dental anomalies in familial hypophosphatasia, *J Periodont Res* 32:375-380, 1997.

281. Fiocchi C: Inflammatory bowel disease: etiology and pathogenesis, *Gastroenterology* 115:182-205, 1998.

282. Habtezion A, Silverberg MS, Parkes R et al: Risk factors for low bone density in Crohn's disease, *Inflamm Bowel Dis* 8:87-92, 2002.

283. Brandtzaeg P: Inflammatory bowel disease: clinics and pathology—Do inflammatory bowel disease and periodontal disease have similar immunopathogeneses?, *Acta Odontol Scand* 59:235-243, 2001.

284. Lamster IB, Rodrick ML, Sonis ST, Falchuk ZM: An analysis of peripheral blood and salivary polymorphonuclear leukocyte function, circulating immune complex levels and oral status in patients with inflammatory bowel disease, *J Periodontol* 53:231-238, 1982.

285. Van Dyke TE, Dowell VR, Offenbacher S et al: Potential role of microorganisms isolated from periodontal lesions in the pathogenesis of inflammatory bowel disease, *Infect Immun* 53:671-677, 1986.

286. Flemmig TF, Shanahan F, Miyasaki KT: Prevalence and severity of periodontal disease in patients with inflammatory bowel disease, *J Clin Periodontol* 18:690-697, 1991.

287. Segal AW, Loewi G: Neutrophil dysfunction in Crohn's disease, *Lancet* 2:219-221, 1976.

288. Karrer S, Landthaler M, Schmalz G: Ehlers-Danlos type VIII. Review of the literature, *Clin Oral Investig* 4:66-69, 2000.

289. Perez LA, Al-Shammari KF, Giannobile WV, Wang HL: Treatment of periodontal disease in a patient with Ehlers-Danlos syndrome. A case report and literature review, *J Periodontol* 73:564-570, 2002.

290. Hartsfield JK, Kousseff BG: Phenotypic overlap of EDS types IV and VIII, *Am J Med Genet* 37:465-470, 1990.

291. Terezhalmy GT, Riley CK: Clinical images in oral medicine. Encephalotrigeminal syndrome (Sturge-Weber disease), *Quintessence Int* 31:62-63, 2000.

292. Cohen MM Jr: Perspectives on craniofacial asymmetry. VI. The hamartoses, *Int J Oral Maxillofac Surg* 24:195-200, 1995.

293. Mendieta C, Reeve CM: Periodontal manifestations of systemic disease and management of patients with systemic disease, *Curr Opin Periodontol* 18-27, 1993.

294. Cohen PS, Meltzer JA: Strawberry gums: a sign of Wegener's granulomatosis, *JAMA* 246:2610-2611, 1981.

295. Israelson H, Binnie WH, Hurt WC: The hyperplastic gingivitis of Wegener's granulomatosis, *J Periodontol* 52:81-87, 1981.

296. Klokkevold PR, Mealey BL, Carranza FA: Influences of systemic disease and disorders on the periodontium. In Newman MG, Takei HH, Carranza FA, editors: *Carranza's clinical periodontology*, Philadelphia, 2002, WB Saunders.

32 Effect of Periodontal Infection on Systemic Health and Well-Being

Sara G. Grossi, Brian L. Mealey, and Louis F. Rose

PERIODONTAL DISEASE AS A BIOFILM INFECTION

Periodontal diseases involve the inflammatory destruction of tooth-supporting tissues in response to bacteria in subgingival plaque. Dental plaque (supragingival and subgingival) is a microbial biofilm, that is, "matrix enclosed bacterial populations adherent to one another and to surfaces or interfaces"[1] (see Chapter 6). Bacterial growth in biofilms, unlike growth in a planktonic state, is aimed at growth and survival of the bacterial community as a whole. As such, bacteria growing in biofilms have developed sophisticated mechanisms to escape clearance either by the host or by antimicrobials. Bacteria growing in these complex biofilms are resistant to phagocytosis and killing by the host's immune system and to the effects of antimicrobial drugs. In this manner, bacterial biofilms are able to escape natural surveillance and clearance mechanisms, are preserved, and sustain continuous growth. Socransky and coworkers[2] described the organization of dental plaque biofilms as conglomerates of "microbial complexes," whereby microbial species in dental plaque exist in communities that relate to one another in a specific fashion, referred to as "red, orange, yellow and green complexes" (Fig. 32-1) (see Chapter 4). Cluster and community ordination analysis, including 13,000 plaque samples from 185 patients with periodontal conditions ranging from health to disease, revealed that *Actinomyces naeslundii* 2 (*Actinomyces viscosus*) appears closely related to members of the "yellow complex" (*Streptococcus sanguis, Streptococcus mitis, Streptococcus gordonii* and *Streptococcus intermedius*), "green complex" (*Eikenella corrodens, Capnocytophaga gingivalis, Capnocytophaga sputigena*), and "purple complex" (*Veillonella parvula, Actinomyces odontolyticus*), and appear to colonize the subgingival sulcus first. Thus, these organisms are associated with gingival health and are detected in healthy periodontal sites. These complexes are followed by members of the "orange complex" consisting of *Eubacterium nodatum, Peptostreptococcus micros*, and species from the genera *Fusobacterium, Prevotella*, and *Campylobacter* (Fig. 32-1). Members of the orange complex are associated with gingivitis and more specifically with the presence of gingival bleeding. The orange complex, in turn, is associated with the "red complex" consisting of *Porphyromonas gingivalis, Tannerella forsythensis* (formerly *Bacteroides forsythus*), and *Treponema denticola*. These organisms are found in significantly greater numbers in diseased sites, sites with deeper pockets, and more advanced lesions.[3] Notably, these three organisms are commonly detected together in subgingival plaque samples. Thus, it appears that in the structure of the dental plaque biofilm there is a succession in microbial colonization with a dramatic shift in flora from health to disease and establishment of a gram-negative anaerobic flora in sites with periodontal pocketing.[2]

One of the salient features of bacteria growing in biofilm is the complex communal physiology, allowing

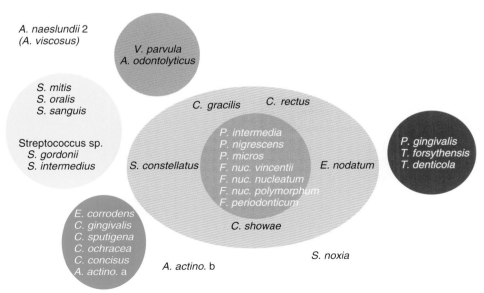

Figure 32-1. Microbial complexes in subgingival biofilms. A total of 13,261 plaque samples from 185 subjects diagnosed as periodontally healthy, well-maintained elderly or with adult periodontitis were analyzed using checkerboard DNA-DNA hybridization. Microbial species exist in the subgingival biofilm in the specific complexes depicted in the figure. (*Redrawn from Socransky S, Haffajee AD, Cugini MA et al: Microbial complexes in subgingival plaque,* J Clin Periodontol 25:134-144, 1998.)

for the survival of the entire microbial community. Coaggregation of *P. gingivalis* with other gram-negative or gram-positive organisms is mediated by specific outer membrane proteins, and as such, plays an important role in the maintenance of the subgingival biofilm. Bacteria growing in biofilms are notoriously resistant to clearance mechanisms such as phagocytosis and killing by the host's immune system or by antimicrobial drugs. This unique feature of bacterial biofilms underscores the recurrent nature of periodontal disease and the difficulty in eliminating periodontal infection. Probably the most significant consequence of bacteria growing on biofilms is the constant shed of bacterial products and byproducts into the neighboring environment. Significant virulence factors able to evade the host's clearance mechanisms and to participate in tissue destruction have been identified in *P. gingivalis*.[4] They include a number of inhibitors of PMN chemotaxis and phagocytosis, capsule, fimbriae, and outer membrane proteins. In addition, bacteria within the subgingival biofilm are continuously releasing cell surface products into the gingival sulcus. The ulcerated pocket epithelium becomes a significant portal of entry of oral bacteria and their products into the general circulation. With apical and lateral extension of the bacterial biofilm along the root surface, the subgingival space becomes a niche of gram-negative organisms with the potential to seed oral bacteria at distant sites and into the general circulation in small and major blood vessels. The total surface area of periodontal ligament membrane in a complete dentition has been compared with the size of the palm of an adult hand. Thus, the potential for distant seeding of oral infections is ever present. In this manner, periodontal biofilm infection contributes not only to local inflammation resulting in destruction of tooth supporting structures, but to systemic inflammation as well.

PERIODONTAL BIOFILM INFECTION AND CHRONIC SYSTEMIC INFLAMMATION

A number of chronic conditions such as atherosclerosis, coronary heart disease (CHD), rheumatoid arthritis, type 2 diabetes, obesity, osteoporosis, and periodontal disease share a common pathophysiologic feature: chronic, sustained, exacerbated inflammatory response to a given stimulus. This exacerbated response is marked by increased production of proinflammatory cytokines, initially secreted to provide clearance of invading organisms and to repair tissue damage. This exacerbated proinflammatory response may result in excessive tissue damage rather than repair. A significant finding has been the determination that monocyte-derived cytokines such as tumor necrosis factor–α (TNF-α) and interleukins (IL-1β, IL-6, and IL-8) may be released in response to a series of

stimuli secondary to periodontal infection.[5] One of these potential stimuli, the endotoxin lipopolysaccharide (LPS) from gram-negative bacteria, is present in subgingival biofilm. LPS and other bacterial components can activate synthesis and secretion of these cytokines and an inflammatory cascade that, in turn, contributes to systemic inflammation, either through a direct action on blood vessel walls, or indirectly by inducing the liver to produce acute phase proteins.[6,7] LPS from the cell walls of these gram-negative organisms has both endotoxic and immunologic activities. Specifically, *P. gingivalis* LPS is a potent inducer of IL-1β, TNF-α, prostaglandin E$_2$ (PGE$_2$), and matrix metalloproteinases.[5] The LPS and the inflammatory cytokines present in periodontal disease may also increase expression of leukocyte adhesion molecules such as inflammatory cell adhesion molecule or vascular cell adhesion molecule by endothelial cells.[8-11]

Evidence indicates that *P. gingivalis* has the ability to invade endothelial cells. *P. gingivalis* can actively adhere to and invade bovine heart cells and aortic endothelial cells.[12] Studies in animal models have shown that *P. gingivalis* LPS and its outer membrane vesicles are able to induce macrophages to engorge low density lipoprotein (LDL) to form large "foam cells" (an important characteristic of cardiovascular disease), monocyte chemotaxis from endothelial cells, and oxidation of LDL.[13] Thus, LPS and cell surface products from *P. gingivalis* are able to recruit inflammatory cells into major blood vessels; activate the inflammatory cascade by direct effect on these inflammatory cells and secrete inflammatory mediators such as IL-1β and TNF-α on the vascular endothelium; and promote smooth muscle proliferation, platelet aggregation, fatty degeneration, and deposition on the vessel wall (Fig. 32-2). This cascade of events serves to narrow the

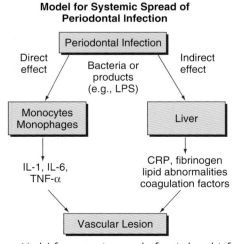

Figure 32-2. Model for systemic spread of periodontal infection and effects on vasculature.

vessel lumen and inhibit normal blood flow. In addition, proteolytic enzymes from *P. gingivalis* released in large quantities can activate factor X, prothrombin, and protein C, promoting a thrombotic tendency. Some investigators have proposed a direct effect on systemic inflammation of some of the bacteria found in dental plaque, which enter the bloodstream during episodes of dental bacteremiae.[14,15] The oral gram-positive bacteria *S. sanguis* and the periodontal pathogen *P. gingivalis* have been shown to induce platelet activation and aggregation through the expression of collagen-like, platelet aggregation–associated proteins. The aggregated platelets may contribute to hypercoagulability and thrombosis, thus leading to thromboembolic events. Therefore, presence of these microorganisms in the bloodstream, derived from an oral source such as the periodontium, may increase the risk for thrombus formation and subsequent release of an embolus.

LPS and other cell wall products from periodontal bacteria can indirectly stimulate the liver to produce the acute phase protein known as C-reactive protein (CRP). The acute phase response is part of innate immunity and is the initial response to a bacterial challenge. This highly reactive enzyme can, in turn, promote deposits on injured blood vessels if secreted in excess (Fig. 32-2). Specifically, CRP binds to damaged cells, fixes complement, and activates neutrophil chemotaxis. Moderately increased serum levels of CRP constitute a systemic marker of inflammation, a documented risk factor for cardiovascular disease. Increased levels of CRP have been proposed as a marker to predict future myocardial infarction and stroke. Significantly increased levels of CRP have been demonstrated in patients with chronic periodontitis.[16] These increased CRP levels have been associated with body mass index, an indicator of obesity (a condition also associated with excessive inflammatory response), and periodontal disease in otherwise healthy middle-aged adults.[17] Furthermore, levels of CRP in patients with periodontitis are related to the severity of periodontal disease and level of infection with *P. gingivalis*, *T. forsythensis*, and *P. intermedia*, thus implying a gradient of periodontal infection and systemic inflammation.[18] People with periodontitis are also at risk for having increased levels of circulating fibrinogen.[19,20] Increased fibrinogen is a risk factor for acute events such as myocardial infarction and stroke, because fibrinogen is associated with coagulation and with increased blood viscosity. The net effect of increased CRP and fibrinogen levels, especially when accompanied by increased platelet aggregation and narrowing of the blood vessel lumen, is an increased risk for major cardiovascular and cerebrovascular events.

Direct evidence for the role of periodontal infection in systemic inflammation comes from the identification of periodontal pathogens in human carotid atheromas.[21]

About 70% of atheromatous lesions removed from the carotid arteries of patients undergoing carotid endarterectomy had bacteria in the atheroma; 44% had one or more periodontal pathogens.[21] Additional direct evidence that infection with *P. gingivalis* contributes to systemic inflammation comes from animal studies. *P. gingivalis* activates the acute phase response, increases blood lipid levels, and enhances atheroma lesion formation in mice. Infection of mice with *P. gingivalis* leads to calcification of aortic atherosclerotic plaques, with the amount of calcification increasing with the length of exposure to *P. gingivalis* infection. Therefore, the subgingival biofilm infection is a constant reservoir of LPS and other toxic bacterial products, which likely contribute to and sustain systemic inflammation and promote lesions in blood vessel walls.

Evidence suggests that the presence of periodontitis dramatically increases the risk for endotoxin being transferred to the systemic circulation. Increased endotoxin levels in the vasculature can initiate the proinflammatory responses discussed earlier, resulting in changes to the vasculature. For example, one study showed that after chewing gum, there was a fourfold increase in the incidence of endotoxemia (endotoxin in the bloodstream) in patients with severe periodontitis compared with subjects with only mild or moderate periodontitis.[22] Not only was the risk for endotoxemia greater, but the quantitative level of endotoxin was more than fourfold greater in the patients with periodontitis than in those subjects without periodontitis. Thus, the simple act of chewing can induce bacteria and their products such as endotoxin to enter the bloodstream, and the risk for this event is much greater in patients with periodontitis.

PERIODONTAL INFECTION AND CARDIOVASCULAR DISEASE

Tobacco smoking and high levels of LDL or "bad" cholesterol have long been associated with cardiovascular disease. More recently, increased levels of CRP have been identified as important risk factors for myocardial infarction, increasing its risk twofold to fivefold. A large body of evidence supports the hypothesis that periodontal disease is associated with cardiovascular risk factors including CRP and plasma fibrinogen. Using data from the Third National Health and Nutrition Examination Survey (NHANES III), a large epidemiologic study of the U.S. population, investigators found that individuals with periodontitis have increased systemic levels of CRP and fibrinogen after adjustment for dental calculus, ethnicity, education, sex, age, family size, poverty index, body mass index, family history of myocardial infarction, diabetes, and tobacco and alcohol use.[19,20] This has been confirmed by others who showed that CRP levels were increased in patients with periodontal disease as compared with periodontally healthy individuals.[16,23] This increase was not associated with seropositivity to *Chlamydia pneumoniae*, cytomegalovirus, or *Helicobacter pylori* in subjects with periodontal disease, thus eliminating these organisms not associated with periodontitis as the probable cause of the increase in CRP levels.[23] Furthermore, treatment of periodontal patients is associated with a reduction of CRP levels 1 year after therapy.[16] Antiinfective periodontal therapy, such as scaling and root planing and administration of subgingival doxycycline as an adjunct to scaling and root planing, results in a reduction in levels of CRP and fibrinogen to normal levels.[24] In addition, periodontal maintenance therapy aimed at reducing levels of subgingival *P. gingivalis* maintains the levels of CRP and fibrinogen within normal values over time. Mechanical periodontal therapy combined with subgingival administration of minocycline reduced levels of CRP and TNF-α in patients with increased risk for atherosclerosis.[25] Results from these studies have quite significant implications for management of periodontal infections in patients with periodontal disease and increased risk for cardiovascular disease. In this chapter, the evidence supporting an association between periodontal disease and cardiovascular disease is reviewed in relation to the different types of cardiovascular diseases.

Periodontal Infection and Atherosclerosis

Atherosclerosis, the primary cause of death and disability in the United States, is one of the chronic conditions associated with hyperinflammatory states. Atherogenesis is a multifactorial process resulting when endothelial cells and smooth muscle cells are subjected to excessive extracellular stimuli. Histologically, atherosclerotic plaques resemble healing inflammatory lesions, from which Dr. Russell Ross proposed a "response to injury" hypothesis for their formation.[26] Of great significance in the pathogenesis of atherosclerosis are endothelial dysfunction, lipid deposition and oxidation in the subendothelial space, leukocyte chemotaxis, proliferation of smooth muscle cells, and, finally, plaque rupture. Intraplaque inflammation has been proposed to play a role in thinning of the fibrous cap, plaque rupture, and thrombosis and to precipitate the clinical events leading to myocardial infarction, unstable angina, stroke, and transient ischemic attacks. Recently, the theory of chronic inflammation in atherosclerosis and plaque rupture has gained considerable interest, both from the basic and applied research point of view, as well as patient management. Most of the newly developed drugs to manage cardiovascular disease exhibit significant antiinflammatory effects.

Direct evidence for the role of periodontal infection in atherosclerosis comes from the identification of periodontal pathogens in human carotid atheromas.[21] Fifty carotid atheromas obtained at endarterectomy were analyzed for the presence of bacterial 16 S rDNA by polymerase chain reaction using synthetic oligonucleotide probes specific for the periodontal pathogens *Actinobacillus actinomycetemcomitans*, *Tannerella forsythensis* (*Bacteroides forsythus*), *P. gingivalis*, and *Prevotella intermedia*. Of the specimens, 30% were positive for *Tannerella forsythensis* (*B. forsythus*), 26% were positive for *P. gingivalis*, 18% were positive for *A. actinomycetemcomitans*, and 14% were positive for *P. intermedia*. *Chlamydia pneumoniae* DNA was detected in 18% of these atheromas. *C. pneumoniae* has long been associated with atherosclerosis. These studies suggest that periodontal pathogens may be present in arteriosclerotic plaques where, like other infectious organisms such as *C. pneumoniae*, they may play a direct role in the development and progression of atherosclerosis.

Nuclear factor-kappa B (NF-κB) is an inducible nuclear transcription factor that controls multiple aspects of the inflammatory response. Stimulation of cells with various inflammatory stimuli (LPS, TNF-α, and IL-1β) results in nuclear translocation and transcription of NF-κB. In turn, NF-κB is responsible for macrophage activation and regulation of smooth muscle cell proliferation. A mechanistic pathway to explain the relation of periodontal infection and atherosclerosis is through constant activation of NF-κB by stimuli such as LPS, TNF-α, and IL-1β from chronic periodontal infection. This activation of NK-κB up-regulates macrophages and induces them to secrete large quantities of proinflammatory cytokines, which further exacerbates inflammatory effects on the blood vessel wall.

Another potential linking mechanism between periodontal disease and atherosclerosis involves immune responses that result in production of antibodies to periodontal bacteria, including antibodies to bacterial heat shock proteins that cross-react with heat shock proteins of the heart. These autoreactive antibodies to heat shock proteins are found in patients with periodontal disease and may contribute to atheroma formation.[27,28]

The clinical association between periodontal diseases and atherosclerosis has been evaluated by using coronary angiograms. In one study, there was a significant association between the severity of periodontal disease assessed radiographically and the degree of coronary atheromatosis.[29] In another study, the extent and severity of periodontitis were significantly greater in people with stenosis of one or more epicardial arteries compared with individuals without arterial stenosis.[30] However, when the data were adjusted to account for the effects of age and smoking, factors common to both periodontal disease and cardiovascular disease, the relation between the diseases was no longer statistically significant. This study serves to point out an important factor that must be considered when examining the evidence that relates periodontal diseases to other systemic conditions; namely, the confounding that may occur when risk factors are shared by the various diseases. For example, smoking and diabetes are risk factors for periodontitis and CHD. In determining the relation between periodontitis and CHD, it is important to understand the smoking status and diabetes status of the subjects examined in the various studies to ensure that the relation is between the two diseases and not between risk factors for those diseases. This is generally done through statistical analysis of the data, using tests that can account for such confounding factors and can provide support that a given risk factor (such as periodontal disease) is independent of other known risk factors (such as smoking).

Periodontal Infection and Coronary Heart Disease (Myocardial Infarction)

There is extensive evidence associating inflammatory factors such as CRP and fibrinogen with CHD. Systematic reviews of prospective studies demonstrate highly statistically significant associations between increased white blood cell counts and increased levels of acute phase proteins such as fibrinogen and CRP with a subsequent risk for cardiovascular disease.[31] Increased CRP levels have been suggested to be valuable prognostic indicators of the risk for cardiovascular events.[32,33] Periodontal infections may be associated with increased risk for atherosclerotic processes such as coronary artery disease and strokes, in part by their association with increased levels of CRP, as discussed earlier.

A series of case–control and cross-sectional studies have shown a significant association among various indexes of poor dental health and CHD.[34-38] For example, Arbes and colleagues[37] evaluated the association between periodontal disease and CHD in NHANES III and found that the odds for a history of heart attack increased with the severity of periodontal disease. With the greatest severity of periodontal disease, the odds ratio was 3.8 (95% confidence interval [CI]; 1.5 to 9.7) as compared with no periodontal disease after adjustment for co-risk factors for periodontal disease and heart disease such as age, sex, race, poverty, smoking, diabetes, high blood pressure, body mass index, and serum cholesterol. This study confirmed the association seen in other cross-sectional studies and also demonstrated a gradient response with high levels of periodontal disease associated with greater prevalence of reported heart attack. However, consistent with other cross-sectional studies, these results point merely to an association, because no temporal sequence is established. Data from longitudinal studies is needed to establish a temporal sequence between periodontal disease and heart disease.

Longitudinal studies suggest that indicators of poor periodontal health precede cardiovascular events.[39-43] Data from 9760 men and women examined in the first NHANES study (NHANES I) and again in its 16-year Epidemiological Follow-up Study showed that periodontal disease was a significant predictor of subsequent CHD disease.[39] There was a 70% increase in the risk for hospitalization or death from a CHD-related event in individuals younger than 50 years who had periodontitis compared with similarly aged people without periodontitis. Again, the association was independent of all important co-risk factors. In addition to the consistent association between periodontal disease and heart disease, there appears to be a biologic gradient between periodontal infection and incidence of CHD. In an assessment of 921 men 21 to 80 years old who were free of CHD at baseline and were then followed for a period of approximately 18 years, investigators found a dose relation between various levels of bone loss (20%, 40%, 60%, and 80%) and cumulative incidence of angina and myocardial infarction[41] (Fig. 32-3). A similar gradient was observed for fatal coronary disease and mean alveolar bone loss, again independent of all important co-risk factors. These longitudinal studies, in which the presence of periodontal disease is known to have preceded the CHD-related events, provide support for the concept that periodontal disease is a risk factor for CHD.

The association of specific subgingival periodontal organisms with myocardial infarction has been assessed.[44] In this study, 97 nonfatal myocardial infarction cases were compared with 233 control subjects. The adjusted odds ratio (95% CI) for myocardial infarction was 2.99 (1.40 to 6.35) for the presence of *Tannerella forsythensis* (*B. forsythus*) and 2.52 (1.35 to 4.70) for *P. gingivalis*. These findings support the notion that specific pathogenic bacteria found in periodontal disease may also be associated with myocardial infarction.

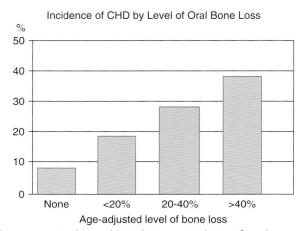

Figure 32-3. Gradient relation between incidence of total coronary heart disease and different levels of alveolar bone loss. (*Adapted from Beck J et al: Periodontal disease and cardiovascular disease.* J Periodontol *67:1123-1137, 1996.*)

Periodontal Infection and Cerebrovascular Disease (Stroke)

Case–control studies have shown poor dental health to be associated with an increased risk for cerebrovascular ischemia (CVA) and stroke.[34] In men younger than 50 years, 25% of patients who experienced a stroke had significant dental disease, compared with only 2.5% of control patients without cerebrovascular disease. Grau and colleagues[45] examined the dental status, including dental caries, periodontitis, and endodontic lesions, of more than 300 patients with CVA, brain infarction, and transient cerebral ischemia. An increased risk for CVA (odds ratio 2.60 [95% CI; 1.18 to 5.70]) was associated with periodontitis and periapical lesions. The risk for CVA was not associated with dental caries. Analysis of NHANES I data showed that periodontal disease was a significant risk factor for nonhemorrhagic stroke, but not for hemorrhagic stroke.[46] Nonhemorrhagic stroke is associated with atherosclerotic change and narrowing of the major arteries, whereas hemorrhagic stroke is generally associated with aneurysm formation and rupture. The relative risk for nonhemorrhagic stroke was 1.41 (95% CI; 1.30 to 3.42) for periodontitis, indicating a significant increased risk for stroke in patients with periodontitis. These associations were seen for white and black men and women. Periodontal disease was also associated with nonhemorrhagic stroke in the Physicians Health Study with similar odds ratios (1.33; 95% CI; 1.03 to 1.70).[47] The finding that periodontal disease was not associated with hemorrhagic stroke in this national sample strengthens the association and points to mechanistic pathways that account for this association. That is, periodontitis increased the risk for those cerebrovascular events that are associated with narrowing of the arteries, and there is substantial evidence that periodontal infection may impact atherosclerosis. Conversely, there is no evidence that periodontal infection is associated with the mechanisms responsible for aneurysm formation, and likewise no clinical evidence that periodontal disease is associated with nonhemorrhagic stroke.

PERIODONTAL INFECTION AND DIABETES MELLITUS

Diabetes mellitus is a disease of dysregulation of carbohydrate and lipid metabolism following the inability of the pancreas to secrete insulin (type 1 diabetes) or a deficiency in insulin action or sensitivity (type 2 diabetes) (see Chapter 31). Type 2 diabetes is by far the most common type of diabetes, accounting for almost 90% of diabetes cases. The prevalence of diabetes mellitus is increasing at alarming rates worldwide, entirely because of the increase in type 2 diabetes. This is mostly related to an epidemic increase in its primary risk factor: obesity.

In the United States alone, the figures are staggering with a 30% increase, to the point of being considered the most significant lifestyle epidemic of modern times. This diabetes epidemic, as it has been defined, carries with it a significant burden to society in terms of morbidity, mortality, and associated health care costs.

A large body of evidence supports the concept that diabetes is a risk factor for periodontal diseases (see Chapter 31 for detailed discussion). The following discussion is focused on the ways in which periodontal diseases may affect the diabetic condition.

Effect of Periodontal Infection on Diabetes Mellitus

Periodontitis has been determined to be a potential risk factor for poor glycemic control in patients with diabetes. In a longitudinal study of patients with type 2 diabetes who demonstrated good glycemic control at baseline, 37% of subjects with severe periodontitis showed a worsening of glycemic control over time, compared with only 11% of subjects without severe periodontitis.[48] Notably, in this study, the presence of periodontal disease was known to have preceded the worsening of blood sugar control. Further evidence for a relation between periodontal infection and diabetic control can be obtained through studies of other diabetic complications, such as retinopathy, nephropathy, and macrovascular complications such as cardiovascular, cerebrovascular, and peripheral vascular disease. In one such study, patients with diabetes and severe periodontitis were shown to have a much greater incidence of macrovascular complications during a 1- to 11-year period than did a control population of patients with diabetes but without periodontitis.[49] Only 21% of patients without periodontitis had one or more macrovascular complications, compared with 82% of patients with severe periodontitis.

Periodontal therapy in patients who also have diabetes may have a beneficial impact on glycemic control and periodontal health. More than 40 years ago, the benefit of periodontal therapy was recognized in a group of young people with type 1 diabetes who also had severe periodontitis.[50] After these patients received treatment, which included systemic antibiotics, extraction of periodontally hopeless teeth, scaling and root planing, and gingivectomy when indicated, there was a reduction in the amount of insulin needed to control blood sugar levels. More recently, the combination of scaling and root planing plus systemic doxycycline therapy (100 mg/day for 14 days) was shown to improve glycemic control in conjunction with improvement in periodontal health.[51] Interestingly, in this study, those patients who had minimal improvement in periodontal health after therapy also showed no improvement in glycemic control. In a randomized, placebo-controlled, clinical trial of periodontal therapy in subjects with type 2 diabetes, the combination of scaling and root planing plus systemic doxycycline was associated with short-term improvement in glycemic control; conversely, scaling and root planing combined with a placebo (i.e., without adjunctive antibiotic therapy) was not associated with significant changes in glycemic control.[52] This study suggests that antibiotic therapy using systemic tetracycline antibiotics such as doxycycline may be an important component of periodontal treatment for these patients. Other research would support this contention. For example, in studies of people with diabetes and periodontal disease in which periodontal therapy consisted only of mechanical debridement (scaling and root planing), without systemic antibiotic therapy, there has been no demonstrated beneficial effect on glycemic control.[53-55] Many of the patients in these studies already had good glycemic control at the baseline examinations; therefore, one might expect less dramatic changes in glycemic control with any type of therapy. Although routine use of systemic antibiotics is not justified for most patients with periodontitis, patients with diabetes may constitute one group in whom such therapy is indicated. The effect of periodontal therapy on diabetic control is more likely to be evident in patients who have more advanced periodontitis and poorer glycemic control before therapy, compared with patients who have less severe periodontitis and better glycemic control before treatment.

Mechanisms of Interaction between Periodontal Infection and Diabetes Mellitus

The mechanisms by which periodontal infection influences glycemic control have not yet been fully elucidated. However, evidence from studies of other systemic conditions provides important clues. It is clear that systemic infections such as viral or bacterial respiratory infections have a major impact on glycemic control because they increase insulin resistance.[56,57] Virtually every cell in the body (except brain cells) has cell surface insulin receptors that act as loading elements signaling the cells' need for glucose uptake. When energy requirements are increased or if blood glucose levels are increased, insulin receptors are displayed on the cell surface and glucose is loaded and transported intracellularly. In this manner, excess glucose is removed from circulation and stored intracellularly, mostly in adipose tissue. Cells can become resistant to the action of insulin. When they do, the pancreas increases production of insulin in an attempt to "force" glucose into the cells. This is known as *insulin resistance.* Tissues affected the most by insulin resistance include the liver, muscle, and adipose. As a result of the compensatory increase in insulin production, there is a state of prolonged hyperinsulinemia. Increased levels of insulin have a direct damaging effect on coronary arteries contributing to atheromatous plaque formation, abnormalities in lipid metabolism, and hypercoagulability.

Some of these abnormalities include increased production of fibrinogen, high levels of triglycerides (the body's main fat storage particles), and decreased levels of high-density lipoprotein. Individuals affected by insulin resistance also will exhibit hyperlipidemia, increased cholesterol, and triglycerides. Increase in circulating lipids leads to excessive lipid oxidation, deposition of these oxidized fractions on the vascular wall, and atherosclerosis.

Because systemic infections increase the resistance of the tissues to the action of insulin, the pancreas must then increase insulin secretion to overcome the insulin resistance. In individuals with type 1 diabetes, who produce no endogenous insulin, such insulin resistance requires the injection of increased amounts of insulin. In patients with type 2 diabetes, who already have increased insulin resistance, increased resistance associated with infection serves to further exacerbate hyperglycemia. Importantly, insulin resistance persists in the tissues even after the patient recovers from the systemic illness; tissue sensitivity to insulin often does not return to normal for many weeks or months after the illness.

It is possible that periodontal infection results in similar increases in insulin resistance, which would then result in poorer glycemic control. Periodontal therapy, aimed at reducing the microbial bioburden and associated inflammation, may serve to restore insulin sensitivity and thereby improve glycemic control.[58,59] In this way, periodontal infection is related to another important risk factor for type 2 diabetes: obesity.

Obesity is a leading cause of insulin resistance, a condition that is becoming more and more prevalent in the Western world and is a significant risk factor for type 2 diabetes mellitus, hypertension, and cardiovascular disease. A significant association was found between obesity and periodontal disease in young adults.[60] Adipocytes, once believed to be essentially fat storage cells, have been identified as extremely metabolically active cells. Adipocytes are highly active in production of molecules important in regulating energy expenditure such as leptin and adinopectin. Adipocytes also are active in production of TNF-α. Blood levels of TNF-α are increased in obese patients and are decreased after weight loss. They also are increased in people with diabetes, especially in those with periodontal disease. Monocytes from patients with diabetes produce 24 to 32 times the level of TNF-α when stimulated by periodontal pathogens than do monocytes from subjects without diabetes.[61] Dumping of TNF-α into the systemic circulation in patients with diabetes may contribute to insulin resistance, and periodontal therapy may reduce the levels of circulating TNF-α and reduce the index of insulin resistance.[62]

TNF-α is an antagonist to the cell surface insulin receptor substrate (IRS-1). It inhibits phosphorylation and translocation of the insulin receptor.[63,64] In doing so,

TNF-α blocking of the insulin receptor inhibits intracellular glucose transport and insulin action, contributing to insulin resistance. Recent evidence suggests that chronic periodontal infection also contributes to insulin resistance.[65] Chronic up-regulation of TNF-α in response to LPS and other cell surface toxins from bacteria in the subgingival biofilm is likely a mechanism contributing to the state of insulin resistance in individuals at risk. Figure 32-4 presents a model proposing how periodontal infection and chronic up-regulation of inflammatory cytokines in response to periodontal bacteria aggravates the state of insulin resistance, precipitating and sustaining metabolic abnormalities. This will, in turn, predispose susceptible individuals to either type 2 diabetes or cardiovascular disease. Thus, excess circulating insulin, as occurs in insulin-resistant states, may function as a common link between chronic periodontal infection and worsening of systemic conditions such as cardiovascular disease or type 2 diabetes. Systemic inflammation and excessive synthesis and secretion of TNF-α appear to be possible mechanisms accounting for the two-way relation between diabetes mellitus and periodontal disease.

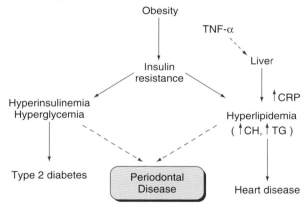

Figure 32-4. Model to describe insulin resistance as a possible mechanism common to periodontal infection and systemic complications such as type 2 diabetes and cardiovascular disease. Insulin resistance (often initiated or exacerbated by obesity) results in hyperinsulinemia and hyperglycemia, which worsens glycemic control. Hyperglycemia may then increase the risk for periodontal disease. Insulin resistance is also associated with hyperlipidemia (*CH*, cholesterol; *TG*, triglycerides). Increased tumor necrosis factor (TNF-α) levels associated with obesity may result in increased C-reactive protein (CRP) production by the liver, further exacerbating hyperlipidemia. Increased lipid levels, particularly low-density lipoprotein and triglyceride, increase the risk for heart disease and may play a role in the pathogenesis of periodontal disease.

PERIODONTAL INFECTION, PRETERM BIRTH, AND LOW BIRTH WEIGHT

Preterm birth (PTB) infants born before the thirty-seventh week of gestation and low birth weight (LBW) infants born at term but weighing less than 2500 g are significant perinatal problems in all developed countries. In the United States alone, this accounts for 6% to 9% of all births and 70% of all perinatal deaths. Substantial morbidity and long-term neurologic sequelae are also associated with LBW, resulting in great costs to the individual, family, and society. Traditional treatment for PTB has been mostly symptomatic–that is, the use of drugs to arrest premature contractions. Despite widespread use of such drugs, there has been no decrease in LBW or PTB in the last 20 years. Therefore, attempting to understand the underlying causes leading to more specific therapies is the more desirable approach. Evidence points to symptomatic genital infections as a primary etiologic factor for PTB. Nongenital infections such as acute pyelonephritis and pneumonia also have been recognized as causes of PTB. Some other known risk factors include smoking, drug or alcohol use during pregnancy, low socioeconomic status, diabetes, and poor prenatal care. Although one or more risk factors is present in most cases of PTB/LBW, none of the known risk factors is present in about 25% of cases.[66] In recent years, subclinical and chronic infections such as periodontal disease have been proposed to play a role in premature birth, and they significantly increase the risk for both LBW and PTB.

The mechanism explaining the hypothesis of chronic infection and premature birth is that microorganisms or their products and toxins, such as LPS, enter the uterine cavity either through the ascending route in genitourinary tract infections or through the circulation in nongenital infections. Once the microorganisms or their products have gained access to the uterine cavity, they can stimulate an inflammatory cytokine cascade, with increased production of proinflammatory mediators such as IL-1β and TNF-α. These eventually lead to elevated prostaglandin synthesis, which causes uterine muscle contraction, cervical dilation, and premature rupture of membranes.

Three lines of evidence support the infectious theory of PTB. Studies in animal models have shown that bacteria and their products are able to induce PTB. Positive cultures of amniotic fluid and membranes are often detected in patients with PTB, and antibiotic treatment has decreased the number of PTB in some clinical trials. Bacterial vaginosis, the most common vaginal disorder in women of reproductive age, is a known risk factor for preterm labor, premature rupture of membranes, and LBW.[67] In bacterial vaginosis, the normal vaginal microflora predominated by facultative lactobacilli is replaced by more anaerobic organisms, many of which produce potent endotoxins (LPS). Presence of these organisms in the chorioamnion may result in the inflammatory cascade discussed earlier, resulting in preterm labor and rupture of membranes. Treatment of bacterial vaginosis with metronidazole in pregnant women has been shown to decrease PTB rates when compared with treatment with a placebo.[68] Women who have preterm labor often have culture-positive amniotic fluid, even when no clinical infection is evident. Usually, the organisms cultured are those associated with genitourinary tract infections such as bacterial vaginosis. But in some occasions, organisms not normally found in the genitourinary tract are cultured. It is possible that these organisms colonized the chorioamnion from a hematogenous route. In women with periodontitis, the oral cavity may be a source of such organisms. In animal models, oral organisms such as *P. gingivalis* implanted subcutaneously have been shown to result in increased amniotic TNF-α and PGE_2 levels.[69] This infection caused a decrease in fetal birth weight and an increase in fetal deaths.

The findings from animal studies have resulted in examination of the effects of periodontal infection on pregnancy outcomes in humans. In a case–control study of 93 women having a LBW delivery and 31 women having normal birth weight delivery, investigators determine that the women with LBW delivery had significantly more severe clinical attachment loss.[70] In fact, the presence of severe periodontitis resulted in a 7.5-fold increased risk for LBW, a greater risk factor than smoking or alcohol use during pregnancy. These results have been confirmed in a large prospective study of more than 1300 women who were examined at 21 to 24 weeks gestation.[71] The presence of generalized periodontitis at this point in gestation was associated with a marked increase in risk for PTB (odds ratios, 4.45 to 7.07). Periodontal disease at antepartum and both the incidence and progression of periodontal disease during pregnancy are associated with greater incidence of PTB and smaller birth weight for gestational age after adjusting for race, parity, and the neonate's sex.[72] The increased risk for LBW and PTB in women with periodontitis also has been confirmed in populations from other countries.[73,74] As the severity of periodontal disease increases, the birth weight and gestational age at delivery decrease.[74]

In utero exposure of the fetus to periodontal microorganisms or their products is demonstrated by a 2.9-fold increase in cord blood immunoglobulin M (IgM) titers to these organisms in preterm neonates compared with neonates delivered at term.[75] In addition, maternal IgG antibody to periodontal organisms appeared protective against both fetal exposure and PTB. No significant differences in the frequency of putative periodontal pathogens were seen between preterm and full-term mothers.

Intervention trials have been performed to determine whether periodontal treatment during gestation can affect pregnancy outcome in women with periodontitis. In one such study, the incidence of PTB or LBW was 1o.1% in women with periodontal disease who did not receive periodontal therapy until after parturition.[76] Conversely, women who received scaling and root planing during the second trimester followed by frequent prophylaxis until delivery had a PTB or LBW rate of only 1.8%. These results are similar to a study in which pregnant women with periodontitis who had scaling and root planing during pregnancy had a lower rate of PTB (o.8%) compared with women who did not receive periodontal treatment until after parturition (6.3%).[77] Taken together, these studies indicate that women who have periodontitis are at increased risk for adverse pregnancy outcomes, and that treatment of the periodontal condition with mechanical debridement and oral hygiene instruction may reduce the risk for such outcomes. The potential public health implications of these findings are incalculable.

PERIODONTAL DISEASE AND RESPIRATORY DISEASES

The upper respiratory tract often contains microorganisms derived from the nasal, oral, and pharyngeal areas. The lower airway is usually free of microorganisms. Pneumonia is an inflammation of the lung tissue caused by bacteria, fungi, or viruses. Pneumonia may be either community acquired or hospital acquired (also called *nosocomial pneumonia*). Most cases of community-acquired bacterial pneumonia are caused by aspiration of oropharyngeal organisms such as *Streptococcus pneumoniae, Haemophilus influenzae,* and *Mycoplasma pneumoniae.*[78] Community-acquired bacterial pneumonia has a low mortality rate and generally responds well to treatment. There is no evidence that periodontal disease or oral hygiene alters the risk for community-acquired pneumonia.

Conversely, hospital-acquired pneumonia has a mortality rate of about 25%.[79] Hospital-acquired pneumonia is not caused by the same organisms that cause community-acquired pneumonia; rather, it usually results from infection with organisms that do not normally colonize the oropharynx, such as *Klebsiella pneumoniae, Pseudomonas aeruginosa, Staphylococcus aureus,* and *Escherichia coli.* These organisms, called *potential respiratory pathogens* (PRPs), are generally found in the gastrointestinal tract, but may be passed into the oropharynx through esophageal reflux. If subsequently aspirated, the PRPs may initiate pneumonia. Oral colonization with PRPs increases during hospitalization, and the longer a patient is hospitalized the greater their prevalence.[80-82] A patient with PRPs colonizing the mouth and oropharynx is at increased risk for pneumonia. Bacterial plaque associated with the teeth can serve as reservoirs for PRPs, particularly during prolonged hospitalization. Poor oral hygiene is common in hospitals or nursing home settings, especially in patients who are quite ill.[80,83] Colonization of dental plaque and the oral mucosa by PRPs is much more common in patients in the intensive care unit compared with patients in an outpatient dental clinic setting.[82,84] The risk for pneumonia was found to be nine times greater in patients in the intensive care unit whose dental plaque was colonized by PRPs compared with those not colonized by these organisms.[85]

A number of intervention studies have shown that improved oral hygiene measures can reduce the incidence of hospital-acquired pneumonia. Application of the antimicrobial chlorhexidine to the teeth, gingiva, and other oral mucosal surfaces has been shown to significantly decrease the risk for pneumonia, especially in patients who are on ventilators.[86,87] In a systematic review of the evidence, Scannapieco and coworkers[88] determined that oral hygiene interventions can reduce the rate of hospital-acquired bacterial pneumonia by approximately 40%.

Chronic obstructive pulmonary disease (COPD) encompasses emphysema and chronic bronchitis and is characterized by obstruction of air flow. Tobacco smoking is the primary risk factor. In COPD, the mucous glands of the bronchi enlarge, and inflammatory cells such as neutrophils and macrophages accumulate within the lung tissue. Because COPD and periodontal diseases are both chronic inflammatory diseases and they share certain pathophysiologic features, the relation between the two diseases has been investigated. Large epidemiologic studies have revealed a significant association between COPD and poor oral hygiene, alveolar bone loss, and smoking.[89,90] In an analysis of data from the NHANES III study, patients with COPD had significantly more clinical attachment loss than did subjects without COPD.[91] These studies demonstrate an association between periodontal diseases and COPD, but they do not show causation. Additional longitudinal studies would be required to validate the associations, and intervention trials are needed to determine if periodontal therapy can reduce the risk for COPD.

CONCLUSION

It is important when examining the relations between periodontal diseases and various systemic conditions for the clinician to consider the public health ramifications of such relations. For example, the associations between periodontal diseases and CHD-related events, although statistically significant, are relatively moderate. That is, the extent to which periodontal disease affects the risk for an event such as myocardial infarction is likely to be somewhat less than smoking or increased LDL levels. However, even a slight to moderate increase in risk, when it is associated with a disease such as cardiovascular disease, can have major public health impact. Because cardiovascular diseases are so prevalent in the population, a slight increase in risk may account for literally millions of new cases. The same can be said for the economic costs of such as association. The costs associated with diabetes, low birth weight, cardiovascular and cerebrovascular events, and respiratory infections are high. Identification of risk factors for such conditions may allow intensified efforts at controlling those risk factors and hopefully reducing the incidence and prevalence of these conditions.

Treatment of periodontal diseases has evolved to a model similar to the medical model of disease management. The whole arena of periodontal medicine is directed toward treating periodontal disease as one would any other risk factor. When an overweight patient with hypertension and increased LDL cholesterol levels sees his or her physician, the physician treats these risk factors for acute cardiovascular and cerebrovascular disease. Treatment of stroke and myocardial infarction is directed toward treatment of the factors that put the patient at risk for such events in the first place. The patient may be placed on a diet and exercise regimen conducive to cardiovascular health. Medications may be prescribed to improve blood pressure and decrease cholesterol levels. Likewise, periodontal therapy is directed toward treatment of periodontal infection as a modifiable risk factor for a number of systemic conditions. No claims are made that treatment of a patient's periodontal disease will eliminate the risk for having a stroke or a myocardial infarction. Rather, periodontal treatment is presented as another means of managing a modifiable risk factor for those conditions.

Patient education and education of our professional colleagues is critical. Subgingival biofilms, as in periodontal infection, are self-maintaining, self-perpetuating, microbial communities, and as such are a continuous source of bacterial products and toxins into the surrounding gingival tissues and general circulation. The continuous spillover of bacterial toxins into the circulation results in chronic activation of the inflammatory cascade, leading to chronic inflammation at distant sites and tissues including inflammatory cell infiltrates of the blood vessel walls. The chronic up-regulation of inflammatory cytokines by periodontal bacteria appears to contribute significantly to increased insulin resistance, which, in turn, aggravates the inflammatory abnormalities on the blood vessel walls. The systemic spread of periodontal infection underscores the need for specific treatment of the subgingival biofilm infection. Evidence from treatment of chronic periodontal infection in patients at high risk for systemic complications such as diabetes, cardiovascular disease, or LBW indicates that effective elimination of subgingival infection has the potential to reduce the systemic spread of this oral infection in patients at high risk. In some patients, a combined treatment approach may be needed—that is, the use of antibiotics combined with mechanical removal of biofilm infection. Clearly, there is a need for patient-based treatment, targeted to both the host and the microbial pathogen. Additional research will undoubtedly strengthen this knowledge base and become the basis for clinical practice and patient management. The ultimate goal is evidence-based treatment of periodontal infection in patients at risk for systemic spread to reduce the burden of oral disease and ameliorate the morbidity associated with these chronic diseases.

REFERENCES

1. Darveau RP, Tanner A, Page RC: The microbial challenge in periodontitis, *Periodontol 2000* 14:12-32, 1997.

2. Socransky SS, Haffajee AD, Ximenez-Fyvie LA et al: Ecological considerations in the treatment of Actinobacillus actinomycetemcomitans and Porphyromonas gingivalis periodontal infections, *Periodontol 2000* 20:341-362, 1999.

3. Kojima T, Yasui S, Ishikawa I: Distribution of Porphyromonas gingivalis in adult periodontitis patients, *J Periodontol* 64:1231-1237, 1993.

4. Holt S, Kesavalu L, Walker S, Genco CA: Virulence factors of Porphyromonas gingivalis, *Periodontol 2000* 20:168-238, 1998.

5. Lindemann R, Economou J, Rothermel H: Production of interleukin-1 and tumor necrosis factor by human peripheral monocytes activated by periodontal bacteria and extracted lipopolysaccharides, *J Dent Res* 67:1131-1135, 1988.

6. Castell JV, Andus T, Kunz D, Heinrich PC: Interleukin-6: the major regulator of acute-phase protein synthesis in man and rat, *Ann NY Acad Sci* 557:87-101, 1989.

7. Gauldie J, Richards C, Northemann W et al: IFNb2/BSF2/IL-6 is the monocyte-derived HSF that regulates receptor-specific acute phase gene regulation in hepatocytes, *Ann NY Acad Sci* 557:46-59, 1989.

8. Beutler B, Cerami A: Cachectin: more than a tumor necrosis factor, *N Engl J Med* 316:379-385, 1987.

9. Bevilacqua MP, Pober JS, Majeau GR et al: Recombinant tumor necrosis factor induces procoagulant activity in cultured human vascular endothelium: characterization and comparison with the actions of interleukin-1, *Proc Natl Acad Sci USA* 83:4533-4537, 1986.

10. Pober JS: Cytokine-mediated activation of vascular endothelium: physiology and pathology, *Am J Pathol* 133:426-433, 1988.

11. Tewari A, Buhles WC, Starnes HF: Preliminary report: effects of interleukin-1 in platelet counts, *Lancet* 936:712-714, 1990.

12. Deshpande RG, Khan MB, Genco CA: Invasion of aortic valve and heart endothelial cells by *Porphyromonas gingivalis*, *Infect Immun* 66:5337-5343, 1998.

13. Kuramitsu HK, Qi M, Kang IC, Chen W: Role of periodontal bacteria in cardiovascular disease, *Ann Periodontol* 6:41-47, 2001.

14. Herzberg MC, Brintzenhofe KL, Clawson CC: Aggregation of human platelets and adhesion of *Streptococcus sanguis*, *Infect Immun* 39:1457-1469, 1983.

15. Herzberg MC, Meyer MW: Effects of oral flora on platelets: possible consequences in cardiovascular disease, *J Periodontol* 67(Suppl):1138-1142, 1996.

16. Ebersole JL, Machen RL, Steffen MJ, Willmann DE: Systemic acute-phase reactants. C-reactive protein and haptoglobin, in adult periodontitis, *Clin Exp Immunol* 107:347-352, 1997.

17. Slade GD, Ghezzi EM, Heiss G et al: Relationship between periodontal disease and C-reactive protein among adults in the Atherosclerosis Risk in Communities study, *Arch Intern Med* 163:1172-1179, 2003.

18. Noack B, Genco RJ, Trevisan M et al: Periodontal infections contribute to elevated systemic C-reactive protein level, *J Periodontol* 72:1231-1236, 2001.

19. Wu T, Trevisan M, Genco RJ et al: Examination of the relation between periodontal health status and cardiovascular risk factors: serum total and high density lipoprotein cholesterol, C-reactive protein, and plasma fibrinogen, *Am J Epidemiol* 15:273-282, 2000.

20. Slade GD, Offenbacher S, Beck JD et al: Acute-phase inflammatory response to periodontal disease in the US population, *J Dent Res* 79:49-57, 2000.

21. Haraszthy V, Zambon JJ, Trevisan M et al: Identification of periodontal pathogens in atheromatous plaques, *J Periodontol* 71:1554-1560, 2000.

22. Geerts SO, Nys M, DeMol P et al: Systemic release of endotoxins induced by gentle mastication: association with periodontitis severity, *J Periodontol* 73:73-78, 2002.

23. Loos BG, Craandiji J, Hoek FJ et al: C-reactive protein and other markers of systemic inflammation in relation to cardiovascular diseases are elevated in periodontitis, *J Periodontol* 71:1528-1534, 2000.

24. Alibhai Z, Grossi SG, Ho A et al: Effect of periodontal treatment on systemic inflammatory mediators, *J Dent Res* 81(Spec Iss A):498, 2002 (abstract).

25. Iwamoto Y, Nishimura F, Soga Y et al: Antimicrobial periodontal therapy decreases serum C-reactive protein, tumor necrosis factor-alpha, but not adinopectin levels in patients with chronic periodontitis, *J Periodontol* 74:1231-1236, 2003.

26. Ross R: Atherosclerosis—an inflammatory disease, *N Engl J Med* 340:115-126, 1999.

27. Wick G, Schett G, Amberger A et al: Is atherosclerosis an immunologically mediated disease? *Immunol Today* 16:27-33, 1995.

28. Sojar HT, Glurich I, Genco RJ: Heat shock protein 60-like molecule from *Bacteroides forsythus* and *Porphyromonas gingivalis*: molecular mimicry, *J Dent Res* 77(IADR Abstracts):#275, 1998 (abstract).

29. Mattila K, Valle MS, Nieminen MS et al: Dental infections and coronary atherosclerosis, *Atherosclerosis* 103:205-211, 1993.

30. Malthaner SC, Moore S, Mills M et al: Investigation of the association between angiographically defined coronary artery disease and periodontal disease, *J Periodontol* 73:1169-1176, 2002.

31. Danesh J, Collins R, Appleby P, Peto R: Association of fibrinogen, C-reactive protein, albumin, or leukocyte count with coronary heart disease: meta-analyses of prospective studies, *JAMA* 279:1477-1482, 1998.

32. Pietila K, Harmoinen A, Hermens WT et al: Serum C-reactive protein and infarct size in myocardial infarct patients with a closed versus an open infarct-related coronary artery after thrombolytic therapy, *Eur Heart J* 14:915-919, 1993.

33. Liuzzo G, Biasucci LM, Gallimore JR et al: The prognostic value of C-reactive protein and serum amyloid A protein in severe unstable angina, *N Engl J Med* 331:417-424, 1994.

34. Syrjanen J, Peltola J, Valtonen V et al: Dental infection associated with cerebral infarction in young and middle aged men, *J Intern Med* 225:179-184, 1989.

35. Mattila K, Nieminen M, Valtonen V et al: Association between dental health and acute myocardial infarction, *Br Med J* 298:779-782, 1989.

36. Paunio K, Impivaara O, Tiesko J, Maki J: Missing teeth and ischemic heart disease in men aged 45-64 years, *Eur Heart J* 14(suppl k):54-56, 1993.

37. Arbes Jr SJ, Slade GD, Beck JD: Association between extent of periodontal attachment loss and self-reported history of heart attack: an analysis of NHANES III Data, *J Dent Res* 78:1777-1782, 1999.

38. Genco RJ: Periodontal disease and risk for myocardial infarction and cardiovascular disease, *Cardiovasc Rev Reports* 19(3):34-40, 1998.

39. DeStefano F, Anda RF, Kahn HS et al: Dental disease and risk of coronary heart disease and mortality, *Br Med J* 306:688-691, 1993.

40. Mattila KJ, Valtonen VV, Nieminen M, Huttunen JK: Dental infection and the risk of new coronary events: prospective study of patients with documented coronary artery disease, *Clin Infect Dis* 20:588-592, 1995.

41. Beck J, Garcia R, Heiss G et al: Periodontal disease and cardiovascular disease, *J Periodontol* 67:1123-1137, 1996.

42. Joshipura KJ, Rimm EB, Douglass CW et al: Poor oral health and coronary heart disease, *J Dent Res* 75:1631-1636, 1996.

43. Morrison HI, Ellison LF, Taylor GW: Periodontal disease and risk of fatal coronary heart and cerebrovascular diseases, *J Cardiovasc Risk* 6:7-11, 1999.

44. Genco RJ, Wu TJ, Grossi SG et al: Periodontal microflora related to the risk for myocardial infarction: a case control study, *J Dent Res* 78(Sp Iss):457, 1999 (abstract).

45. Grau AJ, Buggle F, Ziegler C et al: Association between acute cerebrovascular ischemia and chronic recurrent infection, *Stroke* 28:1724-1729, 1997.

46. Wu T, Trevisan M, Genco RJ et al: Periodontal disease and risk of cerebrovascular disease. The First National Health and Nutrition Examination Survey and its follow-up study, *Arch Intern Med* 160:2749-2755, 2000.

47. Joshipura KJ, Hung HC, Rimm EB et al: Periodontal disease, tooth loss and incidence of ischemic stroke, *Stroke* 34:47-52, 2003.

48. Taylor GW, Burt BA, Becker MP et al: Severe periodontitis and risk for poor glycemic control in patients with non-insulin-dependent diabetes mellitus, *J Periodontol* 67:1085-1093, 1996.

49. Thortesson H, Hugoson A: Periodontal disease experience in adult long-duration insulin-dependent diabetics, *J Clin Periodontol* 16:215-223, 1989.

50. Williams RC, Mahan CJ: Periodontal disease and diabetes in young adults, *JAMA* 172:776-778, 1960.

51. Miller LS, Manwell MA, Newbold D et al: The relationship between reduction in periodontal inflammation and diabetes control: a report of 9 cases, *J Periodontol* 63:843-848, 1992.

52. Grossi SG, Skrepcinski FB, DeCaro T et al: Treatment of periodontal disease in diabetics reduces glycated hemoglobin, *J Periodontol* 68:713-719, 1997.

53. Aldridge JP, Lester V, Watts TLP et al: Single-blind studies of the effects of improved periodontal health on metabolic control in Type 1 diabetes mellitus, *J Clin Periodontol* 22:271-275, 1995.

54. Christgau M, Pallitzsch KD, Schmalz G et al: Healing response to non-surgical periodontal therapy in patients with diabetes mellitus: clinical, microbiological and immunological results, *J Clin Periodontol* 25:112-124, 1998.

55. Smith GT, Greenbaum CJ, Johnson BD et al: Short-term responses to periodontal therapy in insulin-dependent diabetic patients, *J Periodontol* 67:794-802, 1996.

56. Yki-Jarvinen H, Sammalkorpi K, Koivisto VA et al: Severity, duration and mechanism of insulin resistance during acute infections, *J Clin Endocrinol Metab* 69:317-323, 1989.

57. Sammalkorpi K: Glucose intolerance in acute infections, *J Intern Med* 225:15-19, 1989.

58. Grossi SG, Genco RJ: Periodontal disease and diabetes mellitus: a two-way relationship, *Ann Periodontol* 3:51-61, 1998.

59. Mealey BL: Diabetes mellitus. In Rose LF, Genco RJ, Mealey BL, Cohen DW, editors: *Periodontal medicine*. Toronto, Ontario, Canada, 2000, BC Decker Publishers.

60. Al-Zahrani MS, Bissada NF, Borawskit EA: Obesity and periodontal disease in young, middle-aged and older adults, *J Periodontol* 74:610-615, 2003.

61. Salvi GE, Collins JG, Yalda B, et al: Monocytic TNF-α secretion patterns in IDDM patients with periodontal diseases, *J Clin Periodontol* 24:8-16, 1997.

62. Nishimura F, Iwamoto Y, Mineshiba J et al: Periodontal disease and diabetes mellitus: the role of tumor necrosis factor-alpha in a 2-way relationship, *J Periodontol* 74:97-102, 2003.

63. Ling PR, Bistrian BR, Mendez B, Istfan NW: Effects of systemic infusions of endotoxin, tumor necrosis factor, and interleukin-1 on glucose metabolism in the rat: relationship to endogenous glucose production and peripheral tissue glucose uptake, *Metab Clin Exp* 43:279-284, 1994.

64. Kanety H, Feinstein R, Papa MZ et al: Tumor necrosis factor alpha-induced phosphorylation of insulin receptor substrate-1 (IRS-1). Possible mechanism of suppression of insulin-stimulated tyrosine phosphorylation of IRS-1, *J Biol Chem* 270:23780-23784, 1995.

65. Nishimura F, Murayama Y: Periodontal inflammation and insulin resistance—lessons from obesity, *J Dent Res* 80:1690-1694, 2001.

66. Offenbacher S, Jared HL, O'Reilly PG et al: Potential pathogenic mechanisms of periodontitis-associated pregnancy complications, *Ann Periodontol* 3:233-250, 1998.

67. Hill GB: Preterm birth: associations with genital and possibly oral microflora, *Ann Periodontol* 3:222-232, 1998.

68. Morales WJ, Schorr S, Albritton J: Effect of metronidazole in patients with preterm birth in preceding pregnancy and bacterial vaginosis: a placebo-controlled double-blind study, *Am J Obstet Gynecol* 171:245-247, 1994.

69. Collins JG, Windley III HW, Arnold RR et al: Effects of a *Porphyromonas gingivalis* infection on inflammatory mediator response and pregnancy outcome in the golden hamster, *Infect Immun* 62:4652-4361, 1994.

70. Offenbacher S, Katz V, Fertik G et al: Periodontal disease as a possible risk factor for preterm low birth weight, *J Periodontol* 67:1103-1113, 1996.

71. Jeffcoat MK, Geurs NC, Reddy MS et al: Periodontal infection and preterm birth: results of a prospective study, *J Am Dent Assoc* 132:875-880, 2001.

72. Offenbacher S, Lieff S, Bogess KA et al: Maternal periodontitis and prematurity. Part I: Obstetric outcome of prematurity and growth restriction, *Ann Periodontol* 6:164-174, 2001.

73. Lopez NJ, Smith PC, Gutierrez J: Higher risk of preterm birth and low birth weight in women with periodontal disease, *J Dent Res* 81(1):58-63, 2002.

74. Romero BC, Chiquito CS, Elejalde LE, Bernardoni CB: Relationship between periodontal disease in pregnant women and the nutritional condition of their newborns, *J Periodontol* 73:1177-1183, 2002.

75. Madianos PN, Lieff S, Murtha AP et al: Maternal periodontitis and prematurity. Part II: Maternal infection and exposure, *Ann Periodontol* 6:175-182, 2001.

76. Lopez NJ, Smith PC, Gutierrez J: Periodontal therapy may reduce the risk of preterm low birth weight in women with periodontal disease: a randomized controlled trial. *J Periodontol* 73:911-924, 2002.

77. Jeffcoat MK, Hauth JC, Geurs NC et al: Periodontal disease and preterm birth: results of a pilot intervention study, *J Periodontol* 74:1214-1218, 2003.

78. Ostergaard L, Anderson PL: Etiology of community-acquired pneumonia. Evaluation by transtracheal aspiration, blood culture, or serology, *Chest* 104:1400-1407, 1993.

79. Craven DE, Steger KE, Barber TW: Preventing nosocomial pneumonia: state of the art and perspectives for the 1990s, *Am J Med* 91(suppl B):s44-s53, 1991.

80. Scannapieco FA, Mylotte JM: Relationships between periodontal disease and bacterial pneumonia, *J Periodontol* 67:1114-1122, 1996.

81. Limeback H: Implications of oral infections on systemic diseases in the institutionalized elderly with a special focus on pneumonia, *Ann Periodontol* 3:262-275, 1998.

82. Russell SL, Boylan RJ, Kaslick RS et al: Respiratory pathogen colonization of the dental plaque of institutionalized elders, *Spec Care Dentist* 19:1-7, 1999.

83. Beck JD: Periodontal implications: older adults, *Ann Periodontol* 1:322-357, 1996.

84. Scannapieco FA, Stewart EM, Mylotte JM: Colonization of dental plaque by respiratory pathogens in medical intensive care patients, *Crit Care Med* 20:740-745, 1992.

85. Fourrier F, Duvivier B, Boutigny H et al: Colonization of dental plaque: a source of nosocomial infections in intensive care unit patients, *Crit Care Med* 26:301-308, 1998.

86. DeRiso AJ, Ladowski JS, Dillon TA et al: Chlorhexidine gluconate 0.12% oral rinse reduces the incidence of total nosocomial respiratory infection and nonprophylactic systemic antibiotic use in patients undergoing heart surgery, *Chest* 109:1556-1561, 1996.

87. Fourrier F, Cau-Pottier E, Boutigny H et al: Effects of dental plaque antiseptic decontamination on bacterial colonization and nosocomial infections in critically ill patients, *Intensive Care Med* 26:1239-1247, 2000.

88. Scannapieco FA, Bush R, Paju S: Associations between periodontal diseases and risk for nosocomial bacterial pneumonia and chronic obstructive pulmonary disease: A systematic review *Ann Periodontol* 8:54-69, 2003.

89. Scannapieco FA, Papandonatos GD, Dunford RG: Associations between oral conditions and respiratory disease in a national sample population, *Ann Periodontol* 3:251-256, 1998.

90. Hayes C, Sparrow D, Cohen M et al: Periodontal disease and pulmonary function: the VA longitudinal study, *Ann Periodontol* 3:257-261, 1998.

91. Scannapieco FA, Ho AW: Potential associations between chronic respiratory disease and periodontal disease: analysis of National Health and Nutrition Examination Survey III, *J Periodontol* 72:50-56, 2001.

33 Medications Impacting the Periodontium

Sebastian G. Ciancio, Brian L. Mealey, and Louis F. Rose

Patients seeking periodontal therapy often have diseases or conditions for which medications are prescribed. Although these prescribed medications benefit the overall health of the patient, consideration must be given to the effects of some of these drugs on the severity and management of periodontal diseases. This chapter reviews the medications that directly affect periodontal tissues (gingiva and alveolar bone) or increase the risk for periodontal diseases. A review of medications that may impact the dental management of patients is included in Chapter 37.

MEDICATIONS THAT AFFECT GINGIVAL TISSUE

A number of medications may affect gingival tissue, causing gingival enlargement. These include phenytoin, calcium channel blockers, and cyclosporine. Although phenytoin was the first drug reported to have this effect,[1] gingival enlargement is most commonly associated with calcium channel blockers, because of the widespread use of this class of medications. Hypertension is the most prevalent medical condition reported in epidemiologic studies of the U.S. population,[2] and calcium channel blockers are often prescribed for this condition. Patients taking medications associated with gingival enlargement may need adjunctive plaque-control agents and more rigorous monitoring of the status of the periodontal tissues. Other local factors such as mouth breathing and defective restorations must be considered in the diagnosis and management of medication-induced gingival enlargement.

Drug-induced gingival enlargement may be localized or generalized, and it ranges from mild increase in the size of the interproximal papillary gingiva to severe enlargement of marginal and papillary tissues. In its initial stages, gingival enlargement may appear as fibrotic, pebbly papillae that are only slightly enlarged. These are most often seen in the maxillary and mandibular anterior regions, with posterior papillae less frequently affected (Fig. 33-1). As the condition worsens, the papillae and marginal gingiva may enlarge considerably, as may the marginal gingiva, and may coalesce with adjacent areas of enlargement (Figs. 33-2 and 33-3). In severe cases, the patient's ability to function may be adversely affected (Fig. 33-4, A and B).

Phenytoin

Phenytoin (Dilantin: Parke-Davis [Division of Warner-Lambert Co.]; Morris Plains, NJ) is an anticonvulsant drug commonly used for the prevention of seizures. A common side effect of phenytoin therapy is gingival enlargement, occasionally so severe that it requires surgical intervention. The reported prevalence rate of phenytoin-induced gingival enlargement is about 50% of the estimated two million patients who take this

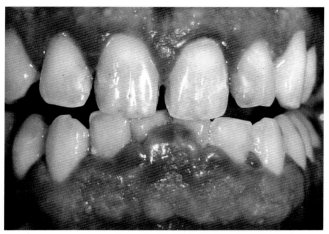

Figure 33-1. Gingival enlargement is localized to the facial and interproximal tissues in the mandibular incisor region. This patient was taking phenytoin (Dilantin; Parke-Davis, Morris Plains, NJ).

medication for prevention of seizures.[3,4] Although the occurrence of gingival enlargement with phenytoin has been well established, the cellular and molecular mechanisms of action are still being fully elucidated.[4] Studies both in vitro and in vivo have demonstrated that macrophages are the predominant cell type in the connective tissue of phenytoin-induced gingival enlargement.[5] Gingival macrophages exposed to phenytoin secrete increased amounts of platelet-derived growth factor-B (PDGF-B).[6] Additional studies have demonstrated that phenytoin regulates macrophage phenotype, expression of the growth factor PDGF-B, and secretion of the proinflammatory cytokine IL-1β in inflamed tissues.[7] In addition, phenytoin may stimulate osteoblast proliferation, differentiation, and maturation leading to bone formation.[8]

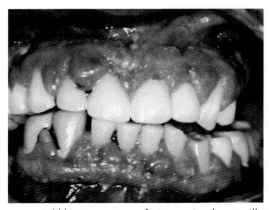

Figure 33-2. Pebbly appearance of tissues in the maxillary and mandibular anterior and premolar areas. Gingival bleeding is indicative of increased inflammation. The patient was taking a calcium channel blocker (nifedipine).

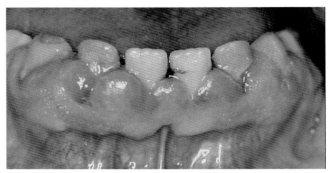

Figure 33-3. Enlargement of the entire zone of keratinized tissue in the mandibular anterior region, extending to the mucogingival junction. The enlargement covers approximately two thirds of the anatomic crowns of the teeth. The patient was taking cyclosporine.

Thus it appears that phenytoin-induced PDGF secretion stimulates proliferation not only of gingival connective tissue cells but also of alveolar bone cells. This effect on bone metabolism could explain in part why patients who take phenytoin tend to have inflamed gingival tissue but do not have much alveolar bone loss compared with an age-matched population.[9] Clinical observations and experimental studies show that phenytoin-induced gingival enlargement is often associated with dental plaque and poor oral hygiene, where accumulation of inflammatory cells such as monocytes and macrophages is increased. This observation has been further supported by studies where patients are enrolled in strict programs of oral hygiene within 10 days of phenytoin therapy and the occurrence of gingival enlargement can be reduced.[10,11]

Calcium Channel Blockers

Calcium channel blockers are antianginal and antihypertensive medications. They inhibit the movement of calcium ions across the membrane of cardiac and arterial muscle cells, resulting in depression of cardiac impulse formation, slowing the velocity of conduction of cardiac impulses, and dilation of coronary arteries, arterioles, and peripheral arterioles. Gingival enlargement has been associated with calcium channel blockers including nifedipine (Procardia: Pratt Pharmaceuticals Division, Pfizer Inc.; New York, NY), verapamil (Calan: G.D. Searle & Co.; Chicago, IL), diltiazem (Cardizem: Marion Merrell Dow Inc.; Kansas City, MO), and felodipine (Plendil: Astra/Merck; Wayne, PA). Studies indicate that gingival enlargement occurs in an average of 30% to 40% of patients taking these medications.[12] Nifedipine is the calcium channel blocker most often associated with gingival enlargement; however, it is also the most frequently prescribed. Theoretically, gingival overgrowth might occur with any of the medications in this class. Histologically, the enlargement associated with nifedipine resembles the inflammatory-type described by Hassell[4] for phenytoin in which numerous inflammatory cells replaced collagen in connective tissue.[13] It appears that nifedipine-induced alterations of the intracellular calcium level in gingival cells, in combination with local inflammatory factors, result in gingival enlargement in some individuals. In a manner similar to phenytoin-induced gingival enlargement, nifedipine-induced enlargement did not recur after gingivectomy when thorough plaque control was maintained.[13] This again supports the significant role of inflammation and dental plaque as important cofactors

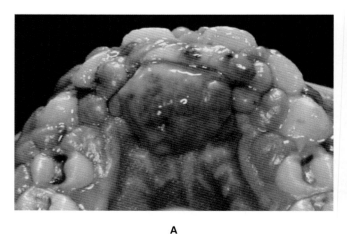

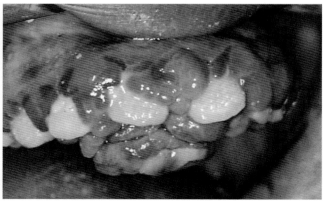

A   B

Figure 33-4. Severe enlargement of facial and palatal tissues in a patient taking phenytoin (Dilantin). **A,** Occlusal view shows severe enlargement interfering with patient speech and function. **B,** Facial view shows inflammatory changes in addition to gingival enlargement. Proper oral hygiene is impossible for this patient.

modulating drug-induced gingival enlargement.[14] Furthermore, a clinical study suggests that nifedipine-induced gingival enlargement can be reversed with aggressive oral hygiene treatment and switching antihypertensive therapy to isradipine, a different dihydropyridine derivative with low incidence of gingival enlargement.[15]

Regardless of the molecular mechanisms of drug-induced gingival enlargement, the role of dental plaque in aggravating the inflammatory response and the clinical presentation of this medication-induced condition cannot be overemphasized. Thus patients receiving these medications need to be placed in effective and rigorous programs of oral hygiene and dental plaque control. This is a critical message that the dental community needs to communicate to medical students and also physicians in practice.

Cyclosporine A

Cyclosporine is an immunosuppressant drug widely prescribed to control rejection of solid organ transplantation and autoimmune disease with or without low doses of systemic corticosteroid. Gingival enlargement also has been reported as a common side effect of cyclosporine treatment with a prevalence of 25 to 40 percent.[16-18] The occurrence of cyclosporine-induced gingival enlargement has been studied in humans[19] and experimental animals,[20] as well as the in vitro cellular response to the drug.[21]

Although the exact histopathologic mechanism of gingival enlargement is not fully elucidated, the role of local etiologic factors and cyclosporine dosage are of great significance. Three major lines of evidence support the histopathology of cyclosporine-induced gingival enlargement, namely dose-related, plaque-associated, and direct effects on cellular targets. A positive correlation was found among cyclosporine dose, plasma levels of the drug, and severity of gingival enlargement in 100 patients during the first 6 months after heart, liver, or kidney transplantation.[22] In a longitudinal study, cyclosporine-induced gingival enlargement was present in 21% of adult patients with multiple sclerosis and was associated with cyclosporine levels greater than 400 ng/ml.[23] In addition, retention of dental plaque appears to magnify the severity of gingival enlargement.[24] Although intensive plaque control does not appear to prevent the development of cyclosporine-induced gingival enlargement, it does improve the gingival condition.[25] Thus dental plaque appears to be a cofactor in the development of cyclosporine-induced gingival enlargement.

A third line of evidence in the pathogenesis of this condition is related to direct effects of the drug on specific cell populations and on the extracellular environment. Cultured monocytes/macrophages exhibit a significant increase in PDGF-B in response to cyclosporine stimulation.[26] An inflammation-independent increase in the growth factor PDGF-B and the proinflammatory cytokine IL-1β is observed in hyperplastic tissues.[7] Furthermore, a specific subpopulation of PDGF-B–producing, proliferative macrophages is activated after stimulation by cyclosporine.[7] Cyclosporine-induced gingival enlargement may be, in large part, caused by disturbance of the intricate balance between synthesis and degradation of the extracellular matrix of the gingival tissues.[27,28] Production of collagen by gingival fibroblasts is normally balanced by the breakdown of existing collagen through production of matrix metalloproteinase (MMP) enzymes. Cyclosporine appears to decrease production of these collagen-degrading enzymes, allowing an accumulation of collagen and resultant gingival enlargement. It is likely that a combination of drug dosage, plaque, and direct cellular effects are operative in the pathogenesis of this condition.

Management of cyclosporine-induced gingival enlargement is complicated by the lack of substitute medications. The major drug alternative, tacrolimus, can be substituted in some cases by the patient's physician, although cyclosporine and tacrolimus each have specific indications for use. Drug-indued gingival enlargement is uncommon in patients taking tacrolimus.[29,30]

Early intervention can prevent or minimize severe gingival problems associated with cyclosporine.[25] As with other drugs causing gingival enlargement, meticulous plaque control early on in therapy can minimize the enlargement, although the impact of plaque control may be less impressive with cyclosporine than with phenytoin or calcium channel blockers. It is recommended that patients be placed on strict oral hygiene programs before the onset of transplant surgery, rather than waiting until the medication treatment is begun.

MEDICATIONS WITH HOST MODULATING EFFECTS

Evidence suggests that the host immunoinflammatory response to the bacterial challenge posed by periodontal pathogens is a significant component of the net tissue destruction seen in periodontal diseases. The understanding of the host–parasite interactions leading to chronic inflammation and destruction of periodontal tissues has led the way to a novel concept—that is, modulation of the host response to periodontal infection. Such host modulation may be directed toward decreasing the susceptibility of the patient to periodontal destruction, as well as treating that destruction when it occurs. Therefore, although it is clear that periodontal diseases are fundamentally infectious in nature and that treatment will rely heavily on an antimicrobial approach, a new approach toward preventing and treating periodontal diseases is emerging. This approach targets the immunoinflammatory response and is often called host modulation therapy.

A number of medications can be included within the category of host modulating agents. The two major categories are nonsteroidal antiinflammatory drugs (NSAIDs) and inhibitors of MMPs.

Nonsteroidal Antiinflammatory Drugs

Local inflammation from the host response to periodontal bacteria results in tissue destruction and production of free arachidonic acid, which can be metabolized through the cyclooxygenase (COX) pathway. Cyclooxygenase-1 (COX-1) is the constitutive form of COX. COX-1 has clear physiologic functions and is protective to cells, including those of the gastric system. Cyclooxygenase 2 (COX-2) is the inducible isomer, which is up-regulated by proinflammatory cytokines and is involved in inflammation.[31] Prostaglandins, especially prostaglandin E_2, are final products of the COX pathway, amplifying inflammation. Expression of COX-2 enzyme has been induced during experimental periodontitis in the rat model and has been demonstrated to play an important role in gingival inflammation and alveolar bone destruction.[32] Induction of COX-2 and production of prostaglandin E_2 in periodontal ligament cells also has been reported in alveolar bone resorption associated with occlusal trauma.[33] NSAIDs block COX production and reduce prostaglandin synthesis. NSAIDs have been evaluated as inhibitors of alveolar bone resorption. A number of NSAIDs including ibuprofen,[34] flurbiprofen,[35] indomethacin,[36] and naproxen[37] have been shown to inhibit gingivitis and ligature-induced periodontitis in animal models. Selective inhibition of COX-2 also has been shown to reduce alveolar bone resorption in ligature-induced periodontitis in experimental animals.[38]

The effects of NSAIDs in human periodontal tissues are less clear.[35,39,40] These agents have been used systemically and topically.[41] Although some reduction in bone loss rates over time have been seen with systemic NSAIDs, the effect lasts only as long as the patient continues taking the drug, requiring chronic drug administration. Further studies are needed before incorporation of these host modulating agents into daily clinical practice.

Adverse effects of prolonged use of NSAIDs include gastrointestinal upset and bleeding and hepatic alterations. Although these adverse effects are seen fairly frequently with nonselective COX inhibitors, selective COX-2 inhibitors have less frequent adverse effects. Selective COX-2 inhibitors are proving to be widely prescribed for management of chronic inflammatory conditions and chronic pain. Therefore dentists should be familiar with the effects of these drugs on periodontal tissues.

Inhibitors of Matrix Metalloproteinases

MMPs are a family of proteolytic enzymes secreted by a number of periodontal cells: recruited (neutrophils, macrophages) and resident cells (epithelial, fibroblast, osteoblast, osteoclast). The primary functions of MMPs are the degradation of extracellular matrix components (collagen, laminin, fibronectin), therefore they are important in tissue remodeling. Although periodontal pathogens produce MMPs, including collagenase, endogenous (host) MMPs are primarily responsible for tissue destruction associated with periodontal disease. Synthetic MMP inhibitors extensively studied include the family of tetracycline antibiotics, which inhibit host-derived MMPs by mechanisms independent of their antimicrobial properties.[42,43] Tetracyclines appear to inhibit MMP activity and extracellular matrix destruction by nonantimicrobial mechanisms, including chelation and inhibition of latent forms of these proteases enzymes.[44,45] Tetracyclines inhibit the release of collagenase by polymorphonuclear leukocytes and inhibit collagenase activity.[43] In so doing, they can increase host resistance to connective tissue destruction.

Subantimicrobial doses of the tetracycline antibiotic doxycycline have been used in treatment of patients with chronic periodontitis. The dose of doxycycline in this drug (20 mg) is below the effective antibiotic dose level; therefore, the agent has no antimicrobial effect. Subantimicrobial dose doxycycline is designed to be used for its potent anti-MMP effects, decreasing the levels of host collagenase and other proteolytic enzymes within the periodontal tissues. This agent has been associated with greater probing depth reduction when used in conjunction with scaling and root planing, compared with scaling and root planing alone.[46] The safety of subantimicrobial dose doxycycline also has been demonstrated.[47] More extensive study of subantimicrobial dose doxycycline is warranted to determine its place in the periodontal treatment armamentarium.

MEDICATIONS THAT CAUSE XEROSTOMIA

Xerostomia, or dry mouth, is a side effect of approximately 400 medications.[48] Xerostomia is most commonly seen in patients using antihypertensives, analgesics, sedatives, tranquilizing agents, antihistamines for allergies, and drugs for Parkinson's disease. Dentists must consider whether the xerostomia is caused by medications or some other health condition. For example, xerostomia also is seen in patients with Sjögren syndrome, endocrine disorders, nutritional deficiencies, stress, or depression. Xerostomia is common in patients who have undergone radiation therapy or chemotherapy. Clinicians also need to recognize the possibility that complaints associated with perceived salivary dysfunction may be psychogenic.[49] In each case, the cause of the xerostomia needs to be understood to avoid prescribing unnecessary treatment.

Xerostomia is a concern of dental professionals for several reasons. First, oral candidiasis is one of the major side effects of drugs that dry the mouth. Candidiasis associated with xerostomia may be subtle and may affect the gingival tissues. Gingival candidiasis may present as gingivitis that does not resolve after mechanical debridement of the teeth to remove plaque and calculus. Second, xerostomia increases the risk for caries, especially smooth surface and root caries. Root caries may be difficult to restore and may require periodontal surgical therapy to gain access to affected root surfaces. Finally, patients with dentures may have severe denture retention problems as a consequence of decreased saliva.

For patients with xerostomia, a number of products can be applied to the root surfaces for both sensitivity and anticaries effects, such as the fluoride varnish Duraphat (Colgate-Palmolive; New York, NY) and Fluor Protector C (Ivoclar Vivodent Inc.; Amherst, NY). Other professional fluoride products, such as PreviDent 5000 Plus, a prescription dentifrice, have been shown to be beneficial for daily use in patients with xerostomia. Fluoride mouth rinses available over-the-counter are beneficial. Saliva substitutes can be used to a limited extent, in addition to sugarless lozenges, and prescription medications such as pilocarpine. However, topical agents are preferable because of the many side effects that can develop with systemic products.

MOOD-ALTERING MEDICATIONS

Mental health conditions such as depression and bipolar disorder can affect oral health.[50,51] Likewise, some of the medications used to treat these disorders have effects that may exacerbate oral disease. For example, many serotonin reuptake inhibitors result in significant xerostomia, with all of the potential adverse oral effects described earlier.[52]

Antianxiety and antidepressant drugs are some of the most widely prescribed medications currently in use, and it is likely that dental health professionals will encounter on a daily basis patients taking these drugs. Some medications used to treat anxiety and depression are also used to manage headaches, obesity, and other conditions. In patients who are depressed or anxious, the medications often elevate their moods. Conversely, in patients who are not experiencing depression, such as patients receiving treatment for headaches, these medications may depress their moods. Drugs that are used to treat hypertension decrease blood pressure, but they may also have slightly depressive effects in some patients. Commonly used antihypertension medications with such effects include Vasotec (Merk & Co.; West Point, PA) (enalapril), Capoten

(Bristol-Meyers; New York, NY) (captopril), and Norvasc (Pfizer Labs; New York, NY) (amlodipine).

Mood-altering medications can reduce patient self-motivation to perform oral hygiene. They can compromise the manner and frequency with which patients use toothbrushes, interdental cleaning aids, mouth rinses, and other oral hygiene products. They also make it more difficult for the clinician to motivate patients by giving them a "care less" attitude about daily activities, including performing adequate oral hygiene. The astute clinician must be aware of these potential drug effects. Patients who take mood-altering medications may need more frequent dental recall visits. They also may need adjunctive oral hygiene products that help make home oral hygiene easier and more effective. (See Chapter 13.)

CONCLUSION

Medications can have many adverse effects on a patient's oral health. Therefore dentists must find new approaches to diagnosing and treating patients. Manufacturers, clinicians, and researchers need to guide practitioners and patients to the products that will best help them in their overall oral and systemic health.

We all have a role in solving these medication-related dental problems. Pharmaceutical manufacturers must design medications with delivery mechanisms and composition that are not harmful to patients' oral health. Dental practitioners must be aware of the potential effect that some medications may have on the patient's dental caries and periodontal disease, and they must develop the appropriate treatment plans accordingly. Patients must understand the need for informing their health professionals, both medical and dental, of their medical conditions and the medications they take regularly. Patients must also understand the importance of using medications in the prescribed manner. Finally, physicians, dentists, and pharmacists must warn patients about all possible side effects, including those that affect the oral cavity, associated with any prescription or over-the-counter medication that they recommend to patients.

REFERENCES

1. Aas E: Hyperplasia gingivae diphenylhydantoinea, *Acta Odontol Scand* 21(suppl):34-48, 1963.
2. Grossi SG, Zambon, JJ, Ho AW et al: Assessment of risk for periodontal disease I. Risk indicators for attachment loss, *J Periodontol* 65:260-267, 1994.
3. Stinett E, Rodu B, Grizzle WE: New developments in understanding phenytoin-induced gingival hyperplasia, *J Am Dent Assoc* 114:814-817, 1987.

4. Hasell TM, Hefti AF: Drug-induced gingival overgrowth: old problem, new problem, *Crit Rev Oral Biol Med* 2:103-137, 1991.

5. Hall BK, Squire CA: Ultrastructural quantitation of connective tissue changes in phenytoin-induced gingival overgrowth in the ferret, *J Dent Res* 61:942-952, 1982.

6. Dill RE, Miller EK, Weil T et al: Phenytoin increases gene expression for platelet-derived growth factor B chain in macrophages and monocytes, *J Periodontol* 64:169-173, 1993.

7. Iacopino AM, Doxey D, Cutler CW et al: Phenytoin and cyclosporine A specifically regulate macrophage phenotype expression of platelet-derived growth factor and interleukin-1 in vitro and in vivo: possible molecular mechanism of drug-induced gingival hyperplasia, *J Periodontol* 68:73-83, 1997.

8. Nakade O, Baylink DJ, Lau K-HW: Phenytoin at micromolar concentration is an osteogenic agent for human-mandibular-derived bone cells in vitro, *J Dent Res* 74(1):331-337, 1995.

9. Hall WB: Dilantin hyperplasia: a preventable lesion, *J Periodont Res* 4:36-37, 1969.

10. Ciancio SG: Medications as risk factors for periodontal disease, *J Periodontol* 67:1055-1059, 1996.

11. Ciancio SG, Yaffe SJ, Catz CC: Gingival hyperplasia and diphenylhydantoin, *J Periodontol* 43:411-414, 1972.

12. Seymour RA: Calcium channel blockers and gingival overgrowth, *Br Dent J* 170:376-379, 1991.

13. Nishikawa SJ, Tada H, Hamasaki A: Nifedipine-induced gingival hyperplasia: a clinical and in vitro study, *J Periodontol* 62:30-35, 1991.

14. Nuki K, Cooper SH: The role of inflammation in the pathogenesis of gingival enlargement during the administration of diphenylhydantoin sodium in cats, *J Periodont Res* 7:102-110, 1972.

15. Westbrook P, Bednarczyk E, Carlson M et al: Regression of nifedipine-induced gingival hyperplasia following switch to a same class calcium channel blocker, isradipine, *J Periodontol* 68:645-650, 1997.

16. Ratteischak-Plüss EM, Hefti A, Lörtcher R, Thiel G: Initial observation that cyclosporine-A induces gingival enlargement in man, *J Clin Periodontol* 10:237-246, 1983.

17. Stone C, Eshenaur A, Hassell T: Gingival enlargement in cyclosporine treated multiple sclerosis patients, *J Dent Res* 68:285-289, 1989.

18. Palestine AG, Nusenblatt RB, Chan CC: Side effects of systemic cyclosporine in patients not undergoing transplantation, *Am J Med* 77:652-656, 1984.

19. Pernu HE, Pernu LMH, Knuuttila MLE, Huttunen KRH: Gingival overgrowth among renal transplant recipients and uraemic patients, *Nephrol Dial Transplantl* 8:1254-1258, 1993.

20. Kitamura K, Morisaki I, Adachi C: Gingival overgrowth induced by cyclosporine A in rats, *Arch Oral Biol* 35:483-486, 1990.

21. Bartold PM: Regulation of gingival fibroblast growth and synthetic activity by cyclosporine-A in vitro, *J Periodont Res* 24:314-321, 1989.

22. Somacarrera ML, Hernández G, Acero J, Moskow BS: Factors related to the incidence and severity of cyclosporine-induced gingival overgrowth in transplant patients, *J Periodontol* 65:671-675, 1994.

23. Hefti AF, Eshenaur AE, Hassell TM, Stone C: Gingival overgrowth in cyclosporine A treated multiple sclerosis patients, *J Periodontol* 65:744-749, 1994.

24. Fu E, Nieh S, Wikesjö UME: The effect of plaque retention on cyclosporine-induced gingival overgrowth in rats, *J Periodontol* 68:92-98, 1997.

25. Seymour RA, Smith DG: The effect of a plaque control program on the incidence and severity of cyclosporine induced gingival changes, *J Clin Periodontol* 18:107-110, 1991.

26. Nares S, Ng MC, Dill RE et al: Cyclosporine A upregulates platelet-derived growth factor B chain in hyperplastic human gingiva, *J Periodontol* 67:271-278, 1996.

27. Hyland PL, Traynor PS, Myrillas TT et al: The effects of cyclosporine on the collagenolytic activity of gingival fibroblasts, *J Periodontol* 74:437-445, 2003.

28. Cotrim P, deAndrade CR, Martelli-Junior H et al: Expression of matrix metalloproteinases in cyclosporine-treated gingival fibroblasts is regulated by transforming growth factor-β1 autocrine stimulation, *J Periodontol* 73:1313-1322, 2002.

29. Hood KA: Drug-induced gingival hyperplasia in transplant recipients, *Prog Transplant* 12:17-21, 2002.

30. McKaig SJ, Kelly D, Shaw L: Investigation of the effect of FK506 (tacrolimus) and cyclosporin in gingival overgrowth following paediatric liver transplantation, *Int J Paediatr Dent* 12:398-403, 2002.

31. DeWitt DL, Meade EA, Smith WL: PGH synthase isoenzyme selectivity. The potential safer anti-inflammatory drugs, *Am J Med* 95:40S-44S, 1993.

32. Lohinai Z, Stachlewitz R, Szekely AD et al: Evidence for the expression of cyclooxygenase-2 enzyme in periodontitis, *Life Sci* 70:279-290, 2001.

33. Schimizu N, Ozawa Y, Yamaguchi M et al: Induction of COX-2 expression by mechanical tension force in human periodontal ligament cells, *J Periodontol* 69:670-677, 1998.

34. Williams RC, Jeffcoat MK, Howell TH et al: Ibuprofen: an inhibitor of alveolar bone resorption in beagles, *J Periodont Res* 23:225-229, 1988.

35. Williams RC, Jeffcoat MK, Howell TH et al: Altering the course of human alveolar bone loss with the nonsteroidal anti-inflammatory drug flurbiprofen, *J Periodontol* 60:485-490, 1989.

36. Williams RC, Jeffcoat MK, Howell TH et al: Indomethacin and furbiprofen treatment of periodontitis in the beagle: effect on alveolar bone loss, *J Periodont Res* 22:403-407, 1987.

37. Howell TH, Jeffcoat MK, Goldhaber P et al: Inhibition of alveolar bone loss in beagles with the NSAID naproxen, *J Periodont Res* 26:498-501, 1991.

38. Holzhausen M, Rossa Jr C, Marcantonio Jr E et al: Effect of selective cyclooxygense-2 inhibition on the development of ligature-induced periodontitis in rats, *J Periodontol* 73:1030-1036, 2002.

39. Jeffcoat MK, Page RC, Reddy MS et al: Use of digital radiography to demonstrate the potential of naproxen as an adjunct in the treatment of rapidly progressive periodontitis, *J Periodont Res* 26:305-311, 1991.

40. Reddy MS, Palcanis KG, Barnett ML et al: Efficacy of meclofenamate sodium (Meclomen) in the treatment of rapidly progressive periodontitis, *J Clin Periodontol* 20:635-640, 1993.

41. Jeffcoat MK, Reddy MS, Haigh S et al: A comparison of topical ketorolac, systemic flurbiprofen, and placebo for inhibition of bone loss in adult periodontitis, *J Periodontol* 66:329-338, 1995.

42. Golub LM, Lee HM, Lehrer G et al: Minocycline reduces gingival collagenolytic activity during diabetes: preliminary observations and a proposed new mechanism of action, *J Periodont Res* 18:516-526, 1983.

43. Golub LM, McNamara TF, D'Angelo G et al: A non-antimicrobial chemically-modified tetracycline inhibits mammalian collagenase activity, *J Dent Res* 66:1310-1314, 1987.

44. Golub LM, Evans RT, McNamara RF et al: A non-antimicrobial tetracycline inhibits gingival matrix metalloproteinases and bone loss in *Porphyromonas gingivalis*- induced periodontitis in rats, *Ann NY Acad Sci* 732:96-100, 1994.

45. Golub LM, Lee H, Ryan ME et al: Tetracyclines inhibit connective tissue breakdown by multiple non-antimicrobial mechanisms, *Adv Dent Res* 12:12-26, 1998.

46. Caton J, Ciancio SG, Blieden TM et al: Treatment with subantimicrobial dose doxycycline improves the efficacy of scaling and root planing in patients with adult periodontitis, *J Periodontol* 71:521-532, 2000.

47. Ciancio SG, Ashley R: Safety and efficacy of sub-antimicrobial-dose doxycycline therapy in patients with adult periodontitis, *Adv Dent Res* 12:27-31, 1998.

48. Butt GM: Drug-induced xerostomia, *J Can Dent Assoc* 57:391-393, 1991.

49. Cohen G, Mandel I, Kaynar A: Salivary complaints: a manifestation of depressive mental illness, *NY State Dent J* 56(10):31-33, 1990.

50. Friedlander AH, Freidlander IK, Marder SR: Bipolar I disorder: psychopathology, medical management and dental implications, *J Am Dent Assoc* 133:1209-1217, 2002.

51. Friedlander AH, Friedlander IK, Gallas M, Velasco E: Late-life depression: its oral health significance, *Int Dent J* 53:41-50, 2003.

52. Boyd LD, Dwyer JT, Papas A: Nutritional implications of xerostomia and rampant caries caused by serotonin reuptake inhibitors: a case study, *Nutr Rev* 55:362-368, 1997.

34

Effect of Tobacco Smoking and Alcohol Use on Periodontal Diseases

Sara G. Grossi

ORAL AND SYSTEMIC EFFECTS OF CIGARETTE SMOKING AND ALCOHOL USE

Alcohol and tobacco are frequently used together and scientific research supports the popular observation that "smokers drink and drinkers smoke." Approximately 70% of alcoholics are heavy smokers (smoke >20 cigarettes/day) compared with 10% of the general population. Likewise, smokers are 1.3 times more likely to consume alcohol compared with nonsmokers. Despite increasing public awareness of the risks associated with tobacco and alcohol use and education programs to discourage their use, cigarette smoking and alcohol consumption remain highly prevalent among the adult population, high school students, and even pre-teens. The unfortunate consequence is that many of these children will go on to become chronic users of cigarettes, alcohol, or both, placing themselves at significant risk for a multitude of health consequences from long-term use of either of these two drugs. Few youths appreciate the addictive properties of nicotine and alcohol or the health consequences of their use.

Smoking and excessive alcohol use are risk factors for cardiovascular disease, obstructive lung disease, and some forms of cancers. Notably, two of these conditions, cardiovascular disease and chronic pulmonary obstruction, also are associated with periodontal disease (see Chapter 32). The risks for cancer of the oral cavity, throat, or esophagus for individuals who smoke and drink are greater than the sum of the individual risks; that is, the relative risks for oral and throat cancer are 7 times greater for smokers, 6 times greater for drinkers, and 38 times greater for smokers/drinkers compared with nonsmokers and nondrinkers. Cigarette smoking continues to be the leading cause of death in the United States. From 1995 to 1999, more than 440,000 deaths/year in the United States alone were attributed to smoking. Likewise, alcohol abuse contributes to a significant amount of mortality and morbidity in U.S. society. Indeed, the economic costs of alcohol abuse can be estimated, although not measured precisely. These costs come in various forms—first and foremost, loss to society because of premature death from alcohol use, loss from treating alcohol-related medical conditions, loss in productivity in the workplace, and costs from treatment of fetal alcohol syndrome. Additional costs to society are health-related costs of alcohol abuse to family life; effects on spouses, children, and family members; and costs involving the criminal justice system, social welfare system, and property losses. Periodontal diseases, the most common chronic infections of humankind, are yet one more health consequence of tobacco smoking and alcohol use. Therefore, thorough assessment of smoking and alcohol use as part of the overall periodontal examination is fundamental for adequate diagnosis and development of a treatment plan. As discussed later in this chapter, success of periodontal therapy depends greatly on appropriate identification and modification of these two important factors contributing to disease severity and progression.

EVIDENCE SUPPORTING SMOKING AND ALCOHOL AS RISK FACTORS FOR PERIODONTAL DISEASE

Early studies on the association of smoking and periodontal disease reported that the negative effect of tobacco smoke on the periodontium was mostly because of effects on oral hygiene and accumulation of local factors.[1,2] Thus, it was expected or justified that smokers would present with more severe periodontal destruction, because they also exhibited greater amounts of local factors; that is, dental plaque and calculus. Consequently, for decades tobacco smoking was largely ignored or overlooked as a significant factor in periodontal disease. A major milestone in periodontal research was the recognition of periodontal disease as multifactorial and that specific risk factors modulate the susceptibility of the host to periodontal infection and affect disease clinical outcome and severity.[3] The identification in the early 1990s of cigarette smoking as quite possibly the most significant risk factor for periodontal disease triggered a considerable amount of research examining the relation between smoking and periodontal disease. As a result, observational studies rather consistently reported that cigarette smoking increases the severity of periodontitis measured either as pocket depth or clinical attachment level independent of oral hygiene status.[4-11] These large-scale studies established unequivocally that tobacco smoking increases the overall risk for severe periodontal disease by 2.8 times compared with nonsmokers independent of the confounding effects of dental plaque and calculus (Fig. 34-1). The effect of cigarette smoking on clinical attachment level is clinically evident with 10 cigarettes/day or more, and each extra cigarette smoked daily increases gingival recession values by 2.3%, pocket depth by 0.3%, and attachment loss values by 0.5%.[6] In addition, the negative effect of cigarette smoking on the periodontium is cumulative and dose dependent. The severity of attachment loss is directly related to the amount of smoking measured either as pack-years (Fig. 34-2)[5] or number of cigarettes per day (Fig. 34-3)[9]—that is, the more cigarettes smoked per day and the longer the individual has smoked, the more severe the level of attachment loss. A similar dose–response relation is seen between amount of cigarette smoking and severity of alveolar bone loss.[12-14] Cigarette smoking significantly increases the risk for tooth loss by 70%,[15] as well as the risk for being totally edentulous.[16] The overwhelming evidence gathered in the

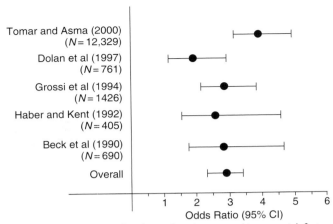

Figure 34-1. Summary of evidence for tobacco smoking as a risk factor for periodontal disease. *Bars* indicate the 95% confidence intervals for the depicted odds ratios. Summary data from the individual cited references. All studies demonstrate that tobacco use is an independent risk factor for the presence of periodontitis.

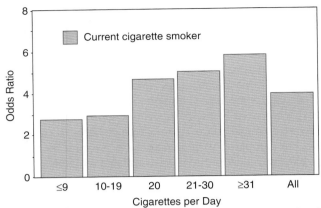

Figure 34-3. Dose-dependent effect of cigarette smoking and risk for periodontal disease. Among current cigarette smokers there was a significant dose response between number of cigarettes per day and presence of periodontitis. (*Adapted from Tomar S, Asma S: Smoking-attributable periodontitis in the United States: findings from the NHANES III, J Periodontol 71:743-751, 2000.*)

1990s dispelled the confusion and established definitively that cigarette smoking is an independent risk factor for periodontal disease. Although most of the evidence supporting tobacco use as a risk factor for periodontal disease is from cigarette smoking, cigar and pipe use also are significant risk factors for loss of periodontal attachment and for total edentulism.[8,10,17] This fact supports the notion that no tobacco product is safe or free of significant health risks.

In a manner similar to tobacco smoking, early studies assessing the effect of alcohol on periodontal tissues suggest that periodontal disease was the result of self-neglect and increased accumulation of dental plaque.[18] Again, similar to tobacco use, for a number of years alcohol use

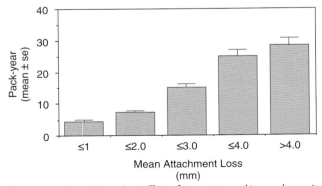

Figure 34-2. Dose-dependent effect of cigarette smoking and severity of attachment loss. For every 10 pack-year increment, there is a 1-mm increase in mean attachment loss. (*Adapted from Grossi SG, Zambon JJ, Ho AW et al: Assessment of risk for periodontal disease. I. Risk indicators for attachment loss, J Periodontol 65:260-267, 1994.*)

was overlooked as an independent factor contributing to periodontal disease. A cross-sectional study of 780 Finnish subjects 55 years of age and older showed that alcohol consumption of 3.5 drinks or more per week was significantly related to pocket depth greater than 3 mm after adjusting for smoking and tooth brushing frequency.[19] The role of alcoholism and cirrhosis also was examined in relation to periodontal disease. Presence of cirrhosis was significantly associated with increased attachment loss, after controlling for smoking and oral hygiene.[20] The Erie County Study, a study to determine risk factors for periodontal disease, included alcohol use as one of the potential risk factors.[21] Alcohol consumption was significantly related to clinical attachment loss and gingival bleeding independent of the confounding effects of plaque and periodontal microorganisms. Indeed, individuals consuming 5 or more drinks/week were 65% more likely to have greater gingival bleeding and 36% more likely to have severe clinical attachment loss compared with those consuming less than 5 drinks/week.[21] The effect of alcohol on periodontal disease was further examined in the third National Health and Nutrition Epidemiological Survey (NHANES III), a large epidemiologic study of health in the United States.[22] Analysis of the data obtained from this sample representative of the entire U.S. population supported the results from the Erie County Study that alcohol use is significantly associated with more severe attachment loss, and demonstrated that similar to tobacco smoking and periodontal disease, the association between alcohol and severity of periodontitis was dose dependent. The odds for severe periodontitis increased with increasing numbers of alcoholic drinks per week (Fig. 34-4) independent of

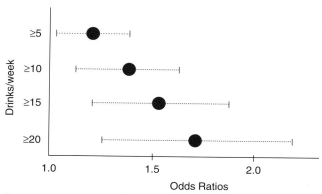

Figure 34-4. Association between alcohol consumption and clinical attachment loss. *Bars* indicate 95% confidence intervals for the depicted odds ratios. Odds ratios and their 95% confidence intervals were derived from multiple logistic regression analysis adjusting for age, sex, race, education, smoking, diabetes, and gingival bleeding. (*Adapted from Tezal M, Grossi SG, Ho AW, Genco RJ: Alcohol consumption and periodontal disease: the third National Health and Nutrition Survey,* J Clin Periodontol 2004 [in press].)

the confounding effects of age, sex, education, income, smoking, and visits to the dentist.[22] However, unlike cigarette smoking, where no amount of smoking is associated with health or is considered safe, moderate alcohol consumption appears to have protective effects for certain chronic diseases, such as cardiovascular disease. Although

a protective effect for moderate or social drinking and periodontal disease has not been observed, this level of drinking does not appear to increase the risk for periodontal disease; there is simply no difference compared with nondrinkers.

Although all criteria required for the definition of cigarette smoking as a risk factor for periodontal disease have been fulfilled,[23] the evidence for alcohol use increasing the risk for periodontal disease is only at the level of observational cross-sectional studies; that is, purely an *association* has been established between alcohol consumption and greater severity of periodontal attachment loss. Therefore, tobacco smoking is indeed a true risk factor, whereas alcohol use is a risk indicator for periodontal disease prevalence and severity. Longitudinal and treatment studies are needed to establish alcohol use as a true risk factor for periodontal disease.

Mechanisms of Tobacco and Alcohol Toxicity to the Periodontium

Another important research question arising from the substantial evidence implicating smoking as an etiologic factor for periodontal disease is whether the toxic effect of tobacco smoke on the periodontium is a local or systemic one. The answer to this question is not one or the other, but both; that is, local *and* systemic mechanisms account for tobacco's toxicity to the periodontium (Fig. 34-5). There are at least 2550 known compounds in tobacco and

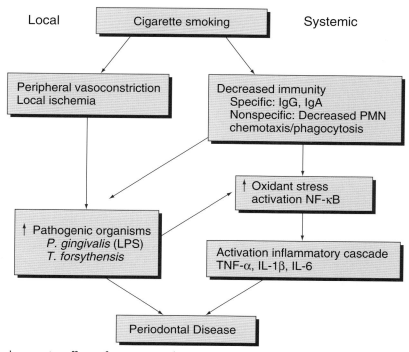

Figure 34-5. Mechanisms for the negative effects of cigarette smoking on periodontal tissues. Diagrammatic representation of local and systemic effects of cigarette smoking leading to severe periodontal disease.

more than 4000 compounds in tobacco smoke. Primary tobacco biohazards include at least 43 carcinogens such as the nicotine nitrosamines and alpha-emitting radionuclides such as Polonium 210. Tobacco smoke contains carbon monoxide, thiocyanate, herbicide, fungicide and pesticide residues, tars, and many other substances that promote disease and impair body functions. Toxic substances in tobacco smoke affect virtually every cell type of the periodontium. First and foremost, smoking has an immunosuppressive effect on the host, adversely affecting host–parasite interactions. Polymorphonuclear leukocyte motility, chemotaxis, and phagocytosis are significantly reduced in smokers.[24-27] Thus, this important first line of defense against subgingival bacteria is compromised in smokers. Specific immunity also is compromised, as demonstrated by reductions in antibody production, especially opsonizing IgG_2 and immunoregulatory T-cell subset ratios.[28,29] In this manner, both innate and acquired immune mechanisms are compromised in current smokers, allowing periodontal bacteria to escape host clearance and establish themselves as subgingival inhabitants. Cigarette smoking increases bacterial adhesion to epithelial cells[30] and has a differential effect on bacterial colonization, favoring growth of gram-negative bacteria.[31] In addition, alterations in the subgingival environment, such as decreased oxygen tension, allow, in turn, the overgrowth of an essentially anaerobic flora and overgrowth of opportunistic pathogenic microbial species (Fig. 34-5).[32,33] Periodontal pocket oxygen tension (PO_2) was significantly less in smokers compared with nonsmokers and was not influenced by gingival oxygen sufficiency.[34]

Studies of experimental gingivitis report that smokers developed greater dental plaque accumulation compared with nonsmokers.[2] Observational studies also report greater levels of dental plaque, calculus, and oral debris in smokers.[1] The unfortunate conclusion from these early studies is that smoking had an effect primarily on calculus, oral debris, and poor oral hygiene. Indeed, for approximately two decades, this conclusion dominated clinical practice. The specific effect of smoking on subgingival microorganisms did not become evident until the research methodology clearly distinguished between current smokers, former smokers, and never smokers, and accounted for varying amounts of smoking. Controlling for the severity of periodontal disease, current smokers were 3.1 times more likely to be infected with *Actinobacillus actinomycetemcomitans*, 2.3 times more likely to be infected with *Bacteroides forsythus* (now reclassified as *Tannerella forsythensis*), and 1.5 times more likely to be infected with *Porphyromonas gingivalis* than were former and never smokers with comparable levels of disease.[35] In a manner similar to the risk for severity of attachment loss, a biologic gradient was observed also for the risk for

infection with periodontal organisms; that is, the risk for being colonized with one of the specific periodontal pathogens increases with increasing amount of cigarette smoking. An increased risk for periodontal infection was evident in 21- to 35-year-old periodontitis-free subjects.[36] The number of bacterial species recovered from subgingival plaque was proportional to the number of pack-years smoked. Periodontitis-free subjects who had smoked 5 or more pack-years were 18 times more likely to be infected by pathogenic bacteria than periodontitis-free nonsmokers.[36] Current smoking also was associated with significantly greater numbers of *P. gingivalis*, *T. forsythensis*, and *C. recta* in subjects with early-onset periodontitis.[37] A significant positive relation was demonstrated between smoking and frequency of colonization by the periodontal pathogens *P. gingivalis*, *T. forsythensis*, and *Treponema denticola*.[38,39] All three organisms are members of the so-called red complex, whose members have been considered as etiologic factors in periodontal disease, and were significantly more prevalent in current smokers compared with nonsmokers.[40] In summary, current smokers are significantly more likely to be infected with pathogenic periodontal bacteria and have a greater number of bacterial species compared with former or nonsmokers with comparable levels of periodontal disease. The number of pathogenic periodontal bacteria in current smokers increases with increasing number of cigarettes smoked per day. This direct local effect of smoking on subgingival bacteria has great significance in the outcome of periodontal therapy, especially with regard to removal of subgingival infection in current smokers.

Cigarette smoking also was associated with increased levels of TNF-α in crevicular fluid compared with nonsmokers.[41] Neutrophil elastase activity, levels of prostaglandin E_2 (PGE_2), and matrix metalloproteinase-8 (MMP-8) were increased in smokers compared with nonsmokers.[42-44] Nicotine, in addition, up-regulates lipopolysaccharide-mediated monocyte secretion of PGE_2 and IL-1β.[45] Generation of free oxygen radicals from neutrophils also is increased in smokers compared with nonsmokers. Levels of metallothionein, a free radical scavenger, are increased in gingival tissues of smokers compared with nonsmokers.[46] This increased defense against free radicals in gingival tissue of smokers suggests that inflammation is much greater in smokers compared with nonsmokers regardless of periodontal status. Therefore, smoking appears to favor a pathogenic subgingival flora, decreases specific immunity against periodontal organisms, and also aggravates the inflammatory cascade in response to this chronic infection, leading to greater severity of periodontal disease and impaired wound healing (Fig. 34-5).

Several studies have demonstrated the absorption of nicotine in periodontal tissues. Nicotine has been detected on root surfaces of smokers with periodontal disease.[47] Cotinine, the major metabolite of nicotine, is found in serum, saliva, and gingival crevicular fluid of smokers.[48] Fibroblasts exposed to nicotine have shown reduced proliferation, migration, and attachment to root surfaces.[30,49,50] In addition, fibroblasts have been shown to nonspecifically bind and internalize nicotine.[51] This could, in turn, result in an alteration of cell metabolism including collagen synthesis and protein secretion.

Biologic plausibility for mechanisms of alcohol toxicity on periodontal tissues bears some similarities to those for tobacco smoke. First, alcohol is a well recognized toxic compound and, similar to tobacco smoke, has a negative effect on periodontal tissue by decreasing host defense mechanisms. Neutrophil function and activity is reduced in excessive alcohol users. In addition, impaired host defense appears also to be associated with altered cytokine production and altered T-lymphocyte functions.[52,53] Complement activity also is reduced, and clotting mechanisms such as prothrombin production and vitamin K activity are altered. Bone metabolism, with increased bone resorption and decreased bone formation, also is affected. Wound healing is decreased with specific decreases in vitamin B complex and total protein. In summary, cigarette smoking and alcohol consumption appear to trigger a cycle of impaired immune response, anaerobic subgingival infection, and connective tissue cytotoxicity leading to greater severity of periodontal disease and impaired wound healing.

CIGARETTE SMOKING AND RESPONSE TO PERIODONTAL THERAPY

Another milestone in periodontal research during the 1990s was the overwhelming number of studies supporting the negative effects of cigarette smoking on response to periodontal therapy. Scientific evidence has demonstrated that virtually all modalities of periodontal therapy are less predictable and have poorer outcomes in smokers compared with nonsmokers, indicating that smoking impairs periodontal wound healing. The shadow of confusion and uncertainty has been lifted, and we now know conclusively that cigarette smoking is not only a major risk factor for periodontal disease, but adversely affects the response to therapy as well.

Nonsurgical Therapy

Periodontal intervention studies consistently demonstrate that smokers have a less favorable response to nonsurgical periodontal therapy compared with nonsmokers. The short-term clinical outcomes of periodontal therapy— that is, reduction in pocket depth and gain in clinical attachment level—are significantly reduced in current smokers compared with nonsmokers.[54-56] All these

studies combined former smokers and never smokers into the "nonsmoker" study group. One clinical trial examined the effect of nonsurgical therapy in smokers compared with former and never smokers.[57] The clinical response of former smokers to mechanical periodontal therapy was comparable to never smokers and was significantly better than that of current smokers, providing indirect evidence of the benefits of smoking cessation in restoring the host's healing capacity to levels comparable to never smokers. The greatest differences between smoking groups were evident in sites with initially deep probing depths—that is, probing depths of 5 or more mm. On average, current smokers reported 0.8 mm less reduction in mean pocket depth at 3 months after nonsurgical therapy. Not only did current smokers show a reduced clinical response to nonsurgical therapy, the microbial response also was significantly impaired. Current smokers continued to harbor subgingival *T. forsythensis* and *P. gingivalis* after scaling and root planing (SRP) compared with former and never smokers.[57] Prevalence of *T. forsythensis*, *Peptostreptococcus micros*, and *C. recta* were significantly greater in current smokers after nonsurgical therapy compared with nonsmokers.[56] This suggests once again that current smoking promotes a gram-negative anaerobic flora and that mechanical periodontal therapy is less successful at significantly reducing this pathogenic flora in smokers compared with nonsmokers.

Nonsurgical Therapy Combined with Topical or Systemic Antibiotics

To compensate for the poorer treatment response of smokers to SRP, randomized clinical trials have investigated the potential benefit of adjunctive local or systemic antibiotics. In a manner similar to SRP alone, systemic metronidazole 200 mg three times a day for 7 days combined with SRP, or subgingival application of 25% metronidazole gel combined with SRP, resulted in less reduction in pocket depth in smokers compared with nonsmokers.[58] Paralleling the poorer short-term outcome to SRP alone, smokers exhibited, on average, 0.7 mm less reduction in pocket depth compared with nonsmokers, regardless of topical or systemic administration of adjunctive metronidazole. A poorer long-term (5 years) clinical response to SRP and systemic metronidazole was seen in smokers compared with nonsmokers.[59] The poorer clinical response, defined as persistence of inflamed sites with probing depth of 5 or more mm, was accompanied by persistence of subgingival infection with *A. actinomycetemcomitans*, *P. gingivalis*, *P. intermedia*, and spirochetes.[59] A study comparing three different systems of antibiotic delivery, including 2% minocycline gel, 25% tetracycline fibers, and a 25% metronidazole gel, reports similar adverse outcomes for current smokers.[55] Again, mean pocket depth reduction was in the order of

0.8 mm less in smokers compared with nonsmokers.[55] Interestingly, the clinical response to SRP combined with subgingival doxycycline was no different for smokers and nonsmokers; however, in the group treated with SRP alone, smokers again responded less favorably than nonsmokers.[60] Doxycycline and other antibiotics of the tetracycline family have been shown to inhibit activation of latent MMPs and to neutralize products of the neutrophil oxidative burst.[61,62] As such, doxycycline may counteract some of the deleterious effects of cigarette smoking on activation of the inflammatory cascade and healing process.

Surgical and Regenerative Therapy

Current cigarette smoking impairs wound healing after surgical periodontal therapy to a greater extent than after nonsurgical therapy. Smokers who underwent periodontal surgery with either modified Widman flap or mucoperiosteal flap reflection had significantly less reduction in pocket depth and gain in clinical attachment levels compared with nonsmokers.[63] A difference of 1 mm in reduction of pocket depth or gain in attachment between smokers and nonsmokers was observed in sites with initial probing depths of 7 or more mm.[64] Pocket depth reduction and gain in alveolar bone after modified Widman flap surgery also was greater in former and never smokers compared with current smokers.[65,66] Smokers also had significantly less gain in clinical attachment at 1, 2, and 5 years after flap surgery and grafting with demineralized freeze-dried bone allografts compared with nonsmokers.[67] Cigarette smoking also has been associated with a reduced healing response after guided tissue regeneration therapy in deep intrabony defects.[67,68] An 80% failure rate in treatment of furcation defects using regenerative therapy has been seen in smokers.[69] The long-term (5 years) response to guided tissue regeneration surgery also is dependent on smoking status. In a longitudinal study, 100% of the patients showing loss of attachment over time were current smokers.[70] Current smoking also decreases the percentage of root coverage that takes place after soft tissue grafting.[71] Treatment of gingival recession with guided tissue regeneration was again impaired in smokers compared with nonsmokers.[72] Smokers showed significantly less reduction in gingival recession and root coverage (57%) compared with nonsmokers (78%). In summary, current smoking is by far the most significant factor responsible for impaired periodontal wound healing and poor clinical outcome after flap and regenerative surgery.

Implant Therapy

With the ever increasing use of dental implants to replace missing teeth, a number of studies have examined factors associated with implant success and failure. Cigarette smoking has been identified as a significant factor associated with implant failure at different stages of the implant procedure. Current smokers were 2.6 times more likely to have an implant failure between the time of implant uncovering and the time of restorative loading.[73] Current smokers had the greatest implant failure rate in all regions of the mandible or maxilla; however, the greatest differences in implant failure rates between smokers and nonsmokers are seen in the maxilla. Statistically significant differences were seen in the anterior maxilla where smokers had a 16.8% failure rate versus 3.6% in nonsmokers.[73,74] Implant failure rates for smokers were significantly greater than nonsmokers when examined based on the number of implants that failed and on the number of patients who had one or more implant failures.[75] It must be stated, however, that implant therapy can be successful in smokers. In some of the studies cited earlier, implant success rates in smokers were approximately 93%, whereas in nonsmokers, the success rates were close to 97%. Thus, although the failure rate in smokers (7%) was significantly greater than that in nonsmokers (3%), the large majority of implants placed in smokers were successful.

Smoking may influence postimplant surgery healing and the long-term health of periimplant tissues. Current smokers had more problems with periimplant soft tissue health[76] and greater bleeding scores[77] compared with nonsmokers. In a 15-year prospective study of mandibular implant prostheses, current smoking was more strongly associated with marginal bone loss around implants than was poor oral hygiene.[78] Of current smokers undergoing intraoral bone grafting and simultaneous implant placement, 80% showed impaired wound healing, defined as loss of bone or implant, compared with only 10% of nonsmokers.[79] In a manner similar to severity of periodontal attachment loss, incidence of minor and major complications after implant therapy was significantly associated with both the amount and duration of smoking.[80] Similar to the response to nonsurgical periodontal therapy, smokers who followed a smoking cessation protocol in the 8-week period after implant placement had implant failure rates significantly less than current smokers and comparable to never smokers.[81] These results suggest once again the significant benefit to be gained from discussing with patients the oral health risks associated with smoking and encouraging them to enroll in a smoking cessation program.

Periodontal Maintenance Therapy and Need for Retreatment

The effect of cigarette smoking on long-term response to periodontal maintenance therapy also has been investigated. Independent studies consistently report that smokers have a less favorable response to maintenance compared with nonsmokers.[55,63,82] Only a small percentage of patients showed a high incidence of sites breaking down, and they were mostly smokers.[83] Again, a biologic gradient was seen between smoking and long-term response to periodontal maintenance; that is, heavy smokers (i.e., >20 cigarettes/day) responded less favorably than light smokers (≤20 cigarettes/day) to long-term maintenance.[82] These studies again report the encouraging finding that former smokers respond to maintenance in a manner similar to those who never smoked. Of the patients diagnosed with refractory periodontitis or failure to respond to conventional periodontal therapy, 90% were current smokers.[27] Thus, not only does smoking result in reduced response to all modalities of periodontal treatment and less favorable outcome, susceptibility to recurrence and need for retreatment also are increased. Again, the case is made for the importance of incorporating smoking counseling and assistance in smoking cessation as an integral procedure in any dental practice.

ALCOHOL USE AND ITS RELATION TO PERIODONTAL THERAPY

No studies have examined the effect of alcohol on healing of periodontal tissues after therapy. However, indirect evidence supporting a negative effect of chronic alcohol use on periodontal healing comes from a study of reduced healing of buccal mucosal ulcers.[84] Acetaldehyde, a toxic intermediate in the metabolism of alcohol, has significant toxicity even at low doses. Acetaldehyde has shown cytotoxicity on buccal epithelial cells and human gingival fibroblasts.[85] Although much more research is needed in this area, current findings support the possibility of a negative effect of chronic alcohol use on periodontal healing as well.

SMOKING CESSATION AND ALCOHOL COUNSELING IN THE PERIODONTAL OFFICE

The reasons for providing clinical tobacco and alcohol intervention services in the dental office are compelling.[86] Overwhelming evidence indicates that tobacco is harmful to oral health and that smoking status is an important factor in the outcome of all modalities of periodontal therapy. Although the evidence for alcohol and periodontal disease is less abundant compared with tobacco smoking, one cannot dispute the harmful effect of chronic alcohol use on oral health. Thus, helping patients to quit smoking and to reduce alcohol use is not only professionally indicated, it is an ethical obligation. Smoking cigarettes kills half of those who smoke regularly, and half of those who die of a tobacco-related disease will die prematurely, losing, on average, two decades of life. Chronic alcohol

abusers are at increased risk for chronic diseases, depression, and premature death. Clinical tobacco and alcohol intervention services are cost-effective. Long-term tobacco users develop chronic conditions that often become time-consuming patient management problems. Smokers and drinkers are often ill, frequently leading to problems with appointments, medical considerations, and significantly greater risk for requiring emergency visits for acute problems.

Dentist's Role in Treating Nicotine Addition and Chronic Alcohol Abuse

Of all health professionals, dentists are without a doubt the ones with the greatest chance to significantly encourage and affect the patient's desire to want to quit smoking.[87] First and foremost, a concrete and tangible ill consequence of tobacco smoking (periodontal disease) is at hand for the patient to consider. The presence of periodontal pockets, tooth mobility, suppuration, and other problems offer the dentist the unique opportunity to connect the patient's smoking habit to a disease process that has already taken place, as opposed to the eventual possibility of a life-threatening condition in some distant future. Thus, the patient is confronted with a health consequence of tobacco smoking that is a reality rather than a probability. Second, a patient sees the dentist far more often than he or she sees a physician. Third, dentists are among health professionals most trusted and respected by patients, and whose opinions and recommendations are most valued. A randomized clinical trial reports a smoking cessation of 13% in a group of patients receiving periodontal treatment, oral hygiene instruction, and advice in smoking cessation compared with 5% cessation in the nontreatment control group.[88] Many professional organizations have developed support systems that help clinicians to integrate cessation services into their practices. For example, several dental organizations have adopted tobacco-related clinical policies. The American Dental Association has published and distributed a guide to therapeutics titled "Tobacco Counseling for the Control and Prevention of Oral Disease," established a service code for tobacco counseling (01320), and included tobacco questions in its standard Health History Form. Educational guidelines have been developed for dental education institutions. Such infrastructure developments ease the integration of clinical tobacco intervention services into practice.[89,90]

A practical routine should be integrated into every clinical practice. Basic steps are known as the "5 As": Ask, Advise, Assess, Assist, and Arrange (Box 34-1). First proposed by Glynn and Manley[91] of the National Cancer Institute, the steps have remained the core of successful clinical programs for smoking cessation programs. These steps have been adapted to allow management of alcohol

Ask	All your patients about tobacco use
Advise	Tobacco users to quit
Assess	Tobacco users' willingness to quit
Assist	Tobacco users in developing a quit plan
Arrange	Tobacco-users' follow-up contact

reduction programs (Box 34-2). The basic steps are detailed in the following sections.

Ask

Identify the tobacco and alcohol use status of every patient: "Do you use tobacco?" and "Do you consume alcohol?" This information should be considered a vital sign. Inquiry can be integrated within existing patient questionnaire systems. Inasmuch as nicotine dependency is chronic and relapsing, it is important to ask this question at every encounter. Tobacco and alcohol users must be asked about the duration and intensity of their use, past experience with quitting, and especially about their desire to stop: "How interested are you in quitting now?" and "How interested are you in reducing your alcohol consumption?"

Advise

The advising step focuses on building patient's motivation to be tobacco- and alcohol-free. Although brief and simple, building motivation is one of three basic clinical intervention services. Commend never-users and ex-users on the wisdom of their behavior.

First, advise all tobacco/alcohol users in clear language that you think they should quit tobacco use and quit or reduce alcohol consumption. Patients place great weight on such advice by clinicians.

Second, associate use with existing patient oral and periodontal conditions. When possible, show the patient his or her own tobacco-related conditions; for example, a deep infrabony defect, a furcation involvement, tooth mobility, or suppurating pocket. Patients should understand the

Ask	All your patients about alcohol use
Advise	Heavy alcohol users to reduce alcohol use
Assess	Heavy alcohol users' willingness to reduce alcohol use
Assist	Heavy alcohol users in developing an alcohol-reduction plan
Arrange	Heavy alcohol users' follow-up contact

health and oral risks of tobacco use. Showing them existing lesions brings the reality of tobacco- and alcohol-related disease into the *present*. Discuss with the patient the increased risk for oral and throat cancer in smokers and drinkers. Point to mucosal lesions to demonstrate the patient's alcohol-related conditions.

Assess

Assess the patient's willingness to quit smoking or to reduce alcohol use. Ask each patient for his or her own reasons for wanting to quit smoking or alcohol use. Expressing those reasons helps strengthen them, even though many have little to do with health. The patient's reasons provide clues on which the clinician can add motivating ideas and perspectives that help dispel unwarranted hesitancy. Emphasize the benefits of eliminating these habits in terms that are specific to each patient's interests, circumstances, and culture.

Many patients will not be interested in quitting or abstaining immediately, but the "Advise" step strengthens the decision-making process that individuals must progress through to initiate a behavior change. The discussion clarifies in the patient's mind the opinion of a respected individual. Discussion helps individuals who are generally interested in quitting to begin thinking more seriously about what they are doing to themselves and about their prospects for living tobacco- and alcohol-free. A clinician's advice to quit can trigger the decision to act. The patient's desire for successful and enduring clinical therapy can influence his or her desire to quit.

Patients who are not interested in quitting at the moment should be offered assistance in the future: "When (not 'if') you are ready, I'll be glad to help." In addition, patients should be given motivational literature that is appropriate to their interests, circumstances, and, if possible, culture.

Assist

Although Ask, Advise and Assess are routine steps for all tobacco and alcohol users, the Assist step is used with a subset of patients who are ready to quit or to reduce alcohol use. This step focuses on helping patients cope with the quitting process. The clinician acts as a caring, skilled facilitator because, of course, the primary responsibility remains with the individual who must quit.

The most basic component of the Assist phase is to set an actual quit date. The clinician asks the patient who has decided to quit to set a specific date. Once the patient has set a date, the clinician should suggest that the patient inform friends and family members of that date. This will enable them to become an integral part of the patient's support system. The patient should plan, and the support network should reinforce, the removal of all tobacco or alcohol products from the patient's home, work, car, or other accessible sites. The clinician can provide literature on the quitting process. Such booklets are readily available from organizations such as the National Cancer Institute and American Heart Association. They describe coping strategies, motivational tools, and methods to manage the effects of cessation, such as nicotine withdrawal and weight gain.

Arrange

Establish a schedule for follow-up contacts, either in person or by telephone. This is a key component to cessation. Although some increase in patient quit rates can be anticipated from a single encounter, long-term abstinence is dramatically improved (threefold to fourfold) when there is timely follow-up.

The recommended postquit date follow-up contact schedule is four to seven contacts over a 3-month period. The first follow-up contact should be within 2 weeks of the quit date, preferably within the first week. The second, third, and fourth contact should be near the end of the first, second, and third months.

Providing clinical intervention services requires a team approach. Clinic personnel, the office environment, and the management system need a few simple adjustments for services to be provided efficiently, effectively, and pleasantly. First, an individual, usually not the primary care provider, needs to be responsible for the service operation. All members of the clinical team need to understand the objectives and methods used. The Ask step is usually managed by reception/receiving staff, including recording of the patient's tobacco use status. This is verified when other vital signs are taken and initial workup is begun. Diagnosis and treatment planning must include the Advice step. Assist often is begun by the primary clinician or other provider. Other staff may provide more detailed help for the patient who commits to a quit date and may ensure that the Arrange step is done so that follow-up will occur.

CONCLUSION

Substantial evidence supports the concept that tobacco smoking has a profound negative effect on periodontal disease severity, prevalence, incidence, and progression. Chronic alcohol abuse may also be associated with periodontal diseases. Tobacco smoking has a negative effect in all forms of periodontal therapy, leading to less favorable treatment outcomes, in the short- or long-term, or both. Tobacco smoking and chronic alcohol abuse also have a profound negative effect on the health and well-being of users, society, and clinical practice. Tobacco use and alcohol abuse are preventable negative lifestyle habits. Adoption of scientifically sound clinical tobacco cessation and alcohol reduction services is a professional obligation, a moral imperative, and a practical matter. Three to five minutes of cessation assistance integrated into other clinical services is a potentially life-saving service that benefits patients, community, and practice. Periodontal health and prognoses for periodontal therapy substantially improve when patients quit smoking and reduce alcohol consumption.

REFERENCES

1. Sheiham A: Periodontal disease and oral cleanliness in tobacco smokers, *J Periodontol* 42:259-263, 1971.
2. Bastian RJ, Wait IM: Effect of tobacco smoking on plaque development and gingivitis, *J Periodontol* 49:480-482, 1978.
3. Genco RJ: Risk factors for periodontal diseases, *J Periodontol* 67:1041-1049, 1996.
4. Haber J, Wattles J, Crowley M et al: Evidence for cigarette smoking as a major risk factor for periodontitis, *J Periodontol* 64:16-23, 1993.
5. Grossi SG, Zambon JJ, Ho AW et al: Assessment of risk for periodontal disease. I. Risk indicators for attachment loss, *J Periodontol* 65:260-267, 1994.
6. Martinez-Canut P, Lorca A, Magan R: Smoking and periodontal disease severity, *J Clin Periodontol* 22:743-749, 1995.
7. Dolan T, Gilbert G, Ringelberg M et al: Behavioral risk indicators of attachment loss in adult Floridians, *J Clin Periodontol* 24:223-232, 1997.
8. Albandar J, Streckfus C, Adesanya M, Winn D: Cigar, pipe and cigarette smoking as risk factors for periodontal disease and tooth loss, *J Periodontol* 71:1874-1881, 2000.
9. Tomar S, Asma S: Smoking-attributable periodontitis in the United States: findings from the NHANES III, *J Periodontol* 71:743-751, 2000.
10. Beck J, Koch G, Rozier R, Tudor G: Prevalence and risk indicators for periodontal attachment loss in a population of older community-dwelling blacks and whites, *J Periodontol* 61:521-528, 1990.
11. Haber J, Kent RL: Cigarette smoking in a periodontal practice, *J Periodontol* 63:100-106, 1992.
12. Grossi SG, Genco RJ, Machtei EE et al: Assessment of risk for periodontal disease. II. Risk indicators for alveolar bone loss, *J Periodontol* 66:23-29, 1995.
13. Mullally B, Breen B, Linden G: Smoking and patterns of bone loss in early-onset periodontitis, *J Periodontol* 70:394-401, 1999.
14. Hildebolt C, Pilgram T, Crothers N et al: Alveolar bone height and postcranial bone mineral density: negative effects of cigarette smoking and parity, *J Periodontol* 71:683-689, 2000.
15. Randolph W, Ostir G, Markides K: Prevalence of tooth loss and dental service use in older Mexican Americans, *J Am Geriatr Soc* 49:585-589, 2001.
16. Krall E, Hughes B, Papas A, Garcia R: Tooth loss and skeletal bone density in healthy postmenopausal women, *Osteoporosis Int* 4:104-109, 1994.

17. Jette AM, Feldman HA, Tennstedt S: Tobacco use: a modifiable risk factor for dental disease among elderly, *Am J Public Health* 83:1271-1276, 1993.

18. Larato DC: Oral tissue changes in the chronic alcoholic, *J Periodontol* 43:772-773, 1972.

19. Sakki TK, Knuutila MLE, Vimpari SS, Hartikainen MSL: Association of lifestyle and periodontal healh, *Community Dent Oral Epidemiol* 23:155-158, 1995.

20. Novacek G, Plachetzky U, Potzi R et al: Dental and periodontal disease in patients with cirrhosis: role of etiology of liver disease, *J Hepatol* 22:576-582, 1995.

21. Tezal M, Grossi SG, Ho AW, Genco RJ: The effect of alcohol consumption on periodontal disease, *J Periodontol* 72:183-189, 2001.

22. Tezal M, Grossi SG, Ho AW, Genco RJ: Alcohol consumption and periodontal disease: the third National Health and Nutrition Survey, *J Clin Periodontol* 2004 (in press).

23. Gelskey SC: Cigarette smoking and periodontitis: methodology to assess the strength of evidence in support of a causal association, *Community Dent Oral Epidemiol* 27:16-24, 1999.

24. Kenney EB, Kraal JH, Saxe SR, Jones J: The effect of cigarette smoke on human oral polymorphonuclear leukocytes, *J Periodont Res* 12:223-234, 1977.

25. Fredriksson MI, Figueredo CM, Gustafsson A et al: Effect of periodontitis and smoking on blood leukocytes and acute-phase proteins, *J Periodontol* 70:1355-1360, 1999.

26. Corberand J, Laharraghe P, Nguyen F et al: In vitro effect of tobacco smoke components on the function of normal human polymorphonuclear leukocytes, *Infect Immun* 30:649-655, 1980.

27. MacFarlane GD, Herzberg MC, Wolff LF, Hardie NA: Refractory periodontitis associated with abnormal polymorphonuclear leukocyte phagocytosis and cigarette smoking, *J Periodontol* 63:908-913, 1992.

28. Tew JG, Zhang J-B, Quinn S et al: Antibody of the IgG2 subclass, *Actinobacillus actinomycetemcomitans* and early-onset periodontitis, *J Periodontol* 67(Suppl):317-322, 1996.

29. Costabel U, Bross KJ, Reuter C et al: Alterations in immunoregulatory T-cell subsets in cigarette smokers: a phenotypic analysis of bronchoalveolar and blood lymphocytes, *Chest* 90:39-44, 1986.

30. Venditto MA: Therapeutic considerations: lower respiratory tract infections in smokers, *J Am Osteopath Assoc* 92:897-900, 1992.

31. Ertel A, Eng R, Smith S: The differential effect of cigarette smoke in the growth of bacteria found in humans, *Chest* 100:628-630, 1991.

32. Loesche WJ, Gusberti F, Mettraux G et al: Relationship between oxygen tension and subgingival bacterial flora in untreated human periodontal pockets, *Infect Immun* 42:659-667, 1983.

33. Mettraux G, Gusberti F, Graf H: Oxygen tension (pO2) in untreated human periodontal pockets, *J Periodontol* 55:516-521, 1984.

34. Hanioka T, Tanaka M, Takaya K et al: Pocket oxygen tension in smokers and non-smokers with periodontal disease, *J Periodontol* 71:550-554, 2000.

35. Zambon JJ, Grossi SG, Machtei EE et al: Cigarette smoking and subgingival infection, *J Periodontol* 67:1050-1055, 1996.

36. Shiloah J, Patters MR, Waring MB: The prevalence of pathogenic periodontal microflora in healthy young smokers, *J Periodontol* 71:562-567, 2000.

37. Kamma JJ, Nakou M, Baehni PC: Clinical and microbiological characteristics of smokers with early onset periodontitis, *J Periodont Res* 34:25-33, 1999.

38. Kazor C, Taylor GW, Loesche WJ: The prevalence of BANA-hydrolyzing periodontopathic bacteria in smokers, *J Clin Periodontol* 26:814-821, 1999.

39. Darby I, Hodge P, Riggio M, Kinane D: Microbial comparison of smoker and non-smoker adult and early-onset periodontitis patients by polymerase chain reaction, *J Clin Periodontol* 27:417-424, 2000.

40. Haffajee A, Socransky S: Relationship of cigarette smoking to attachment level profiles, *J Clin Periodontol* 28:283-295, 2001.

41. Bostrom L, Linder LE, Bergstrom J: Smoking and crevicular fluid levels of IL-6 and TNF-alpha in periodontal disease, *J Clin Periodontol* 26:352-357, 1999.

42. Soder B: Neutrophil elastase activity, levels of prostaglandin E2, and matrix metalloproteinase-8 in refractory periodontitis sites in smokers and non-smokers, *Acta Odont Scand* 57:77-82, 1999.

43. Pauletto NC, Liede K, Nieminen A et al: Effect of cigarette smoking on oral elastase activity in adult periodontitis patients, *J Periodontol* 71:58-62, 2000.

44. Ryder MI, Fujitaki R, Lebus S et al: Alterations of neutrophil L-selectin and CD18 expression by tobacco smoke: implications for periodontal diseases, *J Periodont Res* 33:359-368, 1998.

45. Payne JB, Johnson GK, Reinhardt RA et al: Nicotine effects on PGE2 and IL-1 beta release by LPS-treated human monocytes, *J Periodont Res* 31:99-104, 1996.

46. Katsuragi H, Hasegawa A, Saito K: Distribution of metallothionein in cigarette smokers and non-smokers in advanced periodontitis patients, *J Periodontol* 68:1005-1009, 1997.

47. Cuff MJ, McQuade MJ, Scheidt MJ et al: The presence of nicotine on root surfaces of periodontally diseased teeth in smokers, *J Periodontol* 60:564-569, 1989.

48. McGuire JR, McQuade MJ, Rossman JA et al: Cotinine in saliva and gingival crevicular fluid of smokers with periodontal disease, *J Periodontol* 60:176-181, 1989.

49. Tanur E, McQuade MJ, McPherson JC et al: Effects of nicotine on the strength of attachment of gingival fibroblasts to glass and non-diseased human root surfaces, *J Periodontol* 71:717-722, 2000.

50. Raulin LA, McPherson JC III, McQuade MJ, Hanson BS: The effect of nicotine on the attachment of human fibroblasts to glass and human root surfaces in vitro, *J Periodontol* 59:318-325, 1988.

51. Hanes PJ, Schuster GS, Lubas S: Binding, uptake and release of nicotine by human gingival fibroblasts, *J Periodontol* 62:147-152, 1991.

52. Szabo G: Consequences of alcohol consumption on host defense, *Alcohol Alcohol* 34:830-841, 1999.

53. Christen AG: Dentistry and the alcoholic patient, *Dent Clin North Am* 27:341-361, 1983.

54. Preber H, Begström J: The effect of non-surgical treatment on periodontal pockets in smokers and nonsmokers, *J Clin Periodontol* 13:319-323, 1986.

55. Kinane DF, Rafvar M: The effects of smoking on mechanical and antimicrobial periodontal therapy, *J Periodontol* 68:467-472, 1997.

56. Van Winkelhoff AJ, Bosch-Tijhof CJ, Winkel EG, van der Reijden WA: Smoking affects the subgingival microflora in periodontitis, *J Periodontol* 72:666-671, 2001.

57. Grossi SG, Zambon J, Machtei EE et al: Effects of smoking and smoking cessation on healing after mechanical periodontal therapy, *J Am Dent Assoc* 128:599-607, 1997.

58. Palmer RM, Matthews JP, Wilson RF: Non-surgical periodontal treatment with and without adjunctive metronidazole in smokers and non-smokers, *J Clin Periodontol* 26:158-163, 1999.

59. Soder B, Nedlich U, Jin LJ: Longitudinal effect of non-surgical treatment and systemic metronidazole for 1 week in smokers and non-smokers with refractory periodontitis, *J Periodontol* 70:761-771, 1999.

60. Ryder MI, Pons B, Adams D et al: Effects of smoking on local delivery of controlled-release doxycycline as compared to scaling and root planing, *J Clin Periodontol* 26:683-691, 1999.

61. Ramamurthy NS, Vernillo A, Greenwald RA et al: Reactive oxygen species activate and tetracyclines inhibit rat osteoclast collagenase, *J Bone Mineral Res* 8:1247-1253, 1993.

62. Golub LM, Sorsa T, Lee HM et al: Doxycycline inhibits neutrophil (PMN)-type matrix metalloproteinases in human adult periodontitis gingiva, *J Clin Periodontol* 22:100-109, 1995.

63. Ah MK, Johnson GK, Kaldahl WB et al: The effect of smoking on the response to periodontal therapy, *J Clin Periodontol* 21:91-97, 1994.

64. Scabbia A, Cho KS, Sigurdsson TJ et al: Cigarette smoking negatively affects healing response following flap debridement surgery, *J Periodontol* 72:43-49, 2001.

65. Preber H, Bergström J: Effect of cigarette smoking on periodontal healing following surgical therapy, *J Clin Periodontol* 17:324-328, 1990.

66. Bostrom L, Linder L, Bergström J: Influence of smoking on the outcome of periodontal surgery, *J Clin Periodontol* 25:194-201, 1998.

67. Rosen PS, Marks MH, Reynolds MA: Influence of smoking on long-term clinical results of intrabony defects treated with regenerative therapy, *J Periodontol* 67:1159-1163, 1996.

68. Tonetti MS, Pini-Prato G, Cortellini P: Effect of cigarette smoking on periodontal healing following GTR in infrabony defects: a preliminary retrospective study, *J Clin Periodontol* 22:229-234, 1995.

69. Rosenberg ES, Cutler SA: The effect of cigarette smoking on the long-term success of guided tissue regeneration: a preliminary study, *Ann R Austral Coll Dent Surg* 12(4):89-93, 1994.

70. Cortellini P, Paolo G, Pini-Prato G, Tonetti MS: Long-term stability of clinical attachment following guided tissue regeneration and conventional therapy, *J Clin Periodontol* 23:106-111, 1996.

71. Miller PD Jr: Root coverage with the free gingival graft: factors associated with incomplete coverage, *J Periodontol* 58:674-681, 1987.

72. Trombelli A, Kim C, Zimmerman G, Wikesjö U: Retrospective analysis of factors related to clinical outcome of guided tissue regeneration procedures in intrabony defects, *J Clin Periodontol* 24:366-371, 1997.

73. Lambert P, Morris H, Ochi S: The influence of smoking on 3-year clinical success of osseointegrated dental implants, *Ann Periodontol* 5:79-89, 2000.

74. Bain CA, Moy PK: The association between the failure of dental implants and cigarette smoking, *Int J Oral Maxillfac Implants* 8:609-615, 1993.

75. Gorman L, Lambert P, Morris H et al: The effect of smoking on implant survival at second-stage surgery: DICRG interim report No. 5, *Implant Dent* 3:165-168, 1994.

76. Weyant R: Characteristics associated with the loss and peri-implant tissue health of endosseous dental implants, *Int J Oral Maxillofac Implants* 9:95-102, 1994.

77. Haas R, Haimböck W, Mailath G, Watzek G: The relationship of smoking on peri-implant tissue: a retrospective study, *J Prosthet Dent* 76:592-596, 1996.

78. Lindquist LW, Carlsson GE, Jemt T: A prospective 15-year follow-up study of mandibular fixed prosthesis supported by osseointegrated implants, *Clin Oral Implant Res* 7:329-336, 1996.

79. Jones JK, Triplett RG: The relationship of cigarette smoking to impaired intraoral wound healing: a review of evidence and implications for patient care, *J Oral Maxillofacial Surg* 50:237-240, 1992.

80. Schwartz-Arad D, Samet N, Samet N, Mamlider A: Smoking and complications of endosseous dental implants, *J Periodontol* 73:153-157, 2002.

81. Bain CA: Smoking and implant failure-Benefits of a smoking cessation protocol, *J Oral Maxillfac Implants* 11:756-759, 1996.

82. Kaldahl WB, Johnson GK, Patil KD, Kalkwarf KL: Levels of cigarette consumption and response to periodontal therapy, *J Periodontol* 67:675-681, 1996.

83. Kaldhal WB, Kalkwarf KL, Patil KD et al: Long-term evaluation of periodontal therapy: II. Incidence of sites breaking down, *J Periodontol* 67:103-108, 1996.

84. Slomiany BL, Piotrowsky J, Slomiany A: Suppression of endothelin-converting enzyme-1 during buccal mucosal ulcer healing: effect of chronic alcohol ingestion, *Biochem Biophys Res Commun* 271:318-322, 2000.

85. Vaca CE, Nilsson JA, Fang JL, Grafstrom RC: Formation of DNA adducts in human buccal epithelial cells exposed to acetaldehyde and methylglyoxal in vitro, *Chem Biol Interact* 108:197-208, 1998.

86. Tomar SL, Husten CG, Manley MW: Do dentists and physicians advise tobacco users to quit? *J Am Dent Assoc* 127:259-265, 1996.

87. Dolan TA, McGorray SP, Grinstead-Skigen CL, Mecklenburg RE: Tobacco control activities in U.S. dental practices, *J Am Dent Assoc* 128:1669-1679, 1997.

88. MacGreggor ID: Efficacy of dental health advice as an aid to reducing cigarette smoking, *Br Dent J* 180:292-296, 1996.

89. Mecklenburg RE: Tobacco: addiction, oral health, and cessation, *Quintessence Int* 29:250-252, 1998.

90. Somerman M, Mecklenburg RE: Cessation of tobacco use. In Ciancio SG, editor: *ADA guide to dental therapeutics*, Chicago, 1998, ADA Publishing Company, 505-516.

91. Glynn TJ, Manley MW: *How to help your patients stop smoking: a National Cancer Institute manual for physicians.* U.S. Department of Health and Human Services, Public Health Service, National Institutes of Health, NIH Publication No. 90-3064, 1989.

35 Selected Soft and Hard Tissue Lesions With Periodontal Relevance

Alfredo Aguirre and Jose Luis Tapia

SOFT TISSUE LESIONS
Desquamative Gingivitis
Reactive Nodular Lesions of the Gingiva
Peripheral Odontogenic Lesions
Benign Lesions of the Gingiva
Malignant Lesions of the Gingiva
Metastatic Gingival Lesions

HARD TISSUE LESIONS
Odontogenic Lesions
Nonodontogenic Lesions

MISCELLANEOUS
Giant Cell Fibroma
Retrocuspid Papilla
Gingival Fibrous Nodule
Langerhans Cell Disease
Oral Focal Mucinosis
Gingival Hyperplasia Associated With Plasminogen Deficiency (Amyloid-like gingival hyperplasia)
Verruciform Xanthoma
Gingival Salivary Gland Choristoma
Wegener's Granulomatosis

The soft and hard periodontal tissues are susceptible to not only inflammatory changes but also benign and malignant conditions. The clinical presentation of soft tissue lesions affecting the periodontium may generate diagnostic challenges for the dentist. The formulation of a sound differential diagnosis is essential for proper patient management. Although most of the soft tissue lesions affecting the periodontium can be accurately diagnosed at the microscopic level with conventional laboratory procedures, sometimes histochemistry, immuno-histochemistry, or immunofluorescence evaluations are needed to arrive at a precise diagnosis. In bone lesions that affect the periodontium, imaging studies in combination with microscopic evaluation of a biopsy specimen are essential to render a precise diagnosis.

The purpose of this chapter is to provide an overview of selected soft and hard tissue conditions that have periodontal relevance. When appropriate, algorithms developed to facilitate the diagnostic process are presented.

SOFT TISSUE LESIONS

Desquamative Gingivitis

The term chronic desquamative gingivitis (DG) describes a peculiar condition characterized by intense erythema, desquamation, and ulceration of the free and attached gingiva. Although 50% of DG cases are localized exclusively in the gingiva, it is not unusual to see additional oral involvement.[1] The term *desquamative gingivitis* is rather unspecific and comprises a gingival response associated with a variety of conditions.[2-5]

Approximately 75% of DG cases have a dermatologic origin and are mainly associated with mucous membrane pemphigoid (MMP), lichen planus (LP), and, to a lesser degree, pemphigus vulgaris (PV) in more than 95% of the cases.[1,6] However, chronic ulcerative stomatitis (CUS), bullous pemphigoid, linear IgA disease, lupus erythematosus, and dermatitis herpetiformis can also present as DG.[7]

Therefore to properly diagnose the condition responsible for DG, clinical examination coupled with a thorough medical history and routine histologic and immunofluorescence studies are warranted.[8] Immunofluorescence analysis include both direct (DIF) and indirect (IIF) studies. DIF is performed on biopsies of tissue specimens that are placed into a special medium (not formalin). Immunofluorescent staining is directly visualized in the microscopic sections. IIF is performed on serum from a patient's blood specimen and detects circulating antibodies. Despite a thorough evaluation, the cause of DG remains elusive in up to one third of the cases.[9] Although the differential diagnosis of DG is extensive, the current discussion is limited to four conditions: erosive LP, MMP, PV, and CUS. However, the histologic, DIF, and IIF features of other lesions that may present clinically as DG are found in Table 35-1. Figure 35-1 illustrates an approach to elucidate the genesis of DG.

Lichen Planus

LP is a relatively common, chronic cutaneous condition. Oral lichen planus (OLP) presents in 0.1% to 4% of the population.[10] Most of the patients with OLP are middle-aged and older women (2:1 ratio of females to males), and children are rarely affected. There are several clinical forms of OLP such as reticular, patch, atrophic, erosive, and bullous forms; the most common are the reticular and erosive subtypes. Typically, the buccal mucosae show reticular and asymptomatic bilateral lesions. Up to 10% of patients with OLP have lesions restricted to the gingival tissue, which may occur as keratotic, erosive/ulcerative, vesicular/bullous, or atrophic subtypes (Fig. 35-2).[11]

Microscopically, hyperkeratosis, hydropic degeneration of the basal layer, "saw-toothed" configuration of the rete ridges, and a dense "bandlike" infiltrate primarily of T lymphocytes in the lamina propria are observed (Fig. 35-3). Colloid bodies (Civatte bodies) may be seen at the epithelium–connective tissue interface. DIF of both lesional and perilesional OLP biopsy specimens reveal "shaggy" deposits of fibrin in the basement membrane zone, along with immunoglobulin-staining colloid bodies in the upper areas of the lamina propria (Fig. 35-4). IIF is negative in LP. A clinical–histopathologic–immunofluorescence correlation has to be made to arrive at a diagnosis of LP. Lupus erythematosus, CUS, cicatricial pemphigoid, PV, and linear IgA disease should be included in the differential diagnosis of erosive LP.

The erosive, bullous, or ulcerative lesions of OLP are treated with high-potency topical steroids (for example, 0.05% fluocinonide ointment applied to lesions three times daily). Alternatively, systemic steroids can also be used but require close follow-up by a dermatologist because of their potentially deleterious side effects. It is important to closely follow-up patients with a diagnosis of erosive LP because the malignant potential of OLP is still a controversial issue.[12-16]

Mucous Membrane Pemphigoid (Cicatricial Pemphigoid)

MMP (also known as cicatricial pemphigoid) is a chronic, vesiculobullous autoimmune disorder that predominantly affects women in their fifth decade of life, and occasionally young children.[17] As the name implies, MMP predominantly affects a variety of mucous membranes; however, in about 20% of cases, the skin may also be involved. The target antigens identified in MMP include the bullous pemphigoid antigens 1 and 2 (BPAg1 and BPAg2), laminins 5 (epiligrin) and 6, type VII collagen, β_4-integrin subunit, and additional unknown proteins.[18,19]

TABLE 35-1   Histologic and Immunofluorescence Findings in Lesions Presenting as Desquamative Gingivitis

DISEASE	HISTOLOGIC FINDINGS	DIF FINDINGS	IIF FINDINGS
• Lichen planus	• "Saw-tooth" epithelial rete ridges; liquefaction degeneration of basal epithelial cell layer; dense "bandlike" infiltration of lymphocytes in lamina propria; presence of Civatte bodies (colloid bodies) at interface of connective tissue and epithelium	• Fibrillar deposits of fibrin at junction of epithelium and connective tissue (basement membrane zone); immunoglobulin staining of colloid bodies	• Negative
• Mucous membrane pemphigoid (cicatricial pemphigoid)	• Subepithelial cleft; basal epithelial layer remains intact and attached to epithelium	• Linear deposits of C3 at basement membrane zone; may also have linear deposits of IgG antibody	• IgG antibody to basement membrane zone antigens present in about 10% of cases
• Bullous pemphigoid	• Subepithelial cleft; basal epithelial layer remains intact and attached to epithelium	• Linear deposits of C3 at basement membrane zone; may also have linear deposits of IgG antibody	• IgG antibody to basement membrane zone antigens present in up to 70% of cases
• Pemphigus vulgaris	• Intraepithelial cleft above basal layer; basal epithelial cells remain attached to underlying connective tissue and "row of tombstones"; acantholysis present; may have acantholytic "Tzanck cells" within the cleft	• IgG antibody deposits in intercellular spaces of epithelium; often have deposits of C3 intercellularly as well	• IgG antibody to intercellular antigens present in 90% to 100% of cases in later stages of disease
• Chronic ulcerative stomatitis	• Similar histologically to lichen planus (see above)	• IgG antibody deposits within nuclei of basal epithelial cells; fibrin deposits at junction of epithelium and connective tissue	• Stratified epithelium-specific antinuclear antibody present
• Lupus erythematosus	• Hyperkeratosis; degeneration of epithelial basal cell layer; inflammatory infiltrate concentrated in perivascular areas	• IgG or IgM antibody deposits at junction of epithelium and connective tissue; C3 deposits may also occur	• ANA present in more than 95% of patients with systemic lupus, and in 60% to 90% of patients with subacute lupus; ANA generally absent from patients with chronic cutaneous lupus
• Epidermolysis bullosa acquisita	• Similar histologically to pemphigoid (see above)	• Linear deposits of IgG antibody and C3 at basement membrane zone	• IgG antibody to basement membrane zone antigens present in about 25% of cases
• Erythema multiforme	• Liquefaction degeneration of upper layers of epithelium, with intraepithelial microvesicles and necrotic keratinocytes; acanthosis; pseudoepitheliomatous hyperplasia; degeneration of basement membrane zone; dense inflammatory infiltrate in lamina propria, with edema	• Negative	• Negative

ANA, Antinuclear antibody; DIF, direct immunofluorescence; IIF, indirect immunofluorescence.

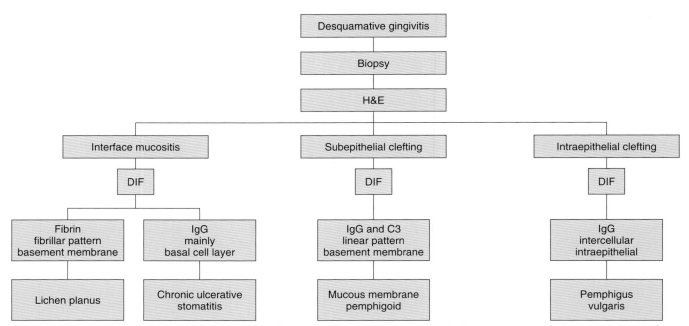

Figure 35-1. Desquamative gingivitis. Illustration of the diagnostic steps required to accurately diagnose a patient with signs of "desquamative gingivitis."

Currently, at least five subtypes of MMP—oral pemphigoid, antiepiligrin pemphigoid, anti-BP antigen mucosal pemphigoid, ocular pemphigoid, and multiple antigens pemphigoid—are recognized.[17] An important aspect of MMP is ocular involvement that warrants referral to an ophthalmologist for evaluation. Symblepharon, ankyloblepharon, and vesicular lesions on the conjunctiva may eventually produce severe scarring, corneal damage, and blindness.[20]

DG is the most typical oral presentation and is characterized by the presence of areas of gingival erythema,

desquamation, and ulceration (Fig. 35-5).[21,22] In addition, numerous vesiculobullous lesions may occur elsewhere in the mouth.[22] Rupture of the vesiculobullous lesions leave serpiginous ulcerations that may take 3 weeks or longer to heal.

Microscopically, subepithelial clefting occurs with separation of the epithelium from the underlying lamina propria, leaving an intact basal layer. A mixed inflammatory infiltrate consisting of lymphocytes, plasma cells, neutrophils, and scarce eosinophils is observed in the stroma (Fig. 35-6). Direct immunofluorescence reveals

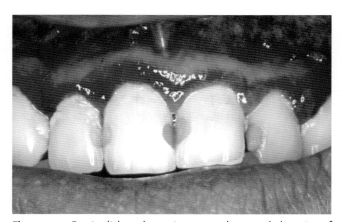

Figure 35-2. Erosive lichen planus. Intense erythema and ulceration of the gingiva with a delicate reticular white pattern that is more obvious in the interdental gingiva of #9 and #10.

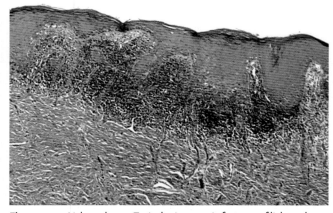

Figure 35-3. Lichen planus. Typical microscopic features of lichen planus with prominent interface mucositis in a "bandlike" configuration and "saw-tooth" rete pegs.

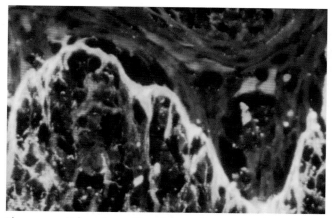

Figure 35-4. Lichen planus. Direct immunofluorescence shows a strong signal of fibrin deposition in the epithelial basement membrane with a characteristic linear-fibrillar pattern.

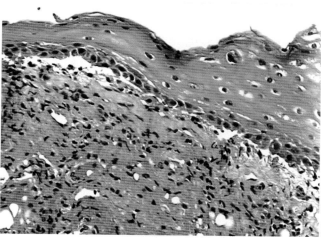

Figure 35-6. Microscopic features of mucous membrane pemphigoid. Small subepithelial clefting resulting from a clean detachment of the epithelium from the subjacent connective tissue. The basal cell layer remains attached to the epithelium.

deposits of IgG and C3 restricted to the basement membrane (Fig. 35-7). Less than 25% of patients show positive IIF finding.[23] PV, bullous pemphigoid, bullous LP, dermatitis herpetiformis, linear IgA disease, erythema multiforme, herpes gestationis, and epidermolysis bullosa acquisita should be considered in the differential diagnosis of MMP.

When the oral lesions of MMP are confined to the gingival tissues, vacuum-formed custom trays can be used for delivery of fluocinonide (0.05%) or clobetasol propionate (0.05%) three times a day.[17] Meticulous oral hygiene is essential to decrease the gingival inflammatory response. It is not uncommon for extreme gingival recession with ensuing dentinal hypersensitivity to develop in

patients with MMP. To alleviate root surface sensitivity and to improve esthetics, connective tissue grafting has been used successfully after the MMP lesions are eradicated and under control.[24] Referral to a dermatologist is indicated for recalcitrant, unresponsive lesions that require systemic corticosteroids. Currently, the drug of choice is dapsone (25 to 200 mg daily). However, caution should be exercised in elderly patients and patients with G6PD deficiency, where this drug is contraindicated. Alternative effective therapeutic agents include sulfamethoxypyridazine, sulfapyridine, tetracyclines, and

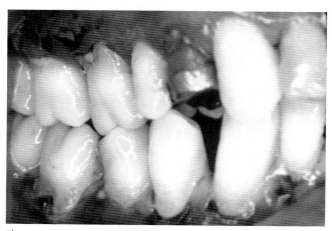

Figure 35-5. Mucous membrane pemphigoid. Large areas of ulceration and erythema that clinically present as "desquamative gingivitis." This clinical appearance also could be seen with lichen planus and pemphigus, reinforcing the need for histologic and immunofluorescence studies to determine a diagnosis.

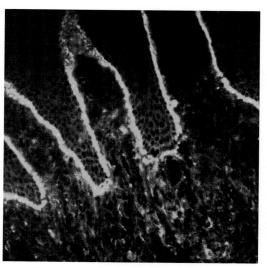

Figure 35-7. Direct immunofluorescence of mucous membrane pemphigoid. Characteristic deposition of C3 along the basement membrane. The subepithelial cleft occurs in this region of C3 deposition.

nicotinamide.[18,20,25,26] Close follow-up of the patients is warranted because all these medications have serious potential side effects. All patients with a diagnosis of MMP should be referred to a physician for ophthalmologic examination.

Pemphigus Vulgaris

PV is an autoimmune blistering disease characterized by the presence of circulating IgG antibodies against the cadherin-type adhesion molecules desmoglein 3 (Dsg3) and desmoglein 1 (Dsg1).[27] PV is a potentially lethal chronic condition with a 10% mortality rate and predilection for women after the fourth decade of life.[28] Rarely, PV may present in young children and even newborns.[28-30]

Oral lesions are the first sign of the disease in approximately 60% of patients and may present one year or more before the cutaneous lesions.[31] The oral lesions of PV range from small vesicles to large bullae that have an ephemeral life. The Nikolsky sign is positive in PV.[32] This clinical test is performed by using either an air syringe to blow air on the perilesional tissue or by gently rubbing the perilesional tissue with a finger. If the surface layer of mucosa separates from the underlying tissue, the patient is said to exhibit a positive Nikolsky sign. This sign may be positive not only in PV, but in other desquamative lesions as well. Once the bullae rupture, the lesions coalesce to form extensive areas of ulceration. The soft palate is the site most frequently affected followed by, in descending order of frequency, the buccal mucosa, tongue, and lower labial mucosa. Rarely, the only manifestation of PV may be manifested as *desquamative gingivitis* (Fig. 35-8).[33]

Microscopically, PV lesions demonstrate a characteristic intraepithelial clefting above the basal cell layer with a characteristic "tombstone" appearance to the basal cells and acantholysis.[34,35] Rounded acantholytic "Tzanck cells" are often visible in the cleft.[36] The subjacent stroma usually exhibits a mild to moderate chronic inflammatory cell infiltrate. DIF of perilesional unfixed, frozen sections gives a strong intercellular and intraepithelial IgG signal (Fig. 35-9). IIF is less sensitive than DIF and may be negative in early stages of the disease. Nevertheless, in most cases, the IIF titers are valuable to monitor disease activity and thus have prognostic value. If the oral lesions of PV are restricted to the gingival tissues, the differential diagnosis should include erosive LP, MMP, linear IgA disease, and CUS.

PV is treated with systemic corticosteroids.[31] Tapering of the medication is done as soon as possible to minimize its side effects. "Steroid-sparing" therapies combine small doses of steroids plus any of the following: azathioprine, cyclophosphamide, cyclosporine, dapsone, gold, methotrexate, photoplasmaphoresis, or plasmaphoresis.[23] Topical antifungal medication may be needed to eliminate iatrogenic *Candidiasis*, which often arises when topical steroids are used intraorally.[37] Meticulous oral hygiene and periodontal care are essential for the overall management of patients with PV. Patients in the maintenance phase may require prednisone before professional oral prophylaxis and periodontal surgery.[28]

Chronic Ulcerative Stomatitis

CUS presents mainly in women in their fourth decade of life as chronic oral erosions and ulcerations, with only few cases exhibiting concurrent cutaneous lesions.[38-40]

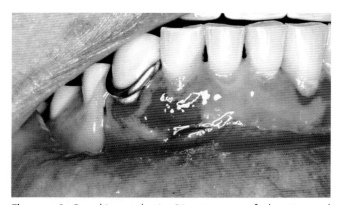

Figure 35-8. Pemphigus vulgaris. Discrete areas of ulceration and hemorrhage are seen on the attached and marginal gingiva. This clinical appearance of desquamative gingivitis could also be seen with other diseases described in this chapter.

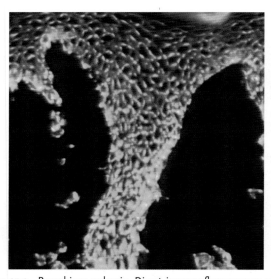

Figure 35-9. Pemphigus vulgaris. Direct immunofluorescence reveals an intraepithelial and intercellular deposition of IgG that involves the entire thickness of the epithelium. The "split" occurs within the epithelium and distinguishes this disease from lichen planus and pemphigoid.

The oral lesions consist of small blisters and erosions with surrounding erythema and pain mainly on the gingiva and the lateral border of the tongue. A clinical diagnosis of DG is not unusual for these patients. A remarkable similarity with erosive LP is seen at the microscopic level where hyperkeratosis, acanthosis, liquefaction of the basal cell layer and areas of subepithelial clefting are consistently seen. The subjacent lamina propria contains a lymphohistiocytic infiltrate in a "bandlike" configuration. DIF of normal and perilesional tissues reveal the presence of stratified epithelium-specific antinuclear antibodies, consisting of deposits of IgG with a speckled pattern, mainly in the basal epithelial cell layer. In addition, fibrin deposits are visualized at the epithelial–connective tissue interface. IIF studies also reveal the presence of circulating stratified epithelium-specific antinuclear antibodies. Because CUS is clinically similar to other desquamative lesions, erosive LP, PV, cicatricial pemphigoid, linear IgA disease, bullous pemphigoid, and lupus erythematosus must be included in the clinical differential diagnosis. DIF and IIF studies are needed to arrive at a correct diagnosis.

Mild cases of CUS are treated with topical steroids (fluocinonide, clobetasol propionate). Alternatively, topical tetracycline may also be used. Clinical improvement is observed with topical medications, but recurrences are common.[41] A high dose of systemic corticosteroids may be used to achieve transient remission. Hydroxychloroquine sulfate at a dosage of 200 to 400 mg/day seems to be the treatment of choice to produce a long-lasting remission.[42-44] Unfortunately, the initial response to chloroquine may end after several months or years of treatment.[38] In those cases, a combined therapeutic approach (small doses of corticosteroids and chloroquine) might be indicated.

Reactive Nodular Lesions of the Gingiva

The gingival mucosa is continuously facing a wide variety of challenges. The response of the gingival tissues to pathogenic factors such as dental plaque, calculus, ill-fitting prosthetic devices, and thermal and chemical agents may lead to reactive, hyperplastic changes. These changes are distinctive and can be segregated into four clinical lesions: fibrous hyperplasia, pyogenic granuloma, peripheral ossifying fibroma, and peripheral giant cell lesion. Although these lesions may show subtle clinical features that permit their clinical distinction, microscopic examination is imperative because of the different biologic behavior that they exhibit. In addition, biopsy is warranted because peripheral odontogenic lesions, benign, malignant, metastatic neoplasms, and a variety of other lesions may clinically resemble reactive nodular lesions of the gingiva. Figure 35-10 shows an algorithm illustrating a number of selected conditions that must be segregated.

Reactive Fibrous Hyperplasia (Peripheral fibroma, traumatic fibroma, irritation fibroma, focal fibrous hyperplasia)

Peripheral fibroma is typically an asymptomatic, dome-shaped nodule with either a sessile or pedunculated base. The nodule is usually less than 1.0 cm in diameter and exhibits a smooth surface with a pale pink color.[45] If traumatized, the surface may ulcerate and alter the typical pale pink color of the lesion.

At the microscopic level, the peripheral fibroma is surfaced by parakeratinized stratified squamous epithelium with or without focal hyperkeratinization. The main feature of the specimen is the presence of hyperplastic collagen fibers arranged in intersecting fascicles with a varied amount of blood capillaries.[46,47] This lesion is managed by surgical excision and has an excellent prognosis with a low recurrence rate.

Pyogenic Granuloma (florid granulation tissue, exuberant granulation tissue, pregnancy tumor)

Pyogenic granuloma is a nodular, purple to red, hemorrhagic circumscribed friable polypoid lesion that bleeds easily and is often ulcerated (Fig. 35-11).[45] Microtrauma from toothbrushing and local irritants such as dental plaque and calculus seem to be the etiologic factors of this condition.[48] Pyogenic granuloma is painless, occurs mainly in women during the second and fifth decades of life and usually in the anterior mandibular or maxillary gingiva.[49,50] The so-called pregnancy tumor is a clinical term used to identify a pyogenic granuloma that occurs in pregnant women.[51]

Microscopically, this lesion exhibits ulceration of the surface epithelium and, characteristically, a fibroendothelial proliferation of the stroma amidst acute and chronic inflammatory cells (Fig. 35-12).[46]

Surgical excision is the preferred treatment of choice, with removal of local irritants to prevent recurrence. For pregnancy tumor, a conservative approach is recommended. In the absence of significant esthetic or functional problems, or both, the lesion should not be excised because it may resolve after parturition. Local irritants such as plaque and calculus should be removed. Those lesions failing to resolve should be surgically excised. Follow-up of the patient is needed because pyogenic granuloma exhibits a tendency to recur.

Peripheral Ossifying Fibroma

Peripheral ossifying fibroma usually presents as a polypoid, pink lesion in the interdental papilla (Fig. 35-13).[45] Clinically, this lesion may be impossible to distinguish from a pyogenic granuloma (Fig. 35-11). In some cases, an astute clinician may make a clinical diagnosis of peripheral ossifying fibroma by taking a periapical film of the suspicious area that reveals the presence of radiopacities

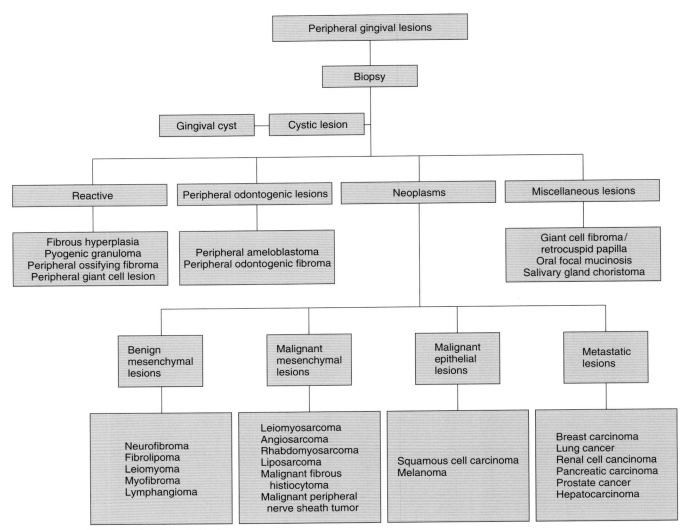

Figure 35-10. Selected peripheral gingival lesions.

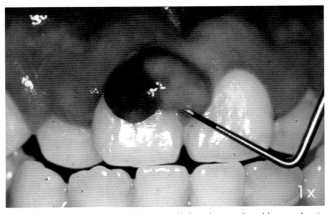

Figure 35-11. Pyogenic granuloma. Nodular ulcerated and hemorrhagic lesion involving the attached and marginal gingiva of a young woman. (*Courtesy Dr. Maria de los Angeles Limonchi, Acapulco, Mexico.*)

in the gingival lesion. However, calcifications within the lesion may not always be visible radiographically. Peripheral ossifying fibroma may appear from the first to the sixth decade of life with a peak incidence in the second decade of life. About 60% of the cases involve the anterior segment of the dental arch with a 1:1 ratio between the mandibular and the maxillary gingivae and a definite predilection for female over male individuals (4:1).[49]

Microscopically, the surface epithelium may or may not be ulcerated, but if it is, associated granulation tissue is observed. The main microscopic feature is the presence of either bone metaplasia or dystrophic calcification in the fibrous connective tissue stroma of the lesion (Fig. 35-14).[52] When strands and islands of odontogenic epithelium are found in the stroma of the specimen, the diagnosis of peripheral odontogenic fibroma is appropriate.

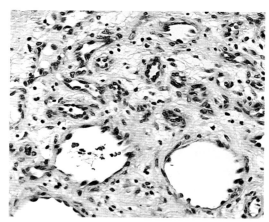

Figure 35-12. Pyogenic granuloma. Numerous blood capillaries of various calibers are seen amidst a proliferating fibrous connective tissue with interspersed inflammatory cells.

Surgical excision down to the periosteum and periodontal ligament with thorough root planing is the mainstay of treatment for peripheral ossifying fibroma.[53,54] However, an 8% to 20% recurrence rate is typically observed and justifies follow-up of the patient.[49,55]

Peripheral Giant Cell Lesion

Peripheral giant cell lesion presents as a gingival nodule with a sessile base and a red to purple discoloration that may sometimes produce displacement of teeth (Fig. 35-15).[56] In rare occasions, it may be seen in the alveolar mucosa of edentulous areas.[57] The lesion is not always as dramatic as that in Figure 35-15, and it is often indistinguishable clinically from a pyogenic granuloma (Fig. 35-11) or a peripheral ossifying fibroma (Fig. 35-13). Local etiologic factors such as trauma, calculus, food debris, and ill-fitting dental restorations/prosthesis seem

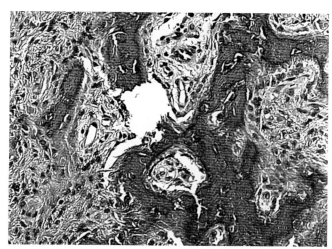

Figure 35-14. Peripheral ossifying fibroma. The presence of considerable amounts of bone metaplasia separates peripheral ossifying fibroma from pyogenic granuloma.

to play a significant role in the development of this lesion.[58]

Close to 60% of the peripheral giant cell lesions are confined to the anterior segment of the jaws with an equal distribution between maxilla and mandible. They can occur from the first to the eighth decade of life with a mean age of 35 years. A 2:1 female-to-male ratio is routinely observed.[49] Radiographic evidence of superficial resorption of the subjacent alveolar bone is common.[56]

Microscopically, the surface epithelium may or may not show areas of ulceration. The underlying fibrous connective tissue exhibits the presence of conspicuous,

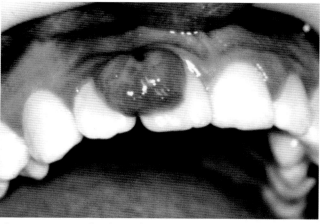

Figure 35-13. Peripheral ossifying fibroma. Nodular erythematous lesion with a pedunculated base on the buccal gingiva of the central and lateral maxillary incisors.

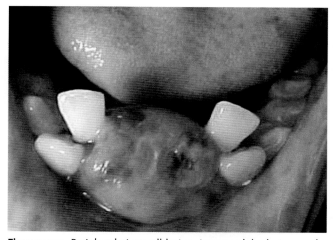

Figure 35-15. Peripheral giant cell lesion. Large nodular lesion on the anterior mandibular gingiva with focal areas of bluish discoloration. The lesion has produced migration of the anterior mandibular teeth. (*Courtesy Dr. Beatriz Aldape, Universidad Nacional Autonoma de Mexico, Mexico City, Mexico.*)

distinct nodules of multinucleated giant cells amidst spindle mesenchymal cells and numerous vascular channels (Fig. 35-16).[59] In some cases, the nodules may be confluent. Hemosiderin granules, hemorrhage, and, in some occasions, dystrophic calcifications, osteoid, and even frank bone metaplasia may also be observed. In those cases, the presence of multinucleated giant cells helps distinguish this lesion from the peripheral ossifying fibroma, where such cells may be absent, or present only in small numbers.

Surgical excision is the treatment of choice for peripheral giant cell lesions. A 10% recurrence rate is typical and thus warrants follow-up of the patient to monitor proper healing.[49]

Peripheral Odontogenic Lesions

Although a rare occurrence, the gingival tissues of the maxilla and mandible have the potential to develop any type of peripheral odontogenic cysts or tumors. There are no particular features that may aid to render an accurate clinical diagnosis for any of the peripheral odontogenic cysts or tumors. It is only after examination of a biopsy specimen that the identity of the lesion is unveiled. This chapter discusses only the most common of the rather infrequent peripheral lesions: gingival cyst and peripheral ameloblastoma.[60-62]

Gingival Cyst

The gingival cyst of adults is a rare odontogenic lesion with a slight predilection for men in their fifth to sixth decade of life. The majority of these lesions (75%) are located in the labial attached or free gingiva of the mandible in the premolar–canine–incisor area.[63]

Clinically, a single, small raised lesion reminiscent of a vesicle shows a bluish discoloration. Interestingly, this bluish discoloration with fluid content is suggestive of mucocele (Fig. 35-17). However, gingival tissues do not normally contain minor salivary glands and only rarely are ectopic gingival salivary glands observed. Typically, radiographs of the area show only normal structures.[64] On rare occasions, multiple unilateral or bilateral gingival cysts may be present.[65]

Microscopically, the gingival cyst is typically lined by a thin epithelium with or without focal intraluminal budding and a noninflamed cyst wall. Surgical excision is the preferred treatment, and, in some cases, superficial saucerization of the alveolar bone may be seen during surgery.[66] If incompletely excised, recurrence of the lesion is feasible.

Peripheral Ameloblastoma

Peripheral ameloblastoma presents as a painless, sessile growth with a firm consistency. The surface is usually smooth and similar in color to the surrounding mucosa, but in some cases it has been described as erythematous, papillary, or even warty (Fig. 35-18). In rare occasions, the lesion is ulcerative rather than exophytic.[67] Peripheral ameloblastomas are about 1 cm in diameter, and they occur more frequently in men during the fifth and sixth decades of life.[61] Close to 60% of peripheral ameloblastomas occur in the mandibular, canine, and incisor gingiva and, distinctly, half of them are located in the lingual gingiva of the canine–premolar area.[62]

The microscopic features of peripheral ameloblastoma are identical to those seen in the central ameloblastoma. The most common histologic patterns are the follicular and acanthomatous patterns (Fig. 35-19).[60,68]

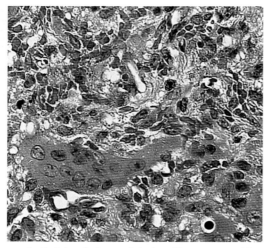

Figure 35-16. Peripheral giant cell lesion. Numerous multinucleated giant cells of the osteoclastic type are seen amidst a vascularized stroma and extravasated red blood cells.

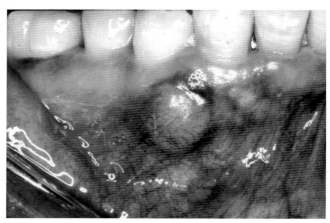

Figure 35-17. Gingival cyst. Classic presentation of a gingival cyst in the anterior mandible as a fluid-filled mass with a bluish discoloration. Racial pigmentation is also observed in this patient.

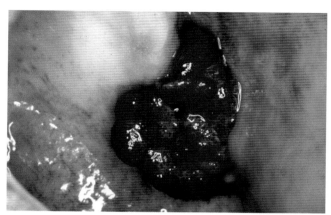

Figure 35-18. Peripheral ameloblastoma. Hemorrhagic polypoid soft tissue mass on the maxillary edentulous alveolar border. The right side of the figure shows the left buccal mucosa; on the left side, part of the hard and soft palate are observed. The patient reported that a dentist had diagnosed the lesion as a "pyogenic granuloma" and that two neighboring molars were extracted with the hope of eliminating the lesion.

Surgical excision with adequate margins is the treatment of choice. Recurrence (rate: 16% to 19%) is thought to be caused by incomplete removal. Although the prognosis is excellent, long-term follow-up is warranted because recurrences may take place several years later, even in cases of adequate surgical removal.[60] In addition, some peripheral ameloblastomas may show malignant potential and long-term follow-up is indicated in view of a report of a squamous cell carcinoma arising in a conventional peripheral ameloblastoma.[69,70]

Benign Lesions of the Gingiva

Papillary Epithelial Lesions

A variety of conditions with a papillary and verruco/papillary appearance may present in the gingival tissues. Figure 35-20 illustrates selected conditions that require microscopic examination to be diagnosed with accuracy.

Human Papillomavirus Warts. Human papillomavirus (HPV), a small DNA virus with more than 100 subtypes, can induce oral lesions.[70-73] Depending on clinical, histologic, and in situ hybridization studies, HPV warts of the oral cavity can be segregated into squamous papilloma, verruca vulgaris, and condyloma acuminatum.

Clinical distinction of squamous papilloma from verruca vulgaris can be difficult at times.[74] However, oral verruca vulgaris is most common in children and young adults, whereas squamous papilloma appears often during the third to fifth decades of life.[74-78] Squamous papilloma can affect any oral surface but the most common sites in order of decreasing frequency are: soft and hard palate, tongue, lips, and gingiva.[75] For verruca

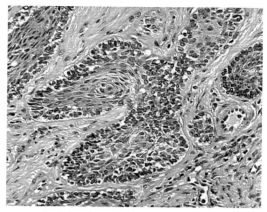

Figure 35-19. Peripheral ameloblastoma. Islands of ameloblastic epithelium showing polarization, hyperchromatism, and vacuolization of the cytoplasm of basal cells are shown. The ameloblastic epithelium originated from the surface gingival epithelium.

vulgaris, the most common sites in order of decreasing frequency are: the vermillion border, lips, hard and soft palate, tongue, buccal mucosa, and gingiva.[74,78,79] Clinically, both lesions have a white papillary surface (Fig. 35-21).[75,80] However, a "cauliflower" appearance is more typical of a verruca vulgaris.

Microscopically, both lesions consist of papillary vascularized fibrous connective tissue cores surfaced by hyperkeratinized stratified squamous epithelium (Fig. 35-22). Focal cellular atypia and koilocytes (HPV-altered epithelial cells) may be present in the epithelium.[75,76] However, verruca vulgaris exhibits rete pegs with distinctive bending inward, toward the center of the specimen, a feature not shown by squamous papilloma.[74,76,79,81] In situ hybridization studies have demonstrated the presence of HPV subtypes 6 and 11 in squamous papilloma and subtypes 2, 4, and 40 in verruca vulgaris.[76,80] Surgical excision is the preferred treatment for both conditions and recurrence is uncommon.[76]

Condyloma acuminatum is a sexually transmitted disease with a slight predilection for teenagers and young adults where HPV subtypes 2, 6, 11, 53, and 54 are commonly identified.[82-84] Upper lip, lingual frenum, dorsum of the tongue, lower lip, ventral part of tongue, and gingiva (in decreasing order of frequency) are the most common locations for condyloma acuminatum.[85] Single or multiple oral lesions may be observed.[84] The early stages of oral condyloma acuminatum consist of multiple small, fleshy nodules that proliferate and eventually coalesce.[86] Long-standing oral condylomas are larger than squamous papilloma and verruca vulgaris and exhibit a broad-base and a fleshy surface with blunted papillary projections.[76]

Microscopically, oral condyloma acuminatum shows papillary projections covered by stratified squamous epithelium with prominent acanthosis, deep crypts lined

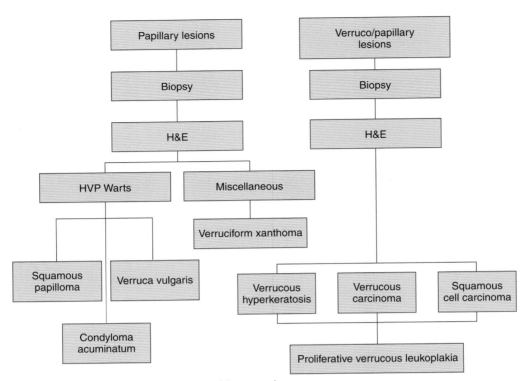

Figure 35-20. Selected papillary and verruco-papillary lesions of the gingival tissue.

with parakeratin, and increased mitotic activity with koilocytes in the upper spinous cell layer. The rete pegs are often bulbous.[85] The mainstay of treatment for intraoral condyloma is surgical excision; however, topical podophyllin and laser ablation have also been advocated.[76]

Mesenchymal Exophytic Lesions

A number of benign mesenchymal tumors may develop on the gingival tissues. They are usually asymptomatic (unless traumatized), exophytic, sessile nonulcerated lesions with the same color as the adjacent gingival tissues. A number of cases with a diverse cell lineage such as neurofibroma, fibrolipoma, leiomyoma, myofibroma, and bilateral symmetric lymphangiomas of the gingiva have been documented in the literature.[87-94]

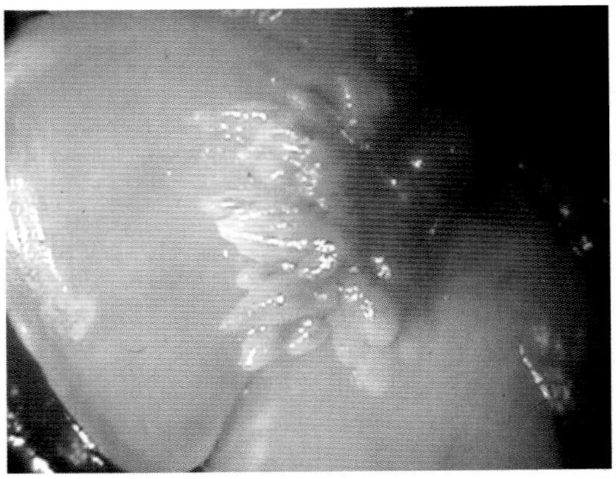

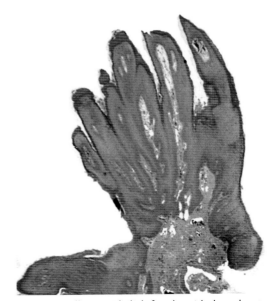

Figure 35-21. Typical warty appearance of a papilloma situated in the palatal gingiva between the maxillary central incisors.

Figure 35-22. Papillary epithelial fronds with hyperkeratosis and connective tissue cores.

It is practically impossible to make an accurate clinical diagnosis of any type of benign mesenchymal tumor of the gingiva because all of them exhibit clinical features that are similar to conventional inflammatory lesions. Microscopic examination of these lesions is indispensable to establish a proper diagnosis and suitable management.

Malignant Lesions of the Gingiva

Proliferative Verrucous Leukoplakia

In 1985, Hansen[95] described for the first time a unique form of leukoplakia in a cohort of 30 patients. Because of its clinical appearance, consisting of expanding, verrucous white lesions, the term *proliferative verrucous leukoplakia* (PVL) was used.[96] A total of 80% of patients with PVL are women, with a mean age of 65 years. The mean age at the time of diagnosis for men is 49 years.[96] A significant absence of risk factors is observed in patients with PVL.

Clinically, the early lesions of PVL appear as a deceptive solitary homogeneous leukoplakia (Fig. 35-23). Despite its innocuous appearance, the leukoplakia recurs and relentlessly spreads over time resulting in diffuse, multifocal, and exophytic or verrucous type of oral lesions.[97] The most common site is the buccal mucosa followed by the gingiva and the tongue. However, the gingiva exhibits the greatest malignant transformation rate, usually 7 years after the initial diagnosis.

At the microscopic level, an array of changes occur over time and range from simple hyperkeratinization, verrucous hyperplasia, verrucous carcinoma, and at the end of the spectrum, invasive squamous cell carcinoma (Fig. 35-24).[97]

Surgical eradication and laser vaporization of the lesions is difficult given the widespread nature of the condition, and render disappointing results with repeated recurrences. In cases in which PVL may be associated

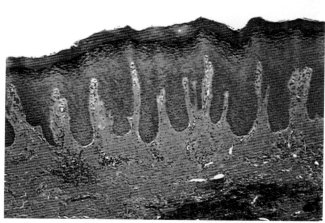

Figure 35-24. Proliferative verrucous leukoplakia. Verrucous hyperkeratosis with prominent granular cell layer and elongated rete pegs.

with HPV, a combination of surgery and a synthetic antiviral seem to be promising.[98] Close follow-up of the patients with early aggressive treatment and regular long-term follow-up are warranted.[99]

Squamous Cell Carcinoma

Squamous cell carcinoma is the most common malignancy of the oral cavity and oropharynx. Every year, 31,000 new cases of oral cancer are diagnosed in the United States. The gingiva (alveolar ridge included) is the third most common site for intraoral squamous cell carcinoma and represents about 15% to 25% of the oral epithelial malignancies.[100-102] Mandibular gingival squamous cell carcinomas are more common than their maxillary counterparts (2:1 ratio) and characteristically exhibit a wide spectrum of clinical presentations, sometimes deceptively mimicking innocuous inflammatory conditions (Fig. 35-25).[101,103,104]

Microscopically, infiltrative cords, islands, and sheets of malignant keratinocytes invade the connective tissue and exhibit cellular pleomorphism, hyperchromatism, and aberrant mitosis. The well differentiated squamous cell carcinomas show keratin pearl formation that facilitate their identification, whereas the poorly differentiated carcinomas may have to be subjected to immunocytochemical examination to be properly diagnosed (Fig. 35-26).

Early diagnosis and treatment of squamous cell carcinoma of the gingiva leads to a 77% 5-year survival rate (stage I). In contrast, only 24% 5-year survival rates are observed in advanced stages (stage IV).[105] Thus biopsy of gingival lesions that fail to resolve within 2 weeks is warranted.[106] Gingival mandibular carcinomas exhibit a tendency to invade the underlying alveolar bone; however,

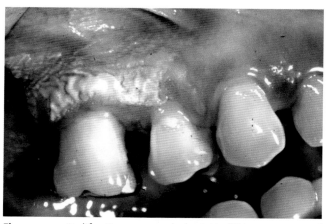

Figure 35-23. Proliferative verrucous leukoplakia. White verrucous and corrugated lesion with distinct borders.

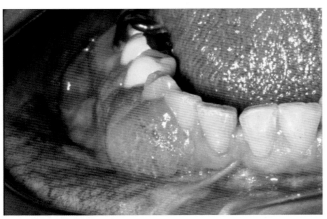

Figure 35-25. Squamous cell carcinoma. Nodular mass on the mandibular right gingiva exhibiting a deceptively innocuous appearance. Results of a biopsy revealed the presence of a squamous cell carcinoma. (*Courtesy Dr. Carl Allen; Ohio State University, Columbus, Ohio.*)

the size of the tumor is more important than mandibular invasion in predicting local disease control.[107]

The mainstay of treatment for gingival squamous cell carcinoma is surgical resection with or without postoperative radiotherapy.[108] Flow cytometry can be used to determine cellular phenotypic presentations (diploid and aneuploid cells). The presence of a large percentage of aneuploid signals in a squamous cell carcinoma heralds a poor prognosis.[109]

Melanoma

Melanomas originate from two types of neural crest cells: melanocytes and nevus cells. Melanocytes are dendritic cells that reside in the epithelium and show contact inhibition. In contrast, nevus cells reside in the subjacent connective tissue and tend to aggregate in clusters. Oral melanoma accounts for 0.5% of all oral malignancies.[110]

Although the most common site for oral melanoma is the palate (40%), gingival melanomas represent close to one third of these tumors. Oral melanoma is more frequent in men than in women and is diagnosed during the fifth to sixth decade of life (age range, 40 to 90 years).[111,112] Clinically, oral melanoma may exhibit three presentations: either a pigmented macule, a pigmented nodule with or without areas of ulceration, or a nodule with similar color to the surrounding oral mucosa (amelanotic melanoma) (Fig. 35-27). When the clinical presentation is a pigmented macule, lesions that should be included in the differential diagnosis include amalgam tattoo, oral melanotic macule, junctional nevus, and melanoma. (Fig. 35-28). It is not unusual for the nodular gingival melanoma to be asymptomatic and to be preceded by an area previously occupied by a long-standing (months to years) pigmented macule. Alternatively, oral melanoma may appear de novo as a rapidly growing mass.[111] Although the presence of pigmentation in a rapidly growing mass is an ominous sign suggestive of melanoma that will certainly prompt the clinician to take a biopsy, the lack of pigmentation of some melanomas (amelanotic melanoma) may not alert the practitioner to the seriousness of this lesion. Thus any rapidly growing lesion, either pigmented or not, requires a biopsy without delay.[112]

Microscopically, the pigmented nodular type of melanoma is the most common (73%), consisting of proliferating atypical, pleomorphic, spindle-shaped, or epithelioid tumor cells containing melanin with frequent mitotic figures.[113,114]

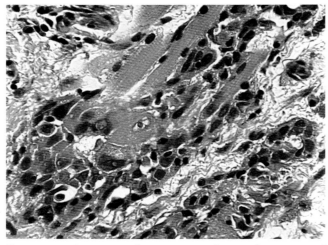

Figure 35-26. Squamous cell carcinoma. High magnification view of pleomorphic keratinocytes infiltrating striated muscle fibers.

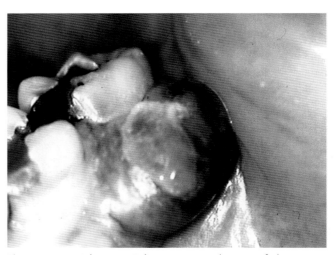

Figure 35-27. Melanoma. Solitary pigmented mass of the gingiva representing a vertical growth of a melanoma.

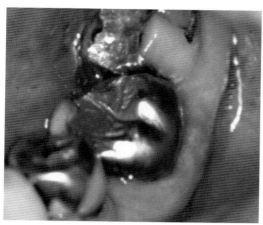

Figure 35-28. Amalgam tattoo. Prominent pigmentation of the attached and marginal gingiva next to a large amalgam restoration.

The treatment of choice for oral melanoma is surgical excision with adequate negative margins. Radiotherapy and chemotherapy are palliative interventions that may be used in addition to the surgical excision.[110,115] The prognosis for gingival melanoma is quite poor and the 5-year survival rate stands at 18%. The survival rate is negatively affected by the presence of lymph node involvement at the time of diagnosis.[110]

Sarcomas

Intraoral soft tissue sarcomas (STS) are extremely rare, and there is an even greater paucity of STS affecting the periodontal tissues.[116] Consequently, there is little clinical information regarding their occurrence. Most of the knowledge available in the literature about STS has been derived from case reports. Usually, STS are diagnosed in patients older than 20 years with no sex predilection.

Cases of malignant peripheral nerve sheath tumor, angiosarcoma, rhabdomyosarcoma, leiomyosarcoma, liposarcoma, fibrosarcoma, and malignant fibrous histiocytoma have been reported involving the periodontium, especially the gingival tissues.[116-129] Clinically, oral STS are exophytic, infiltrative masses that may exhibit rapid growth and may or may not be painful.[116]

Because the clinical features are not specific, the precise final diagnosis is based on the histologic features of the tumor. Distant metastasis of intraoral STS is not uncommon.[116]

Metastatic Gingival Lesions

Metastasis to the gingival tissues is uncommon.[130] However, more than half (55%) of the metastases restricted to the oral soft tissues involve the gingiva.[131,132]

Clinically, some gingival metastatic lesions present as asymptomatic benign pink enlargements, whereas other lesions may closely simulate localized inflammatory reactive lesions that are misdiagnosed as pyogenic granuloma, giant cell granuloma, or peripheral fibroma.[133] A more ominous presentation includes rapidly growing exophytic, erythematous, or hemorrhagic masses that may be pedunculated or sessile, rubbery to firm or fixed (Fig. 35-29). They usually exhibit large areas of ulceration producing marked halitosis and, in some cases, paresthesia of the lower lip. An equal distribution of mandibular and maxillary gingival metastatic lesions is observed.[131] Circulating malignant cells show a proclivity to becoming entangled in the rich capillary network of the chronically inflamed gingiva.[134] This notion is suggested by the observation that in 79% of dentate patients the oral metastases were located on the gingiva, whereas in edentulous patients, the metastases were located mainly in the tongue and the alveolar mucosa.[131]

A biopsy is necessary to unveil the metastatic character of a gingival lesion.[135] Microscopic examination of the excised gingival tissue reflects the cytologic features of the primary tumor. Large cell carcinoma of the lung, osteosarcoma, angiosarcoma, Ewing's sarcoma, choriocarcinoma, multiple myeloma, hepatocellular carcinoma, transitional cell carcinoma, renal cell carcinoma, pancreatic carcinoma, prostate adenocarcinoma, breast carcinoma, neurosarcoma, and malignant fibrous histiocytoma have been reported as primary malignancies capable of producing metastasis to the gingival tissues.[130,132-146]

Removal of gingival metastases is warranted because of the discomfort and bleeding that they produce.[132] The prognosis for these patients is grim; death usually occurs a few months after the diagnosis of metastasis to the gingiva.[147]

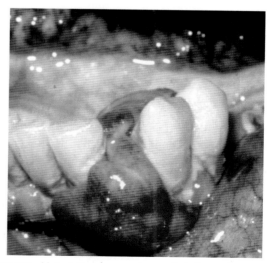

Figure 35-29. Metastatic adenocarcinoma. Lobular erythematous and hemorrhagic mass in the left mandibular gingiva. An incisional biopsy revealed a metastatic adenocarcinoma.

HARD TISSUE LESIONS

Similar to the gingival tissues, the mandible and maxilla are prone to development of odontogenic and nonodontogenic lesions. Imaging studies and microscopic examination play a central role in the proper diagnosis and management of these lesions. Figure 35-30 illustrates a selected number of bone lesions that must be separated on the basis of their microscopic characteristics.

Odontogenic Lesions

Cysts

The list of central odontogenic cysts and tumors is extensive. Several comprehensive review articles and monographs on odontogenic cysts and tumors have been published.[148-150] This section deals with a selected number of central odontogenic lesions that may present clinical or radiographic features affecting periodontal structures.

Buccal Bifurcation Cyst. A variant of odontogenic cysts with specific clinical and radiographic features is the buccal bifurcation cyst. Clinically, a completely erupted and vital molar tooth presents buccal tipping of the crown, which is readily seen with an occlusal film. The most commonly affected tooth is the mandibular first molar, and less frequently the mandibular second molar.[151] Imaging studies reveal the presence of a unilocular radiolucency at the bifurcation of a molar tooth (Fig. 35-31).

Microscopically, a cystic process with epithelial lining may or may not present chronic inflammation. Enucleation of the cyst with preservation of the involved teeth is the preferred treatment.[152]

Lateral Periodontal Cyst. The lateral periodontal cyst (LPC) is an odontogenic cyst that originates from rests of dental lamina.[153] LPC is more common in adults during the fifth to seventh decades of life. This lesion shows no sex predilection.

The majority of these lesions are located in the mandibular canine to premolar areas and are usually discovered during a routine radiographic examination.[154] An important aspect that allows their segregation from inflammatory odontogenic cysts is that the neighboring teeth are vital.[155] Expansion of the buccal or lingual alveolar plate with normal-appearing or slightly blanching surface mucosa may be observed in some cases. Pain is not a common feature of LPC. Radiographically, a well defined oval to teardrop, corticated radiolucency flanks two contiguous teeth, along their lateral root surfaces and between the alveolar crest and the root apices (Fig. 35-32).[156]

Microscopically, a single cystic cavity lined by a thin layer of epithelium with focal budding is seen alternating with clear, glycogen-rich cells (Fig. 35-33). Nests of dental lamina rests are also seen in the cyst wall. A conspicuous absence of inflammatory cells is typical of LPC. The botryoid odontogenic cyst is a variant of LPC that exhibits a gross, radiographic, and microscopic polycystic appearance.[157] The lesion may appear like a cluster of grapes radiographically and histologically. Unlike LPC, the botryoid odontogenic cyst exhibits the potential to recur.[158]

Because other types of cysts and neoplasms may mimic the clinical and radiographic presentation of LPC, it is important to establish the final diagnosis of LPC on the basis of histopathologic, radiographic, and clinical information.[159] Complete surgical removal of LPC with preservation of the neighboring teeth is the most appropriate treatment.

Odontogenic Keratocyst. The odontogenic keratocyst (OKC) originates from remnants of dental lamina, occurs during the second and third decades of life, and affects the mandible twice as much as the maxilla. The most common location for OKC is the posterior body of the mandible and the ramus. Swelling or pain, or both, may be the only manifestations of OKC.[160] OKC typically presents as a corticated unilocular radiolucency, although multilocular radiolucencies have been reported. In some occasions, the unilocular radiolucency is located between the roots of vital premolar mandibular teeth, thus simulating the radiographic presentation of a conventional LPC (Fig. 35-34).

Microscopically, a cystic lining of highly uniform thickness, usually 6 to 8 layers in thickness, is surfaced by parakeratin with a corrugated profile and palisading of the basal cells (Fig. 35-35). Detachment of the epithelium from the subjacent connective tissue and absence of rete pegs are seen.[161] Inflammation is characteristically absent in the cystic connective tissue wall. However, if secondarily inflamed, the typical microscopic features of OKC are lost.

Surgical removal with peripheral ostectomy is recommended because of the 10% to 30% recurrence rate that OKC exhibits.[162] Some authors advocate the use of Carnoy's solution before enucleation of the cyst.[163]

Tumors

Ameloblastoma. Ameloblastoma is the second most common odontogenic tumor and originates from any sort of odontogenic epithelium including dental lamina rests, epithelial rests of Malassez, reduced enamel epithelium, and cystic epithelial lining. Ameloblastoma exhibits no sex predilection and occurs in the mandible and the maxilla of adults at about their fourth decade of life.[164] Most ameloblastomas occur in the mandibular molar area, are usually asymptomatic, and are discovered during a routine radiographic examination or during the exploration of a painless jaw swelling.

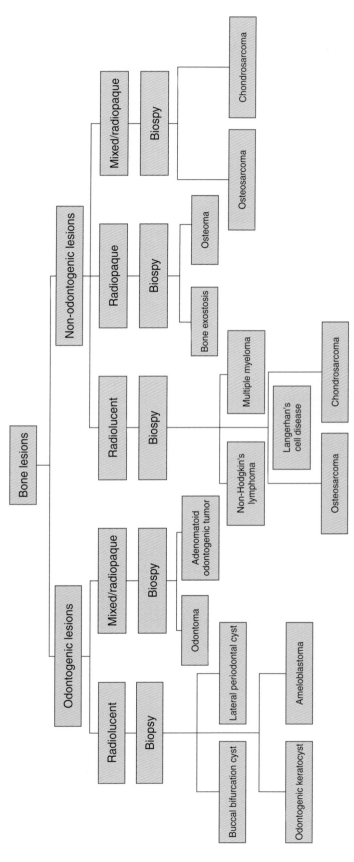

Figure 35-30. Selected odontogenic and nonodontogenic bone lesions.

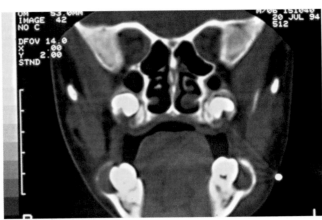

Figure 35-31. Buccal bifurcation cyst. Computed tomography scan showing bilateral radiolucencies involving the bifurcation of the first mandibular molars. (*Courtesy Dr. Lee Slater, Armed Forces Institute of Pathology, Washington, D.C.*).

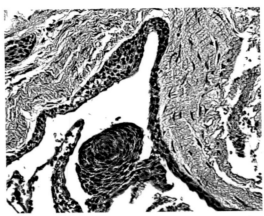

Figure 35-33. Lateral periodontal cyst. The cystic space is lined by a thin epithelium with focal intraluminal budding.

Radiographically, ameloblastomas present as unilocular or multilocular corticated radiolucencies; however, the most common radiographic presentation of ameloblastoma is a unilocular radiolucency with corticated borders.[165] When ameloblastoma presents in the mandible in an interradicular location in the area of premolars, distinction of LPC and OKC can only be done through microscopic examination of the lesion.

Microscopically, ameloblastoma exhibits a variety of patterns, but the more common ones are the follicular and plexiform types. Palisading and nuclear hyperchro-

matism with reverse polarization and vacuolization of basal cells characterize ameloblastoma.[166] Surgical excision with margins free of tumor is the treatment of choice.[167] Conservative treatments such as enucleation and curettage are unacceptable and result in extremely high recurrence rates.[164]

Adenomatoid Odontogenic Tumor. Adenomatoid odontogenic tumor is typically identified in the anterior jaws (mainly in the maxilla) of young individuals usually in their second decade of life. A definitive predilection for female individuals is observed.[168]

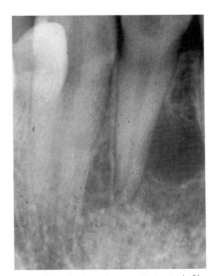

Figure 35-32. Lateral periodontal cyst. Periapical film showing an interradicular corticated radiolucency that has produced separation of neighboring teeth.

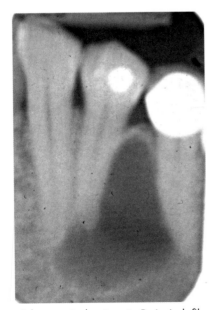

Figure 35-34. Odontogenic keratocyst. Periapical film showing an interradicular corticated radiolucency that simulates the radiographic findings of lateral periodontal cyst. (*Courtesy Dr. Jeffrey Meltzer, Fayetteville, N.Y.*)

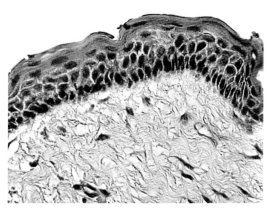

Figure 35-35. Odontogenic keratocyst. Classic microscopic features of odontogenic keratocyst with very uniform thickness of epithelial lining, corrugated parakeratinization, and palisading of the basal cell layer.

This lesion is characterized by a painless swelling with radiographic evidence of the presence of a unilocular radiolucency that sometimes shows focal radiopacities and is associated with an impacted tooth. However, some adenomatoid odontogenic tumors may present as an interradicular, unilocular radiolucency in the anterior jaws mimicking a LPC.[169]

Microscopically, typical ductlike structures alternate with spindle-shaped to cuboidal epithelial cells that form nests or rosette-like structures with interspersed eosinophilic amorphous material and scattered calcifications (Fig. 35-36).[170] The adenomatoid odontogenic tumor is treated by simple enucleation and the prognosis is excellent with no recurrences anticipated.[162]

Odontoma. Odontoma is the most common odontogenic tumor.[171] Two types of odontomas are recognized. The compound odontoma is characterized by the presence of hard and soft dental tissues that have a tendency to recreate the shape of teeth (denticles). In contrast, complex odontoma is the result of a haphazard configuration of hard and soft dental tissues. Compound odontomas exhibit a predilection for the anterior maxilla, whereas complex odontomas are usually located in the posterior areas of the maxilla and mandible.[172]

The majority of odontomas are associated with an unerupted tooth and are diagnosed during childhood and adolescence in the course of a routine radiographic examination. Radiographically, an odontoma in an early stage appears as a well defined radiolucency. However, once mineralization is established, compound odontomas exhibit radiopaque toothlike structures surrounded by a peripheral thin radiolucency (Fig. 35-37). The complex odontoma consists of a radiopaque mass.

Microscopically, enamel matrix, dentin, pulp, and reduced enamel epithelium are observed. Enucleation is the preferred treatment and the prognosis is excellent.

Nonodontogenic Lesions

Benign

Bone Exostosis. Exostoses are localized peripheral overgrowths of bone. Depending on their location in the jaws, they are identified as torus mandibularis (lingual mandibular plate) or torus palatinus (hard palate). Sometimes, several bony overgrowths occur on the vestibular alveolar bone and are simply called multiple exostosis (Fig. 35-38).

A peculiar condition consisting of bone exostosis has been reported to occur in some patients after undergoing either a skin graft vestibuloplasty or an autogenous free gingival graft.[172-174] A slowly growing exostosis develops at the recipient site of the gingival graft. A definitive

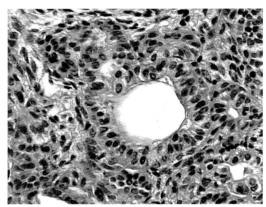

Figure 35-36. Adenomatoid odontogenic tumor. Figure illustrates two characteristic ductlike structures composed of cuboidal epithelial odontogenic cells.

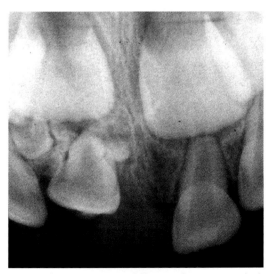

Figure 35-37. Odontoma. Periapical film reveals a compound odontoma associated with the crown of a central incisor.

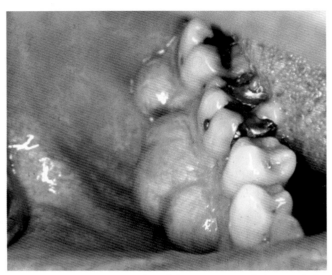

Figure 35-38. Exostosis. Multinodular exostosis of the vestibular alveolar bone. On palpation, its bony nature is confirmed.

female sex predilection is characteristic of this condition, which usually presents in the canine–premolar area of the mandible or maxilla.

Microscopically, the bone exostosis consists of lamellar or woven bone, or both, surrounded by fibrous connective tissue with or without scarce inflammatory cells.[175,176] Surgical removal of this lesion is indicated if interference with a removable prosthetic appliance occurs or if esthetic concerns emerge.[177] Patients receiving a free gingival graft should be informed about the potential for development of a bone exostosis at the surgical site.[176]

Osteoma. Osteomas of the jaw bones are usually diagnosed in the second to fourth decade of life during a routine radiographic examination and are more common in the mandible.[178] Radiographically, they appear as radiopaque masses and well defined lesions. The presence of multiple osteomas in the mandible may represent the first sign suggesting a diagnosis of Gardner syndrome.[179]

Microscopically, osteomas consist of either dense lamellar bone with scarce connective tissue stroma or lamellar trabecular bone with accompanying fibrofatty marrow. Surgical excision is reserved only for symptomatic cases and the prognosis is excellent.

Malignant

Osteosarcoma. Osteosarcoma is a malignant tumor characterized by the direct formation of bone or osteoid tissue by the tumor cells.[180] Although the literature seems to indicate that osteosarcomas of the jaws have a slight female sex predilection, some series report a greater incidence in male individuals.[180-183] Osteosarcoma of the jaws can appear throughout a wide age spectrum, but it is usually diagnosed during the third to fourth decade of

life, and it seems to affect mandible and maxilla at similar rates.[184] More specifically, the body of the mandible is the most frequent primary site for osteosarcoma, followed by the symphysis, angle, and ascending ramus. In the maxilla, the alveolar ridge and the maxillary antrum are the most frequent sites.[185]

Clinically, swelling, pain, and paresthesia are the most common signs and symptoms.[186] Paresthesia is an ominous symptom that is associated with a poor prognosis.[187] The typical scenario involves a rapidly growing firm or hard tumor that may cause loosening and migration of the teeth.[183] In some cases, swelling without pain or accompanying neural deficit may be the only complaint.[186] A variant of osteosarcoma, the so-called juxtacortical osteosarcoma, can arise on the alveolar bone of dentate patients and may mimic the clinical appearance of "pyogenic granuloma."[188]

Radiographically, osteosarcoma presents as radiolucent, radiopaque, or mixed lesions. Most osteosarcomas show a mixed (radiopaque–radiolucent) density with irregular margins and only a small number shows well defined borders without cortication. The classic "sunburst" appearance of osteosarcoma may be seen in about half of the cases.[189] A symmetric widening of the periodontal ligament space is a significant feature of osteosarcoma. This finding may present as the initial radiographic sign in close to a third of osteosarcomas of the jaws and is best demonstrated with periapical films. If the periodontal ligament widening affects all the teeth, scleroderma (systemic sclerosis) should be considered in the differential diagnosis. The mandibular canal may show indistinct and irregular borders when the tumor is in close proximity to it. A comprehensive radiographic assessment including periapical, occlusal, and panoramic films can be extremely valuable to establish an early diagnosis of osteosarcoma.[182,189]

Microscopically, osteosarcoma is composed of malignant stromal cells that form osteoid or primitive bone. A predominance of a fibroblastic, osteoblastic, or chondroblastic component may be observed in osteosarcoma.[185]

Surgical excision is the treatment of choice. Hemimandibulectomy is recommended for lesions of the ascending ramus. For body of the mandible and parasymphyseal tumors, a wide surgical excision with clear surgical margins greater than 5 mm is imperative to improve 5-year survival rates. For maxillary tumors, maxillectomy with orbital preservation is preferred.[181] Five-year survival rates range from 10% to 85%.[181] Patients receiving coadjuvant chemotherapy seem to have better survival rates.[187]

Chondrosarcoma. Chondrosarcoma is a malignant tumor characterized by the formation of cartilage by the tumor cells.[190] Chondrosarcoma of the jaws presents equally in male and female individuals with a peak incidence in the third to fifth decades of life and shows predilection for the maxilla.[191,192] The most common sign of chondrosarcoma is the presence of an enlarging mass that produces cortical expansion with concomitant resorption and exfoliation of neighboring teeth.[192,193]

The typical radiographic appearance consists of an ill-defined radiolucency with mottled areas of calcification. Sometimes, a "sunburst" pattern similar to that seen in osteosarcoma is observed. In addition, widening of the periodontal membrane of teeth involved by the tumor may be demonstrated in periapical radiographs.[193]

At the microscopic level, chondrosarcoma shows identifiable cartilage with different degrees of maturation, cellularity, nuclear pleomorphism, and binucleation, with a distinctive lobular pattern of growth.[194]

The preferred treatment for chondrosarcoma of the jaws is radical surgery. Although chondrosarcomas are slow growing and metastasize later in their course, they are locally aggressive and exhibit a 5-year survival rate that ranges from 32% to 80%.[193,194] Long-term follow-up is warranted as some chondrosarcomas may recur 10 to 20 years later.[192,193]

Lymphoma. Lymphomas are malignant neoplasms of the lymphoreticular system that can be divided into two main categories: Hodgkin's disease, characterized by the presence of Reed-Sternberg cells, and non-Hodgkin's lymphoma (NHL).[195] Hodgkin's lymphoma rarely presents in the oral cavity, and thus is not discussed in this section.

The head and neck represent the second most common site for primary extranodal NHL.[196,197] Most cases of NHL in the oral cavity are secondary rather than primary lesions. However, when the oral cavity is the primary site, NHL tends not to spread to other sites.[198] NHL of the oral cavity is most commonly diagnosed in adults after the sixth decade of life and shows a 2:1 male-to-female ratio.[199,200] The favored intraoral soft tissue sites for NHL are the palate and gingiva.[199] Clinically, a mass or an ulcerated mass similar to squamous cell carcinoma or salivary gland tumor is observed.[201] However, NHL may also appear as a benign swelling.

When intraosseous, NHL exhibits an ill-defined radiolucency with alveolar bone loss and tooth mobility that may resemble aggressive periodontitis or periodontal abscesses.[195,201,202] Perforation of the cortical bone with ensuing swelling, pain, numbness, and an exophytic soft tissue mass is observed in long-standing central lesions.[201]

At the microscopic level, NHL is segregated into follicular and diffuse types. A variety of immunocytochemical probes have revealed that most NHLs have a B-cell make-up and only a minority are T-cell lymphomas.[200,203] The treatment of lymphoma varies according to the type of tumor. Radiotherapy, chemotherapy, and surgery are commonly used.[198]

Multiple Myeloma. Multiple myeloma is a malignant neoplasm characterized by a monoclonal proliferation of plasma cells involving multiple bone sites that is accompanied by increased levels of immunoglobulins in serum or light chains in urine (Bence Jones protein). Serum electrophoretic analysis reveals a monoclonal expansion of either IgG- or IgA-producing cells.[204,205] Multiple myeloma occurs most frequently in adults after their fourth decade of life, mainly in African-Americans, and exhibits a slight male sex predominance.[206,207]

Multiple myeloma may affect any bone, but the vertebrae, ribs, skull, pelvis, jaw bones, femur, clavicles, and scapulae are the most commonly affected sites.[208] Jawbone involvement often occurs in advanced stages of the disease and is more common in the posterior mandible and the premolar and molar region.[205,208,209] Although an asymptomatic swelling of the mandible is the most common sign, pain, numbness, mobility of the teeth, a gingival mass, and pathologic fractures are not uncommon.[205,209]

Radiographically, multiple "punched out" osteolytic lesions are observed.[205] Multifocal areas of alveolar bone loss may resemble periodontal disease.[208] Sometimes, solitary bone lesions (plasmacytoma) or soft tissue lesions (extramedullary plasmacytoma) may present without bone marrow involvement. Nevertheless, they may progress, eventually involve the bone marrow, and follow the typical course of multiple myeloma.[206]

A not uncommon complication of multiple myeloma is amyloidosis, which may result in macroglossia.[210] Chemotherapy is the treatment of choice for multiple myeloma. The prognosis is poor with a 5-year survival rate of only 25%.[207]

MISCELLANEOUS

Giant Cell Fibroma

Giant cell fibroma is a lesion commonly seen in young individuals with definitive predilection for the mandibular gingival tissues.[211] This lesion is usually pedunculated and presents a nodular surface.

The microscopic features are characteristic and consist of hyperplastic fibrous connective tissue with interspersed large stellate and multinucleated fibroblasts that conglomerate mainly in the vicinity of the epithelial–connective tissue interface but can be seen throughout the lesion.[212] Simple surgical excision is the preferred treatment.[213]

Retrocuspid Papilla

The retrocuspid papilla is a small sessile (occasionally pedunculated) nodular lesion on the lingual gingiva, adjacent to the mandibular canine, usually 1 mm below the free gingival margin.[214] The retrocuspid papilla is bilateral, asymptomatic, more common in children and young adults, and, in some cases, it may disappear with age. The mean age at the time of diagnosis is around 26 years. This lesion displays a firm consistency, pinkish-white color, and measures approximately 0.5 cm in diameter.

Microscopically, a striking resemblance to giant cell fibroma is observed.[215] This lesion is considered by most authors to be a "normal variation," whereas others deem it an hamartomatous condition.[216]

Once a sound clinical diagnosis is established on the basis of bilateral distribution, clinical appearance, and location, biopsy is unnecessary. However, in those few cases where the retrocuspid papilla exhibits a reddish discoloration, biopsy is warranted to rule out a pathologic process.[215]

Gingival Fibrous Nodule

Gingival fibrous nodule represents a variation of normal oral structures. Clinically, single or multiple asymptomatic nodules, 2 to 4 mm in diameter, are located on the anterior labial mucogingival region. They exhibit white-pink to pink color and are firm but not bony hard.

Microscopically, these nodules consist of hyperplastic dense fibrous connective tissue with sparse fibroblasts and scattered lymphocytes. The differential diagnosis of gingival fibrous nodule includes fibroma, papilloma, focal epithelial hyperplasia, multiple hamartomas, gingival cyst, and exostosis.[217] Because this is a variation of normal oral structures, no treatment is indicated and a biopsy is necessary only if there is clinical uncertainty.

Langerhans Cell Disease

Langerhans cell histiocytosis is a proliferative disorder of the reticuloendothelial system with a suspected underlying neoplastic etiology.[218,219] Langerhans cell histiocytosis includes three clinical entities: Letterer–Siwe disease (acute disseminated histiocytosis), Hand–Schüller–Christian disease (chronic disseminated histiocytosis), and eosinophilic granuloma (chronic localized histiocytosis).[220] These variants have different clinical features but considerable overlap is observed among them. The following discussion focuses on the oral involvement of eosinophilic granuloma.

Eosinophilic granuloma may present as a monostotic or polyostotic bone disorder, and rarely it may be restricted to oral soft tissues, mainly the gingiva.[218,221-223] Pain, jaw swelling, and tooth mobility are common clinical features.[220,221] Radiographically, a "scooped-out" radiolucency with well defined borders is typically observed.[224] Severe destruction of the supporting alveolar bone can produce displacement of the teeth and may mimic advanced periodontal disease.[220] In extreme cases,

the radiologic appearance of teeth "floating in air" is observed.[221] Oral soft tissue involvement is usually manifested as swelling or ulceration of the gingiva.[218,223]

The microscopic features of eosinophilic granuloma consist of sheets of mononuclear cells with pale cytoplasm and vesicular lobulated nuclei with a "coffee bean" appearance (Langerhan's cells) and abundant eosinophils. The definitive diagnosis of eosinophilic granuloma requires the identification of Langerhan's cells by either immunohistochemistry (CD1 or S-100 antisera) or electron microscopy (cytoplasmic Birbeck's granules).[225]

Therapeutic interventions include surgery, radiation, or chemotherapy. Intralesional injection of corticosteroids (prednisone) in solitary lesions has been reported to be effective.[218,226] The prognosis for eosinophilic granuloma is good. However, long-term follow-up is mandatory, because progression and dissemination of the disease with subsequent visceral involvement can occur and has a poor prognosis.[227]

Oral Focal Mucinosis

Oral focal mucinosis is an uncommon condition of unknown etiology.[228] This condition occurs in a wide age range (16 to 61 years) with a mean age around 40 years and exhibits a 2:1 female-to-male ratio. A marked predilection for gingival tissues is characteristically seen.[229] Oral focal mucinosis appears as a smooth surface nodular mass that rarely may exhibit a lobular surface and that it is usually clinically diagnosed as a "fibroma." This lesion is asymptomatic and varies in size from 0.3 to 2.0 cm, but most are about 1 cm in diameter.

Microscopically, oral focal mucinosis is characterized by the presence of a localized area of myxomatous connective tissue that may or not be circumscribed by a dense fibrous connective tissue stroma. A homogeneous mucinous material separating collagen fibrils interspersed with fusiform, stellate, or ovoid fibroblasts occupies the core of the myxomatous area.[230] Histochemical stains suggest that the mucinous material is hyaluronic acid produced by fibroblasts.

The treatment for oral focal mucinosis is surgical excision. The prognosis is excellent and no recurrence has ever been reported.

Gingival Hyperplasia Associated With Plasminogen Deficiency (Amyloid-like gingival hyperplasia)

Plasminogen is the precursor of plasmin, the main fibrinolytic enzyme, which plays an important role in wound healing. A quantitative or qualitative deficiency of plasminogen results in the accumulation of fibrin in the oral mucosa, in particular, in the gingival tissues. This condition has a predilection for female individuals and is clinically characterized by gingival enlargement composed of nodules, papules, plaques, and ulcerations (Fig. 35-39).[231,232] Although these lesions usually develop within the first two decades of life, there is a report of an individual developing the typical gingival lesions at age 59 years.[233] A small number of these patients may show synchronous ligneous ("woodlike") conjunctivitis.[234]

Microscopically, the stratified squamous epithelium is acanthotic with hyperplastic rete pegs, severe neutrophilic exocytosis, and ulceration. The papillary lamina propria contains numerous pools of acellular, eosinophilic, homogeneous material that stains positively for fibrin with Fraser–Lendrum histochemical stain and antifibrin antibodies with direct immunofluorescence.[233,235]

Surgical excision of the enlarged tissue followed by meticulous oral hygiene is the preferred treatment. Unfortunately, the excised lesions show a tendency to recur swiftly. Replacement therapy with lys-plasminogen holds great promise once it becomes widely available.[236]

Verruciform Xanthoma

Verruciform xanthoma is a benign and uncommon lesion of unknown etiology with predilection for the masticatory mucosa. At least one third of verruciform xanthomas occur in the gingival tissues.[237] Typically, this lesion is small (0.2 to 2.0 cm), asymptomatic, and has a "warty" surface of normal to slightly reddish or gray color, usually with a sessile base.[238,239] Most patients with verruciform xanthoma are middle-aged individuals in their fourth to fifth decades of life.

Microscopically, the lesion shows a verrucous surface with hyperkeratinization that extends down in a cryptic pattern among elongated rete pegs. The uniformity of depth of the rete pegs is quite distinctive and the papillary lamina propria is filled by characteristic foamy macrophages.[238] Simple surgical excision is the treatment of choice.[240]

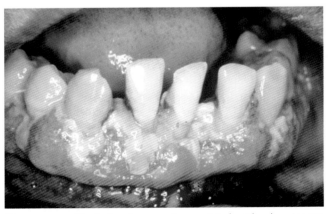

Figure 35-39. Gingival enlargement associated with plasminogen deficiency. Gingival enlargement with ulcerations.

Gingival Salivary Gland Choristoma

The presence of normal-appearing tissue in an abnormal location is known as choristoma. A number of gingival salivary gland choristomas have been documented. They present as sessile or pedunculated smooth nodular lesions on the attached gingival tissues. The subjacent bone is intact as indicated by the appropriate imaging studies.

Microscopic examination reveals the presence of fibrous connective tissue containing mucous producing acinar cells and associated excretory ducts. This lesion is managed surgically and has an excellent prognosis with no recurrences ever reported.[241-244]

Wegener's Granulomatosis

Wegener's granulomatosis (WG) is a systemic disease of unknown etiology characterized by the formation of necrotizing granulomas of lower and upper respiratory tract, generalized necrotizing vasculitis of small arteries and veins, and necrotizing glomerulonephritis.[245] WG has no sex predilection and it is more common in white individuals. WG occurs in a wide age range with a mean age of about 40 years.[246-248]

Three clinical variants of WG have been described: classic, limited, and superficial. The classic form of WG affects upper and lower respiratory tracts exhibiting rapid disseminated necrotizing vasculitis that without treatment progresses and may lead to kidney failure and death.[245,249] The limited variant of WG is characterized also by upper and lower respiratory tract lesions, but without a fatal renal outcome.[249] The superficial variant affects only mucosal or cutaneous tissues. Although this variant of WG may also evolve to pulmonary or renal involvement, or both, it shows a slow progression and better prognosis.[249]

Oral lesions are the initial manifestation in about 6% to 13% of patients with WG. Alternatively, the oral lesions may appear concurrently with or shortly after upper respiratory tract, pulmonary, and renal involvement.[245,247,250] The oral lesions consist of a characteristic focal or generalized gingival enlargement with a red granular surface referred to as "strawberry gums or strawberry gingivitis" (Fig. 35-40).[247,250] The gingival enlargement usually begins in the interdental papilla and eventually produces periodontal destruction and tooth loss.[247,251] WG patients may also present ulcers, especially in the palate (by extension from a nasal involvement), poor healing of extraction sites, and oral-antral fistulae.[250] Rare salivary gland involvement has also been reported.[252,253]

Microscopically, the oral lesions consist of a mixed infiltrate of acute and chronic inflammatory cells with microabscess formation and occasional multinucleated giant cells. In addition, necrotizing vasculitis, hemorrhage, pseudoepitheliomatous hyperplasia, or epithelial ulceration are also present.[250] Although these microscopic

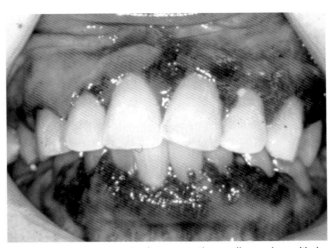

Figure 35-40. Wegener's granulomatosis. The maxillary and mandibular gingiva show the classic "strawberry gingivitis" associated with Wegener's granulomatosis.

features are unspecific, evaluation by immunofluorescence of cytoplasmic neutrophil anticytoplasmic autoantibodies in the patient's serum has been proven to be highly specific for WG.[254]

WG is best treated with the systemic administration of prednisone and cyclophosphamide.[248] Intralesional infiltration with corticosteroids has been reported to induce a prompt resolution of gingival lesions.[247] Early diagnosis and treatment of WG greatly improves its prognosis. Therefore familiarity with the oral manifestations of WG is crucial.

REFERENCES

1. American Academy of Periodontology Position Paper: Oral features of mucotaneous disorders, *J Periodontol* 74:1545-1556, 2003.
2. Nisengard RJ, Neiders M: Desquamative lesions of the gingiva, *J Periodontol* 52:500, 1981.
3. Laskaris G, Demetrou N, Angelopoulos A: Immunofluorescent studies in desquamative gingivitis, *J Oral Pathol* 10:398, 1981.
4. Rogers RS, Sheridan PJ, Jordon RC: Desquamative gingivitis: clinical, histopathologic and immunopathologic investigations, *Oral Surg* 42:316, 1976.
5. Sklavounou A, Laskaris G: Frequency of desquamative gingivitis in skin diseases, *Oral Surg Oral Med Oral Pathol* 56:141, 1983.
6. Valliant L, Chauchaix-Barthes S, Hüttenberger B et al: Desquamative gingivitis: retrospective analysis of 33 cases, *Ann Dermatol Venereol* 127:381, 2000.
7. Scully C, Porter SR: The clinical spectrum of desquamative gingivitis, *Semin Cutan Med Surg* 16:308, 1997.

8. Yih WY, Maier T, Kratochvil FJ, Zieper MB: Analysis of desquamative gingivitis using direct immunofluorescence in conjunction with histology, *J Periodontol* 69:678, 1998.
9. Rees TD: Adjunctive therapy. In Proceedings of the World Workshop in Clinical Periodontics. Chicago, 1989, The American Academy of Periodontology, pp X1-X31.
10. Scully C, Beyli M, Ferreiro MC, et al: Update on oral lichen planus: etiopathogenesis and management, *Crit Rev Oral Biol Med* 9:86, 1998.
11. Scully C, El-Kom M: Lichen planus: review and update on pathogenesis, *J Oral Pathol* 14:431, 1985.
12. Holmstrup P: The controversy of a premalignant potential of lichen planus is over, *Oral Surg Oral Med Oral Pathol* 73:704, 1992.
13. Eisenberg E: Lichen planus and oral cancer: is there a connection between the two?, *J Am Dent Assoc* 123:104, 1992.
14. Eisenberg E, Krutchkoff DJ: Lichenoid lesions of oral mucosa. Diagnostic criteria and their importance in the alleged relationship to oral cancer, *Oral Surg Oral Med Oral Pathol* 73:699, 1992.
15. Silverman S, Shachi B: Oral lichen planus update: clinical characteristics, treatment responses, and malignant transformation, *Am J Dent* 10:259, 1997.
16. Lozada-Nur F: Oral lichen planus and oral cancer: is there enough epidemiologic evidence?, *Oral Surg Oral Med Oral Pathol Oral Radiol Endod* 89:265, 2000.
17. Scully C, Carrozzo M, Gandolfo S et al: Update on mucous membrane pemphigoid. A heterogeneous immune-mediated subepithelial blistering entity, *Oral Surg Oral Med Oral Pathol Oral Radiol Endod* 88:56, 1999.
18. Chan LS, Razzaque A, Anhalt GJ, et al: The first international consensus on mucous membrane pemphigoid. Definition, diagnostic criteria, pathogenic factors, medical treatment and prognostic indicators, *Arch Dermatol* 138:370, 2002.
19. Challacombe SJ, Setterfield J, Shirlaw P et al: Immunodiagnosis of pemphigus and mucous membrane pemphigoid, *Acta Odontol Scand* 59:226, 2001.
20. Fleming TE, Korman NJ: Cicatricial pemphigoid, *J Am Acad Dermatol* 43:571, 2000.
21. Shklar G, McCarthy PL: The oral lesions of mucous membrane pemphigoid. A study of 85 cases, *Arch Otolaryngol* 93:354, 1971.
22. Gallagher G, Shklar G: Oral involvement in mucous membrane pemphigoid, *Clin Dermatol* 5:19, 1987.
23. Nisengard R: Periodontal implications: mucocutaneous disorders, *Ann Periodontol* 1:401, 1996.
24. Lorenzana ER, Rees TD, Hallmon WW: Esthetic management of multiple recession defects in a patient with cicatricial pemphigoid, *J Periodontol* 72:230, 2001.
25. Wojnarowska F, Kirtschig G, Khumalo N: Treatment of subepidermal diseases, *Clin Derm* 19:768, 2001.

26. Chan LS: Mucous membrane pemphigoid, *Clin Derm* 19:703, 2001.

27. Scully C: Pemphigus vulgaris: update on etiopathogenesis, oral manifestations, and management, *Crit Rev Oral Biol Med* 13:397, 2002.

28. Robinson JC, Lozada-Nur F, Frieden I: Oral pemphigus vulgaris: a review of the literature and a report on the management of 12 cases, *Oral Surg Oral Med Oral Pathol Oral Radiol Endod* 84:349, 1997.

29. Chowdhury MM, Natarajan S: Neonatal pemphigus vulgaris associated with mild oral pemphigus vulgaris in the mother during pregnancy, *Br J Dermatol* 139:500, 1998.

30. Weston WL, Morelli JG, Huff JC: Misdiagnosis, treatments and outcomes in the immunobullous diseases in children, *Pediatr Dermatol* 14:164, 1997.

31. Siegel MA, Balciunas BA: Oral presentation and management of vesiculobullous disorders, *Sem Dermatol* 13:78-86, 1994.

32. Mignogma MD, Lo Muzio L, Bucci E: Clinical features of gingival pemphigus vulgaris, *J Clin Periodontol* 28:489, 2001.

33. Lamey PJ, Rees TD, Binnie WH et al: Oral presentation of pemphigus vulgaris and its response to systemic steroid therapy, *Oral Surg Oral Med Oral Pathol* 74:54, 1992.

34. Lever WF: Pemphigus, *Medicine* 32:1, 1953.

35. Combes FL, Canizares O: Pemphigus vulgaris, a clinicopathological study of one hundred cases, *Arch Dermatol Syph* 62:786, 1950.

36. Casiglia J, Woo SB, Ahmed AR: Oral involvement in autoimmune blistering diseases, *Clin Dermatol* 19:737, 2001.

37. Lozada-Nur F, Miranda C, Maliski R: Double-blind clinical trial of 0.05% clobetasole propionate ointment in orabase and 0.05% fluocinonide ointment in orabase in the treatment of patients with vesiculoerosive diseases, *Oral Surg Oral Med Oral Pathol* 77:598, 1994.

38. Chorzelski TF, Olszewska M, Jarzabek-Chorzelska M, Jablonska S: Is chronic ulcerative stomatitis an entity? Clinical and immunological findings in 18 cases. *Eur J Dermatol* 8:261, 1998.

39. Lewis JE, Beutner EH, Rostami R: Chronic ulcerative stomatitis with stratified epithelium-specific antinuclear antibodies, *Int J Dermatol* 35:272, 1996.

40. Worle B, Wollenberg A, Schaller M, et al: Chronic ulcerative stomatitis, *Br J Dermatol* 137:262, 1997.

41. Lorenzana ER, Rees TD, Glass M: Chronic ulcerative stomatitis: a case report, *J Periodontol* 71:104, 2000.

42. Beutner EH, Chorzelski TP, Parodi A et al: Ten cases of chronic ulcerative stomatitis with stratified epithelium-specific antinuclear antibody, *J Am Acad Dermatol* 24:781, 1991.

43. Church LF Jr, Schosser RH: Chronic ulcerative stomatitis associated with stratified epithelial specific antinuclear antibodies. A case report of a newly described disease entity, *Oral Surg Oral Med Oral Pathol* 73:579, 1992.

44. Jaremko WM, Beutner EH, Kumar V, et al: Chronic ulcerative stomatitis associated with a specific immunologic marker, *J Am Acad Dermatol* 22:215, 1990.

45. Layfield LL, Shopper TP, Weir JC: A diagnostic survey of biopsied gingival lesions, *J Dent Hyg* 69:175, 1995.

46. Anneroth G, Sigurdson A: Hyperplastic lesions of the gingiva and alveolar mucosa. A study of 175 cases, *Acta Odontol Scand* 42:75, 1983.

47. Zain RB, Fei YJ: Fibrous lesions of the gingiva: a histopathologic analysis of 204 cases, *Oral Surg Oral Med Oral Pathol* 70:466, 1990.

48. Vilmann A, Vilmann P, Vilmann H: Pyogenic granuloma: evaluation of oral conditions, *Br J Oral Maxillofac Surg* 24:376, 1986.

49. Eversole LR, Rovin S: Reactive lesions of the gingiva, *J Oral Pathol* 1:30, 1972.

50. Bhaskar SN, Jacoway JR: Pyogenic granuloma. Clinical features, incidence, histology, and results of treatment: report of 242 cases, *J Oral Surg* 24:391, 1966.

51. Daley TD, Nartey NO, Wysocki GP: Pregnancy tumor: an analysis, *Oral Surg Oral Med Oral Pathol* 72:196, 1991.

52. Walters JD, Will JK, Hatfield RD, et al: Excision and repair of the peripheral ossifying fibroma: a case report of 3 cases, *J Periodontol* 72:939, 2001.

53. Kendrick F, Waggoner WF: Managing a peripheral ossifying fibroma, *J Dent Child* 63:135, 1996.

54. Cuisia ZES, Brannon RB: Peripheral ossifying fibroma. A clinical evaluation of 134 pediatric cases, *Pediatr Dent* 23:245, 2001.

55. Flaitz CM: Peripheral giant cell granuloma: a potentially aggressive lesion in children, *Pediatr Dent* 22:232, 2000.

56. Kfir Y, Buchner A, Hansen LS: Reactive lesions of the gingiva. A clinicopathological study of 741 cases, *J Periodontol* 51:655, 1980.

57. Katsikeris N, Kakarantza E, Angelopoulos P: Peripheral giant cell granuloma. Clinicopathological study of 224 new cases and review of 956 reported cases, *Int J Oral Maxillofac Surg* 17:94, 1988.

58. Giansanti JS, Waldron CA: Peripheral giant cell granuloma: review of 720 cases, *J Oral Surg* 27:787, 1969.

59. Philipsen HP, Reichart PA, Nikai H, et al: Peripheral ameloblastoma: biological profile based on 160 cases from the literature, *Oral Oncol* 37:17, 2001.

60. Buchner A, Sciubba JJ: Peripheral epithelial odontogenic tumors: a review, *Oral Surg Oral Med Oral Pathol* 63:688, 1987.

61. Batsakis JG, Hicks MJ, Flaitz CM: Peripheral odontogenic tumors, *Ann Otol Rhinol Laryngol* 102:322, 1993.

62. Nxumalo TN, Shear M: Gingival cyst in adults, *J Oral Pathol Med* 21:309, 1992.

63. Bell RC, Chauvin PJ, Tyler MT: Gingival cyst of the adult: a review and a report of eight cases, *J Can Dent Assoc* 63:533, 1997.

64. Giunta JL: Gingival cysts in the adult, *J Periodontol* 73:827, 2002.

65. Buchner A, Hansen LS: The histomorphologic spectrum of the gingival cyst in the adult, *Oral Med Oral Surg Oral Pathol* 48:532, 1979.

66. Cairo F, Rotundo R, Ficarra G: A rare lesion of the periodontium: the gingival cyst of the adult. A report of three cases, *Int J Periodontics Restorative Dent* 22:79, 2002.

67. Gurol M, Burkes EJ: Peripheral ameloblastoma, *J Periodontol* 66:1065, 1995.

68. Gardner D: Peripheral ameloblastoma, *Cancer* 39:1625, 1977.

69. Tajima Y, Kurokada-Kawasaki M, Ohno J et al: Peripheral ameloblastoma with potentially malignant features: report of a case with special regard to its keratin profile, *J Oral Pathol Med* 30:494, 2001.

70. Baden E, Doyle JL, Petriella V: Malignant transformation of peripheral ameloblastoma, *Oral Surg Oral Med Oral Pathol* 75:214, 1993.

71. Giovannelli L, Campisi G, Lama A, et al: Human papillomavirus DNA in oral mucosal lesions, *J Infect Dis* 185:833, 2002.

72. Terai M, Takagi M, Matsukura T: Oral wart associated with human papillomavirus type 2, *J Oral Pathol Med* 28:137, 1999.

73. Syrjanen S, Puranen M: Human papillomavirus infections in children: the potential role of maternal transmission, *Crit Rev Oral Biol Med* 11:259, 2000.

74. Green TL, Eversole LR, Leider AS: Oral and labial verruca vulgaris: clinical, histologic and immunohistochemical evaluation, *Oral Surg Oral Med Oral Pathol* 62:410, 1986.

75. Abbey LM, Page DG, Sawyer DR: The clinical and histopathologic features of a series of 464 oral squamous cell papillomas, *Oral Surg Oral Med Oral Pathol* 49:419, 1980.

76. Bouquot JE, Nikai H: Lesions of the oral cavity. In Gnepp DR, editor: *Diagnostic surgical pathology of the head and neck*, Philadelphia, 2001, WB Saunders, p 202.

77. Adler-Storthz K, Newland JR, Tessin BA et al: Human papillomavirus type 2 DNA in oral verrucous carcinoma, *J Oral Pathol* 15:472, 1986.

78. Premoli-de-Percoco G, Galindo I, Ramirez JL: Detection of human papillomavirus-related oral verruca vulgaris among Venezuelans, *J Oral Pathol Med* 22:113, 1993.

79. Chen YK, Hsue SS, Lin LM et al: Oral verruca vulgaris, *Quintessence Int* 33:162, 2002.

80. Ward KA, Napier SS, Winter PC, et al: Detection of human papilloma virus DNA sequences in oral squamous cell papillomas by the polymerase chain reaction, *Oral Surg Oral Med Oral Pathol Oral Radiol Endod* 80:63, 1995.

81. Padayachee A: Human papillomavirus (HPV) types 2 and 57 in oral verrucae demonstrated by in situ hybridization, *J Oral Pathol Med* 23:413, 1994.

82. Neville BW, Damm DD, Allen CM, Bouquot JE, editors: Epithelial pathology. In *Oral & maxillofacial pathology*, ed 2, Philadelphia, 2002, WB Saunders, pp 318.

83. Sykes NL Jr: Condyloma acuminatum, *Int J Dermatol* 34:297, 1995.

84. Suskind DL, Mirza N, Rosin D: Condyloma acuminatum presenting as a base of tongue mass, *Otolaryngol Head Neck Surg* 114:487, 1996.

85. Zunt SL, Tomich CE: Oral condyloma acuminatum, *J Dermatol Surg Oncol* 15:591, 1989.

86. Swan RH, McDaniel RK, Dreiman BB: Condyloma acuminatum involving the oral mucosa, *Oral Surg Oral Med Oral Pathol* 51:503, 1981.

87. Shimoyama T, Kato T, Nasu D, et al: Solitary neurofibroma of the oral mucosa: a previously undescribed variant of neurofibroma, *J Oral Sci* 44:59, 2002.

88. McDaniel RK, Adcock JE: Bilateral symmetrical lymphangiomas of the gingiva, *Oral Surg Oral Med Oral Pathol* 63:224, 1987.

89. Josephson P, van Wyk CW: Bilateral symmetrical lymphangiomas of the gingiva. A case report, *J Periodontol* 55:47, 1984.

90. Montgomery E, Speight PM, Fisher C: Myofibromas presenting in the oral cavity: a series of 9 cases, *Oral Surg Oral Med Oral Pathol Radiol Endod* 89:343, 2000.

91. Salgado R, Gallichio M, Gastaldoni R, et al: Myofibroma of the gingiva: report of a case with immunohistochemical and ultrastructural study, *J Clin Pediatr Dent* 24:75, 1999.

92. Baden E, Doyle JL, Lederman DA: Leiomyoma of the oral cavity: a light microscopic and immunohistochemical study with review of the literature from 1884 to 1992, *Oral Oncol Eur J Cancer* 30B:1, 1994.

93. Graham GS, Brannon RB, Houston GD: Fibrolipoma of the gingiva. A case report, *J Periodontol* 59:118, 1988.

94. Yamamoto H, Takagi M, Otake S: Leiomyoma of the right lower gingiva: a case and a review of the Japanese literature, *J Oral Maxillofac Surg* 41:671, 1983.

95. Hansen LS, Olson JA, Silverman S: Proliferative verrucous leukoplakia. A study of 30 patients, *Oral Surg Oral Med Oral Pathol* 60:285, 1985.

96. Silverman S, Gorsky M: Proliferative verrucous leukoplakia. A follow-up study of 54 cases, *Oral Surg Oral Med Oral Pathol Oral Radiol Endod* 84:154, 1997.

97. Batsakis JG, Suarez P, El-Naggar AK: Proliferative verrucous leukoplakia and its related lesions, *Oral Oncol* 35:354, 1999.

98. Femiano F, Gombos F, Scully C: Oral proliferative verrucous leukoplakia (PVL): open trial of surgery compared with combination therapy using surgery and methisoprinol in papillomavirus-related PVL, *Int J Oral Maxillofac Surg* 30:318, 2001.

99. Zakrzewska JM, Lopes V, Speight P: Proliferative verrucous leukoplakia. A report of ten cases, *Oral Surg Oral Med Oral Pathol Oral Radiol Endod* 82:396, 1996.

100. Silverman S: *Oral cancer*, Hamilton, Ontario, Canada, 1998, BC Decker, pp 1-2.

101. Makridis SD, Mellado JR, Freedman AL et al: Squamous cell carcinoma of the gingiva and edentulous alveolar ridge: a clinicopathologic study, *Int J Periodontics Restorative Dent* 18:292, 1998.

102. Barasch A, Gofa A, Krutchkoff DJ, Eisenberg: Squamous cell carcinoma of the gingiva. A case series analysis, *Oral Surg Oral Med Oral Path Oral Radiol Endod* 80:183, 1995.

103. Wallace ML, Neville BW: Squamous cell carcinoma of the gingiva with an atypical appearance, *J Periodontol* 67:1245, 1996.

104. Aguirre A, Tapia JL, Ciancio S, Coniglio J: Serendipitous diagnosis of protein S deficiency, *J Periodontol* 73:1197, 2002.

105. Soo KC, Spiro RH, King W et al: Squamous carcinoma of the gums, *Am J Surg* 156:281, 1988.

106. Kirkham DB, Hoge HW, Sadeghi EM: Gingival squamous cell carcinoma appearing as a benign lesion: report of case, *J Am Dent Assoc* 111:767, 1985.

107. Overholt SM, Eicher SA, Wolf P, et al: Prognostic factors affecting the outcome in lower gingival carcinoma, *Laryngoscope* 106:1335, 1996.

108. Gomez D, Faucher A, Picot V, et al: Outcome of squamous cell carcinoma of the gingiva: a follow-up study of 83 cases, *J Cranio Maxillo Surg* 28:331, 2000.

109. Cotran RS, Kumar V, Collins T: *Robbins pathologic basis of disease.* Philadelphia, 1999, WB Saunders, pp 119, 324.

110. Hicks MK, Flaitz CM: Oral mucosal melanoma: epidemiology and pathobiology, *Oral Oncol* 36:152, 2000.

111. Ardekian L, Rosen DJ, Peled M: Primary gingival malignant melanoma. Report of 3 cases, *J Periodontol* 71:117, 2000.

112. Gorsky M, Epstein JB: Melanoma arising from the mucosal surfaces of the head and neck, *Oral Surg Oral Med Oral Pathol* 86:715, 1998.

113. Lopez-Graniel, Ochoa-Carrillo FJ, Meneses-Garcia A: Malignant melanoma of the oral cavity: diagnosis and treatment experience in a Mexican population, *Oral Oncol* 35:425, 1999.

114. Rapini RP, Golitz LE, O'Greer R: Primary malignant melanoma of the oral cavity. A review of 177 cases, *Cancer* 55:1543, 1985.

115. Tanaka N, Amagasa T, Iwaki H: Oral malignant melanoma in Japan, *Oral Surg Oral Med Oral Pathol* 78:81, 1994.

116. Gorsky M, Epstein JB: Head and neck and intra-oral soft tissue sarcomas, *Oral Oncol* 34:292, 1998.

117. Guglielmotti MB, Pena C, Dominguez FV: Malignant schwannoma of the gingiva, *Int J Oral Maxillofac Surg* 16:492, 1987.

118. Quinn JH, McConnell HA Jr, Leonard GL: Multifocal angiosarcoma of the gingiva: report of case, *J Oral Surg* 28:215, 1970.

119. Albright CR, Shelton DW, Vatral JJ: Angiosarcoma of the gingiva: report of case, *J Oral Surg* 28:913, 1970.

120. Munoz M, Monje F, Alonso del Hoyo JR: Oral angiosarcoma misdiagnosed as a pyogenic granuloma, *J Oral Maxillofac Surg* 56:488, 1998.

121. Kaloyannides TM: Pleomorphic rhabdomyosarcoma of the gingiva: report of a case, *Oral Surg Oral Med Oral Pathol* 27:150, 1969.

122. Peters E, Cohen M, Altini M, Murray J: Rhabdomyosarcoma of the oral and paraoral region, *Cancer* 63:963, 1989.

123. Piscioli F, Leonardi E, Scappini P: Primary angiosarcoma of the gingiva. Case report with immunohistochemical study, *Am J Dermatopathol* 8:430, 1986.

124. Nikitakis NG, Lopes MA, Bailey JS et al: Oral leiomyosarcoma: review of the literature and report of two cases with assessment of the prognostic and diagnostic significance of immunohistochemical and molecular markers, *Oral Oncol* 38:201, 2002.

125. Goldschmidt PR, Goldschmidt JD, Lieblich SE: Leiomyosarcoma presenting as a mandibular gingival swelling: a case report, *J Periodontol* 70:84, 1999.

126. Poon CK, Kwan PC, Yin NT: Leiomyosarcoma of gingiva: report of a case and review of the literature, *J Oral Maxillofac Surg* 45:888, 1987.

127. Muzio LL, Favia G, Farronato G, et al: Primary gingival leiomyosarcoma. A clinicopathological study of 1 case with prolonged survival, *J Clin Periodontol* 29:182, 2002.

128. Piattelli A, Di Alberti L, Favia GF: Liposarcoma involving the periodontal tissues. A case report, *J Periodontol* 71:322, 2000.

129. Bras J, Batsakis JG, Luna MA: Malignant fibrous histiocytoma of the oral soft tissues, *Oral Surg Oral Med Oral Pathol* 64:57, 1987.

130. Ellis GL, Jensen JL, Reingold IM: Malignant neoplasms metastatic to gingivae, *Oral Surg Oral Med Oral Pathol* 44:238, 1977.

131. Hirshberg A, Leibovich P, Buchner A: Metastasis to the oral mucosa: analysis of 157 cases, *J Oral Pathol Med* 22:385, 1993.

132. Piattelli A, Fioroni M, Rubini C: Gingival metastasis from a prostate adenocarcinoma: report of a case, *J Periodontol* 70:441, 1999.

133. Buchner A, Begleiter A: Metastatic renal cell carcinoma in the gingiva mimicking a hyperplastic lesion, *J Periodontol* 51:413, 1980.

134. Scipio JE, Murti PR, Al-Bayaty HF et al: Metastasis of breast carcinoma to mandibular gingiva, *Oral Oncol* 37:393, 2001.

135. DeCourten A, Irle C, Samson J: Metastatic transitional cell carcinoma of the urinary bladder presenting as a mandibular gingival swelling, *J Periodontol* 72:688, 2001.

136. Suzuki K, Yoshida H, Onizawa K: Metastatic osteosarcoma to the mandibular gingiva: a case report, *J Oral Maxillofac Surg* 57:864, 1999.

137. Yoshii T, Muraoka S, Sano N, et al: Large cell carcinoma of the lung metastatic to the mandibular gingiva, *J Periodontol* 73:571, 2002.

138. Win KKS, Yasuoka T, Kamiya T: Breast angiosarcoma metastatic to the maxillary gingiva. Case report, *Int J Oral Maxillofac Surg* 21:282, 1992.

139. McGlumphy EA, Zysset MK, Montgomery MT: Ewing's sarcoma metastatic to the gingiva, *J Oral Maxillofac Surg* 45:444, 1987.

140. Nespeca JA, Sass JK: Choriocarcinoma metastatic to maxillary gingiva, *J Oral Surg* 38:534, 1980.

141. Lee SH, Huang JJ, Pan WL: Gingival mass as the primary manifestation of multiple myeloma. Report of two cases, *Oral Surg Oral Med Oral Pathol Oral Radiol Endod* 82:75, 1996.

142. Wedgwood D, Rusen D, Balk S: Gingival metastasis from primary hepatocellular carcinoma. Report of a case, *Oral Surg Oral Med Oral Pathol* 47:263, 1979.

143. Toth BB, Fleming TJ, Lomba JA: Angiosarcoma metastatic to the maxillary tuberosity gingiva, *Oral Surg Oral Med Oral Pathol* 52:71, 1981.

144. Allen CM, Miloro M: Gingival lesion of recent onset in a patient with neurofibromatosis, *Oral Surg Oral Med Oral Pathol Oral Radiol Endod* 84:595, 1997.

145. McMurria H, Handlers JP, Abrams AM: Malignant fibrous histiocytoma, myxoid variant metastatic to the oral cavity. Report of a case and review of the literature, *Oral Surg Oral Med Oral Pathol* 51:156, 1981.

146. Stecher JA, Mostofi R, True LD: Pancreatic carcinoma metastatic to the mandibular gingiva, *J Oral Maxillofacial Surg* 43:385, 1985.

147. Hirshberg A, Buchner A: Metastatic tumors to the oral region. An overview, *Eur J Cancer B Oral Oncol* 31:355, 1995.

148. Regezi JA, Kerr DA, Courtney RM: Odontogenic tumors: analysis of 706 cases, *J Oral Surgery* 36:771, 1978.

149. Shear M: Developmental odontogenic cysts. An update, *J Oral Pathol Med* 23:1, 1994.

150. Kramer IRH, Pindborg JJ, Shear M: *Histological typing of odontogenic tumours.* Berlin, 1992, Springer-Verlag.

151. David LA, Sandor GK, Stoneman DW: The buccal bifurcation cyst: is non-surgical treatment an option?, *J Can Dent Assoc* 64:712, 1998.

152. Pompura JR, Sandor GK, Stoneman DW: The buccal bifurcation cyst: a prospective study of treatment outcomes in 44 sites, *Oral Surg Oral Med Oral Pathol Oral Radiol Endod* 83:215, 1997.

153. Wysocki GP, Brannon RB, Gardner DG: Histogenesis of the lateral periodontal cyst and the gingival cyst of the adult, *Oral Surg Oral Med Oral Pathol* 50:327, 1980.

154. Fantasia JE: Lateral periodontal cyst. An analysis of forty-six cases, *Oral Surg Oral Med Oral Pathol* 48:237, 1979.

155. Angelopoulou E, Angelopoulos AP: Lateral periodontal cyst. Review of the literature and report of a case, *J Periodontol* 61:126, 1990.

156. Cohen DA, Neville BW, Damm DD: The lateral periodontal cyst. A report of 37 cases, *J Periodontol* 55:230, 1984.

157. Gurol M, Burkes EJ, Jacoway J: Botryoid odontogenic cyst: analysis of 33 cases, *J Periodontol* 66:1069, 1995.

158. Phelan JA, Kritchman D, Fusco-Ramer M, et al: Recurrent botryoid odontogenic cyst (lateral periodontal cyst), *Oral Surg Oral Med Oral Pathol* 66:345, 1988.

159. Carter LC, Carney YL, Perez-Pudlewski D: Lateral periodontal cyst. Multifactorial analysis of a previously unreported series, *Oral Surg Oral Med Oral Pathol Oral Radiol Endod* 81:210, 1996.

160. Myoung H, Hong S, Hong SD, et al: Odontogenic keratocyst: review of 256 cases for recurrence and clinicopathologic parameters, *Oral Surg Oral Med Oral Path Oral Radiol Endod* 91:328, 2001.

161. Brannon RB: The odontogenic keratocyst: a clinicopathologic study of 312 cases. Part II: Histologic features, *Oral Surg Oral Med Oral Pathol* 43:233, 1977.

162. Regezi JA, Sciubba JJ, Jordan RCK: Cyst of the jaws and neck. In Regezi JA, Sciubba JJ, Jordan RCK, editors: *Oral pathology. Clinical pathologic correlations,* St. Louis, Mo., 2003, Elsevier Science, pp 254, 277.

163. Zhao YF, Wei JX, Wang SP: Treatment of odontogenic keratocysts: a follow-up of 255 Chinese patients, *Oral Surg Oral Med Oral Pathol Oral Radiol Endod* 94:151, 2002.

164. Reichart PA, Philipsen HP, Sonner S: Ameloblastoma: biological profile of 3677 cases, *Eur J Cancer B Oral Oncol* 31B:86, 1995.

165. Kim SG, Jang HS: Ameloblastoma: a clinical, radiographic, and histopathologic analysis of 71 cases, *Oral Surg Oral Med Oral Pathol Oral Radiol Endod* 91:649, 2001.

166. Vickers RA, Gorlin RJ: Ameloblastoma: delineation of early histopathologic features of neoplasia, *Cancer* 26:699, 1970.

167. Bonn GE, DeBoom GW: Multilocular radiolucent area of the posterior mandible, *J Am Dent Assoc* 116:393, 1988.

168. Melrose RJ: Benign epithelial odontogenic tumors, *Semin Diagn Pathol* 16:271, 1999.

169. Philipsen HP, Reichart PA: Adenomatoid odontogenic tumour: facts and figures, *Oral Oncol* 35:125, 1999.

170. Courtney RM, Kerr DA: The odontogenic adenomatoid tumor. A comprehensive study of twenty new cases, *Oral Surg Oral Med Oral Pathol* 39:424, 1975.

171. Budnick SD: Compound and complex odontomas, *Oral Surg Oral Med Oral Pathol* 42:501, 1976.

172. Siegel WM, Pappas JR: Development of exostoses following skin graft vestibuloplasty. Report of a case, *J Oral Maxillofac Surg* 44:483, 1986.

173. Pack ARC, Gaudie WM, Jennings AM: Bony exostosis as a sequela to free gingival grafting: two case reports, *J Periodontol* 62:269, 1991.

174. Hegtvedt AK, Terry BC, Burkes EJ: Skin graft vestibuloplasty exostosis, *Oral Surg Oral Med Oral Pathol* 69:149, 1990.

175. Czuszak CA, Tolson GE, Kudryk VL: Development of an exostosis following a free gingival graft, *J Periodontol* 67:259, 1996.

176. Echeverria JJ, Montero M, Abad D: Exostosis following a free gingival graft, *J Clin Periodontol* 29:474, 2002.

177. Otero-Cagide FJ, Singer DL, Hoover JN: Exostosis associated with autogenous gingival grafts: a report of 9 cases, *J Periodontol* 67:611, 1996.

178. Moshref M, Ebrahimi B, Hafez MT: Periosteal compact osteoma, *Oral Surg* 58:743, 1984.

179. TakeuchiT, Takenoshita Y, Kubo K, et al: Natural course of jaw lesions in patients with familial adenomatosis coli (Gardner's syndrome), *Int J Oral Maxillofac Surg* 22:226, 1993.

180. Slootweg PJ, Müller H: Osteosarcoma of the jaw bones: analysis of 18 cases, *J Maxillofac Surg* 13:158, 1985.

181. Doval DC, Kumar RV, Kannan KS et al: Osteosarcoma of the jaw bones, *Br J Oral Maxillofac Surg* 35:357, 1997.

182. Bennett JH, Thomas G, Evans AW: Osteosarcoma of the jaws: a 30-year retrospective review, *Oral Surg Oral Med Oral Pathol Oral Radiol Endod* 90:323, 2000.

183. Gorsky M, Epstein JB: Craniofacial osseous and chondromatous sarcomas in British Columbia. A review of 34 cases, *Oral Oncol* 36:27, 2000.

184. El-Mofty SK, Kryakos M: Soft tissue and bone lesions. In Gnepp DR, editors: *Diagnostic surgical pathology of the head and neck*, Philadelphia, 2001, WB Saunders, p 560.

185. Batsakis JG: Osteogenic and chondrogenic sarcomas of the jaws, *Ann Otol Rhinol Laryngol* 96:474, 1987.

186. Chindia M: Osteosarcoma of the jaw bones, *Oral Oncol* 37:545, 2001.

187. August M, Magennis P, Dewitt D: Osteogenic sarcoma of the jaws: factors influencing prognosis, *Int J Oral Maxillofac Surg* 26:198, 1997.

188. Piattelli A, Favia GF: Periosteal osteosarcoma of the jaws, *J Periodontol* 71:325, 2000.

189. Givol N, Buchner A, Taicher S: Radiological features of osteogenic sarcoma of the jaws. A comparative study of different radiographic modalities, *Dentomaxillofac Radiol* 27:313, 1998.

190. Garrington GE, Collet WK: Chondrosarcoma. I. A selected literature review, *J Oral Pathol* 17:1, 1988.

191. Weiss WW, Bennett JA: Chondrosarcoma: a rare tumor of the jaws, *J Oral Maxillofac Surg* 44:73, 1986.

192. Hackney FL, Aragin SB, Aufdemorte TB, et al: Chondrosarcoma of the jaws: clinical findings, histopathology, and treatment, *Oral Surg Oral Med Oral Pathol* 71:139, 1991.

193. Garrington GE, Collet WK: Chondrosarcoma. II. Chondrosarcoma of the jaws, *J Oral Pathol* 17:12, 1988.

194. Saito K, Unni KK, Wollan PC: Chondrosarcoma of the jaw and facial bones, *Cancer* 76:1550, 1995.

195. Hokett SD, Cuenin MF, Peacock ME, et al: Non-Hodgkin's lymphoma and periodontitis. A case report, *J Periodontol* 71:504, 2000.

196. Economopoulos T, Asprou N, Stathakis N, et al: Primary extranodal non-Hodgkin's lymphoma in adults: clinicopathological and survival characteristics. *Leuk Lymphoma* 21:131, 1996.

197. Hanna E, Wanamaker J, Adelstein D et al: Extranodal lymphomas of the head and neck. A 20-year experience, *Arch Otolaryngol Head Neck Surg* 123:1318, 1997.

198. Neville BW, Damm DD, Allen CM, Bouquot JE, editors: Hematologic disorders. In *Oral & maxillofacial pathology*, ed 2, Philadelphia, 2002, WB Saunders, pp 519, 521.

199. Takahashi H, Tsuda N, Tezuka F, Okabe H: Primary extranodal non-Hodgkin's lymphoma of the oral region, *J Oral Pathol Med* 18:84, 1989.

200. Takahashi H, Fujita S, Okabe H, et al: Immunophenotypic analysis of extranodal non-Hodgkin's lymphomas in the oral cavity, *Pathol Res Pract* 189:300, 1993.

201. Regezi JA, Sciubba JJ, Jordan RCK: Lymphoid lesions. In Regezi JA, Sciubba JJ, Jordan RCK, editors: *Oral pathology. Clinical pathologic correlations.* St. Louis, Mo., 2003, Elsevier Science, p 225.

202. Abdelsayed RA, Sangueza O: Refractory localized "periodontitis," *Oral Surg Oral Med Oral Pathol Oral Radiol Endod* 93:394, 2002.

203. Regezi JA, Zarbo RJ, Stewart JC: Extranodal oral lymphomas: histologic subtypes and immunophenotypes (in routinely processed tissue), *Oral Surg Oral Med Oral Pathol* 72:702, 1991.

204. Cotran RS, Kumar V, Robbins SL: Diseases of white cells, lymph nodes, and spleen. In Cotran RS, Kumar V, Robbins SL, editors: *Pathologic basis of disease*, ed 5, Philadelphia, 1994, WB Saunders, p 665.

205. Lee SH, Huang JJ, Pan WL: Gingival mass as the primary manifestation of multiple myeloma: report of two cases, *Oral Surg Oral Med Oral Pathol Oral Radiol Endod* 82:75, 1996.

206. Pisano JJ, Coupland R, Chen SY: Plasmacytoma of the oral cavity and jaws: a clinicopathologic study of 13 cases, *Oral Surg Oral Med Oral Pathol Oral Radiol Endod* 83:265, 1997.

207. Neville BW, Damm DD, Allen CM, Bouquot JE, editors: Hematologic disorders. In *Oral & maxillofacial pathology*, ed 2, Philadelphia, 2002, WB Saunders, pp 526, 527.

208. Petit JC, Ripamonti U: Multiple myeloma of the periodontium. A case report, *J Periodontol* 61:132, 1990.

209. Witt C, Borges AC, Klein K: Radiographic manifestations of multiple myeloma in the mandible: a retrospective study of 77 patients, *J Oral Maxillofac Surg* 55:450, 1997.

210. Van der Waal RI, Van de Scheur MR, Huijgens PC et al: Amyloidosis of the tongue as a paraneoplastic marker of plasma cell dyscrasia, *Oral Surg Oral Med Oral Pathol Oral Radiol Endod* 94:444, 2002.

211. Savage NW, Monsour PA: Oral fibrous hyperplasias and the giant cell fibroma, *Aust Dent J* 30:405, 1985.

212. Weathers DR, Callihan MD: Giant-cell fibroma, *Oral Surg Oral Med Oral Pathol* 37:374, 1974.

213. Houston GD: The giant cell fibroma. A review of 464 cases, *Oral Med Oral Path Oral Surg* 53:582, 1982.

214. Hirschfield I: The retrocuspid papillae, *Am J Orthod* 33:447, 1974.

215. Buchner A, Merrell PW, Hansen LS: The retrocuspid papilla of the mandibular lingual gingiva, *J Periodontol* 61:586, 1990.

216. Everett FG, Hall WB, Bennett JS: Retrocuspid papillae, *Periodontics* 3:81, 1965.

217. Giunta JL: Gingival fibrous nodule, *Oral Surg Oral Med Oral Pathol Oral Radiol Endod* 88:451, 1999.

218. Milian MA, Bagan JV, Jimenez Y et al: Langerhans' cell histiocytosis restricted to the oral mucosa, *Oral Surg Oral Med Oral Pathol Oral Radiol Endod* 91:76, 2001.

219. Willman CL, Busque L, Griffith BB et al: Langerhans'-cell histiocytosis (histiocytosis X): a clonal proliferative disease, *N Engl J Med* 331:154, 1994.

220. Gorsky M, Silverman S Jr, Lozada F, Kushner J: Histiocytosis X: Occurrence and oral involvement in six adolescent and adult patients, *Oral Surg Oral Med Oral Pathol* 55:24, 1983.

221. Hartman KS: Histiocytosis X: a review of 114 cases with oral involvement, *Oral Surg Oral Med Oral Pathol* 49:38, 1980.

222. Bottomley WK, Gabriel SA, Corio RL, Jacobson RJ: Histiocytosis X: report of an oral soft tissue lesion without bony involvement, *Oral Surg Oral Med Oral Pathol* 63:228, 1987.

223. Cleveland DB, Goldberg KM, Greenspan JS et al: Langerhans' cell histiocytosis: report of three cases with unusual oral soft tissue involvement, *Oral Surg Oral Med Oral Pathol Oral Radiol Endod* 82:541, 1996.

224. Dagenais M, Pharoah MJ, Sikorski PA: The radiographic characteristics of histiocytosis X. A study of 29 cases that involve the jaws, *Oral Surg Oral Med Oral Pathol* 74:230, 1992.

225. Emile JF, Wechsler J, Brousse N et al: Langerhans' cell histiocytosis. Definitive diagnosis with the use of monoclonal antibody O10 on routinely paraffin-embedded samples, *Am J Surg Pathol* 19:636, 1995.

226. Jones LR, Toth BB, Cangir A: Treatment for solitary eosinophilic granuloma of the mandible by steroid injection: report of a case, *J Oral Maxillofac Surg* 47:306, 1989.

227. Howarth DM, Gilchrist GS, Mullan BP et al: Langerhans cell histiocytosis: diagnosis, natural history, management, and outcome, *Cancer* 85:2278, 1999.

228. Iezzi G, Rubini C, Fioroni M: Oral focal mucinosis of the gingiva: case report, *J Periodontol* 72:1100, 2001.

229. Buchner A, Merrel PW, Leider AS: Oral focal mucinosis, *Int J Oral Maxillofac Surg* 19:337, 1990.

230. Tomich CE: Oral focal mucinosis. A clinicopathologic and histochemical study of eight cases, *Oral Surg Oral Med Oral Pathol* 38:714, 1974.

231. Gokbuget AY, Mutlu S, Scully C et al: Amyloidaceous ulcerated gingival hyperplasia: a newly described entity related to ligneous conjunctivitis, *J Oral Pathol Med* 26:100, 1997.

232. Günham Ö, Celasun B, Perrini F et al: Generalized gingival enlargement due to accumulation of amyloid-like material, *J Oral Pathol Med* 23:423, 1994.

233. Suresh L, Aguirre A, Kumar V et al: Recurrent recalcitrant gingival hyperplasia and plasminogen deficiency: a case report. *J Periodontol* 74: 1508-1513, 2003.

234. Scully C, Gokbuget AY, Allen C et al: Oral lesions indicative of plasminogen deficiency (hypoplasminogenemia), *Oral Surg Oral Med Oral Pathol Oral Radiol Endod* 91:334, 2001.

235. Günhan Ö, Günhan M, Berker E: Destructive membranous periodontal disease (ligneous periodontitis), *J Periodontol* 70:919, 1999.

236. Schott D, Dempfle CE, Lierman A, et al: Homozygous plasminogen deficiency-treatment and prevention of blindness by long-term replacement therapy with lys-plasminogen, *Ann Hematol* 74:85, 1997.

237. Oliveira PT, Jaeger RG, Cabral LAG et al: Verruciform xanthoma of the oral mucosa. Report of four cases and a review of the literature, *Oral Oncol* 37:326, 2001.

238. Miller AS, Elszay RP: Verruciform xanthoma of the gingiva: report of six cases, *J Periodontol* 44:103, 1973.

239. Nowparast B, Howell FV, Rick GM: Verruciform xanthoma. A clinicopathologic review and report of fifty four cases, *Oral Med Oral Surg Oral Pathol* 51:619, 1981.

240. Allen CM, Kapoor N: Verruciform xanthoma in a bone marrow transplant recipient, *Oral Med Oral Surg Oral Pathol* 75:591, 1993.

241. Brannon RB, Houston GD, Wampler HW: Gingival salivary gland choristoma, *Oral Surg Oral Med Oral Pathol* 61:185, 1986.

242. Ide F, Shimura H, Saito I: Gingival salivary gland choristoma: an extremely rare phenomenon, *Oral Surg Oral Med Oral Pathol* 55:169, 1983.

243. Moskow BS, Baden E: Gingival salivary gland choristoma. Report of a case, *J Clin Periodontol* 13:720, 1986.

244. Ledesma-Montes C, Fernandez-Lopez R, Garces-Ortiz M et al: Gingival salivary gland choristoma, *J Periodontol* 69:1164, 1998.

245. Eufinger H, Machtens E, Akuamoa-Boateng E: Oral manifestations of Wegener's granulomatosis. Review of the literature and report of a case, *Int J Oral Maxillofac Surg* 21:50, 1992.

246. Hoffman GS, Kerr GS, Leavitt RY et al: Wegener granulomatosis: an analysis of 158 patients, *Ann Intern Med* 16:488, 1992.

247. Lilly J, Juhlin T, Lew D: Wegener's granulomatosis presenting as oral lesions: a case report, *Oral Surg Oral Med Oral Pathol Oral Radiol Endod* 85:153, 1998.

248. Fauci AS, Haynes BF, Katz P: Wegener's granulomatosis: prospective clinical and therapeutic experience with 85 patients for 21 years, *Ann Intern Med* 98:76, 1983.

249. Allen CM, Camisa C, Salewski C: Wegener's granulomatosis: report of three cases with oral lesions, *J Oral Maxillofac Surg* 49:294, 1991.

250. Cohen RE, Cardoza TT, Drinnan AJ et al: Gingival manifestations of Wegener's granulomatosis, *J Periodontol* 61:705, 1990.

251. Patten SF, Tomecki KJ: Wegener's granulomatosis: cutaneous and oral mucosal disease, *J Am Acad Dermatol* 28:710, 1993.

252. Vanhauwaert BG, Roskams TA, Vanneste SB: Salivary gland involvement as initial presentation of Wegener's disease, *Postgrad Med J* 69:643, 1993.

253. Kavanaugh AF, Huston DP: Wegener's granulomatosis presenting with unilateral parotid enlargement, *Am J Med* 85:741, 1988.

254. Neville BW, Damm DD, Allen CM, Bouquot JE, editors: Hematologic disorders. In *Oral & maxillofacial pathology*, ed 2, Philadelphia, 2002, WB Saunders, p 300.

36

Medical and Dental History

Robert E. Schifferle, Brian L. Mealey, and Louis F. Rose

A thorough evaluation of the patient's dental and medical history is fundamental for accurate diagnosis, appropriate treatment planning, and proper management of the patient's periodontal condition. The importance of obtaining and evaluating a complete medical and dental history cannot be overemphasized. There is a rapidly growing segment of the population whose physical or psychosocial problems may complicate dental treatment. The elderly or medically compromised patient may require special consideration before undergoing dental treatment. Identification of potential systemic disorders is a prerequisite to assessing the impact of such conditions on dental care. The significance of medical history and current medical status to periodontal diagnosis and treatment planning is even more relevant in light of the substantial evidence linking periodontal disease to systemic conditions (see Chapters 31 and 32). It is through this information that the clinician is made aware of previous or current medical conditions, which may directly affect the severity and extent of periodontal disease and the ability to treat the patient's periodontal needs. In addition, a major goal of dental care is to provide a safe treatment environment and to prevent in-office medical emergencies. Medically compromised patients present the greatest risk for such emergencies. The medical history and physician consultation, when indicated, provide the best means of preventing perioperative medical emergencies in the dental office.

Taking the medical and dental history includes eliciting information regarding the patient's past and current medical and dental status. This is done by administering a questionnaire to the patient, where systemic health is self-reported, followed by interviewing the patient. The degree of effectiveness in eliciting and gathering information on the medical status depends both on the clarity of the questionnaire administered and the quality of communication between the dentist and the patient. It is important to determine the patient's reason for seeking dental care by eliciting his or her chief complaint (Box 36-1). Establishing the chief complaint allows the dentist's initial focus to be on what the patient perceives to be his or her main problem. Although patients are typically asking the clinician to resolve their chief complaint, the dentist first needs to evaluate the patient health as a whole. It is through a thorough assessment of the information obtained that the health care provider makes a decision to either treat the patient's presenting symptom immediately or to first investigate the medical status further.

MEDICAL HISTORY

The goal of the medical history evaluation is to assess all physiologic systems and to identify all prescription and nonprescription medications being taken by the patient.[1,2]

Box 36-1   Establishing the Patient's Chief Complaint

Questions to ask include:
- Is there a problem?
- Is the problem acute or chronic?
- If the problem is chronic, what is the duration of the problem?
- Is the patient experiencing pain? If so, what is the level of severity? (A visual analog scale of 1 to 10 or 1 to 100 may be useful for determining the degree of pain.)
- Does the patient have a sense of urgency?
- Has the patient received prior treatment for this problem?

The clinician must critically evaluate the patient's medical history and determine its relevance and impact on the care that is needed. If the patient is undergoing treatment for any current illnesses or medical conditions, it is generally of greater relevance to treatment than past illnesses, although this may not always be true depending on the nature of the past condition.

History taking is a technique for eliciting subjective information. These data are organized logically to convey the patient's physical and emotional status. Diagnosis of a specific systemic condition may require consultation with a physician. Approximately 25% of patients in population studies of dental schools require medical consultation.[2] The medical history puts the physical and dental examination into perspective by supplying information that should alert the clinician to suspected abnormalities. A proper evaluation of the patient includes recording a complete medical history, recording appropriate findings from physical examination, ordering and interpreting laboratory studies, when indicated, and initiating medical consultation as needed.

Recording the Medical History

The two basic steps in obtaining a medical history include a written questionnaire and a personal interview. Both steps are an absolute requirement. The personal interview augments the written questionnaire; significant findings may be elicited by a detailed interview, even in patients whose written questionnaire is essentially negative. The questionnaire helps the patient recall frequently used medications and various symptoms that may indicate an underlying systemic disorder. It can also assist the dentist in focusing the personal interview and identifying areas to explore in further depth. The questionnaire, completed in privacy, can alleviate embarrassment in answering questions related to habits or addictions, sexual preferences or risks for sexually transmitted diseases, and other sensitive topics. The dentist must always keep patient confidentiality and sensitivity in mind when conducting the personal interview.

In some dental practices, the medical and dental history forms are sent to the patient for completion before the first appointment. By receiving the form before the first visit a patient may have access to information that may not be available to them if they were filling out the form in the waiting room. The information that they may need to look up includes their physician's name, address, and phone number; a list of medications that they are currently taking with appropriate dosages; a list of any drug allergies; and the dates of prior illnesses and hospitalizations. If the patient arrives at the dental office with a completed form with all of this information at the initial visit, it provides the dentist with an ideal starting point for a verbal interview to ensure that it is safe to proceed with dental examination and treatment.

Medical and dental history forms are available from the American Dental Association (Fig. 36-1) and from numerous private companies, or one may prefer to prepare an individualized form tailored to their specific practice. This form should include biographical data such as the patient's name, address, weight, age, sex, social security number, and emergency contacts, along with an assessment of his or her own medical health and dental health. This "self-assessment" of health will provide the practitioner with another means by which to assess the patient's readiness and capability of having dental treatment performed. The name, address, and telephone number of the patient's physician should be obtained, along with any medical treatment being received, the reasons for treatment, the frequency of care, and the time elapsed since the last visit to the physician. The medical history and evaluation should be updated during each maintenance visit after active periodontal therapy (e.g., every 3 to 6 months). During protracted periods of active therapy, frequent updates are also indicated, because the patient's physical condition can change significantly between visits.

A list of current medications, dosages, and their indications should be obtained. The dentist should determine if the medication is being used for a chronic condition or for a current or acute need. Self-medication with herbs, vitamins, and over-the-counter products should be assessed because they can interfere with other medications or treatment, and a patient may not report self-medication unless specifically asked.

Social History/Habits

Taking a social history may assist in determining the patient's response to the demands of daily life. The social history may help explain the patient's attitudes toward his or her health problems and the dentist's treatment

recommendations. For example, an alcoholic patient may be unwilling to follow recommendations about diet and oral health regimens. Patients should be questioned regarding alcohol and recreational drug use including what is consumed, frequency of use, and quantity. Patients who abuse these substances may be poor risks for certain types of treatment, because of either the acute effects of these drugs or the long-term effects of chronic abuse.

Tobacco use is a lifestyle habit with direct impact on the successful outcome of treatment of periodontal disease, and it is an important part of the social history (see Chapter 34). Tobacco use is an important risk factor in the prevalence, severity, and progression of periodontitis.[3] Information on tobacco use should not be restricted to a simple "yes" or "no" answer. The medical history should include specific questions on type of tobacco product used—for example, cigarettes, cigars, pipe, or smokeless tobacco, or any combination of these different products—and the frequency of use, both in terms of number of times per day and years of use. This will give the dentist information on the severity of the nicotine dependency of the patient and also will allow an estimate of the possible outcome of different modalities of periodontal therapy. Patients should be counseled on the risks of tobacco use and on its detrimental effect on periodontal health and on any periodontal therapy rendered. Thus patients should be asked specific questions on their desire to quit using tobacco and on any past efforts to quit.

Review of Systems

A review of medical systems should be performed to clarify any positive responses from either the questionnaire or from the verbal interview. Questions that may be useful for a review of the cardiovascular and cerebrovascular systems are included in Box 36-2. The medical history should specifically ask about each of these conditions, and follow-up questions should be asked during the interview.[4] Data should include how long the condition has been present and what limitations the patient may have as a result of that condition. Cardiac conditions should be assessed and may or may not require additional consultation with the patient's physician, but it is desirable to investigate the relevance of the condition before treatment.

If there is a history of stroke, the type of stroke, the time since the stroke, history of repeated strokes, and the level of deficit and recovery should be determined. If there is a history of ischemic stroke, patients frequently have some degree of medically necessary anticoagulation. It may be necessary to obtain information on their International Normalized Ratio (INR) values before treatment to assess the possibility of bleeding (see Chapter 37). It is likely that the level of anticoagulation necessary for scaling and root planing would be different from that which would be

ADA. American Dental Association
www.ada.org

Medical Alert:	Condition:	Premedication:	Allergies:	Anesthesia:	Date:

HEALTH HISTORY FORM

Name: _____ Home Phone: ( )_____ Business Phone: ( )_____
　　　LAST　　　　　FIRST　　　　MIDDLE

Address: _____ City: _____ State: _____ Zip Code: _____
　　　P.O. BOX or Mailing Address

Occupation: _____ Height: _____ Weight: _____ Date of Birth: _____ Sex: M ☐ F ☐

SS#: _____ Emergency Contact: _____ Relationship: _____ Phone: ( )_____

If you are completing this form for another person, what is your relationship to that person? _____

　　　　　　　　　　　　　　　　　　　　　　　　　　　　　　　NAME　　　　　　　　RELATIONSHIP

For the following questions, please (X) whichever applies, your answers are for our records only and will be kept confidential in accordance with applicable laws. Please note that during your initial visit you will be asked some questions about your responses to this questionnaire and there may be additional questions concerning your health. This information is vital to allow us to provide appropriate care for you. This office does not use this information to discriminate.

DENTAL INFORMATION

	Yes	No	Don't Know
Do your gums bleed when you brush?	☐	☐	☐
Have you ever had orthodontic (braces) treatment?	☐	☐	☐
Are your teeth sensitive to cold, hot, sweets or pressure?	☐	☐	☐
Do you have earaches or neck pains?	☐	☐	☐
Have you had any periodontal (gum) treatments?	☐	☐	☐
Do you wear removable dental appliances?	☐	☐	☐
Have you had a serious/difficult problem associated with any previous dental treatment?	☐	☐	☐

If yes, explain:

How would you describe your current dental problem? _____

Date of your last dental exam: _____

Date of last dental x-rays: _____

What was done at that time? _____

How do you feel about the appearance of your teeth? _____

MEDICAL INFORMATION

	Yes	No	Don't Know
If you answer yes to any of the 3 items below, please stop and return this form to the receptionist.			
Have you had any of the following diseases or problems?			
Active Tuberculosis	☐	☐	☐
Persistent cough greater than a 3 week duration	☐	☐	☐
Cough that produces blood	☐	☐	☐
Are you in good health?	☐	☐	☐
Has there been any change in your general health within the past year?	☐	☐	☐
Are you now under the care of a physician?	☐	☐	☐

If yes, what is/are the condition(s) being treated? _____

Date of last physical examination: _____

Physician: _____
NAME　　　　　　　　　PHONE

ADDRESS　　　CITY/STATE　　　ZIP

NAME　　　　　　　　　PHONE

ADDRESS　　　CITY/STATE　　　ZIP

	Yes	No	Don't Know
Have you had any serious illness, operation, or been hospitalized in the past 5 years?	☐	☐	☐

If yes, what was the illness or problem? _____

	Yes	No	Don't Know
Are you taking or have you recently taken any medicine(s) including non-prescription medicine?	☐	☐	☐

If yes, what medicine(s) are you taking?

Prescribed: _____

Over the counter: _____

Vitamins, natural or herbal preparations and/or diet supplements: _____

	Yes	No	Don't Know
Are you taking, or have you taken, any diet drugs such Pondimin (fenfluramine), Redux (dexphenfluramine) or phen-fen (fenfluramine-phentermine combination)?	☐	☐	☐
Do you drink alcoholic beverages?	☐	☐	☐

If yes, how much alcohol did you drink in the last 24 hours?

In the past week? _____

	Yes	No	Don't Know
Are you alcohol and/or drug dependent?	☐	☐	☐
If yes, have you received treatment? (circle one) Yes / No			
Do you use drugs or other substances for recreational purposes?	☐	☐	☐

If yes, please list:

Frequency of use (daily, weekly, etc.): _____

Number of years of recreational drug use: _____

	Yes	No	Don't Know
Do you use tobacco (smoking, snuff, chew)?	☐	☐	☐
If yes, how interested are you in stopping? (circle one) Very / Somewhat / Not interested			
Do you wear contact lenses?	☐	☐	☐

PLEASE COMPLETE BOTH SIDES

Figure 36-1. American Dental Association medical history form.

Continued

Are you allergic to or have you had a reaction to?

	Yes	No	Don't Know
Local anesthetics	❏	❏	❏
Aspirin	❏	❏	❏
Penicillin or other antibiotics	❏	❏	❏
Barbiturates, sedatives, or sleeping pills	❏	❏	❏
Sulfa drugs	❏	❏	❏
Codeine or other narcotics	❏	❏	❏
Latex	❏	❏	❏
Iodine	❏	❏	❏
Hay fever/seasonal	❏	❏	❏
Animals	❏	❏	❏
Food (specify) _____	❏	❏	❏
Other (specify) _____	❏	❏	❏
Metals (specify) _____	❏	❏	❏

To yes responses, specify type of reaction.
_____
_____
_____

	Yes	No	Don't Know
Have you had an orthopedic total joint (hip, knee, elbow, finger) replacement?	❏	❏	❏

If yes, when was this operation done? _____

If you answered yes to the above question, have you had any complications or difficulties with your prosthetic joint?
_____

	Yes	No	Don't Know
Has a physician or previous dentist recommended that you take antibiotics prior to your dental treatment?	❏	❏	❏

If yes, what antibiotic and dose? _____
Name of physician or dentist*: _____
Phone: _____

WOMEN ONLY

	Yes	No	Don't Know
Are you or could you be pregnant?	❏	❏	❏
Nursing?	❏	❏	❏
Taking birth control pills or hormonal replacement?	❏	❏	❏

Please (X) a response to indicate if you have or have not had any of the following diseases or problems.

	Yes	No	Don't Know
Abnormal bleeding	❏	❏	❏
AIDS or HIV infection	❏	❏	❏
Anemia	❏	❏	❏
Arthritis	❏	❏	❏
Rheumatoid arthritis	❏	❏	❏
Asthma	❏	❏	❏
Blood transfusion. If yes, date: _____	❏	❏	❏
Cancer/Chemotherapy/Radiation Treatment	❏	❏	❏
Cardiovascular disease. If yes, specify below:	❏	❏	❏

___Angina   ___Heart murmur
___Arteriosclerosis   ___High blood pressure
___Artificial heart valves   ___Low blood pressure
___Congenital heart defects   ___Mitral valve prolapse
___Congestive heart failure   ___Pacemaker
___Coronary artery disease   ___Rheumatic heart
___Damaged heart valves   disease/Rheumatic fever
___Heart attack

	Yes	No	Don't Know
Chest pain upon exertion	❏	❏	❏
Chronic pain	❏	❏	❏
Disease, drug, or radiation-induced immunosurpression	❏	❏	❏
Diabetes. If yes, specify below:	❏	❏	❏

___Type I (Insulin dependent)   ___Type II

	Yes	No	Don't Know
Dry Mouth	❏	❏	❏
Eating disorder. If yes, specify: _____	❏	❏	❏
Epilepsy	❏	❏	❏
Fainting spells or seizures	❏	❏	❏
Gastrointestinal disease	❏	❏	❏
G.E. Reflux/persistent heartburn	❏	❏	❏
Glaucoma	❏	❏	❏

	Yes	No	Don't Know
Hemophilia	❏	❏	❏
Hepatitis, jaundice or liver disease	❏	❏	❏
Recurrent Infections	❏	❏	❏
If yes, indicate type of infection: _____			
Kidney problems	❏	❏	❏
Mental health disorders. If yes, specify: _____	❏	❏	❏
Malnutrition	❏	❏	❏
Night sweats	❏	❏	❏
Neurological disorders. If yes, specify: _____	❏	❏	❏
Osteoporosis	❏	❏	❏
Persistent swollen glands in neck			
Respiratory problems. If yes, specify below:	❏	❏	❏

___ Emphysema   ___ Bronchitis, etc.

	Yes	No	Don't Know
Severe headaches/migraines	❏	❏	❏
Severe or rapid weight loss	❏	❏	❏
Sexually transmitted disease	❏	❏	❏
Sinus trouble	❏	❏	❏
Sleep disorder	❏	❏	❏
Sores or ulcers in the mouth	❏	❏	❏
Stroke	❏	❏	❏
Systemic lupus erythematosus	❏	❏	❏
Tuberculosis	❏	❏	❏
Thyroid problems	❏	❏	❏
Ulcers	❏	❏	❏
Excessive urination	❏	❏	❏
Do you have any disease, condition, or problem not listed above that you think I should know about?	❏	❏	❏

Please explain: _____

NOTE: Both Doctor and patient are encouraged to discuss any and all relevant patient health issues prior to treatment.

I certify that I have read and understand the above. I acknowledge that my questions, if any, about inquiries set forth above have been answered to my satisfaction. I will not hold my dentist, or any other member of his/her staff, responsible for any action they take or do not take because of errors or omissions that I may have made in the completion of this form.

_____   _____
SIGNATURE OF PATIENT/LEGAL GUARDIAN   DATE

FOR COMPLETION BY DENTIST

Comments on patient interview concerning health history: _____

Significant findings from questionnaire or oral interview: _____

Dental management considerations: _____

Health History Update: On a regular basis the patient should be questioned about any medical history changes, date and comments notated, along with signature.

Date	Comments	Signature of patient and dentist
_____	_____	_____
_____	_____	_____

©2002 American Dental Association   S500

Figure 36-1. cont'd.

| Box 36-2 | Pertinent Questions Relative to Cardiovascular and Cerebrovascular Disease |

Does the patient have a history of any of the following:
- Myocardial infarction (heart attack)
- Angina (chest pain)
- Bypass surgery
- Congestive heart failure
- Heart valve defects
- Mitral valve prolapse
- Heart murmur
- Rheumatic heart disease
- Hypertension
- Coronary artery disease
- Implantable pacemaker
- Implantable defibrillator
- Cerebrovascular accident (stroke)
- Transient ischemic attack

needed for surgical therapy. Frequent interaction with the patient's physician may be required for treatment of these patients.

Respiratory concerns that should be addressed when taking a medical history are in Box 36-3. A positive response to questions about these conditions warrants additional investigation.[2] For example, if the patient has asthma, what induces the reaction? How often does the patient have an asthma attack? Does the attack respond readily to treatment? If the patient has emphysema, is supplemental oxygen required? If a patient is positive for tuberculosis and the disease is active, this may contraindicate treatment other than palliative or emergency care. Active tuberculosis requires the provider to use special mask protection to prevent inhalation of the infective agent. If the patient is under medical treatment for any of these conditions, what is the patient being treated with, for how long, and what is the current disease status? If there is

| Box 36-3 | Pertinent Questions Relative to Respiratory Disease |

Does the patient have a history of any of the following:
- Asthma
- Emphysema
- Chronic bronchitis
- Chronic obstructive pulmonary disease (COPD)
- Upper respiratory disease
  - Sinusitis
  - Hay fever
  - Seasonal allergies
- Tobacco use

any uncertainty about the patient's respiratory status, a physician consult is indicated.

For upper respiratory problems, the dentist should ascertain the frequency and severity of the condition, and if any etiologic factors, such as dust, mold, or pollen are associated with the condition. The influence of upper respiratory conditions and their relation to facial pain could be of importance in the differential diagnosis of a patient's chief complaint. The symptomatology of a sinus infection may closely mimic odontogenic pain, and a history of previous sinusitis may assist the dentist in arriving at a correct diagnosis and avoiding treatment errors. The presence of chronic sinusitis may also be a relative contraindication for sinus elevation procedures.

A major risk factor in the progression of periodontal disease is a history of diabetes mellitus[2,5,7] (see Chapter 31). Signs of diabetes mellitus should be evaluated in patients that deny a history of the disease. If the patient confirms the presence of some of these signs, such as thirst, fatigue, increased frequency of urination, and loss of weight in a nondieting situation, a referral to the physician may be indicated. Patients who report a positive family history of diabetes mellitus and exhibit any of the above signs and symptoms should be referred immediately for physician evaluation of possible undiagnosed diabetes. In patients with a history of diabetes, the presence of either type 1 or type 2 diabetes should be determined (see Chapter 37). The method of control of their blood glucose and medication dose should be determined. The methods could include diet, oral medication, insulin, or a combination of these methods. The dentist should review the patient's level of glycemic control, the frequency of blood sugar testing, and the range of blood glucose values obtained. It is common for the dentist to contact the patient's physician for an objective assessment of the patient's metabolic control.

For hepatic disease, the dentist should inquire about any episodes of jaundice or hepatitis. If a positive response is obtained, the clinician should determine what type of hepatitis was contracted, when it occurred, whether the patient is a carrier, and the treatment provided. Because the liver is responsible for the production of numerous clotting factors, there may be a need to evaluate for possible bleeding concerns during treatment (see Chapter 37). The dentist should also exercise caution in prescribing medications metabolized by the liver such as aspirin, acetaminophen, ibuprofen, tetracycline, and metronidazole.

Patients may have a history of either osteoarthritis or rheumatoid arthritis. These patients often are being treated with nonsteroidal antiinflammatory drugs or steroids, or both. Nonsteroidal antiinflammatory drugs could lead to increased bleeding because of their effects on platelets. Steroid use may induce adrenal suppression, mask oral infection, or impair wound healing.[2] The increased stress of an acute oral infection, odontogenic pain, or significant dental treatment may induce an adrenal crisis. The physician should be consulted for patients taking steroids on a long-term basis, or patients taking high doses of steroids even on a short-term basis. Patients with arthritis should be questioned as to their ability to perform adequate oral hygiene. They may have difficulty in holding a toothbrush or using dental floss, and instruction on proper use of dental aids may be needed to help them obtain optimal oral hygiene. For patients with symptomatic arthritis, appointments may need to be kept short and the patient allowed to make frequent changes in position.

Renal disease can manifest itself as a variety of conditions.[8] These could range from a history of kidney stones (renal calculi) to end-stage renal failure. Because the kidney is involved in excretion of many medications, one must be certain that the patient will adequately eliminate any medication prescribed, to avoid any undesirable complications. Caution should be used with the recommendation of any nephrotoxic medications.

Joint replacement is being seen at an increasing frequency with more than 100,000 major joint prostheses being placed annually. Microbial infection is the major cause of prosthetic joint failure. It is necessary to determine what joints have been replaced, the reason why this was indicated, the length of time since placement, and any cautions the patient has received from the physician. It is generally recommended that the patient be premedicated before dental procedures that may induce bleeding for at least the first 2 years after joint replacement.[9] The organisms most frequently implicated in infection are *Staphylococcus aureus* and *Staphylococcus epidermidis*, which are rare inhabitants of the oral flora. If there is any uncertainty, the patient's physician should be contacted for clarification and/or recommendations in providing treatment.

Bleeding disorders may manifest during a broad range of conditions[2] (see Chapter 37). The bleeding tendency could be caused by hereditary conditions such as hemophilia or von Willebrand's disease, an autoimmune disease such as thrombocytopenia, liver problems such as cirrhosis, or by design such as a patient on daily aspirin or warfarin (Coumadin) therapy. Patients should be questioned about possible bleeding problems. Have they received transfusions for their problem. If yes, was it one instance or more frequently? When they cut themselves, can they stop the bleeding themselves or do they need medical assistance? If they are on anticoagulant therapy, do they receive frequent monitoring and do they know their current INR value? The underlying cause of the bleeding tendency should be ascertained and the level of treatment that may be provided may best be determined by consultation with their physician. With appropriate medical management, most periodontal therapy can be provided to these patients.

A patient may have a past or current history of cancer (Box 36-4). Depending on the type of cancer and the treatment provided, there is a wide variation in the effect it may have on dental treatment (see Chapter 37).[2,10-13] Cancer of the head and neck treated with radiation may greatly limit what treatment can be provided. Xerostomia often develops in these patients, with an increased incidence of dental caries, and osteoradionecrosis also may develop. Periodontal surgical therapy may be contraindicated in these patients. Cancer located at distant sites may have a minimal to a major influence on dental care. The immune status of the patient and the type of treatment administered to control the cancer can impact dental treatment and its results. The dentist should obtain information on the type of cancer, the staging, and the treatment. Did the patient receive chemotherapy, radiation therapy, or a combination of approaches? If the patient received radiation therapy for head and neck cancer, it is critical to determine the total radiation dose and the exact anatomic locations that were irradiated. The physician should be consulted to obtain this information. The physician can also help in determining the appropriate timing for dental treatment if the patient is receiving active cancer treatment.

More and more patients are seeking dental treatment while also being treated with immunosuppressive medications (see Chapter 37). Some have received organ transplants and are being treated to prevent tissue rejection, whereas others could be receiving treatment for an autoimmune disease. It is important to know what medications are being prescribed and what level of immunosuppression is present. Is the patient more

---

Box 36-4   Pertinent Questions Relative to Cancer Therapy

Has the patient had radiation therapy?
    What was the total radiation dose?
    Exactly what regions were irradiated?
    Will dental treatment be performed in the irradiated area? Will this dental treatment increase the risk for osteoradionecrosis?
    How long ago was the radiation treatment done?
Has the patient had chemotherapy?
    How long has it been since the last chemotherapy treatment?
    Is the patient still under active chemotherapy?
    Is there an increased risk for oral infection?
        What is the patient's white blood cell count?
        What is the patient's absolute neutrophil count?
    Is there an increased risk for oral bleeding?
    What is the patient's platelet count?

susceptible to infection and will he or she require pre-medication for dental care? Is there a greater risk for bleeding? What side effects could develop that are detrimental to oral health? For example, patients being treated with cyclosporine are at a greater risk for development of gingival enlargement. These are just some of the questions that can be evaluated in consultation with the patient's physician.

Patients should be asked about the presence of any current infections and what treatment is being provided to treat the infection. Infections could range from acute respiratory infection, to chronic osteomyelitis, to sexually transmitted diseases, to human immunodeficiency virus infection. An entire gamut of infection is possible, and knowledge of current or past infections and past and present treatment helps provide appropriate care.

Female patients may present with circumstances unique to their sex. The dentist should be informed when the patient is pregnant or nursing. This could modify dental treatment in a variety of ways.[2] Exposure to radiation should be minimized in pregnant patients. The use of medications is often modified in women who are pregnant or are nursing. Women may also be using oral contraceptive therapy. Pregnancy or use of oral contraceptives may modify the patient's response to plaque leading to an increase in gingival inflammation (see Chapter 31). Knowing that a woman is pregnant early in gestation allows the dentist to provide a thorough periodontal examination and appropriate care to reduce the presence of periodontal pathogens and level of periodontal inflammation, possibly decreasing the risk for adverse pregnancy outcomes[14,15] (see Chapter 32).

A history of any allergies should be obtained and reviewed for their ability to modify dental treatment. The clinician should determine if there are any allergies to environmental agents, medications, local anesthetics, iodine, or latex. The type of reaction that occurred with respect to the allergen should be elicited. Some responses may be caused by a side effect and may not be a true allergy, whereas others may indeed be a serious allergic reaction. Patients should be questioned about the presence of hives or itching, any difficulty breathing, and the presence of any anaphylactic reaction. Any medication used previously to treat reactions or relieve symptoms should be determined and documented in the patient's dental chart.

Review of Medications

The patient should provide the dentist with a list of current medications. This should include all prescription medication, over-the-counter medication, vitamins, and herbal preparations. The indication for each medication should be determined and medications should be reviewed for their possible influence on dental care. Patients can

then be advised of possible interactions or influences of their medications on their dental health and care. Likewise, any potential interactions between medications currently being taken by the patient and those the dentist considers prescribing can be determined.

DENTAL HISTORY

After obtaining an adequate medical history, the clinician can then proceed to the dental history. A detailed dental history will help to better define treatment approaches to the patient's dental needs by evaluating his or her past dental care along with the current dental concerns and perceptions. Again the initial focal point is evaluation of the patient's chief complaint. Was the patient referred for treatment? If so, by whom and for what specific reasons? Additional information should be obtained about any history of dental treatment and about the patient's level of compliance. Does the patient have any history of oral injury, serious oral infection, or radiation therapy to the head and neck region? If there is a history of extractions, were there any problems with pain, bleeding, infection, or anesthesia? Positive responses will require additional data gathering. Were the teeth extracted because of caries, periodontal problems, or some other reason? Has the patient worn prostheses to replace missing teeth? If so, is the patient still wearing these prostheses? If not, why not? Was the patient dissatisfied with the function or esthetics of the prostheses? When discussing past dental experiences, the dentist should determine if past experiences were pleasant or unpleasant, and if the patient has been satisfied with prior treatment. If the patient has seen 10 dentists in the past 10 years and none of them was "good," it is highly likely that the twelfth dentist will find out that the eleventh dentist was also poor. By knowing the patient's past experiences and current expectations, the clinician can better develop an individualized approach to the patient's treatment.

Past periodontal therapy and current oral hygiene practices should be evaluated. For oral hygiene evaluation, what do the patients use to clean their teeth, how frequently and for how long? Do they brush for 10 seconds or for 10 minutes? The effectiveness of their oral hygiene habits can be confirmed visually during the initial examination. Does the cleanliness of their mouth seem to be in agreement with their methods of oral hygiene and does the stated time allotted to oral hygiene seem reasonable for the observed clinical appearance? For past periodontal therapy, what was the nature of treatment, how long ago was the treatment, were they satisfied with their past care, and how readily did they comply with the previous dentist's treatment recommendations? Did they receive maintenance therapy? If yes, with what recall frequency, and with what level of compliance? What is their impression of their current periodontal health? Are they aware of increased bleeding when flossing, drifting teeth, increased mobility, recession, or pain, or do they feel that their status is stable or showing improvement? Patients' answers will help the dentist to plan the course for their future care.

The patient should be asked about the presence or absence of tooth hypersensitivity. If the teeth are sensitive, the patient could have a restorative, endodontic, or periodontal problem, or a combination of problems. Is the observed pain elicited by cold, hot, sweets, or other stimuli? Is the pain transient or persistent? If persistent, is it of a long or short duration? Is the sensitivity localized to a given tooth or teeth, or is it more generalized in nature?

The patient should be asked about episodes of clenching or bruxism, which can be confirmed by the presence of wear facets, fremitus, and other patterns of mobility. Other parafunctional habits that may be uncovered by questioning and examination could include using teeth as tools, such as holding pins, biting thread or fingernails, or opening bottles. Can the patient open as widely as they would like or do they have concerns about being able to open adequately during dental visits? The patient should be asked about past cold sores or herpetic lesions and about canker sores or aphthous ulceration. If positive response is obtained, the dentist should ask about the frequency and locations of the lesions, and if the patient is aware of any trigger that could lead to lesion recurrence.

Patients should be questioned about changes in their overall stress level and any changes in their daily routines.[16] Do they feel that stress has affected their oral health? Has stress affected any other behaviors such as alcohol or tobacco use? The dentist should attempt to discover the value that the patient places on maintaining his or her teeth and oral health. Patients who are not concerned about losing many or all of their teeth would most likely agree to a different treatment plan than patients who want to maintain all of their teeth. Finally, the dentist should look for familial trends in oral disease patterns or health behaviors. Does the patient have parents and/or siblings with a history of periodontal disease? If yes, were they treated and how successful was their care?

In summary, to provide the best periodontal treatment to our patients, dentists, dental hygienists, and ancillary personnel must know their patients. We should know their medical and dental history, and update these on a frequent basis. We should know what the patient expects from treatment and at what end-point they wish to arrive. By first getting to know each patient through his or her medical and dental history, we will be able to develop and individualize the proper treatment plan for that patient. This will better allow both the patient and the dentist to achieve their desired goals in the provision of periodontal care.

REFERENCES

1. Jolly DE: Evaluation of the medical history, *Dent Clin North Am* 38:361-380, 1994.
2. Mealey BL: Periodontal implications. Medically compromised patients, *Ann Periodontol* 1:256-321, 1996.
3. Tonetti MS: Cigarette smoking and periodontal diseases: etiology and management of diseases, *Ann Periodontol* 3:88-101, 1998.
4. Rose LF, Mealey B, Minsk L, Cohen DW: Oral care for patients with cardiovascular disease and stroke, *J Am Dent Assoc* 133:37s-44s, 2002.
5. Grossi S, Genco R: Periodontal disease and diabetes mellitus, *Ann Periodontol* 3:51-61, 1998.
6. Mealey BL: Diabetes mellitus. In Rose LF, Genco RJ, Mealey BL, Cohen DW, editors: *Periodontal medicine*, Toronto, 2000, BC Decker Publishers.
7. Mealey BL: Diabetes and periodontal disease: two sides of a coin, *Compend Contin Educ Dent* 21:943-956, 2000.
8. Ziccardi VB, Saini J, Demas PN, Braun TW: Management of the oral and maxillofacial surgery patient with end-stage renal disease, *J Oral Maxillofac Surg* 50:1207-1212, 1992.
9. Seymour RA, Whitworth JM: Antibiotic prophylaxis for endocarditis, prosthetic joints, and surgery, *Dent Clin North Am* 46:635-651, 2002.
10. Semba SE, Mealey BL, Hallmon WW: The head and neck radiotherapy patient: part 1—oral manifestations of radiation therapy, *Compend Contin Educ Dent* 15:250-260, 1994.
11. Mealey BL, Semba SE, Hallmon WW: Dentistry and the cancer patient: part 1—oral manifestations and complications of chemotherapy, *Compend Contin Educ Dent* 15:1252-1261, 1994.
12. Semba SE, Mealey BL, Hallmon WW: Dentistry and the cancer patient: part 2—oral health management of the chemotherapy patient, *Compend Contin Educ Dent* 15:1378-1387, 1994.
13. Mealey BL, Semba SE, Hallmon WW: The head and neck radiotherapy patient: part 2—management of oral complications, *Compend Contin Educ Dent* 15:442-458, 1994.
14. Jeffcoat MK, Geurs NC, Reddy MS et al: Current evidence regarding periodontal disease as a risk factor in preterm birth, *Ann Periodontol* 6:183-188, 2001.
15. Lopez NJ, Smith PC, Gutierrez J: Periodontal therapy may reduce the risk of preterm low birth weight in women with periodontal disease: a randomized controlled trial, *J Periodontol* 73:911-924, 2002.
16. Genco RJ, Ho AW, Kopman J et al: Models to evaluate the role of stress in periodontal disease, *Ann Periodontol* 3:288-302, 1998.

37

Periodontal Treatment of the Medically Compromised Patient

Terry D. Rees and Brian L. Mealey

Many patients seeking treatment from dental health professionals have systemic conditions that may alter the provision of dental care. This may result from changes in overall systemic stability of the patient and in the patient's ability to tolerate dental therapy. Furthermore, patients may be taking a variety of medications as part of their medical management that may affect oral health and dental treatment. While Chapter 31 focuses on systemic conditions affecting the periodontum, this chapter reviews conditions that may require alterations in the normal pathways and practices of dental therapy.

HORMONAL CONSIDERATIONS

Dental Treatment of the Patient with Diabetes

Proper dental management of patients with diabetes requires a thorough understanding of the diagnostic testing and medical management currently in use. Patients with undiagnosed diabetes may present with one or more signs and symptoms (Box 37-1). The diagnosis of diabetes is based on the presence of these clinical signs and symptoms together with specific laboratory findings. The diagnostic guidelines were most recently published by the American Diabetes Association in 2003 (Box 37-2).[1] Under these guidelines, the primary laboratory tests used for diagnosis of diabetes are the fasting glucose and casual (nonfasting) glucose. The diagnosis of diabetes is not made until the patient has exceeded threshold glucose levels on two separate occasions. Urinary glucose analysis is no longer used in establishing the diagnosis of diabetes. If the clinician suspects that a patient has undiagnosed diabetes, the patient should be asked questions related to the classic signs of diabetes such as:

- How many times do you get up to go to the bathroom at night? (polyuria)
- Does your mouth often feel dry? Do you often feel thirsty, even shortly after you've had something to drink? (polydipsia)
- Do you get hungry again not long after you've eaten? (polyphagia)
- Have you had any changes in your vision recently?
- Have you lost weight recently or had any unexplained weight loss in the past?

If any of these questions further substantiate a suspicion of diabetes, the patient should be referred for appropriate laboratory testing and physician consultation.

When a patient is known to have diabetes, the clinician must establish the degree of glycemic control before beginning periodontal therapy. Patients with diabetes and periodontal disease respond well to periodontal therapy when their blood glucose is well controlled.[2,3] In fact, the patient with well controlled diabetes should generally receive the same type of periodontal therapy that would

Box 37-1 | Signs and Symptoms of Undiagnosed or Poorly Controlled Diabetes

- Polydipsia (excessive thirst)
- Polyuria (excessive urination)
- Polyphagia (excessive hunger)
- Unexplained weight loss
- Changes in vision
- Weakness, malaise
- Irritability
- Nausea
- Dry mouth
- Ketoacidosis*

Ketoacidosis is usually associated with severe hyperglycemia and occurs primarily in type 1 diabetes.

Box 37-2 | Criteria for Diagnosis of Diabetes

Diabetes may be diagnosed by any one of three laboratory methods. Whatever method is used *must be confirmed on a subsequent day* by using any one of the three methods:

1. Symptoms of diabetes plus casual (nonfasting) plasma glucose ≥200 mg/dl. Casual glucose may be drawn at any time of day without regard to time since the last meal.
2. Fasting plasma glucose ≥126 mg/dl. Fasting is defined as no caloric intake for at least 8 hours.
3. Two-hour postprandial glucose ≥200 mg/dl during an oral glucose tolerance test. The test should be performed using a glucose load containing the equivalent of 75 g anhydrous glucose dissolved in water.*

Categories of fasting plasma glucose (FPG) include:
1. FPG <110 mg/dl = normal fasting glucose
2. FPG ≥110 mg/dl and <126 mg/dl = impaired fasting glucose
3. FPG ≥126 mg/dl = provisional diagnosis of diabetes (must be confirmed on subsequent day)

Categories of 2-hour postprandial glucose (2hPG) include:
1. 2hPG <140 mg/dl = normal glucose tolerance
2. 2hPG ≥140 mg/dl and <200 mg/dl = impaired glucose tolerance
3. 2hPG ≥200 mg/dl = provisional diagnosis of diabetes (must be confirmed on subsequent day)

From American Diabetes Association: Report of the expert committee on the diagnosis and classification of diabetes mellitus, Diabetes Care 26(suppl 1):s5-s24, 2003.
*The third method is not recommended for routine clinical use.

be appropriate for a patient without diabetes. Conversely, when glucose control is poor, the response to periodontal therapy is often poor as well.[4] For this reason, the patient with poorly controlled diabetes should receive treatment for acute periodontal problems, but should not have extensive therapy until blood glucose is controlled. Research has shown that thorough debridement through scaling and root planing may not only improve periodontal health, but may also improve glycemic control in many patients with diabetes. (See Chapter 32.) This is most likely to occur in a patient with poorly controlled diabetes who receives scaling and root planing in combination with systemic tetracycline antibiotics, such as doxycycline, for 14 days.[5-8]

How does the clinician establish the degree of glycemic control? Asking the patient how well controlled he or she is can be worthwhile; however, this method often provides an inaccurate assessment. The best method of determining glycemic control in a known diabetic patient is through the glycated, or glycosylated, hemoglobin assay (also called the glycohemoglobin test).[8] This test allows determination of blood glucose status over the 30 to 90 days before collection of the blood sample. This is in contrast to the fasting and casual plasma glucose tests, which provide a determination of glucose levels at only a single moment in time; namely, at the time the blood sample is collected. As glucose circulates in the bloodstream, it becomes attached to a portion of the hemoglobin molecule on red blood cells. The greater the plasma glucose levels over time, the greater the percentage of hemoglobin that becomes glycated. There are two different glycated hemoglobin assays in use: the hemoglobin A1 test (HbA1) and the hemoglobin A1c test (HbA1c), with the HbA1c being used most often. Because these tests measure two different portions of the hemoglobin molecule, the normal range for the test results differs. The normal HbA1 is less than approximately 8%, whereas the normal HbA1c is less than 6.0% (Box 37-3). The American Diabetes Association recommends that individuals with diabetes attempt to achieve a target HbA1c of less than 7%, whereas an HbA1c greater than 8% suggests that a change in patient management may be needed to improve glycemic control.[9] The HbA1C assay

became available as an at-home test in 2002. If at-home use becomes widespread, it will simplify assessment of this important parameter of glycemic control.

Self-blood glucose monitoring has revolutionized patient management of diabetes.[10] Development of small, handheld glucometers has allowed the patient with diabetes to take much greater control of his or her disease. Glucometers use a small drop of capillary blood from a finger-stick sample to assess glucose levels in seconds to minutes (Figs. 37-1 through 37-3). Almost all patients with diabetes that use insulin have a glucometer, as do many taking oral agents. There are a variety of different glucometers available. The frequency with which the patient tests his or her blood glucose depends on that patient's individual treatment regimen. Some patients test once a day or even less often. Others, especially those taking insulin, test multiple times each day. As a general rule, more intensively managed patients with diabetes use self-blood glucose monitoring more frequently than less intensively managed individuals.

Medical management of diabetes involves a combination of diet, exercise, weight reduction, and medications. The goal of diabetic management is to maintain blood glucose levels as near to the normal range as possible. Several long-term studies have clearly documented the tremendous reduction in diabetic complications that can be achieved through good glucose management.[11-16] Patients with diabetes are now much more rigorously controlled than they were before these studies. The oral health care provider must have a clear understanding of each individual patient's medical regimen to provide safe and proper dental care.

Box 37-3	Evaluation of Glycemic Control in Patients with Diabetes Using HbA1c	
≤6%	Normal	
<7%	Good glycemic control	
7% to 8%	Moderate glycemic control	
>8%	Suggest action to improve glycemic control	

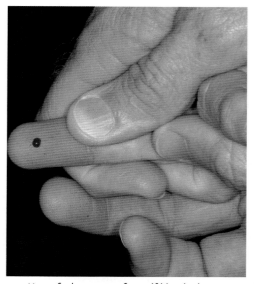

Figure 37-1. Use of glucometer for self-blood glucose monitoring. A lancet is used to prick the finger and a small drop of blood is obtained.

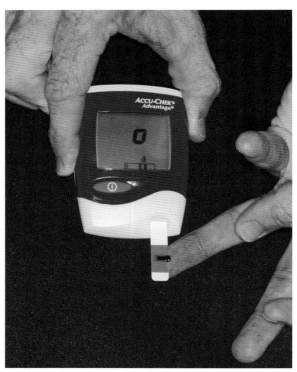

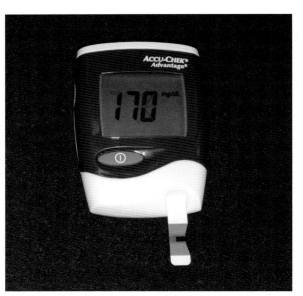

Figure 37-3. Use of glucometer for self-blood glucose monitoring. The glucometer takes several seconds to determine blood glucose, and the value is displayed on the screen. In this case, the blood glucose is 170 mg/dl.

Figure 37-2. Use of glucometer for self-blood glucose monitoring. Drop of blood is placed on a strip inserted into the glucometer.

In particular, the clinician must know exactly which medications the patient takes to control his or her diabetic condition. All patients with type 1 diabetes take insulin by injection, as do many with type 2 (Table 37-1). Insulins are classified as rapid-, short-, intermediate-, or long-acting.[8,17] Each type of insulin has its own time of onset, peak activity, and duration. In addition, the pharmacodynamics of insulins vary widely among individuals. Oral agents are commonly used in management of diabetes. There are five major classes of oral agents: sulfonylureas, biguanides, meglitinides, thiazolidinediones, and alpha-glucosidase inhibitors (Table 37-2). The mechanism of action differs among these drug classes, as does the propensity for patients taking them to develop hypoglycemia—episodes of low blood glucose that can be life threatening.

Periodontal treatment of the patient with diabetes depends on both the periodontal diagnosis and on the patient's degree of glycemic control. Patients with gingivitis should receive thorough home care instructions and complete debridement of the teeth. The response to therapy may not be as favorable in patients with poor glycemic control (HbA1c >10%) as it is in those with better control (HbA1c <8%). Patients with poorly controlled diabetes may continue to exhibit gingival redness and bleeding, despite improved plaque control.

For patients with periodontitis, the type of periodontal therapy is highly dependent on glycemic control (Fig 37-4). Once a diagnosis of periodontitis has been established, the clinician should determine the level of glycemic control through evaluation of recent glycated hemoglobin values and physician consultation, as indicated. If the

TABLE 37-1	Types of Insulin			
TYPE OF INSULIN	INSULIN CLASSIFICATION	ONSET OF ACTIVITY	PEAK ACTIVITY	DURATION OF ACTIVITY
• Lispro/Aspart	Rapid-acting	15 min	30-90 min	<5 hr
• Regular	Short-acting	30-60 min	2-3 hr	4-12 hr
• NPH	Intermediate-acting	2-4 hr	4-10 hr	14-18 hr
• Lente	Intermediate-acting	3-4 hr	4-12 hr	16-20 hr
• Ultralente	Long-acting	6-10 hr	12-16 hr	20-30 hr
• Glargine	Long-acting	6-8 hr	"Peakless" (has no peak in activity)	>24 hr

TABLE 37-2   Oral Agents for Diabetes Management

AGENT CLASS/ACTION	DRUGS IN CLASS	RISK FOR HYPOGLYCEMIA
• Sulfonylureas (stimulate pancreatic insulin secretion)	• Glyburide	High
	• Glipizide	High
	• Glimepiride	Low
	• Tolbutamide	Moderate
	• Tolazamide	Moderate
• Biguanides (block production of glucose by liver; improve tissue sensitivity to insulin)	• Metformin	Very low
• Meglitinides (stimulate rapid pancreatic insulin secretion)	• Repaglinide	Low
	• Nateglinide	Low
• Thiazolidinediones (improve tissue sensitivity to insulin)	• Rosiglitazone	Very low
	• Pioglitazone	Very low
• α-Glucosidase inhibitors (slow absorption of carbohydrate from gut; decrease postprandial peaks in glycemia)	• Acarbose	Low
	• Miglitol	Low
• Combination agents	• Glucovance (metformin combined with glyburide; Bristol-Meyers Squibb; Princeton, NJ)	Moderate
	• Metaglip (metformin combined with glipizide; Bristol-Meyers Squibb; Princeton, NJ)	Moderate
	• Avandamet (metformin combined with rosiglitazone; GlaxoSmithKline; London, UK)	Very low

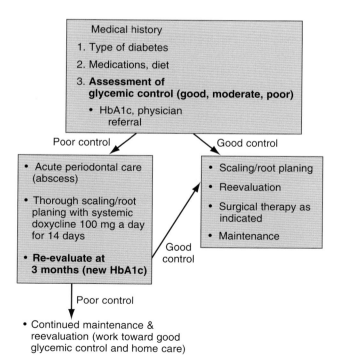

Figure 37-4. Pathways of periodontal therapy for patients with diabetes.

patient has well controlled diabetes (HbA1c <8%), periodontal therapy can generally be provided in a fashion similar to a nondiabetic person with periodontitis. This includes nonsurgical, surgical, and maintenance care. During maintenance, it is important for the clinician to not only assess the state of the periodontium, but also to continuously evaluate the patient's glycemic control. Once a relationship has been established with a patient and his or her physician, this is a simple matter of obtaining HbA1c values whenever they are accomplished. Comparison with past values can provide knowledge of the stability of the patient's diabetic condition. A patient with diabetes and periodontitis has two chronic diseases, each of which impacts on the other. Therefore, ongoing assessment of both diseases is critical to successful patient management. Because periodontal therapy usually involves multiple office visits over extended periods, the dentist and hygienist are in the perfect position to encourage patient compliance and control.

If diabetes is poorly controlled (HbA1c >10%), therapeutic pathways may need modification. The clinician should provide treatment for any emergent periodontal condition, such as a periodontal abscess. If an infection is associated with systemic signs or symptoms such as increased temperature or lymphadenopathy, a systemic antibiotic also may be indicated. Management of acute lesions should be followed by thorough scaling and root planing to remove plaque and calculus. A systemic antibiotic such as doxycycline (100 mg/day for 14 days), used in combination with scaling and root planing, may help improve glycemic control. Meticulous plaque control should be emphasized, as should the importance of improving glycemic control. Physician consultation is often indicated to describe for the physician the extent of the patient's periodontal condition and any therapy planned. After scaling and root planing, a period of 2 to 3 months should be allowed before reevaluation. At this time, the periodontal condition should be assessed for response to initial debridement. Home care should be evaluated. In patients who require further periodontal therapy, another HbA1c should be requested to determine any changes between initial therapy and reevaluation. The clinician must recall that the HbA1c evaluates glucose control over a 30- to 90-day period. Therefore, at least 60 days should be allowed to lapse between evaluations of HbA1c. If glycemic control remains poor, the patient should be placed on frequent maintenance intervals, with continued periodontal supportive care given. Glycemic control can be evaluated periodically in consultation with the physician to determine the patient's glycemic status. Only when glycemic control has improved should further periodontal therapy, such as surgical care, be considered. Otherwise, the response to treatment may be less than favorable.

The patient with moderate glycemic control (HbA1c between 8% and 10%) presents a treatment planning challenge. As with all patients, acute periodontal problems should be managed and thorough debridement should be accomplished. The clinician must pay particular attention to the patient's response to scaling and root planing and home care instruction. If the patient responds well to initial therapy and surgical treatment is indicated, the clinician should perform this treatment carefully. Smaller areas of surgical access may be indicated, allowing extended healing periods before proceeding with other areas of surgery. In this way, the individual patient response to surgical care can be determined.

The use of dental implants in patients with diabetes has not been thoroughly evaluated. Although there is some evidence in animals that poorly controlled diabetes can decrease the degree of osseointegration of dental implants,[18-20] there are no human data to support this contention. Human clinical studies have demonstrated slightly greater long-term failure rates for dental implants among patients with diabetes compared with individuals without diabetes, but the results were not definitive.[21,22] Until further evidence is presented, it is recommended that good glycemic control be established before dental implant placement.

In addition to the level of glycemic control, important considerations related to periodontal therapy for patients with diabetes include diet modification, stress reduction, and appointment timing. Periodontal treatment may result in postoperative discomfort that can limit dietary intake. To the patient with diabetes, food is medicine, and dietary intake is closely matched to medication regimens. Any changes in the ability to eat must be taken into account by the patient and clinician. Whereas some patients with diabetes are very knowledgeable about modification of diet and medications, others are not. Consultation with the physician may be indicated.

Stress reduction and adequate pain control also are important. Stressful situations increase production of endogenous catecholamines and cortisol, which increase blood glucose levels. Minimizing patient apprehension, providing profound anesthesia, and reducing postoperative discomfort through use of analgesics will help reduce fluctuation in blood glucose levels.[23]

Appointment timing is often a function of the patient's medication regimen. Although some have recommended seeing patients with diabetes in the morning, this may not be an appropriate schedule for all patients. When possible, appointments should be timed so that they do not coincide with peak insulin activity. This decreases the risk for perioperative hypoglycemia. The clinician should review the patient's medication regimen to establish when these peaks will occur. In some cases, however, it is difficult to avoid peak insulin activities because they are not always predictable. In these cases, the clinician simply needs to be aware of the potential for hypoglycemia.

Prevention of perioperative hypoglycemia is paramount when providing dental care to the patient with diabetes. Signs and symptoms of hypoglycemia range from mild to severe (Box 37-4). Although hypoglycemia may occur in patients taking oral agents such as sulfonylureas, it is much more common in those using insulin. The intensified treatment regimens for diabetes currently in use

Box 37-4	**Signs and Symptoms of Low Blood Glucose Levels (Hypoglycemia)**

- Confusion
- Agitation
- Anxiety
- Sweating
- Shakiness
- Tremors
- Tachycardia
- Dizziness
- Feeling of "impending doom"
- Seizures
- Loss of consciousness

increase the risk for hypoglycemia about threefold compared with regimens common in the past.[24,25] Signs and symptoms of hypoglycemia are most common when blood glucose levels decrease to less than 60 mg/dl, but may occur at greater levels in patients with chronic poor metabolic control.

The two best means of preventing hypoglycemia are patient questioning and assessment of capillary blood glucose. Before each dental appointment, patients should be asked what medications they have taken in the last 12 hours, what they have had to eat that day, and when they last checked their blood glucose. They also should be questioned about any history of hypoglycemic episodes. One of the most common causes of hypoglycemia in the dental office is a patient taking their normal medication regimen, but then reducing or eliminating a meal before the appointment. Because several medications increase insulin levels, including sulfonylureas and injected insulin, the patient must not skip meals or snacks that they would normally consume. To have an accurate, up-to-the-minute assessment of blood glucose, patients with diabetes should be instructed to bring their glucometers to the dental office. Before treatment, patients can assess their blood glucose in a matter of seconds (Figs. 37-1 through 37-3). If they are at or near the lower limits of normal blood glucose (about 70 to 90 mg/dl), patients can be given carbohydrates orally to increase the glucose level before commencing treatment. Likewise, if symptoms of hypoglycemia develop in the patient during the appointment, they can immediately assess their blood glucose level using their glucometer.

If hypoglycemia develops during dental treatment, it should be treated immediately (Box 37-5). If the patient is able to take food by mouth, about 15 g oral carbohydrates should be given. If the oral route cannot be used, emergency drugs may include 50% dextrose given intravenously, or 1 mg glucagon given intravenously, intramuscularly, or subcutaneously. Glucagon causes immediate release of stored glucose from the liver into the bloodstream. The patient should respond to either agent within 10 to 15 minutes, and should check the blood glucose again to confirm recovery. The patient should then remain in the office for approximately 1 hour to ensure stability before release.

Puberty, Pregnancy, and Oral Contraceptives

Puberty

Periodontal changes associated with alterations in human sex hormone levels have been recognized for many years (see Chapter 31). A surge of the sex hormones estrogen, progestin, or more rarely, testosterone, may induce an exaggerated response to the presence of bacterial plaque resulting in development of erythematous, edematous,

---

Box 37-5   **Treatment of Perioperative Hypoglycemia**

- Establish blood glucose with patient's glucometer, if possible
- If patient can take food by mouth, give approximately 15 g of carbohydrate:
  - 4 to 6 ounces of fruit juice or sugared soda
  - 3 to 4 teaspoons of table sugar
  - Glucose tablets (carried by many patients with diabetes) or hard candy
- If patient cannot take food by mouth and intravenous access is present:
  - 25 to 30 ml of 50% dextrose (D50) given intravenously
  - 1 mg glucagon given intravenously
- If patient cannot take food by mouth and intravenous access is *not* present:
  - 1 mg glucagon given intramuscularly or subcutaneously
- Monitor patient for 1 hour
- Call emergency medical services if patient does not respond

---

hemorrhagic, hyperplastic gingivitis in circumpubertal adolescents. The condition appears to stabilize after the body adjusts to the new hormone levels, and there is no evidence that this hyperplastic gingivitis leads to periodontitis if effective plaque control is established and maintained.

When pubertal gingivitis occurs, several therapeutic decisions are required. Because the condition generally represents an edematous response, nonsurgical periodontal debridement and establishment of meticulous oral hygiene is the preferred treatment. In more severe cases, microbial culturing, the use of antimicrobial mouthrinses, and local delivery of antimicrobial agents may be beneficial.[26] Occasionally, the degree of gingival enlargement may be sufficient to hamper normal occlusal function, and surgical intervention may be required if the patient fails to respond to more conservative therapy. The patient should be managed closely during this period, and conservative treatment should be provided as often as necessary to sustain a relatively good level of periodontal health. After stabilization of peripubertal gingival changes, reevaluation is indicated to determine if acceptable gingival contours have been reestablished. If not, surgical intervention may be necessary to eliminate sites in which the improper contours may create an esthetic concern or the potential for impairment of localized plaque control.

Pregnancy

Hyperplastic, edematous, erythematous, easily bleeding gingivitis with or without an increase in occurrence of pyogenic granuloma (pregnancy tumor) in response to the presence of minor irritants such as subgingival calculus or a faulty restoration margin may develop in patients who are pregnant. The gingival response usually begins during the second month of pregnancy when hormonal increases first become evident. It peaks during the eighth month, and subsequently begins to diminish in severity. This coincides with the peak during the eighth month of progesterone and subsequent reduction of hormonal levels during the ninth month and postpartum. On many occasions, gingivitis and any pyogenic granulomas present return to prepregnancy levels a few months after parturition. These transient changes may occur without an increase in plaque levels being noted before, during, or after the pregnancy.[27]

Gingivitis associated with pregnancy tends to occur most commonly on the facial marginal gingiva and interdental papillae. Increased tooth mobility has been noted, perhaps as a result of the inflammatory process or as a result of increased levels of relaxin, a water-soluble polypeptide hormone found in the corpus luteum during pregnancy. Relaxin appears to contribute to relaxation of the pubic symphysis. It has been hypothesized that this substance also exerts its effect on the connective tissue fibers of the periodontal ligament.[28] Increased periodontal pocket depths have been reported in animals and by case report in humans, but this is not a common finding.[29] Evidence indicates that advanced periodontal disease in pregnant patients may result in an increased risk for neonates with low birth weight and premature births (see Chapter 32). Consequently, periodontal health and appropriate periodontal therapy are extremely important during pregnancy. Women with periodontal health before pregnancy can generally sustain that health by preventive periodontal therapy and effective oral hygiene procedures. Others with periodontitis that precedes their pregnancy may require extensive scaling and root planing, frequent recall intervals, and excellent home care. Except in acute situations, it is generally believed that nonsurgical periodontal therapy is the preferred treatment. However, in event of acute infection, surgical intervention may create a smaller risk than allowing the infection to continue unabated.[30]

Several therapeutic principles have evolved regarding dental and periodontal management of patients who are pregnant. The medical history should include information regarding complications during the pregnancy, previous miscarriages or early delivery, and any signs or symptoms suggestive of potential miscarriage or premature delivery. Medical consultation may be necessary if extensive periodontal therapy is required. Effective oral hygiene measures should be initiated as soon as possible and maintained throughout the pregnancy.[26]

It is usually recommended that any necessary dental treatment be provided during the second trimester.

The organogenesis occurring during the first trimester may cause the fetus to be especially susceptible to environmental stimuli. Most pregnant individuals are uncomfortable in the dental chair during the third trimester, and, in the later stages of this trimester, the patient may be especially prone to premature delivery. However, emergency dental treatment should be provided whenever necessary.

Conservative periodontal therapy may be provided during pregnancy, and should include scaling and root planing in the patient with periodontitis or severe gingival inflammation, but elective periodontal procedures usually can be postponed until after delivery. Cardiac output and heart rate are increased during pregnancy, and as the size of the uterus increases the patient is susceptible to developing the supine hypotension syndrome if reclined in the dental chair. This is the result of partial blockage of venous return through the vena cava, and it may be associated with decreased perfusion of the fetus. This syndrome can be avoided by placing the patient on her left side during dental treatment or by raising the right hip several inches. Pressure on the diaphragm in the supine position may increase the risk for patient or fetal hypoxia. For these reasons, the supine position in the dental chair should be avoided, and the patient should remain semi-reclined.

The dental practitioner should remain aware that several systemic complications can develop in the pregnant patient and be alert to signs and symptoms suggestive of these. Gestational diabetes mellitus may occur in individuals who are at risk for this condition, and increased renal clearance associated with pregnancy may necessitate greater doses of some drugs to achieve optimal therapeutic levels. At the same time, it is important to remember that most drugs cross the placental barrier and may also be present in breast milk. Most drug reference texts classify prescription drugs regarding their relative safety for use during pregnancy. Such a reference should be available in all dental offices.

Judicious use of local anesthetic agents such as lidocaine with 1:100,000 epinephrine is safe during pregnancy, but excessive quantities of anesthetics could affect the physiologic state of the fetus. Certain other drugs should be avoided. Penicillin and cephalosporin may be used if necessary, but tetracyclines can have adverse fetal effects that may result in tooth discoloration. Prolonged tetracycline use may inhibit bone growth and fetal development. Although some mycin drugs are generally safe for use in pregnancy, clarithromycin is not, and erythromycin estolate should be avoided because it can induce hepatotoxicity. The effects of amoxicillin, antibiotics containing clavulanic acid, and metronidazole have not been adequately studied in humans and are generally avoided.[25]

If short-term pain medication is necessary in managing a dental condition, acetaminophen is usually considered the drug of choice. However, its safety in humans has not been extensively studied.[31] In most instances, it is prudent to confer with the patient's physician before prescribing any medication other than a local anesthetic.

Some controversy exists regarding the safety of taking dental radiographs for pregnant individuals. Extensive exposure to radiation can be quite harmful to the developing fetus. However, dental radiographic equipment does not emit large quantities of radiation, and safety precautions have been established for dentistry. As a rule of thumb, elective radiographs should be avoided. However, radiographs necessary for diagnosis or management of a dental condition or emergency may be obtained safely, provided a lead apron shield is used.

Oral contraceptives

Oral contraceptives consist of various combinations of female sex steroid hormones that mimic pregnancy. In the past, use of oral contraceptives has occasionally resulted in gingival changes suggestive of pregnancy gingivitis, often in the first months after initiation of the drug. In recent years, however, the sex steroid hormone levels of oral contraceptives have been markedly reduced and it is currently not known whether the newer agents adversely affect gingival response to bacterial plaque. Some reports suggest that chronic gingivitis may occur in association with long-term use of the drug. Other studies have reported, however, that the associated susceptibility to gingivitis diminishes over time.[32] If gingivitis does occur in conjunction with these agents, appropriate periodontal therapy should be provided. Effective oral hygiene measures, more frequent recall intervals, and professional scaling and debridement should be sufficient to control the gingival condition; and the patient is a candidate for any necessary invasive periodontal therapy. An increased incidence of alveolar osteitis (dry socket) has been reported to occur after extractions in women using oral contraceptives.[33] This issue is somewhat controversial and additional studies are needed.

It has been suggested that administration of antibiotics to individuals taking oral contraceptives could lead to unwanted "break-through" pregnancy. The drugs indicted include antihistamines; anticonvulsants; some analgesics; and antibiotics such as penicillin, ampicillin, rifampicin, or tetracyclines. However, this risk may have been overstated. Evidence for and against this concept is primarily anecdotal and the practitioner must decide whether to forewarn female patients about this possible risk. If the decision is made to do so, the patient should be encouraged to use alternative or multiple forms of birth control during the menstrual cycle in which the antibiotics were taken.[26,30,33,34] A recent position statement

by the American Dental Association (ADA) recommends that women who use oral contraceptives should be advised of the potential risks if antibiotics are prescribed. They also should be encouraged to maintain compliance with oral contraceptives when using antibiotics concurrently and advised to seek medical advice regarding use of an additional nonhormonal method of contraception.[35]

Adrenocortical Insufficiency/Corticosteroid Medications

Impaired function of the adrenal cortex (hypoadrenalism) can have profound effects on the ability of the host to withstand emotional or physical stress. The condition may be precipitated by a number of systemic disorders including blood dyscrasias, lupus erythematosus, Sjögren syndrome, progressive systemic sclerosis, Crohn's disease/inflammatory bowel disease, and AIDS.[36] In addition, reduced adrenal cortex function may result from administration of large dosages of immunosuppressive drugs or prolonged use of these drugs even in low dose.[37,38]

Patients afflicted with impaired adrenal gland function may be in danger of developing systemic toxemias from localized infections, such as periodontal diseases.[39] It seems logical to assume that individuals with adrenal suppression may be more susceptible to localized periodontal disease because of suppression of the host immune response. Currently, however, periodontal disease has not been found to be more common or severe in individuals receiving long-term immunosuppressive drugs than in the general population.[40] However, immune suppression may mask the clinical signs and symptoms of gingivitis and periodontitis while subtle clinical attachment loss occurs.[41]

Severe adrenal insufficiency (Addison's disease) may induce hyperpigmentation of the skin and oral mucosa. In the oral cavity, the lips, buccal mucosa, palate, gingiva, and ventral surface of the tongue may be affected.[42] When these clinical changes are noted, the cause should be evaluated before performing extensive dental/periodontal treatment. Other conditions may cause similar hyperpigmented oral lesions including pregnancy (melasma), smoking, excessive supplementation of female sex hormones, and oral contraceptives.[43,44] Some drugs such as tetracycline, silver compounds, and azathioprine also can precipitate these changes. Drug-induced hyperpigmentation is probably most commonly associated with the administration of azathioprine to patients with AIDS. However, AIDS itself may cause adrenal cortex hypofunction.[43] In the presence of this type of oral hyperpigmentation, definitive periodontal treatment should not be initiated until the presence or absence of hypoadrenalism has been determined.

Prolonged or high dose-administration of corticosteroids may induce a reduction in production of adrenocorticotropic hormone secretion leading to atrophy of the adrenal cortex.[45] In general, any patient who has received a glucocorticoid dose equivalent to 20 mg or more of prednisone daily for more than 5 days is at risk for adrenal suppression. Lower dosage levels that are closer to the physiologic range may also induce suppression, but a longer treatment time is required.[46] If adrenal suppression is present, it may adversely influence the ability of an affected individual to withstand emotional or physical stress to include periodontal therapy, especially surgical procedures. Occasionally, a stressful event can induce adrenal shock and even death.

Other adverse effects of high-dose or long-term systemic corticosteroid therapy may include secondary diabetes mellitus, hypertension, osteoporosis, gastrointestinal ulcers, and impaired wound healing.[25] The dental practitioner should be alert for signs and symptoms of these conditions among patients receiving this medication.

Several management principles have been suggested when providing dental therapy to individuals who are receiving corticosteroid therapy. Medical consultation is important to fully understand the underlying condition that afflicts the patient, the degree of control achieved by the drug regimen and the need for corticosteroid supplementation when these individuals receive dental treatment. Some have suggested that individuals who take exogenous steroids and who require periodontal or other oral surgical procedures should receive corticosteroid supplementation immediately before the procedure. Although there is little danger in following this proposed protocol, it may not always be necessary. Patients receiving low dose, long-term steroid therapy may be at risk for adrenal shock. For example, 5 mg prednisone is the equivalent of the 25 to 30 mg cortisol normally produced by the body on a daily basis.[47,48] Consequently, reduced adrenal steroid output might occur at this dosage and cortisol reserves may not be present. In this event, corticosteroid supplementation may be indicated. Conversely, individuals receiving daily dosages of 10 mg or more of prednisone (or its equivalent) theoretically have an adequate corticosteroid load to withstand most stressful dental situations and supplementation may not be required.[48] It is imperative, however, that the proposed treatment and planned management of adrenal function be discussed with the patient's physician and medical permission acquired.[46]

Thyroid Dysfunction

Thyroid hormones regulate the biochemical activities of most body tissues. Their release is controlled by release of thyroid-stimulating hormone (thyrotropin) from the anterior pituitary gland and by the intrathyroidal iodine level. Release of thyroid-stimulating hormone is largely determined by circulating thyroid hormone levels in blood (homeostatic feedback mechanism). Thyroxine and other thyroid hormones contribute greatly to maintenance of metabolic homeostasis. The body is adversely affected by either an excess or deficiency of these hormones.

Hyperthyroidism

Hyperthyroidism accelerates metabolic activity and may initiate an acute response under emotional or physical stress. The most common cause is Graves disease (diffuse toxic goiter). The condition usually occurs in middle-aged individuals and it is far more common in women than men (5:1). Affected individuals may demonstrate extreme nervousness, anxiety, emotional instability, proptosis (exophthalmos), eyelid lag, loss of weight, alopecia, or heat intolerance accompanied by excessive perspiration. The cardiovascular system may be significantly affected and individuals may experience heart murmur, tachycardia, hypertension, and increased pulse pressure (widening between systolic and diastolic sounds). In untreated or severe cases, cardiac enlargement may occur.[49]

In managing hyperthyroid patients with periodontal diseases, treatment should be performed with great caution because individuals with uncontrolled hyperthyroidism are subject to a severe exacerbation known as thyroid storm. This may be precipitated by superimposed infection, surgery, or stress. It is characterized by severe manifestations of conditions associated with hyperthyroidism, and if not controlled can lead to dehydration, shock, and even death.

Dental patients who display signs and symptoms suggestive of undetected or uncontrolled hyperthyroidism should be referred to a physician for evaluation as quickly as possible. Elective treatment procedures should be deferred pending medical evaluation, and treatment in the hospital environment should be considered if emergency invasive dental care is needed. General anesthesia may be appropriate.

Individuals with a history of hyperthyroidism should be carefully questioned about their disease, including its etiology and severity. Medical consultation should be obtained if extensive periodontal therapy is anticipated.

Dental infections may precipitate a thyroid crisis; therefore, optimal oral health is a highly desirable goal. Infections, including those present in severe periodontal disease, should be controlled with antibiotics and other conservative, noninvasive methods until medical stability has been achieved. The presence of comorbid conditions such as heart disease or diabetes mellitus should be taken under consideration when planning treatment. Dental treatment should be provided in short, minimally stressful appointments. Adequate preoperative sedation may be necessary for the anxious patient and epinephrine is contraindicated in local anesthetics and gingival retraction cord. Vital signs should be closely monitored throughout the dental procedure.[50,51]

Hypothyroidism

Hypothyroidism (myxedema) also has a predilection for female individuals (6:1 over males). It is characterized by lack of production of thyroid hormones. The most common etiologic factor is chronic thyroiditis (Hashimoto's thyroiditis) or ablative therapy for hyperthyroidism. Secondary hypothyroidism may result from pituitary hypofunction. It may also be drug induced or result from radiation therapy to the head and neck. The condition is far more common than hyperthyroidism, and a large number of individuals older than 50 years receive thyroid supplementation because of evidence of the disease. The signs and symptoms of myxedema vary widely, but it is characterized by a lack of energy, lethargy, mental dullness, weight gain, and nonpitting edema of tissues. The skin may be scaly and dry. Sensitivity to cold is common.

Hypothyroidism has been associated with increased incidence of dental diseases, but this effect may relate to the mental dullness and lethargy of the affected patient. Xerostomia is often present, possibly increasing susceptibility to caries and periodontitis. There are no contraindications to dental treatment including implant placement in the controlled patient.[52,53] However, bleeding diatheses may occur in individuals with moderate to severe hypothyroidism, sometimes secondary to acquired von Willebrand's disease. Consequently, blood studies may be appropriate before surgical procedures and the affected patient managed as described for others with hemorrhagic diatheses. Patients suspected of having undiagnosed or poorly controlled hypothyroidism should be referred to a physician for diagnosis, evaluation, and control. Currently, there is no cure for hypothyroidism, although thyroid hormone supplementation is successful in controlling the disease. Conversely, the dental practitioner should be alert for evidence of possible overdosing with synthetic thyroid hormones that could lead to signs and symptoms suggestive of hyperthyroidism.

Hyperparathyroidism

The parathyroid glands serve in coordination with vitamin D to control calcium levels in bone and extracellular fluids. Primary hyperparathyroidism occurs when an excess of parathyroid hormone is produced as a result of a parathyroid adenoma, hyperplasia, or malignancy. Secondary hyperparathyroidism occurs when renal dysfunction leads to excessive calcium or magnesium excretion in urine and retention of serum phosphorus. This initiates a reactive parathyroid hyperplasia. Both primary and secondary hyperparathyroidism lead to the leaching of calcium from bone reservoirs in an effort to maintain physiologic homeostasis between serum calcium and phosphorus.[54]

In the oral cavity, hyperparathyroidism may result in development of a multilocular, radiolucent jaw lesion (the brown tumor of hyperparathyroidism) that is indistinguishable radiographically or histologically from a central giant cell granuloma.[55] The reduced calcium levels in bone associated with primary or secondary hyperparathyroidism may make the patient more susceptible to rapid alveolar bone destruction in the presence of plaque-induced periodontitis, but it does not directly induce loss of marginal alveolar bone.[56] Mobility and drifting of teeth has been described in the absence of significant periodontal disease; consequently, occlusal appliances or fixed splints may be indicated.

Periodontal treatment for individuals with primary hyperparathyroidism should be deferred until the condition is corrected. However, chronic secondary hyperparathyroidism may develop in patients with renal disease. In these individuals, periodontal therapy should be provided as necessary to prevent excessive periodontal destruction or tooth loss. Conservative therapy is preferred, excellent oral hygiene is essential to success, and frequent maintenance recall visits are usually required. Minimally invasive surgical therapy can be provided if necessary to arrest the periodontal disease process. Prophylactic antibiotics may be considered to minimize the effect of orogenic bacteremias.

HEMATOLOGIC CONDITIONS

Coagulation Disorders

Postsurgical hemorrhage or even prolonged and excessive bleeding after scaling and root planing procedures are occasional complications of periodontal therapy. Although generally manageable with conservative measures, it is desirable to avoid this complication. In most cases, an adequate medical/dental history will identify patients with a potential bleeding diathesis. Most hemorrhagic incidents are related to local factors occurring as a part of the treatment received. However, there are a number of drugs and systemic conditions that may be associated with prolonged or excessive hemorrhage. These should be identified in advance of treatment whenever possible.[57,58]

Hemostasis occurs through a complex mechanism of platelet aggregation to form a clot, activation of the coagulation factor cascade to strengthen the clot, and, finally, clot degradation. Any condition that disrupts this mechanism can result in excessive or prolonged bleeding.

As a rule, patients suspected of having a bleeding disorder can be evaluated using only a few clinical and laboratory procedures. A thorough medical history can lead to a proper diagnosis in the majority of patients. Certain laboratory tests are helpful in screening patients for a deficiency of clotting factor(s), a platelet deficiency or dysfunction, or other systemic disorders that might interfere with adequate blood clotting. A complete blood count with differential will help identify platelet deficiencies; the Ivy bleeding time or a platelet function analyzer will identify abnormalities in platelet aggregation; and a prothrombin and partial thromboplastin test will help evaluate patients for deficiencies in the extrinsic and intrinsic clotting factors.[59] The results of these tests may necessitate medical consultation before definitive periodontal therapy to rule out specific bleeding disorders.[60] Table 37-3 illustrates the use of screening laboratory tests for hemorrhagic disorders.

This section describes several diseases most often associated with clotting factor deficiencies and discusses principles of management in the dental office. These management principles can be modified to compensate for other factor deficiencies. Management of the patients with liver disorders is discussed in a separate section and patient management of those receiving anticoagulant therapy is discussed in the section on cardiovascular diseases.

Hemophilia

Hemophilia A is the most common type of hemophilia. It occurs because of a deficiency of the intrinsic clotting factor VIII (antihemophilic globulin). It is transmitted as a sex-linked (X-linked) recessive trait that is carried by female individuals, although they are only rarely afflicted with the disease. Susceptible male offspring, however, often have the deficiency. If undetected, this condition can be life threatening.

Hemophilia B occurs because of a deficiency in clotting factor IX (plasma thromboplastin component). It also is inherited as an X-linked recessive trait and is more commonly found in male individuals, although female individuals may also be affected.

Management principles are the same for these two variants of hemophilia. Medical consultation should be sought. The diseases are considered to be relatively mild

if 30% or more of the circulating factor levels are present, but supplementation with the appropriate factor often is indicated before dental therapy. This may be accomplished by the use of fresh frozen plasma. However, recombinant factor VIII or IX reduces the potential for posttransfusion viral infections. It is important that excellent oral health is achieved and maintained in afflicted individuals. Effective oral hygiene is an essential component in reaching this goal, but plaque removal should be as atraumatic as possible. A soft bristle toothbrush is preferred, and flossing should be performed carefully to prevent tissue laceration.

Even conservative periodontal therapy may place the hemophiliac at risk for excessive hemorrhage. Scaling and root planing and injection of local block anesthesia can result in severe bleeding unless factor supplementation is accomplished before treatment. Even then, gentle probing and debridement is preferred. If the patient has mild deficiency, it may be more appropriate to remove local irritants progressively in short, multiple appointments to avoid inducing a bleeding diathesis. One should be prepared to manage postoperative hemorrhage using local hemostatic agents such as oxidized cellulose soaked in thrombin or fibrin sealant.[61] Administration of clot-stabilizing agents, such as desmopressin acetate or aminocaproic acid, may be an acceptable alternative to factor supplementation.

Most surgical procedures should be performed in the hospital in close coordination with the patient's hematologist. Ideally, some means should be available for estimating the volume of blood loss during and after the procedure. Preoperative and postoperative hematocrit and hemoglobin assessments may be of some benefit in evaluating hypovolemia.

Care should be taken after surgery to avoid administration of analgesic agents such as aspirin, nonsteroidal antiinflammatory drugs, or even acetaminophen because of their potential to prolong postoperative hemorrhage.[62,63]

TABLE 37-3	Laboratory Testing for Bleeding Disorders			
PLATELET COUNT	**IVY BLEEDING TIME**	**PT**	**PTT**	**SUSPECTED DIAGNOSIS**
Decreased	Prolonged	Normal	Normal	Thrombocytopenia
Normal	Prolonged	Normal	Normal	von Willebrand's disease
Normal	Prolonged	Normal	Normal	Drug induced
Normal	Normal	Abnormal	Normal	Factor VII deficiency
Normal	Normal	Normal	Abnormal	Hemophilia A or B
Normal	Normal	Abnormal	Abnormal	Liver disease

Modified from Rees TD: Dental management of the medically compromised patient. In McDonald RE, Hurt WC, Gilmore HW, Middleton RA, editors: Current therapy in dentistry, vol 7, St. Louis, 1980, Mosby, p. 12.
PT, prothrombin time; PTT, partial thromboplastin time.

von Willebrand's disease

von Willebrand's disease is sometimes referred to as vascular hemophilia. It is transmitted by an autosomal gene to both sexes. A deficiency or abnormality in von Willebrand factor (vWF) alters platelet adherence and aggregation and can lead to a prolonged bleeding time. The factor also may complex with factor VIII and interfere with its activation. This creates clinical features similar to hemophilia. In most instances, the deficiency is relatively mild, although patients with severe deficiency may experience spontaneous gingival bleeding, epistaxis, and ecchymosis.

Patients with von Willebrand's disease may or may not be aware of their condition. It is the most common of the inherited bleeding disorders, and it should be suspected in individuals who report previous moderate to severe postoperative bleeding after periodontal surgical or non-surgical procedures.

For invasive dental procedures, the vWF should ideally be greater than 80% of normal. This can be achieved with factor supplementation. However, in more severe cases, patients may also benefit from administration of desmo-pressin acetate, which stimulates release of endogenous vWF from endothelial cells. Supplemental doses of vWF or desmopressin may be required after surgery to ensure clot stabilization. Aminocaproic acid mouthrinses also can be used for this purpose.[57,60]

Thrombocytopenia

Thrombocytopenia is a decrease in the number of circulating platelets caused by decreased cell production or increased destruction, or both. It may be precipitated secondary to use of myelosuppressive drugs or radiation therapy for treatment of neoplasias, or it may represent an idiopathic hypersensitivity to various drugs including salicylates, barbiturates, phenylbutazone, sulfonamides, meprobamate, diphenhydramine, ethanol, antiepileptics, diuretics, or nonsteroidal antiinflammatory drugs. It may also be induced by infection or myelodysplastic conditions such as aplastic anemia or leukemia. Hypersplenism can result in accelerated destruction of platelets, inducing the deficiency. Interestingly, thrombocytopenia often is idiopathic.

Normal platelet count ranges from 150,000 to 400,000 cells/mm³. Platelet deficiencies can induce spontaneous bleeding when the count decreases to less than 10,000/mm³. However, essential periodontal procedures, including surgery, can usually be performed when the platelet count exceeds 50,000/mm³.

Medical treatment is directed toward identification and elimination of the etiologic factors, when possible, and with infusion of packed platelets as necessary. Elective dental procedures should be deferred until the condition improves. Emergency care should be provided in the hospital with close medical–dental coordination.

Individuals who have slowly progressive or partially controlled thrombocytopenia may receive routine dental care after medical consultation. The dental care should be directed toward elimination of oral conditions that might predispose to hemorrhage. These include faulty restorations, carious lesions, or calculus accumulations. Small areas should be treated and local hemostatic agents used to control bleeding. Oral hygiene should be meticulously maintained using gentle toothbrushing and flossing and frequent oral prophylaxis. The drugs used in treatment of the platelet disorder should be taken under consideration. For example, systemic corticosteroids are often used for idiopathic thrombocytopenia. Patients taking these medications may be predisposed to oral infection and their response to physical or emotional stress may be compromised.[25,62]

Blood Dyscrasias

Red blood cells

Patients seeking periodontal therapy may be affected by deficiency in red blood cells (erythrocytes). This deficiency may be especially likely in elderly or malnourished individuals. In some cases, anemia may be associated with oral manifestations such as glossitis, cheilitis, or pallor of the mucous membranes. However, most often the periodontium is not affected.[64] In general, anemia is a manifestation of a variety of underlying red blood cell disorders. It may occur because of blood loss, iron deficiency, decreased production of erythrocytes (pernicious anemia and folic acid deficiency), increased destruction of red blood cells (hemolytic anemia), or defective red blood cells (sickle cell anemia). Periodontal surgical procedures may be contraindicated in patients who are severely anemic because abnormal bleeding and delayed wound healing may occur. When the condition is suspected the patient should be referred to his or her physician for evaluation or screening laboratory tests should be performed. These usually include a complete blood count with differential, hemoglobin, and hematocrit.

Hemolytic anemia. Although rare, hemolytic anemia may be precipitated by drugs such as dapsone, aspirin, phenacetin, chloramphenicol, sulfonamides, and methylene blue, especially if the individual taking the drugs has an enzymatic deficiency of red blood cells. The most common of these is glucose-6-phosphate dehydrogenase (G6PD) deficiency. This X-linked recessive trait has been reported to be present in approximately 10% of black male individuals. Under drug-induced oxidant stress, hemolysis may occur. Occasionally, the red blood cell destruction is not self-limiting and can even be fatal. Hemolysis may also be precipitated by dental infection and the dentist should manage patients with G6PD deficiency with great caution.[60]

Sickle cell anemia and sickle cell trait. Sickle cell anemia may also induce hemolysis. The condition results from abnormalities in the hemoglobin molecule (hemoglobin S) leading to malformation of erythrocytes under oxidant stress. It occurs almost exclusively in black individuals, and those with a severe form of the disease may die in childhood. In sickle cell disease, more than 75% of hemoglobin is the S form, whereas in sickle cell trait, 20% to 50% of hemoglobin is the S type. Afflicted individuals with more than 50% normal hemoglobin (type A) may often be asymptomatic unless exposed to hypoxia or increased blood pH. In this event, an increase in formation of hemoglobin S occurs and may result in hemolysis or blood stasis.[65]

Clinical manifestations of sickle cell anemia may include pallor, jaundice, and cardiac failure. When abnormal erythrocytes plug blood vessels, ischemic necrosis may result. This tissue destruction may occasionally include periodontal structures. In the oral cavity, sickle cell disease may result in delayed tooth eruption in children and dentinal hypoplasia. Bone marrow hyperplasia may occur, causing formation of a thin trabecular pattern in the jaws with the trabeculae aligned in horizontal rows. Skull radiographs may reveal coarse trabeculae aligned perpendicular to the outer plate (the "hair on end" effect).[65,66] The dentist is more likely to encounter individuals who carry the sickle cell trait than individuals with sickle cell anemia. In patients with the sickle cell trait, sickling crisis is much less likely, but can occasionally occur, especially at greater altitudes. Dental treatment should not be performed during periods of exacerbation, and elective periodontal surgical procedures should not be scheduled unless the patient's normal hemoglobin is 70% or more. General anesthesia is contraindicated as are any drugs likely to induce respiratory depression. Carefully administered nitrous oxide/oxygen conscious sedation may maintain adequate tissue oxygenation, but the patient should be monitored with a pulse oximeter or other device to ensure stability. Treatment procedures should be brief and infiltration with local anesthetics with vasoconstrictors should be used with extreme caution to prevent ischemic necrosis peripheral to the injection site. In surgical procedures, every effort should be made to obtain complete soft tissue coverage of wound sites because osteomyelitis is a risk in this patient population.[60,66]

Dental and periodontal infections can initiate a sickling crisis, therefore good oral health is imperative. If surgical procedures are performed, prophylactic antibiotic coverage as recommended by the American Heart Association (AHA) is probably indicated. Renal and hepatic dysfunction may be present; therefore, penicillin is probably the drug of choice in patients who are not allergic, because any antibiotic taken is likely to remain in the blood system for a prolonged period and penicillin is one of the least toxic antibiotics available.[60]

Aplastic anemia. Aplastic anemia is an acute myelogenous disease that causes defective formation or deficiency of most blood cells formed in the bone marrow. It is characterized by susceptibility to infection and hemorrhage. Patients with this disorder should be managed as described later for the individual with acute leukemia.

White blood cells

As discussed in Chapter 31, deficiency or defective formation of white blood cells may have a profound adverse effect on periodontal health. Quantitative deficiencies (neutropenia, agranulocytosis) may significantly impact the patient's ability to ward off infections including gingivitis and periodontitis. Functional leukocyte disorders (Chediak–Higashi syndrome, chronic granulomatous disease, leukocyte adhesion deficiency, and others) may have a similar effect. The underlying systemic disorder may vary from mild to severe. The severity of the disorder may represent the greatest determinant of the dentist's ability to control plaque-induced periodontal destruction.[67,68] Dental therapy is directed toward management of oral lesions and preservation of the teeth and supporting structures. Good oral hygiene must be meticulously maintained. Frequent maintenance intervals with prophylaxis and gentle scaling and root planing are usually appropriate. Although clearcut therapy protocols have not been established, it is recommended that antibiotics such as tetracyclines, amoxicillin plus clavulanic acid, or a combination of amoxicillin and metronidazole should be prescribed before or during periodontal treatment procedures. However, it may be more appropriate to use microbial culture and sensitivity testing to select the most effective antibiotic. Administration of low-dose tetracycline or local delivery of intrasulcular antibiotics or antimicrobials may be beneficial, although the usefulness of these agents has not yet been adequately evaluated.[69] At a minimum, prophylactic antibiotic coverage is indicated during invasive periodontal therapy. Some reports suggest that early removal of teeth with severe periodontal lesions may alter the oral microbial flora and improve the prognosis for remaining teeth.[68] Currently, the appropriateness of implant placement in this patient population is unknown.

Leukemia. Acute leukemia may run a rapid course and often only palliative treatment can be provided. However, when possible, oral health assessment and management should be accomplished before initiation of medical therapy.[69] Gingival enlargement is a common finding, often induced by infiltration of malignant cells or by soft tissue hemorrhage.[70] Oral infections are found in approximately one third of individuals with acute or active chronic leukemia. Oral mucosal lesions are also common as an adverse effect of chemotherapy. Before and after chemotherapy, oral mycotic (fungal) infections should be controlled, and the use of topical anesthetics or warm, mildly alkaline mouthrinses may help to make patients more comfortable. Every effort should be made to maintain good oral health, but gingival bleeding and infection are a constant threat. The frequency and severity of infections increase with the duration and severity of granulocytopenia. Patients with leukemia should be encouraged to maintain optimal oral health. Often, however, the course of dental treatment is affected by the patient's overall health status and only conservative therapy can be provided. Any dental disease likely to cause infection or gingival irritation should be managed before medical therapy whenever possible. Gingival inflammation, faulty restorations, and subgingival calculus can precipitate gingival bleeding that may be difficult to control. Careful coordination with the patient's hematologist is necessary. Advance knowledge of the patient's blood cell levels may necessitate that fresh frozen plasma or packed platelets are administered before dental therapy. If unanticipated bleeding occurs, local measures such as applied pressure on the site, use of local hemostatic agents such as oxidized cellulose, or the application of topical thrombin should be attempted. Individuals with acute leukemia may undergo chemotherapy or bone marrow transplantation (BMT). These individuals require special care as discussed extensively later in this chapter.

Chronic leukemias are more likely to occur in individuals older than 40 years. They represent approximately one third of all reported leukemias. Any cell type may be involved, but the cells are generally more mature and some cell function may be retained. The condition progresses more slowly and periods of remission may occur with or without medical treatment. Consequently, individuals with chronic leukemia may anticipate a reasonably normal lifestyle and lifespan.

Periodontal treatment should be avoided in patients with chronic leukemia during periods of exacerbation. If emergency care is necessary, tissue lacerations should be avoided. Aspirin, other nonsteroidal antiinflammatory drugs, and acetaminophen should not be prescribed because these drugs may adversely affect platelet function. Dental treatment can be performed during periods of remission. The criteria for remission should be determined by the hematologist. During remission, all potential local irritants should be removed and conservative periodontal therapy performed. Prophylactic antibiotic coverage should be considered and it is probably required if the absolute granulocyte count decreases to less than 1500/mm³.[60]

CARDIOVASCULAR DISEASES

Remarkable strides have been made in recent years in the prevention, diagnosis, and treatment of cardiovascular diseases (CVDs). Despite this progress, these diseases continue to be the most serious and common health problem in the United States. Sudden cardiac arrest takes more than 350,000 adult lives each year and more than 6,000,000 Americans are estimated to have hypertension. The evolution of newer diagnostic and treatment techniques, the increase in the geriatric population in the United States, and the increase in the number of dentate elderly individuals clearly indicate that the dental practitioner will be expected to provide periodontal therapy for an ever-expanding number of individuals with CVD.

Although a causal relation between poor periodontal health and the risk for CVD has not been established, evidence does suggest that individuals with CVD may have more advanced dental/periodontal disease than age- and sex-matched control subjects[71] (see Chapter 32). Successful periodontal management of any patient with CVD is dependent on acquiring a thorough medical history, being aware of signs and symptoms of CVD, routine monitoring of vital signs in the dental office, adherence to accepted treatment principles, and appropriate medical consultation. This section provides practical information regarding safe and effective periodontal therapy for individuals with a variety of CVDs.

Rheumatic Fever and Rheumatic Heart Disease

Rheumatic fever is a streptococcal infection that most commonly affects children between the ages of 5 and 15 years. It is characterized by onset of a sore throat followed a few weeks later by an acute febrile illness and pain in multiple joints of the body. The disease usually lasts from 6 to 12 weeks and after-effects are minimal. Acute cardiac inflammation may occur in approximately 50% of afflicted individuals, and in some instances an autoimmune phenomenon is induced by antibodies against the streptococcal microorganisms that are cross-reactive with valvar (valvular) tissue of the heart. As an aftermath to this cross-reactivity, vegetative valvar lesions representative of chronic rheumatic heart disease may gradually but progressively develop. Rheumatic heart disease features progressive fibrosis, calcification, stenosis, and incompetence (regurgitation) of heart valves, especially the mitral or aortic valves. It was once considered to be the most likely cause of valvar heart damage in young individuals, but timely use of antibiotics and other treatment modalities have markedly reduced the incidence in

Western countries. Presence of rheumatic heart disease with valvar lesions and chronic valvar regurgitation may lead to congestive heart failure and also place the afflicted patient at risk for acute or subacute infectious endocarditis (IE). These conditions are discussed later in this section.[72]

Congenital Heart Defects

Congenital heart defects currently represent the most common type of heart disease in children. They occur in approximately 1% of live births. Although the condition was often fatal in the past, new developments in cardiac surgical interventions have markedly improved the prognosis for individuals born with these defects.

Congenital defects may affect portions of the heart or adjacent vessels. The cause is unknown but a genetic etiology is suspected, although embryonically acquired rubella and cytomegalovirus infections may also be implicated. Failure of the heart to perform its physiologic function may lead to death, whereas cyanosis and clubbing of the fingers are described in those who survive without surgical repair. Pulmonary hypertension may occur and the right ventricle may become hypertrophic.

Ventricular septal defects result in inappropriate backflow from the left to the right ventricle leading to right ventricular hypertrophy. Atrial septal defects are the most common form of congenital heart deformities. Fortunately, these defects have minimal effect on heart function, although they may lead to embolus formation and also ultimately result in right ventricular hypertrophy.

Patent ductus arteriosus is an opening between the aorta and pulmonary artery. The condition is associated with both systolic and diastolic murmurs, and the risk for IE is great. Pulmonary stenosis interferes with normal blood flow to the lungs and leads to breathlessness and subsequent right ventricular failure.

Coarctation of the aorta results in hypotension of the lower portion of the body, whereas the head, neck, and upper body experience hypertension. This occurs because the narrowing of the aorta is usually found beyond the origin of the subclavian arteries. In this condition, development of an aneurysm is a constant threat.

The tetralogy of Fallot represents multiple congenital defects, specifically ventricular septal defects, pulmonary stenosis, improper blood flow into the aorta, and compensatory right ventricular hypertrophy. If the condition is not surgically corrected, heart failure is a common outcome.

Valvar calcifications may occur as the result of the presence of congenital defects and further promote the risk for endocarditis for this group of individuals. Congenital conditions such as ventricular septal defects, pulmonary stenosis, the tetralogy of Fallot, and a patent ductus arteriosus previously presented the patient with a grim prognosis because of heart failure or infective endocarditis. Currently, however, with successful cardiac surgery, patients often can anticipate a normal life expectancy. Appropriate dental management of patients who have experienced these defects is discussed in the section regarding IE.

Congenital mitral valve prolapse is inherited as an autosomal dominant trait. It is a genetically derived condition of the chordae tympanae of the mitral valve that can result in incomplete valve closure. It may occur in otherwise healthy individuals, but it is also a characteristic feature of Marfan syndrome, the Ehlers-Danlos syndromes, and panic disorder. It may be more common among young female than male individuals.[72]

If untreated, congenital cardiac defects may lead to early death dependent on the severity of the condition. In milder cases, tooth eruption may be delayed, enamel hypoplasia is evident, and the teeth are often malposed. IE is a constant risk, and bleeding may occur after invasive dental procedures because of abnormal platelet function and increased fibrinolytic activity. In contrast, individuals with surgically repaired congenital defects usually can anticipate a normal or near normal life expectancy, although in some cases an increased risk for development of IE persists throughout life.[73]

Congestive Heart Failure

Congestive heart failure (CHF) occurs when the heart muscle is unable to pump an adequate supply of oxygenated blood to the body. It most commonly occurs as a result of coronary artery disease, hypertension, valvar heart disease, diabetes mellitus, or cardiomyopathy.[74] The condition may induce ventricular arrhythmias and sudden death. Heart transplantation may be the only way to cure the disease, but new treatment techniques help assure significant prolongation in life of individuals with CHF.

Signs and symptoms of undiagnosed or poorly controlled CHF include shortness of breath at rest or with minimal exercise, cyanosis, and nocturnal heart pain (angina).[75] Patients with poorly controlled CHF are not candidates for elective dental treatment and any necessary emergency dental care should be as conservative as possible (analgesics and antibiotics). In some cases, dental treatment should only be performed in the hospital environment.

Currently, it is often possible for patients to achieve and sustain satisfactory levels of cardiac output and prolonged life. In this circumstance, some individuals may be candidates for elective periodontal therapy, to include surgical procedures, with some modifications to the dental treatment protocol. Dental appointments should be short and every effort should be made to establish a nonstressful treatment environment. This may require the use of conscious sedation or relaxation techniques, or both. Supplemental oxygen should be available as needed, and the dental chair should be positioned in an upright or semi-reclined position to ensure that peripheral blood returns to the central circulation and that the decompensated myocardium is not further impaired.[76]

The goal of medical treatment of CHF is to increase contractile force of the heart muscle to increase cardiac output. To achieve this, most patients with CHF are treated with diuretics or with various combinations of digitalis, diuretics, beta-blocking agents, calcium channel–blocking agents, and angiotensin-converting enzyme inhibitors. The dental practitioner should familiarize himself or herself with the potential side effects of these drugs and remain alert for signs and symptoms suggestive of adverse drug effects. These may include altered cardiac rhythm, anorexia, diarrhea, fatigue, headache, dizziness, or delirium.[75]

The long-term use of calcium channel–blocking agents may result in gingival enlargement (see Chapter 33). Available evidence suggests that drug-induced gingival enlargement occurs in association with inadequate plaque control and every effort should be made to ensure that the patient maintains excellent oral hygiene and that he or she is scheduled for frequent periodontal maintenance visits.[77,78]

Cardiac Arrhythmias

Cardiac arrhythmias may be caused by reversible physiologic events such as hypoxia, diminished or excess serum potassium levels, or electrolyte imbalances. Most arrhythmias, however, are associated with conditions such as myocardial ischemia, hypertension, valvar heart disease, or CHF.[79]

Sudden cardiac arrest is a constant threat in individuals with severe arrhythmia. Prevention of sudden cardiac arrest has markedly improved, however, with the early use of automated external cardiodefibrillator devices, and it is strongly suggested that these devices be available in the dental office.[80]

Patients with chronic arrhythmias are frequently maintained with antiarrhythmic drugs such as amiodarone, beta-blocking agents, and calcium channel–blocking agents. Adverse effects of these drugs may include blood dyscrasias, xerostomia, and gingival enlargement, any of which may be associated with poor periodontal health.[77]

The proper protocol for use of local anesthetics containing vasoconstrictor agents is controversial in this patient population and in those with hypertension and some other types of CVD. Vasoconstrictors (epinephrine, levonordefrin) may occasionally increase blood pressure or even induce ventricular arrhythmias if used in excessive quantity. It is beyond the scope of this text to fully address this issue, but adherence to certain principles can help to avoid a medical crisis during dental treatment. Vasoconstrictors are desirable in local anesthetics to facilitate profound anesthesia and prevent release of endogenous epinephrine by the patient. However, the quantity of vasoconstrictor administered should be carefully controlled. Intraosseous and intraligamental injections with local anesthetics containing vasoconstrictors are contraindicated.[81] Local anesthetics should be slowly and carefully administered using aspiration to prevent an untoward reaction, and it is probably prudent to limit the total epinephrine administered to 0.04 mg per dental appointment. This is the equivalent of 2 carpules of lidocaine with 1:100,000 epinephrine or 4 carpules of 1:200,000 epinephrine. For obvious reasons this precaution limits invasive periodontal therapy to small areas and short appointments.[82]

Placement of implanted cardiac pacemakers has become common in treatment of cardiac arrhythmias. The devices are usually placed in the upper chest wall and inserted into the heart chambers through the transvenous route. These devices are often inserted into both the atrium and ventricle (dual chamber). The presence of these devices creates a slightly increased risk for IE, but the AHA does not recommend prophylactic antibiotic coverage when performing dental procedures for these patients.[83]

In rare instances, cardiac pacemakers may be disrupted by external electromagnetic fields. Patients with these devices should avoid exposure to powerful magnets, and magnetic resonance imaging is contraindicated. The function of older, poorly shielded pacemakers may be disrupted by airport security devices and even cellular telephones.[84] It is important, therefore, for the dental practitioner to determine the type of pacemaker and when it was placed. Newer pacemakers are shielded against the adverse effects of minor external electrical fields. One study, however, evaluated the effect of 14 electrical dental devices on shielded pacemakers. The authors report that electrosurgical equipment, ultrasonic instrument baths, and magnetorestrictive ultrasonic instruments may slightly disrupt pacemaker function if used in close proximity to the implanted device. Should this occur, the external device should be removed or disconnected. If this is done, the pacemaker will return to normal function.[85]

Automatic implanted cardioverter defibrillators are often used to manage patients with persistent cardiac arrhythmias, and combination pacemaker/defibrillator devices may be beneficial. Individuals with these implanted devices are not considered to be at increased risk for IE and prophylactic antibiotic coverage is not required for invasive dental procedures unless other risk factors are present.[83]

In most instances, the presence of implanted pacemakers or defibrillators is not considered to be a contraindication to dental treatment. It is probably prudent to exercise some precautions when treating individuals with implanted defibrillators. These devices are programmed to provide an electrical shock to the patient in event of a ventricular arrhythmic event that cannot be stopped by a cardiac pacing function. When shocked, patients are likely to experience an involuntary movement that could lead to injury to themselves or to the dentist. The dentist and patient should discuss this before treatment. If an arrhythmic event occurs, newer defibrillator models will attempt to reverse the arrhythmia by a pacing mechanism. This usually lasts from 10 to 20 seconds and the shock mechanism is not activated unless the pacing has failed to stop the dysrhythmia. Patients are usually aware when they are experiencing an arrhythmic episode and they should forewarn the dentist in time to remove dental instruments before the shock, should it occur. It is prudent to use a mouth prop when performing dental treatment to provide further protection for the patient and dentist. If possible, a local anesthetic without vasoconstrictor should be used. However, to prevent discomfort and release of endogenous epinephrine, a local anesthetic containing a vasoconstrictor often is necessary. However, the total dose of 0.04 mg per appointment should not be exceeded, as discussed earlier.[86]

Ischemic Heart Disease (Coronary Artery Disease)

Ischemic heart disease is the leading cause of sudden death in the United States. It can occur at any age and may induce atrial or ventricular fibrillation, angina pectoris, or myocardial infarction (MI).[74] The underlying condition represents a narrowing of one or more of the coronary arteries because of atherosclerotic plaque formation as a result of vascular injury. This injury may be derived from a variety of etiologic factors, possibly including long-standing severe periodontitis.[71,87]

Angina pectoris

Angina pectoris is the result of a discrepancy between the oxygen demands placed on the myocardium and the ability of the coronary arteries to meet these demands. It most commonly occurs because of narrowing of the lumen of the coronary arteries and is characterized by a sensation of pain or pressure in the retrosternal area. This discomfort may radiate into the shoulder, arms, or side of the neck, mouth, and face.[88] Consequently, angina pectoris may occasionally be mistaken for pain of dental origin.

Stabile angina is defined as pain from exertion, and it usually subsides with rest or administration of vasodilator drugs such as nitroglycerin. Patients with diagnosed stabile angina are often treated with drugs such as nitrates, calcium channel–blocking agents and beta-blocking agents.

Dental patients with stabile angina can usually receive routine periodontal therapy to include necessary surgical procedures. This is predicated, however, on the use of a stress reduction protocol. Appointments should be short, and late morning or early afternoon appointments are preferred. This represents a change from previous dental protocols that called for early morning appointments. The change is based on the observation that endogenous epinephrine may increase the risk for vascular constriction and that endogenous epinephrine levels peak during the early morning hours. Local anesthetics containing a vasoconstrictor are probably indicated in treating these patients to prevent an increase of endogenous epinephrine levels. However, the quantity of vasoconstrictor administered should be controlled as described for other CVDs.

If angina occurs during dental treatment, the procedure should be terminated and the patient placed in a semi-supine position; 100% oxygen should be administered, and a 0.32- or 0.4-mg nitroglycerin tablet placed sublingually. Previous recommendations suggest that the patient's own nitroglycerin would be best to use. However, nitroglycerin has a relatively short shelf-life and it may be more appropriate to use tablets from the dental office medical emergency kit provided it is being properly maintained and expired drugs are being replaced in a timely manner.

Nitroglycerin should be repeated at 5-minute intervals if pain persists, but the minimal dose required should be used because excessive amounts of the drug may induce hypotension. Pain that persists for longer than 15 to 20 minutes or other signs and symptoms of MI dictate that the patient be transferred to the hospital emergency room. These signs and symptoms may include diaphoresis, nausea, syncope, or hypertension.[86]

Throughout the course of managing the medical emergency, vital signs should be monitored and oxygen administered. If pain is severe or if the patient is extremely anxious, 5 to 10 mg morphine sulfate may be given intravenously. In event of cardiac arrest, resuscitative measures should be initiated to include application of automatic external cardiofibrillation. External cardiofibrillation should not be administered to a conscious patient.[89]

Unstable angina is an intermediate stage between stabile angina and MI. The patient may experience chest pain and radiating pain at rest and there may be an increase in the frequency and/or severity of angina. Unstable angina may not be responsive to nitrates. Afflicted patients are not candidates for routine dental care, and emergency dental treatment should be provided only after medical consultation. Use of local anesthetics with vasoconstrictors is generally contraindicated, and the hospital is usually the best site for performing necessary dental therapy.[88]

Variant angina (Prinzmetal's angina) may occur in an otherwise healthy heart as a result of coronary artery spasm. The condition is usually quickly relieved by administration of nitrates, but life-threatening arrhythmias may accompany the angina. Coronary artery spasm may be idiopathic, but it also has been reported to occur in association with cocaine abuse. The emergency steps described above are appropriate for variant angina, and definitive dental care should be deferred until the etiologic factor is identified and controlled. Vasoconstrictors should be used with extreme caution in patients known to have this type of angina.[86]

Myocardial Infarction

MI occurs when the coronary arteries are markedly occluded, with possible necrosis of the portion of the myocardium distal to the point of blockage. Thrombus formation is a common cause and thrombus breakup may place the patient at risk for a cerebrovascular event. Patients usually describe the discomfort associated with MI as a severe crushing substernal pain that may radiate to the neck, jaws, or left arm. The greatest risk associated with MI is ventricular fibrillation, and most deaths occur within 12 hours of the event. Individuals who have survived an MI are at increased risk for recurrence for the first 6 months after the event. Consequently, elective dental therapy is usually contraindicated during this period, although emergency dental care can probably be safely provided, if necessary.[90]

Six months after an MI, routine dental care can usually be provided, but physician consultation is recommended. A stress reduction protocol should be followed to include a calm relaxing atmosphere within the dental office, profound local anesthesia, and conscious sedation, if indicated. Vital signs should be closely monitored. Once again, the dental practitioner should be alert for signs and symptoms of adverse drug reactions or interactions.

Hypertrophic Cardiomyopathy

Hypertrophic cardiomyopathy is a genetically derived condition featuring significant heart muscle enlargement, reduced cardiac output, restricted movement of the septal leaflets of the heart valves, and susceptibility to cardiac arrest. Exercise-induced sudden death may occur and afflicted patients should be treated with caution in the dental office. Patients with cardiomyopathy are at risk for infective endocarditis, and appropriate prophylactic antibiotic coverage is indicated for any invasive periodontal procedures. Medical consultation is imperative before treating patients with this condition. Profound local anesthesia is needed before dental treatment, but

epinephrine should be used with caution. Nitroglycerin or other vasodilating drugs are contraindicated.[91] Consequently, early activation of the medical emergency response system may be necessary if the patient develops medical complications. Oxygen should be administered if the patient develops cardiac symptoms and the practitioner must be prepared to administer cardiopulmonary resuscitation if necessary.

Valvar (Valvular) Heart Disease

Many pathologic processes can damage heart valves in individuals of all ages. Congenital heart defects, rheumatic fever, Kawasaki's disease, systemic lupus erythematosus, ischemic heart disease, and mitral valve prolapse may create valve defects or create blood turbulence that can put the individual at risk for IE. Even heart transplantation may place patients at risk for IE caused by calcification or scarring of heart valves. IE itself may cause valve damage and anyone with a history of IE should be considered at risk for recurrence.[83,92]

Individuals with damaged heart valves are at increased risk for heart failure, cardiac arrhythmias, and IE. Consequently, dental patients with a history of any of the conditions mentioned above should be carefully questioned regarding any known adverse cardiac effects from their disease or disorder. Under ideal circumstances, any patient who reports a medical history of heart murmur should obtain medical evaluation before making decisions regarding dental treatment.[72] Echocardiographic examination or magnetic resonance imaging are very accurate in identifying valve defects that require prophylactic antibiotic coverage before invasive dental procedures including most periodontal therapy.

Mitral valve prolapse is a common condition that occurs when the valve leaflets have lost their tissue tone, resulting in incomplete valve closure. It is common in the general population, especially in young women, and previous use of the weight control drug combination fenfluramine-phentermine may create a low risk for mitral valve prolapse. Currently, individuals with mitral valve prolapse are only considered to require prophylactic antibiotic coverage for dental procedures if regurgitation (heart murmur) is detected.[93]

Infectious Endocarditis

Blood-borne microorganisms may lodge on damaged heart valves or perivalvar endocardium inducing an IE that is potentially life threatening. Individuals with prosthetic heart valves are at the greatest risk should this occur, because of the potential loss of the artificial valve.[94] In an effort to minimize the risk from bacteremias during dental treatment, the AHA has developed guidelines concerning dental management of patients at risk.[83] Invasive dental treatment procedures that involve manipulation of oral soft tissues and bleeding may induce transient bacteremias and theoretically increase the potential for developing IE. These invasive procedures include periodontal therapy such as pocket probing, scaling and root planing, surgical therapy, and the administration of intraligamental local anesthetics. Even the use of oral irrigators or air-abrasive polishing devices has been reported to induce transient bacteremias and, at least theoretically, may increase the risk for IE.[95]

Transient bacteremias also occur in conjunction with daily activities such as bowel movements, tooth brushing, and chewing.[72,96] This has caused some individuals to question the necessity for prophylactic antibiotic coverage for dental procedures. It would appear to be far more imperative that individuals at risk achieve and sustain a high level of periodontal health. This concept is supported by the observation that bacteremias are more frequent and severe in the presence of periodontal infection.[25,66,97]

In 1997, the AHA revised its recommendations for dental management of patients at risk for IE. Prophylactic antibiotic coverage is recommended for certain dental treatment procedures in individuals at risk for IE. Notably, the AHA recommendations specifically address prevention of IE associated with exposure to *Streptococcus viridans*, an organism commonly found in the oral cavity. Decisions regarding the risk from bacteremias by putative periodontal pathogenic microorganisms are left to the dental practitioner.[83] At the time of this publication, it is anticipated that the AHA will soon publish new guidelines indicating a further reduction in conditions in which prophylactic antibiotic coverage is required.

The AHA recommends rinsing with an antimicrobial agent such as chlorhexidine gluconate or povidone-iodine before manipulating periodontal tissues, but long-term home use of these rinses is not recommended because resistant strains of oral microorganisms might develop.[83]

According to the AHA, any periodontal or other dental procedure likely to induce significant bleeding should be preceded by prophylactic antibiotics in patients at risk for IE. If multiple dental appointments are required, an interval of 9 to 14 days between appointments is recommended to reduce the risk for antibiotic resistance. Low-risk dental procedures usually do not require antibiotic coverage, but if unanticipated bleeding should occur during dental treatment, administration of antibiotics within 2 hours of the procedure may offer some protective benefit.[83]

Professional judgment is often required in managing at-risk patients with periodontal disease. Tetracyclines often are prescribed in treatment of some types of periodontitis, but they are contraindicated for prophylactic use in prevention of IE. Some authorities suggest that patients with periodontal infection induced by tetracycline-susceptible organisms such as *Actinobacillus*

actinomycetemcomitans might be best treated using a 2-week course of tetracyclines, followed by a 1-week delay period, and then periodontal therapy using the AHA-recommended antibiotics.[98] Perhaps another more appropriate antibiotic regimen would be to add metronidazole to the amoxicillin recommended by the AHA. This regimen should offer prophylactic protection for IE, yet also be effective against putative periodontal pathogens.

In recent years, a variety of locally delivered timed release antimicrobial substances have been developed for use in periodontal therapy.[99] Several of these products are new to the dental market since the AHA recommendations of 1997. At that time the AHA recommended prophylactic antibiotic coverage when these materials were used because of the possibility of creating a transient bacteremia during insertion. Currently, however, there are no case reports or studies describing IE complications from these procedures. Insertion of some newer, locally delivered agents is far less invasive than for previous devices, and the risk for creating significant bacteremias appears to be quite low.

As discussed earlier, patients with prosthetic heart valves have a high morbidity and mortality rate if IE occurs.[72] Consequently, these individuals require certain special considerations. Ideally all potential oral foci of infection should be eliminated before placement of the prostheses. Unfortunately, this is not always possible because many of these individuals have serious heart conditions before surgical placement of the prosthesis. Routine periodontal or other dental treatment is not recommended for 6 months after valve prosthesis placement, and periodontal health is essential for the lifetime of the patient.[83] Boxes 37-6 and 37-7 outline the degree of risk for IE associated with specific diseases or disorders; Boxes 37-8 and 37-9 provide outlines for dental procedures that do or do not require prophylactic antibiotic coverage according to the AHA. Table 37-4 summarizes the AHA recommendations for specific prophylactic antibiotic regimens.

Anticoagulant Therapy

Patients with prosthetic heart valves and those who are at risk for thromboembolic events often receive anticoagulant therapy administered either during the acute phase of their condition or for their lifetime.[83] In addition, many people take aspirin daily to prevent intravascular clotting, and a number of other drugs are also available that specifically alter platelet aggregation. A daily dose level up to 325 mg aspirin is not usually associated with significant hemorrhage. It is probably prudent, however, to have the dental outpatient discontinue aspirin, nonsteroidal antiinflammatory drugs, ticlopidine, clopidogrel bisulfate, tirofiban, low molecular weight heparin, or

---

Box 37-6   Cardiac Conditions Requiring Antibiotic Prophylaxis Before Periodontal Therapy

High Risk

- Prosthetic cardiac valves
- Previous infective endocarditis
- Complex congenital cardiac defects
- Systemic/pulmonary shunts

Moderate Risk

- Acquired valvar dysfunction
- Hypertrophic cardiomyopathy
- Mitral valve prolapse *with* regurgitation
- Noncomplex congenital cardiac defects

Modified from Dajani A, Taubert KA, Wilson W et al: Prevention of bacterial endocarditis. Recommendations of the American Heart Association, Circulation 96:358-366, 1997. First published in JAMA 277:1794-1801, 1997.

Box 37-8   Dental Procedures That May Induce Significant Bacteremias

- Extractions
- Implant placement
- Tooth reimplantation
- Periodontal procedures likely to cause bleeding (including surgery, scaling and root planing, and probing)
- Endodontic surgery or instrumentation beyond the root apex
- Intraligamentary injections
- Placement of subgingival antibiotic fibers or strips*

Modified from Dajani A, Taubert KA, Wilson W et al: Prevention of bacterial endocarditis. Recommendations of the American Heart Association, Circulation 96:358-366, 1997. First published in JAMA 277:1794-1801, 1997.
*Statement does not address placement of other types of subgingival antimicrobial agents.

---

other platelet aggregation inhibitors for 1 week before a significantly invasive periodontal procedure and for 2 days afterward.[25,58]

Although heparin and low molecular weight heparin are sometimes used in management of outpatients receiving hemodialysis, in individuals with valve prostheses, warfarin (coumarin) remains the most commonly used outpatient anticoagulant drug. Warfarin inhibits use of vitamin K, and therefore has a depleting effect on the vitamin K–dependent clotting factors II (prothrombin), VII, IX, and X.[58,100]

The dosage of warfarin varies according to the extent to which the patient requires prevention of coagulation. Serum levels are monitored by measurement of prothrombin time using the International Normalized Ratio (INR). Prothrombin levels in an outwardly healthy patient have an INR value of 1.0. In most cases, therapeutic levels range from 2.0 to 3.5.[58] The higher the INR, the greater the risk for bleeding complications. Home use INR monitoring devices are available to enable the patient to self-evaluate their levels daily and to sustain target INR levels.[101]

Before periodontal treatment it is important for the dental practitioner to be aware of the INR of patients taking warfarin. Current evidence indicates that limited periodontal surgical procedures and extractions can be

---

Box 37-7   Cardiac Conditions Not Requiring Antibiotic Prophylaxis Before Periodontal Therapy

- Secundum atrial septal defects
- Surgically repaired septal defects without residua beyond 6 months
- Previous coronary artery bypass
- Mitral valve prolapse with *no* regurgitation
- Physiologic or functional heart murmurs
- Previous rheumatic fever or Kawasaki disease without valvar damage
- Cardiac pacemakers and automatic implanted cardioversion defibrillators

Modified from Dajani A, Taubert KA, Wilson W et al: Prevention of bacterial endocarditis. Recommendations of the American Heart Association, Circulation 96:358-366, 1997. First published in JAMA 277:1794-1801, 1997.

Box 37-9   Dental Procedures That Create a Low Risk for Bacteremias

- Restorative procedures with or without placement of retraction cord
- Injection of local anesthetics
- Rubber dam placement
- Suture removal
- Placement or adjustment of orthodontic appliances
- Placement or adjustment of removable prosthodontic appliances
- Dental impressions
- Treatment with topical fluorides
- Oral radiographs
- Shedding of primary teeth

Modified from Dajani A, Taubert KA, Wilson W et al: Prevention of bacterial endocarditis. Recommendations of the American Heart Association, Circulation 96:358-366, 1997. First published in JAMA 277:1794-1801, 1997.

TABLE 37-4	Recommendations for Antibiotic Prophylaxis	
SITUATION	AGENT	REGIMEN
• Standard prophylaxis	• Amoxicillin	• Adults: 2.0 g; Children: 50 mg/kg orally 1 hour before procedure
• Unable to take oral medications	• Ampicillin	• Adults: 2.0 g intramuscularly or intravenously; Children: 50 mg/kg intramuscularly or intravenous 30 min before procedure
• Allergic to penicillin	• Clindamycin	• Adults: 600 mg; Children: 20 mg/kg orally 1 hour before procedure
	or	
	• Cephalexin or Cefadroxil	• Adults: 2.0 g; Children: 50 mg/kg orally 1 hour before procedure
	or	
	• Azithromycin or Clarithromycin	• Adults: 500 mg; Children: 15 mg/kg orally 1 hour before procedure
• Allergic to penicillin and unable to take oral medications	• Clindamycin	• Adults: 600 mg; Children: 20 mg/kg intravenously 30 minutes before procedure
	or	
	• Cefazolin	• Adults: 1.0 g; Children: 25 mg/kg intramuscularly or intravenously 30 min before procedure

Reproduced with permission from Dajani A, Taubert KA, Wilson W et al: Prevention of bacterial endocarditis. Recommendations of the American Heart Association. JAMA 277:1794-1801, 1997. First published in Circulation 96:358-366, 1997. Copyright 1997 American Heart Association.

performed without significant postoperative bleeding at an INR range of 1.0 to 3.0. Greater INR levels may result in some increase in hemorrhage, but localized bleeding is usually manageable by using atraumatic surgical techniques, achieving adequate wound closure, application of postsurgical pressure, and application of topical clotting agents such as foamed gelatin, oxidized cellulose, thrombin, or synthetic collagen. When performing emergency treatment for patients with high INR levels (4.0 to 5.0), tranexamic acid oral rinses may be effective in further controlling hemorrhage. Certain antibiotics (tetracycline, erythromycin, clarithromycin, and metronidazole) are contraindicated in these patients because their use may increase the likelihood of hemorrhage.[102]

Conservative periodontal therapy including surgery that is expected to result in mild to moderate bleeding can be performed on patients receiving anticoagulants with the cooperation of the patient's physician. Reduction of the INR level to less than 3.0 should enable uneventful periodontal treatment. It is generally not advisable to stop the anticoagulant altogether. The physician may suggest a reduced dosage, and it may take between 3 and 5 days to achieve the target INR because of the long half-life of warfarin. It is prudent to have the patient check his or her INR level on the day of treatment to ensure that the desired reduction has been achieved. The decreased level should be sustained for 24 to 48 hours after surgery. Because it takes several days to return to the normal level of anticoagulation after resumption of warfarin, many practitioners have the patient resume taking their warfarin the same day as the periodontal surgery. In event of prolonged postoperative bleeding, blood transfusion, infusion of packed platelets, or infusion of fresh frozen plasma is occasionally necessary.[58,102]

Hypertension

High blood pressure is endemic in the United States with an estimated 15% to 20% of adults being affected.[103] Hypertension is one of the leading risk factors for CVD, stroke, and end-stage renal disease.[104] It has been estimated that one third of individuals with hypertension are not aware of their condition and that one-third are not compliant with prescribed treatment. Consequently, dental health care workers may play an important role in detecting and assisting in managing individuals with hypertension. Monitoring vital signs should be a routine component of dental practice, especially for patients undergoing surgical procedures or conscious sedation. All patients previously identified as having hypertension should be monitored at each dental appointment, and emergency dental therapy should be as conservative as possible for uncontrolled or untreated hypertensive individuals. In contrast, there are no contraindications to providing dental care for patients with well controlled hypertension.

In a series of reports, the Joint National Committee on Prevention, Detection, Evaluation and Treatment of high blood pressure has established guidelines and clarified definitions regarding blood pressure findings.[103,105] Increase of either systolic or diastolic blood pressure is of concern. Individuals with a systolic blood pressure of 120 to 139 mm Hg or a diastolic reading of 80 to 89 mm Hg are now classified as prehypertensive and health-promoting lifestyle modifications are recommended when applicable. However, in individuals older than 50 years, a systolic pressure greater than 140 mm Hg is a more important risk factor for CVD. Hypertension is considered to be present if the blood pressure reaches or exceeds 140 mm Hg systolic or 90 mm Hg diastolic. Values should be averaged from at least two follow-up visits after baseline measurements to establish the diagnosis or to determine the need for medical referral from a dental office. An individual reading in excess of 160 systolic/100 diastolic mm Hg (hypertension stage 2) should warrant immediate medical referral, whereas emergency care should be provided for individuals with blood pressure levels of 180 systolic or 110 diastolic mm Hg or greater (hypertension stage 3) (Box 37-10).

Individuals who are taking antihypertensive medication should be considered hypertensive even if their blood pressure readings are within normal range. Multidrug therapy is common, although a report indicates that diuretic monotherapy may often be at least as effective as combined drug regimens currently in use.[105] Postural hypotension is one of the unwanted side effects of antihypertensive medications and dental patients who have been reclined should first have their chair returned to the upright position, be allowed to sit quietly for a minute or so, then stand carefully while being observed. Illicit

drugs such as cocaine or amphetamines or prescribed drugs such as mineralocorticoids and anabolic steroids may increase blood pressure readings. When possible, individuals who take these drugs should be identified in the dental office and treated with care.[104]

Considerable controversy exists regarding the use of vasoconstricting agents in local anesthetics administered to patients with hypertension. Available evidence indicates that the judicious use of vasoconstrictors is permissible unless the systolic blood pressure exceeds 180 mm Hg or the diastolic blood pressure exceeds 110 mm Hg.[104,106] As discussed previously, however, the quantity of local anesthetic with vasoconstrictor should probably be limited to 0.04 mg epinephrine or its equivalent per appointment. Several reports indicate that epinephrine in local anesthetics does not significantly alter blood pressure levels but, notably, minimal dosages of epinephrine were used in all of these studies.[86,107,108]

Treatment principles for the patient with hypertension include profound local anesthesia, adequate aspiration to prevent intravascular injection, application of psychosedation techniques, and use of conscious sedation, if necessary. Outpatient general anesthesia is not recommended and epinephrine should not be used on retraction cord. The primary goal of management of the patient with hypertension in the dental office is to prevent undue increase in the patient's baseline blood pressure values.[25,109]

Vascular Stents

Angioplasty with insertion of vascular stents has assumed an increasingly important role in management of individuals with coronary artery disease. Although medical consultation is indicated for dental patients with stents, their presence alone is not a contraindication to dental treatment. Prophylactic antibiotic coverage is not necessary, although some cardiologists recommend prophylaxis if emergency dental treatment is necessary within the first 4 to 6 weeks after insertion of the stent. Individuals with coronary artery stents may take anticoagulant medications for the remainder of their lifetime. In that event, the therapeutic modifications discussed earlier would apply.[110,111]

Heart Transplantation

Heart transplantation has become a relatively routine therapeutic procedure in management of a variety of cardiovascular conditions including those discussed in this section. No firm dental management protocols have been established, however, for individuals who receive heart transplants. Whenever possible, periodontal and dental health should be achieved before transplantation, although the underlying cardiac condition may limit the type of dental therapy that can be provided.[86]

Box 37-10	Classification of Adult Blood Pressure
Optimal	<120 systolic/<80 diastolic
Prehypertensive	120-139 systolic/80-89 diastolic
Hypertension	
Stage 1	140-159 systolic/90-99 diastolic
Stage 2	≥160 systolic/≥100 diastolic

From: The seventh report of the Joint National Committee on Prevention, Detection, Evaluation, and Treatment of High Blood Pressure, Bethesda, MD, 2003. National Institutes of Health/National Heart, Lung, and Blood Institute. NIH Publication 03-5233. (See reference 103.)

Postoperative complications are common in heart transplant recipients and infection is a constant risk, in part because of the use of antiinflammatory and immunosuppressive drugs necessary to prevent organ rejection.[112] Therefore, periodontal health may be extremely important to recipients, yet the immunosuppressive drugs may mask early signs and symptoms of infection. Meanwhile, if cyclosporine is used to prevent organ rejection, the risk for gingival enlargement is present.[86] For these reasons, meticulous oral hygiene and a frequent recall periodontal maintenance schedule is indicated. Prophylactic antibiotic coverage is probably indicated for the first 6 months after organ placement in all recipients, whereas those who do not achieve maximal cardiac function or who experience other complications may continue to require prophylactic coverage. The guidelines established by the AHA are probably sufficient unless more stringent antibiotic usage is requested by the patient's cardiologist.

Cerebrovascular Accidents

Stroke and other cerebrovascular accidents (CVAs) can occur at any age. However, the pathophysiologic changes associated with age create a greater risk among the elderly.[113,114] Stroke occurs when blood flow to the brain is blocked, causing ischemia and loss of function of the affected area.[25] Transient ischemic attacks (TIAs) represent a milder form of CVAs in which ischemia causes temporary disorientation or loss of memory or speech. Although these episodes are not life threatening, they may serve as a warning of pending stroke.[115,116]

CVAs may occur in two fashions: (1) disruption of a cerebral blood vessel with ensuing cerebral hemorrhage and formation of a subdural hematoma; or (2) blockage of a cerebral artery by thromboemboli related to coronary artery disease or carotid artery stenosis. Hypertension is the most frequent cause of hemorrhagic stroke, whereas coronary artery disease, atrial fibrillation, carotid artery stenosis, chronic thrombophlebitis, or drug-induced intravascular clotting are associated with thromboembolic or calcific blockage of cerebral blood vessels.[117] Severe periodontal disease has been linked to an increased incidence of stroke, but no cause and effect association has been established[113,118,119] (see Chapter 32).

The dentist has a responsibility for detecting individuals at risk for CVAs or those with signs or symptoms suggestive of stroke. Patients with a history of CVAs or those with diabetes mellitus, cardiac or peripheral vascular disease, or hypertension should be carefully observed during dental therapy. Women who take oral contraceptives may also be at increased risk, as are those who experience chronic atrial fibrillation. Panographic radiographs may be of particular value in detecting the presence of carotid artery stenosis.

Signs and symptoms of stroke range from mild pain or loss of extremity function to sudden death. If an individual survives the original acute episode he or she may experience complete or partial recovery, although the patient may continue to be at risk for recurrence. Facial paralysis may create difficulty in chewing and swallowing of food. This may lead to a significant alteration in diet and possible nutritional deficiency. Food particles may accumulate in the oral cavity, leading to an increased susceptibility to dental caries, periodontal disease, and halitosis. These oral problems may be compounded by medications that the patient takes that are associated with xerostomia.[25]

Dental office management of patients after a CVA or patients who are at high risk for such an incident includes the following:

1. Medical consultation should be sought, as necessary.
2. Careful monitoring of vital signs is important. Do not treat if alarming signs or symptoms of a CVA are evident.
3. Elective dental procedures should be avoided during the recovery phase but oral health is of great importance during the poststroke phase. Patients may have a heightened gag reflex so optimal head positioning and adequate aspiration are essential.
4. Maintain the patient in a calm, comfortable, pain-free mode. Avoid stressful episodes in the dental office and use conscious sedation when appropriate. Deep sedation or general anesthesia should be avoided because these may induce pronounced hypotension that may lead to further cerebral ischemia if vessels of the brain are already occluded.
5. Consider medications the patient may be taking. Patients at high risk or after stroke often receive potent anticoagulant medications on a daily basis and may be at increased risk for posttreatment hemorrhage after periodontal therapy. The principles described for management of patients using anticoagulants apply.[119]
6. Maintain the best possible state of oral health. Individuals with partially occluded cerebral vessels may be at increased risk for development of brain abscesses. Some case reports suggest that these abscesses may occasionally be associated with microorganisms commonly found in severe periodontal disease. This risk appears to be relatively minor but use of prophylactic antibiotics should be considered. If the decision is made to prescribe antibiotics, the recommendations of the AHA would be appropriate. Currently, no controlled studies have been reported that link periodontal diseases to brain abscesses.[120]
7. Assist the patient with oral physiotherapy. Stroke victims may have facial paralysis or weakness and loss of manual dexterity. Anxiety and depression are common in this patient population. This may lead to a reduction in motivation to perform routine preventive

oral hygiene measures. Long-term use of antimicrobial mouthrinses may be indicated, and special oral hygiene devices such as electric toothbrushes, specifically modified manual toothbrushes, floss holders, or mechanical flossing instruments and oral irrigation devices may be beneficial. In severely afflicted individuals, daily oral hygiene measures must be performed by care providers. Frequent recall visits are essential whenever circumstances permit.[59,109]

PROSTHETIC JOINT REPLACEMENT

In recent years, prosthetic joint replacement for damaged body joints has become common in medical practice. Currently, it is feasible to prosthetically replace virtually any joint of the body. Patients undergoing total joint replacement surgery are at risk for postsurgical infection that could lead to rejection of the prosthesis and other complications including death. The incidence of surgically related infections has been markedly reduced, however, by administration of perioperative prophylactic antibiotics. To further decrease this risk, good dental and periodontal health is important to minimize orogenic bacteremias.

Late infections of total joint replacements is also a risk, and some case reports suggest that bacteremias associated with dental treatment may have caused prosthetic joint infection by the hematogenous route.[121] Currently, however, no scientific evidence has been presented to support this concept. Nevertheless, maintenance of good oral health is theoretically important in minimizing the risk from oral bacteremias and this should be emphasized to patients with total joint replacements. In view of the low risk for joint infection from dental bacteremias, some authorities suggest that the risks associated with prophylactic administration of antibiotics exceed the risk for prosthetic joint infection.[122]

Delayed prosthetic joint infections are most frequently caused by gram-positive staphylococci (*Staphylococcus epidermidis* and *Staphylococcus aureus*) or by *Pseudomonas aeruginosa*, a gram-negative organism. These organisms are not common inhabitants of the oral cavity and they are rarely, if ever, found as components of transient bacteremias associated with dental treatment. In addition, those microorganisms commonly found in orogenic bacteremias do not present a great risk for inducing late joint prosthesis infection.[25]

In an effort to resolve this controversy, a panel of experts from the ADA and the American Association of Orthopedic Surgeons have issued advisory statements, most recently in 2003.[123,124] The panel concluded that antibiotic prophylaxis for dental treatment is not necessary for individuals with orthopedic pins, plates, or screws; it also is not indicated for most dental patients with total

joint replacements. However, maintenance of effective oral hygiene and oral health is important in individuals who undergo total joint replacement and for some high-risk individuals who have previously received joint prostheses. This serves to minimize significant bacteremias that occur in conjunction with dental or periodontal infections or daily life events (bowel movement, chewing, bruxing, toothbrushing, and flossing).[83]

Because it is at least theoretically possible that oral bacteremias may contribute to infection of recently placed joint prostheses, the advisory panel recommended prophylactic antibiotic coverage for dental treatment *within 2 years after joint replacement*. After that time, if no replacement complications have occurred, routine dental antibiotic prophylaxis is probably not necessary. Dental antibiotic prophylaxis should still be considered, however, for patients with a history of joint replacement infection or for those with a compromised immune system. The latter would include patients with inflammatory joint disease or those who have received radiation therapy or who are taking immunosuppressive drugs. Other circumstances that may warrant dental antibiotic prophylaxis include malnutrition, blood dyscrasias, HIV infection, diabetes mellitus, and active malignancies.

Invasive dental procedures may place patients at greater risk for bacteremias and subsequent joint infection. These procedures include extractions, periodontal therapy, implant placement, tooth reimplantation, and other procedures previously identified by the AHA as creating a greater risk for infective endocarditis.[83] If the decision is made that dental prophylactic antibiotic coverage is appropriate, cephalexin, cephradine, or amoxicillin, 2 g orally 1 hour before the dental procedure, are recommended if the patient is not allergic to penicillin. In event the patient is unable to take oral medication, administration of 1 g cefazolin or 2 g ampicillin intramuscularly or intravenously is suggested. Individuals allergic to penicillin may receive 600 mg clindamycin orally or intravenously 1 hour before the dental procedure.[124]

PERIODONTAL DISEASE IN HIV-INFECTED INDIVIDUALS

The incidence and severity of oral lesions associated with HIV infection appears to have diminished in recent years with the advent of highly active antiretroviral therapy (HAART). However, this therapy is associated with severe adverse effects and not all HIV-infected patients can tolerate the drugs. In addition, some medical experts advocate withholding HAART until the infected individual becomes significantly immunocompromised. As a result of these factors, the dental practitioner must still be prepared to recognize and treat common oral lesions associated with a compromised immune status.[125,126]

As discussed in Chapter 31, certain periodontal diseases (linear gingival erythema [LGE], necrotizing ulcerative gingivitis [NUG], and necrotizing ulcerative periodontitis [NUP]) occur more frequently in severely immunocompromised individuals, whereas plaque-induced periodontitis may or may not be more common or severe in these individuals. Nonetheless, all practitioners should expect to encounter some HIV-positive patients with periodontal disease.

Treatment concepts do not necessarily differ in an immunocompromised patient. However, the goals of therapy may vary depending on the patient's overall health status. HIV-associated mucosal diseases should be controlled when possible, and acute dental and periodontal infections should be eliminated. Oral health is important to the patient's well-being, and dental evaluation and treatment should be a routine component of medical management of individuals with HIV infection.

Universal precautions and strict adherence to proper infection control procedures are mandatory for all patients in keeping with the recommendations of the Centers for Disease Control and Prevention and the ADA.[127,128] Just as with any other medically compromised individual, the overall health status of an HIV-infected patient is potentially of importance in making therapeutic decisions. For example, a severely immunocompromised patient with AIDS who is in the hospital is not a candidate for elective periodontal surgical procedures. However, if this same patient has advanced periodontitis, transient bacteremias associated with chewing, performance of oral hygiene measures, or bruxing could have a significant impact on his or her systemic health. Consequently, HIV-infected individuals should be educated regarding the importance of periodontal health to their overall health and they should be encouraged to seek periodontal care, if needed, early in the progression of their underlying systemic disease.

This discussion is limited to management of the HIV-positive individual likely to be encountered as a dental outpatient. Such individuals may or may not be aware that they are infected with HIV. Consequently, the dental practitioner must remain alert for the oral signs and symptoms of a compromised immune system (see Chapter 31).

Several authorities have offered guidelines for proper evaluation and management of individuals known to be HIV-posititive.[125,126,128] It is important to know the $CD4^+$ T4 lymphocyte level and viral load of the patient and the length of time in which he or she has been known to be HIV-positive. Marked changes in CD4 counts and viral load may be especially important in patient evaluation. In many instances, individuals with a stable but low CD4 count will be able to undergo periodontal treatment without difficulty. No significant delay in wound healing or increased risk for postoperative infection need

be anticipated.[128] In contrast, a high viral load (greater than 50,000) may indicate that the patient's health status is deteriorating and that the patient is potentially at increased risk for opportunistic infections.[129-131]

Current and previous medical treatment for HIV or the myriad of opportunistic diseases associated with HIV should be reviewed. It is especially important to be informed if the patient has a history of previous or current drug abuse, chronic hepatitis B or C, thrombocytopenia, neutropenia, or adrenocorticosteroid insufficiency. It is equally important to know the medications the patient is taking to identify possible adverse oral reactions to the medications and to avoid adverse drug interactions during dental treatment. New drugs for treatment of HIV infection often become available and the dental practitioner should seek a source of information regarding these drugs and their potential adverse effects. Close coordination with the patient's physician is important and medical laboratory testing may be indicated to monitor the patient's health status.[126,132]

A careful and complete oral examination will determine the dental and periodontal treatment needs of the patient and will detect mucosal lesions, adverse drug reactions, or evidence of other systemic diseases. Acute periodontal and dental infections must be managed and every effort made to assist the patient in achieving good oral health. Conservative nonsurgical periodontal therapy is a treatment option for most HIV-positive individuals and elective procedures including periodontal surgery and placement of dental implants can be safely and effectively performed for many individuals, depending on their overall health status. Decisions regarding elective periodontal therapy require the informed consent of the patient and appropriate medical consultation.

If the patient is periodontally healthy, maintenance recall intervals can be consistent with those associated with routine periodontal treatment protocols. However, it is often desirable to encourage periodontal maintenance recall visits at short intervals (2 to 3 months) and to treat any progressing or recurring periodontal disease as aggressively as the patient's health status will allow. Systemic antibiotic therapy should be used with caution to minimize the risk for development of antibiotic resistant microorganisms or opportunistic fungal infections that may cause severe illness in these individuals. If antibiotic therapy is required, it may be appropriate to also prescribe an antifungal agent such as nystatin oral suspension as a preventive measure.

Despite the progress in medical management of HIV-positive individuals, the presence of this condition may have a profound psychological impact on the patient.[133] Coping with AIDS or HIV infection may cause excessive anxiety or depression, or both, and many HIV-positive individuals are taking prescription antianxiolytic or antidepressant drugs. Occasionally, the emotional strain of the patient may manifest as irritability or anger with the dentist or dental staff, and all dental care providers should demonstrate empathy and concern regarding the patient's situation. It is imperative that dental treatment be provided in a calm, relaxed atmosphere and physically or emotionally stressful dental procedures may require application of conscious sedation techniques.

Dentists should be prepared to interact with HIV-infected individuals who are unaware of their disease status. It is important to remember that early diagnosis and treatment of HIV infection can markedly affect the quality of life and life expectancy of infected individuals, and the dentist should be prepared to advise and counsel patients regarding the process by which testing can be obtained. Individuals with oral lesions suggestive of HIV infection should be informed of these findings and testing should be encouraged. Although self-testing or anonymous testing in public health facilities is available, it may be best to encourage testing in a physician's office or other facility where immediate counseling can be provided if the tests are positive. It is, however, within the purview of the dentist to request appropriate testing provided specific informed consent is obtained.

As previously discussed, some periodontal conditions are more common in HIV-positive individuals, although the same conditions also occur in the general population. LGE may occur as a separate inflammatory condition or in conjunction with NUG. It has been reported to be refractory to treatment, although spontaneous remission may occur. The condition often can be successfully managed, however, using conservative, nonsurgical periodontal therapy. The involved gingival area(s) should be thoroughly scaled and polished. Subgingival irrigation with chlorhexidine or povidone-iodine has been recommended and meticulous oral hygiene should be encouraged. Evidence suggests that LGE may sometimes represent an unusual manifestation of oral candidiasis.[134] Consequently, if lesions are not responsive to conservative periodontal therapy, a course of treatment with topical or systemic antifungal agents, or both, may be indicated. Patients with LGE should be placed on a frequent periodontal maintenance program until the condition is controlled.

The incidence of NUG appears to increase among HIV-positive individuals or others with a compromised immune system. However, treatment of the condition is consistent with that recommended for any patient with NUG. NUG is extremely painful, which must be taken into consideration during therapy. At the initial visit, the affected areas should be gently debrided after application of a topical anesthetic agent. The patient should be encouraged to rinse frequently with warm water, chlorhexidine, or another antimicrobial mouthrinse twice daily. Use of tobacco, alcohol, and spicy condiments should be avoided. Metronidazole or amoxicillin may be prescribed if the patient is experiencing moderate to severe soft tissue destruction, lymphadenopathy, fever, or other symptoms of toxemia. If antibiotics are used, topical or systemic antifungals may also be prescribed to prevent secondary candidiasis. Metronidazole has a narrow spectrum, which targets gram-negative anaerobes, precisely those organisms commonly found in NUG, and is thus less likely to cause secondary fungal overgrowth.

Treatment scheduling recommendations vary markedly in the dental literature. However, the best effect appears to be achieved if the patient is seen daily or every other day with treatment repeated until patient comfort is achieved. As healing progresses, plaque control procedures can be gradually reintroduced. The gingival destruction produced by NUG may result in gingival deformities that can cause difficulty in plaque removal. This may promote recurrence of the acute infection and/or chronic gingivitis or periodontitis. Consequently, reevaluation is necessary approximately 4 to 6 weeks after therapy. If permanent tissue damage has occurred, further therapy may be necessary.[126]

NUP should be treated as early as possible to prevent irreversible loss of periodontal structures and ultimate extraction of the involved teeth. Therapy should include local debridement, scaling and root planing as necessary, and in-office irrigation with chlorhexidine gluconate or povidone-iodine. Meticulous oral hygiene should be encouraged and chlorhexidine mouthrinse prescribed for home use during the initial phase of therapy. If necessary, metronidazole should be prescribed. When possible, periodontal defects should be surgically corrected after control of the acute phase of the condition.[126,129,130]

Necrotizing ulcerative stomatitis is a severely destructive, acutely painful condition that may result in extensive damage to oral soft tissues and underlying bone. The condition may represent an extension of NUP that involves adjacent soft tissue and results in osseous exposure.[129,135,136] Necrotizing ulcerative stomatitis should be treated aggressively with an antibiotic such as metronidazole, with antimicrobial mouthrinses, and by surgical removal of necrotic bone to promote adequate wound healing.[129,135]

It should be emphasized that plaque-induced gingivitis or periodontitis or necrotizing oral diseases can occur in otherwise healthy individuals. However, these diseases may also serve as harbingers of decreasing immune competency and their presence may occasionally represent the first evidence that an individual is HIV-positive. Medical consultation is probably indicated when the patient's HIV status is unknown or he or she is not currently receiving medical care.

PERIODONTAL MANAGEMENT OF THE PATIENT WITH CANCER

In recent years significant improvements have occurred in medical management of patients with cancer, and posttreatment life expectancy has continued to increase. This, coupled with improved diagnostic techniques and increased emphasis on early cancer detection, suggests that the dentist will be called on with increasing frequency to treat patients currently undergoing cancer treatment or with a history of cancer treatment. Ironically, the incidence of death from oral cancer has not been markedly reduced, suggesting that there must be more emphasis on early cancer detection by all health care providers.

General principles of dental management of cancer patients are straightforward. Under ideal conditions, the dentist should be consulted before initiation of cancer therapy. Patients with cancer may be scheduled to undergo chemotherapy, radiation therapy, BMT, surgical excision, or combinations of these procedures, and oral health is an important component in improving morbidity and mortality rates. Interceptive dental treatment should be accomplished to ensure that dental foci of infection are eliminated before cancer therapy and to promote dental health during and after treatment.[137]

At the initial evaluation, the dentist should perform a complete clinical and radiographic examination, obtain a complete medical and dental history, and evaluate the patient's level of oral hygiene. It is important that the dentist be aware of the cancer treatment plan including information regarding the diagnosis and staging of the condition, and the type and timing of the planned cancer therapy. The patient's dental awareness should be evaluated, together with his or her motivation and ability to perform effective oral hygiene measures. Baseline dental and periodontal charting should be recorded, and existing oral pathoses should be eliminated to the extent possible. Nutritional counseling should be provided, if needed, to enable the patient to avoid an increase in incidence of dental caries and soft tissue trauma and to minimize the adverse effects of xerostomia that may result from the cancer therapy.[138]

If circumstances allow, prophylactic procedures and any needed periodontal scaling and root planing should be performed before cancer therapy. Faulty dental restorations should be replaced, repaired, or the involved teeth extracted to prevent subsequent soft tissue irritation or periapical infection in the midst of the cancer therapy. Periodontally questionable or hopeless teeth and those with advanced caries should be extracted or endodontically treated, as appropriate, before cancer treatment. When possible, extractions should be performed 1 week or longer before initiation of the cancer therapy to ensure adequate wound healing. Extractions should be

as atraumatic as possible, sharp osseous ledges should be reduced, and maximal soft tissue closure achieved. Elective periodontal surgery should be avoided because it requires a prolonged healing period and maintenance of meticulous oral hygiene measures during healing. Patients receiving cancer therapy may or may not be permitted to continue with their routine oral hygiene protocol depending on the type of therapy they will receive.[139]

The Irradiated Dental Patient

Radiation is cytotoxic to malignant cells and also to normal cells in the area(s) of exposure. This is a limiting factor in the radiation dosage administered at one time; therefore, therapy is usually performed at intervals (fractionalization) to maximize cancer cell death yet minimize damage to normal tissues. Radiotherapy may be administered by an external beam or by implantation of radioactive substances into the tissue requiring treatment. The unit of measure of radiation exposure is the centigray (cGy), and head and neck exposure is often fractionalized at a rate up to 1000 cGy per week, with a total exposure of 5000 to 6000 cGy. This dosage often results in significant complications. Severe dermatitis and loss of hair follicles may occur on exposed external facial areas, and oral mucositis, xerostomia, and loss of taste sensation (dysgeusia) are common. Loss of vascularity of bone and soft tissue may ensue, and fibrosis and trismus of the muscles of mastication may follow. Damaged oral tissues may become hyperpigmented (postinflammatory hyperpigmentation) and these tissues are very susceptible to opportunistic infections with fungal, viral, or bacterial microorganisms.[139,140]

Radiation mucositis features dry, erythematous, and possibly ulcerated soft tissues. It usually appears 5 to 7 days after radiation therapy and its severity increases in relation to the total radiation dose received. Dental management of mucositis is usually palliative in nature. Rinsing with lukewarm saline or sodium bicarbonate (5%) in water may be of some benefit, and use of a soothing mixture of kaolin and diphenhydramine (Benadryl) is sometimes recommended. However, a systematic review of the literature reported that most topical agents are of little benefit in reducing discomfort from mucositis. Only allopurinol mouthwash and vitamin E were reported to be of weak benefit in a review of randomized controlled studies.[141] Topical anesthetic agents such as lidocaine hydrochloride may partially reduce discomfort. All sources of soft tissue irritation or infection should be eliminated if this has not been accomplished before initiation of radiotherapy. Patients should be advised to avoid use of irritating substances such as alcohol, tobacco products, or spicy foods. Some authorities have recommended the use of mouthrinses containing chlorhexidine gluconate or 0.5% povidone-iodine solution to reduce risk for secondary infection. However, commercially available chlorhexidine mouthrinses contain alcohol and their use may increase patient discomfort. Povidone-iodine is contraindicated in individuals with a history of allergy to iodine.

Oral candidiasis is a frequent complication of mucositis and xerostomia. It may present in its classic pseudomembranous, hyperplastic, or atrophic forms, but atypical ulcerations may also occur. Candidal sepsis may occasionally be fatal. Treatment and prevention of oral candidiasis may be accomplished using topical antifungal agents such as nystatin, clotrimazole, amphotericin B, or fluconazole, whereas systemic antifungal drugs such as ketoconazole, fluconazole, itraconazole, or amphotericin B may also be indicated.[141,142]

In the past, some authorities have recommended curtailment of most oral hygiene procedures immediately after head or neck radiation therapy to reduce the risk for tissue injury. However, the need for maintenance of optimal oral health is obvious and effective oral hygiene is essential to this goal. It may be necessary, however, to resort to the use of gentle oral hygiene measures such as dental sponges or mouthrinses, immediately after radiation therapy, with a gradual return to routine oral hygiene measures. Postradiation outpatients should be encouraged to maintain oral hygiene using ultrasoft toothbrushes, mild toothpastes, and dental floss.

Gingiva is sensitive to irradiation and postradiation gingival recession has been reported in the absence of significant periodontal inflammation. Dental or periodontal infections may pose a significant risk for patients after irradiation. Hypovascularity (obliterative endarteritis) may cause soft tissue ischemia and compromise wound healing. In addition, the risk for osteoradionecrosis is increased. Osseous hypovascularity can result in severe osseous destruction in the presence of periodontal infections. Susceptibility to osteoradionecrosis may persist for the life of the patient.[143]

After recovery from the immediate effects of radiation therapy, the cautious use of nonsurgical therapy is permissible in the area(s) of exposure. Great care should be taken to treat the tissues gently. If extractions are necessary in the zone of irradiation, the use of hyperbaric oxygen therapy is strongly recommended. However, routine periodontal therapy including surgery can be performed in portions of the dental arches outside the zone of radiation.[144]

Trismus of the muscles of mastication may result as a consequence of radiation-induced hypovascularity. Once present, it may be irreversible and patients should be strongly encouraged to perform prophylactic muscle stretching exercises before, during, and after radiation therapy.[145]

Salivary gland function may be permanently impaired if the glands are located within the zone of radiation focus.

This is especially likely if total radiation exceeds 6000 cGy. Two drugs, pilocarpine and cevimeline, have been demonstrated to increase salivary output in some patients after irradiation, especially if prescribed for use before and during the therapy.[146] Under ideal circumstances, initial baseline salivary flow should be evaluated before prescribing the agents to assess their benefit or lack thereof. Alcohol, tobacco products, and caffeine-containing products should be avoided. Artificial salivary substitutes may be of some benefit for patient comfort and patients should be encouraged to consume copious quantities of water.[147]

Xerostomia may result in an increased tendency for plaque accumulation and also a decrease in the pH of residual saliva. These factors markedly increase susceptibility to dental caries and extensive preventive effort should be made. Soft, custom-made, dental carrier trays may be useful to deliver topical fluorides to the natural dentition. Some evidence indicates that neutral sodium fluoride may be preferred to partially neutralize salivary acidity. Patients should adhere to a bland semi-soft diet that is not acidic or cariogenic. If necessary, foods can be thinned with sauces, milk, or gravy to facilitate swallowing.

The Dental Patient Receiving Chemotherapy

Chemotherapeutic drugs may be used alone or in combination with radiation, surgery, or BMT to destroy or suppress malignant cells. Because these agents may also destroy normal tissue cells that are metabolically active, the kidneys, heart, skin, immune system, and the gastrointestinal track (including the oral cavity) may be adversely affected. Oral tissues are continually exposed to injury (physical, chemical, thermal, and microbial) and the mouth is often the primary site of complications associated with chemotherapy.[148]

Xerostomia, dysphagia, altered taste perception, mucositis, soft tissue ulceration, and infection are common adverse oral effects. Onset of mucositis usually occurs within 5 to 7 days of initiation of therapy and the condition may last for days to weeks. Lesions may be more severe and last longer if combination drug therapy or chemoradiotherapy is used. However, some newer anticancer drugs do not induce the degree of mucositis previously experienced by many patients. Chemotherapy-associated mucositis should be managed palliatively as described earlier for radiation-induced mucositis.[25,149]

Gingivitis may be the second most common oral complication, perhaps as the result of secondary pancytopenia associated with drug-induced myelosuppression. Symptoms of myelosuppression may include gingival hemorrhage and increased susceptibility to infections. This condition may profoundly affect decisions regarding oral hygiene procedures and periodontal therapy. Viral infections are common during the most severe stages of myelosuppression, and severe oral ulceration or even disseminated viral infections with agents such as herpes simplex virus are not uncommon. Oral ulcers should be cultured for viral, bacterial, or fungal origin and treated appropriately once the causative agent is identified.[25,148]

Dental management of the patient receiving chemotherapy is similar to that of the patient receiving head and neck radiation therapy. However, chemotherapy is usually administered for 3 to 5 days with recovery intervals of 21 to 28 days before the next therapy. This provides a window in which dental treatment can be safely rendered during the latter stages of the recovery interval. Drug-induced thrombocythemia and leukocytopenia are a constant concern, and careful coordination is required between the dentist and the patient's oncologist. The state of the patient's drug-induced thrombocytopenia may determine the appropriate time for performing any necessary nonsurgical periodontal therapy. Some authorities recommend curtailment of oral hygiene measures when platelet counts decrease to less than 50,000/mm^3, whereas others suggest that gentle oral hygiene measures may be continued as long as the platelet count is greater than 20,000/mm^3. Any ensuing gingival hemorrhage can usually be controlled using local measures such as pressure, placement of a periodontal dressing, or application of topical hemostatic agents. Prolonged gingival bleeding may require platelet supplementation.[150]

Leukocytopenia may predispose a chemotherapy patient to orogenic bacteremias that may lead to sepsis and even death. Consequently, periodontal therapy and vigorous mechanical cleaning should be avoided when the white blood cell count is less than 2000 cells/mm^3 or the absolute granulocyte count is less than 1500 cells/mm^3. If emergency periodontal therapy is required, prophylactic antibiotic coverage is indicated after consultation with the patient's oncologist to select the most appropriate antibiotic. Many cancer therapy protocols require the cessation of all oral hygiene measures at this point, although several authorities believe that the risk for plaque-associated bacteremia necessitates continuation of gentle oral hygiene measures throughout the cancer therapy. These may include wiping of the teeth using cotton swabs or sponges and/or the use of brushing sticks (toothettes) dipped in an antimicrobial agent such as chlorhexidine digluconate. Gentle, frequent professional removal of plaque and calculus often is indicated to assist the patient in maintaining optimal oral hygiene and oral health.[151,152]

Some chemotherapeutic agents may have a neurotoxic effect on peripheral, autonomic, or central nerves. Plant alkaloids such as vincristine sulfate are more commonly associated with this effect and may induce oral pain that mimics pain of periodontal or dental origin. In the event that this occurs, the condition should be managed by use of analgesic medications. Neurologic effects generally subside after chemotherapy has been completed.

Bone Marrow Transplantation

Bone marrow transplantation (BMT) is used for individuals with hematologic malignancies or conditions that are unresponsive to chemotherapy or radiation alone. It is often the treatment of choice for leukemia, lymphoma, multiple myeloma, neuroblastoma, some solid tumors, several types of anemia, and other conditions.[148,153]

Whenever possible, BMT grafts are taken from the patient's own marrow (autologous graft) or from an identical twin (syngeneic graft). Often, however, the BMT is obtained from any donor whose marrow cells are reasonably histocompatible with the patient's marrow (allogenic graft). Weak histocompatibility between the donor and patient may result in development of graft-versus-host disease (GVHD), a condition in which the new donated marrow cells attempt to reject the host.

Before BMT, chemotherapy and total body irradiation are used to destroy the patient's malignant marrow cells. This chemoradiation therapy is usually performed 1 to 2 weeks before marrow transplantation. The BMT recipient is extremely susceptible to opportunistic infections immediately after chemoradiation and infusion of donor marrow cells (pancytopenic phase). The patient is usually isolated for 3 to 4 weeks until adequate engraftment has taken place and host defenses are partially reestablished with the absolute neutrophil count exceeding 500 cells/mm^3.[153] However, neutropenia may continue to place the patient at risk for 1 to 2 months.[148] During the pancytopenic and recovery phase, the patient is at risk from even minor infections. Consequently, the importance of minimizing potential oral sources of infection cannot be overstated.[154]

During the pancytopenic phase, the BMT patient may experience severe ulcerative oral mucositis and xerostomia.[155-157] The patient is also highly susceptible to fungal, viral, and bacterial infections including infection with microorganisms commonly found in periodontal diseases.[157-159] Patients may be especially susceptible to NUG and necrotizing stomatitis. When marrow suppression is severe, these conditions are probably best treated with an antibiotic such as metronidazole. During early recovery (neutropenic phase), gentle debridement, removal of necrotic bone, use of chlorhexidine mouthrinses, antibiotics, and frequent recall intervals should be used after consultation with the patient's oncologist.[148]

GVHD is a potentially life-threatening immunologic phenomenon that may affect up to 45% of BMT patients. Acute lesions usually occur within the first month after engraftment. Target organs include the liver, lungs, and gastrointestinal tract. The exocrine glands, skin, and mucosa also may be affected, and the oral cavity is usually involved. Oral signs and symptoms are similar to those encountered in lupus erythematosus, lichen planus, scleroderma, or Sjögren syndrome.[160] GVHD is classified as chronic if signs and symptoms persist for longer than 100 days, but chronic GVHD also may appear *de novo* several months to years after engraftment.[148]

Diagnosis of GVHD is based on abnormal liver function tests or the appearance of skin and mucosal lesions. A wide variety of oral changes may occur ranging from mild mucosal erythema to severe mucositis. Gingivitis, desquamation of oral tissues, ulcerations, and xerostomia are common.[161] Occasionally, a salivary retention phenomena results in formation of saliva-filled vesicles. Atypical pyogenic granulomas may occur in response to trauma.[148,162]

Immunosuppressant drugs such as cyclosporine, tacrolimus, or mycophenolate mofetil are usually prescribed in patients with BMT to prevent and treat GVHD. Among these drugs, only cyclosporine has been found to induce gingival enlargement in patients with inadequate dental plaque control. Cyclosporine also is associated with an increased incidence of skin and oral squamous cell carcinoma, lymphoma, and Kaposi sarcoma.[163-165]

Drug-induced gingival enlargement is managed by discontinuation of the causative drug when possible, surgical therapy, and establishment of meticulous oral hygiene techniques and frequent maintenance recall visits. However, for reasons that have not yet been elucidated, drug-induced gingival overgrowth rarely occurs in BMT patients.

Periodontal management before and after BMT is consistent with that described for other patients with cancer who receive radiation or chemotherapy.[166] Brushing and flossing usually should be sustained until white blood cell and/or platelet counts decrease to less than the minimally acceptable levels (1500 absolute neutrophils/mm³ or 20,000 platelets/mm³). At this point, cotton swabs, gauze sponges, soft sponge sticks, and chlorhexidine rinses are appropriate for oral cleansing until sufficient recovery of marrow cells has been achieved.[148,164,167] Patients are then managed as described for individuals receiving chemoradiation therapy. Oral GVHD can usually be controlled using topical and/or systemic corticosteroids and other immunosuppressant drugs, and by maintenance of meticulous oral hygiene coupled with frequent dental visits.[160]

RENAL DISEASE

Several diseases of the kidney can result in serious complications including end-stage renal disease (ESRD) and organ failure. The classic phases of kidney dysfunction include inflammation, fibrosis, atrophy, and failure. Acute glomerulonephritis was once the leading cause of renal failure. It may result from infection, complement deficiency, adverse reaction to medications, or other reasons. It also has been described secondary to infective endocarditis or infected ventroatrial shunts.[168] The syndrome of kidney degeneration (nephrotic syndrome) features marked edema, proteinuria, hypoalbuminemia, and increased susceptibility to infection. It may occur in association with systemic conditions such as amyloidosis, systemic lupus erythematosus, diabetes mellitus, and severe or progressive hypertension.

ESRD and renal failure may result in retention of blood urea nitrogen, creatinine, and other metabolic waste products. This uremic syndrome is characterized by azotemia (increased nitrogen-type waste products in the blood) and metabolic acidosis. It may cause secondary CVDs, neuropathy, encephalopathy, osteoporosis, hyperparathyroidism, and bleeding disorders.[169] It may also feature development of grey to bronze discoloration of skin and deposition of a fine white uremic powder (uremic frost) on skin and mucosa.[170]

Oral manifestations of renal failure include an increase in deposition of salivary calculus; a decreased caries rate (because of increased salivary urea nitrogen); severe xerostomia; spontaneous gingival hemorrhage; secondary candidiasis; other fungal, bacterial, or viral infections; increased mobility of teeth; increased periodontal destruction in the presence of periodontal diseases; and tooth loss. ESRD in children may result in enamel hypoplasia and brown discoloration of the teeth coupled with narrowing of dental pulps.[171] Secondary hyperparathyroidism associated with ESRD may initiate deposition of granular calcific deposits in oral soft tissues. Osteopenia reduces the radiographic density of bone (ground glass appearance) and increases susceptibility to jaw fractures.[171,172]

Patients with renal failure are not candidates for dental therapy other than necessary emergency treatment. If teeth must be extracted, delayed wound healing should be expected and any condition that is conducive to bacteremia can result in serious, life-threatening complications. In addition, several drugs used in dentistry may induce acute renal failure and create a risk for individuals known to have renal disease. These drugs include acyclovir, acetaminophen, aminoglycoside antibiotics, tetracyclines, and sulfonamides. Ironically, this creates a situation in which periodontal diseases and their treatment may place the patient at serious risk. Consequently, periodontal health and meticulous oral hygiene measures may be essential to patient survival.[173]

Patients with reversible or irreversible ESRD may be managed by hemodialysis. This procedure is designed to eliminate or minimize accumulation of uremic nitrogen and other waste products in blood and to regulate acid-base balance. The procedure is performed every 2 to 3 days and may require 3 to 5 hours per session. Vascular access is necessary and heparinization is required to prevent blood clotting and disruption of blood flow during the procedure. During hemodialysis the patient's blood is passed from the patient's body through a filtering membrane and back into the blood system after purification. In emergency situations this is accomplished by placement of a double lumen catheter into the femoral, internal jugular or subclavian vein. Often, however, an arteriovenous shunt is created in the arm by anastomosis of the radial artery and cephalic veins.[174]

In contrast to hemodialysis, peritoneal dialysis is accomplished by creation of abdominal ports and infusion of the dialysate solution into the peritoneal cavity. After a sufficient time has passed, the toxic waste products are collected. This procedure may be performed on a continuous or periodic basis and it offers several advantages. For example, it can be performed at home, heparin is not needed, and blood pressure is not affected as it is with hemodialysis. The primary complication of this dialysis method is infection of the port. On occasion, this infection has been caused by putative periodontal pathogens.[174,175]

Long-term hemodialysis has a mortality rate of 20% to 25%, with various CVDs (stroke, MI, hypertension, IE) and sepsis representing the most frequent complications. Currently, the procedure often is used as a temporary measure before organ transplantation from a suitable donor.[174]

Renal transplantation is a highly successful means of managing ESRD provided the organ donor and recipient share compatible blood and antigen types. Immunosuppressant drugs are required to prevent organ rejection, with the quantity and duration dependent on the degree of donor–recipient type matching. On occasion, these drugs may be used for life. This places the recipient at risk for toxemia from bacterial, viral, and fungal infections. Graft rejection is the ultimate complication, although CHF, hypertension, IE, or cardiac arrhythmias are among the leading causes of posttransplant death.[176]

Oral complications are most often related to the medications used to prevent organ rejection. A variety of oral infections may occur, yet they often do not present with the typical features associated with their presence.[177] Cyclosporine remains the antirejection drug used most often, although use of alternative agents such as tacrolimus, sirolimus, mycophenolate mofetil, and others is increasing. Cyclosporine may influence gingival enlargement but this has not yet been reported in conjunction with other immunosuppressants. Genetic susceptibility may influence the severity of cyclosporine-related gingival enlargement, when it occurs.[178] Long-term use of cyclosporine also has been associated with development of opportunistic infections, oral hairy leukoplakia, and increased susceptibility to oral malignancies including lymphoma, squamous cell carcinoma, and Kaposi sarcoma.[179]

Dental Management

No firm protocols have been established for dental management of individuals with chronic or end-stage renal disease, or for recipients of renal transplants. Potential medical complications usually can be identified by a thorough medical and dental history and evaluation of vital signs, coupled with medical consultation and appropriate laboratory screening tests. Oral infections including periodontal diseases may place the patient with renal disease at risk and appropriate measures should be taken to eliminate or to decrease this risk.[173,180] Dental therapy must be closely coordinated with the patient's physician. Heparin is a short-acting anticoagulant administered during the hemodialysis procedure to facilitate blood flow and elimination of toxic waste products. Heparin administration and the periodic elimination of toxic waste products may significantly influence the timing of invasive dental procedures including periodontal therapy. It is usually recommended that periodontal treatment be performed the day after hemodialysis to minimize the risk for systemic infection, although postoperative hemorrhage may result from residual heparin accumulation. Care should be used in prescribing medications that are metabolized in the kidney because the drugs will be retained in the bloodstream for prolonged periods and may reach toxic levels. These drugs include analgesic agents such as aspirin and most nonsteroidal antiinflammatory drugs. Acetaminophen, codeine, and local anesthetics are metabolized in the liver and therefore are safe to use. Some antibiotics such as aminoglycosides, tetracyclines, and polypeptides (bacitracin and polymyxin) are potentially nephrotoxic, and potassium penicillin should be avoided to avoid excessively high serum potassium salt levels. Conversely, other forms of penicillin are well tolerated. Although non–potassium-containing penicillins are metabolized in the kidney, accumulation of high quantities of these drugs in serum is generally not toxic.[171,180]

Monitoring of vital signs is a recognized standard for dental therapy. One should be cautious, however, with patients receiving dialysis. If these individuals have an anastomosis site in an arm, care must be taken to avoid trauma to the area, and the portal should not be used to administer intravenous drugs. In addition, *blood pressure measurements and injection of intravenous or intramuscular drugs are contraindicated in that arm.*[171,181]

Whenever possible, the dentist should participate in treatment planning for individuals scheduled to receive dialysis or organ transplantation. Ideally, all potential oral foci of infection should be eliminated or controlled. Hopeless and questionable teeth should be extracted, although endodontic therapy may be appropriate on some occasions without placing the patient at undue risk. Effective oral hygiene measures should be taught and reinforced, and antiseptic mouthrinses such as those containing chlorhexidine gluconate may be beneficial.

Oral infections can be life threatening unless detected and treated early in their course. Any oral lesion suggestive of infection should be evaluated by appropriate measures including cytologic examination, culture, and/or biopsy, when indicated.[173] It should be remembered that immunosuppressant drugs may suppress and mask the usual signs and symptoms of infection and inflammation including clinical evidence of active periodontal disease.[169]

Dental or periodontal therapy should be conservative and noninvasive when possible, especially for the first 3 months after transplantation. If invasive procedures are required, prophylactic antibiotic coverage should be considered using the recommendations of the AHA in prevention of IE. Infective endocarditis may occur in transplant patients who do not have a history of valvar damage.[171] Currently, however, there are no clinical studies that validate the benefits of prophylactic antibiotic coverage in this patient population.

LIVER DISEASE

Hepatic disease is of growing concern in medicine. In recent years, there has been a marked increase in the incidence of both acute and chronic hepatic disease, and the conditions are often associated with severe complications. Acute hepatitis may be caused by various viruses (hepatitis A, B, C, D, E, F, and G), toxins, or drugs, and it may or may not be reversible. Acute hepatitis is characterized by malaise, fatigue, nausea, vomiting, and possibly jaundice. Gradual recovery usually occurs after viral hepatitis, but chronic infections may persist. Infection with the hepatitis B virus (HBV) may lead to chronic liver disease, liver failure, and malignant transformation in a small but significant number of infected adults and in the majority of infected children. The virus may be transmitted by means of the fecal-oral and parenteral routes. In recent years, the incidence of HBV infection has been reduced in developed countries because of development of an anti-HBV vaccine and application of universal protective methods in the health professions. In addition, improved treatment methods have served to reduce the potential for transition into chronic liver disease.[173,182]

In contrast, the incidence and significance of hepatitis C virus (HCV) infection has continued to increase. This virus is primarily transmitted parenterally, and, currently, no vaccine has been developed. Blood transfusion was once the major source of transmission; however, this risk has been markedly reduced by screening potential blood donors to identify HCV carriers. HCV may also be transmitted by intravenous drug abuse and occupational exposure to blood and blood products among health care professionals. Coinfection with HIV may markedly influence the severity of HCV-related illness.[183] A growing amount of evidence indicates that HCV may be sexually transmitted, and transfer of the virus by household exposure has been suggested.

Signs and symptoms of acute hepatitis C infection may include fever, jaundice, malaise, nausea, vomiting, and fatigue, but asymptomatic infection also is common. Urticaria, cutaneous and oral lichen planus, and Sjögren syndrome may sometimes represent a marker for undiagnosed hepatitis C infection.[184] Hepatitis D appears to occur only as a coinfection with HBV and its presence may contribute to a fulminant hepatitis. In the United States it is found most often in intravenous drug users. Hepatitis E virus may be responsible for acute or chronic disease in developing countries. The existence of the hepatitis F virus has not been clearly confirmed but hepatitis G may be present as a coinfection with HCV.[185] Recently, a previously unidentified transfusion-transmitted viral hepatitis has been reported in a Japanese population but its role in inducing chronic hepatitis is unclear.[186]

The application of universal infection control precautions has assured that individuals with acute infectious hepatitis can be safely treated in the dental office. However, regardless of its etiology, acute hepatitis may markedly impair liver function and elective dental treatment should be deferred until the patient has been medically evaluated and cleared for dental treatment.[185,187,188]

Chronic liver disease may occur as a result of acute infection, as an autoimmune phenomenon, because of adverse reactions to a variety of prescription or illicit drugs, and because of alcohol abuse. Chronic liver disease is defined as hepatic inflammation of more than 6 months in duration. When signs and symptoms are present they may include fatigue, malaise, jaundice, and abdominal pain. Serum aminotransferase levels may be increased and many patients using drugs associated with liver damage are monitored periodically with liver function tests to ensure early detection of adverse reactions.[188-190] Evidence suggests an association between chronic HCV infection and oral lichen planus. Although this association varies in certain geographic locations, patients with oral lichen planus who are unresponsive to established treatment measures should be considered for HCV screening.[191]

Liver cirrhosis is characterized by scarring and fatty infiltration of liver tissues. It may markedly disrupt normal liver function. Although the condition is traditionally associated with alcohol abuse, it may also result from acetaminophen overdose, abuse of illicit drugs, or as an adverse reaction to a wide variety of prescription medications.

Because of the potential risk from invasive periodontal treatment procedures in individuals with liver cirrhosis or end-stage hepatic disease (ESHD), the prudent practitioner should remain alert to clinical features suggestive of the condition. No specific clinic signs or symptoms have been identified that are indicative of liver damage. However, some clinical features should elevate the practitioner's suspicions regarding possible excessive use of alcohol by the patient. These features include palmar erythema, spider nevi, rhinophyma, skin bronzing, and alcohol halitosis. Additional signs such as angular cheilitis or loss of papillae on the dorsum of the tongue may suggest an associated nutritional deficiency.[173,190]

Liver transplantation represents the standard of care for individuals with many types of ESHD. Posttransplant dental management is similar to that described for management of individuals receiving renal transplants. Compromised liver function may be a continuing finding after transplantation, and transplant recipients are at risk for graft rejection or potentially fatal systemic sepsis. Despite these potential complications after transplantation, the 5-year survival rate exceeds 80%.

Dental Management

Individuals with severe liver disease should be treated with caution in dental practice. Medical consultation is strongly recommended to determine the extent of liver damage and to discuss possible contraindications to dental treatment. The liver is the site of metabolism of many drugs, including some that are often used in conjunction with dental treatment. Agents such as acetaminophen, narcotics, local anesthetics, benzodiazepines, barbiturates, and some antibiotics such as erythromycin and ampicillin are retained in the blood system for prolonged periods if liver function is defective, and the potential for toxic overdose is increased. In the presence of liver disease, alternative drugs should be considered or normal dosages reduced to minimize this risk.[173]

Individuals with liver disease are also at risk for excessive bleeding because several coagulation factors (II, VII, IX, and X) are manufactured in the liver. Thrombocytopenia may also occur because of secondary bone marrow cell suppression. Clot fibrinolysis may be accelerated, possibly affecting wound stabilization and healing.

Patients with liver dysfunction who are scheduled for invasive periodontal or other surgical procedures should be screened using appropriate blood tests to anticipate and prevent possible bleeding complications (Table 37-3). These tests should include a complete blood count with differential, platelet count, bleeding time, prothrombin time, and partial thromboplastin time.[192] Abnormal test results may warrant medical consultation and

modification of the proposed therapeutic plan. It is important that precautions be taken to minimize the likelihood of postsurgical hemorrhage. Wound sites should be kept relatively small, and close tissue approximation with adequate suture placement is desirable. Firm pressure should be applied to the surgical site and the use of local hemostatic agents may be indicated. If extensive bleeding is anticipated, an oral rinse containing tranexamic acid may be beneficial.[193] In individuals with ESHD and diminished platelet production, routine periodontal surgical procedures can usually be performed as long as the platelet count remains greater than 50,000/mm^3.[62]

Abnormal protein metabolism and accumulation of toxic levels of serum ammonia is a major concern in patients with a failing liver. In a worse case scenario, ammonia accumulation is associated with seizures, encephalopathy, coma, or death. The dental practitioner should be alert for early signs or symptoms of ESHD. These may include marked personality changes, mood alterations, confusion, and tonic or clonic muscle hyperactivity. Even in early states of organ failure, increased levels of serum metabolic end products may interfere with normal healing.[172]

Compromised liver function may result in accumulation of varying amounts of fluid in the peritoneal cavity (ascites). This may increase the risk associated with periodontal infection if extensive orogenic bacteremias occur. The risk for orogenic infection may also be greater in individuals taking immunosuppressant drugs to prevent organ transplant infection and rejection.

The need for prophylactic antibiotic coverage during invasive dental procedures is controversial in patients with hepatic disease or liver transplants. There are no controlled studies that affirm that prophylactic antibiotics decrease the likelihood of systemic sepsis or organ infection in this patient population. If the decision is made to use antibiotic coverage, the recommendations of the AHA regarding prevention of bacterial endocarditis are most often suggested.[192]

It should be clear, however, that untreated oral infections may increase the potential for life-threatening systemic sepsis in all individuals with organ transplants who are taking immunosuppressant medications. Consequently, affected individuals and their physicians must be aware of the importance of good oral health to survival. Hopeless and questionable teeth should be extracted, although endodontic therapy appears to be feasible, if needed, without undue risk to the patient. Surgical or nonsurgical periodontal therapy should be performed as necessary to achieve oral health. Patients must be instructed in performance of effective oral hygiene procedures, and a periodontal recall system should be established sufficient to maintain maximal oral health. In most instances 2- to 3-month recall intervals appear to be satisfactory.

DISEASES OF THE RESPIRATORY SYSTEM

Acute Upper Respiratory Tract Infections

Dental patients often present for treatment with partial upper airway obstruction or acute upper respiratory infections (URI). These may include the common cold, influenza, tonsillitis, enlarged adenoidal tissue, sinusitis, allergic rhinitis (hay fever), or other conditions. Although these conditions do not necessarily preclude dental treatment, it may be important to take their presence under consideration when caring for affected individuals. The application of the universal occupational safety precautions recommended by the ADA and the Centers for Disease Control and Prevention will protect the practitioner, the dental staff, and other patients from contracting infectious diseases.[194] However, the use of prescribed or over-the-counter medications by patients to treat their URI may impact on dental therapy. Antihistamines and nasal decongestants may cause xerostomia. In addition, these drugs may adversely interact with analgesics or sedatives that may be used as a part of dental therapy. For example, antihistamines can potentiate the response to analgesics, sedative, or tranquilizers. In addition, excessive use of nasal decongestants may increase the risk for hypertension, and ephedrine use may result in an exaggerated response to local anesthetics containing epinephrine or other vasoconstrictor agents.

When patients with URI seek dental care, the practitioner should question them carefully regarding the signs and symptoms they are experiencing and any medications they are taking. The patient should be observed for evidence of active infection such as sinusitis, tonsillitis, laryngitis, or streptococcal throat infection, and medical referral should be provided if appropriate.

Patients who are experiencing drug-induced xerostomia should be cautioned to avoid mouthrinses with high alcohol content and to use sugarless gum, salivary substitutes, and frequent sips of water. If the patient must frequently take xerostomia-inducing medications, the daily use of home fluoride products is probably indicated for their anticaries effects.[192]

Maxillary sinusitis pain may simulate dental pulpitis or periapical abscess in maxillary posterior teeth. The operator should be cautious to avoid overly zealous dental treatment in this situation. Panographic radiographs are of benefit in identifying the maxillary sinus cloudiness often associated with severe sinusititis.[60]

URI often necessitates mouth breathing in afflicted patients. The superficial xerostomia induced by this may result in localized gingivitis, most commonly in the maxillary anterior facial region. Thorough professional debridement and excellent daily home care will help to alleviate the gingivitis, but the patient may also require topical application of lubricating agents such as petroleum jelly or lubricating gels. Currently, there is little evidence that mouth breathing gingivitis can be eliminated, but the condition can usually be controlled sufficiently to prevent development of periodontitis.[195,196]

Patients with URI who have to breath through their mouth may encounter some difficulty when receiving dental treatment. It is important that the airway remains open throughout the procedure. The use of a rubber dam or throat pack is contraindicated for this reason, as is nitrous oxide/oxygen conscious sedation.

Pulmonary Diseases

Special treatment considerations may be required for the patient with asthma or chronic obstructive pulmonary diseases (COPD) such as emphysema or chronic bronchitis. Epidemiologic data suggest that there is an association between poor periodontal health and COPD, but the nature of this relation is yet to be determined.[197]

Patients with asthma may experience bronchial spasm as a result of allergic reactions to drugs such as aspirin or some local anesthetics, food, or even oral hygiene products and dental restorative materials.[198] Symptoms may include wheezing, coughing, and labored breathing. Emotional or physical stress and viral infections may also trigger such a reaction, as can certain medications such as aspirin. This means that the patient with asthma is at constant risk for experiencing a severe asthmatic attack in the dental office. In this event, use of an inhaled corticosteroid or a beta-agonist such as albuterol is widely recommended.[199] A typical dose of albuterol is 2 puffs a few minutes apart and 1 or 2 additional puffs if the patient does not respond well within 5 minutes.[62] If available, a pulse oximeter can be used to monitor oxygen saturation. The dentist must have an oxygen source and injectable epinephrine available in the event that the symptoms do not subside. Epinephrine at a concentration of 1:1000 can be administered subcutaneously or intramuscularly. Preloaded syringes that contain 0.6 ml of this dilution are available. The preferred quantity to be administered is 0.2 to 0.4 ml per injection and the same dosage can be repeated if necessary at 30- to 60-minute intervals. It is probably inappropriate to assume that improvement from emergency treatment has adequately controlled the attack. More serious exacerbation may be imminent and patients may require transportation to the hospital for follow-up monitoring and care as necessary.[200]

Frequent use of corticosteroid or beta-agonist inhalers tends to dry oral mucosa and to make the patient susceptible to candidiasis. Patients who use these inhalers also may be susceptible to dental caries and periodontal disease, and excellent oral hygiene coupled with frequent maintenance visits is imperative.[201]

COPD is characterized by difficulty in obtaining adequate oxygenation and perfusion of body tissues during normal breathing. It may occur secondary to chronic bronchitis or emphysema, or both. The result may be development of cyanosis, cardiac enlargement, and tissue edema. Compensatory erythrocytosis may also occur that can interfere with normal blood coagulation. Oxygen depletion may be worsened by episodes of emotional stress or bronchial edema.

Chronic bronchitis is often associated with smoking and it may induce a productive mucous-producing cough. Emphysema represents a distention of the alveolar spaces of the lungs and it is often the aftermath of chronic bronchitis. Symptoms include wheezing, dyspnea, and cough. Individuals with emphysema may require constant oxygen supplementation, another circumstance that can induce xerostomia and its concurrent oral problems.

A thorough medical history is essential and medical consultation may be necessary in dental management of patients with asthma or COPD. A stress reduction protocol should be applied and sedatives or tranquilizers may be useful to ensure patient comfort and to prevent apprehension. Carefully administered conscious sedation using midazolam or other tranquilizing agents appears to be safe for the individual with asthma, but inhalation sedation is usually contraindicated because it may interfere with oxygenation and precipitate an acute asthmatic attack.[202] Treatment procedures should be short and every effort must be made to maintain a patent airway. Barbiturates and narcotics or other central acting drugs should be used with caution because they may depress the respiratory centers of the brain and further endanger respiratory efficiency.

Special attention should be paid to control of hemorrhage during invasive dental or periodontal procedures. Excessive bleeding may interfere with breathing comfort. Adequate suctioning and minimal use of water or saline spray is an important consideration for individuals at risk.[203] In addition, alterations in the clotting mechanism is possible in emphysemic individuals. Consequently, blood studies are often indicated before performing surgical periodontal procedures. As a minimum, bleeding time and clotting tests should be requested along with a complete blood count with differential and platelet aggregation tests.

Tuberculosis

Tuberculosis is caused by the bacillus, *Mycobacterium tuberculosis*. Typically it gives rise to a granulomatous disease that can affect several systems of the body. The incidence of tuberculosis is low in developed countries of the world, but the prevalence of the disease has increased since the onset of the HIV/AIDS epidemic. Individuals with compromised immunity for any reason are at increased risk, as are institutionalized patients.[204]

There are at least five types of tubercle bacilli, all of which are capable of causing infection in humans. Pulmonary tuberculosis is usually contracted by inhalation of infected sputum droplets. Primary exposure to the tubercle bacilli may lead to subclinical infection but only about 10% of those exposed develop the disease. Individuals with the infection may remain asymptomatic for years, and then the infection will be activated (secondary tuberculosis).[204] Tuberculosis is a life-threatening disease, but early symptoms may be very mild. These symptoms include weight loss, easily fatigability, mild cough, and anorexia. Later, the classic symptoms of persistent cough and bloody sputum can develop in the infected individual. Once the infection is present, it can be spread to bone and the genitourinary tract by the hematogenous route.

Oral lesions are rare, but they can be acquired either by primary inoculation or by spread of the pulmonary disease. Lesions most commonly manifest as painless ulcerations on the dorsum of the tongue. Other sites include the palate, gingiva, tooth extraction sockets, buccal mucosa, and lips. Tubercular osteomyelitis can develop from direct spread of surface oral lesions.

Diagnosis is usually made on the basis of medical history, physical examination, sputum culture, chest radiography, and a positive delayed hypersensitivity (tuberculin) skin reaction. The tuberculin test may remain positive in individuals with a history of exposure to the organism, and positive sputum culture remains the most reliable means of diagnosis. Tuberculosis is usually managed by long-term administration of two or more chemotherapeutic drugs. These most commonly include isoniazid, rifampin, ethambutol thiacetazone, paraaminosalicylic acid, pyrazinamide, and ethionamide. The patient is considered infectious until sputum cultures are negative.[205]

With the advent of AIDS and other conditions that compromise the immune system, a number of nontuberculosis mycobacterial infections have become relatively common. These may include the *Mycobacterium avium-intercellular* complex, *Mycobacterium chelonae*, *Mycobacterium kansasii*, and *Mycobacterium scrofulaceum*. Ulcerative oral lesions are uncommon with these infections, and diagnosis is made by culture of the organisms from tissue biopsy. *M. scrofulaceum* is associated with tuberculous infection of cervical lymph glands (scrofula).[204]

Tuberculosis is of concern in dental and medical practice because the organism(s) is very resistant to surface disinfectants, and routine infection control personal protective gear will not always prevent cross-infection of the practitioner, the staff, or other patients.[194,206] Face shield masks are recommended for maximum protection against aerosol-associated infections. Protective respirators should be worn when treatment is provided for individuals ill with the pulmonary form of the disease and treatment in an isolated, hospital environment is appropriate. Despite these precautions, infection of health care workers in tuberculosis treatment facilities is common. In addition, with the advent of HIV/AIDS, multidrug-resistant forms of the mycobacteria have evolved. As a preventive measure, many health care facilities now require biannual tuberculin testing for all employees. Anyone who tests positive must receive multidrug therapy even if they remain asymptomatic. Failure to do so can result in loss of treatment privileges or employment.[207]

Despite these cautionary statements, it should be noted that the disease has not reached epidemic proportions in the United States, and routine dental/periodontal care generally can be provided for individuals with a history of tuberculosis who have been successfully treated and released into the general population.

DRUG ABUSE

Mood-altering drugs have been used since ancient times as components of religious ceremonies, to increase endurance, to relieve hunger and fatigue, for relaxation, and for medical purposes. Cocaine was once used in dentistry as a local anesthetic, and alcohol in low doses is sometimes recommended for prevention of heart disease and to reduce stress. Unfortunately, however, mood-altering drugs are most commonly used for social purposes and their excessive use has plagued mankind for at least 2000 years.

The illicit use of drugs has reached staggering proportions in the United States. It has been reported that more than 25,000,000 Americans have used cocaine or heroin at least once, yet alcohol and cannabis (marijuana, hashish) use is even more common.[208,209] At least 150 drugs have been identified as substances of abuse and artificial "designer" drugs are continually being created. Drugs of abuse can be classified as stimulants, depressants, hallucinogens, and solvents or inhalants. The dental practitioner is extremely likely to be asked to provide dental care for individuals who are addicted to or who use illicit drugs or alcohol. In addition, a high percentage of users of mood-altering drugs also use tobacco products.[208]

Many medical disorders are more common in individuals who abuse drugs, including AIDS, hepatitis, liver failure, pulmonary disease, skin infections, venereal diseases, diabetes mellitus, gastrointestinal disorders, and CVDs.[208] For example, acute cocaine toxicity may induce a variety of CVDs such as angina pectoris, MI, and death.

Illicit drugs have been associated with adverse oral manifestations. Opiates (e.g., heroin, cocaine, OxyContin), stimulants (e.g., amphetamines), sedatives (e.g., barbiturates), hallucinogens (e.g., Peyote), cannabis, and alcohol all may induce xerostomia, potentially leading to an increased susceptibility to accumulation of bacterial plaque, dental caries, and periodontal diseases.[210]

Controlled release oxycodone hydrochloride currently is a major drug of abuse because of its intense, rapid, and prolonged effect.[211] The dental practitioner should remain alert for signs and symptoms associated with a physiologic need for opiates, including rhinorrhea, increased lacrimation, and dilated pupils.

Hallucinogenic or stimulant drugs include lysergic acid diethylamide (LSD), mescaline, (Peyote), phencyclifin (PCP), psilocybin, and a variety of "designer" drugs. These substances generally do not induce a physiologic addiction, although a psychologic need may develop. Drugs of this nature may induce a toxic psychosis leading to bizarre behavior, inordinate excitement, or panic attacks.[212] A wide variety of these drugs have become popular among teenagers and young adults because of their stimulant and euphoric effects. The abuse of "designer" or "club" amphetamines such as 3,4-methylenedioxymethamphetamine (MDMA; Ecstasy, Adam), 3',4-methylenedioxyamphetamine (MDA; Love), 3,4-methylenedioxyethylamphetamine (MDEA; Eve), prolintane, and 10% nitrite psilocybin is increasing on a worldwide basis, and polydrug use of designer agents and alcohol is common and dangerous.[213] For example, Ecstasy may induce severe water intoxication. Death has been reported due to subsequent ingestion of as little as one glass of water.[214] Other reports link Ecstasy with acute aortic dissection and facial acneiform dermatosis. Ketamine (an anesthetic), gamma-hydroxybutyrate (GBA), and flunitrazepam (Rohypnol—a fast acting benzodiazepine) are the drugs most often associated with "date rape."[215]

Cannabis (marijuana, hashish, hashish oil) may be the most frequently used illicit drug in the Unites States. It induces euphoria and it may be smoked as a cigarette or in a pipe. The active ingredient of cannabis is delta-9-tetrahydrocannabinol (delta9-THC), and potency of the substance is dependent on the THC concentration. Sinsemilla is a form of marijuana with an especially high THC content, and it has been suggested that the THC concentration in cannabis products has gradually increased in recent years.[216] This may result in increased adverse side effects when this drug is used. It is known that excessive and prolonged use of cannabis may impair the immunologic system. Reduced mental function and memory loss also have been reported, and cannabis contains nearly twice as many potential carcinogens as equivalent amounts of tobacco. Prescription of marijuana, however, has been promoted by some to alleviate pain and anxiety among terminally ill individuals with cancer or AIDS.

Cannabis use is associated with xerostomia, edema and erythema of the uvula, leukoplakia, oral cancer, and even gingival enlargement. Use of normal amounts of local anesthetics, retraction cord, and other dental agents containing epinephrine may exaggerate the sympathomimetic effects of individuals who are under the influence of cannabis and may induce tachycardia and peripheral vasodilation. It has been suggested that dental patients who acknowledge frequent use of cannabis should be advised to discontinue its use for a least 1 week before dental treatment.[208]

Cocaine use and abuse has been described throughout recorded history. The drug possesses local anesthetic properties when applied to mucous membranes. It is available as a white crystalline powder that can be absorbed through the mucous membranes of the oral cavity, nasal passages, vagina, or rectum. It also may be mixed with liquid and injected subcutaneously or intravenously. Perhaps it is most frequently used today when prepared in solid form (crack) and smoked. Cocaine abuse may induce severe psychosis (delirium, paranoia, anxiety, depression, or schizophrenia). Atypical angina, myocardial ischemia, MI, and death have been reported as a result of cocaine overdose or its use in combination with other drugs.

Application of cocaine to mucous membranes may induce mucosal irritation and even ischemic necrosis if used in excess. Resultant ulceration or perforation of the nasal septum has been reported, and similar effects can occur when the substance is applied to oral tissues. Long-term oral use has been associated with epithelial desquamation, with gingival erythema and ulceration and with irreversible destruction of alveolar bone.[217,218]

Stimulants such as amphetamines are sympathomimetic agents and they may induce tachycardia, vasoconstriction, elevated blood pressure, vasculitis, and renal failure. Amphetamine derivatives may be available by prescription (diethylpropion, phendimetrazine tartrate) or over-the-counter (ephedrine) as appetite suppressants and to prevent sleepiness.

Methamphetamines can be swallowed, injected intravenously, or smoked (ice, crystal, MDMA, Ecstasy, XTC, Adam, Eve, Love). Symptoms of intoxication include headache, nausea, tremor of extremities, anorexia, and dilated pupils.

Nitrous oxide is a mood-altering inhalant sometimes abused to achieve euphoria. It may be a major drug of abuse among dentists and others who have access to equipment necessary to administer nitrous oxide/oxygen conscious sedation. However, the substance is also used as a propellant in whipping cream and other products and its abuse is relatively common in younger individuals. On occasion, uncontrolled inhalation has been associated with peripheral nerve damage, mitotic

poisoning of bone marrow, psychosis, and mental impairment.[219]

Alcoholism is a chronic, progressive, and potentially fatal malady that is associated with numerous adverse effects on body systems and in the oral cavity. Ingestion of alcohol induces a transient stimulant effect, followed by central nervous system depression. Susceptibility to excessive use of alcohol may be inherited or precipitated by psychologic factors such as loneliness and depression. Alcohol abuse is one of the leading causes of liver disease, nutritional deficiency, white blood cell anomalies, bleeding diatheses, diminished immune system function, and CVDs. Fetal alcohol syndrome may be found in children of mothers who consume excessive amounts of alcohol during pregnancy. This syndrome is characterized by growth retardation, mental retardation, and facial developmental anomalies. The use of alcohol during pregnancy also is associated with premature births and delivery of neonates with low birth weight. The harmful effects of alcohol are compounded if the expectant mother also uses tobacco products.[220]

Skin conditions such as spider angiomata and acne rosacea may be associated with excessive alcohol ingestion, and the presence of associated hepatic disease may induce a yellow or dirty gray pigmentation of the skin (biliary melanoderma).

Excessive alcohol ingestion may cause drying or inflammation of oral tissues resulting in a magenta hued discoloration. Involuntary tongue tremor may occur. Salivary gland function may be impaired and asymptomatic enlargement of the parotid or submandibular salivary glands has been described. Candidal infection and angular celitis may be related to nutritional deficiency and xerostomia.[221] It is likely that the cellular changes associated with alcohol abuse may predispose this group of individuals to periodontal disease and destruction, but this has not been adequately studied.[222] It is clear, however, that alcoholism is often associated with increased incidence of dental caries, periodontal diseases, and tooth loss, possibly because of indifference to performing effective oral hygiene measures and failure to seek dental treatment.[220,222,223] Alcoholic patients may develop increased tolerance to local anesthetics and to agents used in conscious sedation. This patient group may also be especially prone to delayed wound healing and postoperative bleeding or infection.

Dental Management

The prudent dental practitioner should remain alert for signs or symptoms of possible substance abuse among patients from all walks of life. Written health questionnaires and verbal interviews should provide patients with the opportunity to identify an existing or past drug-related problem. It is appropriate to question patients regarding the possibility of misuse of mood-altering drugs of all types. If past or current drug use is acknowledged, the patient should be questioned regarding the substance(s) used, whether the use is current, and any known adverse physical effects.[224]

Patients who abuse drugs may be more anxious than the general population regarding dental treatment and this may prompt them to use their drug of preference before a dental appointment. In this event, awareness of signs and symptoms of drug intoxication and avoidance of a medical emergency in the dental office become the issues of primary importance. Local anesthetics containing epinephrine or another vasoconstrictor should be administered with caution if the practitioner is suspicious that cocaine or a related substance has been used. If emergency treatment is necessary, benzodiazepine conscious sedation may be appropriate because these drugs are often used in management of cocaine toxicity.[208,225]

When possible, elective dental surgical procedures should be avoided in alcoholic patients. If misuse of alcohol is suspected, some screening blood tests may be appropriate before scheduling the patient. A complete blood count with differential along with platelet count, prothrombin time, and partial thromboplastin time may be useful to detect the potential for postsurgical hemorrhage. A screening blood panel for liver disease should include total serum protein, serum albumin, and liver transaminase enzymes. Individuals with abnormal blood test results should be referred to their physician for evaluation before extensive dental procedures. Although laboratory blood testing may be important in individuals who are alcoholics to prevent complications to dental treatment, these tests are unreliable in identifying individuals who misuse alcohol. Careful questioning of the patient appears to be the most reliable means of detecting alcohol misuse, but no clear diagnostic methodology currently exists.

Analgesics should be used cautiously in current or past users of drugs of abuse, especially if they experience physiologic adverse effects. Aspirin, acetaminophen or nonsteroidal antiinflammatory drugs may be contraindicated in individuals with gastrointestinal disorders, liver dysfunction, or blood dyscrasias. Pain medication should be prescribed only in the amount necessary to achieve patient comfort. In event of severe pain, the use of a mild narcotic agent such as codeine may be necessary. Should this be required, use of the medication should be carefully monitored by a family member or responsible friend. Intravenous conscious sedation or administration of nitrous oxide/oxygen sedation should be avoided when possible because of their potential to induce significant depression of cardiovascular and respiratory function.[225,226]

Individuals affected by drug-induced xerostomia should be advised to avoid the use of mouthrinses containing alcohol. It has also been suggested that use of mouthrinses with high alcohol content might precipitate relapse in abstaining alcoholic patients or those with a history of polydrug use that includes alcohol. This concept has not been adequately studied to date. Other measures to control xerostomia include copious ingestion of water, avoidance of substances that contain caffeine (coffee, tea, colas), use of sugarless chewing gum, and chewing of healthy firm foods such as raw carrots and celery to stimulate natural salivary flow. Notably, however, ingestion of water by an individual under the influence of amphetaminelike substances may result in severe water intoxication and possible death.

Artificial saliva substitutes may be of some benefit if used frequently, and two systemic drugs (pilocarpine and cevimeline) have been reported to increase salivation in some individuals. These drugs, however, should only be prescribed after careful evaluation of the patient's overall health status and with knowledge of other medications currently being taken.

Parenteral drug users are at increased risk for HIV and hepatitis B and C infections. IE is more common among this group, and causative microorganisms may include those not commonly associated with occurrence of IE. Appropriate infection control methods should be used in dental practice to minimize the risk for transmission, to others and the dental practitioner should be thoroughly versed regarding the signs and symptoms of these diseases.

It is usually possible to manage the dental needs of patients who abuse drugs by application of the principles described above. Consideration of the overall health status of the patient is important to ensure safe dental treatment and close medical/dental corporation is essential in management. Periodontal treatment may sometimes be limited to nonsurgical therapy, but surgical therapy is not contraindicated for all patients in this category. Maintenance of a high level of personal oral hygiene must be emphasized, and recall intervals should be established as necessary to sustain oral health.[208,227,228]

REFERENCES

1. American Diabetes Association: Report of the expert committee on the diagnosis and classification of diabetes mellitus, *Diabetes Care* 26(Suppl 1):s5-s24, 2003.

2. Christgau M, Palitzsch KD, Schmalz G et al: Healing response to non-surgical periodontal therapy in patients with diabetes mellitus: clinical, microbiological, and immunological results, *J Clin Periodontol* 25:112-124, 1998.

3. Westfelt E, Rylander H, Blohme G et al: The effect of periodontal therapy in diabetics. Results after 5 years, *J Clin Periodontol* 23:92-100, 1996.

4. Tervonen T, Karjalainen K: Periodontal disease related to diabetic status. A pilot study of the response to periodontal therapy in type 1 diabetes, *J Clin Periodontol* 24:505-510, 1997.

5. Miller LS, Manwell MA, Newbold D et al: The relationship between reduction in periodontal inflammation and diabetes control: a report of 9 cases, *J Periodontol* 63:843-848, 1992.

6. Grossi SG, Skrepcinski FB, DeCaro T et al: Treatment of periodontal disease in diabetics reduces glycated hemoglobin, *J Periodontol* 68:713-719, 1997.

7. Grossi SG, Genco RJ: Periodontal disease and diabetes mellitus: a two-way relationship, *Ann Periodontol* 3:51-61, 1998.

8. Mealey BL: Diabetes mellitus. In Rose LF, Genco RJ, Mealey BL, Cohen DW, editors: *Periodontal medicine*, Toronto, Ontario, 2000, BC Decker Publishers.

9. American Diabetes Association: Tests of glycemia in diabetes. *Diabetes Care* 26(suppl 1):S106-S108, 2003.

10. Mealey BL: Impact of advances in diabetes care on dental treatment of the diabetic patient, *Compend Contin Educ Dent* 19:41-58, 1998.

11. Diabetes Control and Complications Trial Research Group: The effect of intensive treatment of diabetes on the development and progression of long-term complications in insulin-dependent diabetes mellitus, *N Engl J Med* 329:977-986, 1993.

12. Diabetes Control and Complications Trial Research Group: Progression of retinopathy with intensive versus conventional treatment in the Diabetes Control and Complications Trial, *Ophthalmology* 102:647-661, 1995.

13. Diabetes Control and Complications Trial Research Group: Effect of intensive diabetes management on macrovascular and microvascular events and risk factors in the Diabetes Control and Complications Trial, *Am J Cardiol* 75:894-903, 1995.

14. Diabetes Control and Complications Trial Research Group: Lifetime benefits and costs of intensive therapy as practiced in the diabetes control and complications trial, *JAMA* 276:1409-1415, 1996.

15. U.K. Prospective Diabetes Study (UKPDS) Group: Intensive blood-glucose control with sulphonylureas or insulin compared with conventional treatment and risk of complications in patients with type 2 diabetes (UKPDS 33), *Lancet* 352:837-853, 1998.

16. U.K. Prospective Diabetes Study (UKPDS) Group: Effect of intensive blood-glucose control with metformin on complications in overweight patients with type 2 diabetes (UKPDS 34), *Lancet* 352:854-865, 1998.

17. Mealey BL, Klokkevold PR, Otomo-Corgel J: Periodontal treatment of medically compromised patients. In Newman MG, Takei HH, Carranza FA, editors: *Carranza's clinical periodontology*, Philadelphia, 2002, WB Saunders.

18. Nevins ML, Karimbux NY, Weber HP et al: Wound healing around endosseous implants in experimental diabetes, *Int J Oral Maxillofac Implants* 13:620-629, 1998.

19. Takeshita F, Iyama S, Akuyawa Y et al: The effects of diabetes on the interface between hydroxyapatite implants and bone in rat tibia, *J Periodontol* 68:180-185, 1997.

20. Takeshita F, Murai K, Iyama S et al: Uncontrolled diabetes hinders bone formation around titanium implants in rat tibiae. A light and fluorescence microscopy, and image processing study, *J Periodontol* 69:314-320, 1998.

21. Olson JW, Shernoff AF, Tarlow JL et al: Dental endosseous implant assessments in a type 2 diabetic population: a prospective study, *Int J Oral Maxillofac Implants* 15:811-818, 2000.

22. Morris HF, Ochi S, Winkler S: Implant survival in patients with type 2 diabetes: placement to 36 months, *Ann Periodontol* 5:157-165, 2000.

23. Diabetes Control and Complications Trial Research Group: Epidemiology of severe hypoglycemia in the Diabetes Control and Complications Trial, *Am J Med* 90:450-459, 1991.

24. Diabetes Control and Complications Trial Research Group: Hypoglycemia in the Diabetes Control and Complications Trial, *Diabetes* 46:271-286, 1997.

25. Mealey BL: 1996 World Workshop in Clinical Periodontics. Periodontal implications: medically compromised patients, *Ann Periodontol* 1:256-321, 1996.

26. Otomo-Corgel J, Steinberg BJ: Periodontal medicine and the female patient. In Rose LF, Genco RJ, Mealey BL, Cohen DW, editors: *Periodontal medicine*, Toronto, Ontario, 2000, BC Decker Publishers.

27. Mealey BL, Moritz AJ: Hormonal influences: effects of diabetes mellitus and endogenous female sex steroid hormones on the periodontium, *Periodontol 2000* 32:59-81, 2003.

28. Nocozisis JL, Nah-Cederquiest HD, Tuncay OC: Relaxin affects the dentofacial sutural tissues, *Clin Orthod Res* 3:192-210, 2000.

29. Miyasaki H, Yamashita Y, Shirahama R et al: Periodontal condition of pregnant women assessed by CPITN, *J Clin Periodontol* 20:21-30, 1991.

30. Rees TD, Hallmon WW: Endocrine disorders. In Wilson TG Jr, Kornman KS, editors: *Fundamentals of periodontics*, ed 2, Chicago, 2003, Quintessence Publishing.

31. Gill EF, Contos MJ, Peng TC: Acute fatty liver of pregnancy and acetaminophen toxicity leading to liver failure and postpartum liver transplantation. A case report, *J Reprod Med* 47:584-586, 2002.

32. Preshaw PW, Knutsen MA, Mariotti A: Experimental gingivitis in women using oral contraceptives, *J Dent Res* 80:2011-2015, 2001.

33. Sweet JB, Butler DP: Increased incidence of postoperative localized osteitis in mandibular 3rd molar surgery

associated with patients using oral contraceptives, *Am J Obstet Gynecol* 127:518-519, 1977.

34. Barnet ML: Inhibition of oral contraceptive effectiveness by concurrent antibiotic administration—a review, *J Periodontol* 56:18-20, 1984.

35. American Dental Association: Council on Scientific Affairs. Antibiotic interference with oral contraceptives, *J Am Dent Assoc* 133:880, 2002.

36. Stanford TW, Rees TD: Acquired immune suppression and other risk factors/indicators for periodontal disease progression, *Periodontol 2000* 32:118-135, 2003.

37. Levin C, Maibach HI: Topical corticosteroid-induced adrenocortical insufficiency: clinical implications, *Am J Clin Dermatol* 3:141-147, 2002.

38. Bugajski J, Gadek-Michalska A, Bugajski AJ: A single corticosterone pretreatment inhibits the hypothalamic-pituitary-adrenal responses to adrenergic and cholinergic stimulation, *J Physiol Pharmacol* 52:313-324, 2001.

39. Ammatuna P, Campisi G, Giovannelli L et al: Presence of Epstein Barr virus, cytomegalovirus and human papillomavirus in normal oral mucosa of HIV-infected and renal transplant patients, *Oral Dis* 7:34-40, 2001.

40. Gleissner C, Willerhausen B, Kasser U, Bolten WW: The role of risk factors for periodontal disease in patients with rheumatoid arthritis, *Eur J Med Res* 18:387-392, 1998.

41. Seymour G: Importance of the host response in the periodontium, *J Clin Periodontol* 18:421-426, 1991.

42. Kim HW: Generalized oral and cutaneous hyperpigmentation in Addison's disease, *Odontostomatol Trop* 11:87-90, 1998.

43. Langford A, Pohle HD, Gelderblom H et al: Oral hyperpigmentation in HIV-infected patients, *Oral Surg Oral Med Oral Pathol* 67:301-307, 1989.

44. Resnik S: Melasma induced by oral contraceptive drugs, *JAMA* 199:601-605, 1967.

45. Calabria-Quilez JL, Grau-Garcia-Moreno D, Silverstre-Donat FJ, Hernandez-Mijares A: Management of patients with adrenocortical insufficiency in the dental clinic, *Med Oral* 8:207-214, 2003.

46. Axelrod L: Perioperative management of patients treated with glucocorticoids, *Endocrinol Metab Clin North Am* 32:367-383, 2003.

47. Shapiro R, Carroll PB, Tzakis AG et al: Adrenal reserve in renal transplant recipients with cyclosporine, azathioprine, and prednisone immunosuppression, *Transplantation* 49:1011-1013, 1990.

48. Glick M: Glucocorticosteroid replacement therapy: a literature review and suggested replacement therapy, *Oral Surg Oral Med Oral Pathol* 67:614-620, 1989.

49. Federman DD: Endocrinology-Thyroid. In Dale DC, Federman DD, editors: *Scientific American medicine*, New York, 1997, WebMD Corporation.

50. Pinto A, Glick M: Management of patients with thyroid disease, *J Am Dent Assoc* 133:849-858, 2002.

51. Rees TD: Systemic factors in periodontal disease. In Newman HN, Rees, TD, Kinane DF, editors: *Diseases of the periodontium*, Northwood, England, 1993, Science Reviews Limited.

52. Van Steenberghe D, Jacobs R, Desnyder M et al: The relative impact of local and endogenous patient-related factors on implant failure up to the abutment stage, *Clin Oral Implants Res* 13:617-623, 2002.

53. Attard NJ, Zarb GA: A study of dental implants in medically treated hypothyroid patients, *Clin Implant Dent Relat Res* 4:220-231, 2002.

54. Federman, DD: Endocrinology-Parathyroid. In Dale DC, Federman DD, editors: *Scientific American medicine*. New York, 1998, WebMD Corporation.

55. Shang ZJ, Li ZB, Chen XM et al: Expansile lesion of the mandible in a 45-year-old woman, *J Oral Maxillofac Surg* 61:621-673, 2003.

56. Frankenthal S, Nakhoul F, Machtei EE et al: The effect of secondary hyperparathyroidism and hemodialysis therapy on alveolar bone and periodontium, *J Clin Periodontol* 29:479-483, 2002.

57. Basi DL, Schmiechen NJ: Bleeding and coagulation problems in the dental patient. *Dent Clin North Am* 43:457-470, 1999.

58. Little JW, Miller CS, Henry RG, McIntosh BA: Antithrombotic agents: implications in dentistry. *Oral Surg Oral Med Oral Pathol Oral Radiol Endod* 93:544-551, 2002.

59. Bona R: Hemorrhage and bleeding disorders. In Bennett JD, Rosenberg MB, editors: *Medical emergencies in dentistry*, Philadelphia, 2002, WB Saunders.

60. Rees TD: Dental management of the medically compromised patient. In McDonald RE, Hurt WC, Gilmore HW, Middleton RA, editors: *Current therapy in dentistry, vol 7,* St. Louis, 1980, CV Mosby.

61. Soffer E, Ouhayoun JP, Anagnostou F: Fibrin sealants and platelet preparations in bone and periodontal healing, *Oral Surg Oral Med Oral Pathol Oral Radiol Endod* 95:521-528, 2003.

62. Patton LL, Ship JA: Treatment of patients with bleeding disorders, *Dent Clin North Am* 38:465-481, 1994.

63. Bennett JD, Rosenberg MB: Wheezing. In Bennett JD, Rosenberg MD, editors: *Medical emergencies in dentistry*, Philadelphia, 2002, WB Saunders.

64. Rees TD, Glick M, Patters MR et al: Other systemic modifiers. In Wilson TG Jr, Kornman KS, editors: *Fundamentals of periodontics*, ed 2, Chicago, 2003, Quintessence Publishing.

65. Saint Clair de Velasquez Y, Rivera H: Sickle cell anemia oral manifestations in a Venezuelan population, *Acta Odontol Latinoam* 10:101-110, 1997.

66. Cherry-Peppers G, Davis V, Atkinson JC: Sickle-cell anemia: a case report and literature review, *Clin Prev Dent* 14:5-9, 1992.

67. Deas DE, Mackey SA, McDonnell HT: Systemic disease and periodontitis: manifestations of neutrophil dysfunction, *Periodontol 2000* 32:82-104, 2003.

68. Kinane D: Blood and lymphoreticular disorders, *Periodontol 2000* 21:84-93, 1999.

69. Epstein JB: Periodontal disease and periodontal management in patients with cancer. In Rose LF, Genco RJ, Mealey BL, Cohen DW, editors: *Periodontal medicine*, Toronto, Ontario, 2000, BC Decker Publishers.

70. Wu J, Fantasia JE, Kaplan R: Oral manifestations of acute myelomonocytic leukemia: a case report and review of the classification of leukemias, *J Periodontol* 73:664-668, 2002.

71. Meurman JH, Qvarnstrom M, Janket SJ, Nuutinen P: Oral health and health behaviour in patients referred for open-heart surgery, *Oral Surg Oral Med Oral Pathol Oral Radiol Endod* 95:300-307, 2003.

72. Genco RJ, Offenbacher S, Beck J, Rees TD: Periodontal considerations in the patient at risk for infective endocarditis. In Rose LF, Genco RJ, Mealey BL, Cohen DW, editors: *Periodontal medicine*, Toronto, Ontario, 2000, BC Decker Publishers.

73. Bricker SL, Langlais RP, Miller CS, editors: *Oral diagnosis, oral medicine, and treatment planning*, ed 2, Philadelphia, 1994, Lea and Febiger.

74. Blanchaert RH Jr: Ischemic heart disease, *Oral Surg Oral Med Oral Pathol Oral Radiol Endod* 87:281-283, 1999.

75. On behalf of the membership of the advisory council to improve outcomes nationwide in chronic heart failure: Consensus recommendations for the management of chronic heart failure, *Am J Cardiol* 83(suppl 2A):1A-7A, 1999.

76. McCarthy FM: Safe treatment of the post-heart-attack patient, *Compend Contin Educ Dent* 10:598-604, 1989.

77. Rees TD: Drugs and oral disorders, *Periodontol 2000* 18:21-36, 1998.

78. Hallmon WW, Rossmann JA: The role of drugs in the pathogenesis of gingival overgrowth. A collective review of current concepts, *Periodontol 2000* 21:176-196, 1999.

79. Langberg JJ, DeLurgio RG: Ventricular arrhythmias. In Dale DC, Federman DD, editors: *Scientific American medicine*, New York, 1999, Scientific American.

80. Stiell IG, Wells GA, Field BJ et al: Improved out-of-hospital cardiac arrest survival through the inexpensive optimization of an existing defibrillation program: OPALS study phase II, *JAMA* 281:1175-1181, 1999.

81. Replogle K, Reader A, Most R et al: Cardiovascular effects of intraosseous injections of 2 percent lidocaine with 1:100,000 epinephrine and 3 percent mepivacaine, *J Am Dent Assoc* 130:649-657, 1999.

82. Malamed SF: Asthma. In Malamed SF, ed: *Medical emergencies in the dental office*, ed 5, St. Louis, 2000, Mosby.

83. Dajani A, Taubert KA, Wilson W et al: Prevention of bacterial endocarditis. Recommendations of the American Heart Association, *Circulation* 96:358-366, 1997. First published in *JAMA* 277:1794-1801, 1997.

84. Hayes DL, Wang PJ, Reynolds DW et al: Interference with cardiac pacemakers by cellular telephones, *N Engl J Med* 336:1473-1479, 1997.

85. Miller CS, Leonelli FM, Latham E: Selective interference with pacemaker activity by electrical dental devices, *Oral Surg Oral Med Oral Pathol Oral Radiol Endod* 85:33-36, 1998.

86. Rees TD: Periodontal management of the patient with cardiovascular disease. Position paper, American Academy of Periodontology. *J Periodontol* 73:954-968, 2002.

87. Joshipura KJ, Rimm EB, Douglass CW et al: Poor oral health and coronary heart disease, *J Dent Res* 75:1631-1636, 1996.

88. Huttler AM: Ischemic heart disease: angina pectoris. In Dale DC, Federman DD, editors: *Scientific American medicine*, New York, 1995, Scientific American Inc.

89. Cobb LA, Fahrenbruch CE, Walsh TR et al: Influence of cardiopulmonary resuscitation prior to defibrillation in patients with out-of-hospital ventricular fibrillation, *JAMA* 281:182-188, 1999.

90. Cintron H, Medina R, Reyes AA, Lyman G: Cardiovascular effects and safety of dental anesthesia and dental interventions in patients with recent uncomplicated myocardial infarction, *Arch Intern Med* 146:2203-2204, 1986.

91. Marian AJ: Pathogenesis of diverse clinical and pathological phenotypes in hypertrophic cardiomyopathy, *Lancet* 355:58-60, 2000.

92. Miller CS, Egan RM, Falace DA et al: Prevalence of infective endocarditis in patients with systemic lupus erythematosus, *J Am Dent Assoc* 130:387-392, 1999.

93. Wee CC, Phillips RS, Auregemma G et al: Risk for valvular heart disease among users of fenfluramine and dexfenfluramine who underwent echocardiography before use of medication, *Ann Intern Med* 129:870-874, 1998.

94. Pallasch TJ: Antibiotic prophylaxis: theory and reality, *Calif Dent Assoc J* 17:27-39, 1989.

95. Romans AR, App GR: Bacteremia, a result from oral irrigation in subjects with gingivitis, *J Periodontol* 42:757-760, 1971.

96. Friedlander AH, Yoshikaua TT: Pathogenesis, management, and prevention of infective endocarditis in the elderly dental patient, *Oral Surg Oral Med Oral Pathol* 69:177-181, 1990.

97. Carmona IT, Diz Dios P, Scully C: An update on the controversies in bacterial endocarditis of oral origin, *Oral Surg Oral Med Oral Pathol Oral Radiol Endod* 93:660-670, 2002.

98. Slots J, Rosling BG, Genco RJ: Suppression of penicillin-resistant oral Actinobacillus actinomycetemcomitans with tetracycline: considerations in endocarditis prophylaxis, *J Periodontol* 54:193-196, 1983.

99. Wynn RL: Latest FDA approvals for dentistry, *Gen Dentistry* 47:19-22, 1999.

100. Hirsh J, Dalen JE, Deykin D, Poller L: Oral anticoagulants. Mechanism of action, clinical effectiveness and optimal therapeutic range, *Chest* 102(suppl 4):312s-326s, 1992.

101. Sawicki PT: A structured teaching and self-management program for patients receiving oral anticoagulation: a randomized controlled trial, *JAMA* 281:145-150, 1999.

102. Blinder D, Manor Y, Martinowitz U, Taicher S: Dental extractions in patients maintained on continued oral anticoagulant: comparison of local hemostatic modalities, *Oral Surg Oral Med Oral Pathol Oral Radiol Endod* 88:137-140, 1999.

103. National high blood pressure education program: *The seventh report of the Joint National Committee on Prevention, Detection, Evaluation and Treatment of High Blood Pressure,* Bethesda, MD, 2003, National Institutes of Health/ National Heart, Lung and Blood Institute. NIH publication 03-5233.

104. Glick M: New guidelines for prevention, detection, evaluation and treatment of high blood pressure, *J Am Dent Assoc* 129:1588-1594, 1998.

105. National Heart, Lung, and Blood Institute Joint National Committee on Prevention, Detection, Evaluation, and Treatment of High Blood Pressure; National High Blood Pressure Education Program Coordinating Committee: The seventh report of the joint national committee on prevention, detection, evaluation, and treatment of high blood pressure: the JNC 7 report. *JAMA* 289:2573-2575, 2003.

106. Bader JD, Bonito AJ, Shugars DA: A systematic review of cardiovascular effects of epinephrine on hypertensive dental patients. *Oral Surg Oral Med Oral Pathol Oral Radiol Endod* 93:647-653, 2002.

107. Meyer FV: Hemodynamic changes of local dental anesthesia in normotensive and hypertensive subjects, *J Clin Pharmacol Ther Toxicol* 24:477-481, 1986.

108. Muzyka BC, Glick M: The hypertensive dental patient, *J Am Dent Assoc* 128:1109-1120, 1997.

109. Rose LF, Mealey B, Minsk L, Cohen DW: Oral care for patients with cardiovascular disease and stroke, *J Am Dent Assoc* 133(suppl):37S-44S, 2002.

110. Al Suwaidi J, Berger PB, Holmes DR: Coronary artery stents, *JAMA* 11:1828-1836, 2000.

111. Semba CP, Sakai T, Slonim SM et al: Mycotic aneurysms of the thoracic aorta: repair with use of endovascular stent-grafts, *J Vasc Interv Radiol* 9(1 Pt 1):33-40, 1998.

112. Schroeder JS: Cardiac transplantation. In Fauci AS, Braunwald E, Isselbacher KJ, Wilson JD, editors: *Harrison's principles of internal medicine,* ed 14, New York, 1998, McGraw-Hill.

113. Janket SJ, Baird AE, Chuang SK, Jones JA: Meta-analysis of periodontal disease and risk of coronary heart disease and stroke, *Oral Surg Oral Med Oral Pathol Oral Radiol Endod* 95:559-569, 2003.

114. Abbott RD, Curb JD, Rodriquez BL et al: Age-related changes in risk factor effects on the incidence of thromboembolic and hemorrhagic stroke, *J Clin Epidemiol* 56:479-486, 2003.

115. Coutts SB, Simon JE, Hudon ME, Demchuk AM: What is causing crescendo transient ischemic attacks? *Can J Neurol Sci* 30:171-173, 2003.

116. Ricci S: Embolism from the heart in the young patient: a short review, *Neurol Sci* 24(suppl 1):171-173, 2003.

117. Panagiotopoulos K, Toumanidis S, Vemmos K et al: Secondary prognosis after cardioembolic stroke of atrial origin: the role of left atrial and left atrial appendage dysfunction, *Clin Cardiol* 26:269-274, 2003.

118. Joshipura KJ, Hung HC, Rimm EB et al: Periodontal disease, tooth loss, and incidence of ischemic stroke, *Stroke* 34:47-52, 2003.

119. Cundiff DK: Anticoagulants for nonvalvular atrial fibrillation (NVAF)-drug review, *MedGenMed* 5(1):4, 2003.

120. Corson MA, Postlethwaite KP, Seymour RA: Are dental infections a cause of brain abscess? Case reports and review of the literature, *Oral Dis* 7:61-65, 2001.

121. Bartzokas CA, Johnson R, Jane M et al: Relation between mouth and haematogenous infections in total joint replacement, *Br Med J* 309:506-508, 1994.

122. Cawson RA: Antibiotic prophylaxis for dental treatment: for hearts but not for prosthetic joints, *Br Dent J* 304:933-934, 1992.

123. American Dental Association; American Academy of Orthopaedic Surgeons: Advisory Statement: Antibiotic prophylaxis for dental patients with total joint replacement, *J Am Dent Assoc* 128:1004-1008, 1997.

124. American Dental Association; American Academy of Orthopaedic Surgeons. Advisory Statement: Antibiotic prophylaxis for dental patients with total joint replacements, *J Am Dent Assoc* 134:895-898, 2003.

125. Patton LL: HIV disease, *Dent Clin North Am* 47:467-492, 2003.

126. Rees TD: Periodontal management of HIV-infected patients. In Newman MG, Takei HH, Carranza FA, editors: *Clinical periodontology,* ed 9, Philadelphia, 2002, WB Saunders.

127. Molinari JA: Infection control, its evolution to the current standard precautions, *J Am Dent Assoc* 124:569-574, 2003.

128. Glick M: Clinical protocol for treating patients with HIV disease, *Gen Dent* 38:418-425, 1990.

129. Robinson PG: The significance and management of periodontal lesions in HIV infection, *Oral Dis* 8(suppl 2):91-97, 2003.

130. Swindells S, Evans S, Zackin R et al: AIDS Clinical Trial Group 722 Study Group Team, *J Acquir Immune Defic Syndr* 30:154-157, 2002.

131. Patton LL, Shugars DC: Immunologic and viral markers of HIV-1 disease progression: implications for dentistry, *J Am Dent Assoc* 130:1313-1322, 1999.

132. Patton LL, van der Horst C: Oral infections and other manifestations of HIV disease, *Infect Dis Clin North Am* 13:879-900, 1999.

133. Asher RS, McDowell JD, Winquist H: HIV-related neuropsychiatric changes: concerns for dental professionals, *J Am Dent Assoc* 124:80-84, 1993.

134. Velagraki A, Nicolatou O, Theodoridou M et al: Paediatric AIDS—related linear gingival erythema: a form of erythematous candidiasis? *J Oral Pathol Med* 28:178-182, 1999.

135. Horning GM: Necrotizing gingivostomatitis: NUG to noma, *Compend Contin Educ Dent* 17:951-958, 1996.

136. European Community Clearinghouse on Oral Problems Related to HIV Infection and WHO Collaborating Centre on Oral Manifestations of the Immunodeficiency Virus: Classification and diagnostic criteria for oral lesions in HIV infection, *J Oral Pathol Med* 22:289-291, 1993.

137. Chambers MS, Toth BB, Martin JW et al: Oral and dental management of the cancer patient: prevention and treatment of complications, *Support Care Cancer* 3:168-175, 1995.

138. Cacchillo D, Barker GJ, Barker BE: Late effects of head and neck radiation therapy and patient/dentist compliance with recommended dental care, *Spec Care Dentist* 13:159-162, 1993.

139. Engelmeier RL: A dental protocol for patients receiving radiation therapy for cancer of the head and neck, *Spec Care Dentist* 7:54-58, 1987.

140. Jones LR, Toth BB, Keene HJ: Effects of total body irradiation on salivary gland function and caries-associated oral microflora in bone marrow transplant patients, *Oral Surg Oral Med Oral Pathol* 73:670-676, 1992.

141. Worthington HV, Clarkson JE, Eden OB: Interventions for treating oral mucositis for patients with cancer receiving treatment (Chochrane methodology review). In *The Cochrane Library, Issue 4*, 2003. Chichester, UK: John Wiley and Sons, Ltd.

142. Epstein JB, Gorsky M, Caldwell J: Fluconazole mouthrinses for oral candidiasis in postirradiation, transplant, and other patients, *Oral Surg Oral Med Oral Pathol Oral Radiol Endod* 93:671-675, 2002.

143. Toljanic JA, Bedard JF, Larson RA, Fox JP: A prospective pilot study to evaluate a new dental assessment and treatment paradigm for patients scheduled to undergo intensive chemotherapy for cancer, *Cancer* 85:1843-1848, 1999.

144. Mealey BL, Semba SE, Hallmon WW: The head and neck radiotherapy patient. Part 2. Management of oral complications, *Compend Contin Educ Dent* 15:442-458, 1994.

145. Hurst PS: Dental considerations in management of head and neck cancer. *Otolaryngol Clin North Am* 18:573-603, 1985.

146. Fife RS, Chase WF, Dore RK et al: Cevimeline for the treatment of xerostomia in patients with Sjogren syndrome: a randomized trial, *Arch Intern Med* 162:1284-1300, 2002.

147. Liu RP, Fleming TJ, Toth BB, Keene HJ: Salivary flow rates in patients with head and neck cancer 0.5 to 25 years after radiotherapy, *Oral Surg Oral Med Oral Pathol* 70:724-729, 1990.

148. Periodontal considerations in the management of the cancer patient. Committee on Research, Science and Therapy of the American Academy of Periodontology, *J Periodontol* 68:791-801, 1997.

149. Rosenberg SW: Oral care of chemotherapy patients, *Dent Clin North Am* 334:239-250, 1990.

150. Semba SE, Mealey BL, Hallmon WW: Dentistry and the cancer patient. Part 2. Oral health management of the chemotherapy patient, *Compend Cont Educ Dent* 15:1378-1388, 1994.

151. Epstein J, Ransier, Lunn R: Enhancing the effect of oral hygiene with the use of a foam brush with chlorhexidine, *Oral Surg Oral Med Oral Pathol Oral Radiol Endod* 77:242-247, 1994.

152. American Dental Association: *Patients receiving cancer chemotherapy*, Chicago, 1989, American Dental Association.

153. Maxymiw WG, Wood RE: The role of dentistry in patients undergoing bone marrow transplantation, *Br Dent J* 167:229-234, 1989.

154. Barasch A, Mosier KM, D'Ambrosio JA et al: Postextraction osteomyelitis in a bone marrow transplant recipient, *Oral Surg Oral Med Oral Pathol* 75:391-396, 1993.

155. Cutler LS: Evaluation and management of the dental patient with cancer. 1. Complications associated with chemotherapy or bone marrow transplantation, *J Conn State Dent Assoc* 61:268-277, 1989.

156. Dahllof G, Heimdahl A, Modeer T et al: Oral mucous membrane lesions in children treated with bone marrow transplantation, *Scand J Dent Res* 97:268-277, 1989.

157. Schubert MM, Izutsu KT: Iatrogenic causes of salivary gland dysfunction, *J Dent Res* 66(Spec No):680-688, 1987.

158. Peterson DE, D'Ambrosio JA: Nonsurgical management of head and neck cancer patients, *Dent Clin North Am* 38:425-445, 1994.

159. Barrett AP, Schifter M: Antibiotic strategy in orofacial/head and neck infections in severe neutropenia, *Oral Surg Oral Med Oral Pathol* 77:350-355, 1994.

160. Elad S, Orr R, Garfunkel AA, Shapira MY: Budesonide: a novel treatment for chronic graft versus host disease, *Oral Surg Oral Med Oral Pathol Oral Radiol Endod* 95:308-311, 2003.

161. Rhodus NL, Little JW: Dental management of the bone marrow transplant patient, *Compend Contin Educ Dent* 13:1040, 1042-1050, 1992.

162. Wandera A, Walker PO: Bilateral pyogenic granuloma of the tongue in graft-versus-host disease: report of a case, *ASDC J Dent Child* 61:401-403, 1994.

163. Varga E, Tyldesley WR: Carcinoma arising in cyclosporin-induced gingival hyperplasia. *Br Dent J* 171:26-27, 1991.

164. Thomas DW, Seddon SV, Shepherd JP: Systemic immunosuppression and oral malignancy: a report of a case and review of the literature, *Br J Oral Maxillofac Surg* 31:391-393, 1993.

165. Maxymiw WG, Wood RE, Lee L: Primary, multi-focal, non-Hodgkin's lymphoma of the jaws presenting as periodontal disease in a renal transplant patient, *Int J Oral Maxillofac Surg* 20:69-70, 1991.

166. Epstein JB, Stevenson-Moore P: Periodontal disease and periodontal management in patients with cancer, *Oral Oncol* 37:613-619, 2001.

167. Thurmond JM, Brown AT, Sims RE et al: Oral Candida albicans in bone marrow transplant patients given chlorhexidine rinses: occurrence and susceptibilities to the agent, *Oral Surg Oral Med Oral Pathol* 72:291-292, 1991.

168. Remuzzi G, Bertani T: Pathophysiology of progressive nephropathies, *N Engl J Med* 339:1448-1456, 1998.

169. Naylor GD, Fredericks MR: Pharmacologic considerations in the dental management of the patient with disorders of the renal system, *Dent Clin N Am* 40:665-683, 1996.

170. Ferguson GA, Whyman RA: Dental management of people with renal disease and renal transplants, *N Z Dent J* 94:125-130, 1998.

171. DeRossi SS, Glick M: Dental considerations for the patient with renal disease receiving hemodialysis, *J Am Dent Assoc* 127:211-219, 1996.

172. Bookatz BN: Management of oral problems related to kidney disease and dialysis. In McDonald RD, Hurt WC, Gilmore JW, Middleton RA, editors: *Current therapy in dentistry, vol 7*, St. Louis, 1980, CV Mosby.

173. Rees TD: Periodontal considerations in patients with bone marrow or solid organ transplants. In Rose LF, Genco RJ, Mealey BL, Cohen DW, editors: *Periodontal medicine*, Toronto, Ontario, 2000, BC Decker Publishers.

174. Tolkoff-Rubin NE: Dialysis and transplantation. In Dale DC, Federman DD, editors: *Scientific American medicine*. New York, 1996, Scientific American Medicine.

175. Carpenter CB, Lazarus JM: Dialysis and transplantation in the treatment of renal failure. In Fauci AS, Braunwald E, Wilson JO, et al, editors: *Harrison's principles of internal medicine*, ed 14, New York, 1998, McGraw-Hill.

176. McCauley J: Medical complications. In Shapiro R, Simmons RL, Starzl TE, editors: *Complications of renal transplantation*, Stamford, CT, 1997, Appleton and Lange.

177. Al-Mohaya MA, Darwazeh A, Al-Khudair W: Oral fungal colonization and oral candidiasis in renal transplant patients: the relationship to Miswak use, *Oral Surg Oral Med Oral Pathol Oral Radiol Endod* 93:455-460, 2002.

178. Linden GJ, Haworth SE, Maxwell AP et al: The influence of transforming growth factor-beta1 gene polymorphisms on the severity of gingival overgrowth associated with concomitant use of cyclosporin A and a calcium channel blocker, *J Periodontol* 72:808-814, 2001.

179. Boltchi F, Rees TD, Iacopino AM: Cyclosporine A-induced gingival enlargement. A comprehensive review, *Quintessence Int* 30:775-783, 1999.

180. Ziccardi VB, Saini J, Demas PN, Braun TW: Management of the oral and maxillofacial surgery patient with end-stage renal disease, *J Oral Maxillofac Surg* 50:1207-1212, 1992.

181. Eigner TL, Jastak JT, Bennett WM: Achieving oral health in patients with renal failure and renal transplants, *J Am Dent Assoc* 113:612-616, 1986.

182. Belli LS, Silini E, Alberti A et al: Hepatitis C virus genotypes, hepatitis and hepatitis C virus recurrence after liver transplantation, *Liver Transpl Surg* 2:200-205, 1996.

183. Romeo R, Rumi MG, Donato MF, et al: Hepatitis C is more severe in drug users with human immunodeficiency virus infections, *J Viral Hepat* 7:297-301, 2000.

184. Jackson JM: Hepatitis C and the skin, *Dermatol Clin* 20:449-458, 2002.

185. Keeffe EB: Acute hepatitis. In Dale DC, Federman DD, editors: *Scientific American medicine*, New York, 1997, Scientific American Medicine.

186. Takata Y, Tominaga K, Naito T et al: Prevalence of hepatitis viral infection in dental patients with impacted tooth or jaw deformities, *Oral Surg Oral Med Oral Pathol Oral Radiol Endod* 96:26-31, 2003.

187. Lodi, G, Porter SR, Scully C: Hepatitis C virus infection: review and implications for the dentist, *Oral Surg Oral Med Oral Pathol Oral Radiol Endod* 86:8-22, 1998.

188. Keeffe EB: Chronic hepatitis. In Dale DC, Federman DD, editors: *Scientific American medicine*, New York, 1998, Scientific American Medicine.

189. Keeffe EB: Cirrhosis of the liver. In Dale DC, Federman DD, editors: *Scientific American medicine*, New York, 1998, Scientific American Medicine.

190. Podolsky DK, Isselbacher KJ: Major complications of cirrhosis. In Fauci AS, Barunwald E, Wilson JO, et al, editors: *Harrison's principles of internal medicine*, ed 14, New York, 1998, McGraw-Hill.

191. Carrozzo M, Gandolfo S: Oral diseases possibly associated with hepatitis C virus, *Crit Rev Oral Biol Med* 14:115-127, 2003.

192. Little JW, Rhodus NL: Dental treatment of the liver transplant patient, *Oral Surg Oral Med Oral Pathol* 73:419-426, 1992.

193. Purcell CAH: Dental management of the anticoagulated patient, *N Z Dent J* 93:87-92, 1997.

194. Araujo MW, Andreana S: Risk and prevention of infectious diseases in dentistry, *Quintessence Int* 33:376-382, 2002.

195. Wagaiyu EG, Ashley FP: Mouthbreathing, lip seal and upper lip coverage and their relationship with gingival inflammation in 11-14 year-old school children, *J Clin Periodontol* 18:698-702, 1991.

196. Gulati MS, Grewal N, Kaur A: A comparative study of effects of mouth breathing and normal breathing on gingival health in children, *J Indian Soc Pedod Prev Dent* 16:72-83, 1998.

197. Garcia RI, Nunn ME, Vokonas PS: Epidemiologic associations between periodontal disease and chronic obstructive pulmonary disease, *Ann Periodontol* 4:71-77, 2002.

198. Pretorius E: Allergic reactions caused by dental restorative products, *SADJ* 52:330-336, 2002.

199. Sollecito TP, Tino G: Asthma, *Oral Surg Oral Med Oral Pathol Oral Radiol Endod* 92:485-490, 2001.

200. Delbridge T, Domeier R, Key CB: Prehospital asthma management, *Prehosp Emerg Care* 7:42-47, 2003.

201. Coke JM, Karaki DT: The asthma patient and dental management, *Gen Den* 50:504-507, 2002.

202. Kil N, Zhu JF, VanWagnen C, Abdulhamid L: The effects of midazolam on pediatric patients with asthma, *Pediatr Dent* 25:137-142, 2003.

203. Sole ML, Byers JF, Ludy JE, Ostrow CL: Suctioning techniques and airway management practices: pilot study and instrument evaluation, *Am J Crit Care* 11:363-368, 2002.

204. Rivera-Hidalgo F, Stanford TW: Oral mucosal lesions caused by infective microorganisms I. Viruses and bacteria, *Periodontol 2000* 21:106-124, 1999.

205. Scully C, Cawson RA: *Medical problems in dentistry*, ed 3, Oxford, 1993, Wright.

206. Diaz-Guzman LM: Management of the dental patient with pulmonary tuberculosis, *Med Oral* 6:124-134, 2001.

207. Naidoo S, Mahommed A: Knowledge, attitudes, behaviour and prevalence of TB infection among dentists in the western Cape, *SADJ* 57:476-478, 2002.

208. Rees TD: Oral effects of drug abuse, *Crit Rev Oral Biol Med* 3:163-184, 1992.

209. Friedlander AH, Gorelick DA: Dental management of the cocaine addict, *Oral Surg Oral Med Oral Pathol* 65:45-48, 1988.

210. Scheutz F: Five-year evaluation of a dental care delivery system for drug addicts in Denmark, *Community Dent Oral Epidemiol* 12:29-34, 1984.

211. Cone EJ, Fant RV, Rohay JM et al: Oxycodone involvement in drug abuse deaths: a DAWN-based classification scheme applied to an oxycodone postmortem database containing over 1000 cases, *J Anal Toxicol* 27:57-67, 2003.

212. Jamieson MA, Weir E, Rickert VI, Coupey SM: Rave culture and drug rape, *J Pediatr Adolesc Gynecol* 15:251-357, 2002.

213. Gross SR, Barrett SP, Shestowsky JS, Pihl RO: Ecstasy and drug consumption patterns: a Canadian rave population study, *Can J Psychiatry* 47:546-551, 2002.

214. Braback L, Humble M: Young woman dies of water intoxication after taking one tablet of ecstasy. Today's drug panorama calls for increased vigilance in health care, *Lakartidningen* 98:817-819, 2001.

215. Schwartz RH, Milteer R, LeBeau MA: Drug-facilitated sexual assault ("date rape"), *South Med J* 93:558-561, 2000.

216. El Sohly MA, Ross SA, Mehmedic Z et al: Potency trends of delta9-THC and other cannabinoids in confiscated marijuana from 1980-1997, *J Forensic Sci* 45:24-30, 2000.

217. Yukna RA: Cocaine periodontitis, *Int J Periodontics Restorative Dent* 11:72-79, 1991.

218. Mari A, Arranz C, Gimeno X et al: Nasal cocaine abuse and centrofacial destructive process: report of three cases including treatment, *Oral Surg Oral Med Oral Pathol Oral Radiol Endod* 93:435-439, 2002.

219. Murray MJ, Murray WJ: Nitrous oxide availability, *J Clin Pharmacol* 20:202-205, 1980.

220. Glick M: Medical considerations for dental care of patients with alcohol related liver disease, *J Am Dent Assoc* 128:61-70, 1997.

221. Friedlander AH, Marder SR, Pisegna JR, Yagiela JA: Alcohol abuse and dependence. Psychopathology, medical management and dental implications, *J Am Dent Assoc* 134:731-740, 2003.

222. Pitiphat W, Merchant AT, Rimm EB, Joshipura KJ: Alcohol consumption increases periodontitis risk, *J Dent Res* 82:509-513, 2003.

223. Hornecker E, Muuss T, Ehrenreich H, Mausberg RF: A pilot study on the oral conditions of severely alcohol addicted persons, *J Contemp Dent Pract* 15:51-59, 2003.

224. Sainsbury D: Drug addiction and dental care, *N Z Dent J* 95:58-61, 1999.

225. Bullock K: Dental care of patients with substance abuse, *Dent Clin North Am* 43:513-526, 1999.

226. Linderoth JE, Herren MC, Falace DA: The management of acute dental pain in the recovering alcoholic, *Oral Med Oral Surg Oral Pathol Oral Radiol Endod* 95:432-436, 2003.

227. Crossley HL: Management of the active or recovering chemically dependent dental patient, *MSDA J* 39:85-86, 1996.

228. Sandler NA: Patients who abuse drugs, *Oral Surg Oral Med Oral Pathol Oral Radiol Endod* 91:12-14, 2001.

Index

Page numbers followed by f indicate figures; t, tables; b, boxes.